Medical Surgical Nursing

Medical Surgical Nursing

Third Edition

Volume 1

BT Basavanthappa MN (N) PhD

Principal
RajaRajeswari College of Nursing, Bengaluru, Karnataka, India

Former Professor and Principal
Government College of Nursing, Bengaluru, Karnataka, India
PhD Guide for Research Work

Member
Faculty of Nursing, RGUHS, Karnataka, India
Academic Council, RGUHS, Karnataka, India

Examiner
UG, PG and Doctoral Courses on Nursing, Various Universities

Ex-Programme In-Charge
IGNOU, BSc Nursing Course, Karnataka and Goa, India

Life Member
Nursing Research Society of India, New Delhi, India
Trained Nurses Association of India, New Delhi, India

President
RGUHS, Nursing Teachers Association, Karnataka, India

Winner
Bharat Excellence Award and Gold Medal
Vikas Ratan Gold Award
UWA Lifetime Achievement Award
Shree Veeranjaneya "Shrujanashri" Award

JAYPEE The Health Sciences Publisher
New Delhi | London | Philadelphia | Panama

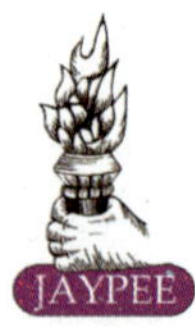

Jaypee Brothers Medical Publishers (P) Ltd

Headquarters

Jaypee Brothers Medical Publishers (P) Ltd
4838/24, Ansari Road, Daryaganj
New Delhi 110 002, India
Phone: +91-11-43574357
Fax: +91-11-43574314
Email: jaypee@jaypeebrothers.com

Overseas Offices

J.P. Medical Ltd
83 Victoria Street, London
SW1H 0HW (UK)
Phone: +44 20 3170 8910
Fax: +44 (0)20 3008 6180
Email: info@jpmedpub.com

Jaypee-Highlights Medical Publishers Inc.
City of Knowledge, Bld. 237, Clayton
Panama City, Panama
Phone: +1 507-301-0496
Fax: +1 507-301-0499
Email: cservice@jphmedical.com

Jaypee Medical Inc.
The Bourse
111 South Independence Mall East
Suite 835, Philadelphia, PA 19106, USA
Phone: +1 267-519-9789
Email: jpmed.us@gmail.com

Jaypee Brothers Medical Publishers (P) Ltd
17/1-B Babar Road, Block-B, Shaymali
Mohammadpur, Dhaka-1207
Bangladesh
Mobile: +08801912003485
Email: jaypeedhaka@gmail.com

Jaypee Brothers Medical Publishers (P) Ltd
Bhotahity, Kathmandu, Nepal
Phone: +977-9741283608
Email: kathmandu@jaypeebrothers.com

Website: www.jaypeebrothers.com
Website: www.jaypeedigital.com

Inquiries for bulk sales may be solicited at: jaypee@jaypeebrothers.com

Medical Surgical Nursing (Volume 1)

First Edition: 2003

Reprint: 2007

Second Edition: 2013

Third Edition: **2015**

ISBN: 978-93-5152-407-6

Printed at Sanat Printers, Kundli

Dedicated to

My Parents
and
my nursing profession
and
my dear students

Preface to the Third Edition

It gives me immense pleasure and satisfaction to introduce third edition of my title *Medical Surgical Nursing*. In offering this text, I remain grateful for the support given to my earlier editions of all my 23 titles on Nursing. Now Medical Surgical Nursing continues to strongly influence by the advancement of science, medicine, surgery and technologies and also changes in social, cultural, and economic environment. So nurses must be updated in their knowledge and skill in decision making, as well as consulting and collaborating with other health care team members. In view of these changes, the text has been fully updated with all the material and added existing new information. An effort has been made to provide the text written at an understandable level with features that help students to understand, apply and practice the challenging content required to function as **full-fledged** nurse. Along with the challenges nurses of today confront with, there are many opportunities to provide skilled, compassionate nursing care in a variety of health care setting, for the patients in the various stages of illness and for patients across the age continuum.

This third edition of the *Medical Surgical Nursing* addresses the concepts and skills needed for adult patient care. With this edition, every chapter has been extensively revised. The context has been updated to reflect the latest available information and the increasing emphasis on wellness and home and community-based care. Many changes are in response to suggestions and comments from faculty and students using the text.

The goal of this book is to provide balanced attention to the art and science of medical surgical nursing. The book focuses on all concepts related to nursing care. So this edition will help nurses be confident in their role, skill, knowledge so that they can be truly with the patients they care for. The present text has been arranged in 22 chapters. In the beginning the chapter briefs about the history of medicine and nursing in India, next explains the concept of nursing process and its application. Chapter 4 introduces human genetics and genomic nursing, and subsequent chapters tell about the immunological problems, responsibilities of nurses in perioperative nursing, critical care and oncological nursing. The remaining chapters have been organized into system-wise disorders, for example, respiratory nursing, gastrointestinal nursing, cardiovascular nursing, neurological nursing, orthopedic nursing, urological nursing, reproductive health nursing, etc.

The features of each chapter include the following:

- The chapters on the system-wise disorders cover the management of specific disorders, and their **pathophysiology, clinical manifestations, assessment and diagnostic findings, medical management and nursing management**. For certain specific disorders, **nursing process** has been applied and nursing care plans have been included, to clarify the nurses' responsibilities in caring for patient with selected disorders, and **nursing care plans** have been provided in tables of certain chapters
- Numbers of relevant **figures** have been provided for better understanding of certain concepts related to concerned disorders and their care
- Some relevant information given in **boxes**, which guides students have precise information about the disorder-related actions, events and education, etc.
- Some important **procedures** have been included in the respective chapters for ready reference
- In appendix **terminology, abbreviations**, and **other important materials** have been included for ready reference.

I hope this text will help nurses and nursing students be confident in their role, skills and knowledge so that they can be truly with the patients they care for. It should be kept in mind that no book can provide all the knowledge, so nurses need to know when working with their patients to make decisions about their care pathway and utilize interventions appropriately. I believe that this book will provide a comprehensive framework to assist in the decision-making process and stimulate nurses' passion for lifelong learning.

I am aware of manifold reasons for errors that might have crept in inadvertently. I shall feel obliged, if such errors are brought to my notice. I sincerely welcome your comments and suggestion and good one will be incorporated in the next edition.

BT Basavanthappa

Preface to the First Edition

It gives me immense pleasure and satisfaction to introduce *Medical Surgical Nursing* to nursing community. In offering this text, I remain grateful for the support given to my earlier titles, i.e. *Community Health Nursing, Nursing Research, Nursing Administration* and *Fundamentals of Nursing.*

I have carefully preserved the aspects of the book that have met with such universal acceptance—its state-of-the-art, scientific-based information, its string, logical and user-friendly organization and easy-to-read style.

Medical Surgical Nursing was developed to provide nursing students with the knowledge and skill they need to become competent, think critically and possess the sensitivity to become caring nurses. Professional nursing practice continues to evolve and adapt to society's changing health priorities. The rapidly changing health care delivery system offers new opportunities for nurses to alter the practice of Medical Surgical Nursing and to improve the way nursing care is given.

In this changing world on health care delivery system, nurses will need a broad knowledge to provide the expert care needed in nursing profession. New efforts to reform health care and guarantee with high quality and cost-effective care are radically transforming the culture of care-giving. I believe that the changes in health care present exciting challenges to nurses and it is felt that there is a need for good nursing texts to assist nurses to meet these challenges globally.

In view of the above changes, the text of *Medical Surgical Nursing* is organized into 19 chapters. Ideally the text is flowed sequentially, but every effort has been made to respect the differing needs of diverse curricula and students. Thus, each chapter stands on its own merit and may be read independently of others. This work is designed to meet the nursing students' requirement as per their respective universities, boards and nursing councils.

I am aware of manifold reasons for errors that might have crept in inadvertently. I shall feel obliged, if such errors are brought to my notice. I sincerely welcome constructive criticism from both the teachers and the students that would help me to enrich myself and good suggestions will be incorporated in the next revised edition.

BT Basavanthappa

Acknowledgments

I owe a great deal of thanks to many who encouraged and supported me with their time and valuable suggestions throughout.

Shri G Basavannappa, Former Minister of Karnataka State, for having initiated and supported me to take up the "Noble Nursing Profession" as my career.

Dr (Mrs) Manjula K Vasundhra, Former Professor and Head, Department of Community Medicine, Bangalore Medical College, who continuously encouraged me to write texts in the field of Nursing since nursing is a major force in Medical and Health Services.

My father Shri Thukkappa, who continues to grace for the progress of my career and all-round development of my personality for the welfare of the community.

My mother Smt Hanumanthamma, who continues to be a bright spot in the lives of all who knew her and whose grace gave me strength to progress in my life.

My wife Smt Lalitha, who gives meaning to my life in so many ways. She is the one whose encouragement keeps me motivated, whose support gives me strength and whose gentleness gives me comfort.

My lovely children BB Mahesh and BB Ganashree, for all the joy they provided me and all the hope that they instill in me and who bear with patience throughout my works of the nursing texts. They keep me young at heart.

Finally, my warmest appreciation goes to Shri Jitendar P Vij (Group Chairman), Mr Ankit Vij (Group President) and Mr Tarun Duneja (Director–Publishing) of M/s Jaypee Brothers Medical Publishers (P) Ltd, New Delhi, India, for sharing my vision for this book and giving me the chance to turn vision into reality.

In addition, I am particularly indebted to the faculty, nurses, student nurses who have put their faith in my titles to assist them on their path of excellence and I also appreciate the many users who have shared their comments and suggestions on the previous editions.

Contents

Volume 1

Volume 2

CHAPTER

1

Brief History of Medicine and Nursing in India

INTRODUCTION

History means "Itihas" in Indian languages. Itihas is combination of three words i.e. Iti + ha + aas. Here, 'Iti' means thus, 'Ha' means positively and 'Aas' means existed or happened. So, 'Itihas' means that it happened or took place. It tells us about the details of the past and real incidents only not of the future. It include the events of the present also. The history of medicine in India goes back through the centuries to about 3000 BC. The beginnings are shrouded in the mist of ancient myths. The experience and concern in health development date back to vedic period between 3000–1400 BC. The Indus Valley Civilization showed relics of planned cities and practice of environmental sanitation. According to Dr Wheeler, on the basis of his research studies from South, Arikamedu (Pondicherry) to North Mohenjo-daro and Harappa, only one culture had been followed. An ideal healthful living of the people, such as every house of Mohenjo-daro and Harappa had separate good water supply. In every backguard of the houses, there was a wide royal street and by the side of the street there was an arrangement of safe drinking water. Actually, this was followed by Dravidians who lived at that time. After the invasion of Aryans, the Dravidian got relegated to South. The specialist of pictograph reader, Father Heras says that it was a fact that ancient people of Mohenjo-daro were proto-Dravidians, a fact also hinted by Sir John Marshall that there was a link between all that is the Dravidian culture, including Mohenjo-daro and Karnataka. The Ayurveda and other system of medicine practised during this time suggests the development of comprehensive concept of health by the ancient sages of India.

Ancient Indian medicine, in fact Hindu medicine, since Hinduism was the only religion existing those days in India, goes back to 6000 years or more. According to Hindu mythology, the creator of the Universe, Lord Brahma, was the first teacher to make a compilation of Ayurvedic texts which he later abridged into eight parts, with medicine (Kayachikitsa) and surgery (Shalya tantra) as the main subjects. It is believed that Brahma propagated this knowledge through Daksha Prajapati who in turn taught this science to the Aswini Kumars (the twin sons of the Sun God). The Aswinis imparted the science to Indra. Up to this time, the knowledge of Ayurveda was known only to celestial personalities. It is believed that it was Lord Indra who passed on this knowledge of Ayurveda, the "science of life", to sages and rishis (mortals), the first pupil being Bharadwaja. He in turn, taught this subject to others including Atreya. He, it is believed, lived in the period 700 – 600 BC and became a renowned teacher at Taxila.

It is believed that in India, the first known writing was recorded in Bramhi script in the third century BC. For centruries in India, knowledge was propagated by word of mouth from Guru (teacher) to Shishya (student) and this situation persisted till the arrival of the Aryans. Information on Egyptian, Babylonian and Greek civilizations has been derived by deciphering hieratic, hieroglyphic and cuneiform writings available through archeological excavations. The excavations of Mohenjo-Daro and Harappa have thrown light on community living and sanitary conditions in ancient Indian civilizations, which even by current standards were commendable. In fact, our present water carriage system of drainage is an improved version of the same. The chief sources of information of ancient Hindu culture and medicine are the four Vedas among which the Rigveda was the earliest and the Atharvaveda, the last. The Atharvaveda believed to have been composed some time in 1200 BC, is the most important source of information on ancient Hindu medicine. All four Vedas are in the form of shlokas (hymns), verses, incantations and rites, used on appropriate occasions to propitiate the respective deity, depending upon the need of the afflicted. The Atharvaveda, a sacred text of Hinduism dating from the Early Iron Age, is the first Indian text dealing with medicine, like the medicine of the Ancient Near East based on concepts of the exorcism of demons and magic. The Atharvaveda also contain prescriptions of herbs for various ailments. The use of herbs to treat ailments would later form a large part of Ayurveda.

Lord Vishnu is also believed to have been associated with ancient medicine. It is said that several sages approached the Lord and begged of Him to help them save humanity from diseases and suffering. In response to their plight and prayers, he ordered the churning of the ocean of milk with the aid of "Vasukis" and "Asuras". Dhanvantari then came out of the ocean with the pot of "Amrita" in his hands. (There is a sculpture of Dhanvantari in the Somanathpur temple in Karnataka) . According to another version, Lord Indra favored and blessed him with knowledge in Ayurvedic medicine. Dhanvantari, in years to come, became a renowned teacher in the art of surgery and taught this subject to his disciples at Varanasi (Kashi). He was considered the "Patron Saint of Surgery" and later elevated to divinity of classical medical wisdom. He lived some time in the 6th century BC.

TRADITIONAL MEDICINE AND SURGERY IN INDIA

Indian medicine is ancient. Its earliest concepts are set out in the sacred writings called the Vedas, especially in the metrical passages of the Atharvaveda, which may possibly dates as far back as the second millennium BC. According to a later writer, the system of medicine called Ayurveda was received by a saint Dhanvantari from Brahma, and Dhanvantari was defined as the god of medicine. In later times, his status was gradually reduced, until he was credited with having been an earthly king who died of snakebite. Legends tell of Dhanvantari's relations with snakes and illustrates the skill with which early Indian practitioners treated snakebite.

The period of Vedic medicine lasted until about 800 BC. The Vedas are rich in magical practices for the treatment of diseases and in charms for the expulsion of the demons traditionally supposed to cause diseases. The chief conditions mentioned are fever, cough, constipation, diarrhea, dropsy, abscesses, seizures, tumors and skin diseases (including leprosy). The herbs recommended for treatment are numerous.

GOLDEN PERIOD OF INDIAN MEDICINE

The golden age of Indian medicine, from 800 BC until about 1000 AD may be termed the Brahmanistic period. It is marked especially by production of the medical treatises known respectively as the Charaka-Samhita and Sushruta-Samhita, attributed respectively to the physician Charaka and Susruta, traditionally a surgeon. Both these works were formerly regarded as being of great antiquity, and hence claims arose for the priority of Indian scientific medicine over its Greek counterpart.

Another school asserted that these works were written many centuries after the beginning of the Christian Era. The most recent estimates place the Charaka Samhita its present form as dating from the 1st century AD, and there were earlier versions. The Sushruta-Samhita probably originated in the last centuries of the pre-Christian Era and became fixed in its present form in the 7th century AD at the latest. Other medical treatises of lesser importance are those attributed to Vagbhata (8th century). All later treatises were based on these works.

Because the Hindus were prohibited by their religion from cutting the dead body, their knowledge of anatomy was limited. The Sushruta-Samhita recommends that a body be placed in a basket and sunk in a river for 7 days. On its removal, the parts could be easily separated without cutting. As a result of these crude methods, the emphasis in Hindu anatomy was given to the bones, and then to the muscles, ligaments and joints. The nerves, blood vessels and internal organs were very imperfectly known.

The Hindus believed that the body contained three elementary substances, microcosmic representatives of the three divine universal forces, which they called spirit (air), phlegm, and bile. These were comparable with the humors of the Greeks. Health depends on the normal balance of these three elementary substances. The spirit has its seat below the navel, the phlegm about the heart, and the bile between the heart and the navel. The seven primary constituents of the body—blood, flesh, fat, bone, marrow, chyle, and semen are produced by the action of the elementary substances. Semen was supposed to be produced from all parts of the body and not from any individual part or organ. Both Charaka and Susruta state the existence of a large number of diseases (Susruta says 1,120). Rough classifications of diseases are given. In all texts "fever" of which numerous types are described, is regarded as important, phthisis (wasting disease, especially pulmonary tuberculosis) was apparently common, and the Hindu physicians knew the symptoms of cases likely to terminate fatally. Smallpox was common, and it is probable that smallpox inoculation was practised.

HINDU WRITINGS ON DIAGNOSIS AND TREATMENT

In diagnosis, the Hindu physicians used all five senses. Hearing was used to distinguish the nature of the breathing, alteration in voice, and the grinding sound produced by the rubbing together of broken ends of bones. They appear to have had a good clinical sense, and their sections on prognosis contain acute references to symptoms that are of grave importance. Magical beliefs still persisted, however, until late in the classical period, the prognosis could be affected by such fortuitous factors as the cleanliness of the messenger sent to fetch the physician, the nature of his conveyance, or the types of persons whom the physician met on his journey to the patient.

Indian therapeutics was largely dietetic and medicinal. Dietetic treatment was important and preceded any medicinal treatment. Fats were mostly used internally and externally. The most important methods of active treatment were referred to as the "five procedures"; the administration emetics, purgatives, water enemas, oil enemas, and sneezing powders, inhalations were frequently employed, as were leeching, cupping and bleeding.

The Indian materia medica was extensive and consisted mainly of vegetable drugs, all of which were from indigenous plants. Charaka knew 500 medicinal plants, and Susruta knew 700. But animal remedies (such as the milk of various animals, bones, gallstones) and minerals (sulfur, arsenic, lead, copper sulfate, gold) were also employed. The physicians collected and prepared their own vegetable drugs. Among those that eventually appeared in western pharmacopoeias are cardamom and cinnamon.

As a result of the strict religious beliefs of the Hindus, hygienic measures were important in treatment. Two meals a day were prescribed with indications of the nature of the diet, the amount of water to be drunk before and after the meal, and the use of condiments. Bathing and care of the skin were carefully prescribed, as were cleaning of the teeth with twigs from neem trees, anointing of the body with oil, and use of eyewashes.

HINDU SURGERY

In surgery, ancient Hindu medicine reached its zenith. Detailed instructions about the choice of instruments and the different operations are given in the classical texts. It has been said that the Hindus knew all ancient operations except the arrest of hemorrhage by the ligature. Their operations were grouped broadly as follows: excision of tumors; incision of abscesses, punctures of collections of fluid in the abdomen; extraction of foreign bodies; pressing out of the contents of abscesses; probing of fistulas; and stitching of wound.

The surgical instruments used by the Hindus have received special attention in modern times. According to Susruta, the surgeon should be equipped with 20 sharp and 101 blunt instruments. The sharp instruments included knives of various patterns, scissors, trocars (instruments for piercing tissues and draining fluid from them), saws and needles. The blunt instruments included forceps, specula (instruments for inspecting body cavities or passages), tubes, levers, hooks and probes. The Susruta Samhita does not mention the catheter, but it is referred to in later writings. The instruments were largely of steel. Alcohol seems to have been used as a narcotic during operations.

Especially in two types of operations the ancient Hindus were outstanding. Stone in the bladder (vesical calculus) was common in ancient India, and the surgeons frequently carried out the operation of lateral lithotomy for removal of the stones. They also introduced plastic surgery. Amputation of the nose was one of the prescribed punishments for adultery, and repair was carried out by cutting from the patient's cheek a piece of tissue of the required size and shape and applying it to the stump of the nose. The results appear to have been tolerably satisfactory, and the modern operation is certainly derived indirectly from this ancient source. The Hindu surgeons, also performed an operation for the cure of anal fistula and in this they were definitely in advance of the Greeks.

In the past, there had been much speculation as to whether the Greek derived any of their medical knowledge from the Hindus. Mid-20th century opinion held that there was certainly intercommunication between Greece and India before the time of Alexander the Great.

CHRONOLOGICAL EVENTS OF HEALTH SCIENCE

A brief description of chronological events related to development of health and medicine in India is given below.

3000 BC: In the Indus Valley Civilization, one finds evidence of well developed environmental sanitation programs such as underground drains public baths, etc. 'Arogya' or 'health' was given high priority in daily life and this concept of health included physical, mental, social and spiritual wellbeing.

2000 BC: Rigveda marks the beginning of the Indian system of medicine. Medicine was considered part of Vedas or scriptures. 'Ayurveda', a science of life and art of living said to be founded by Sage 'Atreya'. Good health implies an ideal balance between tridoshic factors, i.e. wind, bile, phlegm (Vata, Pitta and Kapha) according to Ayurveda. Health promotion and health education were also emphasized by following 'Dinacharya'.

1000 BC: Atharvaveda mentions the twin aims of medical sciences as health and longevity and curative treatment. Hygiene and dietetics are considered important in treatment. Beneficial effects of milk are described in detail.

800 BC: A codification of medical knowledge scattered through vedas by Bhela called Bhela-Samhita.

700 BC: A codification of medical knowledge by Agnivesha, said to be disciple of Atreya, called Agnivesha Samhita became the basis of later Charaka.

700–600 BC: Atreya was an eminent sage and a pupil of Bharadwaja at Taxilla (Taksasila) situated on the banks of the river Sutlej now in Pakistan. He taught medicine and ushered in the age of scientific medicine through his astute observations of symptoms, disease and their correlation. He is rightly known as the "Hippocrates of Ancient Indian Medicine" as well as the "Father of Indian Medicine". Charak was one of his students.

600 BC: A treatise by Kasyapa mainly dealing with pediatrics.

600–500 BC: Dhanvantari at Banaras (Varanasi), became a renowned teacher of surgery and later came to be known as the "Patron Saint of Surgery".

500 BC: 'Chivaravastu', a book written by unknown author is found. It mentions prince Jivika, the court physician of Bimbisara, King of Magadh, as a marvellous physician and surgeon. He is credited with such difficult operations as piercing the skull to operate on the brain, surgery of the eyes, etc. and medical treatment of dropsy, internal tumors and varicose veins.

272–236 BC: King Asoka, a convert to Buddhism, built number of hospitals. More emphasis was laid on the preventive aspects. Doctors, nurses, and midwives were to be trustworthy and skillful. The nurses were usually men and old women. This period saw famous medical schools at Taxila and Nalanda.

237–201 BC: Saint Buddha instituted a state medical system, appointed doctors for every 10 villages on the main roads of India. Pharmaceutical gardens were also maintained.

200–100 BC: Patanjali explored the yoga system of philosophy of men and physical discipline—the starting point of yoga therapy later continued.

100 BC: Charaka Samhita, the first classical exposition of Indian system medicine deals with an almost all the branches of medicine, anatomy, physiology, etiology, prognosis, pathology, treatment procedure, and sequence of medication and an extension Materia Medica for more than 600 drugs. This treatise formed the basis of the Atreya School of Medicine in India, in (100) AD. The qualification of attending nurse, enshrined in the Charaka Samhita, i.e. knowledge of preparation and compounding of drugs for administration, cleverness, devotedness to patient under care and purity of both mind and body.

200–300 AD: Susruta Samhita appears to have been revised by Nagarjuna, laid main emphasis on surgery. This great treatise described more than 300 operations, 43 different surgical processes and 121 different types of instruments. The Materia Medica is also extensive covering more than 650 drugs of animals, plant and mineral origin. This treatise forms the basis of Dhanwantari School (300 AD).

Susruta defines ideal relations of doctor, patient, nurses and medicine as the four feet upon which a cure must rest.

500–600 AD: Vagbhata wrote Astanga Hridaya (8 limbs and heart). The eight limbs refer to the eight traditional branches of Ayurvedic knowledge, i.e. therapeutics, surgery, ENT, mental and superstitious diseases, infantile diseases and treatment, toxicology, arresting physical and mental decay, and rejuvenation or regaining lost virility potency and procreative ability.

This book is the most concise and scientific exposition of Ayurveda. It is in verse form, making it easy to memorise. It incorporates the teachings of the sages Atreya and Dhanvantari and the Rasayana school of medicine. It is distinguished but its knowledge of chemical reactions and laboratory processes. This book has been translated into foreign languages.

600–800 AD: Sodhala (700 AD) two treatises, Gandani-ghraha, a medical treatise and Sodhala a medical lexicon.

Vrudukunta (750 AD) writes Siddayoga, the earliest treatise on Rasa Chikitsa now existing intact. The Rasa Chikitsa system considers mercury as the king of all medicines. Siddayoga explain the various preparations of mercury and other metals, alloys, metallic compounds, salts and sulfur. This school of medicine is called Siddha school. All of them are made of metals, salts and sulfur. It is supposed to be a continuation of the pre-Aryan medical system in India. It is popular in eastern and southern India.

Siddha Nagarjuna Two treatises on the Siddha systems, Rasarathanakara and Arogya Manjari. Madhavacharya (700–800 AD) wrote Madhava Nidana. This is a compilation from the earlier works of Agnivesha, Charaka, Susruta, Vagbhata. It is specially useful as a chemical guide to preparations. It is famous all over India as the best Ayurvedic work on the diagnosis of diseases.

800–1300 AD: A number of treatises were written in India during this period. Arkaprakasha, a book on tincture extraction, Sarangadhara Samhita, Chikitsa Sangraha and Yoga Ratnakara are the better known among them.

The period also witnessed a spirit of writing on the Rasa Chikitsa system. Rasha Hridaya by Govind Vagbhata, Rasaratnakara by Siddha Nityananda, Rasara-Tnasammukta by Vagbhata (another), Rasarnava by Sambhu, Rasendrachintamani by Ramachandra, and Rasendra Choodamani by Somadeva.

1300–1600 AD: Bhavamishra wrote Bhava Prakasha. This is the most renowned Indian treatise during the period. It contains an exhaustive list of diseases and their symptoms and complete list of drugs including many not mentioned in the earlier works. It includes etiology and treatment of syphilis, a disease brought into India by Portuguese seamen.

Other works of this period are Chikitsalaya by Trisata, a manual on diagnosis; Chintamani by Ballbhendra on etiology and diagnosis; and Vaidyamrutha by Moreswara on the treatment of diseases.

Another class of works produced during this period are Medical Lexicons by Madanapala, Nagahari, Bimapala, and Rajavallabha.

1600: East India Company established British Rule in India. Western medicine and surgery started to be practised and became popular in India.

NURSING IN INDIA

Beginning of Modern Nursing

In the past, the progress of nursing in India has been hindered by many difficulties, such as: the low status of women, the system of purdah among Muslim women, the caste system among Hindus, illiteracy, poverty, political unrest, language differences, and the fact that nursing has been looked upon as servant's work.

Since independence in 1947, many changes have taken place and the attitude towards nursing is changing. More women are being educated and many are taking up nursing as their profession.

We have very little information about medicine and nursing in India until the 15th century, when Vasco de Gama came to

India. He set up trading posts on the west coast. Franciscan, Dominican and Jesuit missionaries came to administer the sick and needy. The Portuguese set up European type of dispensaries at Goa and Madras and physicians from Europe were invited to India. One of these, Garcia da Orta, in 1550 wrote 'Simples Drugs of India.'

Military Nursing

Military Nursing was the earliest type of nursing. In 1664, the East India Company helped to start a hospital for soldiers at Fort St. George, Madras. Later, a civilian hospital was built and the medical staff, appoined by the East India Company, served in both hospitals. In 1797 a Lying-in-Hospital was built and in 1854 the government sanctioned a Training School for Midwives. In 1861, through the efforts of Miss Nightingale, reforms in military hospitals led to reforms in civil hospitals. Efforts were made to provide health services for the people of India. This laid the foundation for public health nursing.

Nursing in the military hospitals was of poor quality carried on by male orderlies and menial staff. In 1871 the Government General Hospital, Madras undertook a plan to train nurses. Nurses were brought from England to be in-charge and the first six students were those who had previously received their diploma in midwifery. Later this plan was reversed. General training was taken first followed by a course in midwifery.

In Bombay, among the one of the earliest hospitals is the Jamsetjee Jeejeebhoy Group, the first of which was opened in 1843. Another hospital which was to play an important part in the development of modern nursing in India was the Pestani Hormusji Cama Hospital for women and children, which was founded in 1883 but not opened until 1886.

Provision for the nursing care of patients in these early hospitals was very limited. In the JJ Group, nursing was done by medical students and menials until 1868 when the government invited the Sisters of the Community of All Saints to come from England and take over the work of nursing. Their work was appreciated and the need for training nurses was felt. At this time, it was difficult to get nurses. There were only a few Anglo-Indian and Indian Christian girls working in mission hospitals. The sisters of all saints took the first steps to establish a training school for nurses in this hospital. In 1891, Bai Kashibai Ganpat was the first Indian nurse to come for training. Training was at first 2 years but became 3 years when the Bombay Presidency Nursing Association was established in 1909.

An outstanding graduate of the JJ Group of hospitals was Miss TK Adranvala. After her graduation, she worked as a ward sister, then became assistant Matron under the sisters and finally, superintendent of the hospitals. She held this position until she was asked to accept the position of Nursing Superintendent and Nurse Adviser to the Government of India. She remained in this position until retiring in 1966. She continues active participation in nursing as a WHO representative in Nepal. Miss Adranvala has worked very hard to raise the status of the nursing profession in India. She has given much of her time to the interests of the TNAI having held the office of president for two terms and that of treasurer until she was released at her own request. The nursing profession in India is fortunate to have had such a capable person as Miss Adranvala as its representative in the World Health Organization. She is highly respected by all and many seek her wise counsel.

Mission Hospitals

Mission Hospitals were the first to begin the training of Indians as nurses, very gradually overcoming the prejudices of parents against sending their girls for a training which was felt to be beneath the dignity of decent educated girls. Religion prevented Hindu and Muslim girls from joining at all and so only Christian girls could be trained at first. But for many years, even they felt nursing was an inferior profession.

In the beginning there was no uniformity of courses or educational requirements. About 1907–1910 the North India United Board of Examiners for Mission Hospitals was organized and set up rules for admissions and standards of training and conducted a public examination. On 24th May 1909 the Indian Medical Mission Association granted the Nursing Diploma after examining student by Central Board for Nurses' Training Schools in South India. A few years later the Mid-India and the South India Boards of Nurse examiners were similarly set up. These are Examining Boards of the Nurses' League of the Christian Medical Association of India. The name of the South India Board was changed to 'The Board of Nursing Education, Nurses' League of Christian Medical Association of India branch in 1975.

The Dufferin Fund

Until the late 19th century there were no women doctors and therefore, no care for women except in mission hospitals. This fact was brought to the attention of Queen Victoria. At this time, Lady Dufferin was coming out to India with her husband who was on government service. Queen Victoria instructed Lady Dufferin about the need for medical care for women and children in India and asked her to take a special interest in this problem. Lady Dufferin wrote to her friends and influential people to get financial aid. Thus, in 1885, Lady Dufferin was responsible for starting the 'National Association for supplying Medical Aid by Women to Women of India.' This is commonly called the Dufferin Fund and continues to provide medical education for women, to train nurses and midwives for hospitals and private work, and to improve medical facilities for women.

Between 1890 and 1900, many schools under either missions or government were started in various parts of India. The directors of these schools were English or American. Each school sets up its own pattern of training familiar to the director. There was a need for systematic training of nurses like that given in the Nightingale School in England. Thus, it was that in 1886, money from the Dufferin Fund was made available for this purpose. Miss Atkinson, a Nightingale nurse, was brought out from England to Bombay to set up and be the superintendent of the First Modern Training School for Nurses in India. The school was established in the Cama Hospital for Women and Children in 1891. It began with a one year course but by 1995 it had been extended to 3 years.

The leaders of nursing in India realized that more and better qualified teachers and ward supervisors were needed if standards were to be maintained and nursing was to advance. Hence, courses were set up in several places to give Indian nurses an opportunity to prepare themselves for responsible positions in hospitals and schools of nursing. Post-certificate courses were first offered in nursing administration, supervision and teaching. These originated at the College of Nursing, New Delhi; the College of Nursing, CMC Hospital Vellore and the Government General Hospital, Madras.

The first four-year-basic bachelor degree programs were established in 1946 at the Colleges of Nursing in Delhi and Vellore. This program is now offered in a number of other colleges.

In 1963, the School of Nursing in Thiruvananthapuram instituted the first two year post-certificate bachelor degree program. Other schools have begun this program since that time.

In recent years, as higher education for nurses has developed around the world, courses in India have developed so that the nurse can specialize in almost any subject and continue education through the level of the Master's degree. The first Master's degree course, a two-year postgraduate program was begun in 1960 at the College of Nursing in Delhi (Now Rajkumari Amrit Kaur College of Nursing, New Delhi-110 024). In 1970, many colleges of nursing were started and offering PCBSc Nursing and Basic BSc Nursing courses in various parts of India. In Karnataka, Bangalore University instituted PhD program for nurses in 1991. The author of this book is the first person to get Doctoral degree in Nursing in the State of Karnataka.

Auxiliary Nursing

The use of auxiliary nursing personnel to ease the shortage of professional nurses had been common in some countries when it was first put into practice in India. A two-year program for the Auxiliary Nurse-Midwife was first established in 1951 at St. Mary's Hospital, Tarn Taran in Punjab state. By 1962, there were 263 courses being offered in India. The auxiliary nurse midwife is prepared to practice elementary nursing and full midwifery. She functions primarily in the community rather than the hospital. The practice of the auxiliary nurse-midwife has helped to improve the amount of care given to the patient as well as the health teaching given to the public. In 1977 the ANM course was completely revised by the Indian Nursing Council and expanded to include sociology health education and communication skills and subjects necessary to equip the multipurpose health worker/ ANM to serve effectively as a primary health care worker in the community. Such workers are key persons for achievement of the goal of "Health for all by 2000 AD" to which we in India are committed.

Textbooks on Nursing

One of the handicaps in the development of nursing schools was the lack of textbooks. In other countries, books had been written by doctors and nurses. Some of these were translated into the vernacular for the early schools and colleges. Many English and American textbooks are being used in the schools today. There is a great need for textbooks which have been written by Indian nurses. A beginning had been made in this work and the first 'Textbook for Nurses in India' was printed by the South India Examining Board of the Nurses' League of the Christian Medical Association of India in 1941. The Nurses' League has also directed the publishing of a 'Textbook for Auxiliary Nurse-Midwives', first printed in 1967. This book was completely revised and published in two volumes in 1985 as a 'Textbook for the Health Worker (ANM)' to meet the needs of the health worker. Several manuals related to the basic sciences and nursing have been published by other professional nursing bodies. Although progress has been made in the publication of textbooks by the nurses of India, there remains a wide area of subjects which have not been touched upon and the general need for more and varied textbooks continues. Since a few nursing educator started writing texts on Nursing, to quote, Late Dr (Mrs) Kasturi Sunder Rao wrote text on 'Community Health Nursing', and a few Bombay-based Nurses made an effort to write guides and two books on Nursing. In later part of 1990s onwards the author of this book also has written on Nursing Research (1998), Community Health Nursing (1998), Nursing Administration (2000), Nursing Education (2003), Fundamentals of Nursing (2002), Medical Surgical Nursing (2003), Pediatric Child Health Nursing (2004), Midwifery and Reproductory Health Nursing (2006), Psychiatric Mental Health Nursing (2006), Nursing Theories (2007), Psychology for Nursing (2011), Biostatistics for Nursing and Child Health Nursing. Essential series on, Medical Surgical Nursing, Mental Health Nursing Community Health Nursing, Nursing Research and Statists. Nursing Foundations on the basis of present needs in Indian context and started revision of earlier texts.

Nursing education in India began with very brief periods of training as mentioned in the first part of this chapter. Orderlies and midwives were often chosen for this and were given a period of 2 to 6 months of closely supervised practical experience in general nursing, then called 'sick nursing'. This was training in the hospital, and certificates were given after completion of a training.

The basic program for combined general nursing and midwifery developed rapidly after 1871. The need for theory as well as practical experience was felt. The training for general nursing was extended to 2 years and then 3 years before the student went on for midwifery training. The present basic program for nursing education throughout India consists of a

3½ year program in general nursing and 6 to 7 months in midwifery. Uniformity of training is maintained by recognition of schools which meet the standards and requirements given by the Indian Nursing Council. The basic certificate program now includes all areas of nursing as integrated community health nursing.

Now, most of the states in India started basic BSc Nursing, Postcertificate BSc Nursing and MSc Nursing degree courses in their related universities. And also there in Doctoral degree course in nursing leading to PhD in nursing.

REGISTRATION OF NURSES

As training for nurses, midwives, and health visitors progressed, the need for legislation to provide basic minimum standards in education and training was felt. It was also felt that registration would give greater professional status. For some years, nurses struggled to obtain proper examinations and examiners and registration for nurses. In 1926 Madras State formed the first Registration Council. While most states now have a recognized Registration Council, all do not. It is now possible for the students of all schools in India to be registered in one of the State Registration Councils.

The Indian Nursing Council

The Indian Nursing Council Act was passed by an ordinance on December 31st 1947. The council was constituted in 1949. The purpose of the council is to coordinate activities of the various State Registration Councils, to set up standards for nursing education and to make sure these standards are carried out. Before this time, nurses registered in one state were not necessarily recognised for registration in another. The condition to mutual recognition by the State Nurses Registration Council called reciprocity was possible only if uniform standards of nursing education was maintained. Therefore, the INC was given authority to prescribe curricula for nursing education in all of the states. At the same time, it was given authority to recognize programs of nursing education or refuse recognition. The Indian Nursing Council is not itself a registering body nor examining body but it can enforce its standards by recognizing or refusing to recognize schools. And now, almost all the states of India has their State Nursing Council for example, Karnataka State Nursing Council, etc.

Community Health Nursing

In India, community health nursing had its beginning when the terrible conditions under which children were born were recognized as a cause for the high civilian mortality rate. It was realized that the untrained dais who attended women during delivery must be given training. This was not an easy job as the dais were unwilling to be trained and the patients were very willing to accept the old customary methods and could see no need to change. The first attempts to train dais were carried out by missionaries as early as 1886. In 1900, Lady Curzon brought about the establishment of the Victoria Memorial Scholarship for the purpose of improving safe delivery practices. The need for training a better type of midwife was felt. In this, Madras State led the way when they passed the Madras Registration of Nurses and Midwives Act of 1926.

Slowly the need for trained personnel for maternal and childhealth, as part of community health nursing was felt. To supply this need a Health School for the training of health visitors was started in Delhi in 1918. This has now become the Lady Reading Health School.

A further step forward was taken in 1948, when community health nursing was integrated in the basic program of the new degree courses which were started at the College of Nursing, Delhi and the School of Nursing, CMC Hospital, Vellore under the University of Delhi and Madras respectively.

Since 1953, a post-certificate course in community health nursing has been given at the All India Institute of Hygiene and Public Health in Calcutta. In 1960, a course was established by the Lady Reading Health School in Delhi. Several other schools now offer this program.

To prepare more community health nurses, in 1957 the Government of India selected ten schools of nursing and gave assistance so that they could integrate community health nursing into their basic course. Since that time, recognition of a program of basic nursing education required that community health nursing be integrated into the basic course. Thus, all professional nurses today can function in the hospital and the community at the level of a staff nurse.

Various international organizations, such as WHO, UNICEF and Colombo Plan have assisted by supplying trained personnel and equipment to help in the training of students in the rural field, maternity work and pediatrics.

THE NURSES' RESPONSIBILITY FOR THE FUTURE OF NURSING

Nursing has evolved with the development of civilization of mankind. Nursing encompasses autonomous and collaborative care of individuals of all ages, families, groups and communities, sick or well and in all settings. Nursing includes the promotion of health, prevention of illness, and the care of ill, disabled and dying people. Advocacy, promotion of a safe environment, research, participation in shaping health policy and in patient and health systems management, and education are also key nursing roles. Nursing requires a delicate balance of promoting clients' independence and dependence. Nursing focuses not on illness but rather on the client's response to illness. Nursing promotes health and helps clients move to a higher level of wellness. This aspect of nursing also includes assisting a client with a terminal illness to maintain comfort and dignity in the final stage of life.

Throughout this study of nursing we have seen nursing advance from the kindly ministrations of a mother or a neighbor to the highly organized service of today. In the beginning, individuals were inspired to help one another in distress. This essential care or service still remains but time has brought about changes in our ideas regarding nursing. Today we are not only relieve and give comfort but help our patients to live upto their optimum health. The new emphasis is on health nursing—nursing the mind, the family as a whole and as part of the community with the nurse as the health teacher.

Growing specialization in medicine is resulting in a trend towards increased specialization in nursing. The development of new tests and diagnostic procedures, new medicines and new equipment make specialization even more necessary as the amount of scientific knowledge needed for a certain speciality becomes greater. Developments in other professions also influence trends in the nursing profession. As other members of the health team become more available and more highly specialized, the work of the nurse is changing towards more specific nursing functions. It has also added to the number and kind of professional relationships which must be maintained by the nurse. The power of spiritual factors is becoming of increasing interest as reports of the healing power of spiritual activity such as meditation is receiving more attention. Just as advances in technology tend to take the nurse away from the bedside and a direct relationship with the patient, so these developments are showing the need for a deeper therapeutic relationship between the nurse and the patient. The future will demand a balance of these factors in order to meet the total health needs of the individual and the community. Future trends are likely to show an effort to make this balance.

Nursing is a profession focused on advocacy in the care of individuals, families, and communities in attaining, maintaining, and recovering optimal health and functioning. Nursing is an interpersonal, interactional or partnering, process between the nurse and client with the objective of promoting wellness, preventing illness and giving the client the tools to be able to functions at an optimal level of wellness. Nursing is an art and a science by which people are assisted in learning to care for themselves whenever possible and cared for by others when they are unable to meet their own needs. Nursing promotes health and helps clients move to a higher level of wellness. This aspect nursing also includes assisting a client with a terminal illness to maintain comfort and dignity in the final stage of life.

Many trends leading to professionalism are taking place because of the untiring efforts of nurses dedicated to achieving the aim of becoming a profession. In 1970, WHO recognized Nursing as a profession. It has often been a difficult struggle requiring real courage and vision by nursing leaders in the face of serious obstacles. Today nurses enjoy many rights and privileges, though desired standards are still not achieved in all areas, because nursing leaders have struggled to achieve them. Nurses who are going to be the future leaders have to carry on this work of greater achievement through growing amounts of writing and research.

Nursing today provides an ever widening scope of opportunity for service. With present trends leading towards greater opportunities, varieties of services and growing social and professional recognition, it should be exciting and challenging for nurses to know that all nurses members of this profession since they fulfill the criteria of the profession (for further details please read the authors text on "Nursing Administration").

Medical Surgical Nursing is commonly defined as the nursing care of adults with suspected or diagnosed pathology of physiological function. It encompasses such a large scope that the trend is to subdivide medical-surgical, oncological (cancer) nursing, and only recently have the other specialties been developed.

Currently, all basic nursing programs prepare nurses to practice medical-surgical nursing. Advanced preparation at the master's and doctoral levels is necessary if the nurse wishes to develop expertise and acquire in-depth knowledge in particular aspects or subdivisions of the specialty. These specialties would include intensive care units, the emergency room.

Medical-surgical nursing is the area of practice concerned with the care of adults with predicted or existing physiologic alterations, trauma, or disability. It is the backbone of modern nursing and the practice foundation of virtually all health care institutions.

Traditionally medical-surgical nursing was not considered a specialty area. Rather, practices with a focus on a specific type of health problem within the area of medical-surgical nursing were considered specialties. These included cardiovascular, perioperative, neurologic, gynecologic, infection control and emergency nursing, and practices limited to problems such as wound care, burns, hypertension and diabetes. Today this view has changed. Medical-surgical nursing is now formally recognized as a specialty in its own right, and the focused practice areas are seen as subspecialties.

Now medical-surgical nursing is a nursing specialty area concerned with the care of adult patients in a broad range of settings. Traditionally, medical-surgical nursing was an entry-level position that most nurses viewed as a stepping stone to specialty areas. Medical-surgical nursing is the largest group of professionals in the field of nursing. Advances in medicine and nursing have resulted in medical-surgical nursing evolving into its own specialty. Medicine-surgical nursing is the foundation of all nursing practice. Once upon a time and not so very long ago, all nurse practiced the art and science of nursing on wards, everyone was a medical or surgical nurse - that is where all nursing started. Today many nurses choose to work in the specialty of medical-surgical nursing. Many years ago, a majority of hospital nurses worked on wards, and everyone was a medical-surgical nurse. Today licensed medical-surgical nurses work in a variety of positions, inpatient clinics, emergency departments, nursing administration, outpatient surgical centers, home health care, humanitarian relief work, ambulatory surgical care, and skilled nursing homes. Some military medical-surgical nurses serve on battlefields.

Formal recognition as a specialty means that a practice area meets the criteria for specialty status, which were published in the document titled Recognition of a Specialty Approval of Scope Statements and Acknowledgement of Nursing practice Standards (ANA). The criteria are that the practice area must:

- Be clearly defined and subscribe to the overall purposes and functions of nursing
- Define itself as nursing
- Adhere to the overall licensure requirements of the profession
- Be national or international in scope
- Be able to identify a need and demand for itself
- Have a well-derived knowledge base particular to the practice of the specialty
- Be organized and represented by a national specialty association
- Be concerned with phenomena within the discipline of nursing
- Have defined competencies for the area of specialty practice
- Have existing mechanisms for supporting, reviewing and disseminating research to support its knowledge base
- Have continuing education programs that prepare nurses in the specialty
- Include a substantial number of nurses who devote most of their practice to the specialty.

The nursing profession has adopted standards of practice that describe the responsibilities for which are accountable. All nurses, regardless of education, follow standards of clinical nursing practice to guide their practice. This broad set of standards has two components—standards of care and standards of professional performance. The nursing process and competent level of nursing care are the foundation of the standards of care. The standards of professional performance address expected quality of care, performance appraisal, education, collegiality, ethics, collaboration, research, and resource utilization. Each standard has measurement criteria to demonstrate competent practice.

The Academy of Medical Surgical Nurses, founded in 1991, is an international organization dedicated to fostering excellence in medical-surgical nursing practice. Its mission is to "enhance the clinical expertise, professionalism, and leadership of nurses caring for adults in hospitals, the community, and long-term care".

CHAPTER

2

Nursing Process Application

INTRODUCTION

In the past, nurses have prided themselves on comforting those, who are ill and on executing with precision such tasks as dressing wounds administering medications, and bathing, feeding and ambulating client. Many of these tasks were ordered by doctors and few nurses would have characterized their 'Job' on being independent, scientifically based or creative. Now health care delivery system has changed, and nursing has changed with it. Nurses now work with well and ill clients in all settings. In addition to their role as caregiver, nurses fill specialized roles as care managers—coordinators, teachers, counselors, advocates, nursing administrators, nurse-educators and nurse researchers. Nurses are responsible for a unique dimension of health care "the diagnosis and treatment of human responses to actual or potential health problems" and as such are knowledgeable, competent, and independent professionals who work collaboratively with other health care professionals to design and deliver holistic care.

As the practice of nursing became more complex, nurses began to study the process of nursing to both understand and improve the means nurses used to accomplish their aims. It has been assumed that professional nursing practice is interpersonal in nature. Recognizing the importance and effect of the nurse's relationships with the client/patient professional nurses use this knowledge throughout the nursing process. It is also assumed that professional nurses view human being as holistic, thereby acknowledging that mind and body are not separate but function as a whole. People respond as unique whole beings. What happens is one part of mind or body affects the person as a whole. These assumptions give clue that nursing is interpersonal in nature and the professional nurses view human beings as holistic, give guidance and directions to the use of the nursing process.

NATURE OF NURSING PROCESS

As studied earlier, "nursing is the diagnosis and treatment of human responses to actual or potential problems". The fundamental basis of nursing practice is "Process". Every aspect of practice is affected by an understanding and utilization of nursing practice.

Nursing process is an organized approach to problem-solving and decision-making that describes the intellectual activity of the nurse. It is the accepted methodology for nursing practice. The nursing process is the underlying scheme that provides order and direction of nursing care. It is the essence of profession—nursing practice. It is the 'tool' and methodology of the nursing profession and as such it helps nurses in arriving at decisions and in predicting and evaluating consequences.

The nursing process is a "deliberate, intellectual activity by which the practice of nursing is approached in an orderly systematic manner. Each of these terms for defining the process can be further delineated as follows:

- 'Deliberate' refers to careful, thoughtful and intentional process
- 'Intellectual' refers to the process has rational, knowledgeable, reasonable and conceptional
- 'Activity' refers to state or condition of functioning, initiating, changing and behaving
- 'Orderly' refers to that it is methodological, efficient, and has logical arrangement
- 'Systematic' means to purposeful and pertaining to classification.

The nursing process is a method of making clinical decisions. It is a way of thinking and acting in relation to the clinical phenomena of concern to nurses. Classifically, the nursing

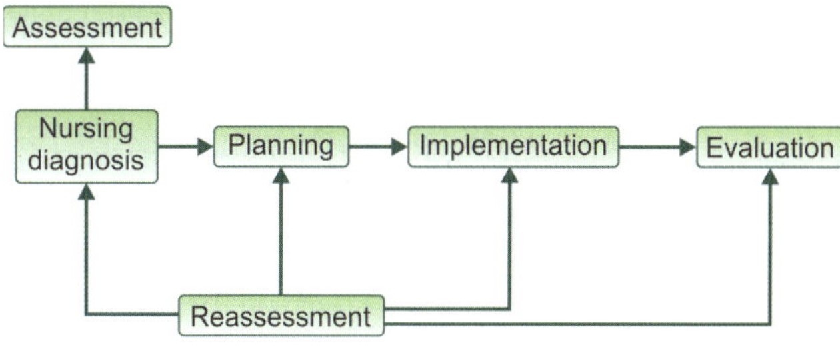

FIG. 2.1: The nursing process

process comprises of five phases or dimensions—assessment, nursing diagnosis, planning, implementation and evaluation. The nursing process is a systematic decision-making model that is cyclic not lineal (Fig. 2.1). By virtue of evaluational phase, the nursing process incorporates a feedback loop that maintains quality control of its decision-making outputs.

The nursing process is indeed a method of solving clinical problems but it is not merely a problem-solving method. Similar to a problem-solving method, the nursing process offers an organized, systematic, approach to clinical problems. Unlike a problem solving method, the nursing process is continuous, not episodic. The five phases constitute a continuous cycle throughout the nurses' moment-to-moment data interpretation and management of patient care. The phases of nursing process being not only continuous, but "interactive" in other words, all phases of the nursing process operate and influence each other and the patient simultaneously. This illustrates interactive nature of the nursing process, wherein each phase represented by a line that intersects with others and converges at point in time to which the nurse attends.

The nursing process was developed as a specific method for applying a scientific approach or a problem-solving approach to nursing practice. Problem-solving approaches are not unique to nursing. For example, health planners have long used a health planning process that is a problem-solving approach aimed at planned social change. Physicians use a specific process for gathering assessment data to make a medical diagnosis. The nursing process deals with problem specific to nurses and their clients/patients. In nursing client/patient may be an individual, family, or community, and the nursing process has been adapted for use with each type of client/patient (Christensen and Kenny 1990).

Students of nursing using the nursing process are learning to behave as professional nurses in practice behave. Since the nursing process is the essence and tool (methodology) of professional nursing practice, student must become familiar with and adopt at using it as their basis of practice. The nursing process also provides a means for evaluating the quality of nursing care given by nurses and assures their accountability and responsibility to the client/patient.

To use the nursing process effectively, nurses need to understand and apply appropriate concepts and theories from nursing, the theological, physical and behavioral sciences and the humanities. These concepts and theories provide a rationale for decision making, judgments, interpersonal relationships and actions. These concepts provide the framework for nursing care.

DEFINITION OF NURSING PROCESS

The nursing process is often defined as the application of critical thinking to client-care activities. In addition, because nursing is a human-caring discipline, other styles of thinking influence nursing decision. Four ways of thinking which include ritual, random, appreciative and critical thinking. *Ritual* thinking underlies the development of habits-actions we perform so often or regularly, that we do them automatically, without conscious decisions. *Random* thinking is the free association of ideas at the unconscious level that can lead to impulsive implementation of the first problem solving solution that comes to mind it can also be creating source of new problem-solving ideas and approaches. *Appreciative* thinking reflects awareness of human values and respect for client's individual needs. *Critical thinking* is based on the acientific method, i.e. the deliberate and systematic use of rational informed thought processes in problem finding and problem solving. It is the key stone of sensible decision making using the nursing process and it yields predictable, repeatable results.

The nursing process can be defined in terms of three major dimensions which include purpose, organization and properties.

Purpose

The primary purpose of the nursing process is to help manage each client care scientifically, holistically and creatively. To do this successfully the nurse needs many intellectual, technical and interpersonal and ethical/legal competencies as well as the willingness to use them creatively when working with the clients to promote wellness, to prevent disease, or illness, to restore health and to facilitate coping with altered functioning.

Organization

The nursing process has traditionally defined as a systematic method for assessing health status, diagnosing health care needs, formulating a plan of care, initiating and implementing plan and evaluating the effectiveness of plan of care. The nursing process consists of five sequential steps or inter-related phases, i.e. assessment, nursing diagnosis, planning implementation, and evaluation. These are considered as organized steps or components or nursing process.

Properties

The nursing process has seven properties, that is, systematic dynamic, interpersonal, flexible, theoretically-based, goal-oriented and universally applicable. Here the various words and phrases have been used to describe the nursing process.

Systematic

The nursing process is a systematic method that directs the nurse and client as together determine the need for nursing care, plan and implement the care and evaluate the results. The steps in this client-centered, goal-oriented process are interrelated each of the five steps preceding it. The process provides a framework that enables the nurse and client to do the following:

- Collect systematically clients' data (assessing)
- Clearly identify client strengths and problem (diagnosing)
- Develop holistic plan of individualized care that specified the desired client goals and related outcomes and the nursing interventions most likely to assist the client to meet those expected outcomes (planning)
- Execute the plan of care (implementing)
- Evaluate the effectiveness of the plan of care in terms of the client goal and achievement (evaluation).

The nursing process directs each step of nursing care in a sequential order/manner. So it is systematic.

Dynamic

The nursing process is dynamic, because it involves continuous change. It is an ongoing process focussed on the changing responses of the client that are identified throughout the nurse-client relationship.

Interpersonal

The nursing process is interpersonal. Always at the heart of nursing is the human being. It is interactive because the interactive nature is based on the reciprocal relationship that occurs between the nurse and the client, family and other health professionals.

Flexible

The nursing process is flexible, because the flexibility of the process may be demonstrated in two contexts.

- It can be adapted to nursing practice and any setting or area of specialization dealing with individuals, groups or communities.
- Its phrases may be used sequentially and concurrently, i.e. the nursing process is most frequently used in sequence, however, the nurse may use more than one step at a time.

Theoretically Based

The nursing process is theoretically based because the process is devised from a broad-based knowledge including the sciences and humanities and can be applied to any other theoretical models of nursing.

Goal-oriented

The nursing process is goal oriented because it offers a means for nurses and clients to work together to identify specific goal related to wellness promotion, disease and illness prevention, health restoration and coping with altered functioning, which are most important to client, and to match them with appropriate nursing actions. Once these are recorded in the plan of care, each nurse can quickly determine the client's priorities and begins nursing with a clear sense of how to proceed. The client benefits from continuity of care and each nurse can move the client close to good achievement.

Universally Applicable

The nursing process is universally applicable the one constant in health care is changed. Once nurses have a working knowledge of the nursing process, they find that they can practice nursing with well or ill persons, young or old, in any type of practice setting. Efforts made by the nurses to master nursing process will result in their possession of a valuable tool that can be used with ease in any nursing situation.

STEPS OF NURSING PROCESS

Nursing process involves five steps which include assessment, nursing diagnosis, planning, implementation and evaluation. In earlier writings about the nursing process, many authors agreed that four phases components, steps or stages were necessary; assessment, including nursing diagnosis or problem identification, planning, intervention or implementation and evaluation. Because nursing diagnosis is the considered essential component of the nursing process, majority of them are accepted as one step in the nursing process. Let us examine in brief of each step.

ASSESSMENT

Assessment is the first phase in the nursing process and has two subphases which include data collection and data analysis or synthesis. Assessment consists of the systematic and orderly collections and analysis of data about the health status of the client/patient for the purpose of making the nursing diagnosis. If incorrect or insufficient assessment leads to incorrect nursing diagnosis which could mean inappropriate planning, implementation and evaluations. Therefore, the importance of accurate assessment cannot be overemphasized. It is vital to the process and is the basis for all other phases. Although assessment is the first phase, it may also occur as reassessment during any other phase of the process when new data are obtained as shown in Figure 2.1.

The systematic and orderly collection of data is essential for the nurse to know if sufficient data have been collected. It also provides a method of quick retrieval of information about the client/patient for auditing professional practice and for doing research. In addition, it serves as a means of communicating information to their health care providers, assessing involves, a thorough, ongoing, comprehensive collection of subjective and objective data of the patient-family-environment, interactions. Such data are obtained via history-taking, observation, physical examination, laboratory data, X-rays and other diagnostic studies. Use of functional health pattern assists in eliciting information concern in nursing. A holistic view during assessment phase ensures that the biological, psychological, social, cultural and spiritual spheres of the client are considered. Any assessment guidelines include the following:

- Biographical data
- A health history including family members
- Subjective data and objective data about current health status including physical examination and reason for contact with health care professional, medical diagnosis, if the client/patient has a medical problem, and results of diagnostic studies
- Social, cultural, and environmental data
- Behaviors that may place a person at risk for potential disease/problems.

By using these guidelines, the data collected are classified into discrete areas that can be compared, contrasted for relationships and clustered during the analysis of data. The current health status of the client is also ascertained through interviewing the client or the person responsible for the client (subjective data) and thorough examination and observation of the client to obtain data that can be seen or measured objectively (objective data). For example, client's description of pain is considered subjective data, whereas vital signs are an example of objective measurement.

By virtue of nursing's unique orientation and commitment to holism, nurses collect an enormous amount of data about a patient's biopsychosocial health status. And by virtue of an array of technophysiologic monitoring devices, nurses process an additional layer of data in the form of physiologic parameter measurements. Consequently, assembling this data base, nurses need some place to file the information as it is collected. Ideally, this storage system would contain compartments, which could keep the data separated and organized. Such system is called as assessment or organizational framework.

Organizational framework can also serve as guides for assessment and their compartments consists of headings corresponding to the attributes the nurse accepts as constituting the nature of human health illness and nursing. In this way, framework helps guide the identification of diagnosis that are within the domain of nursing.

Assessment frameworks are neither new nor unique to nursing. Traditionally nursing used medical assessment framework for the collection and organization of data, but a nursing knowledge base and conceptual orientations become increasingly differentiated and complex, the biologic mechanistic scheme of medicine was found to be insufficiently comprehensive for its use by nurses as a tool for holistic assessment.

- The assessment framework for the generalist medical practice include body systems like cardiovascular, respiratory, neurologic, endocrine metabolic, hematopoietic, integumentory, gastrointestinal, genitourinary, reproductive, and psychiatric.
- The functional health pattern typology developed by Marjory Gordon (1987) are categories of human biologic, psychologic, developmental, cultural, social and spiritual assessment, has gained wide acceptance in nursing service and education systems as assessing framework which includes:
  - Health perception—health management
  - Nutritional—metabolic
  - Eliminations
  - Activity—exercises
  - Sleep—rest
  - Cognitive—perceptual
  - Self-perception—self-concept
  - Role—relationship
  - Sexuality—reproductive
  - Coping—stress tolerance
  - Value—belief
- And Nine human responses revised by NANDA (1986) named NANDA (North American Nursing Diagnostic Association).

Taxonomy I (system of classification that organizes known phenomena into a hierarchic structure and helps direct the discovery of new phenomena). The specifications of a nomenclature and its successor, a taxonomy, is an important preliminary step in building nursing theory and science. The nine human responses patterns of taxonomy I revised are as follows:

1. *Exchanging:* A human response pattern involving mutual giving and receiving.
2. *Communicating:* A human response pattern involving sending messages.
3. *Relating:* A human response pattern involving establishing bonds.
4. *Valuing:* A human response pattern involving the assigning of relative worth.
5. *Choosing:* A human response pattern involving selection of alternatives.
6. *Moving:* A human response pattern involving activities.
7. *Perceiving:* A human response pattern involving reception of informations.
8. *Knowing:* A human response pattern involving the meaning associated with information.

9. *Feeling:* A human response pattern involving the subjective awareness of information.

The selection of any one framework over another, as long as it is designed to organize nursing data is an individual choice.

NURSING DIAGNOSIS

Nursing diagnosis, the second phase of the nursing process is recognized in ANA definition of nursing as the diagnosis and treatment of human responses to actual or potential health problems. The concept of nursing diagnosis, a process whereby nurses interpret assessment data and apply standardized labels to health problems they identify and anticipate treating, is rapidly evolving in clinical and educational settings. Critical attention is being focused on aspects of nursing practice and education that either foster or inhibit the establishment of the discipline nursing as a profession. A traditional reliance on the language and therapeutics of other sciences is inhibiting the establishment of nursing as a free-standing profession. Effort to identify and name the conditions that nurses study and treat, on the other hand, foster nursing professional identity by clarifying its distinct services to society and providing a vehicle for the building of its science.

A nursing diagnosis is a clinical judgment about individual, family or community responses to actual or potential health problems/life processes provide the basis for selection of nursing interventions to achieve outcomes for which the nurse is accountable (NANDA 1990). This diagnostic statement identifies the client's actual or potential health problems deficit or concern, which can be affected by nursing actions. It describes a group of data with interpretation based on the client's ability to meet basic needs. Models for these diagnostic statements have been provided by many authors based on the taxonomy developed by NANDA. For most clients, there will be more than one nursing diagnosis (in medicine also, now there will be more than one medical diagnosis).

Nursing diagnostic statements are derived from the nurse's inferences which are based on the assessed and validated data coupled with nursing, scientific and humanistic concepts and theories. The term 'inference' is very useful in defining nursing diagnosis, because it emphasizes the tentative and assumptive nature of diagnoses. Inference refers to the process of arriving at a conclusion by reasoning from evidence and warns that "if the evidence is slight the term comes close to surmise". In recognizing that element of both judgment and inference are part of nursing diagnosis, one can appreciate the need to limit or control the influence of bias on the part of the nurses and in the act of diagnosing so that the diagnostic conclusion reached is as logical and factually based as possible.

The human response to health and illness situation constitutes the focus of phenomenon, of concern to nurses, and it is the object of nurse's diagnostic activities. As one proceeds through the analysis of data, certain patterns develop and the use of relevant concepts and theories become appropriate. Nursing diagnosis can be considered a client-related behavioral statement that identifies the area for focus of nursing action. A diagnosis may deal with an actual (present-oriented) or a potential (future-oriented) health problem. It is based on conclusion reached in the assessment phase.

Formulating Nursing Diagnosis Statements

Guidelines for use of the taxonomy of approved nursing diagnosis. It is important to recognize that classification of the phenomena to which a profession addresses itself is a sizable and ongoing task. The development and refinement of nursing's nomenclature of health status are in their earliest stages and subject to much revision based on the reserved and clinical reports presented and reviewed at each of NANDA's conferences and by the Diagnosis Review Committee. Work on existing diagnoses also is incomplete. Several have etiologies and defining characteristics yet to be developed, making clinical use difficult and frustrating. Other diagnosis may be deleted from the approved list from conference to conference. Such changes are both necessary and usual in the process of taxonomy development. One has only to look at the system of names describing health problems treated by physicians not many years ago (for example, chilblains consumption, dropsy) to appreciate nursings progress to date.

Guidelines for Diagnostic Labels

Definitions of health problems: Nearly all approved diagnoses have accompanying definitions to better explain the health state they represent. These definitions are important for the student of nursing diagnosis to consider, because they clarify more about the health state than is apparent from the label alone. For example, the definition accompanying the diagnose's fear and anxiety draw a particularly useful distinction between the two problems. Fear is an emotion that has an identifiable source or object that the patient validates, whereas anxiety is an emotion whose source is non-specific or unknown to the patient. Other good examples of such definitions accompany the diagnoses social isolation, powerlessness, altered parenting, and caregiver role strain.

Until definitions accompany all approved diagnoses, it is important for nurses collaborating in care to establish consensus about the meaning and scope of the health problems stated.

Making diagnostic labels specific: Some nursing diagnoses need accompanying qualifiers or specifiers based on the characteristics of the health problem as it manifests itself in a particular patient. For example, the diagnosis fear needs specification as to the object of the patient's particular fear, such as death, pain, disfigurement, or malignancy. Similarly, the diagnosis knowledge deficit needs specification about the content of the deficit, such as use of incentive spirometer, counting the pulse rate or respiratory muscle strengthening exercise. Following is a list of nursing diagnoses needing specification, each with an example of a particular patient circumstance so specified:

- *Fear:* Postoperative pain.
- *Knowledge deficit:* Self-monitoring of oral anticoagulation therapy.
- *Altered peripheral:* Tissue perfusion.
- *Altered nutrition:* Less than body potassium requirements.
- *Altered nutrition:* More than body kilocalorie requirements.
- *Self-care deficit:* Bathing and feeding.
- *Non-compliance:* Prescribed activity restrictions.

Guidelines for Etiologic-related Factors

Making etiologies specific: In many instances, NANDA's etiologies are broad categories or examples needing to be made specific based on characteristics of the health state and the patient being treated. For example, one of several possible etiologies for the diagnosis fluid volume excess is compromised regulatory mechanism. Considering this, the cause of the fluid excess in a particular patient, the nurse needs to specify which regulatory mechanism and in what way compromised (for example, inappropriate ADH secretion by the neurohypophysis) before the diagnosis can be formally stated (disregarding the question of whether the problem is treatable by nurses or needs referral).

Several etiologies needing to be made specific follow-up along with examples of such specification in parentheses:

- Situational crisis (recent diagnosis of terminal illness)
- Psychologic injuring agent (hurtful relationship, verbal abuse)
- Developmental factors (developmental arrest, extremes of age).

Nursing diagnoses as etiologies: Nursing diagnostic labels may rightfully serve as etiologies for other diagnoses.

Examples are anxiety related to knowledge deficit, and activity intolerance related to decreased cardiac output.

Etiologies as the focus of treatment: The treatment plan formulated for a given diagnosis must include interventions aimed at resolution or management of the etiologic factors, as well as the health state. In fact, in some instances nursing treatment is directed exclusively at the etiology of a diagnosis, with the logical expectation that, if the causative factors are reduced in influence, the problem should begin to resolve. This is true especially in instances where a nursing diagnosis has its etiology another nursing diagnosis, consider treatment approaches to the diagnosis. In effective breathing pattern, there is high abdominal incision pain. Predictably, little effectiveness is shown if the interventions are focused solely on reviewing the rationale for slow, deep symmetrical, breathing; demonstrating the technique; and encouraging the patient in its performance without some plan for manipulation of the pain variable.

Medical diagnoses as etiologies: Because, as mentioned, the etiology of a nursing diagnosis becomes a focus of intervention in the management of the overall health state, citing a medical condition or diagnosis as the etiology is conceptually inadvisable if the diagnostic statement is to retain its identity as a health problem primarily resolved by nursing therapies. And yet, many health states of concern to critical care nurse and amenable to their treatment are consequent to medical conditions. Examples are the ineffective airway clearance that results from chronic obstructive pulmonary disease (COPD), and sensory-perceptual alterations that result from coronary artery bypass graft surgery. In these instances the nurse should isolate those aspects of the contributing pathologic state that are modifiable by nursing intervention and cite these factors as aetiologic, for instance, ineffective airway clearance related to thick tracheobronchial secretions, respiratory muscle weakness, and knowledge deficit; effective cough and hydration techniques, and sensory-perceptual alterations related to sensory overload, sensory depression, and sleep pattern disturbance. These diagnostic statements are more clearly worded and provide a much sharper focus for nursing intervention.

Guidelines for Defining Characteristics

Making defining characteristics specific: As with diagnostic labels and statements of etiology, defining characteristics cited for diagnoses are in non-specific form and often need to be modified to reflect the particular situation presented by the patient being diagnosed. For example, the diagnosis impaired gas exchange has one of the possible defining characteristics abnormal blood gases. In the nurses' formulation of this diagnostic statement for clinical use, the specific blood gas value used to diagnose the problem should be cited in the statement (e.g. PO_2: 54 mm Hg and /or PCO_2: 50 mm Hg) versus the non-specific sign category, abnormal blood gases.

Several defining characteristics are cited as following nonspecific form with accompanying examples of proper specification:

- Respiratory depth changes (hypoventilation)
- Blood pressure changes (hypotension)
- Autonomic responses (dilated pupils, tachycardia)
- Altered electrolytes (hypokalemia)
- Change in mental state (confusion, obtundation, apprehension).

Major or critical defining characteristics: Major or critical defining characteristics are designated signs and/or symptoms that must be present for the health problem to be considered present. Major defining characteristics, when applicable, must be present in the nurse's assessment profile to diagnose the corresponding health state with any degree of certainty. For example, the diagnosis unilateral neglect has its major defining characteristic consistent in attention to stimuli on affected side. It is essential, then, that the characteristic be present in the patient's situation (in addition, perhaps, to several other noncritical signs) for the diagnosis of the problem. The assignment of major or critical status to a defining characteristic is based on research or extensive clinical experience in which the signs and symptoms of a health problem are tested for their ability to meet reliably predict the presence of the diagnosis and can therefore be used with confidence by the nurse diagnostician.

Guidelines for Diagnosing High-risk States

Determining a risk state for diagnosis: Predicting a potential health problem in a given patient involves an estimation of probability. The potential for an event, or pattern of response, to occur can truly be said to exist in almost any situation. Consider the high-risk health problems facing the postoperative patient. This risk state includes high-risk for non-compliance with the rehabilitative regimen, high-risk for body image disturbance, high-risk for sleep pattern disturbance, high-risk for ineffective airway clearance, high-risk for constipation and high-risk for aspiration, to name only a few. To state each of these diagnoses on a treatment plan without regard for probabilities and develop desired patient outcomes and interventions for each is pointless.

What should occur is an appraisal of the patient's health status and the identification of risk factors that place him or her at higher risk for the health problem than the general population. For example, all persons recovering from abdominal surgery have high-risk for constipation because of the effects of general anesthesia and narcotic analgesics, manipulation of abdominal viscera, and postoperative immobility. All nurses have a tacit understanding of this risk, and monitoring and intervention are carried out as part of routine nursing care to avert the problem. Hence, there is no need to state the problem.

A patient is at higher risk than the general population of postoperative patient if there is, for example, a history of dependence on laxatives, fluid volume deficit, prolonged immobility, or non-compliance with nursing prescriptions for ambulation. The diagnosis indicating this potential and its risk factors could be stated so that additional and/or more intensified interventions, over those that are routine, can be planned.

Stating high-risk diagnosis: Several of the approved diagnoses address potential dysfunctional status and cite risk factors. Examples of such diagnoses are the following.

Altered Nutrition: High-risk for more than body requirements.

- High-risk for aspiration
- High-risk for disuse syndrome
- High-risk for impaired skin integrity
- High-risk for infection
- High-risk for injury
- High-risk for poisoning
- High-risk for suffocation
- High-risk for trauma
- High-risk for violence.

In addition to those diagnoses formally listed as high-risks, any diagnosis from the approved list can be stated as an at risk problem by simply adding the modifier high-risk to the label. For example, self-esteem disturbance can be written high-risk for self esteem disturbance by virtue of the presence of factors but not yet the actual health problem.

High-risk nursing diagnoses have only two parts to the statement—the health problem at risk and the risk factors (e.g. high-risk for ineffective individual coping, risk factors, malignant biopsy results, absence of interpersonal support system, and history of alcohol abuse).

Guidelines for Stating Wellness Diagnoses

Wellness nursing diagnoses represent clinical judgments regarding an individual, family, or community in transition from a specific level of wellness and functioning to a higher level of wellness and functioning. The terms potential for enhanced (specify) is the designated diagnostic label. Wellness diagnoses are one-part statements, for example, potential for enhanced parenting, potential for enhanced coping.

Diagnostic Reasoning

Diagnostic reasoning is the critical thinking process through which the nurse moves to arrive at a nursing diagnosis. Like any process, it is often orderly and systematic, However, unlike a process, not all of its factors and operations exist in one's conscious awareness. The challenge of refining one's diagnostic reasoning is to bring into awareness the factors and operations that influence the process and are necessary in arriving at an accurate "answer" or diagnosis. Four key components of diagnostic reasonings are collecting and organizing the data base, identifying cues, making inferences, and validating inferences.

Collecting and organizing the data-base: Collecting and organizing a data-base was discussed earlier.

Identifying cues: A cue is a piece of information, a raw fact. Nurses notice and seek cues regarding patients' health status and functioning. Sweaty palms, restlessness, and a heart rate of 102 beats/min are cues. In the process of diagnostic reasoning, cues are the units of information that are collected and recorded for later analysis.

Making inferences: An inference is the assignment of meaning to cues. A nursing diagnosis is an example of an inference. When individual cues are clustered and interpreted collectively, they begin to assume an identity different from what each represents individually. Sweaty palms, restlessness, and a heart rate of 102 beats/min when interpreted as a cluster could now represent anxiety, shock, fear or pain.

Inferences are created, whereas cues exist: The process of creating inferences from cues, therefore, carries with it the risk of error in logic. If the cues sweaty palms, restlessness, and a heart rate of 102 beats/min were grouped and interpreted in a patient, who also manifested gargling respiratory sounds and a rapid shallow breath in pattern and these additional cues were overlooked or ignored by the person assigning meaning to the cluster—the inference might be erroneous, the more probable inference now might be erroneous, the more probable inference now being ineffective airway clearance. Nursing diagnoses are inferences, and defining characteristics and risk factors are the cues that lead to these inferences.

Validating inferences: Once a diagnostic inference is formulated, the nurse will develop and implement a treatment plan designed to resolve or reduce the problem represented by that inference. Erroneous inferences carry, an obvious implication in terms of potential patient harm resulting from treatment of a non-existent health problem or from treatment withheld for a missed diagnostic nursing malpractice. Consequently, it is essential to seek validation of diagnostic interferences before implementing treatments.

Four approaches to the validation of interferences are recommended. First, consult with an authoritative source. This may be a clinical nurse specialist, nurse educator, textbook or published research, for example, seek confirmation of the logical and scientific integrity of your diagnostic statement.

Second, reexamine the cues; could the ones in the diagnostic statement support another diagnosis or only the one chosen? Could the cues from the data base believe not to be a part of the cluster supporting this diagnosis belong to some other cluster, or could several of them, together with cues supporting this diagnosis, suggest an altogether different diagnosis? Third, validate inferences with the patient. Nurses may share with the patient the cluster of cues identified and what is represented. Patients often have remarkable insight into what underlies their pattern of response and can be a great resource in validating the nurse's conclusions. Additionally, people benefit significantly from having their situations reflected back to them.

Indeed, collaborating with the patient in this way may be all the interversion that is necessary. Fourth seek evidence of the reliability of the diagnostic inference from within the appropriate reference group. Do most professional peers conclude the same explanation for the available cues?

These approaches are workable strategies for seeking validation of diagnostic references before the institution of treatment, however the only way to achieve or confirm validation of a diagnosis is to treat the problem and evaluate the outcome. If favorable and predicted outcomes result, strong evidence exists that the problem and its etiology or risk factors and defining characteristics were accurately inferred.

Source of diagnostic error: Much scientific curiosity exists within the nursing profession regarding the diagnostic reasoning process, strategies employed by experts and those used by notices. The following discussion focuses only on the most common type of diagnostic error. The Inferential Leap, and several of the sources. For more in-depth examinations of the skills of clinical problem solving and decision-making, the reader is referred to Gordon, Carneveli, Tanner and Benner.

Inferential leap: As the term implies, the inferential leap involves a jump to a conclusion based on premature termination of the data gathering/data analysis phase of the nursing process. Numerous studies show that this jump to an erroneous conclusion is most frequently made because not all of the variables are known or examined at the time the inference is fomulated. Of interest, the novice often closes the search for cues prematurely, whereas the expert will more often prematurely terminate the analysis of cues.

The novice may close the search for cues prematurely because of a lack of understanding of the scope of the problem to be diagnosed. Diagnose such as disturbance in self-concept and infective individual coping are reported to be at the highest level of abstraction among nursing diagnoses and are, therefore, more difficult to fully grasp, let along discriminate from other diagnostic possibilities. The expert has an advantage in this regard by virtue of a greater breadth of experience, both with the label and the clinical presentation of patients demonstrating the diagnosis.

Professional advantages of nursing diagnosis: Baer assembled from the literature the following statements in advocacy of nursing diagnosis. They are presented here to highlight the advantages nursing diagnosis brings to the profession. Nursing diagnosis does the following:

- Assists in organizing, defining and developing nursing knowledge or scope
- Aids in identifying and describing the domain and scope of nursing practice
- Focus as nursing care on the patient's response to problems
- Prescribes diagnosis-specific nursing interventions that should increase the effectiveness of nursing care
- Facilitates the evaluation of nursing practice
- Provides a framework for testing the validity of nursing interventions
- Provides a standardized vocabulary to enhance intraprofessional and interprofessional communication
- Prescribes the content of nursing curricula
- Provides a framework for developing a system to direct third party reimbursements for nursing services
- Indicates specific rationales for patient care based on nursing assessment
- Leads to more comprehensive and individualized patient care.

In summary, nursing diagnoses are standardized labels that represent clinical judgments made by professional nurses and describe health states resolved primarily by nursing therapies. Nursing diagnosis focuses on nursing assessment and intervention on the human response to altered health states thus constituting a unique, distinct, and imperative component to critical health care. Nursing diagnosis is mandated as part of competent registered nurse performance criteria by most state nurse practice acts, as well as constituting the core of the ANA's formal definition of nursing.

Diagnosing involves the identification of the patients' actual or potential problem, and the etiology or cause of the problem that nurses can independently treat. The most essential and distinguishing feature of any nursing diagnosis is to describe a health condition primarily resolved by nursing intervention or therapies. Nursing diagnosis is a pivotal component of nursing process. On the one hand it is the judgement, conclusion or decision determined by the nurses as a result of the assessing and problem-solving process. It reflects the process involved in gathering analyzing and interpreting the assessment data. On the other hand, nursing diagnosis provides the basis from which patient outcomes are derived and a plan of appropriate nursing interventions is developed and implemented. Put another way, nursing diagnosis emerges from the collection, analysis and interpretation of assessment data, and provides the framework from which the patient's plan of nursing care involves.

Nursing, as a diagnosis-based practice, demands the nurses become expert at assessing patient's needs and problems formulating nursing diagnosis based on that assessment, evolving and implementing, a plan of care and documenting this nursing care process in a manner reflective of the professional, skilled nursing care rendered. It is the only documenting nursing activities that professional practice can be validated and financially rewarded. Nursing diagnosis reflects a patient's problems or unhealthful response and the problem or etiology that nurses can treat independently. It is a definitive statement of an actual or potential problem, alteration or deficit in the life process (i.e. physiologic, psychologic, sociologic, and spiritualism) of an individual. After the nursing diagnosis are identified, they should be ranked in order of priority. This ranking should consider both the clients' and the nurses' opinions. Those areas that have the greatest impact on the client, the family or both should receive particular attention. The nurse should also determine priorities based on past nursing experience and on scientific knowledge of the needs and functions of human beings. Therefore, a continuum of priorities of nursing diagnosis is developed that is based on the degree of threat to the level of wellness of the client.

The nursing diagnosis can be considered a decisive statement concerning the client's nursing needs. It is important to remember that diagnoses are based on the client's concerns as well as an actual or potential problem that may be symptoms of physiological disorder or of behavioral psychosocial or spiritual problem.

Nurses are encouraged to use the nursing diagnostic categories (as listed) in their daily practice when formulating nursing diagnosis. But it should be remembered and noted that nurses need not feel restricted to the use of NANDA's list but rather should be motivated to develop in practice. Other nursing diagnosis which may be submitted included in NANDA's list or to make separate better list of nursing diagnosis. In this way, nurses are able to share their ideas, experiences, logic and creativity. The procreation of nursing language, along with an ever-increasing awareness of the intellectual activity involved in its process and implementation is every nurse's professional responsibility.

PLANNING

Planning is the third phase of the nursing process. The plan for providing nursing care can be described as the determination of what can be done to assist the client. Planning involves the mutual setting of goals and objectives judging priorities and designing methods to resolve actual or potential problems. Two things are accomplished in the planning phase of nursing process, which includes:

- Establishing goals and objectives
- Selection of nursing intervention.

Goals and Objectives

Goals and objectives which are derived from the nursing diagnoses evolve from and are predicted by the problem portion of the nursing diagnoses, and are established for each nursing diagnosis listed. Goals are stated in broad terms to identify effective criteria for evaluating nursing action. These goals pertain to rehabilitation, prevention of complications associated with stressors, the ability of the client to adapt to these stressors, or all three other goals may deal with the achievement of the highest health potential for a client. For example, "Client will have an adquate understanding of basic food groups and their relationship to RDA = Recommeded daily allowance requirements within one month".

Objectives are the short statement of desired or expected outcomes of the client/patient. Objectives are determined from the goals and need to be stated in terms of observable behavior. Objectives should define the conditions under which the expected or desired end behaviors are to occur and should specify the performance level and specific behaviors that will be accepted as evidence that desired outcomes have been met. The behavior in question refers to psychological, physiological, social, cultural and intellectual activities and other observable responses. The desired behavioral outcomes (objectives) should be stated in a manner that everyone can understand without having to seek clarification. The criteria for stating objectives include the following:

Objectives

Objectives should.

- Be written as the patient behaviors or goals. Patient's outcomes reflect those human responses (physiologic, psychologic, emotional) that must occur if the patient problems is to be resolved. Patient outcomes do not reflect goals that the nurse will achieve. The nurse's role is to support and assist the patient to identify and use his/her capabilities and coping mechanisms more effectively in dealing with the problem.
- Be written in precise and consise terms using action verbs.
- Provide directions for care.

- Specify appropriate time frame within which the patient is reassessed and the care plan is reevaluated. This serves to determine the effectiveness of the nursing intervention in assisting the patient to achieve the desired outcome(s).
- Be realistic.
- Be measurable. It is crucial that patient outcomes be stated in measurable terms so that nurses caring for the patient can use the same criteria to evaluate the patient's response to therapy.

Nursing Interventions

The second subphase in nursing care planning is the identification of nursing actions. For each nursing diagnosis, i.e. nursing interventions, nursing interventions evolve from the etiology position of the nursing diagnosis. For learning experiences (learning by doing) each nursing action is based on carefully thought out scientific rationale and specifies what kind of nursing care is to be done to meet the client's problems effectively. Nursing action should be spelled out precisely. These actions are part of the scheme for providing good nursing care. The characteristics of nursing interventions will include the following:

- Determining the nursing intervention requires that the nruses have a strong theoretical and experiential knowledge base. The nurse must be able to establish appropriate rationale for each nursing intervention implemented.
- Nursing interventions need to be specific: Their implementation is directed towards treating the cause and resolving the patient's problems.
- Nursing interventions prescribe nursing treatments, that is, what it is, the nurse must do to treat the etiology (cause) of the patient's problem. Behaviors described by nursing interventions reflect those of the nurse and not necessarily those of the patient.
- Clear and concise documentation of nursing interventions on the patient care plan is essential to communicate the activities and behaviors of the nurses to colleagues and other health care providers.
- In writing the nursing interventions, the care plan needs to be revised systematically in terms of patient's responses and outcomes. Decisions can then be made as to when specific interventions should be revised, updated, renewed or discontinued. Specific dates and time frames should be documented accordingly (please note that specific dates and times are not included in the nursing care plan presented in this text because they need to be individualized for the specific patient).
- Each documented nursing intervention should be dated and signed by the nurse. The nurse's signature is particularly important in terms of accountability and in the sharing of information (feedback), including clarification of goals and rationales underlying care.

Interventions are the power of nursing and a distinct strength, also known as nursing orders or nursing prescriptions which constitute the treatment approach to an identified health alterations. Interventions are selected to satisfy the outcome criteria and prevent or resolve the nursing diagnosis or problem. Planned interventions should provide clarity, specificity, and direction to the spectrum of nurses implementing care of the patients, e.g. "Check vital signs", "measure intake and output". "Monitor heart state", etc.

Nursing interventions are said to be hypotheses established for testing if they contribute to the solution of the problem. It is up to the nurse with the client, the family or both to select appropriate action to produce desired results. In selecting nursing action, it is important to analyze the available options and to determine the probability of success in reaching the objective. Sometimes compromises must be made to provide the best care for the client, and the nurse needs to be aware of this when specifying nursing actions.

The nursing care plan deals with actual or potential problems. Nursing interventions are based on scientific principles and theories of nursing and they need to be specific. The plan serves as a means for resolving the problems and for meeting established goals in an orderly fashion. Also it provides a means for organization, giving direction and meaning to the nursing action used in helping the client, the family or both to resolve the health problems. A plan of action is necessary, because it aids in the efficient use of time. It saves both time and energy by providing essential data for those individuals who are responsible for giving care. Since the clients' condition is continuously changing, the written nursing care plan needs to reflect these changes. Therefore, planning becomes a continuous process based on evaluation and reassessment. The written plan is the most efficient way of keeping all individuals involved in the client's care informed of modification in the plan of nursing care.

Documentation of the patient's nursing care plan reflects the culmination of the problem-solving/decision-making activities of the professional nurse. Such documentation demonstrates the ability of the nurse to apply nursing knowledge to clinical situations and to integrate this knowledge in the implementation of the component of the nursing process.

The nursing care plan (NCP) format is used throughout this text to afford the reader the opportunity to examine the interrelatedness of the components of the process and to appreciate how documentation of language of process which includes problem, reason, objectives, nursing intervention (with rationale) and evaluation.

Problem refers actual or potential problems, stated in the form of nursing diagnosis, which is the product of assessment.

Reason refers to an inference in the diagnostic reasoning. Diagnostic reasoning is the critical thinking process through which the nurse moves to arrive at a nursing diagnosis, which includes the key point of subjective data (client complaints) and objective date (please note that examples of NCP 'reasons', are shown in this chapter: but throughout the text it has not (given/shown) included in nursing care plan presented in the text because they need to be individualized for each patient).

Objectives refer to short statement of derived or expected outcomes of the patient, in the subphase of planning component of nursing process.

Nursing intervention refers to planned interventions which will provide clarity, specificity and direction to the spectrum of nurses implementing care for a patient. Implementation of nursing intervention is the action component of the planning. It is the phase of the nursing process in which the nursing treatment plan is carried out.

Evaluation of the attainment of the exepcted patient outcomes occurs formally at intervals designated in the outcome criteria. Please note that evaluation column is not included in the nursing care plans presented in this text, because they need to be individualized for each patient.

Author used the following 'PRONE' format for nursing care plans when 'P' stands for problem, 'R' stands for reason and 'O' stands for objectives.

Problem	Reason	Objective	Nursing intervention	Evaluation

This is where and 'N' stands for nursing intervention and 'E' stands for evaluation. The sample of nursing care plan with 'PRONE' format are in the end of this chapter.

The sample of nursing care plan have been shown in Tables 2.4 to 2.14 at the end of this chapter.

IMPLEMENTATION

After planning, implementation is the next, or fourth phase of the nursing process. Implementation refers to the actions initiated to accomplish the defined goals and objectives. Implementation is often considered as the actual giving of nursing care. It is putting the plan into action. Other terms used to describe this part of the process are actions or interventions. The words implementation and intervention are not synonymous. Implementation refers to putting a plan into action; intervention speaks to involvement in the affairs of another, a coming between the other and a problematic situation. Therefore, the term implementation seems more appropriate to describe this phase of the process if nursing actions directed towards resolving the problem and meeting the health care needs of the client. It is an ongoing process through which the nurse is reassessing reviewing and modifying the plan of care, and if necessary, seeking assistance in meeting the client's health care needs.

Since the nursing process is interpersonal in nature, it must take place between the nurse and the client. The client may be a person, a group, a family, or even a community. The beliefs that the nurse and the client have about human beings, nurses, and clients and about interactions between nurses and clients will affect the types of actions that both consider appropriate. If human beings are considered unique, then nursing actions should reflect this uniqueness. Therefore, the philosophy of nursing that a nurse develops will affect the nursing actions that he or she uses in meeting the needs of clients. Yura and Walsh (1973) indicated that the implementation phase of the nursing process draws heavily on the intellectual, interpersonal, and technical skills of the nurse. Wilkinson (1992) supports the importance of critical thinking throughout the nursing process. Although the focus is on action, the action is intellectual, interpersonal, and technical in nature.

The implementation phase begins when the nurse considers various alternative actions and selects those most suitable to achieve the planned goals and objectives. Just as goals and objectives have priorities in the plan, actions may also have priorities. Nursing actions may be carried out by the nurse who developed the nursing care plan or by other nurses or nursing assistants. Nursing actions may also be carried out by the client or family. To carry out a nursing action, the nurse refers to the written plan for specific information. Many nursing actions fall into the broad categories of counseling, teaching, providing physical care, carrying out delegated medical therapy, coordination of resources, referral to other sources of help, and therapeutic communication (verbal and nonverbal).

According to the goals and objectives for client, as discussed earlier, several nursing actions could be implemented. For example, under objective 1 (identify the basic food groups from a chart), the following actions could be considered:

1. Establish and agreed upon time when client and her family could meet with the nurse in their home during the next week.
2. Establish a baseline knowledge about the client and the family members' understanding of basic food groups.
3. Take chart and booklets containing information about the basic food groups to client home.
4. Teach family about using the basic good groups for good nutrition (base teaching on information gained from baseline knowledge).
5. Focus on the value of the food groups for each family member based on age, height, weight, and activity.
6. Request a return demonstration in which client and other family members will identify foods by planning the food in a food group and will state why each food group is important.

In Campbell's (1980) study of nursing diagnoses and nursing actions, seven categories of nursing actions were developed. These are assertive hygienic, rehabilitative, supporting, preventive, observational, and educative. Wilkinson (1992) speaks to doing, delegating, and recording. Both point out that almost all nursing actions are initiated by nurses without medical direction. Nurses initiate and carry out all activities that fall within the nursing domain. In the hospital setting, nurses are also asked to assist physicians in carrying out medical prescriptions and to follow institutional policies. Therefore, nurses need to be clear about their dependent and independent functions.

For every nursing action, the client responds as a total person, that is, as a whole, the concept of Holism, which states that a person is more than the sum of that person's parts, means that the nurse may be treating a person's leg but the person will respond as a whole person. The concept is used in thinking about the consequences of any nursing actions. For example, the simple action of turning the patient every 2 hours will have a variety of consequences. Some of these consequences could or should be (i) increased circulation, (ii) improved muscle tone, (iii) improved breathing, (iv) less flatus (gas) in the intestinal track, (v) prevention of pressure sores, (vi) increased or decreased pain, (vii) opportunity for communication with caregiver, (viii) increased ability to socialize with patient in next bed, and (ix) increased or decreased ability to reach articles at bedside. There may be other consequences that could not have been predicted, such as an opportunity to express values or beliefs. Therefore, in planning nursing actions, it is important to consider the cluster of consequences of both positive and negative value that can be expected to occur with and following each action. Using this knowledge will help the nurse select the most appropriate actions. Although not all consequences are predictable for a specific client, it is possible to develop a general knowledge of expected consequences. Knowledge of consequences is an important aspect of the implementation phase of the nursing process. The implementation phase is completed when the nursing actions are finished and the results are recorded against each diagnosis.

EVALUATION

Evaluation is the fifth and final phase of the nursing process. It may be defined as the appraisal of the client's behavioral changes that are a result of the action of the nurse. Although evaluation is considered to be the final phase, it frequently does not end the process. As mentioned earlier in this chapter, evaluation may lead to reassessment, which in turn may result in the nursing process beginning all over again. The main questions to ask in evaluation are: Were the goals and objectives met? Were there identifiable changes in the client's behavior? If so, why? If not, why not? Were the consequences of nursing actions predict? These questions help the nurse to determine which problems have been solved and which problems need to be reassessed and replanned. Unsolved problems cannot be assumed to reflect faulty or inadequate data collection; rather, each part of the nursing process may need to be evaluated to determine the cause of ineffective actions.

The key to appropriate evaluation of nurse-client actions lies in the planning phase of the nursing process. When objectives are described in behavioral terms with clearly stated expected outcomes, it is easy to determine whether or not the nurse-client actions were successful. These objectives become the criteria for evaluating nurse client actions. Just as goals should be mutually set with a client whenever possible, it is also important for the nurse and client to mutually establish the objectives (criteria for evaluation).

According to Wilkinson (1992), evaluation consists of the following five steps:

1. Review the goals or predicted outcomes.
2. Collect data about the client's responses to nursing action.
3. Compare actual outcomes to predicted outcomes and decide if goals have been met.
4. Record the conclusion.
5. Relate nursing plans to client outcomes.

The first three steps are specific to client outcomes. Step 1 has been briefly discussed in relation to the planning phase of the process. In addition to stating the desired behavior change, it is also important for the nurse to decide how the change will be measured (predicted outcome) and when it will be measured.

Step 2 involves the collection of evidence (data). Although data are collected in both assessment and evaluation, the data collected during evaluation are used differently from data collected during assessment. In assessment, data are collected for the purpose of making a nursing diagnosis. In evaluation, data are collected as evidence to determine whether the goals and objectives were met. This is an important difference to note in using the nursing process.

Step 3 in evaluation is the one that is often the most difficult because it is easy to use different measurements in making judgments. For example, if a nurse observed that a client "ate well", would this mean the same thing the client or to another nurse? "Ate well" could be interpreted to mean that the client was able to chew, swallow, and digest the food with no difficulty, or it could refer to the amount and kind of food consumed. Therefore, in evaluation, it is not only important to determine the criteria (objectives) and be specific in predicting outcomes, it is also important to determine the exact way(s) in which evidence is gathered and interpreted to ascertain whether the criteria were met.

When predicted outcomes are not reached, reassessment should occur, and the process begins again. If the evaluation shows that the nurse-client objectives have been met, the nursing process is complete.

Evaluation based on behavioral changes is outcome evaluation. There are two other types of evaluation, both of which are reflected in Wilkinson's two other types of evaluation, both of which are reflected in Wilkinson's (1992) evaluation steps.

Structure evaluation relates to such things as appropriate equipment to assess the client or to carry out the plan and to record evaluation conclusions (Step 4). For example, if the scales were inaccurate, then correct data could not be obtained. Structure evaluation may also relate to the organization within which the nurse works. The nurse may be unable to carry out the nursing process appropriately because of agency limitations on time; this must be considered a part of the evaluation.

Process evaluation which focuses on the activities of the nurse, can be done during each phase of the nursing process, or it may be carried out at the end of the process (Step 5). The following are examples of process evaluation questions that can be used in evaluating each phase of the process.

Assessment

1. Were historical data that might be related to health problems collected?
2. Was a physical examination carried out and the results recorded?
3. Was the analysis logical? Did it make use of the collected data? Were significant findings mentioned in the analysis?

Diagnosis

1. Was the diagnosis based on the analysis?
2. Is the diagnosis a logical conclusion from the data collected?

Planning

1. Are goals and objectives stated?
2. Does the plan rationally follow from the diagnosis?
3. Were goals and objectives mutually established with the client?

Implementation

1. What activities did the nurse carry out?
2. What activities did the client carry out?
3. Were the activities consistent with the objectives?

Evaluation

1. Were the predicted outcomes achieved?
2. What evaluation methods were used?
3. Were the conclusions recorded?

The nurse and the client are responsible for carrying out outcome evaluation. Structure and process evaluations are typically carried out by the nurse, others in nursing administration, or both within an agency.

Note: For more details of "Nursing Process and Health Assessment" Please read author text on "Fundamentals of Nursing (2nd edition)".

HEALTH ASSESSMENT

Health assessment is an integral part of holistic nursing. It provides the basis for nursing process. The nurse works in a variety of settings, seeking information about client's health status. The purposes of the health assessment are to:

- Establish a nurse-client relationship
- Gather data about the client's general health status, integrating physiologic, psychologic, cognitive, socio-cultural, developmental and spiritual dimensions
- Identify clients' strengths
- Identify actual and potential health problems
- Establish a base for the nursing process.

There are two components of health assessment which includes health history and physical assessment.

HEALTH HISTORY

Health history is a collection of subjective and objective data that provides a detailed profile of the client's health status. The subjective data are the symptoms which are indications of illness that are perceived by the patient or client. For example, (pain, nausea, feeling nervous, etc.) The objective data are the signs of illness, as perceived by the examiner, i.e. doctor or nurse. For example, rashes, altered vital signs, visible drainage, etc.

The nurse collects information through interview with the client. An interview is a planned communication. During the assessment, the nurse conducts the interview in a relaxed, unhurried manner in a quiet, private, well-lighted settings. To conduct an effective and informative interview, the nurse must develop interviewing skills, gain the patient's trust, and convey feelings of compassion while remaining objective. The patient must feel the information being given is important to the nurse, the nurse must demonstrate an interest in the patient's state of wellness. The nurse initially establishes trust by introducing himself or herself and asking what name the patient wishes to be called by and then using the name during the interview. An accepting posture in which the nurse is sitting in a relaxed manner at eye level with the patient, will foster trust. A pleasant facial expression will help and eye contacts make the patient feel he has the nurse's full attention. The nurse can enhance communication by using non-judgmental language. The tips of maintaining effective communication are as follows:

Promoting Effective Communication

Maintaining silence: Silence can help the nurse and patient to organize their thoughts. It also enables the nurse to observe the patient more closely.

Listening attentively: Attentive listening allows one to understand an entire message conveyed, verbally and non-verbally. It also facilitates trust.

Conveying acceptance: Acceptance means that one is non-judgmental. Acceptance is not synonymous with agreement; rather, it is a willingness to hear the person's message. One conveys acceptance through positive feedback and making sure verbal and non-verbal cues match.

Asking related questions: Questioning is a direct method of communicating. Asking related questions allows the patient to give information logically. Open-ended questions are useful for eliciting more information from the patient about a subject.

Paraphrasing: It sends feedback to the patient that information has been accurately received.

Clarifying: It helps retain important information. Using examples can clarify abstract ideas. All clarification should be specific.

Focusing: When a discussion becomes vague or ill-defined, focussing directs conversation to a specific topic or issue. It limits the area of discussion to which the patient can respond. The nurse seeks meaning in the patient's message.

Stating observations: Describing a patient's observed behavior can provide feedback as to whether an intended message was received. It can clarify conflicts between verbal and non-verbal cues.

Offering information: It provides a patient with relevant data and prevents one-sided conversations. It is useful for health teaching and helps in decision making.

Summarizing: It is a concise review of main ideas from a discussion. It sets the tone for further interactions. By reviewing a conversation, the participants can focus on key issues and any relevant information previously deleted.

Inhibiting Effective Communication

Giving an opinion: Giving an opinion takes decision making away from the patient. It inhibits spontaneity, stall problem solving, and creates doubt. If offering suggestions, the nurse should stress that they are only options.

Offering false reassurance: Offering false reassurance can do more harm than good. False reassurance may allow the nurse to promise something that will not occur or is unrealistic.

Being defensive: Defensiveness in the face of criticism implies that the patient has no right to an opinion. The patient's concerns often become ignored. Attentive listening helps the patient open up but does not imply agreement.

Showing approval or disapproval: It is judgmental and may halt a conversation. It inhibits the patient's ability to share ideas and make decisions independently. Disapproval can indicate rejection.

Asking why: It may imply an accusation. It can cause resentment, insecurity, and mistrust. If additional information is needed, the nurse can phrase a question to avoid use of "why."

Changing the subject inappropriately: It is rude and shows a lack of empathy. It stalls communication. The patient may then give incomplete or inadequate information.

Forming communication barriers: The barriers by saying something inadvertently that blocks a patient's communication can break down communication. By acknowledging the mistake, the nurse can start the communication process a new.

The health assessment interview also provides information about how the client perceives his or her health status or problems. Although you may not agree with the client's perceptions, it is important to understand these perceptions when planning nursing care.

Any uncertainty about the client's perceptions should be clarified during the interview. Communication techniques such as: direct questioning, or reflecting, or restating the client's comments, may enhance understanding. For example, you can say, I am not certain I understand. Did you mean....?

The Interview Process

The health assessment interview may be formal and structured to collect a wide range of information, or informal and focussed on a specific area of concern. In a formal interview, your primary concern is to establish a comprehensive data base. In an informal interview, you may discuss specific questions with the client while giving nursing care. Assessment through interviewing and questioning should be continuous, ongoing process lasting as long as you and the client interact.

The health care setting may influence the choice of interview topics. In well-child clinics, for example, the interview usually focusses on routine health practices, nutrition, and normal growth and development, whereas in the intensive care unit, data collection focuses on physiological or psychological stability and on maintaining vital functions.

Three interrelated phases constitute an effective interview; the introductory phase, the working phase and the termination phase.

The Introductory Phase

The introductory phase sets the tone and direction of the interview and establishes a mutual understanding of the purpose of the exchange. The purpose of the introductory phase are as follows:

- To establish rapport
- To ensure a comfortable setting
- To define what both parties expect from the interview.

i. *Establishing rapport:* Establishing rapport begins with demonstrating respect for the client as a person with problems, rather than regarding the person as a problem to be solved.

   You should demonstrate respect at the beginning of the interview by extending a cordial greeting, addressing the client by name and then introducing yourself by name. You should not address an adult client with his or her first name unless invited. Offering to shake hands is one way of demonstrating warmth and acceptance.

Non-verbal behaviors, especially on your part, may also help build rapport. Mutual respect best can be expressed when you and the client face each other and maintain eye contact. If possible you should avoid standing over the person, because this may be intimidating. Of course, such a position may be appropriate if you are informally interviewing the person while providing care. If the interview is conducted at the bedside, you should sit beside the bed with the siderail down, leaning slightly toward the person. Non-verbal behaviors such as: expressions of disgust, boredom, or impatience may interfere with establishing rapport or may imply lack of interest.

Beginning the interview with a brief, casual conversation that focuses on the client may help dispel tension or awkwardness. If your comments are predominantly self-centred, the person may feel neglected or unimportant.

ii. *Ensuring comfort:* If possible, you should conduct the interview in a private setting, free from interruptions. When privacy is difficult to maintain, such as in acute care settings, you can at least close the door or wait until other people have left the room before initiating the interview. Pulling the curtains or moving to the corner of the room also helps to promote a sense of privacy, even though these gestures may not necessarily prevent others from hearing what is said.

It is also helpful to demonstrate concern about physical comfort by asking how the client is feeling, whether he or she is comfortable or needs to use the bathroom before proceeding. If the client is in pain or is fatigued, consider postponing the interview.

iii. *Defining expectations:* It is important to clarify what both you and the client expect from the interview and to establish an agreement about the rules and norms of the interview. This process is known as Contracting. You should explain how discussing the person's health concerns will help in planning nursing care and encourage the person to participate in the interview. The client who answers questions, responds honestly, and shares relevant personal information is most likely to benefit from the health assessment interview.

In addition, you should inform the client about other professionals who will see the written account of the interview and the way in which the information will be used. To ensure confidentiality, you should ask if the client does not want certain information recorded.

You may also discuss the length of time the interview will run and the possibility that future sessions may be needed. Finally, you and the client should discuss decision-making. For example, if you intend to make some decisions for the client, the client should be so informed. If you intend to encourage the client to make his or her own decisions, the client should be made aware of the expectation.

The Working Phase

During the working phase of the interview, which is the most time consuming phase, you should collect data that are pertinent to the client's overall health status. Such information will be invaluable in forming an appropriate care plan. Both verbal responses and non-verbal behavior should be recorded. The purposes of the working phase are:

- To collect biographic data
- To collect data pertinent to the client's health status
- To identify and respond to the client's needs.

The Structured interview: It may be used to facilitate data collection during the working phase. Familiarity with the forms before the interview will enable you to concentrate on the client's responses. Formats for structured interviews vary. Traditionally, nurses have followed a medical model in conducting health assessment interviews. However, nursing models are now being used in many settings. The structured interview usually begins with biographic information including name, age and birthdate, sex, address, birth place, marital status, and occupation. Although asking about previously recorded biographic information is unnecessary, you should always review such data, because it is relevant to the person's social identify and self concept.

The next portion of the structured interview concentrates on determining the person's functional status (subsequent chapters discuss specific interview guidelines for each functional area). You can proceed smoothly from one topic to the next by using transitional phrases such as "Now I'd like to discuss how you feel about your sleep habits," or "Now I'd like to ask some questions about your bowel and bladder functions".

The structural interview should proceed from general to specific. Gather general biographic information and data pertaining to health perceptions before discussing sexuality, personal values, and relationships. You must establish trust and rapport before discussing intimate topics.

If the client is reluctant to discuss specific topics, you should provide an opportunity to talk about what he or she feels is most important. Use broad opening statements, such as, "Why don't you begin by telling me what brings you here," or "what's troubling you today?" Once the client has expressed immediate concerns, he or she is more likely to discuss other subjects.

You should view the structured interview as a guide rather than a rigid series of questions that must be asked in a set order. Excessive questioning may undermine rapport, inhibit responses, and encourage the client to assume a passive role of merely answering questions. Applying principles of therapeutic communication rather than direct questioning may result in a more productive interview, as is discussed in more detail in the next section. Such techniques encourage free expression about the topics raised.

Communication is also enhanced when both you and the client speak the same 'language'. The terminology you use should be simple and appropriate and not based on medical jargon.

When necessary, definite terms and structure questions to allow time for the client to respond thoughtfully and meaningfully.

Completing the health assessment interview in one session may not always be possible. If the client shows signs of fatigue or a limited attention span, bring the interview to a close. Trying to continue under these circumstances.

The Termination Phase

The termination phase serves to end the interview. Saying how long the interview will last at the beginning will prevent the client experiencing a sense of premature closure at the end of the interview.

Presummary, summary and follow-up techniques may be incorporated into the termination phase. Presummary involves providing cues to indicate that the interview is coming to an end. For example, you could say, "I see that we only have 10 minutes left. Is there anything else you would like to discuss before our time is up?" or "There are three more questions I'd like to ask." Planning additional interview sessions may be necessary if all relevant topics have not been adequately discussed.

Next, a brief summary of the points covered will allow both you and the client a chance to validate perceptions. Specific plans for follow-up or additional interviewing are discussed at this time.

PHYSICAL ASSESSMENT

The physical examination is usually conducted in a head-to-toe sequence, but can be adapted to meet the need of the client being examined. It offers objective information about the client. The nurse uses the skills of physical assessment to make clinical judgment. The client's condition and response affects the extent of the examination. The accuracy of physical assessment influences the choice of therapies a client receives and the determination of the response to those therapies. Continuity in health care improves when the nurse makes ongoing, objective, and comprehensive assessment. An examination should be designed for the client's needs. If a client is acutely ill, the nurse may assess only the involved body system. A more comprehensive examination conducted when the client feels more at ease and the nurse learns about the client's health status.

Preparation for Physical Assessment

It is very important that some preparation needed for client while conducting physical assessment in the physical environ-ment. Physical examination requires privacy. An examination room should be well-equipped for all necessary procedures. Adequate lighting is needed for proper illuminations of body parts. The room should be sound proof, well-ventilated, and should be warm enough to maintain client's comfort. There should be proper examination table or bed with pad or mattress with necessary articles and linen including small pillow and others.

Client or Patient

Preparation of the client, both psychologically and physiologically also is very important. By which nurse explains to client that body structures will be examined, and asks the client to use toilet to void. For emptying the bladder and bowel, if needed, instruct to collect the specimen required. Physical preparation involves being sure that client is dressed and draped properly.

Equipment

The equipment or instrument needed for examination should be readily available and arranged in order for easy use.

Instruments	Equipment and supplies
• Blood pressure apparatus or sphygmomanometer • Stethoscope • Ophthalmoscope • Snellen's chart • Otoscope • Nasal speculum • Scale with height measurement • Vaginal speculum • Tuning fork • Percussion hammer • Thermometer • Tongue depressor	• Alcohol swabs • Cotton applicators • Disposable pad • Drape or sheet • Gauze dressing (4 and 4) • Gloves (sterile or non-sterile) • Lubricants • Penlight • Flash light and spot light • Safety-pin • Substance for testing smell • Tap measure • Gown for client • Wrist watch with second hand • Paper towels • Swabs and sponge forceps • Specimen container

POSITIONS FOR PHYSICAL EXAMINATION

A number of positions are used during physical assessment, because during examination, the nurse asks client to assume proper positions so that the body parts are accessible and clients stay comfortable. The positions and their uses during physical assessment are as follows:

Sitting Positions

The client may sit upright in a chair or on the side of the examining table or bed. Sitting upright provides full expansion of lungs and provides better visualization of symmetry of upper body parts and facilitates full-lung expansion. It is used to assess the head and neck, posterior and antherior thorax, and lungs, breasts, axillae, heart and upper extremities, and also to take visual signs. If physically weakened, client may be unable to maintain an upright position, may be supine in the bed with the head elevated.

Supine Positions

In supine position, the client lies flat on the back with legs together but extended and slightly bent at the knees. The head may be supported with a small pillow. This is most normally relaxed position. It prevents contracture of abdominal muscles and provides easy access to pulse sites. This position can be used to assess the head and neck, anterior thorax and lungs, breasts, heart, abdomen extremities and peripheral pulses. In this position client becomes short of breath easily, examiner may need to raise the head of the bed.

Dorsal Recumbent Position

In the dorsal recumbent position, the client lies on the back with legs separated, knee bent, and soles of the feet flat on the bed. In this position clients with painful disorders are more comfortable with knees flexed. This position also is used to assess the head and neck, anterior thorax, and lungs, breasts, heart, extremities and peripheral pulse. It is used for client who have difficulty in maintaining supine position. This position should not be used for abdominal assessment because it promotes contraction of abdominal muscle.

Sim's Position

In this, the client lies on either the right or left side. The lower arm behind the body and upper arm is bent at the shoulder and elbow. The knees are both bent, with the uppermost leg more acutely bent. Here the flexion of hip and knee improves exposure of rectal area. This position is used to assess the rectum and vagina. It should not be used for person with joint deformities which may hinder client's ability to bend hip and knee.

Prone Position

In this, the client lies on the abdomen, flat on the bed, with the head turned, to one side. This position is used only to assess extension of hip joint; and can be used to assess the posterior thorax. This position is intolerable for client with respiratory difficulties and difficult in assuming this position for older adults.

Knee Chest Position

Here, the client kneels, using the knees and chest to bear the weight of the body. The body is at 90° angle to the hips, with the back straight, the arm above the head, and the head turned to one side. This position provides maximal exposure to rectal area used to assess. This position is embarassing and uncomfortable. Clients with arthrities or other joint deformities may be unable to assume this position.

Lithotomy Position

In this position, the client is in the dorsal recumbent position with the buttocks at the edge of examining table and the feet supported in stirrup. This position provides maximum exposure of genitalia and facilitates insertion of vaginal speculum, so used to assess rectum and the area of female genitalia and genital tract.

Lithotomy position is also embarrassing and uncomfortable, so examiner minimizes time that the client spends in it. Client is kept well draped. It is uncomfortable for older persons and difficult for clients with severe arthritis or other deformities.

Standing Position

The standing or erect position may be used to assess posture, gait, and balance.

Client's abilities to assume positions will depend on their physical strength and degree of wellness. As stated earlier, some positions may be embarrassing and uncomfortable. Therefore, clients should be kept in these positions no longer than necessary. The examiners explain the positions and assist clients in attaining them. The drapes are adjusted to be sure that the area to be examined is accessible and that no body part is unnecessarily exposed. The nurse chooses the position according to part of body of the client examined on priority wise.

TECHNIQUES OF PHYSICAL EXAMINATIONS

Observation

The basic techniques of physical examination are inspection, palpation, percussion, and auscultation, together referred to as observation. These skills enable you to collect data systematically using the senses of sight, touch, hearing and smell. Physical appearance, behavior, communication patterns, and activity abilities can all be observed, as can a person's environment and events that affect him or her. Observing facial expression for signs of discomfort, detecting odors that indicate infection, listening to chest sounds to determine airway patency, and touching the skin to determine body temperature are all examples of observation.

Inspection

Inspection is systematic and deliberate visual observation to determine health status. Begin the physical examination with a general survey or inspection of the client, including an assessment of age, posture, stature, body weight, grooming and mobility patterns. Next carry out a more thought observation in a head-to-toe fashion. Note the shape and size of the head, hair distribution, general skin condition and facial expressions. Inspect the face for symmetry of eyes and balance of facial expression. While inspecting the neck note visible pulsations, bulges, or venous distension. Inspect the chest and abdomen, noting symmetry, masses, pulsations, skin condition and visible signs of discomfort, such as holding the abdomen. Inspect the lower extremities, noting especially ankle swelling and skin integrity.

Following the general survey, more detailed observations are made as the physical examination progresses to specific body parts or systems. Inspection always precedes palpation, percussion, or auscultation of a particular area. More specific guidelines on examination skills are provided in subsequent chapters.

Effective inspection is facilitated by good lighting and exposure. Occasionally, instruments such as the ophthalmoscope and the otoscope may be used as well.

Palpation

With palpation you rely on the sense of touch to make judgments about (i) the size, shape, texture and mobility of structures and masses; (ii) the quality of pulses; (iii) the condition of bones and joints; (iv) the extent of tenderness in injured areas or structures; (v) skin temperature and moisture; (vi) fluid accumulations and edema and (vii) chest wall vibrations.

Different parts of the hand are used to palpate different types of structures. Breasts, lymph nodes and pulses should be palpated with the fingertips, where nerve endings are most concentrated. The thumb and index fingertips are used to evaluate tissue firmness. Temperature can be quickly assessed with the back of the hand, where temperature sensory nerves are most concentrated and the skin is thin. Vibrations can be felt most strongly with the palm of the hand especially along the metacarpal joints.

Palpitation should be carried out in such a way as to avoid discomfort. Your hands should be warm and the client relaxed to avoid muscle tensing. Palpate painful areas last. The amount of pressure you apply is governed by the type of structure you are examining and the degree to which palpation may cause discomfort. Any expression of distress or pain should prompt you to palpate lightly.

Palpation may be light, deep, or bimanual. Light palpation the safest and least uncomfortable involves exerting gentle pressure with the fingertips of your dominant hand, moving them in a circular motion. Place your hand parallel to the part of the body surface you are examining and extend your fingers to depress the skin surface approximately 0.5 to 0.75 inches (1 to 2 cm). Exert and release fingertip pressure several times over an area. Exerting continuous pressure would tend to dull the tactile discrimination senses.

Deep palpation, which is done after light palpation, is used to detect abdominal masses. The technique is similar to light palpation except that the fingers are held at a greater angle to the body surface and the skin is depressed about 1.5 to 2 inches (4 to 5 cm). A variation of this technique involves placing the fingertips of one hand over the fingertips of the palpating hand. The top hand should press and guide the bottom hand to detect underlying masses.

Bimanual palpation involves using both hands to trap a structure between them. This technique can be used to evaluate the spleen, kidneys, breasts, uterus and ovaries.

Percussion

Percussion involves tapping the body lightly but sharply to determine the position, size, and density of underlying structures, as well as to detect fluid or air in a cavity. Tapping the body creates a soundwave that travels 2 to 3 inches (5 to 7 cm) towards underlying areas. Sound reverberations assume different characteristics depending on the features of the underlying structures. Percussing the right upper abdominal quadrant, for example will usually elicit dull sounds, indicating the presence of the liver, tapping over the lungs should reveal resonant sounds associated with airfilled spaces. Percussion should usually be performed after an area has been palpated.

Three percussion methods can be used: mediate or indirect, immediate, and fist percussion. The method chosen depends on the area to be percussed. Mediate or indirect percussion should be used to percuss the abdomen and thorax, and can be performed by using the finger of one hand as a plexor (striking finger) and the middle finger of the other hand as a pleximeter (the finger being struck). Immediate percussion, used mainly to evaluate the sinuses or an infant's thorax, involves striking the surface directly with the fingers of the hand only. Fist percussion, used to evaluate the back and kidneys for tenderness, involves placing one hand flat against the body surface and striking the back of the hand with a clenched fist of the other hand.

Procedure

Mediate or indirect percussion is the basic technique of percussion and is performed in the following manner:

1. Place the pad of the middle finger of your non-dominant hand firmly against the surface being percussed. The other fingers as well as the heel of this hand, should be raised to avoid contact with the body surface. Hold the finger firmly against the body surface throughout percussion, even when it is not being tapped by the other hand.
2. Use the middle finger of your dominant hand as the plexor. Hold the forearm horizontal to the surface being percussed. Keep the forearm stationary and use wrist motion to make striking movements.

TABLE 2.1: Percussion sounds

Sound	Pitch	Intensity	Quality	Location
Flatness	High	Soft	Extreme dullness	*Normal:* Sternum, thigh *Abnormal:* Atelectatic lung
Dullness	Medium	Medium	Thudlike	*Normal:* Liver, diaphragm *Abnormal:* Pleural effusion
Resonance	Low	Loud	Hollow	*Normal:* Lung
Hyperresonance	Lower than resonance	Very Loud	Booming	*Abnormal:* Emphysematous lung, pneumothorax
Tympany	High	Loud	Musical, drum-like	*Normal:* Gastric air bubble; puffed-out cheek *Abnormal:* Air-distended abdomen

3. Quickly strike the distal phalanx of the finger that is positioned on the body surface with the tips of the finger of the other hand. Use only the wrist to generate motion, and quickly remove the striking hand after percussing to avoid muffling the percussion sound. You may percuss a single area two or three times before moving to the next area. Light tapping is more effective than heavy tapping.
4. Identify the percussion sound. Skillful percussion reveals one of the five percussion sounds, depending on the density of underlying structures, flatness, dullness, resonance, hyperresonance, and tympany (Table 2.1). A flat sound is elicited by percussing over solid masses such as bone or muscle. A dull sound which has a lower pitch than a flat sound, is elicited when high density structures, such as the liver, are percussed. Resonance is a hollow sound heard, for example, by percussing the lung. Hyperresonance is an abnormal sound with a pitch between resonance and tympany, and may indicate an emphysematous lung or pneumothorax. Tympany is a drum-like sound heard over airfilled body parts such as the bowel or stomach.
5. Proceed to the next percussion area. Move from more resonant to less resonant areas, because detecting a change from resonance to dullness is easier than detecting a change from dullness to resonance.

Common Errors in Percussion

The most common errors in performing mediate percussion are as follows:

- Moving the forearm of the dominant hand. Remember, all motion should be generated from the wrist.
- Pressing, the striking finger into the positioned finger. Remove the striking finger immediately after tapping.
- Causing injury to oneself or the client by inadvertently striking the client or your own hand with a long fingernail. The fingernail of the plexor finger should be kept short.
- Falling to hear the percussion note. Eliminate environmental noise including noise caused by bracelets or loose-fitting watches. If the note is still difficult to hear, check your technique.

Auscultation

Auscultation is the skill of listening to body sounds created in the lungs, heart, blood vessels, and abdominal viscera. Auscultation is usually the last technique used during the examination. The sequence usually progresses from inspection to palpation, percussion, and auscultation, except during the abdominal examination, when auscultation is the second step (following inspection).

Immediate auscultation involves placing one's ear directly on the skin, such as over the lung. This method is rarely used because environmental noise frequently interferes with hearing. The usual method is mediate auscultation, for using a stethoscope to detect sounds. The best results are gained using a good quality stethoscope. You should eliminate extraneous poise such as televisions, voices, and equipment sounds before performing auscultation. Do not create noise by moving the stethoscope over the body hair or clothing or by touching the stethoscope tubing.

Auscultated sounds are described in terms of pitch, intensity, duration and quality. Pitch is determined by the frequency of sound vibrations and should be classified as high or low. Intensity refers to the loudness of the sound. Duration refers to how long the sound lasts or how long it takes to occur in relation to a physiological event such as systole. Quality of sound must be described using subjective terms such as tinkling, harsh or blowing. Specific auscultatory guidelines are discussed throughout the test.

SYMPTOM ANALYSIS

Symptoms are detected during the physical examination or identified during the interview. Symptoms that indicate a possible change in physical status include pain, nausea, dizziness, dysphagia, and dyspnea. Such symptoms are systematically evaluated to aid in diagnosing physiological alterations. Evaluate each reported physical symptom according to the following criteria (elicited by questioning the client).

- Onset: When did you first notice the symptom (time and date) was the onset sudden or gradual? Has this symptom occurred at other times in the past? What circumstances precipitated the symptom?

- Location (may be relevant only when the symptom is pain): Where did the pain occur? (ask the client to point to the exact location.) Does the pain radiate?
- Quality: How did you feel when it occurred? How would you describe it?
- Quantity: How intense was the symptom (mild or severe, or rated on a scale of 1 to 10)? Did the symptom interfere with your usual activities, such as: walking, sleeping or talking?
- Frequency and duration: How frequently did the symptom occur and how long did it last?
- Aggravating or alleviating factors: What makes the symptom worse or better?
- Associated factors: Did you notice any other changes when you noticed this symptom? (ask about factors normally associated with the symptom, such as nausea with chest pain).
- Course: How has the symptom changed or progressed over time?

PHYSICAL EXAMINATION INSTRUMENTS

The physical examination is conducted with the aid of several instruments. Some are simple, such as safetypins and cotton wisps used to evaluate sensory function. Others are complex, such as stethoscopes, which are used to evaluate heart tones. Some of the more complex, commonly used physical examination instruments are discussed in this chapter as well as in other chapters. During a complete physical examination, the instruments and equipment listed in display may be used.

Stethoscope

A stethoscope is used to evaluate sounds that are difficult to hear with the human ear, such as: heart, bowel, vascular and lung sounds. The stethoscope transmits sound to the ears while blocking out environmental noise.

The chestpiece of the stethoscope is designed to detect high or low-frequency sounds and consists of two main parts: the diaphragm and the bell. The flat, closed diaphragm filters out low-pitched sounds and is used to detect high-pitched sounds such as lung sounds. Best results are obtained by placing the diaphragm evenly and firmly over the person's exposed skin. Because the diaphragm has a relatively large surface, it transmits acute sounds over a wide area. The diaphragm should be at least 1.5 inches in diameter. Smaller diaphragm pieces are available for examining children.

The open bell portion of the chestpiece is used to detect low-frequency sounds such as diastolic heart murmurs. The bell should be at least 1 inch in diameter. The bell is placed gently on the person's skin. If too much pressure is applied, the bell will function as a diaphragm. Fain sounds may be difficult to detect with the bell because of its relatively small size.

The stethoscope tubing is made of flexible rubber or plastic that is thick enough to block environmental sounds. Double tubes that are less than 12 inches long further enhance sound transmission.

The binaurals are placed in the ears and are positioned to project sound towards the tympanic membrane. The tips of the earpieces approximate the angle of the ear canal, and should fit snugly and comfortably. Manufacturers usually supply several earpieces so that a comfortable pair can be selected.

Doppler Probe

The Doppler probe is used to evaluate blood flow, especially when traditional methods such as pulse palpation or auscultation are inappropriate or ineffective. Common clinical applications include evaluating fetal heart sounds and peripheral pulses such as brachial, radial, femoral, popliteal, dorsalis pedis, and posterior tibial pulses. The Doppler probe or transducer is placed on the skin in order to send a low-energy, high-energy sound beam (ultrasound beam) towards underlying red blood cells. Ultrasound waves are reflected off moving objects, in this case, the red blood cells, and return to the Doppler transducer, which also functions as a receiver. The Doppler probe detects the change in sound frequency as sound is returned and converts the sound into an audible signal. When blood is flowing through the vessel that is being evaluated, a pulsatile sound can be heard.

Doppler probes are available as pencil-shaped probes, flat disks, or stethoscope-like units. Each device usually has an on/off switch and a volume control dial. A small amount of gel can be applied between the end of the Doppler transducer and the client's skin to eliminate air interference. The probe is then placed gently on the skin over the vessel at approximately a 60° angle to the flow within the vessel. Excessive pressure applied to the skin may occlude the vessel.

Ophthalmoscope

An ophthalmoscope is used to inspect internal eye structures. The head of the ophthalmoscope is placed on a battery base, and may be exchanged for an otoscope head. To understand the effective use of this instrument, it is important to become familiar with the structures of the ophthalmoscope head.

Internal eye structures can be viewed by directing a light source toward the person's pupil and looking through the viewing aperture. Light is directed away from the headpiece by a front mirror window. The viewing aperture may be adjusted by turning the aperture selection dial. To see the different apertures available on the ophthalmoscope model, shine the light towards a piece of paper and adjust the aperture selection dial. Usually, the large aperture is selected if pupils are dilated and the small aperture chosen if pupils are constricted. The slit aperture may be used to examine the anterior portion of the eye and evaluate fundal lesion levels. The grid aperture may be used to characterize, locate and measure fundal lesions. The red-free filter or green beam may be used to evaluate the retina and disc, especially for any hemorrhaging, which appears black with this filter, while melanin pigments usually appear gray.

The ophthalmoscope lens can be adjusted to bring the internal eye structures into sharp focus, compensating for nearsightedness or farsightedness of the client or examiner. If necessary, you may wear contact lenses or glasses during the examination if the lens adjustment does not provide sufficient compensation. The lens can be adjusted by rotating the lens selection dial with the index finger while looking through the viewing aperture. At the zero diopter setting on the lens indicator, the lens neither converges or diverges light. The black numbers, obtained by moving the lens selection dial clockwise, have positive values (+1 to +40) and improve visualization if the client is farsighted. The red numbers obtained by counter-clockwise rotation, have negative values (–1 to –20) and improve visualization if the client is nearsighted.

Otoscope

An otoscope is used to inspect the structures of the internal ear. The head of the otoscope should be placed on a battery base and may be exchanged for an ophthalmoscope head.

Internal ear structures should be viewed by looking through the illuminated magnifying lens and speculum. The lens may be displaced to the side so that instruments can be inserted or foreign bodies removed. The size of the speculum should allow maximal visualization with minimal discomfort to the client.

Some otoscopes are equipped with pneumonic devices to introduce a small amount of air against the tympanic membrane, and may be used to evaluate the flexibility of the tympanic membrane.

GUIDELINE FOR HEAD-TO-TOE APPROACH TO PHYSICAL EXAMINATION

General Approach

The physical examination is performed in a systematic manner, such as in a head-to-toe fashion. The guidelines presented here apply to the comprehensive examination of an ambulatory adult. The examination sequence may be modified depending on your preference and the client's condition. Variations are usually recommended when examining persons who are seriously ill or injured, or when examining infants, children, and frail elderly patients.

Preliminary Evaluation

At the beginning of the examination, while the person is ambulatory and before he or she changes into an examining gown, you may evaluate the following:

- Height and weight
- Snellen visual acuity
- Posture and gait
- Cerebellar function.

Sensory Testing

Sensory testing may be performed throughout the examination.

Examination Guidelines for Head-to-Toe Examination

After examination, documentation is necessary; this should be specific, descriptive and objective. The following descriptive terminology suggested for documentation (Table 2.2).

Overall Appearance Inspection

Sex: Male/female

General grooming: Clean? hair combed? make-up?

Position/posturing: Supine? prone? rigid? opisthotonos? erect? slumped?

Body size: Thin? fat? obese? emaciated? flabby? weight proportionate to height? mesomorph? endomorph? ectomorph?

Facial expressions: Smiling? frowning? blank? apathetic?

Body language: Eye contact? no eye contact? arms folded over chest?

Other observations: Restless? fidgeting? lying quietly? listless? trembling? tense?

Skin Inspection and Plapation

Color and vascularity: Pink? tan? brown? dark brown? grayish? pasty? yellowish? flushed? jaundiced?

Turgor and mobility: Elastic? non-elastic? tenting? wrinkles? edematous tight?

Temperature and moisture: Cold? cool? warm? hot? feverish? moist? dry? clammy? oily? sweating? diaphoresis?

Texture: Smooth? rough? fine? thick? coarse? scaly? puffy?

Nails: Clean, manicured? smooth? rough? dry? hard? brittle? splitting? cracking? angle of nail bed? clubbing? curved? flat? thick? yellowing? paronychia? Nail beds and lunulae: pale? pink? cyanotic? red? shape of lunule? blanching? spooning?

Body hair growth: Color? thick? thin? coarse? fine? location and distribution on body? hirsutism?

Skin integrity: Intact? not intact? Lesions, birthmarks, moles, scars and rashes: (describe shape, size and location) nevi? fissures? maculas? papules? pustules? nodules? vullae? cysts? carbuncle? wheals? erythema? excoriation? desquamation? abrations? cherry angiomas? senile lentigines? senile purpura?

TABLE 2.2: Guide for head-to-toe approach to physical examination

	Procedure	What to observe and record
1. Initiate the general survey	• General state of health a. The general survey begins when you first meet the client, in the waiting room or examination room, or while delivering bedside care b. Survey mobility and gait as the person walks into the room c. Continue the general survey as you examine each body region	• Signs of distress such as breathing difficulty, pain • Awareness, behavior, facial expression, mood • Height, weight, nutritional status • Hygiene, grooming, clothes • Skin condition • Odors • Posture, motor activity, physical deformities • Speech pattern • Apparent age vs actual age
With the client seated on the examination table, bed, or chair		
2. Measure vital signs	• Blood pressure • Pulse • Respiratory rate • Body temperature	
3. Examine the head	a. Inspect and palpate the cranium b. Palpate and auscultate the temporal arteries c. Inspect and palpate the face d. Test cranial nerves V and VII e. Inspect the nose and test cranial nerve I	• Hair • Size, shape, and symmetry • Tenderness • Scalp smoothness • Thickening • Tenderness • Bruits • Symmetry • Movements • Tenderness • Nodules • Sinus tenderness • Motor and sensory response • Patency • Septum • Mucosa • Sense of smell
4. Examine the eyes and test vision	a. Inspect and palpate to evaluate external eye structures b. Evaluate visual acuity. Perform near vision new or Sneller-Jaeger chart testing of chart testing of far vision at the beginning of the examination c. Test extraocular muscle function (cranial nerves III, IV and VI) d. Test pupillary reflexes e. Inspect internal eye structure with the ophthalmoscope; darken the room if possible	• Shape and symmetry • Eyelids and eyelashes • Lacrimal glands, puncta, and lacrimal functions • Upper and lower conjunctiva • Lens, cornea, iris, and pupil • Eye chart readings • Peripheral vision • Extraocular eye movements • Eye movement during cover-uncover test • Eye alignment and symmetry • Reaction to light • Accommodation • Retina • Retinal vessels • Optic disc
5. Examine the ears and test hearing	a. Inspect and palpate the external ear b. Evaluate hearing c. Inspect the ear canal and tympanic membrane with the otoscope	• Skin integrity • Structure, alignment and symmetry • Tenderness • Ability to distinguish sounds varying in pitch and intensity • Sound laterelization • Perception of air conduction of sound vs bone conduction • Skin integrity • Obstructions, foreign bodies • Color, light reflection, landmarks and configuration of the tympanic membrane

Contd...

Contd...

	Procedure	What to observe and record
6. Examine the oral cavity	a. Inspect and palpate the outer structures of the oral cavity b. Inspect and palpate the inner structures of the oral cavity c. Test cranial nerves V, IX and XII	• Lips • Jaw • Temporomandibular joint • Parotid glands • Oral mucosa • Tongue • Inner cheek • Hard and soft palates • Oropharynx • Uvula • Motor responses
7. Examine the neck	a. Inspect musculoskeletal structures b. Palpate the lymph nodes c. Inspect and palpate the thyroid gland d. Test neck musculoskeletal function and cranial nerve XI e. Palpate and auscultate the carotid arteries f. Test neck musculoskeletal function and cranial nerve XI g. Palpate and auscultate the carotid arteries	• Alignment • Symmetry • Consistency • Enlargement • Nodules • Tenderness • Consistency • Enlargement • Nodules • Tenderness • Muscle strength and tone • Range of motion • Pulsations • Vascular sounds • Muscle strength and tone • Range of motion • Pulsations • Vascular sounds
8. Examine the upper extremities	a. Inspect the masculoskeletal structure, skin and nails b. Test musculoskeletal function c. Palpate branchial and radial arteries d. Test deep tendon reflexes	• Skin integrity • Muscle mass • Alignment and symmetry • Muscle strength and tone • Range of motion • Pulsations • Motor response
9. Examine the anterior chest	a. Inspect and palpate the breasts and axillae b. Inspect, palpate, percuss, and auscultate the thorax c. Inspect, palpate, and auscultate the precordium	• Skin integrity • Size, shape, and symmetry • Consistency • Skin integrity • Ventilatory pattern • Shape and symmetry • Chest excursion • Vibrations • Percussion tones • Breath sounds • Pulsations • Vibrations • Heart sounds
10. Examine the back	a. Inspect and test musculoskeletal structures b. Perform fist percussion over the spine and kidneys c. Inspect, palpate, percuss and auscultate the posterior thorax	• Spinal alignment • Muscle tone • Range of motion • Tenderness • Same as anterior thorax
Position client supine on the examining table or bed. Elevate the head 30 degrees to inspect the neck veins		

Contd...

Contd...

	Procedure	What to observe and record
11. Inspect the neck veins		• Jugular venous pulsations • Central venous pressure
12. Examine the anterior chest (as above, adding palpation of glandular breast tissue and precordial auscultation in the left lateral position)		
13. Examine the abdomen	a. Inspect, auscultate, palpate and percuss the four abdominal quadrants b. Palpate and percuss specific organs (liver, spleen, kidneys)	• Contour and symmetry • Skin integrity • Bulges • Bowel sounds • Vascular stands • Muscle tone • Masses • Organ characteristics • Percussion tones • Tenderness • Size • Consistency • Tenderness
14. Examine the lower extremities	a. Inspect musculoskeletal structures, skin, and toenails b. Test musculoskeletal function c. Palpate popliteal, posterior tibial, and pedal arteries d. Test deep tendon reflexes and plantar reflex	• Skin integrity • Muscle mass • Alignment and symmetry • Muscle strength and tone • Range of motion • Pulsations • Motor response
Position the female client in the lithotomy position with stirrups		
15. Examine the genitals and pelvis	a. Inspect the external genitals b. Inspect the vagina and cervix c. Palpate the vagina, uterus, and cervix	• Skin integrity • Contour and symmetry • Discharge • Skin integrity • Masses • Discharge • Muscle tone • Position • Size • Consistency and masses
16. Examine the rectum		• Muscle tone • Stool • Tenderness • Masses • Bleeding, discharge
Assist the male client to a standing position		
17. Examine the external genitals	a. Inspect and palpate the peins b. Inspect and palpate the scrotum c. Inspect and palpate for hernias	• Skin integrity • Masses • Discharge • Skin integrity • Size and shape • Testicular descent and mobility • Masses • Tenderness • Bulges
18. Examine the rectum (for male patients, different positions may be used and special attention is given to prostate palpation)		

senile keratoses? seborrheic keratoses? bruises? insect bites? crusts? warts? pimples? blackheads? bleeding? drainage? lacerations? scaly? ulcers? lichenification?

Head Inspection and Palpation

Shape: Round? oval? square? pointed? normocephalic?

Face: Oval? heart-shaped? pear? long square? round? thin? high cheekbones? symmetrical?

Sensation (trigeminal CN V): Sensation on three branches? clenched teeth?

Facial CN VII: Facial expressions, smiles?

Hair: Color and growth coarse? fine? thick? thin? sparse? alopecia? long? short? curly? straight? permed? glossy? shiny? greasy? dry? brittle? stringy? frizzy?

Conditions of scalp: Clean? scaly? dandruff? rashes? sores? drainage?

Masses and lumps: Describe location and shape, measure size.

Eyes Inspection and Palpation

Eyebrows: Color and shape: alignment? straight? curved? thick? thin, sparse? plucked? scaly?

Eyelashes: Long? short? curved? none? artificial?

Eyelids: Dark? swollen? inflamed? red? stye? infected? open and close simultaneously? ptosis? entropion? ectropion? lid lag? xanthomas?

Shape and appearance of eyes: Almond? rounded? squinty? prominent? exophthalmic? sunken? symmetrical? bright? clear? dull? tearing? discharge? (serous? purulent?) exotropia? esotropia? nystigmus? strabismus?

Sclera: White? cream? yellowish? jaundiced? injected? pterygium?

Conjunctiva: Pale pink? pink? red? inflamed? nodules? swelling?

IRIS: Color and shape: round? not round? coloboma? arcus senilis?

Cornea: Clear? milky? opaque? cloudy?

Pupils (Oculomotor-CN III) (Perrla): Size and shape: (measure in mm) round? not round? (describe Equality: symmetrical? anisocoria? right larger than left? left larger than right? convergence? Reaction to light and accommodation? consensual reaction? Extraocular movements (oculomotor), trochlear, abducens, CN III, IV, VI): intact?

Lacrimal glands: Tender? non-tender? inflamed? swollen? tearing?

AIDS: Glasses? contact lenses? prosthesis?

Visual fields (optic-CNII): Intact?

Vision (optic-CNII): Reads newsprint? reports objects across room?

Ears Inspection and Palpation

Pinnae: Size and shape: large? small? in proportion to face? protruding oval? large lobes? small lobes? symmetrical? right larger than left? left larger than right? pinnae irregular? color? skin intact? redness? swelling? tophi? cauliflower ear? furuncles? Darwin's tubercle?

Level in relation to eyes: Top of pinnae level with outer canthus of eyes? top of pinnae lower than outer canthus of eyes? top of pinnae higher than outer canthus of eyes?

Canal: Clean? discharge? (serous? bloody? purulent?) nodules? inflammation? redness? foreign object?

Cilia: Present/absent?

Cerumen: Present/absent? color? consistency?

Tympanic membrane: Color? pearly white? injected? red? inflamed? discharge? cone of light? landmarks? scarring? bubbles? fluid level?

Hearing (Auditory-CN VII): Right-present/absent? left-present/absent? hears watch tick? hears whisper? responds readily when spoken to? Weber: Lateralizes equally? to left? right side? Rinne: Air conduction: bone conduction 2:1? Hearing aid: right/left.

Nose and Sinuses Inspection and Palpation

Size and shape: Long? short? large? small? in proportion to face? flat? broad? broad based? thick? thin? enlarged? nares symmetrical/ asymmetrical? pointed? swollen? bulbous? flaring of nostrils?

Septum: Midline? deviated right? left? perforated?

Nasal mucosa and turbinates: Pink? pale? bluish? red? dry? moist? discharge? (purulent? clear? watery? mucus?) cilia present/absent? rhinitis? epistaxis? polyps?

Patency of nares: (close each side and ask client to breathe) right - patent/partial obstruction/obstructed? left? patent/partial obstruction and obstructed?

Olfactory: (CN I) Correctly identifies odors?

Sinuses: Tender? non-tender? transillumination?

Mouth and Pharynx Inspection

Lips: Color: Pink? red? tam? pale? cyanotic? Shape: Thin? thick? enlarged? swollen? symmetrical? asymmetrical? drooping left side? drooping right side? Condition: Soft? smooth? dry? cracked? fissured? blisters? lesions? (describe)

Teeth: Color and condition: white? yellow? grayish? spotted? stained? darkened? pitting? notched? straight? crooked, protruding? separated? crowded? irregular? broken? notching? peglike? loose? dull? bright? dentulous? malocclusion? caries and fillings: number and location? dental hygiene: clean? not clean?

Breathe odor: Sweet? odorless? halitosis? musty? acetone? foul? fetid? odor of drugs or food? hot? sour? alcohol?

Gums: Pink? firm? swollen? bleeding? sensitive? gingivitis? hypertrophy nodules? irritated? receding? moist? ulcerated? dry? shrunken? blistered? spongy?

Facial and glossopharyngeal (CN VII and IX): Identifies taste? or note?

Tongue: Macroglossia? microglossia? glossitis? geographic? red? pink? pale? bluish? brownish? swollen? clean? thin? thick? fissured? raw? coated? moist? dry? cracked? glistening? papillae?

Hypoglossal (CN XII) Tongue movement: Symmetry? lateral? fasciculation?

Mucosa: Color? leukoplakia? dry? most? intact? not intact? masses? (describe size, shape and location) chancre?

Palate: Moist? dry? color? intact? not intact?

Uvula: Color? midline? remains at midline when saying "ah"? gag reflex present?

Pharynx: Color? petechia? injected? beefy? dysphagia?

Tonsils: Present/absent? cryptic? beefy? size 1 + to 4 + ?

Temporomandibular joint: Fully mobile symmetrical? tenderness? crepitus?

Neck Inspection and Palpation

Appearance: Long? short? thick? thin? masses? (describe size and shape) symmetrical? not symmetrical?

Thyroid: Palpable? nodules? tender?

Trachea: Midline? deviated to right/left?

Lymph nodes: (Occipital-preauricular, postauricular, submental, submaxillary, tonsilar, anterior cervical, posterior cervical, superficial cervical, deep cervical, supraclavicular) non-palpable? tender? lymphadenopathy? shotty? hard? firm?

Thorax and Lungs Inspection, Palpation, Percussion and Auscultation

Respirations: Rate? tachypnea, eupnea, bradypnea? apnea? orthopnea? labored? stertorous? Rhythm: Regular/irregular? inspiration time greater than expiration time? expiration time greater than inspiration time? spasmodic? gasping? orthopneic? gasping? deep? eupnic? shallow? flaring of nostrils with respirations? symmetrical asymmetrical? right thorax greater than left? left throax greater than right? ratio of AP diameter to lateral diameter between 1:2 and 5:7? ribs sloped downward at 45° angle? well? defined costal space? accessory muscles used? pigeon chest? funnel chest? barrel chest? abdominal or chest breather? skin intact? lesions? color? thin? muscular? flabby?

Posterior thorax: Tenderness? masses? Respiratory excursion: Symmetrical? asymmetrical? no respiratory movements on right/left? subcutaneous emphysema? crepitus? fremitus? estimation of level of diaphragm? spine alignment? tenderness? CVA tenderness? resonance? dull? hyperresonance? diaphragmatic excursion 3-5 cm? comparison of one side to the other? suprasternal north located? costochondral junctions tender? chest wall stable? vocal fremitus?

Lung auscultation: Vesicular? bronchovesicular? bronchial? whispered pectroliloquy? adventitious sounds? rales? rhonchi? wheezes? crackles? rub? bronchophony? egophony?

Breasts and Axillae Inspection and Palpation

Breasts: Male? female? present/absent? color? large? small? well developed? firm? pendulous? flat? flabby? symmetrical? asymmetrical? dimpling? thickening? smooth? retraction? peau d'orange? venous pattern? tenderness? masses? (describe) gynecomastia?

Nipples: Present? absent? circular? symmetrical? asymmetrical? inverted? everted? pale? brown? rose? extranipples? discharge? deviation? supernumerary?

Axilla: Shaved/unshaved/odor? masses or lumps? (describe size and shape).

Lymph nodes: (Lateral, central, subscapular, pectoral, epitrochlear) Palpable? tender? shotty?

Heart and Peripheral Vascular Inspection, Percussion, Auscultations and Palpation

Heart: Precordial bulge? abnormal palpations? PMI? thrills? heave or lift with pulsation? S1, loudest at apex? S2 loudest at base? S3? S4? splits? clicks? snap? rub? gallop? Murmurs: systolic? diastolic? holosystolic? harsh? soft? blowing? rumbling? grading 1 through 6? high pitch? medium pitch? low pitch? radiating?

Carotid pulse: Note: Do not check both right and left cartoid pulses simultaneously. Volume: Bounding? forceful? strong? full? weak? feeble? thready? symmetrical? right less than left? left less than right? Rhythm: Regular? irregular? symmetrical? asymmetrical? bruits present? absent?

Apical pulse: Record rate; tachycardia? bradycardia? pounding? forceful, weak? moderate? regular? irregular?

Peripheral pulses: (Do not count rate of these pulses except radial) Record character, volume, rhythm, and symmetry of brachial, radial femoral, popliteal, dorsalis pedis, and posterior tibial pulses. Volume: Full? strong? forceful? bounding? perceptible? imperceptible? weak? thready? symmetrical? asymmetrical? right greater than left? left greater than right? Rhythm: Regular? irregular? symmetrical? asymmetrical? Symmetry: Record as symmetrical? right greater than left or left greater than right? pulse deficit, pulse pressure, BP in both arms, BP lying, sitting and standing if applicable. Jugular venous distention? (record cm above level of sternal angle).

Abdomen Inspection, Auscultation, Percussion, Palpation

Contour: Irregular? protruding? enlarged? distended? scaphoid? concave? sunken? flabby? firm? flat? flaccid?

Skin: Color; intact? not intact? shiny? smooth? scars? lesions? (describe size, shape, and type of lesion) striae? umbilicus?

Bowels sounds: Present? absent? hyperactive? high-pitched tickling? gurgles? borborygmus?

Percussion: Tympanic? dull? flat? (describe where) liver size 6–12 cm? splenic dullness 6–10th rib? ascites?

Palpation: Splenomegaly? hepatomegaly? organomegaly? masses? aotic pulse? diastasis recti? tenderness? bulges? lower pole of kidneys palpable? inguinal or femoral hernia? inguinal nodes? (describe).

Musculoskeletal Inspection and Palpation

Back: Shoulders level? right shoulder higher than left? left shoulder higher than right? alignment? lordosis? scoliosis? kyphosis? ankylosis?

Vertebral column alignment: Straight? lordosis? scoliosis? kyphosis?

Joints: Redness? swelling? deformity? (describe) crepitation? size? symmetry? subluxation? separation? bogginess? tenderness? pain? thickening? nudules? fluid? bulging?

Range of motion: Describe as full, limited or fixed, estimate degree of limitation, assess range of motion of neck, shoulders, elbows wrists, fingers, back, hips, knees, ankles, toes.

Extremities: Compare extremities with each other; describe color and symmetry; temperature; hot, warm, cool, cold, moist, clammy, dry; muscle tone descriptors are firm, muscular, flabby, flaccid, atrophy? fasciculation? tremor?

Lower extremities: Symmetry? (describe any variations from normal abrasions? bruises? swollen? edema? rashes? lesions? (describe) prosthesis? varicose veins?

Genitourinary and Rectum Inspection

Rectum: Hemorrhoids? inflammation? lesions? skin tags? fissures? excoriation? swelling? mucosal bulging? retrocele?

Female genitalia: Pubic hair distribution and color? nits? pediculosis? lesions? nodules? inflammation? swelling? pigmentation? dry? moist? shrivelled, atrophy or full labia? discharge? (describe) odor? asymmetry? varicosities? uterine prolapse? smegma? rash?

Male genitalia: Pubic hair distribution and color? nits? pediculosis? circumcised? uncircumcised? phimosis? epispadias? hypospadius? smegma? priapism? varicocele? cryptorchidism? hydrocele? swelling? redness? chancre? crusing? rash? discharge? (describe) edema? scrotal sack rugated? atrophy?

Neurologic

Describe tics, twitches, paresthesia, paralysis, coordination.

Gait: Balanced? shuffling? unsteady? ataxic? Parkinsonian? swaying? scissor? spastic? waddling? staggering? faltering? swaying? slow? difficult? tottering? propulsive?

Accessory- CN XI: Shrugs shoulder? symmetry?

Reflexes: Report as present or absent.

Coordination: Report as to test done.

Cranial nerves: May be reported here.

Mental Status

Level of alertness: Alert? stuporous? semicomatose?

Orientation: Oriented to time, place and person? confused? disoriented? If confused, check orientation as follows:

Time: Ask client year, month, day, date.

Place: Ask client's residence address, where she/he is now.

Person: Ask client's name, birthday.

Memory: Recent memory: Give client short series of numbers and ask client to repeat those numbers later. Long-term: Ask client to recall some event, that happened several years ago.

Language and speech: Language spoken? Speech: Slurred? slow? rapid? difficulty forming words? aphasia?

Responsiveness: Responds appropriately to verbal stimuli? responds readily? slow to respond?

It is probable that all of the questions in each system will not be included every time you take a history. Nevertheless, some questions regarding each system should be included in every history. These essential races are listed in bold type in the outline that follows. More comprehensive and detailed areas for questions relating to each system are listed afterward and should be included whenever the patient gives positive responses to the first group of questions for that system. Keep in mind that these lists do not represent an exhaustive enumertion of questions that might be appropriate within an organ system. Even more detailed questions may be required, depending on the patient's problem.

General Constitutional Symptoms

Fever, chills, malaise, fatigability, night sweats; weight (average, preferred, present, change, appetite).

Skin

Rash or eruption, pruritus, pigmentation or texture change; excessive sweating, abnormal nail or hair growth.

Skeletal

Joint stiffness, pain, restriction of motion, edema, erythema, heat, bony deformity.

Head

1. *General:* Frequent or unusual headaches, dizziness, syncope, severe injuries.
2. *Eyes:* Visual acuity, blurring, diplopia (double vision), photophobia (abnormal sensitivity to light), pain, recent change in appearance or vision; glaucoma, use of eyedrops or other eye medications, history of trauma or familial eye disease.
3. *Ears:* Hearing loss, pain, discharge, tinnitus, vertigo.
4. *Nose:* Sense of smell, frequency of colds, obstruction, epistaxis, postnasal discharge, sinus pain.
5. *Throat and mouth:* Hoarseness or change in voice; frequent sore throats, bleeding or edema of gums; recent tooth abscesses or extractions; soreness of tongue or buccal mucosa, ulcers; disturbance of taste.

Endocrine

Thyroid enlargement or tenderness, heat or cold intolerance, unexplained weight change, diabetes, polydipsia (excessive thirst), polyuria, changes in facial or body hair, increased fat and glove size, skin striac.

1. *Males:* onset of puberty, erections, emissions, testicular pain, libido, infertility.
2. *Females:*
   a. *Menses:* Onset, regularity, duration of flow, dysmenorrhea, last period, intermenstrual discharge or bleeding, pruritus date of last pap smear, age at menopause, libido, frequency of intercourse, sexual difficulties.
   b. *Pregnancies:* Number of miscarriages, abortions, duration of pregnancy or postpartum period; use of oral or other contraceptives.
   c. *Breasts:* Pain, tenderness, discharge, lumps, mammograms.

Respiratory

Pain relating to respiration, dyspnea, cyanosis, wheezing, cough, sputum (character and quantity), hemoptysis (expectorating blood from respiratory tract, night sweats, exposure to TB; date and result of last chest X-ray examination.

Cardiac

Chest pain or distress, recipitating causes, timing and duration, relieving factors, palpitations, dyspnea, orthopnea (number of pillos needed), edema, claudication (weakness of legs accompanied by cramp-like pain), hypertension, previous myocardial infarction, estimate of excerise tolerance, past ECG or other cardiac tests.

Hematological

Anemia, tendency to bruise or bleed easily, thromboses, thrombophlebitis, any known abnormality of blood cells, transfusions.

Lymph Nodes

Enlargement, tenderness, suppuration to produce purulent (pus) material.

Gastrointestinal

Appetite, digestion, intolerance for any class of foods, dysphagia, heartburn, nausea, vomiting, hematemesis, regularity of bowels, constipation, diarrhea, change in stool color or contents (clay-colored, tarry, fresh blood, mucus, undigested food), flatulence, hemorrhoids, hepatitis, jaundice, dark urine; history of ulcer, gallstones, polyps, tumor; previous X-ray examinations (where, when, findings).

Genitourinary

Dysuria, flank or suprapubic pain, urgency, frequency, nocturia, hematuria, polyuria, hesitancy, dribbling, loss in force of stream, passage of stone; edema of face, stress incontinence, hernias, sexually transmitted disease inquire what kind and symptoms, and list results of serological test for syphilis (STS), if known.

Neurological

Syncope (brief lapse in consciousness caused by transient cerebral hypoixa), seizures, weakness or paralysis, abnormalities of sensation or coordination, tremors, loss of memory unusual frequency, distribution, or severity of headaches, serious head injury in past.

Psychiatric

Depression, mood changes, difficulty concentrating, nervousness, tension, suicidal thoughts, irritability, sleep disturbances.

AN ADVICE TO PUBLIC BY NURSES FOR THEIR CARE

- Taking charge of your own health care, deciding when to see a doctor, when an alternative practitioner might be more appropriate, and what you can handle yourself, is an intelligent, perhaps even necessary approach these days. Unfortunately, there are no easy guidelines—many physicians with years of training and experience often find such decisions difficult. Still, the more you know about how diseases can be treated, the more likely you are to make appropriate choices in managing your own and your family's medical care.

- Thousands of people will die needlessly each year because of denial and delay. Among them are heart attack victims who wait an average of 6 hours to call a doctor, and other people who ignore for months the common warning signs of a major disease such as cancer.

  By contract, those who run to a medical specialist for every ache, pain, and sniffle not only drive up medical costs, but also increase their risk of adverse reactions from overtreatment. The ideal is to find a middle ground based on common sense and knowledge.
- Everyone should have a primary-care physician to oversee and coordinate medical care. This might be a family practitioner, an internist, an osteopath, a pediatrician (for children), or a gynecologist (for women). The doctor may have his or her own practice or be part of a group practice or a clinic. The important thing is that your practitioners know your medical history and have a stake in maintaining your health.

When you are injured or acute illness strikes, always turn first to a conventionally trained medical doctor. These practitioners are the best qualified to treat trauma and other emergencies, infections, diabetes, heart disease, cancer, and other serious illnesses.

If you suffer from a chronic pain syndrome or some other conditions for which conventional medicine can do little, you might be better off seeing an alternative practitioner. And in many cases, you may be the best person to manage your illness, often under the guidance of a medical professional.

When there is problem that demand prompt medical attention, call your local emergency service or get to the nearest emergency room if any of the following develop:

Possible Heart Attack

- Severe pain, light-headedness, fainting, sweating, nausea, or shortness of breath
- Feeling of pain, pressure, fullness, or squeezing in the center chest that lasts more than 2 minutes
- Pain spreading from the center chest to the shoulders, neck, or arms.

Possible Stroke or Mini-stroke

- Sudden weakness or numbness on one side of the body, usually affecting the face, an arm, or leg
- Sudden loss of speech, or difficulty speaking or understanding speech
- Loss of vision or dimness, usually in one eye or half of both eyes
- Unexplained dizziness, unsteady gait, lack of coordination, or falling
- Sudden severe headache unlike any experienced in the past
- Abrupt loss of memory or altered mental abilities.

Possible Shock

- Cold, clammy, and pale skin
- Weakness and light headedness
- Rapid, weak pulse
- Rapid, shallow, and irregular breathing
- Agitation and feeling of apprehension.

Possible Anaphylactic Reaction

- Severe swelling, especially around the eyes, mouth, and face
- Weak, rapid pulse
- Difficulty breathing
- Possible nausea, vomiting, and abdominal cramps
- Bluish tinge to skin and nails
- Confusion, dizziness, possible loss of consciousness.

Possible Internal Bleeding

- Coughing or vomiting up blood, which may look like coffee grounds
- Blood in the stool or urine
- Bleeding from a body opening, such as the ears, nose, or mouth
- Abdominal swelling and tenderness
- Excessive thirst.

Fevers

See a doctor as soon as possible if:

- Body temperature rises to 100.5°F (38°C) in a baby younger than 3 months
- Body temperature rises to 103°F (39.4°C) in a child or adult of any age
- Body temperature rises to 101°F (38.3°C) and stays there for 3 days
- Low-grade fever recurs or persists for two or more weeks
- Fever of any degree is accompanied by severe headache, stiff neck, swelling of the throat, or mental confusion.

Signs and Symptoms

In medical terms, a sign is any visible indication of disease—bleeding, a rash, or swelling, for example. A symptom is something you can feel, such as pain, fever, or nausea, and it may or may not be accompanied by a physical change. The possible causes with signs and symptoms are listed in Table 2.3.

NURSING CARE PLAN OF FEVER–SAMPLES OF NURSING CARE PLAN

Fever is a term used to refer to an evaluation of body temperature above the normal (37.8°C or 38.2°C). Fever may be related to an altered set points of the hypothalemia thermostat mechanism due to excessive heat production (as in hyperthyroidium

TABLE 2.3: Common signs and symptoms

Signs or symptoms	Possible causes
Anxiety	Alcoholism, panic attack, premenstrual syndrome, stress, a thyroid disorder
Belching	Gallbladder disease, indigestion, a malabsorption syndrome
Bleeding and bruises	
Gums	Periodontal disease, leukemia, vitamin deficiency
Eye	Diabetes, high blood pressure
Nose	A clotting disorder, high blood pressure, injury, nasal polyps or tumors
Rectal	Anal fissure, colon cancer or polyps, diverticulitis or other intestinal disorder, hemorrhoids, ulcers
Skin	Allergic reaction, anemia, a blood or clotting disorder, Cushing's syndrome, drug reaction, hemophilia, injury, leukemia
Sputum	Bronchitis, lung cancer, pneumonia, pulmonary embolism, throat infection, tuberculosis
Urine	Bladder infection, urinary tract cancer, kidney stone, prostate disorder
Vagina	Abortion or miscarriage, cancer, a hormonal disorder, infection, menstrual abnormalities, injury, polyps
Vomit	Cirrhosis of the liver, esophageal tear, ulcers
Breathlessness	Anemia, anxiety, asthma, heart disease, hyperventilation, a lung disorder
Confusion	Addiction, alcoholism, Alzheimer's disease or other dementia, drug reaction, head injury, stroke
Constipation	Appendicitis, colon cancer or other bowel disorder, diabetes, diet, drug side effects, inactivity, pregnancy, a thyroid disorder
Coughing	Asthma, bronchitis, common cold, croup, cystic fibrosis, flu, pneumonia
Cyanosis (bluish skin)	A circulatory disorder, congenital heart defect, cystic fibrosis, heart failure, respiratory failure, Raynaud's disease
Delirium	Alcohol or drug abuse, brain tumor or abscess, encephalitis, head injury, heat stroke, meningitis, mountain sickness, poisoning, psychosis, Reye's syndrome
Diarrhea	AIDS, allergies, celiac disease, food poisoning, inflammatory bowel disease, irritable bowel syndrome or other colon disorder, infection, a malabsorption syndrome, traveler's diarrhea
Dizziness	Alcohol or drug abuse, anemia, a brain disorder, cardiac arrhythmia, drug reaction, ear infection, Menière's disease, stroke or mini-stroke, tumor
Fatigue	Anemia, cancer, chronic fatigue syndrome, depression, flu or other infectious disorders, heart disease, hepatitis, mononucleosis, premenstrual syndrome, respiratory disorders
Fever	Abscess, AIDS, appendicitis, cancer, infection (bacterial or viral), medication side effects, rheumatoid arthritis or other autoimmune diseases
Fainting	Anxiety, blood loss, cardiac arrhythmias, heart attack or other heart condition, hyperventilation, hypoglycemia, stroke
Gait changes	Arthritis, a back disorder, multiple sclerosis or other neuromuscular disorder, Parkinson's disease, stroke
Hallucinations	Alcoholism, drug reaction, fever, schizophrenia or other psychotic disorder
Hirsutism	Cancer, Cushing's syndrome, drug side effects, hormonal imbalances, polycystic ovaries or other ovarian disorder
Hoarseness	Anxiety, asthma, bronchitis, cancer, common cold, croup, polyps, smoking, thyroid deficiency
Impotence	Alcoholism, depression, diabetes, drug reaction, multiple sclerosis, hormonal abnormalities, a nerve disorder, surgery for prostate tumors or disease, a thyroid disorder

Contd...

Contd...

Signs or symptoms	Possible causes
Insomnia	Alcohol and caffeine use, anxiety or depression, drug side effects, a thyroid disorder
Intestinal gas	Colic, colon cancer or other bowel disorder, diet, indigestion, a malabsorption syndrome
Itching	Allergies, chickenpox or other rash, dry skin, eczema, fungal or other infection, liver disease, stress, vaginitis
Jaundice	Anemia, blocked bile duct, cirrhosis, hepatitis or other liver disorder, gallbladder disease, a pancreatic disorder, infant prematurity
Loss of appetite	AIDS, anemia, cancer, depression, a digestive disorder, drug reaction, an eating disorder, infection, loss of taste
Mood changes	Alcohol or drug abuse, depression or other psychological disorder, drug reaction, a hormonal disorder, menopause, premenstrual syndrome, psychological stress
Nausea and vomiting	Alcohol abuse, appendicitis, brain injury, drug reaction, ear infection, gallbladder disease, food poisoning, gastritis, glaucoma, heart attack, hepatitis, indigestion, infection, intestinal obstruction, Mènière's disease, morning sickness, motion sickness, ulcers, vertigo
Nightmares	Alcohol or drug abuse, anxiety, depression, fever, post-traumatic stress syndrome
Numbness or tingling	Bell's palsy, carpal tunnel syndrome, a circulatory disorder, neuropathy, Raynaud's disease, shingles
Pain	
Abdomen	Appendicitis, a digestive disorder, gallstones, hepatitis, intestinal disorders menstrual cramps, pelvic inflammatory disease, tubal pregnancy
Back	Arthritis, muscle spasms or strain, osteoporosis, ruptured disk
Chest	Angina, an esophageal disorder, heart attack, heartburn, pleurisy, pneumonia, pneumothorax
Ear	Infection, foreign body
Eye	Conjunctivitis, glaucoma, foreign body, iritis, sinus infection, injury, sty, tumors
Face	Bell's palsy, dental disease, headache, shingles, sinus infection, temporomandibular joint disorder
Foot	Arthritis, bunions, corns or calluses, gout, neuromas, warts
Generalized	Flu, lupus, mononucleosis, rheumatoid arthritis, shingles
Head	Brain tumor, migraine or other type of headache, muscle tension, sinusitis, stroke
Knee	Arthritis, chondromalacia patella, infection, Lyme disease, strain or other injury
Leg	A circulatory disorder, fracture, muscle injury, phlebitis, shin splints
Mouth	Canker sores, cold sores, dental cavities, gum disease, infection
Neck	Arthritis, meningitis, muscle injury slipped disk, stress
Joint/muscle	Arthritis, lupus, strain or sprain, tendinitis
Throat	Cold, flu, laryngitis, strep infection, tonsillitis, quinsy
Painful intercourse	
In males	Penile warts, prostatic or urethral infection
In females	Menopausal dryness, vaginitis, premenstrual syndrome
Palpitations	Anemia, anxiety, caffeine, heart disease, hypoglycemia, menopause, medications, premenstrual syndrome, a thyroid disorder
Rashes	Allergies, drug reactions, eczema, an infectious disease, lupus, rosacea, toxic shock syndrome
Runny nose	Allergies, common cold, sinus infection
Seizures	Brain tumor, drug side effect, cerebral palsy, epilepsy, fever, head injury, hypoglycemia, toxemia of pregnancy, meningitis, poisoning
Speech problems	Alcohol abuse, Alzheimer's disease, Bell's palsy, multiple sclerosis, stroke, Parkinson's disease
Swallowing problems	Anxiety, diphtheria, an esophageal disorder, pharyngitis, strep throat, throat cancer, tonsillitis, quinsy
Sweating	Anxiety, drug reaction, fever, heart attack, infection, menopause, stress, a thyroid disorder
Swelling and lumps	

Contd...

Contd...

Signs or symptoms	Possible causes
Abdominal	Cancer, heart failure, hernias, internal bleeding, intestinal gas, kidney failure liver disease, pregnancy, uterine tumor
Breast	Cancer, fibrocystic condition, mastitis
Generalized	Anaphylactic reaction, drug reaction, heart failure, kidney disease, phlebitis, a liver disorder, thyroid disease
Joints	Arthritis, sprains
Skin or body surface	Abscess, cysts or other benign growths, cancer, edema, enlarged or obstructed lymph glands, ganglion, hives, infection, moles, warts
Taste changes	Bell's palsy, cancer, drug reaction, gum or dental disease, liver disease, loss of smell, pregnancy, a salivary disorder
Thirst	Diabetes, fever, heat exhaustion
Tinnitus (ringing in the ears)	Brain injury or tumor, cold or flu, drug side effects, ear infection, exposure to loud noise, Mènière's disease, earwax build-up, otosclerosis, vertigo
Tremor	Alcoholism, anxiety, Parkinson's disease, a thyroid disorder
Urinary problems	
Discolored urine	Bladder or kidney infection, kidney stones, liver or gallbladder disease, urinary tract cancer
Incontinence	Aging, Alzheimer's disease, a bladder disorder, nerve deterioration, spinal injury, stroke
Urgency	Bladder infection, bladder tumor, diabetes, interstitial cystitis, drug reaction, pregnancy
Painful urination	Bladder infection, gonorrhea or other sexually transmitted disease, kidney infection, kidney or bladder stones, prostatitis, urethritis, vaginitis
Vaginal discharge	Cancer, cervicitis, gonorrhea, vaginitis, pregnancy, premenstrual syndrome
Vision problems	Cataracts, detached retina, glaucoma, iritis, macular degeneration, mini-stroke, retinopathy
Weakness	Anemia, cancer, Guillain-Barré syndrome, heart disease, infection, liver disease, multiple sclerosis, muscular dystrophy, myasthenia gravis, rheumatoid arthritis
Weight changes	
Unexplained gain	Heart failure, kidney disease, liver disease, medications, toxemia of pregnancy, underactive thyroid
Unexplained loss	AIDS, anemia, cancer, diabetes, an eating disorder, infection, an intestinal disorder, malabsorption syndrome, ulcers
Wheezing	Allergies, asthma, bronchitis, emphysema, heart failure, lung disorders

salicylate poisoning, malignant hyperthermias) or due to reduced heat loss (heat stroke, Datura poisoning ectodermal dysplasia). Fever due to infectious diseases is usually to the first mechanism.

Infective agents also called exogenous pyrogens are engulfed by phagocytic leukocytes in the tissues. The inflammatory response triggered by the exogenous agents, agent lead to the production of compounds grouped together as leukotrienes that help the leukocytes, monocytes and macrophages to engulf the infective agent. Activated phagocytic cells produce several polypeptide compounds, such as interleukin-1, cachectin, (also called tumor necrosis factor), interleukin-6 and interseron-α. These compounds are examples of 'endogenous pyrogens' interleukin-1 acts on the arachidonic acid pathway, stimulating the production of prostaglandins by the vascular endothelial cells of the hypothalamus. Increased levels of prostaglandins E2 within the hypothalamus accelerate the "firing rate" of the "cold sensitive" cells in the preoptic anterior hypothalamia nuclei and reduce the activity of the "warm sensitive" cells. This results in the shifting of the set point of the hypothalemia thermostat towards a higher temperature setting. The vasomotor center responds by increasing peripheral vascular tone; cutaneous vasoconstriction decreases heat loss. Shivering thermogenesis may also be initiated. These mechanisms continue until the temperature of blood bathing and the hypothalamic neurons reach the new set point.

Etiology of Fever

Pyrexia of unknown origin (PUO) has been arbitrarily defined as a temperature in excess of 38.3°C (101°F) for a duration of at least 3 weeks, which remains undiagnosed after 1 week of investigation in the hospital. The causes of PUO are as follows:

1. Infections
   - *Pyogenic infections:* Pyogenic abscess, cholangitis, pelvic abscess, liver and subphrenic abscess, diverticular abcess, thrombophlebitis.

- *Vascular infection:* Infective endocarditis, infected vascular access devices.
- *Chronic glomerulomatous infection:* Tuberculosis, atypical mycobacterial infections, fungal infections.
- Other prolonged bacterial, reckettisial, and viral illnesses, brucellosis, chronic meningococcemia.

2. Immune inflammatory diseases: Systemic lupus erythematosus, juvenile rheumatoid arthritis (skin disease), vasculitis including giant cell arteritis.
3. Neoplasms: Primary (renal, pancreas, hepatic, lung, colon), secondary (hepatid secondaries) lymphoid neoplasms.
4. Granulomatous conditions (non-infections): Sarcoidosis.
5. Metabolic and familial conditions: Familial metaranian fever. Fabry's disease.
6. Drug-induced fever.
7. Factitious fever.
8. Undiagnosed fever.

TABLE 2.4: Nursing care plan of patient with fever

Problem	Reason	Objective	Nursing intervention (rationale)	Evaluation
1. Altered comfort related to increased body temperature (infection)	Due to infection • Temperature↑ • Malaise+ • Heart rate↑ • ↑Respiratory rate • ↑WBC count	Patient will have body temperature below 100° F (37.8°C)	• Assess the patient, temperature 4th hourly (to monitor temperature) • Administer antipyretic drugs 4th hourly if ordered (to reduce temperature) • Keep environmental temperature at 70°F (21.1°C) • Avoid heavy layers of clothing or bed covers (to aid in lowering body temperature) • Give tepid sponge bath, after antipyretic therapy (to reduce temperature through evaporation rapidly) • Use skin lotions (to prevent drying) • Change the linen frequently if patient is diaphoretic (to prevent chilling and subsequent rise in body temperature from muscular activity) • Implement appropriate measure (to treat causes of fever)	(Patient response to be written in the column)
2. Risk for fluid volume deficit	• Metabolic rate • Diaphoresis • Decreased oral intake	Patient will have no signs of dehydration	• Assess for rapid respiration and pulse • Assess damp skin, clothing and bed clothing • Assess unwillingness or inability to ingest fluids • Assess signs of dehydration (to determine risk for fluid deficit) • Encourage fluid intake to 3–4 2/day (to replace fluids loss due to fever)	
			• Monitor TPR and BP 4th hourly (to know any indication of hypovolemia) • Administer IV fluids if necessary • Monitor intake and output accurately • Give careful estimate of insensible losses (to evaluate need for replacement)	
3. Risk for altered nutrition: Less than body requirement related to increased caloric need	• Metabolic rate↓ • Oral intake↓	Patient will have no weight loss	• Assess intake and monitor weight daily (to know the risk) • Give high caloric, high proteins, easily digested food and fluidity (to maximize intake and minimize energy expense) • Help patient balance activity and rest to conserve energy (to ensure preferred activity) • Monitor alternate method of nutritional intake, i.e. enteral, parenteral	

↑ = Increased; ↓ = Decreased; + = Present

TABLE 2.5: Nursing care plan of myocardial infarction (MI)

Problem	Reason	Objective	Nursing intervention (rationale)	Evaluation
1. Pain	Imbalance of O_2 supply and demand (write subjective and objective data of pain)	Reducing pain	• Position the patient in bed in Semi-Fowler's position • Handle the patient while providing care, while IV giving taking vital signs, ECG, etc. • Administer oxygen by nasal cannula at 4 L/min • Offer support and reassurance • Administer sublingual nitroglycerin as directed • Monitor TP, heart rate, respiration rate, frequently every 5 minutes • Administer narcotics as prescribed • Obtain basal vital signs • Give IV nitroglycerin as prescribed • Review with patient frequently the importance of the reporting any chest pain, discomfort, without delay	• Pain reduced in semi- Fowler's position • Color improved and patient verbalizes decreased pain • BP remains stable. HR within limits • No signs of bleeding
2. Anxiety	Chest pain (other subjective and objective data)	Alleviating anxiety	• Explain equipment, procedure and need for frequent assessment to patient and family • Explain the visiting hours and importance of limiting number of visitors • Offer family members preferred times and phone unit to check on patient status • Observe autonomic signs of anxiety such as increased HR, BP, RR tremulousness • Administer anti-anxiety agents as prescribed, e.g. diazepam. • Observe adverse effects of sedation such as lethargy, confusion, etc. • Offer touch and massage (may promote relaxation) • Maintain continuity of care (consistency of routine and staff, promote trust and confidence	• Patient and family verbalize understanding • No autonomic signs of anxiety • Verbalizes decrease of anxiety • Cooperation with care and talkative with staff
3. Decreased Cardiac output	(write subjective and objective data)	Cardiac output will improve or maintaining hemodynamic stability	• Monitor BP every 2 hours or as directed • Monitor respiration and lung fields every 2 to 4 hours by auscultating and observing • Evaluate heart rate and heart sounds every 2 to 4 hours or as directed • Administer IV fluids as ordered • Note presence of JVD and liver engorgement • Evaluate major arterial pulses • Take body temperature every 4 hours or as directed • Observe presence of edema • Monitor skin color and temperature • Be alert to change in mental status • Evaluate urine output (30 mL/h) • Monitor life-threatening dysrhythmias • Correct dysrhythmias immediately as directed	
4. Activity intolerance	Insufficient oxygenation and deconditioning effect on bedrest. (+ add subjective and objective data)	Increasing activity tolerance	• Promote rest with following measures: – Minimize environmental noise – Provide comfortable environment temperature – Avoid unnecessary procedures and interruptions – Structure routine care measures including rest – Discuss the patient and family about visiting hours and limiting visitors – Promote restful diversional activities (e.g. reading, listening to music, etc.) – Encourage frequent changes of position gently – Assist the patient with prescribed activities, e.g. change of position, ROM exercises, etc.	

Contd...

Contd...

Problem	Reason	Objective	Nursing intervention (rationale)	Evaluation
5. Risk for injury	"	Prevent bleeding	• Take vital signs every 15 minutes during infusion of thrombolytic agents • Observe the presence of hematomas or skin breakdown in pressure areas sacrum, back, elbows ankles • Be alert verbal complaints of backpain • Observe all punctured sites every 15 minutes • Apply manual pressure to arterial or venous sites of bleeding occurs or use pressure dressings • Observe for blood in stool, emesis, urine and sputum • Minimize venipuncture and arterial punctures • Avoid IM injection • Caution about vigorous tooth brushing • Avoid trauma to patient by gentle handling • Monitor CT, BT, HR% PTT, HCT • Check current blood type and cross match • Administer antacids as directed • Administer IV fluid and transfusion as directed • Monitor changes in mental status • Avoid vigorous oral suctioning (if)	
6. Altered tissue perfusion	"	Maintaining tissue perfusions	• Observe for persistent and/or recurrence of signs and symptoms of MI • Report immediately • Administer oxygen, as directed • Record a 12-load ECG • Prepare patient for possible emergency procedure (catheterization or surgery)	
7. Ineffective individual coping	"	Strengthening coping abilities	• Listen carefully to patient and family to ascertain their clarification • Assist the patient to establish positive attitude towards illness and progress • Manipulate environment to promote restful sleep • Be alert to signs and symptoms of sleep deprivation • Minimize possible emotional response to transfer for ICU	
8. Knowledge deficit R/T care of MI patient		Educate the patient and family for health maintenance and management	• Inform the patient and family members about what has happened to heart • Instruct patient on how to judge the body's response to activity (oxygen requirement, importance of rest, taking pulse, review signs and symptoms) • Design an individual activity progression program for patient as directed – Walk daily gradually increasing distance and time as directed – Avoid activities that tense muscles – Avoid working with arms overhead – Gradually return to work – Avoid extremes in temperature – Do not rush, avoid tension • Tell the patient that sexual relations may be resumed on the advice of health care provider. Usually after exercise tolerance is assessed – If the patient can walk briskly or climb two flights of stairs, can usually resume sexual activity with familial partner – Sexual activity should be avoided after heavy meals, after alcohol or when tired • Advise getting at least 7 hours sleep at each night and take 20–30 minutes rest period in day • Advise limiting visitors	(Patients response to nursing measures, treatment and progress to be written in this column)

Contd...

Contd...

Problem	Reason	Objective	Nursing intervention (rationale)	Evaluation
			• Advise eating 3 to 4 small meals per day • Advise limiting caffeine and alcohol intake • Driving car must be on advice of physician • Teach patient to notify when following symptoms occur: – Chest pain or pressure – Shortening of breath – Unusual fatigue – Swelling of feet and ankles – Fainting and dizziness – Very slow or rapid heart beat • Assist patient to reduce risk for another MI by risk factors modification avoid smoking, reducing high blood cholesterol levels – Reducing high BP, obesity, diabetes, stress, etc. – Control of the condition can be achieved through appropriate measures against obesity, control of serum cholesterol and hypertension and active exercise and physical fitness high dose of vitamin C can effectively reduce the serum cholesterol level in hypercholesterolemia – Long-term use of beta-adrenoceptor blocking drugs can reduce cardiovascular mortality	

TABLE 2.6: Nursing care plan of patient in hypovolemic shock

Problem	Reason	Objective	Nursing intervention (rationale)	Evaluation
1. Hypovolemic shock related to blood loss	Subjective and objective data, e.g. one of the following: • Massive trauma • GI bleeding • Ruptured aortic aneurysm • Surgery • Erosion of vessel from lesion, tubes or other devices • DIC (diminished intravascular coagulation)	• Treat shock • Bring patient to normal level	• Stop external bleeding with direct pressure, pressure dressing tourniquet • Reduce intra-abdominal or retroperitoneal bleeding by applying many tail bandage or prepare for emergency surgery • Administer lactated Ringer's solution or normal saline • Transfuse with fresh whole blood, packed cells, fresh frozen plasma or platelets if no significant improvement with crystalloids • Use non-blood plasma expanders (albumin, dextran) until blood is available • Autotransfusion if appropriate	
2. Shock related to plasma loss	• Burns • Accumulation of intra-abdominal fluid • Malnutrition • Severe dermatitis		• Administer low dose cardiotonics (dopamines) • Administer Ringer's lactate solutions or normal saline • Administer albumin. Fresh frozen plasma or dextran if cardiac output is still low	
3. Shock related to crystalloid loss	• Dehydration • Protracted vomiting or diarrhea • Nasogastric suction		Administer isotonic or hypotonic solution	

Note: When crystallized or colloid solution is administered, proper precautions to be followed and every significant information documented.

TABLE 2.7: Nursing care plan for cardiogenic shock

Problem	Reason	Objective	Nursing intervention (rationale)	Evaluation
1. Cardiogenic shock related to myocardial disease or injury	(Subjective and objective data of one of the following) • Acute MI • Myocardial contusion • Cardiomyopathies	• To rule out hypovolemia • To maintain ventricular filling pressure	• Fluid challenge with up to 300 mL of NS or RL solution to rule out hypovolemia unless CCF or pulmonary edema pressure • Insert CVP (central venous pressure) or pulmonary artery catheter; – Monitor cardiac output, pulmonary pressure – Monitor PCWP (pulmonary capillary wedge pressure) • Administer IV fluids to maintain ventricular filling pressure of 15–20 mm Hg • Administer inotropics (e.g. dopamines or dobutamine) • Administer vasodilators (e.g. sodium nitroprusside) • Administer diuretics (e.g. mannitol or fursemide) • Use cardiotonics (digitalis) beta blockers (propranol) • Use corticosteroids	
2. Shock related to valvular disease or injury	• Ruptured aortic cusp • Ruptured papillary muscles • Ball thrombosis		Same as above (hypovolemia shock)	

TABLE 2.8: Sample nursing care plan for the patient with a carotid artery aneurysm and middle cerebral artery syndrome

Problem	Objective	Nursing interventions	Rationales
Nursing Diagnosis #1			
Alteration in cerebral perfusion, related to: 1. Cerebral infarction with consequent cerebral edema 2. Vasospasm associated with subarachnoid bleeding	Patient will: 1. Maintain cerebral perfusion pressure more than 60 mm Hg; ICP less than 15 mm Hg; mean arterial blood pressure ~80 mm Hg 2. Remain without cardiac dysrhythmias 3. Exhibit intact level of consciousness and mentation: – Oriented to person/ place – Memory intact	• Monitor for signs/symptoms of increasing ICP (Intracranial pressure) – Establish baseline parameters for level of consciousness, mentation, respiratory rate and pattern, pupillary reactions, and sensorimotor function • Maintain the integrity of the ICP monitoring system: – Check for leaks, air; stopcocks in appropriate positions – Perform insertion site care as per protocol • Obtain and record accurate pressure measurements: – Confirm accurate placement of transducer at level of foramen of Monro – Analyze waveforms and pressure readings and identify trends – Calculate and record cerebral perfusion pressure hourly • Implement measures to prevent and/ or reduce ICP: – Maintain proper positioning and body alignment; elevate head of bed; avoid head rotation or flexion on chest	• Initial treatment is focused on stabilizing and supporting intracranial dynamics, and reducing and/or preventing rebleeding. – Baseline measurements are used to compare subsequent responses • ICP monitoring is a highly invasive technique, which places the patient at considerable risk of infection – Inadvertent loss of CSF in the presence of increased ICP can alter intracranial hemodynamics and precipitate herniation – Venting port of transducer should always be at pressure source (i.e. the foramen of Monro). For every inch above or below the pressure source, the pressure reading may be as much as 2 mm Hg off – Trends are more significant in determining status of ICP and intracranial compliance – Allows for optimal venous drainage from cranium via gravity. Prevents jugular vein compression or obstruction • Hypercapnia and hypoxemia predispose to cerebral vasodilation and increased cerebral blood flow

Contd...

Contd...

Problem	Objective	Nursing interventions	Rationales
		• Prevent increase in cerebral blood flow: – Initiate and maintain hyperventilation via mechanical ventilation to maintain $PaCO_2$ at 25–35 mm Hg; PaO_2 more than 80 mm Hg	
Nursing Diagnosis # 2			
Alteration in comfort: Headache, related to: 1. Meningeal irritation 2. Surgical incision	Patient will: 1. Verbalize feeling relieved of pain 2. Demonstrate a relaxed demeanor	• Assess for signs/symptoms of meningeal irritation: – Nuchal rigidity, photophobia, headache, positive Kernig's and Brudzinski's signs • Implement nursing measures to reduce headache and prevent bleeding – Move patient carefully, minimizing head movement or sudden jarring of patient or bed; turn q2h – Dim the patient's bedside light, and maintain a quiet environment with minimal stimuli ◆ Handle patient gently when providing care ◆ Caution patient not to cough, sneeze, or strain • Administer analgesics as prescribed, and monitor effectiveness of medication in relieving pain and relaxing the patient	• Intracranial bleeding is highly irritating to meningeal and brain tissues – Turning helps to mobilize tracheobronchial secretions and redistribute pressure points to maximize circulation – Dimming the lights helps reduce the discomfort of photophobia – These activities cause an increase in ICP • Headache can be excruciating
Nursing Diagnosis #3			
Potential for injury: Seizures, related to: 1. Cranial cerebral insult (cerebral infarction and edema; intracranial bleeding)	Patient will: • Remain seizure free • Maintain serum levels of phenytoin within the acceptable therapeutic range	• Assess/monitor for seizure activity, documenting characteristics: onset, location, type of movement, associated changes in body function • Maintain seizure precautions as per protocol • Administer prescribed anticonvulsants – Monitor serum elvels of phenytoin (dilantin), (serial)	• Craniocerebral insults place the patient at risk of having seizures; anticonvulsant medications are usually prescribed prophylactically
Nursing Diagnosis # 4			
Nutrition, alteration in, less than body requirements, related to: 1. Altered state of consciousness 2. Compromised protective reflexes 3. Ineffective chewing or swallowing 4. Fatigue 5. Depression	1. Patient will maintain an anabolic state: – Body weight within 5% of baseline – Total serum proteins within the acceptable range: albumin 3.5–5.0 g/100 mL 2. Patient will verbalize having an appetite	• Consult with nutritionist to determine caloric and nutritional needs • Initiate prescribed nutritional regimen: – Hyperalimentation; fluid restriction • Monitor response to hyperalimentation: – Intake and output – Laboratory parameters; BUN, creatinine, total protein, and albumin – Daily weight when patient's condition permits • Maintain the integrity of the hyperalimentation system as per unit protocol	• Critical illness increases nutritional needs; these patients can rapidly experience a catabolic state when maintained on intravenous fluid replacement therapy (one liter of dextrose and water contains 600 calories)

Contd...

Contd...

Problem	Objective	Nursing interventions	Rationales
Nursing Diagnosis #5			
Airway clearance, ineffective, related to: 1. Compromised cough 2. Need for minimizing activity of any kind during the acute phase 3. Limited mobility	Patient's airway will remain patent; breath sounds will be normal, without adventitious sounds (e.g., crackles, wheezes, rhonchi)	• Assess breath sounds/adventitious sounds • Suction patient only when absolutely necessary, using meticulous technique – Limit each pass to 10 seconds – Prevent accumulation of secretions • Maintain ventilation and oxygenation as prescribed	• Abnormal breath sounds or the presence of adventitious sounds suggests accumulation and pooling of secretions • Suctioning may increase interacranial pressure – Pneumonia is a frequent complication and usually develops on the paralyzed side (in this case, the right upper and lower lobes). A decrease in thoracic excursion and altered pulmonary hemodynamics are contributory factors
Nursing Diagnosis #6			
Communication impaired, related to: 1. Dysphasia and dysarthria	Patient will: • Demonstrate use of alternative means of communication (e.g., nodding the head, pointing the finger, writing on a tablet, slate board) • Demonstrate ease and comfort when groping for words	• Assess the patient's communication status: – Ask simple questions and determine patient's ability to answer – Evaluate appropriateness of the answer, and the use of words, grammar, and syntax – Evaluate the patient's understanding of the spoken word by asking the patient to follow simple instructions • Loss of the ability to communicate can be devastating. A calm, reassuring approach and supportive manner are essential • Encourage and reassure patient; anticipate needs; verbalize fears, frustrations for patient – Convey acceptance of the patient's behavior • Approach to the patient: – Encourage verbalization – Spend time with patient – Assure patient that speech will improve overtime and with rehabilitation	• Assessment identifies the skills that remain intact • Lesions of the left cerebral hemisphere frequently disturb Broca's area, resulting in an expressive aphasia • Develop a system of communication that facilitates understanding, taking into consideration the patient's deficits – Feeling unhurried may be reassuring as the patient searches for words to express herself
Nursing Diagnosis # 7			
Anxiety, related to: 1. Fear of dying. 2. Potential sequelae related to neurologic deficits	1. Patient will write out needs and concerns on a slate board or tablet 2. Demonstrate relaxed demeanor and perform relaxation techniques as condition permits	• Assess for signs/symptoms of anxiety: – Wide-eyed look, clenched fists, increased heart rate – Identify cause, if possible, and treat • Initiate interventions to reduce anxiety: stay with patient to reassure; verbalize fears/frustrations the patient may be experiencing; indicate acceptance of the patient	• Severe anxiety can aggravate the patient's overall condition. Because Mrs M. is unable to communicate verbally, her anxiety level may be especially high

Note: 'Reason' and 'Evaluation' column not including for want of space and also these may change for patient-to-patient. Users or students are required to include in their case studies

TABLE 2.9: Sample nursing care plan for the patient with spinal cord injury

Problem	Objective	Nursing interventions	Rationales
Nursing Diagnosis #1			
Ineffective breathing pattern: Alveolar hypo-ventilation, related to: 1. Altered ventilatory mechanics: hypoventilation associated with paralysis of intercostal and abdominal muscles	Patient will: 1. Demonstrate effective minute ventilation with trend of improving: – Tidal volume >7 – 10 mL/kg – Respiratory rate <25/min 2. Achieve a vital capacity of >15–25 mL/kg. 3. Verbalize ease of breathing	• Perform a comprehensive respiratory assessment: – Airway potency; rate, rhythm, depth of breathing; chest and diaphragmatic excursion; use of accessory muscles; breath sounds and presence of adventitious sounds • Assess neurologic status: mental status, level of consciousness, status of protective reflexes (cough, gag, swallowing) • Monitor serial pulmonary function tests: Tidal volume, vital capacity • Assess ability to cough and handle secretions	• Major goal of airway management is to establish/maintain adequate alveolar ventilation. – Increased rapid, shallow respirations may signal deterioration of respiratory function • Hypoxia may be reflected by changes in mental status or behavior (restlessness, irritability) • Serial monitoring enables trends to be identified in pulmonary function • Loss of intercostal and abdominal muscles compromises the patient's ability to cough effectively
Nursing Diagnosis #2			
Ineffective airway clearance, related to: 1. Ineffective cough associated with paralysis of intercostal and abdominal muscles 2. Immobility	Patient will: 1. Demonstrate a secretion-clearing cough 2. Maintain arterial blood gas values: – PaO_2 >80 mm Hg – $PaCO_2$~35 – 45 mm Hg – pH 7.35 – 7.45	• Monitor quality, quantity, color, and consistency of sputum; obtain specimen for culture/sensitivity • Implement measures to ensure adequate respiratory function: – Establish and maintain patent airway – Monitor serial arterial blood gases; establish baseline function – Initiate oxygen therapy to maintain arterial blood gases within acceptable range – Initiate measures to handle secretions; provide humidified oxygen; maintain hydration; nasotracheal suctioning only when necessary – Initiate chest physiotherapy when overall condition is stabilized: postural drainage; percussion and vibration; deep breathing and coughing exercises – Instruct in use of incentive spirometry – Use a calm, reassuring approach: anticipate needs, offer explanations, be accessible to patient/family	• Loss of protective reflexes places patient at increased risk of developing aspiration pneumonia • Airway obstruction frequently occurs with spinal cord injury or injuries involving head and neck – Hypoxemia in the spinal cord injured patient is most commonly associated with retained secretions – Suctioning increases risk of infection; suctioning-associated vagal stimulation may precipitate bradycardia in the spinal cord injured patient who may already be bradycardiac – Loosens and dislodges secretions and enhances movement of secretions toward trachea where they may be accessible to removal by coughing/suctioning – Use of incentive spirometry encourages deep breathing, reducing risk of atelectasis – Anxiety is a major problem in the spinal cord injured patient
Nursing Diagnosis # 3			
Cardiac output, alteration in: descreased, related to: 1. Loss of systemic vasomotor tone (neurogenic shock)	Patient's vital signs will stabilize: • BP > 90 mm Hg systolic (or within 10 mm Hg of baseline) • Heart rate ~ 60/min • Body temperature 98.6°F	• Assess cardiovascular function and presence of neurogenic (spinal) shock: – Blood pressure, pulse, body temperature: Skin temperature – Cardiac monitoring for dysrhythmias – Hydration status • Implement measures to stabilize cardiopulmonary function: – Initiate prescribed intravenous therapy ~75–100 mL/h	• Spinal cord injury (T4-6 and above) precipitates spinal shock with loss of sympathetic autonomic reflexes: Loss of systemic tone leads to hypotension; unopposed parasympathetic tone predisposes to bradycardia; interruption of sympathetic innervation underlies hypothermia with impaired temperature regulation

Contd...

Contd...

Problem	Objective	Nursing interventions	Rationales
		– Monitor intake and output – Initiate measures to minimize orthostatic hypotension: apply antiembolic stockings: abdominal binder – Elevate lower extremities at regular intervals	– Orthostatic hypotension results from venous stasis associated with impaired vasomotor tone and skeletal muscle paralysis
Nursing Diagnosis # 4			
Urinary climination, alternation in, related to: 1. Loss of voluntary control of micturition 2. Compromised micturition reflex	Patient will maintain: • Urine output > 30 mL/h • Weight within 5% of baseline • Balanced intake and output • Stable serum electrolytes, BUN, and creatinine • Infection-free urinary tract	• Monitor renal and hydration status: – Specific parameters to assess include body weight (daily), intake/output, serum electrolytes, BUN and creatinine, hematology profile (Hct, Hgb) – Implement straight catheterization protocol using aseptic technique noting amount, color, clarity, and specific gravity of urine – Assess for bladder distention at regular intervals and straight catheterize PRN	• Urinary retention predisposes to complications, such as urinary tract infection, and autonomic dysreflexia • Accurate intake/output and daily weight assist in determining adequacy of renal/urinary function, and fluid balance • Adequate hydration functions to prevent urinary infection and urinary calculi – Adequate renal perfusion maintains filtration and renal function: Hemoconcentration may predispose to electrolyte imbalance; increased blood viscosity may cause thromboembolic complications
Nursing Diagnosis #5			
Skin integrity, impairment of, related to: 1. Immobility 2. Sensory loss	Patient will maintain: • Intact skin with good turgor • Body weight within 5% of baseline	• Maintain skin integrity: – Assess skin carefully q2h for signs of compromised circulation especially at pressure points • Initiate therapeutic regimen: – Turn/position q2h; document rotation of positions – Maintain proper body alignment – Passive ROM exercises – Use of footboard, splints, sheepskin or air mattress, elbow/heel pads – Administer lotion to pressure points – Monitor and evaluate response to therapy • Consult with nutritionist to initiate necessary nutritional regimen	• Pressure ulcer develops when there is lack of movement and distribution of weight; pressure is most concentrated between bone and skin surfaces that support body weight • Implementation of therapeutic regimen maximizes tissue perfusion, prevents venostasis and tissue ischemia – Maintenance of proper body alignment prevents further neurologic damage – Passive ROM exercises help to maintain muscle tone and to improve circulation • Breakdown of body proteins (gluconeogenesis) impairs tissue healing and places the patient at increased risk of pressure ulcer development and infection

TABLE 2.10: Sample nursing care plan for the patient with acute head injury

Problem	Objective	Nursing interventions	Rationales
Nursing Diagnosis #1			
Alteration in cerebral perfusion pressure, related to: 1. Large, right sided acute subdural hematoma	Patient will: 1. Maintain: – Cerebral perfusion pressure > 60 mm Hg – Intracranial pressure <15 mm Hg	• Assess: Level of consciousness, mentation, respiratory rate and pattern, pupillary size and reactivity, sensorimotor function (muscle tone, deep tendon reflexes, posturing)	• Patient responses to increases in ICP can change rapidly from moment to moment; a sustained increase in ICP (>25–30 mm Hg for greater than 15–20 minutes) can compromise cerebral perfusion pressure:

Contd...

Contd...

Problem	Objective	Nursing interventions	Rationales
2. Potential cerebral edema formation	– Arterial blood pressure ~ 80 mm Hg (mean) 2. Exhibit intact level of consciousness and mentation: – Oriented to person, place – Memory intact 3. Demonstrate intact sensorimotor function: – Distinguish pinprick from crude pressure – Purposeful motor response to painful stimulus	– Assess vital signs: BP, pulse, body temperature • Maintain integrity of intracranial monitoring system: Scrupulous hand-washing and aseptic technique; monitor system for leaks, avoid drainage of CSF • Obtain/record pressure readings using appropriate procedure/protocol: – Venting port of transducer at level of foramen of Monro – Monitor waveform configuration/ digital readouts • Implement measures to prevent and/ or reduce ICP: – Maintain proper positioning; elevate head of bed; body in proper alignment – Maintain controlled hyperventilation and oxygenation; prevent accumulation of tracheobronchial secretions; use meticulous suctioning technique • Monitor response to prescribed therapy to reduce cerebral edema: – Diuretic therapy/ hyperosmolar therapy – Corticosteroid therapy – Strict intake and output – Monitor laboratory data: BUN, creatinine, electrolytes, serum osmolality, urine specific gravity	– A rise in BP, widening pulse pressure, and slow-bounding pulse are late occurring signs of increasing ICP • ICP monitoring is a highly invasive system with a high risk of infection: – Maintaining a closed system reduces risk of infection; ensures valid readings – For every inch that the measurement is off, approximately 2 mm Hg is added or subtracted from the digital readout – Monitoring trends provides essential information regarding status of ICP and intracranial compliance – Elevation of head facilitates drainage from cranium via gravity – Hypercapnia causes cerebral vasodilation, increasing intracerebral blood flow – Proper suctioning technique reduces hypoxemia – Fluid restriction coupled with pharmacologic therapy helps to reduce extracellular fluid volume; a mildly dehydrated state is maintained – Craniocerebral insults frequently predispose to diabetes insipidus ◆ Increased serum osmolality helps draw fluid from brain interstitium and reduce cerebral edema
Nursing Diagnosis # 2			
Ineffective breathing pattern, related to: 1. Expanding right-sided acute subdural hematoma with consequent brainstem compression	Patient will: 1. Demonstrate effective breathing pattern: – Respiratory rate < 25/min – Rhythm and depth eupnelc 2. Maintain adequate pulmonary function: – Tidal volume >7–10 mL/kg – Vital capacity >12–15 mL/kg	• Assess respiratory function hourly: – Spontaneous breathing: Rate/ rhythm/ depth – Monitor arterial blood gases (serially) • Implement measures to improve breathing pattern: – Maintain semi-Fowler's position – Maintain nasogastric decompression – Maintain mechanical ventilation and oxygenation: Assess tidal volume and vital capacity at bedside	• Maintenance of adequate ventilation/ oxygenation is imperative because hypercapnia and hypoxemia cause cerebral vasodilation – Allows maximal chest excursion; facilitates drainage of blood and CSF from cranium – Prevents abdominal distention, which can compromise diaphragmatic excursion
Nursing Diagnosis # 3			
Ineffective airway clearance, related to: 1. Compromised protective reflexes (e.g. gag, cough, epiglottal closure) 2. Altered state of consciousness	Patient will: 1. Maintain patent airway: – Normal breath sounds – Absence of adventitious breath sounds (e.g. crackles, wheezes)	• Assess airway patency hourly: – Status of protective reflexes (gag, cough) – Auscultate breath sounds – Assess characteristics of sputum: ◆ Color, tenaciousness, amount, odor – Assess hydration status	• Hypercapnia and hypoxemia increase cerebral blood flow – Compromised protective reflexes place patient at risk of aspiration – Presence of crackles, wheezes, and rhonchi suggests increased pulmonary secretions; or inability to mobilize or clear secretions

Contd...

Contd...

Problem	Objective	Nursing interventions	Rationales
	2. Demonstrate secretion-clearing cough (unless contraindicated by intracranial hypertension)	– Maintain hydration as prescribed ◆ Humidity oxygen administered	– Dehydration causes tracheobronchial secretions to become thick, tenacious, and difficult to clear
Nursing Diagnosis # 4			
Impaired gas exchange, related to: 1. Widespread atelectasis 2. Potential neurogenic pulmonary edema	Patient will: 1. Be alert, oriented to person/place 2. Demonstrate appropriate behavior 3. Maintain optimal arterial blood gases: – $PaCO_2$ ~ 30 mm Hg – PaO_2 > 80 mm Hg – pH ~ 7.35–7.45	• Assess cardiopulmonary function: – Heart rate, skin color – Hemodynamic parameters: Systemic arterial BP, PCWP, cardiac output – Presence of cardiac dysrhythmias • Monitor laboratory data: – Arterial blood gases: ◆ pH ◆ PaO_2, $PaCO_2$ • Calculate $AaDO_2$ • Implement oxygen therapy as prescribed • Implement positive end-expiratory pressure (PEEP) therapy as prescribed Monitor: – ABGs, mixed venous oxygen tension (SVO_2) – Lung compliance – Hemodynamic parameters (PCWP, PAP, CO) • Monitor for complications of PEEP therapy: – Reduction in venous return to the heart and cardiac output; reduction in cerebral perfusion; barotrauma	• Hemodynamic parameters reflect tissue perfusion. Evidence of cyanosis is a late sign of altered perfusion:>5 g hemoglobin are unsaturated: – Hypoxemia is associated with myocardial irritability ◆ Metabolic acidemia is associated with decreased tissue perfusion as the lack of oxygen predisposes to anaerobic metabolism with lactate production ◆ Metabolic acidemia may depress myocardial function predisposing to dysrhythmias – Most closely reflect effectiveness of gas exchange • Alveolar-arterial gradient < 250 to 300 mm Hg with an FIO_2 ~ 60% in the presence of deteriorating pulmonary function is highly suggestive of ARDS: – O_2 concentration should maintain PaO_2 > 60 mm Hg • PEEP therapy maintains airway opening pressure at end-expiration above the atmospheric pressure,thus increasing the FRC (functional residual capacity), preventing airway collapse, and enhancing gas exchange and oxygen transport – Lung compliance is determined by dividing the peak inspiratory pressure (PIP) into the tidal volume – Positive intrathoracic pressures generated reduce venous return via the great veins ◆ Overdistention and rupture of alveoli are major complications of PEEP therapy
Nursing Diagnosis#5			
Potential for injury: Seizures, related to: 1. Cerebral hypoxia associated with an increase in ICP with consequent decrease in CPP 2. Cerebral irritation associated with cerebral trauma with bleeding	Patient will: 1. Remain seizure-free 2. Maintain effective serum levels of phenytoin – Usual serum levels: ~10–20 mg/mL	• Assess characteristics of seizure activity: – Onset, influencing factors, duration – Type of movement: Tonic-clonic – Associated changes in level of consciousness, pupillary size/reactivity – Vomiting, urinary/bowel incontinence • Implement measures to prevent seizure activity:	• Seizure activity can precipitate a significant increase in ICP; it increases cellular metabolism and the oxygen demand; it raises body temperature

Contd...

Contd...

Problem	Objective	Nursing interventions	Rationales
3. Surgical manipulation of fragile brain tissue and meninges		– Avoid activities that cause a substantial sustained increase in ICP (>25–30 mm Hg/15 to 20 minutes) – Monitor for signs/symptoms of meningeal irritation: Nuchal rigidity, photophobia, persistent headache, positive Kernig's and/or Brudzinski's signs • Initiate and maintain seizure precautions: – Oral airway; padded side rails and head-board, side rails in up position, bed in low position – Administer prescribed anticonvulsant therapy – Evaluate patient's response to anticonvulsant therapy (obtain serial blood levels of phenytoin)	
Nursing Diagnosis#6			
Alteration in fluid and electrolyte balance (potential), related to: 1. Aggressive diuretic therapy and corticosteroid therapy 2. Diabetes insipidus	Patient will: 1. Maintain hemodynamic function: – Mean systolic BP ~80 to 100 mm Hg – Heart rate at patient's baseline – Regular rhythm without dysrhythmias 2. Maintain balanced intake/output: – Stable weight (unless contraindicated) – Urine output: > 30 mL, < 200 mL/h – Urine specific gravity: 1.010 to 1.025	• Assess hydration status: – Daily weight if not contraindicated by the presence of a labile ICP – Intake and output – Status of skin/mucous membranes; edema • Implement fluid replacement regimen as prescribed • Monitor for signs/symptoms of diabetes insipidus: – Presence of polyuria, polydipsia – Urine specific gravity ~ 1.005 – Presence of dehydration: poor skin turgor, sunken eyeballs • Monitor laboratory parameters: serum electrolytes, osmolality, BUN, creatinine, hematology profile	• Patients at risk of developing cerebral edema, or an increase in ICP, are maintained in a slightly dehydrated state • Diabetes insipidus may occur secondary to craniocerebral trauma, infection

TABLE 2.11: Nursing care plan for the patient receiving thrombolytic therapy: Streptokinase and tissue plasminogen activator

Problem	Objective	Nursing interventions	Rationales
Nursing Diagnosis #1			
Potential for physiologic injury: Bleeding, related to manipulation of clotting cascade	1. Patient will not have active bleeding as evidenced by: – Stable hematocrit, hemoglobin levels – Guaiac-free stools, secretions – Absence of hematoma, bruising, ecchymosis – Stable blood pressure – Stable mentation	• Perform complete assessment of patient at least every 4 hours including: – Neurologic assessment – Inspection of skin for areas of discoloration – Quality of peripheral pulses – Guaiac results of secretions, excretions – Evaluation of current laboratory values (hemoglobin, hematocrit, PTT, fibrinogen levels) • Monitor vital signs and clinical status every 15–30 minutes until stable, then every 24 hours	• Complete assessment will allow for rapid detection of any possible bleeding complications – Hemoglobin and hematocrit will determine the volume and oxygen-carrying capacity of red blood cells in the circulation. PTT will estimate the blood's ability to clot. Fibrinogen will estimate the amount of coagulation proteins available to make clots • Frequent clinical assessment will allow for rapid detection of bleeding

Contd...

Contd...

Problem	Objective	Nursing interventions	Rationales
		• Inspect insertion sites for bleeding when taking vital signs • Observe for retroperitoneal ecchymosis and severe lower back pain when taking vital signs • Observe for retroperitoneal ecchymosis and severe lower back pain when taking vital signs • Avoid patient care activities that would predispose patient to bleeding or bruising: – Shaving – Venipuncture – Vigorous toothbrushing – Aggressive patient manipulation – Use of non-invasive blood pressure cuffs • Maintain alignment of extremity involved in the procedure and place 5–10 lb sandbag over site • Coordinate blood work if venipuncture is required, or maintain large-bore IV with saline lock for blood sampling • Monitor patient's laboratory work: – Thrombin time – Prothrombin time – Partial thromboplastin time – Fibrinogen split products – Fibrinogen levels – Hematocrit • Hemoglobin • Alert all personnel that patient is anti-coagulated by placing a sign at bedside • If invasive procedures are required avoid noncompressible vessels: – Subclavian vein – Internal jugular vein	• Previous sites of clotting frequently are dissolved during administration of thrombolytic agent • Catheterization via the femoral artery predisposes patient to iliac or femoral dissection • Hemostatic mechanisms are impaired after thrombolytic therapy, preventing rapid resolution of bleeding • Movement of extremity may dislodge newly formed clots. Direct pressure promotes hemostasis • Maintenance of vascular-integrity is critical in preventing uncontrolled bleeding • All indicators of clotting will be prolonged for 6–12 hours after administration of streptokinase – Indicators of bleeding should not decrease during post-procedure period • Increased communication among health care team minimizes risk of complications • Predisposes patient to uncontrolled bleeding
Nursing Diagnosis #2			
Potential of physiologic injury: Bleeding, related to thrombolytic therapy (diminished clotting ability)	1. Patient will remain hemodynamically stable and bleeding will be controlled with minimal blood loss as evidenced by: – No change in blood pressure – No change in hemoglobin, hematocrit levels	• Hold pressure to site for at least 1/2–3/4 hour • Notify physician immediately of any bleeding • Monitor vital signs and document • Be prepared to administer blood products containing clotting factors (FFP, packed RBC, cryoprecipitate) • Administer aminocaproic acid as prescribed, and monitor response to therapy • Administer fluid and plasma expanders	• Hemostasis is prolonged due to manipulation of clotting cycle • Blood pressure will drop and heart rate increase if significant volume loss has occurred • Supplementing clotting cycle is effective in maintaining hemostasis • Aminocaproic acid is a hemostatic agent used to prevent excessive formation of plasmin. This helps to control bleeding caused by thrombolytic agents • May require volume to maintain adequate cardiac output
Nursing Diagnosis #3			
Potential alteration in comfort, related to allergic response (specific to streptokinase only)	Patient will not demonstrate discomfort related to manifestations of an allergic response (i.e. itching, musculoskeletal pain, respiratory distress, fever, anaphylaxis)	• Monitor temperature every 4 hours – Inspect skin every 30 minutes –1 hours for 6 hours, then every 4 hours – If febrile, administer medication that does not affect hemostasis (i.e. acetaminophen)	• Manifestations of allergic response will occur soon after administration of streptokinase as antigen is encountered – Aspirin may contribute to patient's inability to clot

Contd...

Contd...

Problem	Objective	Nursing interventions	Rationales
		• Monitor patient closely if signs/ symptoms of reaction occur and document • Be prepared to administer- corticosteroids, benadryl or life support measures if reaction is severe	• Patient who has recently had exposure to beta-hemolytic streptococcal proteins, will develop a severe response to the therapy
Nursing Diagnosis #4			
Potential alteration in cardiac output, related to dysrhythmias	Patient will remain hemodynamically stable as evidenced by: • Maintenance of MAP greater than 70 mm Hg • Lack of signs and symptoms of decreased cardiac output: Dizziness, nausea, shortness of breath	• Monitor patient's rhythm continuously, noting and documenting any change from baselines • Treat all dysrhythmias with standard protocols, noting patient's response • Reassure patient that this is not unexpected and signals success of the procedure	• Reperfusion dysrhythmias occur frequently after successful thrombolysis • Patients often fear that dysrhythmias mean the procedure has been unsuccessful
Nursing Diagnosis #5			
Potential alteration in tissue perfusion, related to reocclusion of coronary arteries	Patient will remain pain-free or chest pain will be alleviated, with resolution of ECG changes indicative of ischemia, infarction	• Instruct patient to notify nurse immediately at onset of chest pain; reinforce significance of time • Observe patient for nonverbal signs of discomfort • Obtain a 12-lead ECG with any patient discomfort and observe for ischemic changes – Notify physician immediately – Administer standard medications for myocardial ischemia • Prepare patient for possibility of repeat procedure, emergent IABP, or open-heart surgery • Patients may not understand the importance of communicating chest pain or are afraid to admit that the problem has not resolved	• Electrocardiographic indicators of ischemia differentiate true angina from other kinds of discomfort • It may be necessary to revascularize the myocardium by more conventional methods if reocclusion occurs: – Counterpulsation will help with coronary artery perfusion and minimize myocardial demands

TABLE 2.12: Sample care plan for the patient with pulmonary embolism

Problem	Objective	Nursing interventions	Rationales
Nursing Diagnosis #1			
Impaired gas exchange, related to: 1. Altered pulmonary blood flow 2. Ventilation/perfusion mismatching 3. Right-to-left shunting	Patient will maintain optimal arterial blood gas parameters: • pH 7.35–7.45 • PaO_2 > 80 mm Hg • $PaCO_2$ 35-45 mm Hg • HCO_3^- 22–26 mEq/L	• Assess for signs/symptoms of hypoxia, anxiety, tachypnea, dyspnea, air hunger, tachycardia, hypertension, or hypotension • Assess level of fatigue • Monitor arterial blood gas parameters	• A classic sign of a pulmonary embolism is a subtle, mild dyspnea. In the presence of pulmonary infarction associated with an embolism, sudden and severe dyspnea may reflect an underlying total or partial obstruction of pulmonary blood flow • The increased work of breathing may predispose to fatigue; fatigue may result in alveolar hypoventilation with worsening hypoxemia; and it predisposes to hypercapnia

Contd...

Contd...

Problem	Objective	Nursing interventions	Rationales
		• Administer prescribed humidified oxygen therapy – Prepare for intubation	• A metabolic acidemia is often associated with decreased tissue perfusion; the consequent anaerobic metablolism causes a rise in serum lactate levels. Arterial blood gas parameters most closely reflect effectiveness of gas exchange and pH • Oxygenation is effective in the treatment of ventilation/perfusion mismatch – Compromised ventilatory effort, ventilation/perfusion mismatch, and right-to-left shunting may compromise gas exchange sufficiently to require mechanical ventilation
Nursing Diagnosis #2			
Cardiac output, alteration in: Decreased, related to: 1. Pulmonary hypertension 2. Right sided heart failure 3. Decrease in left ventricular end diastolic pressure	Patient will maintain stable hemodynamics: • Heart rate < 100 beats/min • CVP 0–8 mm Hg • PCWP < 25 mm Hg • Cardiac output 4–8 liters/min	• Assess for signs/symptoms of right sided heart failure: Weight gain, imbalance in intake and output; hemodynamic changes—neck vein distention, tachycardia, extra heart sounds (S3 and S4); edematous lower extremities • Administer prescribed medication regimen to treat right heart failure: – Vasopressor therapy, cardiac glycosides, morphine, diuretics, and sedatives – Monitor response to drug therapy	• Pulmonary hypertension is the major hemodynamic disturbance of pulmonary embolism. Hypoxemia, acidemia, and a reduced cross-sectional area of the pulmonary capillary bed contribute to the development of pulmonary hypertension • Therapies are directed towards decreasing myocardial oxygen consumption and demand – Morphine increases systemic venous capacitance; the reduced venous return decreases the work of the heart
Nursing Diagnosis #3			
Tissue perfusion, alteration in, related to: 1. Deep venous thrombosis 2. Pulmonary embolism	Patient will remain without re-current pulmonary embolism as • Absence of pain • Stable vital signs (for patient) • Stable arterial blood gases	• Assess for signs/symptoms of venous thrombosis: Tenderness, warmth, pain, and peripheral arterial disorder – Measure circumference of each extremity at designated point daily – Assess for Homans' sign each shift • Apply antiembolic hose to both lower extremities; remove for 20 min/shift • Assist patient to perform active range of motion exercises each shift unless otherwise contraindicated • Instruct patient to avoid positions that compromise blood flow in the extremities • Encourage deep breathing hourly • Caution to avoid straining, breath-holding, or other Valsalva's maneuver	• Predominantly, pulmonary emboli arise from deep venus thrombosis: Edema in a characteristic manifestation in the presence of disruption in venous blood flow – A positive Homans' sign occurs when pain in the calf is experienced upon dorsiflexion of the foot. It is highly suggestive of venous thrombosis – Periodic removal allows filling of superficial capillaries • Exercise enhances "skeletal-muscular pump," which functions to prevent pooling of blood in the lower extremities (venostasis) and maintains venous return to the heart • Positions that compromise blood flow can cause circulatory stasis • Expands lungs and minimizes atelectasis • Such activities increase risk of dislodging thrombi

Contd...

Contd...

Problem	Objective	Nursing interventions	Rationales
Nursing Diagnosis #4			
Potential for physiologic injury, bleeding, related to anticoagulant therapy	Patient will experience an absence of bleeding: • Stable hematocrit/hemoglobin (for patient) • Stable vital signs • Absence of petechiae, ecchymosis, hematuria, occult blood in stools, or bleeding at invasive sites	• Assess closely for signs/symptoms of bleeding • Teach patient to examine self for signs of bleeding: Petechiae, easy bruising, changes in color of urine or stools • Obtain daily serum coagulation parameters (prothrombin and partial thromboplastin times); monitor closely for desired range • Monitor all invasive sites every shift • Limit puncture sites and blood drawing to only when necessary. – Use only small gauge needles when drawing blood • Teach patient to use an electric razor and to avoid vigorous toothbrushing • Maintain access to protamine sulfate for patients receiving heparin therapy	• Anticoagulant therapy is major treatment in patients with deep venous thrombosis. Major adverse effect of heparin is the risk of bleeding • An average patient may afford early recognition of subtle bleeding • Usual PT/PTT is maintained 1½–2 times the control • Puncture sites and invasive lines will not be able to clot as quickly during anticoagulant therapy. Large hematomas may occur without appropriate application of pressure post-injection and at puncture sites. It may be necessary to apply direct pressure to these sites for as long as 10 minutes followed by application of pressure dressing • Protamine sulfate is the antidote for heparin and should be readily available for administration if necessary

TABLE 2.13: Sample care plan for the patient with myocardial infarction

Problem	Objective	Nursing interventions	Rationales
Nursing Diagnosis #1			
Alteration in comfort, related to: 1. Myocardial ischemia	Patient will verbalize feeling free of pain	• Assess for presence of chest discomfort – Have patient rate discomfort on a scale of 1–10, with 10 being most severe – Notify physician of any episodes of chest pain and take appropriate actions: Obtain vital signs, get a 12-lead ECG • Minimize discrepancy between O_2 supply and demand: – Provide periods of rest – Regulate activities – Maintain a quiet environment	• Continuous assessment of patient to determine verbal and nonverbal cues of pain episodes is essential as patient may be experiencing denial of his condition – Patient may not appear to be in distress, but because he may mask signs of pain as a result of such factors as stoicism and cultural differences, pain may be severe. A scaling system is a more objective tool – Enhanced sympathoadrenal response associated with pain and anxiety may increase heart rate and oxygen demand, and may provoke myocardial ischemia • Goal in treatment is to maximize O_2 supply and minimize O_2 demand
Nursing Diagnosis #2			
Potential for anxiety, related to: 1. CCU environment 2. Newly diagnosed disease	Patient will: 1. Verbalize anxiety and/or fears 2. Demonstrate behavior suggesting decreased anxiety: Relaxed facies and demeanor 3. Heart rate 60–80 beats/minute	• Assess for verbal and nonverbal cues of anxiety – Provide patient/family with information regarding diagnosis, diagnostic procedures • Orient patient and family to CCU environment: Staff, equipment, visiting hours, when and whom to call for information about the patient's condition	• Patient may verbalize he is not feeling anxious but may be demonstrating anxious behavior – Family members can be helpful in relaxing patient but must be included when giving information regarding care • Knowing what to expect assists in coping; family may feel reassured knowing when they can visit or whom to call to get progress reports on the patient's condition

Contd...

Contd...

Problem	Objective	Nursing interventions	Rationales
	4. Blood pressure within 10 mm Hg of baseline	• Sedate as necessary, and monitor response	• Quiet rest and relaxation are essential especially during acute phase when oxygen demands need to be reduced
Nursing Diagnosis #3			
Alteration in cardiac output: Decreased, related to: 1. Dysrhythmias 2. Left ventricular dysfunction	Patient will: 1. Maintain electrophysiologic stability: – Heart rate 60–80 beats/minute – Rhythm: regular 2. Maintain hemodynamic stability: – Blood pressure within 10 mm Hg of baseline – Mental status: Alert, oriented to person, time, and place 3. Skin warm, usual color 4. Urine output greater than 30 mL/h	• Initiate continuous cardiac monitoring. – Monitor rate, rhythm • Treat serious or "warning" dysrhythmias as per unit protocol • Initiate hemodynamic pressure monitoring as prescribed/indicated: Arterial pressure, central venous pressure; PAP, PCWP, CO; should the patient's condition become complicated • Monitor for signs and symptoms of left ventricular dysfunction: Sinus tachycardia, dyspnea, orthopnea, crackles, S3 gallop, jugular venous distention; hypotension, elevated pulmonary pressures, and decreased cardiac output • Initiate treatment protocol should left ventricular dysfunction occur: – Administer vasopressors as prescribed and monitor response to therapy – Administer antidysrhythmics as prescribed and monitor response to therapy – Administer vasodilator therapy and monitor resposne to therapy	• Early detection of serious dysrhythmias allows early treatment and prevention of complications • "Warning dysrhythmias" may precipitate episodes of ventricular tachycardia and/or fibrillation • Rhythm and conduction disturbances may be associated with hemodynamic compromise, particularly in the patient with marginal left ventricular function • Myocardial ischemia and/or infarction predisposes patient to left ventricular dysfunction • Prompt treatment to reduce ischemia and decrease oxygen demand may prevent myocardial injury and necrosis and preserve left ventricular function – Dysrhythmias may reduce cardiac output and compromise coronary artery perfusion – Should left ventricular function become compromised, therapy to reduce preload and afterload may be initiated to reduce the work of the left ventricle and, thus, oxygen demand
Nursing Diagnosis #4			
Coping, potentially ineffective (individual), related to: 1. Diagnosis, and fear of dying 2. Necessary changes in lifestyle, occupation	Patient will: 1. Verbalize feelings of depression, fears about heart disease 2. Use denial as a mechanism to help control fear and anxiety, but not to interfere with ultimate acceptance of diagnosis and rehabilitation	• Assess for signs and symptoms of depression: Withdrawal, insomnia, listlessness, crying, lack of self-esteem, feelings of hopelessness, anorexia • Encourage verbalization of feelings • Assess use of denial as a defense mechanism: – Support appropriate use of denial by the patient • Monitor physiologic parameters (heart rate, blood pressure, pulse) closely during conversations that involve potentially stressful topics	• Depression may interfere with patient's ability to deal realistically with situation, and may compromise recovery • Denial is commonly used by patients who have myocardial infarctions; this mechanism can reduce overwhelming anxiety and enable the patient to progress through the acute phase without further physiologic compromise • Potentially distressful topics include pain, fear of dying, and consequences of death for family members, as well as changes in lifestyle and occupation as may be necessitated by the myocardial infarction – Such topics can cause changes in physiologic parameters and may reflect the patient's coping ability
Nursing Diagnosis #5			
Knowledge deficit regarding: 1. Coronary artery disease	Patient will have knowledge of disease: • Risk factors • Medications • Rest/exercise • Changes in lifestyle • Follow-up care	• Assess knowledge base and learning needs of patient and family – Utilize resources in patient teaching (pamphlets, video tapes, as appropriate) • Document knowledge base, teaching, and patient's response to teaching in progress notes	• Patient has a cardiac history and may have received teaching previously. Assessment of learning needs is essential at this time – Patient may not be ready for teaching while in the CCU, but the foundation for learning can begin • This facilitates continuity of care

TABLE 2.14: Nursing care plan for the patient with neoplastic-related surgery of the head and neck

Problem	Objective	Nursing interventions	Rationales
Nursing Diagnosis #1			
Alteration in breathing pattern, related to: 1. Postoperative tracheostomy	Patient will: 1. Maintain adequate respiratory function: A. Respiratory < 25/ min B. Tidal volume 5–7 mL/kg C. Arterial blood gases: ◆ pH 7.35–7.45 ◆ $PaCO_2$ 35–45 mm Hg ◆ PaO_2>60 mm Hg. 2. Maintain intact neurological function: – Mental status alert and oriented to person, place, and date	• Note preoperative respiratory status and history from records • Assess respiratory status q 4 h include auscultution of anterior and posterior chest, respirations, and arterial blood gases (as indicated) • Tracheostomy care q 4 h (as per institutional guidelines) • Encourage coughing, turning, and deep breathing q 2 h • Encourage use of incentive spirometer • Administer humidified air/oxygen • Keep head of bed elevated 30° • Assess neurological status q 4 h and PRN	• May already be compromised. • To mobilize secretions • To moisten secretions • Note physician recommendations • Changes in level of consciousness may result from decreased oxygen
Nursing Diagnosis #2			
Potential for alteration in hemodynamics and tissue perfusion, related to: 1. Manipulation of major vessels in neck intraoperatively	Patient will: 1. Maintain presurgical circulatory status – Heart rate 60–80/ minute – Rhythm: Regular sinus – Blood pressure within 10 mm Hg of baseline • Hemodynamic parameters within acceptable range (arterial pressure, pulmonary artery and pulmonary capillary wedge pressures) • Usual skin color, skin warm to touch • Brisk capillary refill	• Note preoperative circulatory status and history from records • Assess pulse and blood pressure q 4 h • Encourage range of motion to unaffected extremities q 2 h with assistance • Note color and temperature of extremities PRN and record • Observe for signs and symptoms of phlebitis every shift • Encourage early ambulation • Keep tracheostomy ties loosely applied • Avoid use of excessive dressings on neck and chest as per physician recommendations	• May have history of circulatory problem (e.g. carotid arterial insufficiency, risk of cerebral vascular accident) • Will prevent venous stasis • Will prevent decreased circulation to flaps • Improves visibility of area and facilitates assessment
Nursing Diagnosis #3			
Alteration in fluid balance, related to: 1. Surgical procedure. Patient will:	Patient will: 1. Maintain balanced intake and output, and body weight within 5% of baseline 2. Maintain stable laboratory values: – Serum osmolality 285-295 mOsm/kg – Serum electrolytes within acceptable range – Urine specific gravity: 1.010–1.025	• Assess present fluid balance • Record accurate intakes and outputs and report imbalances • Administer intravenous fluids/blood products as prescribed • Note and record color and type of drainage from drains, EG and NG tubes • Begin tube feedings when indicated	• Note estimated blood loss, in-sensible losses, urine output, intravenous infusions blood products, gastric and wound drainage. Clear fluid from drains may indicate improper placement into lymph channels

Contd...

Contd...

Problem	Objective	Nursing interventions	Rationales
Nursing Diagnosis #4			
Impaired skin integrity, related to: 1. Surgical incision 2. Poor wound healing	Patient will: 1. Not experience an infection at surgical sites 2. Have skin become/ remain intact	• Note preoperative skin integrity from history • Assess skin integrity q 4 h • Assess unaffected areas in neck and chest area for swelling and discoloration • Cleanse incisions as per institutional protocol	• May already be compromised
Nursing Diagnosis #5			
Alteration in body image, related to: 1. Surgical procedure	Patient will: 1. Verbalize feelings about body image changes 2. State ways to adapt to body alterations	• Discuss potential changes in body image preoperatively • Encourage patient to voice feelings, comments, and questions about surgery • Answer questions and reinforce information given by physician • Encourage support from family or significant others • Offer realistic hope whenever possible • Refer patient for additional professional help, when indicated	• Important to assess previous problems, adjustment difficulties, or coping mechanisms

CHAPTER

3

Common Problems of Adult Patient

STRESS AND ITS MANAGEMENT

Stress is a state produced by a change in the environment that is perceived as challenging, threatening or damaging to the persons dynamic balance or equilibrium. There is an actual or perceived imbalance in the person's ability to meet the demands of the new situation. The change or stimulus that evokes this state is the 'Stressor'. The nature of the stressor is variable, an event or change that will produce stress in one person will be neutral for another, and event that may produce at one time and place for one person may not do so for the same person at another time and place. A person appraises and copes with changing situations. The desired goal is adaptation or adjustment to the energy and ability to meet new demands. This is stress-coping process, a compensatory process with physiologic and psychologic components.

Adaptation is a constant, ongoing process that requires a change in structure, function, or behavior so that the person is better suited to the environment. The process involves an interaction between the person and the environment. The outcome depends upon the degree of fit between the skills and capacities of the person and his or her sources of social support, on the one hand and the types of challenges or stressors being confronted on the other. As such adaptation is an individual process with each individual having different levels of ability to cope and/or respond. As new challenges are met, this ability to cope and adapt can change, thereby providing the individual with a wide range of adaptation ability from which to draw. Adaptation goes on throughout the lifespan and during that process, many developmental and situational challenges will be encountered, especially in situations of health and illness. The goal of these encounters is to promote adaptation. In situations of health and illness, this goal is realized by optional wellness.

Theories/Approach to Stress

There were three different theoretical approaches which have been used to define stress in nursing.

1. Stress as response
2. Stress as stimulus
3. Stress as transaction

- The first theory conceptionalizes stress as a response to an environmental stressor. This theory was first proposed by Hans Selye (1956, 1976) who identified/defined "stress as a non-specific response of the body to any demand made upon it, regardless of its nature" Selye referred to these stress-inducing demands as 'stressor'. Stressors can be physical (e.g. noise, burns, running a marathon, infectious disease, pain, etc.) or emotional (e.g. diagnosis of cancer, promotion at work, watching a loved one die, failing an examination, financial loss, winning a beauty contest) and pleasant or unpleasant, as long as they require the individual to adopt. In response to either physical or psychologic stressors, a series of physiologic changes occur. Selye called/labeled this pattern of responses as General Adaptation Syndrome (GAS) (the detailed discussion included in this chapter).
- A second stress theory, views stress as a stimulus that causes a response. This theory originated with Holmes TH, (1967), Rahe RH and Masuda (1967, 1975) who developed a tool to assess the effects of life changes on health. Life changes are defined as conditions ranging from minor violation of law to death of a loved one. They define stress as a stimulus, or the cause of the response. In this context, stress is viewed as external to the individual. In this psychosomal model, life events are measured as predictors of illness. Stress is considered as a predisposing or precipitating factor increasing the individual vulnerability to illness. The life events that make people more vulnerable to illness and their mean values are as follows: (Holmes, Rahe 1967) (Table 3.1).

TABLE 3.1: Life event stressors and their mean value

Sl. No.	Life event stressors	Mean value
1.	Death of spouse	.. 100
2.	Divorce	.. 73
3.	Marital separation from male	.. 65
4.	Detention	.. 63
5.	Death of a close family member	.. 63
6.	Major personal injury or illness	.. 53
7.	Marriage	.. 50
8.	Being fired at work	.. 45
9.	Marital reconciliation with mate	.. 45
10.	Retirement from work	.. 45
11.	Major changes in health of a family member	.. 44
12.	Pregnancy	.. 40
13.	Sexual difficulties	.. 39
14.	Gaining a new family member (through birth, adoption, etc.)	.. 39
15.	Major business readjustment (merger, reorganization, bankruptcy)	.. 39
16.	Major changes in financial state (worse or better than early)	.. 38
17.	Death of a close friend	.. 37
18.	Changing to different line of work	.. 36
19.	Major change in number of arguments with spouse	.. 35
20.	Taking out a mortgage or loan for a major purchase	.. 31
21.	Foreclosure on a mortgage or loan	.. 30
22.	Major changes in responsibilities at work (promotions demotions, transfers)	.. 29
23.	Son or a daughter leaving from home	.. 29
24.	Trouble with in-laws	.. 29
25.	Outstanding personal achievement	.. 28
26.	Spouse beginning or ceasing work outside home	.. 26
27.	Beginning or ceasing normal schooling	.. 26
28.	Major change in living conditions (building new house, deterioration of house or neighborhood)	.. 25
29.	Revision of personal habits (dress, manners, association)	.. 24
30.	Trouble with boss	.. 23
31.	Major change in working hours or conditions	.. 20
32.	Change in residence or changing to a new school	.. 20
33.	Major change in usual type and amount of recreation	.. 19
34.	Major change in social activities	.. 17
35.	Taking out a mortgage or loan for a lesser purchase	.. 17
36.	Major changes in sleeping habit	.. 16
37.	Major changes in number of family get together and eating habits	.. 15
38.	Vacation	.. 13
39.	Christmas or any major festival	.. 12
40.	Minor violation of law (traffic tickets, disturbing peace, etc).	.. 11

The factors that affect are individual response to life events indicating the importance of using a holistic approach when assessing the patient/client.

- A third stress theory focuses on person-environment-transactions and is referred to as the "transaction or interaction" theory. In this, stress is defined as transaction. In the transactive model, there is an exchange or transaction between the person and the environment, which provides feedback to the person-environment-relationship. A proponent of this theory is Richard Lazarus, who emphasized the role of Cognitive Appraisal in assessing stressful situations and selecting coping options. Lazarus and Folkman (1984) defined "Psychologic stress" as a particular relationship between the person and the environment that is appraised by the person as taxing his or her resources and endangering his or her wellbeing.

Lazarus theory focuses on the person-environment-transactions and cognitive appraisal of demands and coping options. Appraisal is a judgment process that includes recognizing the degree of demands or stressors, placed on the individual. The appraisal process also involves the recognition of available resources or options that help when dealing with potential or actual demands.

During primary appraisal, demands are according to the possible impact on the individual wellbeing. Demands can be judged as irrelevant, benign-positive, or stressful. If demands are appraised stressful, they can be classified as representing harm or loss, threat or challenge. Harm or loss demands involve actual damage and threat demand, involve anticipated harm or loss, challenge demand differes from threat and harm or loss because they are viewed as a potential for personal gain or growth.

Secondary appraisal refers to the process of recognizing the coping resources and options that are available. Primary and secondary appraisal often occur simultaneously and interact with each other in determining stress. Cognitive reappraisal is the process of continually relabeling cognitive appraisals. Certain factors influence the labeling of appraisals. Situational factors include the intensity of the external demands, the immediacy of the expected impact and ambiguity. Person-related factors include motivational characteristics, belief systems and intellectual resources and skills.

Appraisal and coping are affected by the internal characteristics of the person. These include health and energy, as well as the person's belief system including existential belief (faith, religious beliefs, commitments or life goals (motivational properties), and the persons own sense of self including self-esteem, control and mastery. They also include knowledge, problem-solving skills and social skills which include ability to communicate and interact with others.

Physiologic Response to Stress

An understanding of the physiological changes associated with stress provide the foundation for the assessment of the client experiencing stress and the implications for health outcomes. The physiologic response to a stressor is a protective and adaptive mechanism to maintain the hemostatic balance of the body. Stressors or demands may be physical; psychologic or social. The body will respond physiologically to both actual or symbolic stressors. The complex processes by which an event is perceived as a stressor and by which the body responds is not fully understood. However, there are three interrelated systems viz. nervous system, endocrine system, immune system.

Nervous System

Neural and hormonal actions to maintain hemostatic balance are integrated by the hypothalamus. Hypothalamus is located in the center of the brain, surrounded by the limbic system and the cerebral hemispheres. It integrates autonomic nervous system mechanism, that maintains the chemical constancy of the internal environment of the body. Hypothalamus participates in both emotional and physiologic response to stressors. This control is significant because most stressors precipitate an emotional reaction. In addition to the hypothalamus, other parts of the CNS including cerebral cortex, limbic system and reticular formations are involved in the neural control of emotions and the physiologic responses to stress. The functions of these structures are closely interrelated.

Cerebral cortex: After an external event has occurred, afferent input is sent to the cerebral cortex via sensory impulses from the peripheral nervous system including the eyes and ears. In stress response, afferent impulses are carried from sensory organs (eyes, ear, nose, skin) and internal sensors (baroreceptors, chemoreceptors) to nerve centers to the brain. Afferent impulses that travel to the cortex from the periphery via the spinal cord (spinothalamic pathway) also activate the reticular formation in the area of the brainstem. The reticular formation then relays input to the thalamus and from the thalamus to the cerebral cortex. The cerebral hemispheres are concerned with cognitive functions, through processes, learning and memory (the limbic system has connection with the both cerebral hemispheres and the brainstem). The network of neurons which is involved with arousal and consciousness is called reticular activating system (RAS). The RAS functions to maintain wakefulness and alertness. The somatic, auditory and visual associative areas and the cerebral cortex receive input from the peripheral sensory fibers and then interpret it. The prefrontal area serves to reduce the speed of the associative functions so that the person has time to evaluate the information in light of the past experiences and future consequences and to plan a course of action. All these functions are involved in the perception of a stressor.

Limbic System

The limbic system, which lies in the inner mid-portion of the brain, near the base includes the septum, cingulate gyrus, amygdala, hippocampus, and anterior muscle of the thalamus. The function of the limbic system is thought to be involved with emotions and behavior. When these structures are stimulated, emotions, feelings, and behaviors can occur that ensure survival and self-preservation such as feeding, sociability and sexuality (drinking, eating, temperature control, reproduction defense and aggression).

The cerebral cortex and limbic system instruct to serve the experiential and executive functions of emotions. Endorphins are found in this system and around, reduce the perception of painful stimuli.

- Reticular formation is also located in between the lower end of the brainstem and the thalamus. It contains the RAS, which sends impulses contributing to the limbic system and to the cerebral cortex and thalamus. In addition to receiving input, from the periphery, the RAS also receives impulses from the hypothalamus, when the RAS stimulates it increases its output of impulses leading to wakefulness. Both physiologic stresses, usually increase the degree of wakefulness.
- Hypothalamus which lies just above the pituitary gland has many functions as given below:
  i. Coordinates impules:
     - Autonomic nervous system
     - Body temperature regulation
     - Food intake
     - Water balance
     - Urine formation
     - Cardiovascular function.
  ii. Secretes releasing factors—regulation of anterior and posterior pituitary hormone.
  iii. Affects behavior:
     - Emotion and alertness.

The hypothalamus receives information regarding traumatic stimuli via the spinothalamic pathway, pressure-sensitive input from the baroreceptors via brainstem, and emotional stimuli via limbic system. Because the hypothalamus secretes peptide hormones and factors that regulate the release of hormones by the anterior pituitary, it is central to the connection between the nervous and endocrine system responding to stress. In addition, the hypothalamus regulates the function of both sympathetic and parasympathetic branches of the autonomic nervous system.

Endocrine System

Once the hypothalamus activated in response to stress, the endoctrine system becomes involved. The sympathetic nervous system stimulates the adrenal medulla to release the hormones epinephrines and the sympathetic nervous system including adrenal-medulla, is referred to as sympathoadrenal response. These hormones prepare the body for the "Fight or flight response" response. This response activated by physical stressors such as hypovolemia and hypoxia, and emotional status, particularly anger, excitement and fear.

The hypothalamus released cortiocotropin releasing hormones (CRH) which stimulates the anterior pituitary to release preopiomelanocortin (POMC). Both adrenocorticotropic hormones (ACTH) and endorphin are derived from POMC. ACTH, in turn stimulates adrenal cortex to synthesize and secretes glucocorticoids, and to a lesser degree aldosterone and androgen. Glucocorticoids in particular, cortisol, are essential for the stress response. Cortisol produces a number of physiologic effects that include increasing the glucose level, potentiatory action of catecholamines on blood vessels and inhibiting inflammatory response. Aldosterone acts to increase sodium reabsorption in the kidney tubules, and as a result increases ECF. During stress, neural stimulation of the posterior pituitory results inthe secretion of ADH which also promotes water reabsorption by the distal and collecting tubules of the kidney.

Stimulation of both the adrenal medulla and cortex results in an increased blood glucose levels. This elevation provides the additional fuel for the increased metabolism needed for fighting or fleeing. The increased cardiac output, due to increased (HR and ECF) increased blood glucose level, and increased metabolic rate make the physical response possible. In addition dilatation of the skeletal muscle blood vessels and the brain provide quick movement and increased alertness.

Immune System

Negative stressors lead to alterations in immune functions in humans through processes involving the hypothalamic-pituitary adrenal axis and the autonomic nervous system that affect immune function. In return, the immune system also affects endocrine and CNS responses. Both corticosteroids and catecholamines are known to suppress immune function. Interleukin-I (which is released by activated macrophages), one type of cytokine, may directly stimulate the release of ACTH and thus initiate the stress response. Glucocorticoids depress the immune system, when these are present in high concentrations, there is a reduction in the inflammatory response to injury or infection. The steps of inflammation process is inhibited, lymphocytes are destroyed in lymphoid tissues and antibody production is decreased. As a result, the ability of the persons to resist infections is reduced.

Selye's Theory of Stress

In 1936, Selye, experimenting with animals, first described a syndrome consisting of the enlargement of the adrenal cortex, shrinkages, and thymus, spleen, lymph nodes and other lymphatic structures and the appearance of deep, bleeding ulcers in the stomach and duodenum. He identified this as a non-specific response to diverse, noxious stimuli. From this, he developed a theory of adaptation to biologic stress, which he titled The General Adaptation Syndrome (GAS).

The General Adaptation Syndrome (GAS) has three phases: Alarm, resistance, and exhaustion. Once the stressor or stimulus is integrated into CNS, multiple responses occur because of activation of the hypothalamic pituitary adrenal axis and autonomic nervous system. The nature of these responses, in which the stimulus and its effects successively cause changes in nervous, endocrine and immune systems is fundamental to understanding the physiologic and behavioral changes that occur in an individual experiencing stress.

Stage of Alarm Reaction

The first stage of the stress response is the alarm reaction of the GAS, in which the individual perceives a stressor physically or mentally and the 'Fight or Flight' response is initiated. When the stressor is of sufficient intensity to threaten the steady of state of the individual, it requires a reallocation of energy so that adaptation can occur. In this stage, the sympathetic fight or flight response is activated with release of adrenal medullary hormones and the ACTH-adrenal cortical response begins. The alarm reaction is defensive and anti-inflammatric but self-limited. This temporarily decreases the individual's resistance and may even result in disease or death, if the stress is prolonged and severe (because it is impossible to live in a continuous state of alarm).

The physical signs and symptoms of the alarm reactions are generally those of sympathetic nervous system stimulation. These signs include increased blood pressure, increased heart and respiratory rate, decreased gastrointestinal motility, pupil dilatation, and increased perspiration. The patient may complain of such symptoms as increased anxiety, nausea and anorexia.

Stage of Resistance

Since it is impossible to live in a continuous state of alarm, the person moves into the second stage, resistance. Ideally, the individual quickly moves from the alarm reaction to the stage of resistance, in which physiologic forces are mobilized to increase the resistance to stress. During this stage, adaptation to noxious stressors occurs. At this time, adaptation may occur, involving modification of the external and internal environment. Resistance is high at this time as compared with the normal state due to increased cortisol activity. The amount of resistance varies among individuals, depending on the level of physical functioning, coping abilities, and total number and intensity of stressors experienced. Although few overt physical symptoms and signs occur in this state as compared with the alarm stage, the person is expending energy in an attempt to adapt. This adaptive energy is limited by the resources of the individual.

Stage of Exhaustion

The stage of exhaustion occurs when all the energy for adaptation has expended. Exhaustion sets in and endocrine activity increases, producing deleterious effects on the body systems (especially circulatory, digestive and immune) that can lead to death. The physical symptoms of alarm reaction may briefly reappear in a final effort by the body to survive. This is exemplified by a terminally ill person who becomes alert and has stronger vital signs shortly, before death. The individual in this stage of exhaustion usually becomes ill and may die if assistance from outside sources is not available. This stage can often be reversed by external sources of adaptive energy such as medications, blood transfusion or psychotherapy. According to Selys, there is also a local adaptation syndrome (LAS). This syndrome includes inflammatory response and repair process that occur at the local site of tissue injury. The LAS occurs in small, topical injuries such as in contact dermatitis. If the local injury were severe enough, the GAS would be activated also.

Nursing Management

The client faces an array of potential stressors, or demands that can have health consequences. The nurse needs to be aware of the situations, that are likely to result in stress and also must assess the client's appraisal of the situations. The major areas that provide the nurse with useful guide in the assessment process include demands, human response to stressors and coping. It is always better to observe the following indices of stress, in which some are psychologic, some are physiologic, some behavioral, and some reflect social behavior and thought process. Some of these reactions may be coping behaviors.

- General irritability, hyperexcitation or depression
- Dryness of the throat and mouth
- Overpowering urge to cry or run and hide
- Easily fatigued, loss of interest
- Floating anxiety—do not know what or why
- Easily startled
- Stuttering or other speech difficulties
- Hypermobility, pacing, moving about, cannot sit still
- GI symptoms—butterflies in the stomach, diarrhea, vomiting
- Change in menstrual cycle
- Loss or excessive appetite
- Increased use of legally prescribed drugs, e.g. tranquilizers
- Accident proneness
- Disturbed behavior
- Pounding of the heart
- Impulsive behavior, emotional instability
- Inability to concentrate
- Feelings of unreality, weakness or dizziness
- Tension, alertness
- Nervous laughter
- Grinding of teeth
- Insomnia
- Perspiring
- Increased frequency of urination
- Muscle tension and migraine, headache
- Pain in the neck and lower back

- Increased smoking
- Alcohol and drug addiction
- Nightmares.

The probable nursing diagnosis in coping-tolerance pattern will be:

- Impaired adjustment
- Caregiver role strain
- Ineffective individual coping: Defensive coping/Ineffective denial
- Ineffective family coping; compromised
- Ineffective family coping; disabled
- Family coping: potential for growth
- Post-trauma response
- Relocation stress syndrome
- Risk for self-harm
- Risk for violence.

And plan the nursing interventions accordingly to the situation or event and stress.

Nursing Interventions in Stress Management

The first step in managing stress is to become aware of its presence. This includes identifying and expressing stressful feelings (as stated above), and the nurse has to assess the stress by keeping an eye on and having been alert for the following signs and symptoms:

- Restlessness
- Depression
- Dry mouth
- Overpowering urge to act out
- Fatigue
- Loss of interest in life activities
- Intense periods of anxiety
- Strong startle response
- Hyperactivity
- Gastrointestinal distress
- Diarrhea
- Nausea or vomiting
- Changes in menstrual cycle
- Change in appetite
- Injury-prone
- Palpitations
- Impulsive behaviors
- Emotional lability
- Concentration difficulties
- Feeling weak or dizzy
- Increased body tension
- Tremors
- Nervous habits
- Nervous laughter
- Bruxism (grinding of teeth)
- Difficulty sleeping
- Excessive perspiration
- Urinary frequency
- Headaches
- Pain in back, neck, or other parts of the body
- Increased use of tobacco
- Substance use or abuse
- Unintentional weight loss or gain.

The role of the nurse is to facilitate and enhance the coping and adaptation. Nursing interventions depend on the severity of the stress experience and demand. The nurse's efforts are directed to life-supporting interventions and to the inclusion of approaches aimed at the reduction of additional stressors to the client. The importance of cognitive appraisal in the stress experience should prompt the nurse to assess if changes in the way the client perceives and labels particular events or situations (cognitive reappraisal) are possible. So the nurse should also consider the positive effects that result from successfully meeting stressful demands. Greater emphasis should also be placed on the part of cultural values and beliefs enhancing or constraining various coping options.

An individual personal resource that aids in coping include health and energy. A health promoting lifestyle provides these resources and buffers or cushions the impact of stressors. Lifestyle or habits that contributed to the risk of developing illness can be reduced or eliminated. Health risk appraisal is an assessment method designed to promote health by examining the individual personal habits and recommending change where health risk is identified. For example, smoking, causes lung cancer and can be prevented by reducing or leaving the habit of smoking.

Coping Enhancement

It is a nursing intervention (and defined as "assisting a patient to adapt to perceived stressors, changes, or threats which interfere with meeting life demands and roles" (McCloskey, Bulechek 1992). After completing a health-risk approach, the nurse could use "Coping enhancement to assist the patient in an analysis of the appraisal and to explore methods to improve the person's coping abilities including appraisal of his or her own personal resources.

The activities of coping enhancement are as follows:

- Appraise the patient's adjustment to change in body image as indicated
- Appraise the impact of the patient's life situations on roles and relationships

- Encourage the patient to identify a realistic description of change in role
- Approve the patient's understanding of the disease process
- Approve and discuss alternative responses to situation
- Use a calm reassuring approach
- Provide an atmosphere of acceptance
- Assist patient in developing an objective appraisal of an event
- Help the client to identify the information he/she made ineterested in obtaining
- Provide factual information concerning diagnosis, treatment and processes
- Provide the patient with realistic choices about certain aspects of care
- Encourage an attitude to realistic hope as a way of dealing with feelings of helplessness
- Evaluate patients decision-making ability
- Seek to understand the patient's perspective of a stressful situation
- Discourage decision-making when patient is under severe stress
- Encourage gradual mastery of the situation
- Encourage patience in developing relationships
- Encourage relationships with persons who have common interests and goals
- Encourage social and community activities
- Encourage the acceptance of limitation of others
- Acknowledge the patient's spiritual/cultural background
- Encourage the use of spiritual resources if desired
- Explore the patient's previous achievements of success
- Explore patient's reason for self-criticism
- Confront patient's ambivalent (anger or depression) feelings
- Foster constructive outlets of anger and hostility
- Arrange situations that encourage patient's autonomy
- Assist patient in identifying positive responses from others
- Encourage the identification of specific life values
- Explore with the patient previous methods of dealing with life problems
- Introduce the patient to persons (or group) who have successfully undergone the same experience
- Support the use of appropriate defense mechanisms
- Encourage verbalization of feelings, perceptions and fears
- Discuss consequences not dealing with guilt and shame
- Encourage the patient to identify own strength and abilities
- Assist patient in identifying appropriate short and long-term goals
- Assist the patient in breaking down complex goals into manageable steps
- Assist the patient in examining available resources to meet the goal
- Reduce stimuli in the environment that could be misinterpreted as threatening
- Appraise patient's needs/desires for social support
- Assist the patient to identify available support systems
- Determine the risk of the patient's inflicting self-harm
- Encourage family involvement as appropriate
- Encourage the family verbalize feelings about ill family member
- Provide appropriate social skills training
- Assist the patient in problem-sloving in a constructive manner
- Instruct the patient on the use of relaxation techniques as needed
- Assist the patient to grieve, and work through the losses of chronic illness and/or disability if appropriate
- Assist the patient to clarify misconceptions
- Encourage the patient to evaluate his/her own behavior.

Relaxation Techniques

Synder (1993) and Egan (1993) identified relaxation technique as the major method used to relieve stress, included in nursing interventions. Commonly used techniques cited were progressive muscle relaxation, relaxation with guided imagery, and Benson's relaxation response. The goal of relaxation training is to produce response that counters the stress response.

- *Progressive muscle relaxation* involves tensing and releasing the muscles of the body in sequence and sensing the difference in feeling. It is best if the person lies on a soft cushion on the floor, in a quiet room, where he can breath easily. Self-taught or instructor-directed exercise that can involve learning to contract and relax muscles in a systematic way beginning with face and ending with feet. This exercise may be combined with breathing exercises that focus on inner-self.
- *Relaxation with guided imagery* is the 'purposeful use of imagination to achieve relaxation and/or direct attention away from undesirable sensations. The nurse helps the person to select a pleasant scene or experience from his or her past. This image serves as the mental device in this technique. As the person sits comfortably and quietly the nurse guides him to review the scene trying to feel and relieve the imagery with all of the senses. A tape recording can be made for description of science or experience the pleasant one.

Benson's Relaxation Response

Benson and Proctor (1984) describe the following steps for this response which include:

Step 1: Pick a brief phrase or word that reflects your basic belief systems.

Step 2: Choose a comfortable position.

Step 3: Close your eyes.

Step 4: Relax your muscle.

Step 5: Become aware of your breathing and start using your selected focus word.
Step 6: Maintain a passive attitude.
Step 7: Continue for a set period of time.
Step 8: Practice the technique twice a day.

The response combines meditation with relaxation.

The other techniques of stress management will also include the following:

- *Thought stopping:* It is a self-directed behavioral approach used to gain control of self-defeating thoughts. When these thoughts occur the individual stops the thought process and focuses on conscious relaxation.
- *Exercises:* Regular exercise, especially, aerobic movement, results in improved circulation, increased release of endorphins on an enhanced sense of wellbeing.
- Humor in the form of laughter, cartoons, funny movies, riddles, audiocassettes, comic books and joke books can be used for both the nurse and patient.
- *Assertive behavior:* Open honest, sharing feelings, desires and opinions in a controlled way. The individual who has control over one's own life is less subject to stress.
- *Social support:* This may take the form of organized support and self-help groups, relationships with family and friends and professional help.

In addition, meditation, breathing techniques, therapeutic touch, music therapy, biofeedback can be used as stress management technique.

PAIN AND ITS MANAGEMENT

Introduction

Pain is a complex, multidimensional phenomenon. Everyone has experienced some types or degrees of pain. Pain prompts people to seek health care more often than any other problem. Pain is one of the most common problems faced by nurses when they are dealing with the patients. And also nurses are in an excellent position to work with the client in pain and to help that client overcome the pain. For which nurse has to earn more knowledge about pain and its management. The nurse has a responsibility to understand the experience of pain and to initiate measures that provide relief or help the client learn to cope. Because, the nurse spends more time with the patient in pain than any other health care professionals and has the opportunity to help relieve pain and its harmful effects. Some of the definitions enhance the nurse's ability to assess the client who is in pain by focusing on specific aspects of the pain experience.

Pain is considered as the fifth vital sign and must be treated effectively in every patient with pain. The effective relief of pain is of great importance to the surgical team. Effective pain relief not only improves the patients feeling of comfort, it also enhances recovery and enhances earlier discharge from hospital. Effective pain management has been shown to promote earlier mobilization, adequate rest, reduced hospital stays, postoperative complications, and costs. Thus, effective pain control requires a multidisciplinary quality improvement team. This team needs to work together to develop and implement a comprehensive evidence-based program for postoperative pain management. However, the measures used for pain relief are still inadequately understood. Various studies have evaluated interventions to improve postoperative pain management and have shown inconsistent results.

Definitions of Pain

1. Pain is defined by McCaffery as "whatever the person experiencing the pain says it is, existing whenever the person says it does". It is subjective experience with no objective measurement.
2. The International Association for the Study of Pain (IASP) defined, "pain is an unpleasant sensory and emotional experience associated with actual or potential tissue damage or it is described in terms of such damage". Pain can be a major factor inhibiting the ability and willingness to recover from illness.
3. Mount Castle defined pain as "that sensory experiences evoked by stimuli that injure or threaten to destroy tissue, defined introspectively by every man as that which hurts".
4. Sternbach defined pain as: (i) An abstract concept which refers to a personal, private-sensation of hurt, (ii) A harmful stimulus that signals current or inpending tissue damage, and (iii) A pattern of responses to protect the organism from harm".

The nursing definition of pain is "whatever bodily hurt, he says it does". The cardinal rule in the care of patients with pain is that all pain is real, even if its cause is unknown.

Nature of pain

As stated earlier pain is whatever the experiencing person says it is and existing whenever the person says or does. This statement/definition makes the client the expert about his or her own pain. Because clinical pain is subjective and no objective measures of it exists, the only people who can accurately define their own pain are experiencing that pain. Although it is subjective in nature, the nurse charged with accurately assessing and helping to relieve the client's pain. To help a client gain relief, that nurse must believe that the pain exists.

Pain is a protective physiological mechanism. A person with a sprained ankle avoids bearing full weight on the foot to prevent further injury. Pain is a warning that tissue damage has occurred. The client who is unable to feel sensation, such as one with spinal cord tumor, is unaware of pain-inducing injuries. Pain is a leading cause of disability. As the average lifespan increases more people have chronic diseases in which pain is a common symptom. In additional medical advance have resulted in diagnostic and therapeutic measures that are uncomfortable. Nurses care daily for clients in pain.

Dimensions/Components of Pain

Pain consists of five components, i.e. affective, behavioral, cognitive, sensory, and physiologic. Affective component includes the emotions related to the pain. Behavioral components include the behavioral responses to the pain. Cognitive components include the beliefs, attitudes, evaluation and goals about the pain, and sensory components include the control how pain is perceived by altering transmission of nociceptive stimuli to the brain, that is, physiologic components of pain. These components are also called as dimensions of pain which help in assessment and management of pain. Pain results from complex interactions among these dimensions and can be understood by considering first the physiologic and thereafter the sensory, affective, behavioral and cognitive dimensions.

Physiology of Pain/Pain Process

Pain is a complex phenomenon. It is a mixture of physical, emotional and behavioral reactions. One way to gain the understanding the pain experience is to conceptualize pain as a process made-up of three physiological steps, i.e. reception, perception and reaction. Examining these steps of the process helps the nurse better understand the pain experience and better treat the client in pain.

(i) Reception of Pain

Reception components involves three major steps: Transduction, transmission and modulation.

Pain Transduction

The strain of events that leads to pain begins where primary afferent nociceptors (PAN) fibers are excited by a variety of stimuli. The stimuli consist of mechanical events such as stretching of organs or pressures, extremes of temperature, i.e. heat or cold, and chemical changes such as ischemia. Specific fibers that react to these stimuli are classified as mechanical, thermal or chemical nociceptors. Fast pain is usually elicited by mechanical and thermal type of receptors (A-delta fibers) whereas slow pain can be elicited by all receptors (C-fibers). Together these fibers referred to as primary afferent nociceptors-primary afferent nociceptors fibers (Fig. 3.1).

Fast pain: It is the pain that occurs in about 0.1 second when painful stimuli are applied. It is often referred to as sharp, prickling, acute or electric pain. It is transmitted through a A-delta fibers. Fast pain is mostly caused by a more superficial stimulus.

Slow pain: It is pain that begins one second or more after stimulation and increases slowly over seconds or minutes.

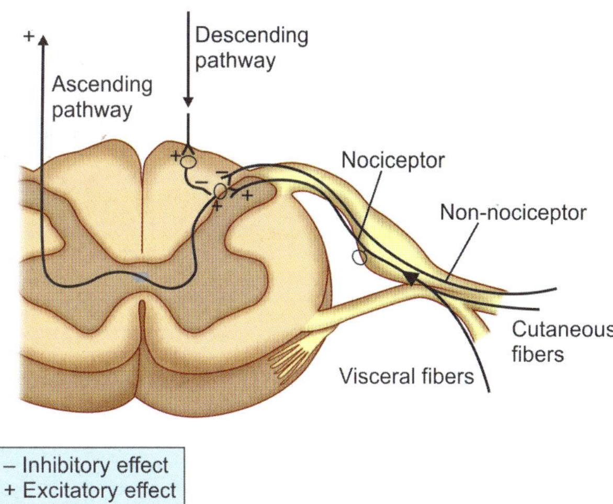

FIG. 3.1: Representative nociception system, showing ascending and descending sensory pathways of the dorsal horn

This pain is also known as burning, aching, throbbing or chronic pain. It is often associated with tissue distraction and is felt in both superficial and deep tissues. It is transmitted through the more primitive type of fibers. A wide variety of chemical substances, including bradykinin, serotinin, histamine, substances of potassium, iron, acids, proteolytic enzymes, prostaglandins, and acetylcholine are significants in slow pain that often follows tissue injury.

Pain Transmission

Once the PAN (primary afferent nociceptors) are stimulated, the impulse they discharge travel as electrical activity to the spinal cord and on to the brain. This electrical activity becomes the experience of pain when it reached the brain. There will be no experience of pain, when/if the neural pathway for these impulses is blocked by surgical cutting or medications which inhibit the activity of pathways fibers or natural methods (endogenous) that block portion/the pain pathways.

Nerve fibers that carry somatosensory information from the body periphery to the spinal cord include A-beta, A-delta, and C fibers. A-type fibers have a myelin sheath that speeds up information transmission. A-delta fibers, transmit pain stimuli, A-beta fibers are larger and carry other sensory information such as touch. C-fibers transmit pain stimuli more slowly because they have no myelin sheath. C-fibers also conduct thermal, chemical and strong mechanical impulses. Pain sensation following stimulation of A-delta fibers differ from that following C-fiber stimulation. A-delta fiber activity is felt more slowly after painful stimulation but the sensation is more constant and continuous. It is persistent, dull and acting and is difficult to localize. These different fibers enter the dorsal root of the spinal cord, which transmits the pain impulses. The fibers separate as they enter the cord and then reform in the dorsal horn. This area receives, transmits and processes sensory

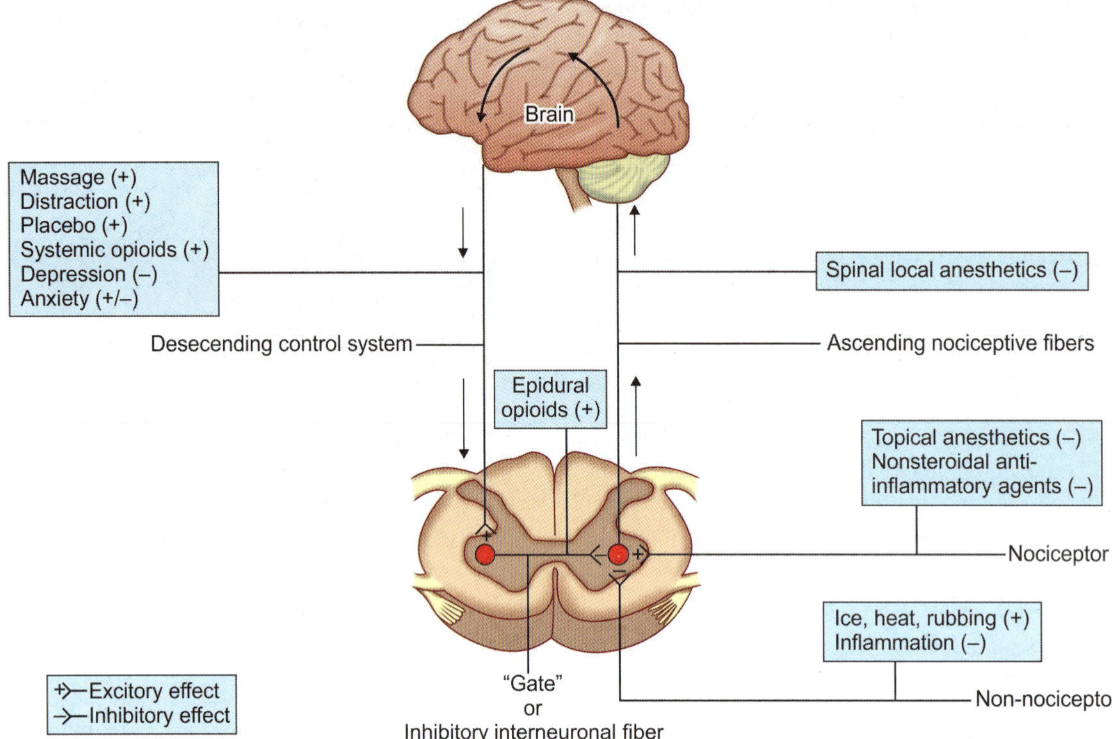

FIG. 3.2: A schematic representation of the gate control system and aspects of the nociceptive system. The nervous system is made up of stimulatory and inhibitory fibers. For example, stimulation of the nociceptor results in the transmission of an impulse that will be interpreted as pain. When it is stimulated, it will stimulate transmission at the next fiber junction (represented as +>–). The interneuronal fiber is an inhibitory neuron (–>–). When it is stimulated, it in turn, inhibits or shuts off transmission at the next junction. So a placebo has a (+) stimulatory effect on the descending control system, which has a stimulatory effect (+) on the interneuronal fiber (–) on the ascending control system. A topical anesthetic has an inhibitory effect (–) on nerve transmission at the nociceptor level, and a spinal anesthetic has the same impact (–) on the ascending nociceptive fibers

impulses. The afferent nociceptors end at the level of the first, second and fifth laminae. The substation gelatinosa is found in the second laminae hypothized to be gating mechanism (Gate control theory) (Fig. 3.2).

Gate control theory: A pain proposed by Melzack and Wall (1965) suggests that pain impulse can be regulated or even blocked by gating mechanisms along with central nervous system. The proposed location of the gates is in the dorsal horn of the spinal cord. Further findings suggested other gates exist (Melzact, denis 1978). When gates are open, pain impulses flow freely. When gates are closed, pain impulses become blocked. Partial opening of the gates may also occur. Small fibers carry most potentially painful impulses. Excitation of C-fibers inhibits gating mechanisms so that pain stimuli flow easily to cortical controls of brain. Large A-fibers pass through the same gating mechanisms. Whether the gates remain open or closed depend on whether competing passages from larger nerve fibers stimulate the gating mechanism. A bombardment of a large fiber sensory impulses such as those from the pressure of the back sub or heat of a warm compress closes the gates to PAN stimuli. Transmission of pain impulses from the spinal cord to the cerebral cortex can be inhibited or facilitated thus altering perception. This gate control theory gives the nurse a conceptual basis for pain relief measures to some extent.

Pain Modulation

There is a great deal of variations in the way clients perceive similarly painful stimuli. The pain modulation system is one reason, thus occurrence of variance. There are variety of mechanisms that contribute modulation are as follows:

Modulation via the dorsal horn: The dorsal horn was once considered a simple relay for impulses, but is now known to contain extremely complex circulatory and multiple biochemical agents that both transmit and modulate nociceptive input. The dorsal horn is now thought to modulate the nociceptive impulses rather than simply receive and transmit these impulses. A high degree of processing of the sensory impulses occurs at this level.

Modulation via descending pathways: The descending serotoninergic inhibitory fibers originate in the periaqueductal gray matter (PAG) of the midbrain and descend downward into the nuclear raphe magnus. Neurons from the PAG project downward into the dorsal horn at the first and fifty lamae levels. The neurotransmitters serotonin and substance P are released into these areas, contributing modulation of pain.

Modulation via endogenous chemicals: Some chemical compounds release by injury or inflammation stimulate nociceptors, for example, histamine, bradykinin, serotonin, substance P and prostaglandin E. Pain may be reduced by medication that block these agents such as steroids, aspirin and other non-steroidal anti-inflammatory drugs (NSAIDs) that reduce inflammation and block prostaglandins. There is also a naturally occurring system within the nervous system called the "analgesia systems".

This analgesia system described by Guyton and Hall has three parts: (i) neurons from the periductal gray area of the mesencephalon and upper pons surrounding the adequate of Sylvius send their signals to (ii) the raphe magnus nucleus, a thin midline nucleous located in the lower pons and upper medulla where the signals are sent down the dorsolateral columns in the spinal cord to (iii) a pain inhibitory complex located in the dorsal horns of the spinal cord. At this point in the system, pain can be blocked.

(ii) Perception of Pain

Pain perception refers to interpretation of the next phase of the pain process. Once the nociceptive input has been received and transmitted, it must be perceived or interpreted. Because every individual perceives and interprets pain based on his or her individual experience, this one point at which pain becomes different for each person. Pain modulation occurs as it is being transmitted. For example, other sensory input will help reduce, the amount of nociceptive information that is transmitting supraspinally.

Pain perception does not depend solely on the degree of physical damage. It is generally agreed both physical stimuli and psychosocial factors influence a person's experience of pain. Although there is little consensus on the specific effects of these factors, it is known that anxiety, experience, attention, expectation and measuring of the situation in which injury occurs affect pain perception. Brain activities such as distraction or anxiety may also affect the severity and quality of the pain experience.

In the past, pain was viewed as a primary sensation and motivational and cognitive processes were believed to influence only our reaction to pain, it now seems apparent that there are mechanisms within the body that can modify pain-related neural impulses even before they are transmitted to the brain. Thus, pain is likely to be determined by a relative balance between the sensory peripheral input and mechanisms of central control (brain) input to gating mechanisms in the spinal cord.

The first point the nurse needs to consider, is the client's pain threshold. This is defined as the lowest intensity of a painful stimulus that is perceived by the client as pain. The pain threshold may vary based on physiologic factors such as inflammation or injury near pain receptors, but essentially it is similar for all people if the central and peripheral nervous system are intact. The second part of pain pertains to the individuals tolerance of pain. Tolerance is different for each person who experiences pain. This may vary within each person based on many subjective factors, such as meaning of pain and the setting. It really refers to the amount of pain the client willing to endure. Some individuals have high tolerance, that is, they can tolerate a lot of pain without distress, whereas others have a very low tolerance. This tolerance will also vary for a given individual depending on a variety of factors that influence pain such as nausea, fatigue and other sensory input. Only the client, not the health care team, can tell the tolerance level. The nurse must remember that pain tolerance can vary from situation to situation or from event to event.

Another aspect that will alter a person's perception of pain is his or her experience with pain. This may be the reason that people incorrectly assume that infants do not have pain. When infants feel pain, it is simply that the infant has no experience with pain and therefore, is unable to interpret it, and cannot communicate what is being felt. The reverse is also true. When a person has a bad experience with pain, the anticipation that future pain may be bad can make any work. There is also a physiologic reason if the pain is in the same area, that is persons with recurrent low back pain actually have a lower pain threshold and that area than persons who have not had low back pain.

(iii) Reaction to Pain

The reaction to pain is the physiological and behavioral responses that occur after pain is perceived. In physiological responses; as pain impulses ascend the spinal cord towards the brain system and thalamus, the automatic nervous system becomes stimulated as part of the stress response. Pain of low to moderate intensity and superficial pain elicits the flight or flight reaction of the general adaptation syndrome. Stimulation of the sympathetic branch of the autonomic nervous system results in physiological responses. If the pain is unrelenting, reverse or deep, typically originating from involvement of the visceral organs (such as with myocardial infarction, and colic from gallbladder or renal stones). The parasympathetic nervous system goes into action. Sustained physiological responses to pain could cause serious harm to an individual. Except in case of severe traumatic pain, which may send a person into shock, most people reach a level of adaptation in which physical signs return to normal. Thus, a client in pain will not always exhibit physical signs.

The behavioral responses of pain may be described in three phases of a pain experience which include anticipation, sensation and aftermath (Mein Hart and McCaffery 1983). Usually anticipation phases occur before pain received except some unforseen painful situations. Anticipation of pain often allows a person to learn about pain and its relief. With adequate instruction and support, client learn to understand pain and control anxiety before it occurs. Nurses play an important role in helping clients during the anticipatory phases with proper guidance, which help clients make aware of unknown and they cope with their discomfort. Sensation of pain occur when pain is felt. The ways that people choose to react to discomfort vary widely. A person's tolerance of pain is the point at which there is an unwillingness to accept pain of greater severity, or duration. The extent to which a person tolerates pain depends on attitudes, motivation and value. Pain threatens physical and psychological well-being. Typical body movements and facial expressions that indicate pain include holding the painful part, bent posture and grimaces. A client may cry moan. Often the client expresses discomfort through restlessness and frequent requests to the nurse. The nurse soon learns to recognize patterns of behavior that reflect pain. Aftermath phase of pain occurs when it is reduced or stopped. Even though the source of discomfort is controlled, a client may still require the nurse's attention. Pain is a crisis. After painful experience client may experience physical symptoms such as chills, nausea, vomiting, anger or depression. If there are repeat episodes of pain, aftermath responses can become serious health problems. The nurse helps clients gain control and self-esteem to minimize fear over potential pain experience.

The individual reaction to pain adds even more variation to the pain process. There are many variable factors in this part of the process, including situation, culture, age, sex, cause of pain, tolerance, value and meaning of pain and various psychological factors such as fear, anxiety and depression.

Factors Influencing Pain

Situation

The situation associated with the pain influence the person's response to it. A person's responses to pain experienced in a formal crowded situations may differ greately from the responses were he or she alone or in a hospital.

Culture

Culture influences how people learn to react to express pain. People respond to pain in different ways. The nurse must neve assume to know how clients will respond. However, an understanding of cultural background, socioeconomic status, and personal attitudes help the nurse more accurately assess pain and its meaning for clients. A young girl in a stoic culture may be allowed to cry because of pain whereas boys are not allowed to cry in some culture.

Age

Age is an important variable that influences pain, particularly in children and older adults. Age may release a client from culturally imposed norms in relation to pain expression. Developmental differences found among these age groups can influence how children and older react to the pain experience. Young children have difficulty in understanding pain and the procedures nurses administer that may cause pain. Young children who have not developed vocabularies also have difficulty verbally describing an expressing pain to parents/caregivers. Cognitively toddlers are unable to recall explanations about pain or associate pain as experiences that can occur in various situation. Older people may assign different meanings to that pain. Pain is often thought by the elderly as natural manifestation of aging.

Sex

Gender may be an important influence in pain. In most cultures boys are expected to show less expression of pain than girls. As they grow older men are also expected to express pain less than that of women.

Meaning of Pain

The meaning of a person's pain is a factor that influences his or her responses to pain. A person will perceive pain differently if it suggests a threat, loss, punishment, or challenges. For example a woman in labor perceives pain differently from a woman expressing pain from a recent back injury or pain caused by childbirth. If the cause is unknown, more negative psychological factors use such as fear, anxiety, etc. Come into play and the pain may be misinterpreted resulting in an inappropriate response. A client copes differently with pain, depending on its meaning.

Anxiety

The degree of anxiety the client is experiencing also may influence the client's response to pain. It is not possible to separate the mind from the body, so pain, always, has both physiologic and psychological components. When anxiety is high, pain is felt greater. Emotionally healthy persons are usually able to tolerate moderate or even severe pain than those whose emotions are less stable.

Fatigue

Fatigue heightens perceptions of pain. This intensifies pain and decreases coping abilities. Pain is often experienced less after a restful sleep than at the end of a long day.

Attention

The degree to which a client focuses on pain can influence pain perception. Increased attention has been associated with increased pain, whereas distraction has been associated with a diminished pain response. This concept is one that nurses apply in various pain relief measures such as relaxation, guided emergency and massage.

Previous Experience

Each person learns from painful experiences. Previous experience does not necessarily mean that a person will accept pain more easily in the future. If a person has had frequent episodes of pain without relief or bouts of severe pain, anxiety or even fear may occur. In contrast if a person had repeated experience of pain, may be better prepared to tolerate or take necessary actions to relieve pain to some extent.

Coping Style

The experience of pain can be lonely, when client experiences pain in health care setting such as hospitals, the loneliness can be unbearable. Frequently, client feels a loss of central pain and an inability to control their environments or the outcome of event's coping style thus influences the ability to deal with pain.

Family and Social Support

Parents and attitudes of significant others also affect pain response. People in pain often depend on family members for support, assistance or protection. An absence of family members or friends can often make the pain more stressful. For children, presence of parents is very essential.

Types of Pain

There are different ways to define types of pain, which include according to onset, duration, severity, modes of transmission, location, causation and causative force. The examples of which are as follows:

- Onset or time of occurrence, e.g. postoperative pain
- Duration, e.g. chronic pain or acute pain
- Severity or intensity, e.g. severe, mild or scored (0 to 10 on a scale)
- Location or source, e.g. superficial, deep or central pain
- Causation, e.g. pain due to receptor stimulation or nerve damage, or psychophysiologic pain
- Causative force or agent, e.g. spontaneous, self-inflicted or other pain.

The common terms used to classify pain are as follows:

Acute Pain

Acute pain is usually of recent onset and is most commonly associated with a specific injury. It is time limited and generally has a defined cause and purpose. It may be mild, moderate or severe in nature and is usually sudden in onset. It occurs abruptly after an injury or disease, persists until healing occurs, and often intensified by anxiety or fear. Acute pain consistently, increasing during wound care, ambulation, coughing and deep breathing. It is described in sensory terms such as sharp, stabbing and shooting. Acute pain indicates that damage or injury has occurred. It draws the attention to the fact that it is occurring and teaches us to avoid similar potentially painful situation. So acute pain is seen as a useful and limiting pain in that indicates injury and motivates the person to get relief by treatment of the pain and usually the cause. Acute pain is usually reversible or controllable with adequate treatment. If no lasting damage occurs or systematic disease exists, acute pain usually decreases as healing occurs; this generally occurs in less than 6 months and usually less than 1 month. Acute pain can be described as lasting from a few second to 6 months, e.g. prick of finger in a second and fracture for 6 months.

Usually the acute pain leads to discomfort, uncomfortable and disturbs the individual in many aspects according to the nature and extent of pain. An unrelieved acute pain can affect the pulmonary, cardiovascular, gastrointestinal, endocrine and immunologic system. It leads to autonomic response that is considered with sympathetic stress response. The significant negative effects are increased heart rate, increased stroke volume, increased blood pressure, increased pupillary dilation, increased muscle tension, decreased gastrointestinal motility, decreased salivary flow (dry mouth). The stress response may increase the patient risk for physiologic disorder (MI, pulmonary infection, thromboembolism, prolonged paralytic ileus) and the psychological disorders which include anxiety and persists. If acute pain is not effectively managed, it may progress to a chronic pain.

Chronic Pain

Chronic pain is a complex physiological and psychological phenomenon that causes varying degrees of disability in a large portion of the population. Chronic pain is constant or intermittent in nature that persists over a period of time. It lasts beyond the expected time and often cannot be attributed to a specific cause or injury. Chronic pain is often defined as pain that lasts for 6 months or more. It may begin as acute pain but it persists over an extended period of time. The pain may be mild, moderate or severe and may be intermittent or continuous.

Chronic pain is classified as malignant or nonmalignant.

Nonmalignant Pain

Chronic pain is usually considered pain that lasts more than 6 months or 1 month beyond the normal end of the condition causing pain and has no forcible and except very slow healing, as with burns, or death. It is continuous or persistent and recurrent. Chronic pain may have an identifiable cause although the cause may be difficult to determine; and is often described using effective terms, such as 'hateful' or 'sickening', and is often much more difficult to treat than acute pain. It is considered useless pain because it is not usually a manifestation of impending damage. For example, severe rheumatic arthritic chronic pain is often frustrating and difficult for a person to live with. It gives no clues about how to lessen it. Clients experiencing continuous and continually recurring chronic pain often become increasingly engrossed by their illness. They may seem fearful, tense, fatigued and depressed. Many persons with an unending chronic pain become withdrawn and isolated. Their pain often exhausts them and their families, physically and emotionally.

Malignant Pain

Malignant pain is considered to have qualities of both acute and chronic pain. It can be of different types. An individual's mental response to pain depends on the duration and possibility and the intensity of the pain. Pain that is constant, continuous and moderate is often described by the client (patient as far more difficult to bear that pain than paroxysmal and intense). The duration of chronic pain includes months and years of pain, not minutes or hours. It is associated withdrawal and despair. Anxiety may give way to depression. Some chronic pain patients/clients learn to adapt and cope with the pain, adjusting their lives.

The sympathetic arousal that may be associated with acute pain diminishes over weeks or months even though the pain itself persists. Sympathetic adaptation occurs over time. The nurse must remember, however, that the absence of expected expression of severe pain does not mean, that the pain is gone. The nurse must depend on the client's description, the manifestations are not expected to find in the clients. Most clients have major effective and behavioral changes when experiencing pain for prolonged period. Such changes may be compounded and chronic pain syndrome can develop. The following are the characteristics of chronic pain syndrome:

- Depressed mood
- Increased or decreased appetite and weight, decreased libido capacity, poor physical tone and increased depression
- Social withdrawal—withdrawal from outside interests and relationship
- Preoccupation with physical manifestation
- Poor sleep and chronic fatigue, leads to inactivity, analgesics, depression.

For example, in cases of cancer pain, arthritis, trigeminal neuralgia, etc. Some clients with chronic pain may not exhibit any of the above mentioned manifestations or they may exhibit only a few. However, once these changes take place, they may become more significant to treatment than the pain's original physical source. Unfortunately, psychosocial implications about pain sometimes reinforce the idea that clients may make too much fuse over that pain.

Superficial Pain

Superficial pain occurs when the receptors in surface tissues are stimulated. Superficial or cutaneous pain is classified into two types:

i. Pain with an abrupt onset and a sharp or stinging quality, and
ii. Pain with a slower onset and burning quality.

Superficial pain may be delineated by having the client point to the painful area. It may occur along each segment representing a portion of the body surface innervated by one dorsal root, a dermatome or skin segment in an area of skin supplied by one dorsal root. Each spinal nerve has dorsal and sensory root. The boundaries of dermatome may appear to be distinct in anatomic drawings, but nerve distribution actually overlaps. Irritation of one posterior root produces pain in adjacent dermatomes. A spinal nerve attaches the spinal cord with two roots anterior and posterior. The anterior root contains efferent nerve fibers that carry impulses from the CNS to the periphery of the body. The posterior root contains afferent nerve fibers that carry impulses from the body's periphery towards CNS. Cutaneous pain is relatively uncomplicated because it is readily localized, that is, which client can indicate exactly where it hurts.

Deep Pain

Deep pain arises from deeper tissues. Deep pain is divided automatically into splanchnic which refers to pain in the viscera and deep somatic refering to pain in deep structures other than the viscera, such as muscle, tendons, joints and periosteum.

Splanchnic Pain

Viscera refers to abdominal viscera. Actually, a viscus (plural viscera) in any of the large interior body organs occupies any body cavity such as the cranial, thoracic, abdominal or pelvic cavities. Visceral pain tends to be diffuse, poorly localized, vague, dull pain. Nerve fibers innervating body organs follows the sympathetic nerves to the spinal cord. This may be the reason why autonomic manifestations (e.g. diarrhea, cramps, sweating, hypertension) frequently accompany visceral pain. Typical visceral pain includes acute appendicitis, cholecystitis, inflammation of the biliary and pancreatic tract, gastroduodenal disease, cardiovascular disease, pleurisy and renal and ureteral colic. Visceral pain is transmitted through the sympathetic and parasympathetic fibers of autonomous nervous system, with the pain being referred to the body surface, often in sites at a distance. Visceral pain also may be sent through the nerve fibers in the parietal pleura, pericardium, or peritoneum and is called parietal pain. Parietal pain is transmitted directly to the spinal nerves, with the pain being felt directly over the painful area. Parietal tissue is well supplied with spinal nerve instead of sympathetic nerves. Pain starting in the parietal tissue is often very sharp.

Deep Somatic Pain

Somatic structures are those of the body wall, such as muscles and bones. Pain in the somatic structures is complicated phenomenon. The main difference between superficial pain and deep pain is difference between cutaneous and deep sensitivity (i.e. the capacity to receive stimulus and respond to them is the difference in nature) of the pain evoked by noxious or harmful stimuli. For example, unlike cutaneous pain, deep pain is poorly localized, may produce nausea, and is frequently associated with sweating and changes in the blood pressure. Deep somatic pain is generally diffuse, less localizable than cutaneous pain. This is because the area supplied by one posterior nerve root (sclerotome) is less well defined than in dermatome and does not correspond with a dermal segment. Also pain from deep structures frequently radiates/spreads from primary site, e.g. pain from lumbar disc is felt along the sciatic nerve.

Somatic structures vary in their sensitivity to pain. Highly sensitive structures include tendons, deep fascia, ligaments, joints, bone periosteum, blood vessels and nerve. Skeletal muscle is sensitive only in stretching and ischemia. Bone and cartilage respond to extreme pressure and chemical stimulation, for example, Rh arthritis, osteomyelitis.

Localized Pain

Localized pain arises directly from the site of the disturbance.

Referred Pain

Referred pain is one which is felt in a part of the body which is remote from the actual point of stimulation. The impulses usually arise in an organ, but the pain is projected to a surface area of the body. Both visceral and somatic pains are usually referred to as segment of skin because visceral fibrosynapse at the level of the spinal cord close to fibers innervating some subcutaneous tissue. A classifical example of referred pain is that associated with 'angina pectoris,' the pain originates in the heart muscle as a result of ischemia, but it may be experienced in the midsternal region, the base of the neck and down the left arm. Similarly, in myocardial infarction, pain is not felt in the heart, but it is felt at left arm shoulder or jaw pain. It may be due to the fibers innervating these areas are close to those innervating the myocardium resulting in the referred pain. Similarly, in pain of appendicitis is often reported by the patient as being in the midline of the abdomen, above the umbilicus whilst the appendix is usually located deep in the abdomen, close by the appendix, on the right side.

Identification of the segment of the spinal cord that is involved, is transmitting referred pain is diagnostically helpful. Pain arising from a deep structure, whether a deep somatic structure or a viscus has a referred segmental distribution or a pattern of pain, determined according to the spinal cord segment supplying to this structure. The sites of referred pain have been shown in Figure 3.3

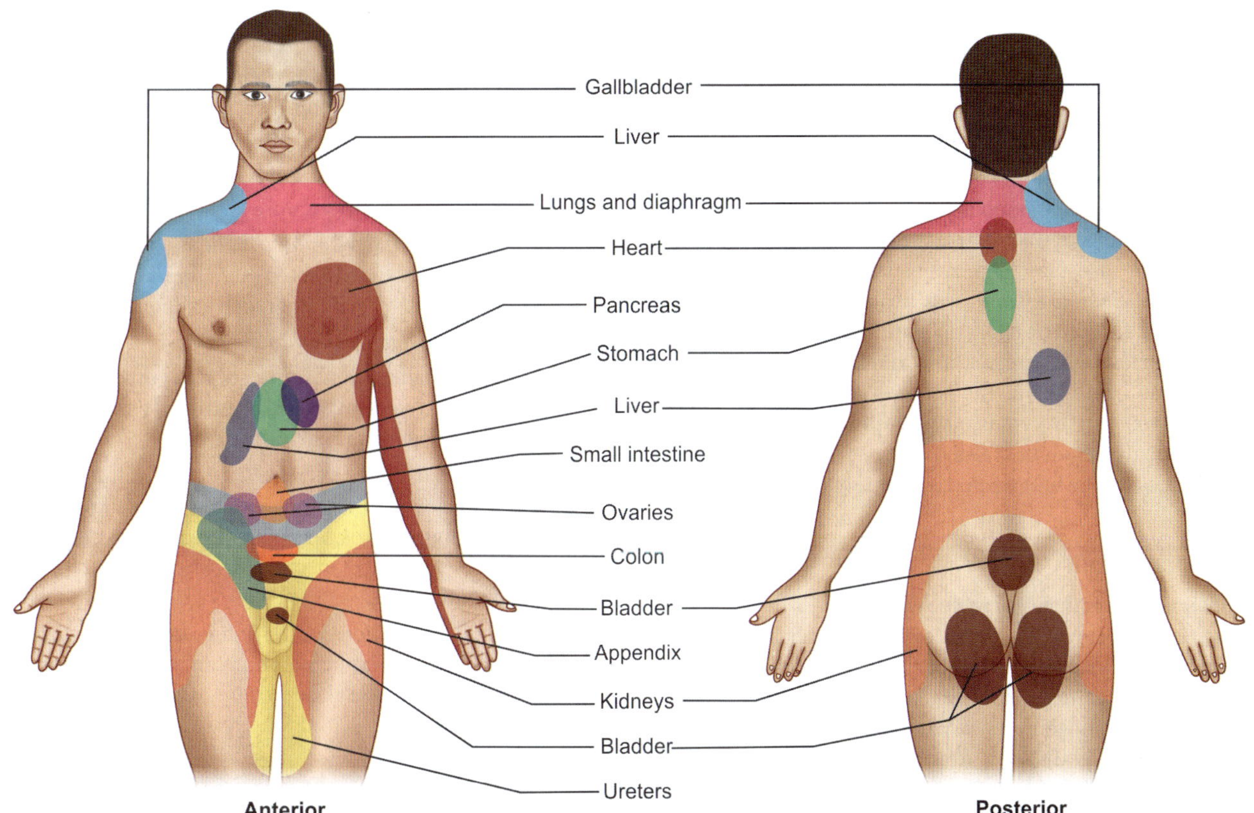

FIG. 3.3: Sites of referred pain

Intractable Pain

Persistent, severe pain that cannot be effectively controlled by the usual medication is referred to as "intractable pain". Intractable chronic pain states, producing prolonged and intense bombardment of the central nervous system are very difficult to bear. The client may become suicidal or at least take no steps to prolong life.

Headache

Headache is the most common type of pain, frequently discomfort experienced by many people, and applies to the pain sensation that is perceived as being in the cranial vault (excluding facial pain, toothache and earache). There are many causes of headache involving both intracranial and extracranial structures. The brain itself is almost insensitive to pain, although the venous sinuses, tentorium, dura, some of the cranial nerves and associated vasculature are pain sensitive. One of the most sensitive areas in the brain is middle meningeal artery. Changes in intracranial pressure, either decrease or increase, may lead to headache, because the pressure changes cause the pain sensitive structures in the head to shift.

There are many types of headache of intracranial origin. Vascular headache is common type of intracranial headache. This headache can be caused by a variety of problems such as: hypertension, sepsis, hypoxia, and various medications. Other causes of intracranial headache include infection, hemorrhage, and changes in intracranial structures. Migraine is also a type of headache of intracranial origin but cause is unknown.

There are many types of headaches of extracranial original which are common and have many causes. Many extracranial structures are sensitive to nociceptive stimuli. These structures include the skin, subcutaneous tissues, muscles, arteries and periosteum of the skull. Problem in the eyes, sinuses, ears, teeth, nose, and jaws also may lead to headache. The mechanisms of these headaches are similar to headaches of intracranial origin. Stimuli such as: traction, distention, dilation and spasms of vessels, irritation of nerves and inflammation of various structures can cause them. The common types of extracranial headache are muscle tension, temporomandibular joint syndrome, ocular sinus, dental and otic.

Headaches can be best treated by first identifying the cause.

Psychogenic Pain

Psychogenic pain is that experience when there is no detectable organic lesion. However, pathology may still be present. Psychogenic pain refers to pain that believed primarily due to emotional factor rather than physiologic dysfunctions. Clients experiencing psychogenic pain have a real pain experience. Psychogenic pain is different from pretended pain. Although psychogenic pain starts without a physical basis, repeated severe stress probably alters the complex physiology of pain transmission, modulation, and perception. The pain the client feels is real to that client and the tension and/or stress the client is feeling may lead to pronounced physiologic changes. When the psychogenic effect of stress, anxiety, fear and anger produces painful alteration in physiology, these can be called "psychophysiologic pain". Psychogenic pain requires that the cause may be found and treated.

Factors Affecting Pain Control

1. *Implementation of pain guidelines:* This method utilizes a group of different interventions provided to the patients using specific pain control guidelines.
2. *Type of surgery:* Some surgeries are more extensive and may cause more pain than other minor surgeries. Thoracic and upper abdominal operations are associated with the most severe pain.
3. *Effect of anesthesia:* Patients may feel less pain in the immediate postoperative period due to the effect anesthesia. However, as the effect anesthesia reduces, the patient may start experiencing more pain.
4. *Preoperative teaching:* Patients who receive good preoperative preparation and instructions on pain expectation and ways to control pain will feel lesser pain than who are suddenly encountered with the painful postoperative period. Appropriate preoperative education can improve expectations, compliance and ability to effectively interact with pain management techniques. Preparing patients in order to understand their responsibilities in pain management is important.
5. *Age of the patient:* Elderly patients request smaller doses of analgesia.
6. *Sex:* Females may report more pain than the males.
7. *Preoperative analgesic use:* Patients who are put on analgesia immediately after the surgery may have lesser pain than those who do not receive adequate analgesia.
8. *Past history of poor pain management.*
9. *Coexisting medical conditions* such as substance abuse or withdrawal, hyperthyroidism, anxiety disorder, affective disorder, hepatic or renal impairments.
10. *Cultural factors and personality:* Some cultures consider pain as a part of life and considers people crying due to pain as a sign of weakness. People from such cultures may report lesser pain than cultures where pain reporting is considered a right.
11. *Individual variation in response and pain threshold:* Patients varies from being intolerant of any discomfort to surprising self-control or patients consider pain to be a normal part of life.
12. *Attitude of the ward staff:* Cooperative and courteous staff tend to induce more satisfaction in pain control methods. Patients are more receptive for pain management techniques from nurses who talk softly and empathetically.

The aims of effective postoperative pain management are to:

- Improve the comfort and satisfaction of the patient
- Facilitate recovery and functional ability
- Reduce morbidity
- Promote rapid discharge from hospital.

JCAHO Pain Management Standards

1. Recognizes patient's right to pain management.
2. Requires regular pain assessment with follow-up.
3. Requires staff competence.
4. Examines policies and procedures for effective pain control.
5. Necessitates patient education.

The WHO pain control ladder can be used as a useful guide in selection of analgesic agents, which includes first administer Aspirin and NSAIDs, if pain unrelieved add local anesthetic and weak opioids, still if pain unrelieved add strong opioids.

Nursing Management of Pain

In the management of pain, nursing has an important role in anticipating and preventing pain, and in supporting clients who have been thorough physically painful experience. Appropriate information effectively communicated can do much to help provide a sense of control and minimizing anxiety. Advance knowledge of the physiological and psychological dimensions of plan provides a challenge for the nurse critically to examine nursing practices in pain assessment and management.

Assessment

Assessment is essential for diagnosis and for planning of pain control measures. Pain is difficult to measure because pain is a subjective experience or phenomena. One of the priorities for adequate treatment of pain is an accurate assessment. The goal of pain assessment is to identify the etiology of the pain; to understand the patient's sensory, affective, behavioral and cognitive pain experience for the purpose of implementing pain management techniques; and to identify the patient's goal for therapy and resources for self-management of the pain. It is the nurse often who is responsible for gathering and documenting assessment data.

Assessment, however, is highly influenced by the client's ability to delineate aspects of the pain experience accurately. If the client cannot communicate clearly (e.g. child, unconscious patient) then this aspects of the pain assessment is altered. Without the subjective information, it is difficult to intervene effectively except by trial and error. Ongoing assessment of pain is useful. This ongoing assessment should include subjective and objective assessment, that is, the individuals' verbal description of the pain and observation of person's behavior.

Each person has a basic human need to be free to pain and discomfort. Humans are motivated to avoid pain. Pain can occur as a result of inadequate satisfaction of other basic human needs. For example, need to eliminate urine not met because urinary stones block the bladder outlet and pain occurs. Part of the nursing assessment is to identify any unmet needs that may contribute to person's pain.

Each person experiences and expresses uniquely and attaches personal meaning or explanations to pain experiences. The personal meanings nurses attach to pain may interfere with the assessment. The personal meanings attached to pain result from personal pain experience throughout life and may arise from a person's individual experience and sociocultural experiences. The cultural and familial role modeling one supposes to teach a child is as the following:

- What pains are appropriate or inappropriate to talk about
- Behavior that is a appropriate or inappropriate when one experiences pain
- Circumstances likely to produce pain, which should therefore be avoided
- Various methods to avoid pain
- Reasons, why one may experience pain such as punishment, testing by supernatural or devine powers, or bad thoughts
- Possible consequence of pain, such as attention or lack of attention from others, imminent death.

A pain experience is also affected by personal factors:

- Pain expectancy (the anticipation of pain)
- Pain experience (willingness to experience pain)
- Pain apprehension (generalized desire to avoid pain)
- Pain anxiety (the anxiety of pain provokes because of its associated mystery, loneliness, helplessness, threat).

Since the pain evokes emotional responses, observation of behavior of the client/patient provides a nurse with understanding of a person's feelings and of what pain means to a particular person. By accepting behaviors and trying to understand their origins, nurses can help individuals experiencing pain. To do this well, nurses must:

- Accurately observe client's behavior
- Listen to all that clients say
- Never judge clients or jump to conclusions.

The perception, pain, is influenced by number of factors, which include integrity of the nervous system, state of consciousness, age, physical states (fatigue, debility, lack of sleep, and prolonged suffering all reduce a client's ability to tolerate pain) and emotional states (worry, fear, and anxiety reduce a person's ability to tolerate pain).

Assessment Process

The assessment process should provide the nurse with understanding of the patient's/client's pain, as well as establishing the nurse as a partner in the patient's search for pain relief. Patient teaching is an integral part of assessment, as information is provided clarifying the nurse's questions or responding to the patient's concern. As the patient discomfort is a source of stress to the family, it is important to involve the family and other members of the patient's network in the pain assessment. If the patient's ability to speak for himself or herself is limited, it is imperative to involve the family.

An accurate history is essential to assess a client's/patient's experience of pain. A detailed system analysis is performed using the following guidelines, to find out various aspects of pain:

Location: The location should be identified as specifically as possible. To determine the location of the patient's pain ask the following questions:

- Where is pain in the body?
- Is the pain internal or on the surface (external)?
- Is the pain always in these areas?
- If the pain is in more than one spot, are the pains equal, or does one trigger the others?
- Is the pain on both sides of your body? If so, is it the same on each side?

The site may be well-defined or diffused or the pain may radiate, involving wider area. To determine the extension and radiation of patient's pain ask the following questions:

- Does the pain extend from where it started? Does it cover a wider area, or can you point to where it is?
- Is there a pattern in which the pain spreads?
- Is the pain on the surface or deep inside?

Observing the pain locations on the patient's body will help localize the sites of pain as well as identify any physical changes at the site such as swelling/or discoloration.

Onset and duration: When the pain first began and how the pain has changed over time should be determined. To determine the onset and pattern of the patient's pain ask the following questions:

- When did the pain begin? Is it a regular pain or does it vary? Does it occur in cycles? For example, sometimes, every day; every month or every spring
- What triggers the pain? Are there specific things that always trigger it? Can you identify particular patterns?
- Does the pain begin suddenly or gradually over time? Is it continuous, or does it vary? Are there separate episodes of pain? If, so, does the pain go away completely between episodes or does it just get better?
- Has the pain pattern changed at all since it began?
- Has your lifestyle changed since the pain began?

To determine the duration of the patient's pain, ask the following questions:

- How long does the pain last? Are you free of pain between episodes?
- Is the pain constant, intermittent or rhythmic?

Character or quality: A description of the pain, using patient's own words is helpful in determining the origin of pain and possible pain relief measures. To determine the character or quality of the patient's pain, ask the client the following question to describe it.

- Is the pain, dull, sharp, throbbing, burning, electric or shooting?

If the patient is unable to provide such descriptions the descriptors used in the McGill-Melzack pain questionnaire can be used.

Exacerbating factors: Often patients may be comfortable at rest, but have difficulty in morning due to pain. Activities which exacerbate the pain should be identified. To determine the factors, that precipitate, aggravate and alleviate the patient's pain, ask the following questions:

- What seems to trigger pain? Can you identify a specific cause or event that always or sometime precedes the pain?
- Does anything alter the pain? Does anything make it worse, such as smoking, drinking alcohol, eating, heat or tension? Is there anything that makes the pain better, such as rest, activity-heat or cold or medications.

Associated manifestations: The impact of pain on the person's physical functioning should be explored. To determine whether there are any manifestations associated with client's pain, ask the following questions:

- Are there any other problems caused by your pain?
- Do you have any nausea/vomiting, restlessness, insomnia, excessive sleeping, or loss of appetite?

Associated manifestations also include profuse perspiration, fainting, inability to perform usual functions, dulling of senses, apathy, clouding of consciousness, disorientation and inability to rest and sleep.

Effect on activities of daily living: To determine how the client's pain affects activities of daily living, ask the following questions:

- Does the pain interfere with work, sleep, driving, eating, school work, sexual relations, housework, social activity or other activity?
- Has the pain caused any changes in your lifestyle?
- When did you last have a good night's sleep?

Intensity: A new pathogenic condition must be ruled out when there is sudden increase in pain intensity, the intensity of the pain can be measured in several ways which are summarized as follows:

- *Visual analogue scale (VAS)*—consists of a 10 cm line vertical or horizontal with one end marked 'no pain' and other 'worst possible pain' (Fig. 3.4).

  Visual analogue scales (VASs) are useful in assessing the intensity of pain (Fig. 3.4). One version of the scale includes a horizontal 10 cm line with anchors (ends) indicating the extremes of pain. The patient is asked to place a mark indicating where the current pain lies on the line. The left anchor usually represents "none" or "no pain", whereas the right anchor usually represents "severe" or "worst possible pain." To score the results, a ruler is placed along the line, and the distance the patient marked from the left of low end is measured and reported in millimeters or centimeters.

Some patients (e.g. children, elderly patients, visually or cognitively impaired patients) may find it difficult to use an unmarked VAS. In those circumstances, ordinal scales, such as a simple descriptive pain intensity scale or a 0 to 10 numeric pain intensity scale, may be used (Fig. 3.4).

The patient marks the line to show where the pain lies. This approach works well for acute pain. It is not useful in chronic pain. Some patients have difficulty in understanding the basic concept involved in it, and may not be able to use the scale at all.

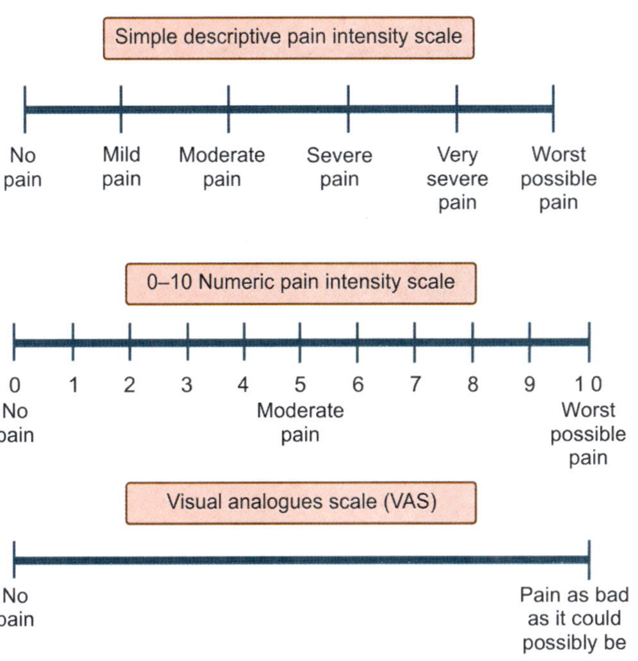

FIG. 3.4: Examples of pain intensity scales

- *Numerical rating scale (NRS)*—typically runs from 0 (no pain) to 10 (unbearable) although 0-5 or 0-7 may be used. Here the patient simply gives a score to indicate that pain level (Fig. 3.5).
- *Verbal descriptor scale (VDS)*—here, a range of words are used to describe the potential spectrum of pain and the patient states which word most accurately reflects how they feel.
- *McGill pain questionnaire*—is complex but reliable and sensitive tool which involves multidimensional measurements of pain with time, the effect it has on the patient, location and intensity of pain.

Faces Pain Scale–Revised

This instrument has six faces depicting expressions that range from contented to obvious distress (Fig. 3.5). The patient is asked to point to the face that most closely resembles the intensity of his or her pain.

To determine the intensity of patient's pain the following should be done:

- Ask, on a scale of 0–10 with '0' being 'no pain' and '10' being 'the worst pain you can imagine' how would you rate your pain now? How would you rate it worst? How would you rate it with activity?
- Note what non-verbal manifestation of pain the client exhibits—grimacing, crying, moaning, sleeping, appearing exhausted, or remaining immobile.

Relief measures: The efficacy of measures used by the patient to relieve pain should be identified. To determine how the patient obtains pain relief, ask the following questions:

- What do you do to relieve the pain (ask about both invasive and non-invasive pain relief measures)?
- What has not worked to relieve your pain?

This includes both those activities suggested by the medical and nursing staff such as the use of analgesic, as well as measures employed by the patient himself, such as distraction,

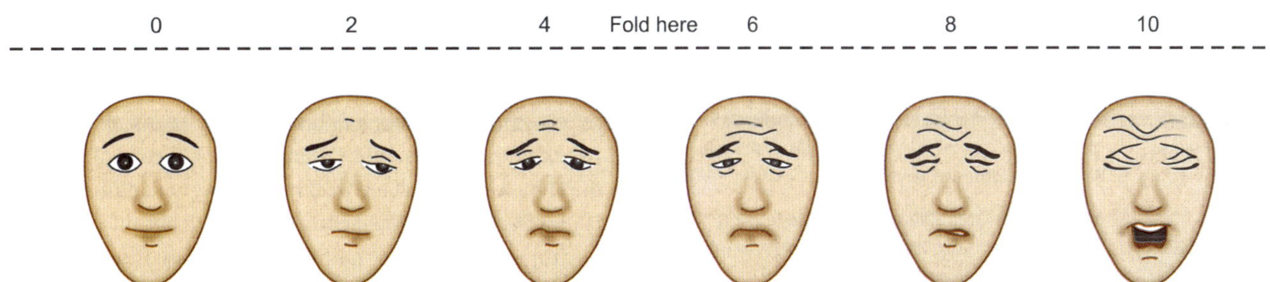

FIG. 3.5: Faces pain scale—revised. This pain scale is especially suited for helping children describe pain. Instructions for using this scale follow: "These faces show how much something can hurt. This face (point to left-most face) shows no pain. The faces show more and more pain (point to each from left to right) up to this one (point to right-most face). It shows very much pain. Point to the face that shows how much you hurt (right now)." Score the chosen face 0, 2, 4, 6, 8, or 10, counting left to right, so 0 = no pain and 10 = very much pain. Do not use words like "happy" or "sad." This scale is intended to measure how children feel inside, not how their face looks

visualization, rubbing, etc. All drugs used by the patients and their dose.

Physical examination: Start the examination by having the patient show where the pain is and describe how it feels. Pain is subjective and the patient himself is an expert about his/her pain, but objective manifestations that observed by nurse and other health care providers give clue to its cause. Objective manifestations of pain can be divided into three categories which include sympathetic responses, parasympathetic responses and behavioral responses.

Sympathetic responses are often associated with minimal to moderate pain intensity or superficial pain. They signify the other body defenses are mobilized and that the fight-or-flight response has begun. Objective manifestations include pallor, increased pulse, increased blood pressure, increased respiration, skeletal muscle tension, dilated pupils and diaphoresis.

Parasympathetic responses are often associated with pain of severe intensity or with deep pain. In this, body defenses may collapse in an attempt to lessen the effects of external threat. Manifestations of parasympathetic response include decreased blood pressure, decreased pulse, nausea and vomiting, weakness, prostration, pallor and loss of consciousness.

The patient may exhibit the behavioral responses in the acute pain as follows (Table 3.2):

- Assume a posture that minimizes pain such as lying rigidly, guarding drawing up the legs, or assuming the fetal position
- Moan, sign, grimace, clench the jaws or fist, become quiet, or withdraw from others
- Blink rapidly
- Cry, appear frightened, exhibit restlessness
- Have a drawn facial expression
- Have twitching muscles
- Withdraw when touched
- Hold or protect the painful area or remain motionless.

Although it is unreasonable to think that the nurse would be performing the detailed assessment constantly with a patient, portions of it are important and should be done at regular intervals.

TABLE 3.2: Behavioral indications of effects of pain

• Vocalization:	Moaning, crying, screaming, gasping, grunting.
• Facial expression:	Grimace, clenched teeth, wrinkled forehead, tightly closed or widely opened eyes or mouth, lip biting, tightened jaw
• Body movement:	Restlessness, immobilization, muscle tension, increased hand and finger movements, pacing activities, rhythmic or rubbing motions, protective movement of body parts
• Social interaction:	Avoidance of conversation, focus only on activities for pain relief, avoidance of social contact, reduced attention span

Nursing Diagnosis

An accurate diagnosis made only after a complete assessment clusters of defining characteristics reveal the nursing diagnosis best fitted to the client/patient condition and needs. The nursing diagnosis should focus on the specific nature of these pains to help the nurse identify the most useful types of interventions for alleviating pain and minimizing its effect on the client's lifestyle and function.

The nursing diagnoses are directly associated with care of patients with pain, i.e. chronic pain. The other nursing diagnoses that may be appropriate because of the effects of pain on other aspects of a patient's life include the following (Table 3.3):

- Anxiety
- Knowledge deficit (specify)
- Body image disturbance
- Altered nutrition
- Colonic constipation
- Impaired physical mobility
- Ineffective family coping, disabling
- Ineffective individual coping
- Powerlessness
- Altered family processes
- Altered role performance
- Fatigue
- Selfcare deficit (specify)
- Fear
- Sexual dysfunction
- Anticipatory grieving
- Sleep pattern disturbance
- Social isolation
- Altered thought process.

Following are the examples of nursing diagnoses for pain:

1. Anxiety related to unrelieved pain.
2. Pain related to physical injury/reduced blood supply to tissue/natural childbirth process.
3. Chronic pain related to chronic physical disability/psychosocial disability/inadequate pain control.
4. Hopelessness related to chronic malignant pain.
5. Ineffective individual coping related to chronic pain.
6. Impaired physical mobility related to musculoskeletal pain/incisional pain.
7. Risk for injury, related to reduced pain reception.
8. Self-care deficit (specify) related to musculoskeletal pain.
9. Sexual dysfunction related to arthritic hip pain.
10. Sleep pattern disturbance related to low back pain.

TABLE 3.3: Nursing care plan for pain relief

Problems	Reasons	Objectives	Nursing interventions	Evaluation
Pain related to abdominal incision movement	Complain of sharp, localized pain over lower abdominal incisions worsening during coughing and movement. Guards abdomen rigidly while turning and breathing deeply	1. Client will achieve control of pain within 24 hours after surgery 2. Patient will initiate movement in bed without painful behavioral cues 3. Client will express relief during PCA infusion	1. Position client anatomically on side with knee flexed and small pillow below legs 2. Have colleagues available to lift client in bed for repositioning. Encourage cient to ask for assistance 3. Explain the purpose of PCA device, method for initiating device and expected response 4. Demonstrate and coach client through relaxation exercise	
Impaired physical mobility related to musculoskeletal pain	Complain of pain, edema manifested by painful movement, decreased range of motions. Loss of muscle strength.	Patient will demonstrate increase in mobility of joints	Place the patient in position of comfort, suggests joints anatomically with pillow or pads and change position every hour: • Assist in ROM exercise • Avoid restrictive clothing • Assist to ambulate as tolerated • Maintain save environment	
Self-care deficit related to pain	Not dressed Not groomed	Patient's independence in self-care activities will increase within the parameters of disability	• Teach self-care activities • Establish and teach routine plan of ADLs • Set goals with patient, encourage short-term easily accomplished goal • Discuss the use of snaps on clothing and slip-on shoes • Encourage verbalization about fears and anxiety of disease process • Deal with behavioral change denial, powerlessness, etc. • Be supportive and kind in setting goals • Encourage independence • Modify environment	
Chronic low-self-esteem related to inability to work	Preoccupation with body changes and verbalization of powerlessness	Patient will verbalize understanding of changes in body image caused by disease process and will begin to exhibit increased confidence in dealing with self-esteem		
Knowledge deficit related to home care management	Having misconception about medication regimen, exercise program and diet			

Planning

For each nursing diagnosis identified, the nurse develops a care plan for the client/patient needs. Together the nurse and patient discuss realistic expectation for pain-relief measures and the degree of pain relief to expect. Objectives of the care are selected on the basis of the nursing diagnosis and client condition. Appropriate measures and therapies are chosen on the basis of the related factor contributing to the patient's pain or health problem.

A critical element in the management of a patient with a pain syndrome is the establishment of a trusting relationship and good rapport with the patient and the family. The patient and the family need to know that the nurse considers the pain significant and understands that pain may totally disrupt a person's life. The nurse's goal is to help the patient cope with the pain by using medications and techniques to help with relaxation, comfort, sense of aloneness and isolation, and protection from depersonalizations and the nurse will help the patient maintain or regain control over the environment. A priority for the nurse caring for a patient with pain is to let it be known that the nurse believes the person has pain and to explain some of the physiologic mechanism of pain.

Nursing actions that promote the establishment of an effective relationship with the person who is experiencing pain and with the family should include the following:

Believe the patient: The patient needs to be able to trust the nurse to believe in the pain's existence. This message can be conveyed verbally to the patient by saying "I know you are in pain". The nurse may need to help the family believe the patient.

Clarify responsibilities in pain relief: Discuss what the nurse is going to do, and what the patient and the family are expected to do.

Respect the patient's response to pain: The nurse should accept the right of the patient to respond to the pain in the necessary manner. The family also needs help in this area. The patient may need help to accept the reasons to pain; the behavior may be less than is expected by the patient and the family.

Collaborate with the patient: The patient should be encouraged to use coping techniques that have been effective in the past. The patient and the family should be helped to participate actively in setting goals for pain relief.

Explore the pain with the patient: The nurse needs to find out the meaning of the pain to the person enduring the pain and to the family.

Be with the patient often: The nurse should act as buffer for the patient and the family during difficult times. The nurse's physical presence may reassure or distract the patient or it may offer variety, thus relieving the pain.

Guidelines for Individualizing Pain Therapy

When providing pain relief measures, the nurse chooses therapies suited to the client's unique pain experience. McCaffery (1979) suggests nine useful guidelines for pain therapy. The following guidelines are relevant, which include nine guidelines of McCaffery.

Establish a relationship of mutual trust: Always believe the client and try to convey concern. An adversial relationship between nurse and client lessens the effectiveness of pain therapies.

Use different types of pain relief measures: Using more than one therapy has an additive effect in reducing pain. In addition, the character of pain may change throughout the day, requiring several different therapies.

Provide pain relief measures before pain becomes severe: It is easier to prevent severe pain than to relieve it after it exists. Giving analgesics half an hour before, client must walk or perform an activity is an example of controlling pain early.

Consider the client's ability or willingness to participate in pain relief measures Some client cannot actively assist with pain therapy because of fatigue, sedation or altered level of consciousness. However, there are variations of pain-relief measures that require little effort, such as relaxation exercises in bed or listening to music as a distraction. The nurse will not relieve pain by forcing an unwilling patient to participate in therapy.

Choose pain-relief measures on the basis of the clients behavior reflecting the severity of pain. It would be poor judgment to administer a patient narcotic if a client has only mild pain. The nurse carefully assesses the client's comments and behavior before choosing pain therapy. Some clients acquire relief from severe pain after using only mild analgesics. Only the client can determine the potency of an effective therapy.

Use measures that the client believes are effective: The client is the expert of pain. The client may have ideas about measures to use (e.g. rubbing lotion on a swollen finger) and times to use them will make pain therapy successful.

If a therapy is ineffective at first, encourage client to try again before abandoning it. Often, anxiety or doubt prevents a therapy from relieving pain, or the measure may require adjustment or practice to become effective. The nurse should be patient and understanding in helping the client learn to use measures that do not afford immediate relief.

Keep an open mind about what may relieve pain: New ways are often found to control pain. There is still much to be learned about the pain experience. Rejecting non-conventional therapies leads to mistrust. The nurse should be sure all therapies are safe.

Keep trying: The nurse can easily become frustrated when efforts at pain relief fail. The nurse should not abandon the client when pain persists but reassess the situation and consider alternative therapies.

Protect the client: A pain therapy should not cause more distress than the pain itself. The nurse always observes the client's response to therapy. The nurse's aim is to relieve pain without disabling the client mentally, emotionally or physically.

Educate the client about the pain: When possible, the nurse should explain the cause of the pain, time of occurrence, duration and quality and ways to gain relief. Education promotes the prevention of pain.

The basic nursing responsibility is protecting the client from harm. One simple way to promote comfort is by removing or preventing painful stimuli. The following measures can be performed by the nurse to assist in pain control:

- Tighten and smooth wrinkled bed linen
- Reposition drainage tubes/other objects on which patient is lying
- Place warm bath blankets for coolness
- Loosen constricting bandages (unless specifically applied as a pressure dressing)
- Change wet dressings
- Position the client in an anatomical alignment
- Check temperature of hot or cold applications including bath water
- Lift client on bed—do not pull. Patient up in bed; handle gently

- Position patient correctly on bed pan
- Avoid exposing skin or mucous membrane to irritants (e.g. diarrheal stool, wound drainage)
- Prevent urinary retention by keeping Foley's catheters patent and free flowing
- Prevent constipation with fluids, diet and exercises.

Nursing Intervention

Nursing interventions for pain relief can be grouped and discussed in two broad categories:

1. Noninvasive or nonpharmocological intervention/pain relief strategy.
2. Invasive interventions/pain relief strategies.

Noninvasive Interventions

The noninvasive techniques which may be offered by the nurses often used as adjuncts to the analgesic regimen, not alternatives.

Trusting relationship: Develop good trusting relationship as already explained.

Alleviate anxiety: To Alleviating anxiety, stay with the client for a while. Allow the client to talk and express feelings and fears. Communicate empathy and willingness to listen. Take measures to relieve anxiety in positive direction according to experience of nurses. With patient with pain, for example, self-directed pain prevention/reduction techniques such as meditation, using therapeutic touch, backrub, applying cool cloth, etc.

Distraction or diversion: It is one of the measures used to pain relief. Distraction helps to focus attention away from the pain and to some extent, any contact the nurse with the patient which is not focused on pain *per se*. Distraction which reduces the conscious awareness of pain usually works with mild pain than severe pain. Distraction may take many forms, viz. occupational therapy, conversation, reading, watching television, listening to radio, meditation, self-hypnosis, biofeedback, and autosuggestion, etc. Distractions serve to increase pain tolerance, that is, it makes the pain more bearable.

Combating anticipatory fears: Anticipatory fears are those fears that occur prior to an experience of pain-producing stimuli. These help prepare clients to meet pain realistically by talking with them about the pain they fear.

Providing physical care: Effective physical nursing care for clients experiencing pain is directed at reducing mechanical, chemical and thermal stressors that lower pain tolerance. This includes protecting patient from local irritations or inflammation such as infection or thrombosis, muscle spasm or muscle strain, interference with local blood supply and venous and lymphatic drainage, distention of hollow visceral organs such as the bowel and bladder and further damage to traumatized tissue.

Non-pharmacological methods of pain control: These methods are sometimes referred to as complimentary pain relief methods. While these methods are not always enough on their own to treat pain, they can be useful in reducing pain when combined with pain medicines and reducing the amount of pain medicine required to control pain. These methods allow patients to have more control over their pain. Some of these methods are:

Physical methods: Commonly used physical agents include applications of cold, massage, rest or immobilization.

TENS: Transcutaneous electrical nerve stimulation (TENS) may be effective in reducing pain and improving physical function. This has been used with varying degrees of success in the management of postoperative pain. Evidence is accumulating that TENS acts by increasing CSF levels of beta-endorphins, together with activating of the "pain gate" by counter irritation.

Extracorporeal shock wave lithotripsy (ESWL): This is a minimally invasive treatment, during and after which a number of patients do not need any analgesia specifically in urological surgeries. Analgesics may be given on demand during and after ESWL because not all patients need pain-relief.

There are several important principles of physical nursing care as follows:

- Identify the source of pain and eliminate or reduce the pain
- Handle sensitive or injured tissue carefully
- Always perform painful procedures when pain-relieving medications are producing their maximal effect
- Check drainage tubes frequently to ensure that they are not caught, stretched, pulled, kinked, or looped and that they are positioned correctly
- Protect the client from fatigue and helping the client to get a good night's sleep
- Be alert to inflammation and ischemia caused by immobilization—take suitable measure to reduce it
- Change the position to relieve muscle spasms, maintain good body alignment of the client
- Use gentle massage and application of heat or cold if needed
- Use dermal stimulation, i.e. application of pressure, acupressure, massage. TENS (transcutaneous electric nerve stimulation), ice massage (massaging area with ice).

Invasive Intervention

Pharmacological methods: These methods involve controlling pain by utilizing pharmacological agents in the form of drugs and analgesia. Although most of the pharmacological agents are used in the postoperative period for controlling post-surgical pain, stress is now being given on the pre-emptive analgesic therapy. This therapy involves the application of opioids, local anesthetic blocks and other analgesic modalities before surgery in an attempt to decrease the intensity and duration of postoperative pain.

Preoperative patient preparation include:

- Patient evaluation
- Adjustment or continuation of medication in order to avoid abstinence syndrome
- Premedication as part of multimodal analgesia
- Behavioral-cognitive interventions for the patient and family with the aim of alleviating anxiety and fear of postoperative pain. This in turn leads to a reduction in the amount of analgesia required postoperatively and better and more efficient pain management.

The techniques used postoperatively generally include intramuscular, subcutaneous, intravenous, oral, rectal, transdermal or transmuscular analgesics; continuous infusions of opioids and/or NSAIDs; patient-controlled administration of opioids and/or NSAIDs; and intermittent boluses and /or continuous infusion of epidural or intrathecal opioids. Following are the pharmacological agents commonly used in the postoperative period:

1. *NSAIDs:* NSAIDs are the most commonly used pain relieving agents. NSAIDs have been the cornerstone of pharmacologic management of pain. They are generally short acting drugs, yet provide good level of pain control for mild to moderate postoperative pain. Thus, they often decrease the need for opioids However, NSAIDs are not sufficient as the sole analgesic agent after major surgery. NSAIDs have several advantages over opioids. They do not have hemodynamic effects, do not cause respiratory depression, or slow gastric emptying or small-bowel transit time. The pharmacy cost of some of them, however, is significantly greater than that of morphine, even by the oral route. IV parecoxib is very expensive. However, NSAIDs may also have some side-effects including renal impairement, increase risk of bleeding, exacerbation of aspirin-induced astham, poor bone or wound healing and GI upset.
2. *COX specific inhibitors:* They have a longer duration of action in comparison to NSAIDs. The molecular biology of COX-2 regulation is consistent with observations that COX-2 expression increases in response to inflammatory stimuli and tissue repair. The new highly-selective COX-2 inhibitors (e.g. rofecoxib, celecoxib) can inhibit prostaglandin synthesis without inhibition of platelet aggregation, and with reduced renal and GI toxicity.
3. *Opioid drugs:* For postoperative pain, the most commonly used opioid drugs are morphine, papaveretum, pethidine, codeine and methadone. Medicines given by mouth cause less discomfort than injections, but they can work just as well. They are inexpensive, simple to give, but there may be a delay in pain relief. Short and long-duration presentations are available. Tramadol has been used extensively in postoperative management. It has proven to be a very weak opioid with an analgesic potency roughly similar to pethidine that is due primarily to non-opioid actions. At low doses, it potentiates opioid actions with low dependency liability. Little respiratory depression occurs unless given in large doses. Opioids can also be given intramuscularly, intravenously or as an epidural agent depending upon the urgency and severity of the pain.
4. *Regional and local analgesia:* Direct injection of local analgesic drugs close to peripheral nerves, major nerve trunks or nerve roots produces analgesia by blocking condution of afferent impulses. Neural blockade with neuraxial administration of local anesthetics and/or opioids has now been established as being an effective means postoperative pain treatment. In some situations, such as major abdominal, orthopedic and thoracic surgery, it has been documented to provide superior pain relief to alternative techniques. Risks of epidural local anesthetics include hypotension, epidural abscess or hematoma, paraplegia, etc. (various other blocks are already discussed under anesthesia).
5. A multimodal approach to pain management takes into account an understanding of the molecular mechanisms of nociceptive pain signaling and peripheral and central sensitization. The concept of multi-modal (balanced) analgesics and routes of administration, which then act in synergy. The combined use of different classes of analgesics and analgesic techniques improves the effectiveness of pain relief after surgery and reduces the maximal dosage and adverse effects. Multi-modal postoperative analgesia may be the pain management technique of choice in elderly patients.
6. *Patient-controlled analgesia (PCA):* Systemic administration of opioids may follow the 'as needed' schedule or 'around-the-clock' dosing. PCA stands for patient-controlled analgesia. It means that the patient can have control over his own pain relief using pain medicines such as morphine or fentanyl. When the patient start to feel uncomfortable, he presses a button attached to a PCA pump. The pump then injects a small dose of the medicine into an intravenous (IV) cannula. However, the dose in each push is adjusted by the health care provider.

The drugs used to relieve pain work by altering pain sensation, depressing pain perception or modifying the patient's response to pain as the nurse has considerable control over and responsibility for the effective use of medicines to reduce pain, knowledge of the drugs used in pain control, their routes of administration and side effects is needed. Examples of analgesic are of four types as follows:

1. Non-narcotic analgesics
   - Acetaminophen (tylenol, atnol)
   - Acetyl salicylic acid (aspirin)
   - Choline magnesium trisalicylate (tritisate)
2. NSAIDs
   - Ibuprofen (brufen)
   - Naproxen (naprosyn)
   - Indomethacin
   - Tolmetin
   - Piroxicam

3. Narcotic analgesics
   - Meperidine
   - Methylmorphine (codeine)
   - Morphine sulfate (morphine)
   - Fentanyl (sublimaze)
   - Butorphanol (butarin)
   - Hydromorphone hydrochloride
4. Adjuvants
   - Amitriptyline
   - Hydroxyzine
   - Caffeine
   - Chlorpromazine
   - Diazepam

There are four types of analgesic as mentioned below which include (i) non-narcotic analgesics, (ii) NSAIDs, (iii) opioids and (iv) adjuvants or coanalgesics. Non-narcotic and NSAIDs provide relief for mild and moderate pain, such as the pain.

MANAGEMENT OF FLUID, ELECTROLYTE AND ACID-BASE IMBALANCES

The cells that make-up body tissues exist in a chemically constant but physiologically dynamic internal environment. Physiologic processes function to regulate this environment so that responses to stimuli minimally affect the body. The chemical consistency achieved through fluid, electrolyte and acid-base balance. Physiologic homeostasis and life itself depends on normal fluid and electrolyte balance and acid-base balance. It is essential to maintain homeostasis. Homeostasis is the term used to describe the ability to maintain internal balance in the presence of external stressors.

The homeostatic mechanisms that regulate fluid and electrolyte balance represent interaction between chemical and physiologic processes. Promoting balance in either a wellness or an illness state can prevent fluid and electrolyte imbalances that may be life-threatening. Nurses have primary professional contact with most clients. In any setting, it is natural for them to play an action role in the prevention, early detection and treatment of fluid and electrolyte imbalances. Now nurses not only have the opportunity, but they have broad base of knowledge of normal physiology and pathology, to assist in the identification of clients at risk and recognizing early manifestations of imbalance and taking measures to correct imbalance through nursing process.

Water Content of the Body or Body Fluid

Water is the primary component of all body fluids. It is the solvent used to transport nutrients to cells and to remove waste products produced by the cellular metabolism. Temperature regulation is assisted by evaporation of water on the body surface. Approxiately 60% of weight in a typical adult is composed of fluids, i.e. water and electrolytes. Factors that influence the amount of body fluids are age, gender, and body content. As a general rule, younger people have a higher percentage of body fluid than that of older people and men have proportionately more body fluid than that of women. Obese people have less fluid than thin people because fat cells contain little water. Adipose tissues contain less water than an equivalent amount of muscle tissue. In an older adult, body water content averages 45 to 55% of the body weight. In the infant, water content averages 70 to 80% of body weight. Therefore, the young are at risk because they have less fluid reserve. Both the very young and very old have a decreased ability to compensate for fluid loss.

Body fluid is located in the two compartments, viz., intracellular space (fluid in the cells) and the extracellular space (fluids outside the cells). Intracellular fluid (ICF) is located (primarily in the skeletal muscle mass) and constitutes 40% of body weight or 70% or two-thirds of the total body fluids/water. Extracellular fluid (ECF) constitutes about 20% of the body weight or 30% or one-third of total body fluids/water. Extracellular fluid (ECF) constitutes about 20% of the body weight or 30% or one-third of total body water. ECF consists of interstitial (between cells and lymph) intravascular (fluid within the cells is plasma), cerebrospinal, and intraocular fluid, as well as secretions of the gastrointestinal (GI) tract. Sometimes, the term 'transcellular', i.e. a product of secretion and diffusion from cells is used to refer to cerebrospinal, pericardial, synovial, intraocular and pleural fluids, sweat and digestive secretions.

ECF transports nutrients, electrolytes and oxygen to cells; carries waste products for excretion; regulates heat; lubricates and cushions, joints and membranes; hydrolizes food for digestive processes, and maintains vascular volume by passing easily through the capillary walls. ICF provides the cell with the internal aqueous medium necessary for its chemical functions. Normally, the fluid volume inside and outside of the cells maintains a steady state due to compensatory responses. 'Fluid spacing' is a term used to classify the distribution of body water. The term 'fluid' is used because more than water is found in these ICF and ECF compartments such as glucose, sodium and potassium. First spacing is a normal distribution of fluid in both the ECF and ICF components. Second spacing refers to an excess accumulation of interstitial fluid (edema). Third spacing occurs when fluids accumulate in areas that normally have no fluid or only a minimum amount of fluid. (For example, of third spacing are, ascitis, sequestration of fluid in the bowel in peritonitis and edema associated with burns).

Water is not only responsible for the body's structure and functions but it is also necessary for the maintenance of equilibrium (homeostasis) and of life itself. Body fluids normally shift between the two major compartments or spaces in an effort to maintain the equilibrium between the spaces. Loss of fluid from the body can disrupt the equilibrium. Sometimes, fluid is not lost from the body, but it is unavailable for use by either ICF or ECF space. Loss of ECF into a space that does not contribute to equilibrium between ICF and ECF is referred to as third space fluid shift. Third spacing is a concern because it takes fluid away from the normal fluid compartments and may produce hypovolemia. An early clue of a third space fluid shift is a decrease in urinary output, despite adequate fluid therapy. Urine output decreases because fluid shift out of the intravascular space; the kidneys that receive less blood flow and attempt to compensate by decreasing urine output. Other signs and symptoms of 'third spacing' that indicates an intravascular fluid volume deficit, include increased heart rate, decreased blood pressure, decreased central venous pressure, edema, increased body weight and imbalance in fluid intake and output. For example, third space occurs in ascitis, burns, massive bleeding into a joint or body cavity.

Physiology

As the primary body fluid, water is the most important nutrient of life, whereas life can be sustained for only a few days without water. The following are the primary functions of water in the body:

- Provide a medium for transporting nutrients to cells and wastes from the cells, and transporting such substances as hormones, enzymes, blood platelets, and red and white blood cells
- Facilitate cellular metabolism and proper cellular chemical functioning
- Act as a solvent for electrolytes and non-electrolytes
- Helps maintain normal body temperature
- Facilitates digestion and promotes elimination
- Act as a tissue lubricant.

Regulation of Body

As water moves through all parts of the body it is constantly being lost. Fluid leaves the body through the kidneys, lungs, skin, and GI tract. To maintain homeostasis, the normal daily loss must be met by the normal daily intake. Hemostasis is a relatively constancy in the internal environments of the body, naturally maintained by adaptive responses and that promote healthy survival. An approximate daily water intake and output of an adult eating 2,500 calories per day are as follows:

Intake		Output	
Route	Gain (mL)	Route	Amount of loss (mL)
Water in food	1,000	Skin	500
Water from oxidation	300	Lungs	350
Water as liquid	1,200	Feces	150
		Kidney	1,500
Total	2,500	Total	2,500

Mechanisms Controlling Fluid and Electrolyte Movement

There are many different processes which control the movement of fluid and electrolytes between the ICF and ECF spaces. These processes include simple diffusion, facilitated diffusion, active transport, osmosis, fluid presence (hydrostatic pressure and oncotic pressure).

Simple Diffusion

Diffusion is defined as the natural tendency of a substance or solutes to move from an area of higher concentration to one of lower concentration. It occurs through the random movement of ions and molecules. It occurs in liquids, gases, and solids. For example, exchange of oxygen and carbon dioxide between pulmonary capillaries and alveoli. Net movement of the molecules stops when the concentrations are equal in both areas. The membrane separating the two areas must be permeable to the diffusing substance for the process to occur. These molecules move without external energy. Diffusion is an efficient mechanism for the movement of molecules in and out of cells. Diffusion does not require energy.

Facilitated Diffusion

Some molecules diffuse slowly into the cell because of the composition of cellular membrane. However, when they are combined with a specific carrier molecule, the rate of diffusion accelerates. Like simple diffusion, facilitated diffusion moves molecules from an area of high concentration to one of low concentration. Glucose transport into the cell is an example of facilitated diffusion. The hormone insulin increases the rate of facilitated diffusion of glucose in most tissues.

Active Transport

Active transport is a process in which molecules move in the absence of a favorable diffusion gradient. In which, the physiologic pump that moves fluid from an area of lower concentration to one of higher concentration. External energy is required for this process because molecules are being moved against a concentration gradient. Active transport requires adenosine triphosphate (ATP) for energy. The energy production of energy depends on oxygen and glucose availability. The concentration of sodium and potassium differs greatly intracellularly and extracellularly. By active transport, sodium moves out of the cell and potassium moves into the cell. The energy source for the sodium-potassium pump is ATP which is produced in the mitochondria. By definition, active transport implies that entry expenditure must take place for the movement to occur against a concentration of gradient.

Osmosis

Osmosis, a special type of diffusion, is the flow of water between two compartments separated by a membrane permeable to water but not to solute. Here the movement of fluid across a semipermeable membrane from an area of low solute concentration to an area of high solute concentration. This process stops when the solute concentrations are equal on both sides of the membrane. In this, water moves from the compartments that is more dilute (has more water) to the side that is more concentrated (has less water). The semipermeable membrane prevents movement of solute particles. Osmosis requires no outside energy sources and stops when concentration differences disappear. In addition to diffusion, osmosis is very important for maintaining the chemical stability of body cells.

Osmotic pressure or force is a term used to describe the movement of water by the process of osmosis. It can be described as a pulling of water. Osmotic pressure is an important factor in the movement of water between fluid compartment, 'osmolarity' and 'osmolality' both measurement of osmotic pressure.

Osmolarity measures to osmotic force of solute per unit of weight of solvent. It reflects the concentration of fluid that affects the movement of water between fluid compartments by osmosis, osmolality measures the solute concentration per kilogram in blood and urine. It is measured in miliosmoles per kg of water (mOsm/kg). The normal osmolality of body fluids between 275 and 295 mmol/kg or mOsm/kg. The major determinants of osmolality are sodium, glucose, and urea with sodium. Increase in the concentration of these substances in the plasma causes fluid movement into plasma because of its increased osmotic pressure.

Osmolality measures the total miliosmols of solutes per unit of a total volume of solution. The number of osmoles, the standard unit of osmotic pressure per liter of solution. It is expressed as miliosmols per liter (mOsm/L) used to describe the concentration of solutes or dissolved particles.

In clinical practice, osmolality is used most oftenly. Serum osmolality may be measured directly through laboratory tests or estimated at the bad side by doubling the serum sodium level or by utilizing the following formula:

$$Na^{+} \times 2 + \frac{\text{Glucose}}{18} + \frac{\text{BUN (blood urea nitrogen)}}{3}$$

= Approximate value of serum osmolality.

In osmotic movement of fluid cells are affected by the osmolality of the fluid that surrounds them. Where fluids are added to the body those that have same osmolality as cell interior are "isotonic" solutions that contain more water than the cell are hypotonic (hypo-osmolar), those with less water than the cell are hypertonic (hyperosmolar).

Fluid Pressure

As a result of pressure, body fluids shift between the interstitial space and the vascular space within the capillary. The pressure in the body fluids are either hydrostatic or oncotic.

Hydrostatic pressure is the force exerted by a fluid against the walls of its container. The heart is a main component in generating pressure in blood vessels. Hydrostatic pressure in the vascular system gradually decreases as the blood moves through the arteries until it is about 40 mm Hg at the arterial end of a capillary. Because of the size of the capillary bed and fluid movement into the interstitium, the pressure decreases to about 10 mm Hg at the venous end of the vessel. Hydrostatic pressure in the capillaries tends to filer fluid out of the vascular compartment into the interstitial fluid.

Oncotic pressure (colloidal osmotic pressure) is an osmotic pressure exerted by colloidal, in solution. In plasma, proteins molecules attract water and contribute to the total osmotic pressure in the vascular system. Unlike electrolytes, the large molecular size prevents proteins from leaving the vascular space through pores in capillary walls. Plasma oncotic pressure is approximately 25 mm Hg. Some proteins are found in the interstitial space, and they exert an oncotic pressure of approximately 1 mm Hg.

The movement of the fluid through a capillary via the above stated two pressures (hydrostatic and oncotic) is called 'filtration'. An example of filtration is the passage of water and electrolytes from the arterial capillary bed to the interstitial fluid. In this instance, the hydrostatic pressure is furnished by the pumping action of the heart. Through filtration absorption or reabsorption resorption will take place. Absorption usually refers to the initial movement of substances such as end products of digestion or medications from organ such as GI tract or tissues such as the muscle, subcutaneous or dermal tissue, buccal or pharyngeal tissues, into the vascular system. Reabsorption refers to movement of water, electrolytes, vitamins, amino acids, glucose, lactate or other essential substances from one compartment, such as the interstitial or renal tubules, back into vascular capillaries. Resorption refers to the process of calcium salts leaving the bone and moving into the blood in an ionized form.

REGULATION OF FLUIDS AND ELECTROLYTES OR HOMEOSTATIC MECHANISM

The body is equipped with remarkable homeostatic mechanisms to keep the composition and volume of body fluid within narrow limits or normal. Organs involved in the homeostatic mechanism or regulation of fluid and electrolytes include hypothalamus, pituitary gland, adrenal gland, kidney, GI tract, parathyroid gland, heart, blood vessels and lungs, etc.

Hypothalamus

Water ingestion in the conscious client is regulated by the thirst receptors located in the hypothalamus. The thirst mechanism is stimulated by the hypotension and increased serum osmolality. In addition, thirst may result from polyuria, fluid volume depletion as small as 0.5% excess sodium intake, hypertonic feedings, and hypertonic IV fluids. Although thirst can be reported and is an important clinical manifestation of fluid imbalances, it is not a true indicator of fluid balance in all persons. The thirst mechanism depressed in the elderly. The desire to consume fluids is also affected by social and psychologic factors not related to fluid balance. A dry mouth will cause the client to drink, even when there is no measurable body water deficit. Water ingestion will equal water excretion in the individual who has free access to water, a normal thirst and ADH mechanism and normally functioning kidneys.

Pituitary Gland

The hypothalamus manufactures a substance known as antidiuretic hormone (ADH) which is stored in vesicle in the posterior pituitary gland and released as needed. ADH which regulates water retention by kidneys. The distal tubules and collecting ducts in the kidneys respond to the ADH by becoming more permeable in water so that water is absorbed into the blood and not excreted. When there is a normal plasma osmolality and normal circulating plasma volume, continued ADH secretion is called syndrome inappropriate anti-diuretic hormone (SIADH). ADH is released in response to many conditions an increase in plasma osmolality, ECF volume depletion, pain, stress, and use of certain medications such as narcotics, barbiturates, and anesthetics. Stress may be physiologic or psychologic. The factors which suppressing ADH include hypo-osmolality of the ECF, increased blood volume, exposure to cold, acute alcohol ingestion, carbon dioxide inhalation, administration of some diuretics, lithium and some anti-psychotic medications. ADH prevents urine production and promotes water reabsorption from the renal tubules. Stimulation of the thirst mechanism and ADH release usually occurs concurrently in response to a body fluid deficit.

Adrenal Gland

ECF volume is maintained by a combinations of hormonal influences. ADH affects only water reabsorption. Hormones released by the adrenal cortex help regulate both water and electrolytes. Two groups of hormones secreted by the adrenal cortex include glucocorticoids and mineralocorticoids. The glucocorticoids primarily have an anti-inflammatory effect and increase serum glucose, whereas mineralocorticoids (e.g. aldosterone) enhances sodium retention and potassium excretion. When sodium is reabsorbed, water follows as a result of osmotic changes. Cortisol is most common 'hormone which are the properties of gluco and minerlocorticoids properties. Adrenocorticotropic hormone (ACTH) from the anterior pituitary is necessary for aldosterone secretions. Hypovolemic is a common clinical condition in which aldosterone is secreted to maintain homeostasis.

Kidneys

The kidneys maintain fluid volume and concentration of urine by filtering the ECF through the glomeruli. Reabsorption and excretion of ECF occurs in the renal tubules in response to ADH, aldosterone and ANP (atrial natriuretic peptides). ANP released from the atria in response to atrial distention, vasoconstriction, or direct cardiac damage. These factors increase the excretion of sodium and water and results in vasodilation. Renal prostaglandins and renal rennin-kinin system also increases sodium excretion. The major function of kidneys in maintaining normal fluid balance include the following:

- Regulation of ECF volume and osmolality by selective retention and excretion of body fluids
- Regulation of electrolytes level in the ECF by selective retention of needed substances and excretion of unneeded substances
- Regulation of pH of ECF by retention of hydrogen ions
- Excretion of metabolic wastes and toxic substances.

Parathyroid Gland

The parathyroid glands embedded in the corners of thyroid gland, regulate calcium and phosphate balance by means of parathyroid hormone (PTH). PTH influences bone resorption, calcium absorption from the intestine and calcium reabsorption from the renal tubules.

GI Tract

Daily water intake and output are between 2,000 and 3,000 mL. The gastrointestinal tract accounts for the most of the water intake, water intake includes fluids, water from food metabolism and water present in solid foods. Lean meal is approximately 70% water whereas the water content of many fruits and vegetables is about 100%. Most of the body water is excreted by kidneys. A small amount of water eliminated by GI tract is feces.

Lungs

The lungs are also vital in maintaining homeostasis. Insensible water loss, which is unavoidable vaporization from the lungs and skin assists in regulating body temperature. Normally, about 900 mL per day is lost. The amount of water loss is increased by accelerated body metabolism, which occurs with increased body temperature and exercise. Through exhalation, the lungs remove approximately 300 mL of water daily in the normal adult.

Heart and Blood Vessels

The pumping action of the heart circulates blood through the kidneys under sufficient pressure for urine to form. Failure of the pumping action interferes with renal perfusion and thus with water and electrolytic regulation.

In addition, neural mechanisms also contribute to the balance of water and sodium. Mechano-receptors and baroreceptors are nerve receptors involved in neural mechanism.

ORGANS THAT MAINTAIN HOMEOSTASIS

Kidneys

- Regulate ECF volume and osmolality by selective retention and excretion of body fluids
- Regulate electrolytic levels in the ECF by selective retention of needed substances and excretion of unneeded substances
- Regulate pH of ECF by excretion or retention of hydrogen ions
- Excrete metabolic wastes (primarily acids) and toxic substances.

Heart and Blood Vessels

- Circulate blood through the kidneys under sufficient pressure of urine to form (pumping action of the heart)
- React to hypovolemia by stimulating fluid retention (stretch receptors in the atria and blood vessels).

Lungs

- Eliminate about 13, 000 mEq of hydrogen ions (H^+) daily, as opposed to only 40 to 80 mEq excreted daily by kidneys
- Act promptly to correct metabolic acid-base disturbance, regulate H^+ concentration (pH) by controlling the level of CO_2 in the ECF as follows:
  - Metabolic alkalosis causes compensatory hypoventilation resulting in CO_2 excretions (increased acidity of the ECF)
  - Metabolic acidosis causes compensatory hyperventilation, resulting in CO_2 excretion (decreased acidity of the ECF)
- Remove approximately 300 mL of water daily through exhalation (insensible water loss) in the normal adult.

Adrenal Glands

- Regulate blood volume and sodium and potassium balance by secreting aldosterone; a mineralocorticoid secreted by the adrenal cortex
  - The primary regulator of aldosterone appears to be angiotensin II which is produced by the reninangiotensin system. A decrease in blood volume triggers this system and increases aldosterone secretion, which causes sodium retention (and thus water retention) and potassium loss
  - Decreased secretion of aldosterone causes sodium and water loss and potassium retention
- Cortisol, another ACTH, has only a fraction of the potency of aldosterone
- However, secretion of cortisol in large quantities can produce sodium and water retention and potassium deficit.

Pituitary Gland

- Stores and releases ADH, which makes the body retain water. Functions of ADH include:
  - Maintains osmotic pressure of the cells by controlling renal water retention or excretion
  - When osmotic pressure of the ECF is greater than that of the cells (as in hypernatremia or hyperglycemia), ADH secretions is increased causing renal retention of water
  - When osmotic pressure of the ECF is less than that of the cells, (as in hyponatremia) ADH secretion is decreased, causing renal excretion of water.
- Controls blood volume (less influential than aldosterone)
  - When blood volume is decreased, an increased secretions of ADH results in water conservation
  - When blood volume is increased, a decreased secretion ADH results in water loss.

Parathyroid Glands

Regulate calcium (Ca^{2+}) and phosphate (PO_4^{-2}) balance by means of PTH; PTH influences bone reabsorption, calcium absorption from the intestines and calcium reabsorption from renal tubules.

- Increased secretion of PTH causes:
  i. Elevated serum calcium concentration
  ii. Lowered serum phosphate concentration
- Conversely, decreased secretion of PTH causes:
  i. Lowered serum calcium concentrate
  ii. Elevated serum phosphate concentrate.

FLUID IMBALANCES

Fluid imbalances occur when the body's compensating mechanisms are unable to maintain homeostatic state. Fluid imbalances may relate to either volume or distribution of water or electrolytes.

Fluid Volume Deficit (FVD)

Fluid volume deficit can be caused by a deficiency in the amount of both water and electrolytes in ECF, but the water and electrolytes proportions remain near normal. The state is commonly known as 'hypovolemia.' Both osmotic and hydrostatic pressure changes for the interstitial fluid into intravascular space. As the interstitial space is depleted, its fluid becomes hypertonic, and cellular fluid is then drawn into the interstitial space, leaving cells without adequate fluid to function properly.

Fluid volume deficit results from the loss of body fluids expecially if fluid intake is simultaneously decreased. The related factors of FVD are:

i. Loss of water and electrolytes, as in:
   - Vomiting
   - Polyuria
   - Diarrhea
   - Fever
   - Excessive laxative use
   - Excessive sweating
   - Fistulas
   - Third-space fluid shifts
   - Gastrointestinal suction.

ii. Decreased intake, as in:
   - Anorexia
   - Inability to gain access to fluids
   - Nausea
   - Inability to swallow fluids
   - Depression.

The main characteristics of fluid volume deficits are:

- Weight loss over short period (except in third-space losses)
- Decreased skin and tongue turger
- Dry mucus membranes
- Urine output less than 30 mL per hour in adult
- Postural hypotension (systolic pressure drops by more than 15 mm Hg when client moves from lying to standing or sitting position)
- Weak, rapid pulse
- Slow-filling peripheral veins
- Decreased body temperature, such as 95° to 98°F (35°C to 36.7°C) unless infection is present
- CVP less than 4 cm H_2O
- BUN elevated out of proportion to serum creatinine
- Specific gravity (urine) high
- Hematocrit elevated
- Flat neck veins in supine position
- Marked oliguria, late
- Altered sensorium.

Nursing Intervention for FVD

1. Assess for presence or worsening of FVD
2. Administer oral fluids if indicated:
   - Consider the client's likes and dislikes when offering fluids
   - If the client is reluctant to drink because of oral discomfort select fluids that are non-irritating to the mucosa, and provide frequent mouth care (offer saline gargle and apply lubricant to lips)
   - Offer fluids at frequent intervals
   - Explain the need for fluid replacement to the client
   - Administer medications if nausea is present, to provide relief before fluids are offered.
3. Consider the following interventions for clients with impaired swallowing:
   - Assess gag reflex and ability to swallow water before offering solid foods; have a suction apparatus on hand
   - Position the client in an upright position with a head and neck flexed slightly forward during feeding (tilting the head backward during swallowing predisposes to aspiration because this position opens the airway)
   - Provide thick fluids or semisolid foods (such as pudding or gelatine). These are more easily swallowed because of their consistency and weight than are thin liquids.
4. If the client is unable to eat and drink, discuss possibility of tube feeding or TPN with the physician.
5. Monitor response to fluid intake, either orally or parenterally.
6. Monitor clients with tendency for abnormal fluid retention (such as renal or cardiac problems) for signs of overload during aggressive fluid replacement.
7. Turn client frequently, apply moisturizing agents to skin.

Sometimes dehydration used as synonym for hypovolemia; technically it is wrong. Dehydration refers only to a decreased volume of water; but water is not decreased without electrolyte charges also. Hydration is the union of a substance with water and is often used to indicate that there is normal water volume in the body.

Fluid Volume Excess

Excessive retention of water and sodium in ECF in near normal proportions results in a condition termed as Fluid volume excess. It is also called "hypervolemia". Overhydration refers only to above-normal amounts of water in extracellular spaces. Malfunction of the kidneys causing an inability to excrete the excesses and failure of the heart to function as a pump resulting in accumulation of fluid in the lungs and dependant parts of the body, are common causes. When water is retained in excessive amount, so as sodium.

Due to increased extracellular osmotic pressure from the retained sodium, fluid is pulled from the cells to equalize the tonicity. By the time intracellular and extracellular spaces are isotonic to each other, an excess of both water and sodium are in ECF, while the cells are nearly depleted The excessive ECF may accumulate in tissue spaces, thus is known as "edema". Edema can be observed around eyes, fingers ankles and sacral space and also accumulate in or around body organs. It may result in a weight gain in excess of 5%. When the excess fluid remains in the intravascular space, the concentration of solids in the blood is decreased.

Interstitial to plasma shift is the movement of fluid from the space surrounding the cells to the blood. This shift, also called hypervolemia is a compensatory response to volume or osmotic pressure changes of the intravascular fluid. Although the body attempts to maintain normal balance in all fluid spaces, the intravascular fluid is usually protected at the expense of interstitial fluid and ICF.

The common related factors which lead to fluid volume excess (FVE) are as follows:

- Compromised regulatory mechanisms such as:
  - Renal failure
  - Congestive heart failure
  - Cirrhosis of liver
  - Cushing's syndrome
- Overzealous administration of sodium containing IV fluids
- Excessive ingestion of sodium containing substances in diet or sodium containing medication.

The characteristics of fluid volume excess will include:

- Weight gain over short period
- Peripheral edema excess of fluid in interstitial space
- Distended neck veins
- Distended peripheral veins
- Slow-emptying peripheral veins
- CVP over 11 cm H_2O
- Crackles and wheezers in lungs
- Polyuria (if renal function normal)
- Ascitis, pleural effusion (when FVE is severe, fluid transuades into body cavities)
- Decreased BUN (due to plasma dilution)
- Decreased hemalocrit (due to plasma dilution)
- Bounding, full-pulse
- Pulmonary edema, if severe.

Nursing Intervention

- Assess the presence or worsening of FVE
- Encourage adherence to sodium restricted diet if prescribed
- Teach client requiring sodium restricitions to avoid over-the-counter drugs without first checking with the health care adviser/nurse
- When fluid retention persists despite adherence to dietary sodium intake, consider hidden sources of sodium, such as water supply or use of water softener
- When indicated, encourage rest period, lying down favors diuresis of edema fluid
- Monitor the client's response to diuretics. Discuss significant findings with physician
- Monitor the rate of parenteral fluids and the client response. Discuss significant finding with physician
- Teach self-monitoring of weight and intake and output measurements to clients with chronic fluid retention (such as those of CCF, renal failure, cirrhosis of liver)
- If dyspnea or orthopnea are present, position the client in semi-Fowler's position to facilitate lung expansion
- Turn and position the client frequently, be aware that edematous tissue is more prone to skin breakdown than in normal tissue.

ELECTROLYTES AND THEIR IMBALANCE

Electrolytes are substances whose molecules dissociate or split into ions when placed in water. These substances are found in ECF and ICF that dissociate into electrically charged particles known as ions. Cations are positively charged ions. For example, sodium (Na^+), potassium (K^+), calcium (Ca^{2+}) and magnesium (Mg^+), hydrogen (H+) ions. Anions are negative charged ions. For example, bicarbonates (HCO_3^-) chloride (Cl^-) and phosphate (PO_4^-) ions and proteins. The ionic charge is termed valence. Cations and anions combine according to their valency.

The concentration of electrolytes can be expressed in milligrams per deciliter (mg/dL), millimeter per liter (mm/L) or milliequivalent per liter (mEq/L). See the normal level of electrolytes in appendix. The role of electrolytes in cellular functions includes the following:

1. Regulation of water distribution, and osmolality
2. Regulation of acid-base balance
3. Transmission of nerve impulses, i.e. neuromuscular activity
4. Contraction of muscles
5. Clotting of blood
6. Enzyme reaction.

Electrolytes

Regulation of Electrolytes

Electrolytes regulate water distribution regulate acid-base balance and maintain a balanced degree of neuromuscular excitability. There are many different kinds of electrolytes in the body. These include sodium (Na^+), potassium (K^+), calcium (Ca^{++}), magnesium (Mg^{2+}), chloride (Cl^-), bicarbonate (HCO_3^-), phosphate (PO_4^-), etc.

Sodium

Sodium is the chief electrolyte of ECF. It moves easily between intravascular and interstitial spaces and moves across cell membrane by active transport. Many chemical reactions in the body are influenced by sodium, particularly in nervous tissue cells and muscle tissue cells.

The functions of sodium are as follows:

- It controls and regulates the volume of body fluids
- It maintains waterbalance throughout the body
- It is the primary regulator of ECF volume
- It influences ICF volume
- It participates in the generation and transmission of nerve impulses
- It is an essential electrolyte in the sodium-potassium pump.

The sources and losses of sodium are:

- An average daily intake is not known; but the average adult intake is eliminated to be between 6 and 15 g and the RDA for sodium for adults is approximately 500 mg for 0.5 g
- Sodium is found in many foods. Particularly, bacon, ham, sausage, catsup, mustard, relish, processed cheese, canned vegetables, bread, cereal, and salted snack food. It is found in table salt (NaCl) which is about 46% sodium
- Sodium excess are eliminated primarily by the kidneys. Small amounts are lost in feces and perspiration.

Regulation of Sodium

- Sodium normally is maintained in the body within a relatively narrow range, and deviations quickly result in a serious health problem
- Salt intake regulates sodium concentrations
- Sodium is conserved through reabsorption in the kidneys, a process of stimulated by aldosterone
- The normal extracellular concentrations of sodium is 135 to 145 mEq/L (mmol/L).

Potassium

Potassium is the major cation of ICF. Potassium and sodium work reciprocally. For example, an excessive intake of sodium results in an excretion of potassium and vice versa. The functions of potassium are as follows:

- It is the chief regulator of cellular enzyme activity and cellular water content
- It plays a vital role in such process as the transmission of electric impulses, particularly in nerve, heart, skeletal, intestinal, and lung tissue; protein and carbohydrate metabolism and cellular building
- It assists in regulation of acid-base balance by cellular exchange with H^+.

The sources and losses are:

- An average daily requirement of K^+ is not known; but an intake of 50 to 100 m Eq daily maintains potassium balance
- A well-balanced diet contains adequate quantities of potassium. Major sources include bananas, peaches, kiwi, figs, dates, appricots, oranges prunes, melons, raising, broccoli, and potatoes. Meat and dairy products also provide adequate amounts of potassium
- Potassium excreted primarily by the kidneys. The kidneys have no effective method of conserving potassium. Therefore, deficits develop readily if excreted in excess without being replaced simultaneously
- Gastrointestinal secretions contain potassium in large quantities. Some is also found in perspiration and saliva.

Regulation of Potassium

- Cellular potassium is conserved by the sodium pump when sodium is excluded
- The kidneys conserve potassium when cellular K^+ is decreased
- Aldosterone secretions trigger potassium excretion in urine
- The normal range for serum potassium is 3.5 to 5 mEq/L.

Calcium

Calcium is the most abundant electrolyte in the body. Up to 99% of the total amount of calcium in the body is found in bones and teeth in ionized form. There is close link between concentration of calcium and phosphorus. The functions of calcium are:

- It is necessary for nerve impulse transmissions and blood clotting
- It is catalyst for muscle contraction. Strength of contractions (especially cardiac muscle contraction) is directly related to the serum concentration of calcium ions
- It is needed for vitamin B_{12} absorption and for its use by body cells. It acts as a catalyst for many cell chemical activities
- It is necessary for strong bones and teeth
- It establishes thickness and strength of cell membrane.

The sources and losses of calcium are:

- The average daily requirements for calcium is about 1 g for adults. Higher amounts are required according to body weight, for children, for pregnant and lactating women, and postmenopausal women
- Calcium found in milk, cheese and dried beans. Some calcium is present in meats and vegetables
- Use of calcium is stimulated by vitamin D. The most active form of vitamin D (calcitriol) promotes calcium absorption and limits calcium excretion when levels are inadequate
- It leaves bones and teeth to maintain normal blood calcium levels if necessary
- It is excreted in urine, feces, bile, digestive secretion and perspiration.

Regulation of Calcium

- When ECF calcium levels decrease, the parathyroid glands increase the secretions of PTH, which acts on bones to increase the release of calcium into the blood and acts on the kidney tubules and the intestinal mucosa to increase the absorption of calcium from the kidneys and the intestine
- A high serum phosphate concentration increases serum calcium; a low serum phosphate concentration decreases serum calcium
- Calcitonin, a hormone secreted by the thyroid gland has an opposite effect of calcium than PTH. Increases in calcitonin reduce the serum calcium concentration primarily by opposing osteoclast bone resorption.

Magnesium

Most of the cation magnesium is found within body cells. It is present in heart, bone, nerve, and muscle tissues. Magnesium is the second most important cation of ICF. The functions of magnesium are as follows:

- It is important for the metabolism of carbohydrates and proteins
- It is important for many vital reactions related to the body's enzymes
- It is necessary for protein and DNA synthesis, DNA and RNA transcription, and translation of RNA
- It maintains normal intracellular levels of potassium
- It serves to help maintain electric activity in nervous membranes and muscle membranes.

The sources and losses of magnesium are:

- The average daily adult requirement for magnesium is about 18 to 30 mEq. Children required larger amount
- Magnesium found in most foods but especially in vegetables, nuts, fish, wholegrains, peas and beans.

Regulation of Magnesium

- Magenesium is absorbed by the intestines and secreted by the kidneys
- Plasma concentration of magnesium range from 1.3 to 2.1 mEq/L with about one-third of that amount bound to plasma proteins.

Chloride

Chloride, the chief extracellular anion, is found in blood, interstitial fluid, and lymph and in minute amounts in intracellular fluid. The functions of chlorides are as follows:

- It acts with sodium to maintain the osmotic pressure of the blood
- It plays a role in the body's acid-base balance
- It is important in buffering action when O_2 and CO_2 exchange in RBCs
- It is essential for the production of HCl in gastric juices
- The average daily requirement of chlorides are unknown. It is found in foods high in sodium, in dairy products and meat.

Regulation of Chloride

- It is normally paired with sodium and excreted and conserved with sodium by the kidneys
- Chloride deficits lead to potassium deficit and vice versa
- Normal serum chloride levels range from 95 to 105 mEq/L.

Bicarbonate

The bicarbonate molecule is an anion. It is the major chemical base buffer within the body and is found in both ECF and ICF. The bicarbonate is essential for acid-base balance. Bicarbonate and carbonic acid constitute the body's primary buffer systems.

Phosphate

The phosphate ion is the major anion in body cells. It is a buffer anion in both ICF and ECF. The functions of phosphate are:

- It helps maintain acid-base balance
- It is involved in important chemical reactions in the body. For example, it is necessary for many B vitamins to be effective; helps promote nerve and muscle action, and plays role as carbohydrate metabolism
- It is important for cell division and for the transmission of heredity traits.

An average daily requirement for phosphorous are similar to those for calcium. It is found in most foods especially in beef, pork, and dried peas and beans. It is metabolized in the same manner as calcium.

Phosphate is regulated by PTH and by activated vitamin D. Calcium and phosphates are inversely proportional and increase in one results in a decrease in the another. The normal range of phosphate is 2.5 to 4.5 mEq/L (mmol/L).

Electrolytes Imbalance

Human body contains quite large volume of water as ICF and ECF and the fluid contains several inorganic ions such as sodium, potassium, chloride, bicarbonate, sulfate, phosphate, calcium and magnesium. The complex mechanism of human life maintains the concentration and volume of the body fluids at a constant level and in general, it is not influenced by dietary intake and metabolism, while kidneys play a vital role in maintaining the balance. When clients present with deficit or excesses of sodium, potassium, calcium, magnesium or phosphate, special nursing care is required. A brief description of the common electrolyte imbalances are as follows:

Hyponatremia

Hyponatraemia refers to a sodium deficit in ECF caused by loss of sodium or a gain of water. It is a condition on lowered level of plasma volume. In this condition, osmotic pressure changes results in ECF, moving into the cells. When this occurs, an examiner's fingerprints tend to remain on the client's skin over the sternum where pressure is applied with the fingers.

The related factors leading to hyponatremia are:

- Loss of sodium as in: Loss of GI fluids, use of diuretics; adrenal insufficiency
- Gains of water as in: Excessive administration of D5W, diseases associated with SIADH; pharmacologic agents that impair renal water excretion
- Hyponatremia or sodium depletion occurs from loss of body fluids through sweating, vomiting, diarrhea, intestinal fistula, dialysis and from aspiration of gastric contents

- Chronic pyelonephritis, chrome uremia, diutretic phase of acute renal failure, diabetic ketoacidosis, cystic diseases of the kidney, and excessive or prolonged use of diuretics results excessive loss of sodium through urine
- Endocrine diseases show as myxedema, Addison's disease, hyperaldosteronism, and uncontrolled diabetes mellitus also leads to sodium depletion
- Excessive loss of sodium can also occur through the skin as in extensive burns, generalized dermatitis, etc. in children, cystic fibrosis.

Sodium is mainly an extracellular ion, and its depletion causes migration of water in the intracellular compartments, making the extracellular fluid hypotonic. Consequently plasma becomes hypo-osmolar and plasma volume falls.

The main characteristics of hyponatremia are:

- Anorexia
- Fingerprint overstrenum
- Nausea and vomiting
- Muscular twitching
- Lethargy
- Seizures
- Confusion
- Coma
- Muscle cramps
- Serum sodium below 135 mEq/L.

This condition presents with tiredness, lethargy, muscular weakness, mental confusion, and in severe cases, convulsions and coma. The skin appears cold, pale and inelastic. Tongue is dry. Reduction in plasma volume causes reduction in cardiac output and results tachycardia fall of blood pressure and raising pulse rate. The eyeballs become soft due to reduced intraocular pressure, urine output is reduced and soon oliguria supervenes and finally leads to uremia. When the plasma serum concentration falls exaggeratedly to 120 mmol/L of blood or less, muscle cramps occur. It can produce acidosis and circulatory failure as complication.

Treatment

Mild cases are treated with frequent drink of water with added sodium chloride or with isotonic (0.9%) saline solution by IV injection. In other cases, 2–4 liters of isotonoic saline solution is given IV infusion over 6–12 hours. More severe cases are treated with 2–3 liters of IV isotonic solution in first 2–3 hours, followed by further 2–5 liters within 24–48 hours. If there is associated water intoxication water intake is restricted to 500–1000 mL in 24 hours. In addition, the client is given treatment for the underlying condition.

Nursing Intervention

- Identify clients at risk for hyponatremia
- Monitor fluid losses and gains. Look for loss of sodium containing fluids, particularly in conjunction with low-sodium-intake
- Monitor presence of gastrointestinal symptoms, such as: anorexia, nausea, vomiting, and abdominal cramping
- Monitor laboratory date for serum sodium levels less than normal
- Check specific gravity of urine
- With clients able to consume a general diet, encourage foods and fluids with high sodium content
- Be familiar with the sodium content of commonly used parenteral fluids. Monitor client with cardiovascular disease receiving sodium-containing fluids closely for sign of circulatory overload such as moist rales in the lungs
- Use extreme caution when administering hypertonic saline solution (3 to 5% NaCl). Be aware that these fluids can be lethal if infused carelessly
- Avoid giving large water supplements to clients receiving isotonic tube feedings, particularly if routes of abnormal sodium loss are present or water is being retained abnormally.

Hypernatremia

Hypernatremia or sodium excess refers to surplus of sodium in ECF that can result from excess water loss or overall excess of sodium. Because of the increased extracellular osmotic pressure, fluids move from the cells, leaving them without sufficient fluid. It is a condition which excess of sodium occurs in the ECF, giving rise to cellular dehydration.

The related factors which lead to hypernatremia are:

- Deprivation of water, most common in those unable to perceive or respond to thirst
- Hypertonic tube feeding with inadequate water supplement
- Increased insensible water loss (as in hyperventilation)
- Ingestion of salt in unusual amounts
- Excessive parenteral administration of sodium-containing solution:
  - Hypertonic saline (3% or 5% NaCl)
  - 7.5% sodium bicarbonate
  - Isotonic saline
- Profuse sweating
- Diabetes insipidus
- Heat stroke
  - Drowning in sea water
- Hypernatremia also occurs when water losses of the body exceed sodium loss as that is seen in diabetes insipidus, marked glycosuria, hypercalcemia, hypokalemia, chronic renal failure, and recovery phase of acute renal failure
- Sodium excess may occur along with water excess when due to inadequate clearance of the kidneys both sodium and water accumulate in the extracellular space, leading to edema, for example, nephrotic syndrome, cardiac failure, nutritional or thiamine deficiency, cirrhosis of liver and in cases of usage of drugs such as corticosteroids, androgens, phenylbutazone, oral contraceptive and carbenoxelone.

It causes retention of sodium, increased volume of ECF and edema in the interstitial compartment.

The main characteristics of hypernatrema are:

- Thirst
- Elevated body temperature
- Tongue dry and swollen, sticky mucus membranes
- In severe hypernatremia:
  - Disorientation
  - Hallucinations
  - Lethargy when disturbed
  - Irritable and hyperreactive when stimulated
  - Focal or grand mal seizures, coma, low blood pressure, tachycardia.
- Serum sodium above 145 mEq/L
- Urinary specific gravity 0.015 provided water loss from non-renal route.

It may produce hyponatremia, hyperglycemia and shock as complication.

Treatment

Management of the condition calls for an immediate attention and treatment instituted within 24–48 hours can avoid occurrence of cerebral edema.

Mild cases are given IV influsion 5% dextrose solution. Other cases need restriction of water and salt by mouth. Management of the condition depends upon the underlying condition.

Diuretics and other measures are taken on the advice of the physician according to condition of patient.

Nursing Intervention

- Identify clients at risk of hypernatremia
- Monitor fluid losses and gains. Look for abnormal losses of water or low water intake, and for large gains of sodium as might occur with ingestion of proprietory drugs with high sodium content. And also consider that prescription drugs may have high sodium content. Of coruse, one should look for excessive intake of high sodium foods
- Monitor changes in behavior such as restlessnes, disorientation and lethargy
- Look for excessive thirst, and elevated body temperature. If present, evaluate in relation to other signs
- Monitor serum sodium level
- Prevent hyponatremia in debilitated clients unable to perceive or respond to thirst by offering them fluids at regular intervals. If fluids intake remains inadequate, consult the physician to plan an alternate route for intake, either by tube feedings or by the parenteral route
- If tube feedings are used, give sufficient water to keep the serum sodium and the BUN level within normal limits.

  Beware that the higher the osmolality of the feeding, the greater the need for water supplements.

Hypokalemia

Hypokalemia refers to a potassium deficit in ECF. When the extracellular potassium level falls, potassium moves from the cell, creating an intracellular potassium deficiency. Sodium and hydrogen ions are then retained by the cells to maintain isotonic fluids. These electrolyte shifts influence normal cellular functioning, the pH of ECF, and function of most of the body systems. Skeletal muscles are generally the first to demonstrate a potassium deficiency. It is a condition associated with depletion of potassium characterized by muscular weakness, leg cramps, apathy, mental confusion and paralysis.

The related factors leading to hypokalemia are:

- It develops from excessive loss of potassium in the urine and stool and from severe water depletion
- Potassium-losing diuretics, i.e. furosemide, thiazide, etc.
- Steroid administration
- Use of carbenicillin, sodium penicillin, amphotericin B
- Hyperaldosteronism
- Hyperalimentations
- Poor intake as in anorexia nervosa, alcoholism, potassium free parenteral fluids
- Osmotic diuresis (as occurs in uncontrolled diabetes mellitus or mannitol administration).

The main characteristics of hypokalemia are:

- Fatigue
- Anorexia, nausea and vomiting
- Muscle weakness
- Decreased bowel motility (intestinal ileus)—Paralytic ileus
- Cardiac arrhythmia
- Increased, i.e. sensitivity to digitalis
- Polyuria, nocturia, dilute urine (if hypokalemia prolonged).

Mild hyperglycemia

- Serum K below 3.5 mEq/L
- Paresthesias or tender muscles
- ECG changes: Fattened T waves, ST segment depressions
- Respiratory hyperventilation.

Treatment

Management of the condition requires adequate management of the underlying conditions.

Nursing Intervention

- Beware of clients at risk for hypokalemia and monitor for its occurrence
- Assess digitalized clients at risk for hypokalemia especially closely for symptoms of digitalis toxicity
- Take measures to prevent hypokalemia when possible
  - Prevention may take the form of encouraging extrapotassium intake for at-risk patient (when the diet allows)

  - When hypokalemia due to abuse of laxatives or diure-tics education of the client may help alleviate the problems.
- Administer oral potassium supplement when prescribed
- Be aware that clients may not need potassium supplements if they are using salt substitutes because these substances usually contains viable amounts of potassium
- Be thoroughly familiar with the critical facts related to administering potassium intravenously.

Hyperkalemia

Hyperkalemia refers to an excess of potassium in ECF. It is a condition with excess of potassium, characterized by conduction defect in the heart and myoneural junction of the muscle.

The related factors which lead to hyperkalemia are:

- Decreased potassium excretions as in
  - Oliguric renal failure
  - Potassium-conserving diuretic usage
  - Hypoaldosteronism
- High potassium intake, especially in presence of renal insufficiency:
  - Improper use of oral potassium supplements
  - Rapid excessive administration of IV potassium
  - High-dose potassium penicillin
  - Foods high in potassium (such as dried apricots)
- Shift of potassium out of cells due to acidosis, tissue trauma, and malignant cell lysis
- Potassium excess also occurs in acute renal failure, severe crush injuries and burns. Severe hemorrhages and adrenal insufficiency
- It is also seen in diabetic keto acidosis.

The main characteristics of hyperkalemia are:

- Vague muscular weakness is usually first sign
- Cardiac arrhythmias, bradycardia and heart block can occur
- Paresthesias of face, tongue, feet and hands
- Flaccid muscle paralysis (spreads from legs to trunk and arms, respiratory muscle may be affected)
- Gastrointestinal symptoms such as nausea, intermittent intestinal colic, or diarrhea may occur
- ECG changes tall, peaked T waves, absent P waves widened QRS complex
- Serum K, above 5.0 mEq/L (mmol/L).

It can produce cardiac arrest, metabolic acidosis and respiratory acidosis as complications.

Treatment

Management of the condition is done by replacement of water loss and correction of electrolyte imbalance. The client is given diet with restricted protein but with as much as fat and carbohydrate and also managing the underlying condition.

Nursing Intervention

- Beware of clients at risk for hyperkalemia and monitor for its occurrence. Hyperkalemia is life-threatening; it is imperative to detect it easily
- Take measures to prevent hyperkalemia when possible by following guidelines for administering potassium safely both intravenously or orally:
  - Follow rules for safe administration of potassium
  - Avoid administration of potassium conserving diuretics, potassium supplements or salt substitutes to client with renal insufficiency
  - Caution client to use salt substitute sparingly if they are taking other supplementary form of potassium or taking potassium-conserving diuretics (example, spironolactone, triamterene, and amiloride)
  - Caution hyperkalemic clients to avoid foods high in potassium content. Some of these are coffee, cocoa, tea, dried fruits, dried beans, wholegrain breads.

Hypocalcemia

Hypocalcemia refers to a calcium deficit in ECF. If the condition is prolonged calcium is taken from bones. This results in osteomalacia, which is characterized by soft and pliable bones. Common signs and symptoms for hypocalcemia include numbness and tingling of fingers, muscle, cramps and tetany.

The related factors leading to hypocalcemia are:

- Surgical hypoparathyroidism (may follow thyroid surgery or radical neck surgery for cancer)
- Malabsorption
- Vitamin D deficiency
- Acute pancreatitis
- Excessive administration of citrated blood
- Primary hypothyroidism
- Alkalotia states (decreased ionized calcium)
- Hyperphosphatemia
- Medullary carcinoma of thyroid
- Hypoalbuminemia (as in cirrhosis, nephrotic syndrome and starvation)
- Hypomagnesemia
- Decreased ultraviolet exposure.

The main characteristics of hypocalcemia will include:

- Numbness-tingling fingers, circumoral region and toes
- Cramps in the muscle of extremities
- Hyperactive deep tendon reflexes (such as patellar and triceps)
- Trousseau's sign
- Chvostek's sign
- Mental changes such as confusion and alteration in mood and memory

- Convulsions, usually generalized but may be focal
- Spasm of laryngeal muscles
- ECG shows prolonged QT interval
- Spasms of muscles in abdomen (can stimulate acute abdo-emergency)
- Total calcium level below 8.5 mg/dL or ionized level below normal (below 50%)
- Hypocalcemic state occurs when calcium loss occurs causing a fall in serum calcium level. This may eventually cause tetany and death
- It is usually asymptomatic and the neurological manifestation develop slowly
- It then gives rise to diffuse encephalopathy, depression and psychosis
- In severe cases there may be laryngiospasm and gen convulsion
- It may also give rise to papilledema and cataract.

Treatment

Most cases respond well to adequate or supplemented calcium and phosphorus. The patient may be given calcium carbonate, 2.52 to 3.78 g daily orally or calcium gluconate 0.5–1.5 g along with calciferol 15.45 µg daily orally. Otherwise, 10 mL of 10% calcium gluconate is given by slow IV. Adequate management and control of predisposing causes can prevent the occurrence of the condition.

Nursing Interventions

- Beware of clients at risk for hypocalcemia and monitor its occurrence
- Be prepared to take seizure-precautions
- Monitor condition of airway closely because laryngeal stridor can occur
- Take safety precautions if confusion is present
- Be aware of factors related to the safe administration of calcium replacement salts
- Educate people in high-risk groups for osteoporosis (especially postmenopausal women not on estrogen therapy). If adequate amounts are not consumed in the diet (as is often the case), calcium supplements should be considered
- Educate people at risk for osteoporosis about the value of regular physical exercise in decreasing bone loss
- To prevent osteoporosis in later years, educate young women about the need for a normal diet to ensure adequate calcium intake. Also discuss the calcium-losing aspects of alcohol and nicotine use.

Hypercalcemia

Hypercalcaemia refers to an excess of calcium in ECF. It presents an emergency situation because this condition often leads to cardiac arrest. It is a condition of excess of calcium and is characterized by polyuria, polydipsia, skeletal muscle weakness and hypertension.

The related factors that lead to hypercalcemia are:

- Hyperparathyroidism
- Malignant neoplastic disease
- Prolonged immobilization
- Large doses of vitamin D or intoxication
- Overuse of calcium containing antacids or calcium supplements thiazide diuretics
- Milk-alkali syndrome
- Sarcoidosis
- It is also seen in person with Paget's disease, myxedema, Addison's disease and osteoporosis in aged persons.

The common features of hypercalcemia are:

- Muscle weakness
- Tiredness, listlessness, lethargy
- Constipation
- Anorexia, nausea, and vomiting
- Decreased memory span, decreased attention span, and confusion
- Polyuria, and polydipsia
- Renal stones
- Neurobic behavior progressing to frank psychosis may occur (reversible with correction of hypercalcemia)
- Cardiac arrest may occur in hypercalcemic crisis
- ECG shows shortened QT interval
- Serum calcium over 10.5 mg/dL
- It may produce renal failure, shock and death in complication.

Treatment

In mild cases, adequate rehydration is often effective. Management of the condition also includes management of the underlying conditions. In other cases, intravenous infusion of isotonic saline is given to promote calciuria. Calcium is also eliminated or maintained in the lower level by giving sodium phosphate 1–2 g orally daily and client is encouraged to take more fluids.

Nursing Intervention

- Be aware of clients at risk for hypercalcemia and monitor its occurrence
- Increase client mobilization when feasible
- Encourage the oral intake of sufficient fluids to keep the client well hydrated
- Discourage excessive consumption of milk products and other high calcium foods
- Encourage adequate bulk in the diet to offset the tendency for constipation
- Take safety precautions if confusion or other mental symptoms by hypercalcemia are present

- Be aware that cardiac arrest can occur in clients with severe hypercalcemia be prepared to deal with this emergency
- Be aware that bones may fracture more easily in clients with chronic hypercalcemia because bone resorption has been excessive, weakening the bony structure. Transfer clients cautiously
- Educate home-bound oncology clients with a predisposition for hypercalcemia and their families, to be alert for symptoms that occur with this condition and to report them to the health care providers before they become severe
- Be alert for signs of digitalis toxicity when hypercalcemia occurs in digitalized clients
- Help prevent formation of calcium renal stones in clients with long-standing hypercalcemia or immobilization by:
  - Forcing fluids to maintain a dilute urine, thus avoiding supersaturation of precipitates
  - Encouraging fluids that yield an acid ash (prune or cranberry milk) because a urinary pH less than 6.5 favors calcium deposits
- Preventing urinary stasis by turning the immobilized client, elevating head of the bed and having the client sit up if this can be tolerated.

Hypomagnesemia

Magnesium is an important and plentiful cation and is essential for many enzymatic system associated with protein, carbohydrate and lipid metabolism.

Hypomagnesemia refers to magnesium deficit. It is condition of low plasma concentration of magnesium, characterized by neuromuscular and CNS hyperirritability.

The related factors which lead to hypomagnesemia are:

- Chronic alcoholism
- Intestinal malabsorption syndrome
- Diarrhea
- Nasogastric suction—prolonged
- Aggressive refeeding after starvation (as in TPN)
- Prolonged administration of magnesium-free IV fluids
- Uncontrolled diabetes mellitus—diabetic ketoacidosis
- Hyper aldosteronism
- Drugs-prolonged use of
  - Diuretics, aminoglycoside, antibiotics (e.g. gentamicin), cisplatin
  - Excessive dose of vitamin-D or calcium supplements
  - Citrate preservative in blood products
- Pancreatitis, thyrotoxicosis, hyperparathyroides
- Severe osteitis fibrosa, PEM.

The common characteristics of hypomagnesemia are:

- It presents with multiple metabolic and nutritional deficiency
- It gives rise to anorexia, lethargy, vomiting, weakness and tetany
- Neuromuscular irritability:
  - Increased reflex
  - Course tremors
  - Positive Chvostek's and Trousseau's signs
  - Convulsions
- Cardiac manifestations will include:
  - Trachyarrhythmias
  - Increased susceptibility to digitalis toxicity
  - ECG changes in severe cases. PR and QT interval prolongation, Widened QRS complex, ST segment depression and T-wave inversion
- Mental changes:
  - Disorientation in memory
  - Mood changes
  - Intense confusion
  - Hallucination
- Serum magnesium level below 1.3 mEq/L.

Treatment

Repletion of the cases are done through magnesium sulfate and chloride. It is customary to give double the amount required because half of magnesium given excreted by the kidneys. The repletion is done gradually and is given orally or intravenously. In severe cases, IV only.

Nursing Intervention

- Be aware client at risk for hypomagnesemia, especially closely for symptoms of digitalis toxicity because a deficit of magnesium predisposes to toxicity
- Be prepared to take seizure precautions when hypomagnesemia, especially closely for symptoms of digitalis toxicity, because a deficit of magnesium predisposes to toxicity
- Monitor condition of airway, because laryngeal stridor can occur
- Take safety precautions if confusion presents
- Be familiar with magnesium replacement salts and factors related to these safe administration
- Be aware that magnesium-depleted clients may experience difficulty in swallowing
- When magnesium deficit is due to abuse of diuretics in laxatives, educating the client may help alleviate problem
- Be aware that most commonly used IV fluids have either no magnesium or relatively small amount. When indicated, discuss the need for magnesium replacement with physicians
- For clients experiencing abnormal losses, but able to consume a general diet, encourage intake of magnesium, rich foods (such as green-leafy vegetables, nuts, legumes and fruits such as bananas, oranges, and grape fruits).

Hypermagnesemia

Hypermagnesaemia refers to a magnesium excess. It can occur especially in end stage renal failure. When kidneys fail to excrete magnesium and excessive amounts are administered therapeutically. It is a condition associated with excess of magnesium and is characterized by muscular weakness and ECG changes.

The related factors which lead to hypermagnesemia are:

- Renal failure (particularly when magnesium containing medication is administered)
- Adrenal insufficiency
- Excessive magnesium administration during treatment of eclampsia
- Hemodialysis with excessively hard water or with dialysate inadvertantly high in magnesium content.

Magnesium has a direct action on the myoneural junction. Its excess creates blockage causing impairment of neuromuscular transmission and that results in diminished excitability of the muscle cells.

The main characteristics of hypermagnesemia are:

- Early signs (serum level of mg of 3 to 5 mEq/L)
  - Flushing and a sense of skin warmth (due to peripheral vasodilation)
  - Hypotension (due to blockage of sympathetic ganglia as well as to direct effect on smooth muscle)
- Depressed respiration
- Drowsiness, hyoactive reflexes and muscular weakness
- Cardiac abnormalities—cardiac arrest may develop
- Weak or absent cry in newborn
- ECG shows prolonged PR interval, widened QRS complex and elevated T-wave amplitude
- Elevated serum magnesium level.

Treatment

In severe cases and also in other cases cardiac and respiratory support are given by IV injection of 10–20 mL of 10% calcium gluconate maintenance of adequate hydration is essential. The client is also given furosemide by IV injection to promote excretion of magnesium. In more severe cases hemodialysis is done.

Nursing Intervention

- Be aware of client at risk for hypermagnesemia and assess for its presence. When it is suspected assess the following parameters:
  - Vital signs: Look for low blood pressure and shallow respirations with periods of apnea
  - level of consciousness: Look for drowsiness, lethargy and coma
- Do not give magnesium containing medication to clients with renal failure or compromised renal function
- Be particularly careful in following 'standing order' for bowel preparation for X-ray because some of these include the use of magnesium citrate
- Caution clients with renal disease to check with their health care providers before taking over the counter-medication
- Be aware of factors related to safe parenteral administration of magnesium salts.

Hypophosphatemia

Hypophosphatemia refers to a below-normal serum concentration of inorganic phosphorous. It is a clinical manifestation of phosphate depletion, characterized by progressive encephalopathy and osteomalacia.

The related factors which lead to hypophosphatemia are:

- Inadequate intake or absorption of phsophorous - malabsorption
- It is associated with vomiting and diarrhea
- Prolonged ingestion of aluminium hydroxide or bicarbonate
- It is also seen in:
  - Prolonged use of glucose insulin, fructose, administrations
  - Refeeding after starvation
  - Hyperalimentation
  - Alcohol withdrawal
  - Diabetic ketoacidosis
  - Respiratory alkalosis
  - Phosphate-binding antacids use
  - Recovery phase after severe burns
  - Use of anabolic steroids
  - Chronic hemodialysis.

The main characteristics of hypophosphatemia are:

- Progressive encephalopathy
- Paresthesias
- Muscle weakness
- Muscle pain and tenderness
- Mental changes, such as apprehension, confusion, delirium coma
- Cardiomyopathy
- Acute respiratory failure
- Seizures
- Decreased tissue oxygenation
- Joint stiffness
- Serum phosphate below 2.5 mg/dL
- Phosphate compounds are present in all normal foods and are essential for metabolism of carbohydrate, protein and fat. They are also responsible for changes, transfer, or depletion occurs from prolonged negative phosphate balance and form chronic malnutrition.

Treatments

Management of the condition includes treatment of the underlying cause, repletion of phosphate, and maintenance of body fluids.

Nursing Intervention

- Identify clients at risk for hypophosphatemia;
  - Severely malnourished clients
  - Alcoholic clients
  - Clients with diabetic ketoacidosis
- Monitor clients at risk for the presence of hypophosphatemia
- Be aware that severely hypophosphatemic clients are thought to be greater risk for infection because of changes in WBCs
- Administer IV phosphate products cautiously
- Be aware that in adults the usual maintenance dose of phosphorous is 10 to 15 mmol/L of TPN solution
- Be aware of the need to introduce hyperalimentation gradually in clients who are malnourished
- Because it is possible to give too much phosphorous when administering phosphate solutions, moniter for signs of hyperphosphatemia and of the salt in which it is administered
- Monitor for diarrhea in clients taking oral phosphorus supplements; consult physician if it persists or is severe
- Mispowdered oral phosphorus supplements with chilled or ice water to make them more palatable.

Hyperphosphatemia

Hyperphosphatemia refers to above-normal serum concentrations of inorganic phosphorous. It is a condition associated with increased level of phosphate and is characterized by hypocalcemia.

The related factors which lead to hyperphosphatemia are:

- Excessive intake of phosphatemia
- Excessive intake of phosphate
- Hypervitaminosis D: Large vitamin D intake
- Acute renal failure
- Chronic renal insufficiency
- Chemotherapy: Particularly for acute lymphoblastic leukemia and lymphoma
- Large intake of milk
- Use of cow's milk in infants
- Excessive intake of phosphate containing laxatives
- Overzealous administration of phosphorous-supplements (oral or IV)
- Excessive use of Fleets Phosphosoda as enema solution particularly in children and people with slow bowel elimination
- Hypoparathyroidism
- Hyperthyroidism.

The main characteristics of hyperphosphatemia are:

- This condition by itself does not give rise to any symptoms but manifested with that of hypocalcemia which includes:
  - Short-term consequences: Symptoms of tetany, such as tingling of fingertips and around mouth, numbness and muscle spasms
  - Long-term consequences: Precipitation of calcium phosphate in non-osseous sites; such as kidneys joints, arteries, skin or cornea
  - Serum phosphate above 4.5 mg/dL.

Treatment

Management of the condition requires correction of underlying condition.

Nursing Intervention

- Identify clients at risk for hyperphosphatemia
- Monitor signs of tetanus and other features of hypocalcemia
- Be aware that soft-tissue calcification can be long-term complication of a chemically-elevated serum phosphate level. Calcification may occur in site such as kidney, arteries, joints
- Administer prescribed oral or IV phosphate supplements cautiously and monitor serum phosphorous levels periodically during their use
- When appropriate, instruct clients that use of phosphate, containing laxatives may result in acute phosphate poisoning
- Beware that phosphate containing enema can result in hyperphosphatemia if used injudiciously, particularly in children and those with slow bowel emptying, instruct clints accordingly
- When low-phosphorus diet is prescribed, instruct clients to avoid foods high in phosphorous content. Such foods include hard cheese or cream, nuts and nut products; whole grain cereals (e.g. bran and oatmeal) dried fruits, dried vegetables; special meats such as kidneys, sardines, and sweet breads and desserts made with milk.

ACID-BASE IMBALANCES

Arterial blood gases (ABGs) are most commonly used to assess and treat acid-base imbalances. Results from venous, blood are only specific for particular extremity or area where the blood was sampled and do not provide information on how well the lungs oxygenating the blood. The pH of plasma indicates balance or impending acidosis or alkalosis. In addition however, a study of the blood oxygen and carbon dioxide gases is important. The partial pressure (indicated by 'p') of these gases, or their tensions are determined by the use of a nomogram, which reflects the chemical and physical activities of two gases. The partial pressure of carbon dioxide $PaCO_2$; for oxygen, it is PaO_2. The "a" indicates an arterial specimen. When the PaO_2 is low, hemoglobin carries less than normal amounts of oxygen, when the PaO_2 is high, the hemoglobin carries more oxygen, oxygen saturation readings (SaO_2) reveal the percentage of O_2 in the blood that combines with hemoglobin. The $PaCO_2$ is influenced almost entirely by respiratory activity. When $PaCO_2$ is low, carbonic acid leaves the body in excessive amounts; When the $PaCO_2$ is high, there are excessive amounts of carbonic acid in the body.

Acid-base imbalance occurs when the carbonic acid or bicarbonate levels become disproportionate. When there is a single primary cause, these disturbances are known as respiratory acidosis or alkalosis and metabolic acidosis or alkalosis. These disturbances are a result of an upset in acid-base balance, as follows:

- Respiratory disturbance alters carbonic acid portion:
  - Respiratory acidosis and alkalosis are the results of respiratory disturbances
  - Compensation occurs to resolve balance in the kidneys by either conserving or excreting more bicarbonate.
- A metabolic disturbance alters the bicarbonate portion.
  - Metabolic acidosis and alkalosis are almost entirely the result of metabolic processes
  - The primary organs for compensation to restore balance are lungs, which either try to conserve or excrete more CO_2 which is available in weakly ionized carbonic acid.

The brief description of management of acid-base imbalances are as follows:

Respiratory Acidosis (Carbonic Acid Excess)

Respiratory acidosis is primary excess of carbonic acid in ECF. Any decrease in alveolar ventilations that result in retention of CO_2 can cause respiratory acidosis. Because the lungs are the source of the problem, they are unable to participate in compensation. As the carbonic acid content increases, the kidney attempts to retain more bicarbonate and increase their hydrogen excretion. It is a clinical state of altered hydrogen excretion. It is a clinical state of altered hydrogen ion concentration characterized by hypoventilation.

RA = high $PaCO_2$ because of alveolar hypoventilations.

The related factors for respiratory acidosis (RA) are:

- Acute respiratory acidosis:
  - Acute pulmonary edema
  - Aspiration of a foreign body
  - Atelectasis
  - Pneumothorax, hemothorax
  - Overdose of sedatives or anesthetic
  - Position on operative room table that interferes with respiration
  - Cardiac arrest
  - Severe pneumonia
  - Laryngospasm
  - Mechanical ventilation improperly regulated
  - Chronic respiratory acidosis
  - Emphysema
  - Cystic fibrosis
  - Advanced multiple sclerosis
  - Bronchiectasis
  - Bronchial asthma.
- Factors favoring hypoventilation:
  - Obesity
  - Tight abdominal binders and dressings
  - Postoperative pain (as in high abdominal or chest incisions)
  - Abdominal distention from cirrhosis or bowel obstruction.

The main characteristics of respiratory acidosis are:

i. Acute respiratory acidosis:
   - Mental cloudiness
     - Ventricular fibrillation may be first sign in anesthetized patient (related to hypokalemia)
   - Dizziness
   - Palpitations
   - Muscular twitching
   - Convulsions
   - Warm flushed skin
   - Unconsciousness
   - Arterial blood gases (ABGs)
     - pH below 7.35
     - $PaCO_2$ over 45 mm Hg (primary)
     - HCO_3^- normal or only slightly elevated.

ii. Chronic respiratory acidosis:
   - Weakness
   - Dull headache
   - Symptoms underlying disease process
   - ABGs
     - pH below 7.35 or within lower limits of normal.
     - $PaCO_2$ over 4.5 mm Hg (primary)
     - HCO_3^- over 26 mEq/L (compensatory).

Treatment

Administer respiratory stimulants, i.e. Nikethamide 2–4 mL of 25% solution by IV repeated every 1 or 2 hours and treating the underlying condition.

Nursing Intervention

- Treatment is directed at improving ventilation; exact measures vary with the cause of inadequate ventilation
- Pharmacological agents are used as indicated. For example, bronchodilators help reduce bronchial spasm; antigiotic for infection
- Pulmonary hygienic measures are used when necessary to rid the respiratory tract of mucus and purulent drainage
- Adequate hydration (2 to 3 L/day) is indicated to keep mucous membranes moist and thereby facilitate removal of secretions. Supplemental oxygen is used as necessary
- A mechanical respirator, used cautiously, may improve the pulmonary ventilation. One must remember that overzealous use of a mechanical respirator may cause rapid excretion of CO_2 that the kidneys will be unable to eliminate excess

bicarbonate with sufficient rapidity to prevent alkalosis and convulsion. For this reason the elevated $PaCO_2$ must be decreased slowly.

Respiratory Alkalosis (Carbonic Acid Deficit)

Respiratory alkalosis is a primary deficit of carbonic acid in ECF. It is the result of the increased alveolar ventilation and therefore, a decrease in CO_2. An increase in respiratory rate and depth causes the CO_2 loss because the CO_2 is excreted faster than normal. Because of the deficit of the CO_2, which is a respiratory stimulant sensed in the medulla of the brain. Depression of cessation of respiration eventually can occur. Because the lungs are the source of the problem, they are unable to participate in compensation. Therefore, kidneys attempt to alleviate the imbalance by increasing bicarbonate excretion and by retaining more hydrogen. Respiratory alkalosis = Low $PaCO_2$ because of alveolar hyperventilation.

It is a clinical disorder of altered hydrogen's ion concentration that is developing from hyperventilation.

The related factors which lead to respiratory alkalosis are:

- Extreme anxiety (most common cause)
- Hypoxemia
- High fever
- Early salicylate intoxication (stimulates respiratory center)
- Gram-negative bacteremia
- CNS lesions involving respiratory center, meningitis, encephalitis
- Pulmonary emboli, pneumonia
- Thyrotoxicosis
- Excessive ventilation by mechanical ventilators
- Pregnancy (high progesterone level sensitizes the respiratory center to CO_2 : Physiologic).

The main characteristics of respiratory alkalosis are:

- The condition presents with anxiety
- Light-headedness (a low $PaCO_2$ causes cerebral vasoconstrictions and thus decreased cerebral blood flow)
- Respiratory symptoms—frequent, deep-sighing, or rapid and deep breathing
- Hyperventilation syndrome, i.e. tinnitus, palpitations, sweating, dry mouth, tremulousness, precordial pain (tightness) nausea and vomiting, epigastric pain, blurred vision, convulsions and loss of consciousness
- ABGs
  - pH over 7.45
  - $PaCO_2$ below 35 mm Hg (primary)
  - HCO_3- under 22 mEq/L (compensatory).

Treatment

Treatment is given by correction of underlying causes.

Nursing Intervention

- If the cause of respiratory alkalosis is anxiety, the client should be made aware that the abnormal breathing practice is responsible for the symptoms accompanying this condition
- Instruct the client to breathe more slowly (to cause accumulation of CO_2) or to breathe in closed system (such as paper bag)
- Usually sedative is required to relieve ventilation in very anxious patients (if alkalosis severe enough to cause fainting, the increased ventilation ceases and respiration reverts to normal)
- Treatment for other causes of respiratory alkalosis is directed at correcting for the underlying problem.

Metabolic Acidosis (Base Bicarbonate Deficit)

Metabolic acidosis is a proportionate deficit of bicarbonate in ECF. The deficit can occur as the remit of an increase in acid components or an excessive loss of bicarbonate. The lungs attempt to increase the CO_2 excretion by increasing the rate and depth of respirations. The kidneys attempt to compensate by retaining bicarbonate and by excreting more hydrogen. If the body is unable to achieve normal balance, the person may lose consciousness as metabolic acidosis increases and death eventually results. Thus

Metabolic acidosis = Low bicarbonate, non-volatile acid present, use of HCO_3^- in disproportionate amounts.

It is a condition of hydrogen ion concentration characterized by rise of hydrogen ion and reduction in plasma bicarbonate level.

The related factors which lead to metabolic acidosis are:

- Normal anion gap related to:
  - Diarrhea
  - Intestinal fistulas
  - Ureter sigmoidostomy
  - Hyperalimentation-vomiting excessively
  - Acidifying drugs (such as ammonium chloride)
  - Renal tubular acidosis (RTA).
- High anion gap related to:
  - Diabetic ketoacidosis
  - Starvational ketoacidosis
  - Lactic acidosis
  - Renal failure
  - Ingestion of toxins (such as salicylates, ethylene glycol, and methanol)
  - Acute alcoholic.

The main characteristics of metabolic acidosis are:

- Headache, confusion, drowsiness
- Increased respiratory rate and depth (may not become clinically evident until HCO_3^- is quite low)
- Nausea and vomiting

- Peripheral vasodilation (may be present, causing warm flushed skin)
- Decreased cardiac output when pH below 7. Bradycardia may be present
- ABGs
  - Fall in pH below 7.35
  - HCO_3^- under 22 mEq/L (primary)
  - $PaCO_2$ under 35 mm Hg (compensatory by lungs)
  - Base excess always negative.
- Hypokalemia frequently present
- Hyperpnea - Kussmaul's respiration
- It eventually produces circulatory shock in complication.

Management

Salt and water repletion, and treating underlying conditions treatment is directed towards correcting the metabolic defect. If the cause of the problem is excessive intake of chloride, treatment obviously focuses on eliminating the source, when necessary, bicarbonate is administered.

Control of the condition requires avoidance of an adequate management of the conditions which gives rise to the condition.

Nursing Intervention

Metabolic alkalosis (base bicarbonate excess)

Metabolic alkalosis is a primary excess of bicarbonate in ECF. This may be the result of excessive acid losses or increased base ingestion or retention. The body attemtps to compensate by retaining CO_2. The respirations become slow and shallow, amid periods of breathing may occur. The kidneys attempt to excrete potassium and sodium with the excessive bicarbonate, and retain hydrogen in carbonic acid. Thus:

Metabolic alkalosis = High bicarbonate (non-volatile acid is lost and it is not using up HCO_3^- or HCO_3^- gained is disproportionate amount).

It is a disorder of hydrogen ion concentration disturbance characterized by hypocalcemia and hypokalemia.

The related factors which lead to metabolic alkalosis are:

- Vomiting or gastric suction
- Hypokalemia
- Hyperaldosteronism
- Cushing's syndrome
- Potassium losing diuretics (e.g. thiazide, furosemide, ethacrynic acid)
- Alkali ingestion (bicarbonate containing antacids)
- Parenteral $NaHCO_3$ administration for cardiopulmonary resuscitation
- Abrupt relief of chronic respiratory acidosis.

The main characteristics of metabolic alkaloids are:

- Irritation and neuromuscular excitation
- Those related to decreased calcium ionization are:
  - Dizziness, tingling of fingers and toes, circumoral paresthesia, carpopedal spasm, hypertonic muscles.
- Depressed respiration (compensatory action by lungs)
- ABGs
  - pH above 7.45, bicarbonate over 26 mEq/L,
  - $PaCO_2$ over 45 mm Hg (compensatory)
  - Base excess always possible.
- Hypokalemia often present
- Serum chloride relatively lower than Na.

Treatment

Correction of the underlying cause is essential for proper management of condition. Treatment is aimed at reversal of the underlying disorder. Sufficient chloride must be supplied to the kidney to absorb sodium with chloride (allowing the excretion of excessive bicarbonate).

Treatment also includes restoration of normal fluid volume by administration of sodium chloride fluids because continued volume depletion serves to maintain the alkalosis.

Nurses wishing to be a role model of self-care behaviors that promote fluid, electrolyte, and acid-base balance should meet the following goals:

The nurse will:

- Daily ingest the quantity and type of fluids (to include six to eight glasses of water) that promote healthy hydration and urinary functioning
- Evaluate use of food diets, diuretics, laxatives, and alcohol, identifying potential risks to health
- Identify situations of high risk for fluid and electrolyte imbalance and intervene appropriately.

CHAPTER

4

Human Genetics and Genomic Nursing

INTRODUCTION

Genomics is the branch of molecular biology concerned with the structure function, evolution, and mapping of genomes. Genotype is the genetic constitution of an individual organism. Genomic is the complete set of genetic material of an organism.

The term 'genetics' has been derived from Greek word "gene" which means "to grow into" or "to become", "Gene" is a unit of heredity, which is transferred from a parent to offspring and is held to determine some characteristics of offspring, in particular, a distinct sequence of DNA forming part of chromosome. The terms 'Genetic' was introduced by **Bateson** in 1906.

Genetic is the scientific study of heredity in which it deals with how specific traits or predispositional one transmitted from parents to offspring. 'Genome' is the total genetic compliment of an individual genotype. Genotype is the genes and variations there in than a person inherits from his or her parents. "Genomics" is the study of human genome including gene sequencing mapping, and function.

Human genetics is the study of the human condition as it is influenced by inherited factors that affect and determine growth and development and that can be transmitted from generation to generation. Furthermore, genetic factors extend beyond the limited view of solely distinct genetic syndromes to encompass influences on health, the occurrence of complex disorders, individual biologic responses to illness, potential treatment and medical management approaches, and strategies for prevention or cure.

Advances in genetic science raise questions as to what is normal and abnormal, when variation is called disease; and when variation should be treated, prevented, or both. Cultural perspectives on when to consider a variation a disease are a source of potential conflict among population group in a diverse world. As knowledge of human variation increases care must be taken to ensure that human rights are not violated.

This tremendous realization is readily apparent through the accomplishments of the Human Genome Project (HGP). One significant goal is to identify the 50,000 to 100,000 human genes. These advances and the associated knowledge will continue to significantly impact the delivery of health care and nursing practice. Genetic evaluations, screening, testing, guided treatment, family counseling, and related legal, ethical, and psychosocial issues will become daily practice for nurses.

Human genome discoveries have ushered in a new era of medicine, genomic medicine, which recognizes that multiple genes work in concert with environmental influences to cause disease. Genomic medicine aims to improve predictions about a persons susceptibility to diseases; the time of onset, extent and eventual severity of diseases; and the treatments or medications likely to be most effective or most harmful. New gene-based strategies for disease detection, management, and treatment have been created, allowing health professionals to tailor care to a person's particular genetic makeup.

Genomic nursing will be a challenging of nursing, in which nurses study and recognize the pattern of inheritance, understand the new technologies of testing and management of gene-based health care services, and applying genetic principles in respective clinical areas of nursing for assessment. diagnosis, planning and intervention of genetic related health needs of the client.

To meet the challenges of genomic nursing, nurses must understand the new technologies and treatments of gene-based health care. Nurses also must recognize that they are a vital link between the patient and health care services; patients often turn to nurses first with questions about a family history of risk factors, genetics information, and genetic tests and interpretations. The incorporation of genetics into nursing means bringing a genetic framework to health assessments, planning, and interventions that supports identification of and response to the changing genetics-related health needs of people.

When obtaining family and health histories, nurses must learn to recognize patterns of inheritance and understand when it is appropriate to consider new gene-based testing and treatment options. The clinical application of genetics principles in medical and surgical nursing, outlines the nurses role in genetic counseling and evaluation, addresses important ethical issues, and provides genetics resources for nurses and patients.

SCOPE OF GENOMIC NURSING

Now genetics is called the new central science of health care. Knowledge about molecular biology is necessary for future health care professionals to understand innovations in diagnosis, treatment and prevention of disease based on genetic information. Nursing with its tradition of holistic care, offers a unique contribution to patients and family trying to make sense of new genetic information for making health decisions. Because nurses serve people throughout the lifespan and across setting, they are in key position to integrate knowledge of genetics influences into health care.

The unique contribution of nursing to genomic medicine is its philosophy of holism. Nurses are ideally positioned to incorporate genetics into the care of patients at all ages and stages of life and in all settings. The holistic view that characterizes nursing takes into account each person's intellectual, physical, spiritual, social, cultural, biopsychologic, ethical and esthetic experiences while addressing genetic information, gene-based testing, diagnosis, and treatment. Thus, knowledge of genetics is basic to nursing practice.

Integrating genetics into nursing practice includes a philosophy of care that recognizes when genetic factors are playing a role or could play a role in a person's health. This means using family history and the results of genetic tests effectively, informing patients about genetics concepts, understanding the personal and societal impact of genetics information, and valuing the privacy and confidentiality of genetics information.

A person's responses to genetics information, genetic testing, or genetics-related conditions may be either empowering or disabling. Genetics information may stigmatize people if it affects how they view themselves or how others view them. Nurses can help individuals and families learn how genetic traits and conditions are passed on within families and how genetic and environmental factors influence health and disease.

Nurses facilitate communication among family members, the health care system, and community resources, and they offer valuable support by virtue of their continuity of care with patients and families. All nurses should be able to recognize when a patient is asking a question related to genetics information and should know how to obtain genetics information by gathering family and health histories and conducting physical and developmental assessments. Being able to recognize a genetics concern allows nurses to provide appropriate genetics resources and support to patients and families.

Essential to a genetic in nursing is the awareness of one's attitudes, experience, and assumptions about genetics concepts and how these are manifested in one's own practice.

The information from HGP about the 3 billion base pairs of the human genome will open the possibility of changes in every aspect of biology and medicine and have a major impact on health care in the future. Much effort is being focused on identifying gene variations. Although as a human species we are 99.9% alike, it may be the 0.1% variation that will help us understand the genetic risk for illnesses. It is hoped that treatment strategies can be devised that are specific to an individuals disease mutation. Another new field of study created by the HGP is the study of how inheritance affects the body's responses to drugs, called *pharmacogenetics*. The hope is that better, safer, and in some cases more powerful drugs can be developed. The information from HGP may influence more areas than we can currently imagine. Because of this, it has focused on issues such as genetic discrimination, privacy, and education. It will continue to look at new issues generated by information about our human genome.

Nurses will increasingly be faced with interpreting genetic information in client histories and diagnostic testing, and with assuming responsibility for protecting client privacy. To better counsel families and to participate likely problems, the nurses needs a fundamental understanding of the principles of genetics and the importance of heredity and the parental environment as etiologic factors in diseases and disorders of childhood. **Key terms for understanding genetics are defined as given below:**

Allele: Any one of two or more alternate forms of a gene at the same location. An allele for each gene is inherited from each parent. Alternative forms of a gene occupying same locus on homologous chromosomes.

Association: Nonrandom cluster of malformations without a specific etiology (e.g. CHARGE or VATER association).

Autosome: Chromosome other than a sex (X or Y) chromosome; in normal human cells there are 22 pairs of autosomes and 2 sex chrosomes.

Carrier: Person who possesses one copy of affected gene and one copy of unaffected gene and is clinically unaffected; however, may have clinically affected offspring because of expansion of mutation, X-linked expression, or recessive paring with the another.

Chromosome aberration: Addition, loss, or structural abnormality of a chrosome; detectable by cytogenetic analysis.

Congenital: Condition present at birth, although may not be apparent; causes may be genetic, nongenetic, environmental, or multifactorial.

Cytogenetics: Study of relationship of microscopic appearance of chrosome and their behavior during cell division to genotype and phenotype of individual.

Deformation: Fetal abnormalities due to extrinsic factors (e.g. uterine position); may also show subsequent defects.

Deoxyribonucleic acid (DNA): Two-stranded molecule that contains the genes or blueprints responsible for the structure and function of living organisms and allows the transmission of genetic information from one generation to the next.

Nuclear DNA (nDNA): Located in the nucleus of the cell; it contains blueprints for the cells that make up the body.

Mitochondrial DNA (mtDNA): Located in the mitochondria or powerhouse of each cell.

Diploid: The number of chromosomes normally present in somatic cells. For humans, that number is 46.

Dominant: A genetic trait that is normally expressed when a person has a gene mutation on one of a pair of chromosomes and the "normal" form of the gene is on the other chromosome.

FISH analysis: Fluorescent in suit hybridization (FISH), a process by which chromosomes or portions of chromosomes are painted with fluorescent molecules; technique is useful for identifying chromosomal microdeletions.

Gamete: One of two cells produced by a gametocyte, male (spermatozoon) and female (ovum), whose union in sexual reproduction initiates development of a new individual.

Genes: Genetic material (DNA) responsible for programming body's physiologic functions and characteristics.

Genome: Complete genetic information of an organism, usually described as total number of base pairs, human genome contains 3 billions base pairs.

Genotype: Genetic constitution that determines the physical and chemical characteristics of an individual.

Germ cell: Sperm or ovum with DNA complement of 23 unpaired chromosomes.

Genetics: The scientific study of heredity; how specific traits or predispositions are transmitted from parents to offspring.

Genome: The total genetic complement of an individual genotype.

Genomics: The study of the human genome, including gene sequencing, mapping and function.

Genotype: The genes and the variations therein that a person inherits from his or her parents.

Haploid: The number of chromosomes present in egg or sperm (gametes); in humans, this is 23.

Human genome project: An international research effort aimed at identifying and characterizing the order of every base in the human genome.

Human genome project: International research project to map each human gene and sequence the human genome.

Imprinting: Phenomenon in which an allele at a given locus is altered or inactivated, depending on whether it is inherited from mother or father; implies a functional difference in genes inherited from the two parents and explains some variation in expression.

Inherited (heritable, hereditary): Genetic transmission of a particular quality or trait from parent to offspring.

Malformation: Morphogenic defect of organ, part of organ, or larger region of the body resulting from intrinsically abnormal developmental process.

Major malformation: Structural abnormality with serious medical, surgical, or cosmetic consequences.

Minor malformation: Has no serious consequences or is normal variation (e.g., extra nipple or umbilical hernia).

Meiosis: Cell division that results in reproductive cells (gametes) containing a complement of 23 unpaired chromosomes.

Meiosis: The reduction division of diploid egg or sperm (germ cells) resulting in haploid gametes (having 23 chromosomes each).

Mitosis: Cell division occurring in somatic cells that normally results in daughter cells with the same number of chromosomes - 46 (diploid).

Mitosis: Cell division resulting in two daughter cells identical to parent cell in chromosome complement (23 pairs) and genetic information.

Monosomy: Missing one of a chromosome pair in normally diploid cells (For example, 45, X females have only one X chromosome).

Mutation: A heritable alteration in the genetic material.

Nondisjunction: The failure of a chromosome pair to separate appropriately during meiosis, resulting in abnormal chromosome numbers in reproductive cells (gametes).

Mitochondrion: Part of the cell that is responsible for converting nutrients into energy as well as many other specialized tasks; own separate and unique DNA; mtDNA is inherited exclusively from the mother.

Monogenetic: Genetic disease caused by single-gene mutation.

Monosomy: Chromosome abnormality in which one chromosome of a pair is missing; most monosomies are nonviable.

Mosaicism: Condition in which an individual harbors two or more genetically distinct cell lines (generally, one cell line is normal and one is abnormal); results from a genetic change after formation of a zygote (i.e. postzygotic event).

Multifactorial: Complex interaction of both genetic and environmental factors that produces an effect on individual.

Mutation: Structural or chemical alteration in genetic material that when changed remains changed and is transmitted to future generations; usually occurs naturally **(spontaneous)**, or can be **induced** by a variety of external agents, or **mutagens**, including temperature, certain chemicals, and radiation.

Mutation: **Hereditary** changes in genetic material; can be either change in single gene or change in chromosome characteristics, gene mutations can be passed from parent to offspring or can be new mutation in an individual, which is then heritable in offspring.

Nondisjunction: Failure of two chromatids or two homologous chromosomes to separate during cell division, so that both members of a pair pass to new cell, resulting in trisomy of that chromosome pair, or monosomy in cell that does not receive chromosome.

Pedigree: Diagram of genetic family tree.

Penetrance: Frequency with which a heritable trait is manifested in individuals carrying gene.

Phenotype: Clinically exhibited physical or chemical characteristics of individual; produced by interaction of environment with genotype.

Polygenic: Inheritance involving many genes at separate loci whose combined, additive effects produce a given phenotype.

Polymorphism: A genetic variation with two or more alleles that is maintained in a population.

Population screening: The application of a test or inquiry to a group to determine if persons in the group have an increased likelihood of a genetic condition or a mutation in a specific gene (e.g. cholesterol screening for hypercholesterolemia).

Predisposition testing: Testing that is used to determine the likelihood that a healthy person with or without a family history of a condition will develop the disorder. Having the gene mutation would indicate that the person has an increased susceptibility to the disorder, but this is not a diagnosis. One example is DNA mutation testing for hereditary breast/ovarian cancer.

Prenatal screening: Testing that is used to identify whether a fetus is at risk for a birth defect such as Down syndrome or spina bifida (e.g. multiple marker maternal serum screening in pregnancy).

Presymptomatic testing: Genetic testing that is used to determine whether persons with a family history of a disorder, but no current symptoms, have the gene mutation. An example of this would be Huntington's disease.

Proband (index case): Affected individual (regardless of sex) through whom family comes to attention of investigator.

Recessive: Refers to a gene that produces its effect (is expressed) only when it is present in homozygous state.

Recessive: A genetic trait that is expressed only when a person has two copies of a mutant autosomal gene or a single copy of a mutant X-linked gene in the absence of another X-chromosome.

Somatic cell: Body tissue cells with DNA complement of 46 chromosomes.

Sporadic: Birth defect or disorder occurring as a new case in a family and not inherited.

Syndrome: Recognized pattern of malformations with a single, specific etiology (e.g. Down syndrome).

Translocation: Transfer of all part of a chromosome to a different chromosome following chromosome breakage; can be balanced, producing no phenotypic effects, or unbalanced, producing severe or lethal effects.

Transcription: The process of transforming information from DNA into new strands of messenger RNA.

Trisomy: Condition in which there are three, rather than two, copies of one chromosome in same cell.

Trisomy: The presence of one extra chromosome in an otherwise diploid chromosome complement—for example, trisomy 21 (Down syndrome).

Variable expression: Variation in the degree to which a trait is manifested; clinical severity.

X-linked: Located on the X chromosomes.

X-inactivation (Lyon hypothesis): In normal female most of genes on one of X chromosomes are inactivated during early embryonic development, such that alleles on active chromosome are allowed full expression.

X-linked: Refers to gene located on X-chromosome and to specific mode of inheritance of such genes.

Zygote: Conjugation of male and female gametes.

HEREDITY IN HEALTH PROBLEMS

Scientists and philosophers have long speculated about heredity and developed theories to explain how traits are transmitted to offspring. Developments in technology and research have increased understanding of genetics, resulting in better understanding of relatively rare diseases such as phenylketonuria (PKU) or hemophilia that are related to mutations of a single gene inherited in families. New technologies and tools allow scientist to characterize inherited metabolic variations that interact over time and lead to common diseases such as cancer, heart disease, and dementia. This transition from genetics to genomics highlights how understanding of single genes and their individual functions has evolved to understanding how multiple genes act and control biologic processes. Most health conditions are now believed to be the result of a combination of genetic and environmental influences.

Contained within the nucleus of every somatic cell in the human body are approximately 35,000–70,000 genes, the genetic material responsible for programming the body's physiologic process and characteristics. These genes are composed of segments of DNA (deoxyribonucleic acid) and are organized into structures called chromosomes, which are visible only during certain stages of cell division. Alterations of a whole chromosome, a part of a chromosome, or even a single gene can manifest as a genetic disorder. Important to this concept is that this alteration or mutation may have been passed from one or both parents and previous generations, or it may be a new alteration in that individual. It is misleading to regard all genetic disorders as having been "passed through the family".

There is probably a genetic component in all disease processes. In some disorders the genetic defect is known; in others the precise nature of the genetic component is more obscure. In some the disorder is apparent at birth; in others the manifestations do not appear for weeks, months, or years (Table 4.1). Some diseases and disorders are determined by the genetic constitution of the individual, such as muscular dystrophy, Marfan's syndrome, and Down syndrome. Other diseases, although genetically determined, do not become clinically apparent until environmental factors precipitate the onset of symptoms. For instance, phenylketonuria is a disorder in which the enzyme to metabolize the protein phenylalanine is lacking. Deleterious effects in the infant are exhibited subsequent to sufficient ingestion of phenylalanine—containing substances, such as milk. Also, the acute symptoms of sickle cell disease are precipitated by certain conditions such as lowered oxygen tension, infection or dehydration.

Another area in which this interplay of genetic and environmental factors is being investigated is cancer genetics. All cancer is genetic in the sense that cancer cells result from a "sporadic" gene malfunction (acquired mutation). However, only 5 to 10% of all cancers are inherited, which means the gene mutation that pre-disposes to cancer development was present in the germline. Therefore the individual is prone to cancerous development much earlier in life.

TABLE 4.1: Characteristic age of onset for manifestations of some genetic disease

Age of onset	Condition
Lethal during prenatal life	Some chromosome aberrations Some gross malformations
Birth	Congenital malformations Chromosome aberrations (e.g. Down's syndrome) Some forms of adrenogenital syndrome Some forms of deafness
Soon after birth	Phenylketonuria Galactosemia Cystic fibrosis (sometimes) Maple-syrup urine disease
Infancy	Sickle cell anemia (sometimes later) Tay-Sach's disease Werding-Hoffman's disease
Early childhood	Cystic fibrosis Duchenne muscular dystrophy Fragile X-syndrome
Near puberty	Limb-girdle muscular dystrophy Some forms of adrenogenital syndrome Turner's syndrome
Young adulthood	Acute intermittent porphyria Hereditary juvenile glaucoma
Variable-onset age	Diabetes mellitus (0 to 80 years) Huntington chorea (15 to 65 years) Myotonic dystrophy (birth to old age)

Other disorders result primarily from environmental factors. These include most infectious diseases and trauma. Development of the disease depends on environmental contact with the etiologic agent, but there is strong evidence to indicate a decided genetic element in the susceptibility to most disease (e.g. tuberculosis, poliomyelitis, and measles in some population).

Genetic diseases can usually be classified into one of the following broad categories according to the hereditary factors that produce the observed effect—cytogenetic, mitochondrial, monogenetic, or multifactorial. Prenatal environmental influences, such as alcohol exposure and placental abnormalities, are also regarded as being within the realm of genetics because these effects can produce congenital structural, functional, or growth defects. In such cases the chromosomes would be normal although anomalies produced might be indistinguishable phenotypically from a genetically determined anomaly. The important difference is that the defects would not be inheritable because they would not have been caused by a genetic mutation.

Genes are central components of human health and disease. Specific genes are associated with specific genetic conditions makes diagnosis possible, even in the unborn. Research demonstrates that many common conditions have genetic causes. Many more associations between genetics, health, and disease are likely be identified with refinement of human genome mapping and sequencing.

Genes and Chromosomes

A persons unique genetic constitution, called a **genotype**, is made up of some 30,000 to 40,000 genes. A person's **phenotype**, the observable characteristics of his or her genotype, includes physical appearance and other biologic, physiologic, and molecular traits. Environmental influences modify every persons phenotype, even phenotypes with a major genetic component.

Human growth, development, and disease occur as a result of both genetic and environmental influences and interaction. The contribution of genetic factors may be large or small. For example, in a person with cystic fibrosis or PKU, the genetic contribution is significant. In contrast, the genetic contribution underlying a persons response to infection may be less important.

A single gene is conceptualized as a unit of heredity. A gene is composed of a segment of **deoxyribonucleic acid (DNA)** that contains a specific set of instructions for marking the protein or proteins needed by body cells for proper functioning. Genes regulate both the types of proteins made and the rate at which proteins are produced. The structure of the DNA molecule is referred to as the double helix. The essential components of the DNA molecule are sugar-phosphate molecules and pairs of nitrogenous bases. Each **nucleotide** contains a sugar (deoxyribose), a phosphate group, and one of four nitrogenous bases: adenine (A), cytosine (C), guanine (G), and thymine (T), a number of nucleotides. The strands are held together by hydrogen bonds between pairs of bases (Figs 4.1 to 4.10).

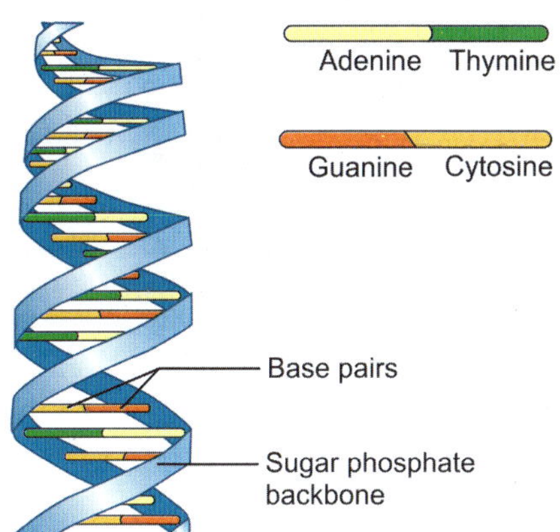

FIG. 4.1: DNA is a double helix formed by base pairs attached to a sugar-phosphate backbone. DNA carries the instructions that allow cells to make proteins. DNA is made up of four chemical bases

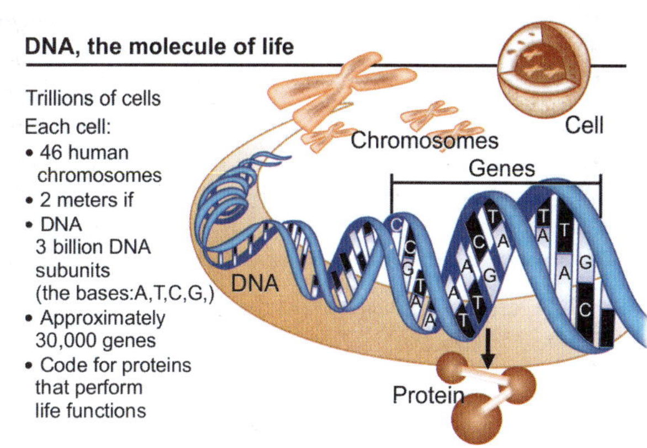

FIG. 4.2: DNA: The molecule of life. Illustrates the embedding of protein codes in base pair sequences of genes on DNA strands of chromosomes in the nucleus of the cell

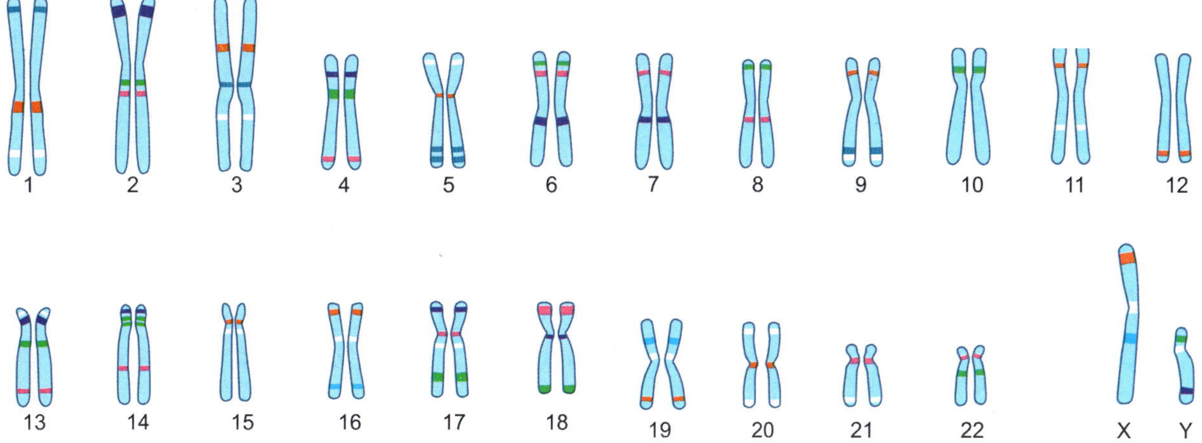

FIG. 4.3: Each human cell contains 23 pairs of chromosomes, which can be distinguished by their size and unique banding patterns. This set is from a male, because it contains a Y chromosome. Females have two X chromosomes

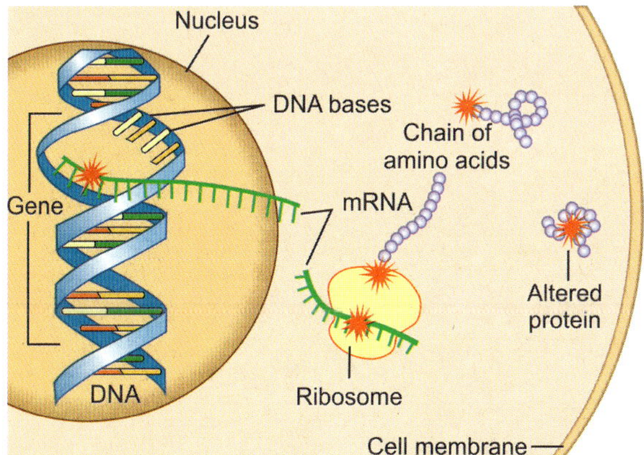

FIG. 4.4: When a gene contains a mutation, the protein encoded by that gene is likely to be abnormal. Sometimes the protein is able to function, although it does so imperfectly. In other cases, it is totally disabled. The outcome depends not only on how the mutation alters the protein's function but also on how vital that particular protein is to survival

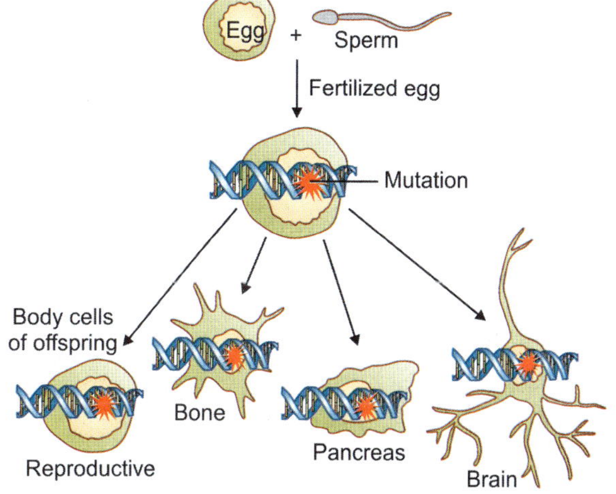

FIG. 4.5: Hereditary mutations are carried in the DNA of the reproductive cells. When reproductive cells containing mutation combine to produce offspring, the mutation is present in all of the offspring's body cells

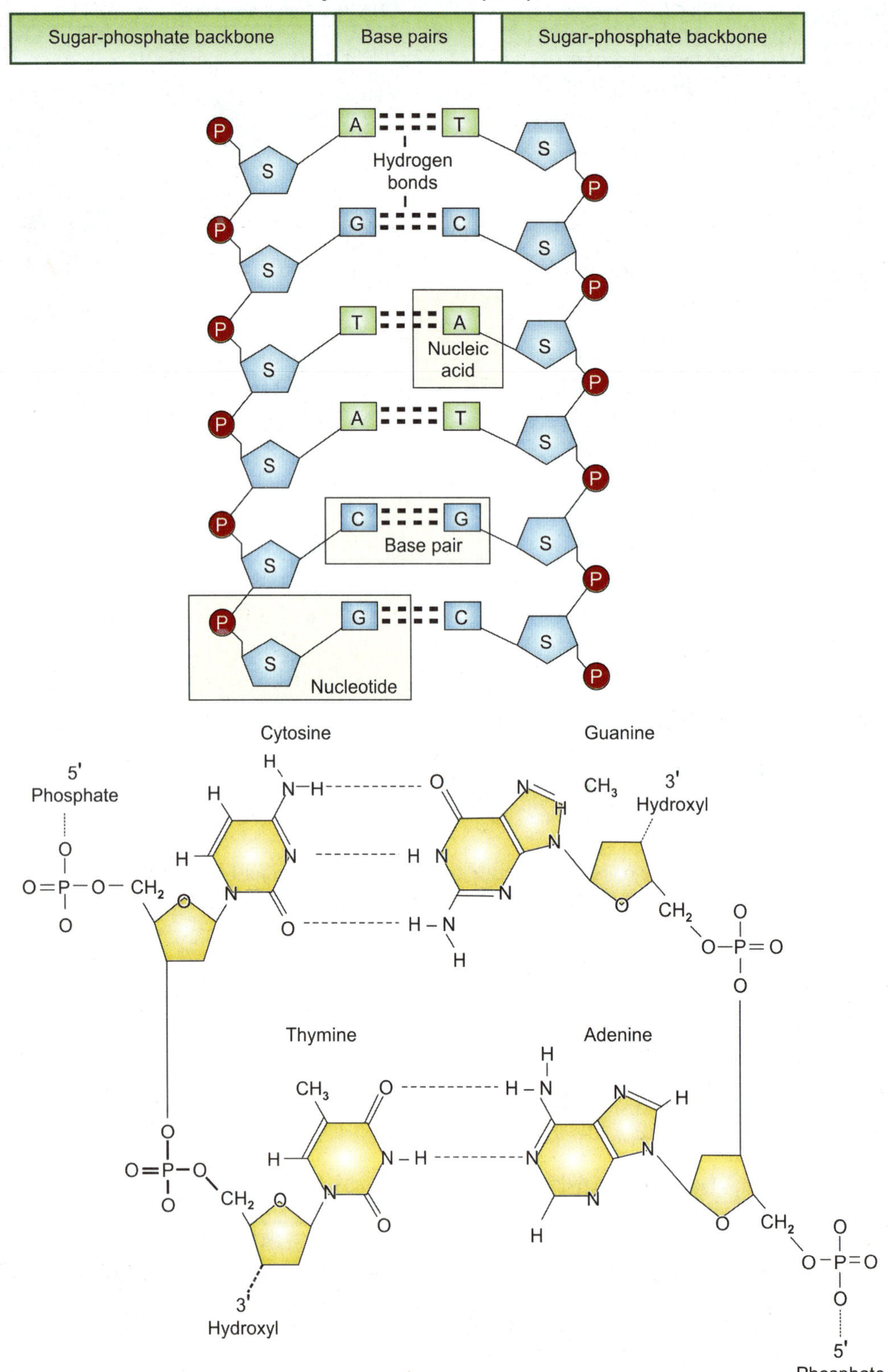

FIG. 4.6: Base pairs of DNA include A, adenine pairs with T, thymine; G, guanine pairs with C, cytosine; P, phosphate; S, sugar

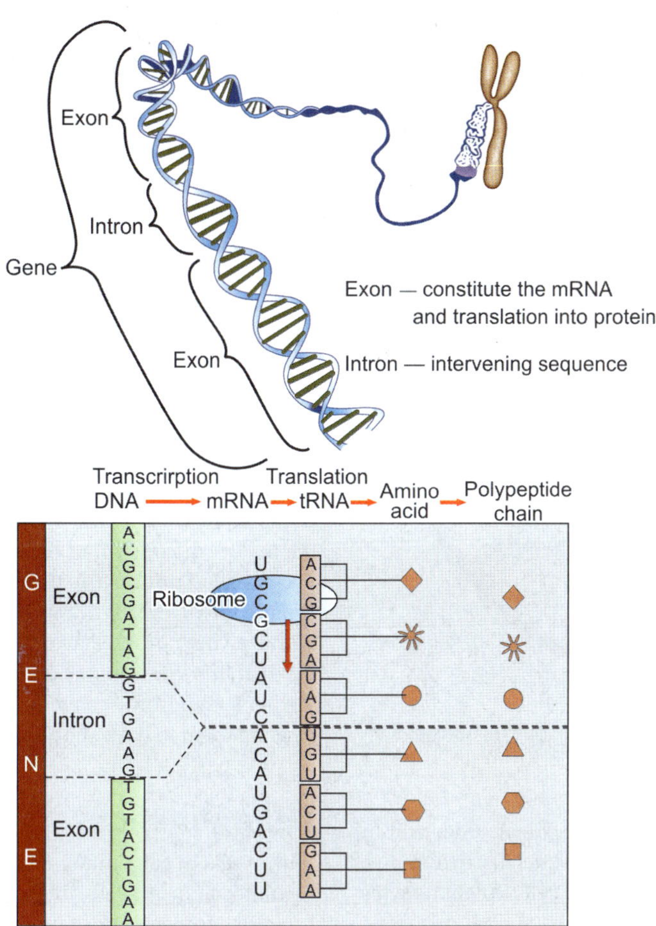

FIG. 4.7: Diagram of genetic components that produce amino acid chains using the script from the DNA base pairs. Messenger RNA carries directions from part of the gene to cell ribosomes where one of 20 possible amino acids are created. Amino acids form proteins. mRNA, messenger ribonucleic acid; tRNA, transfer RNA; A, adenine; G, guanine; C, cytosine; T, thymine; U, uracil

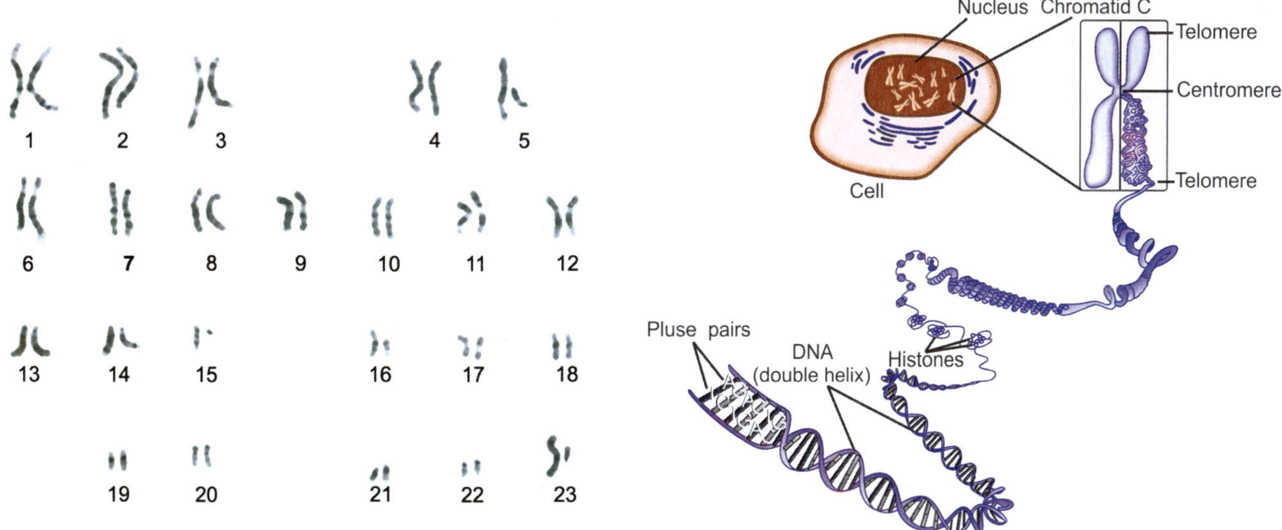

FIG. 4.8: Karyotype. Visual display of the 22 pairs of chromosomes and male sex chromosomes

FIG. 4.9: Chromosome structure in increasing detail from nucleus to base pairs

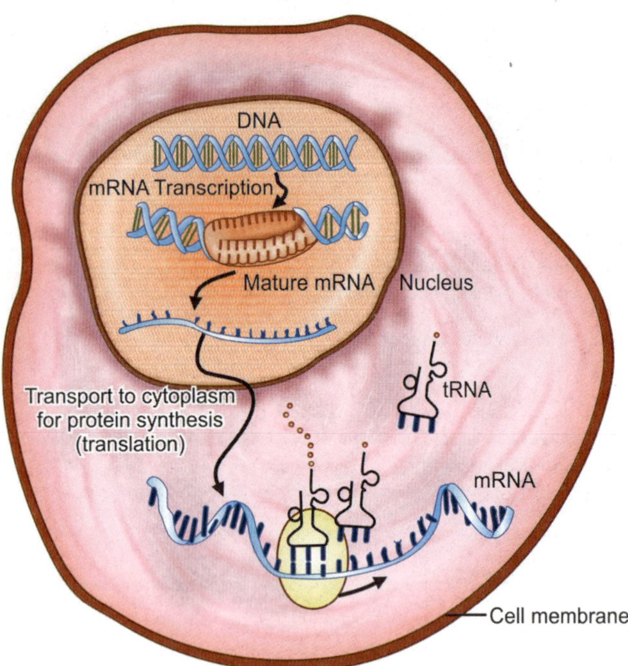

FIG. 4.10: Messenger ribonucleic acid (mRNA); tRNA, transfer RNA

Genes are packaged and arranged in a linear order within **chromosomes**, which are located in the cell nucleus. In humans, 46 chromosomes occur in pairs in all body cells except oocytes (eggs) and sperm, which each contain only 23 chromosomes. Twenty-two pairs of chromosomes, called autosomes, are the same in females and males.

The 23rd pair is referred to as the sex chromosomes. A female has two X-chromosomes, whereas a male has one X- and one Y-chromosome. At conception, each patient normally gives one chromosome of each pair to his or her children. As a result, children receive half of their chromosomes from their father and half from their mother (Fig. 4.3).

Careful examination of DNA sequences from many people shows that these sequences have multiple versions in a population. These different versions, or sequence variations, are called **alleles**. Sequences found in many forms are said to be polymorphic, meaning that there are at least two common forms of a particular gene.

Cell Division

The human body grows and develops as a result of the process of cell division. Mitosis and meiosis are two distinctly different types of cell division.

Mitosis is involved in cell growth, differentiation, and repair. During mitosis, the chromosomes of each cell duplicate. The result is two cells, called daughter cells, each of which contains the same number of chromosomes as the parent cell. The daughter cells are said to be diploid because they contain 46 chromosomes in 23 pairs. Mitosis occurs in all cells of the body except oocytes and sperm.

Meiosis, in contrast, occurs only in reproductive cells and is the process by which oocytes and sperm are formed. During meiosis, a reduction in the number of chromosomes, takes place, resulting in oocytes or sperm that contain half the usual number, or 23 chromosomes. Oocytes and sperm are referred to as **haploid** because they contain a single copy of each chromosome, compared to the usual two copies in all other body cells. During the initial phase of meiosis, as the paired chromosomes come together in preparation for cell division, portions cross over, and an exchange of genetic material occurs before the chromosomes separate. This event, called recombination, creates greater diversity in the makeup of oocytes and sperm.

During meiosis, a pair of chromosomes may fail to separate completely, creating a sperm or oocyte that contains either two copies or no copy of a particular chromosome. This sporadic event, called **nondisjunction**, can lead to either a **trisomy** or a monosomy. Down syndrome is an example of trisomy. People with Down syndrome have three copies of chromosome number 21. Turner's syndrome is an example of monosomy. Girls with Turner's syndrome usually have a single X-chromosome, causing them to have short stature and infertility.

Gene Mutations

Within each cell, many intricate and complex interactions regulate and express human genes. Gene structure and function, **transcription** and translation, and protein synthesis are all involved. Alterations in gene structure and function and the process of protein synthesis may influence a persons health. Changes in gene structure, called **mutations**, permanently change the sequence of DNA, which in turn can alter the nature and type of proteins made (Figs 4.11 and 4.12).

Some gene mutations have no significant effect on the protein product, whereas others cause partial or complete changes. How a protein is altered and its importance to proper body functioning determine the impact of the mutation. Gene mutations may occur in hormones, enzymes, or other important protein products, with significant implications for health and disease. Sickle cell anemia is an example of a genetic condition caused by a small gene mutation that affects protein structure, producing hemoglobin S. A person who inherits two copies of the hemoglobin S gene mutation has sickle cell anemia and experiences the symptoms of severe anemia and thrombotic organ damage resulting from hypoxia.

Other gene mutations may be larger, such as a deletion (loss), insertion (addition), duplication (multiplication), or rearrangement (translocation) of a longer DNA segment. Duchenne muscular dystrophy, an inherited form of muscular dystrophy, is an example of a genetic disorder caused by structural gene mutations such as deletions or duplications in the dystrophin gene. Another type of gene mutation, called a

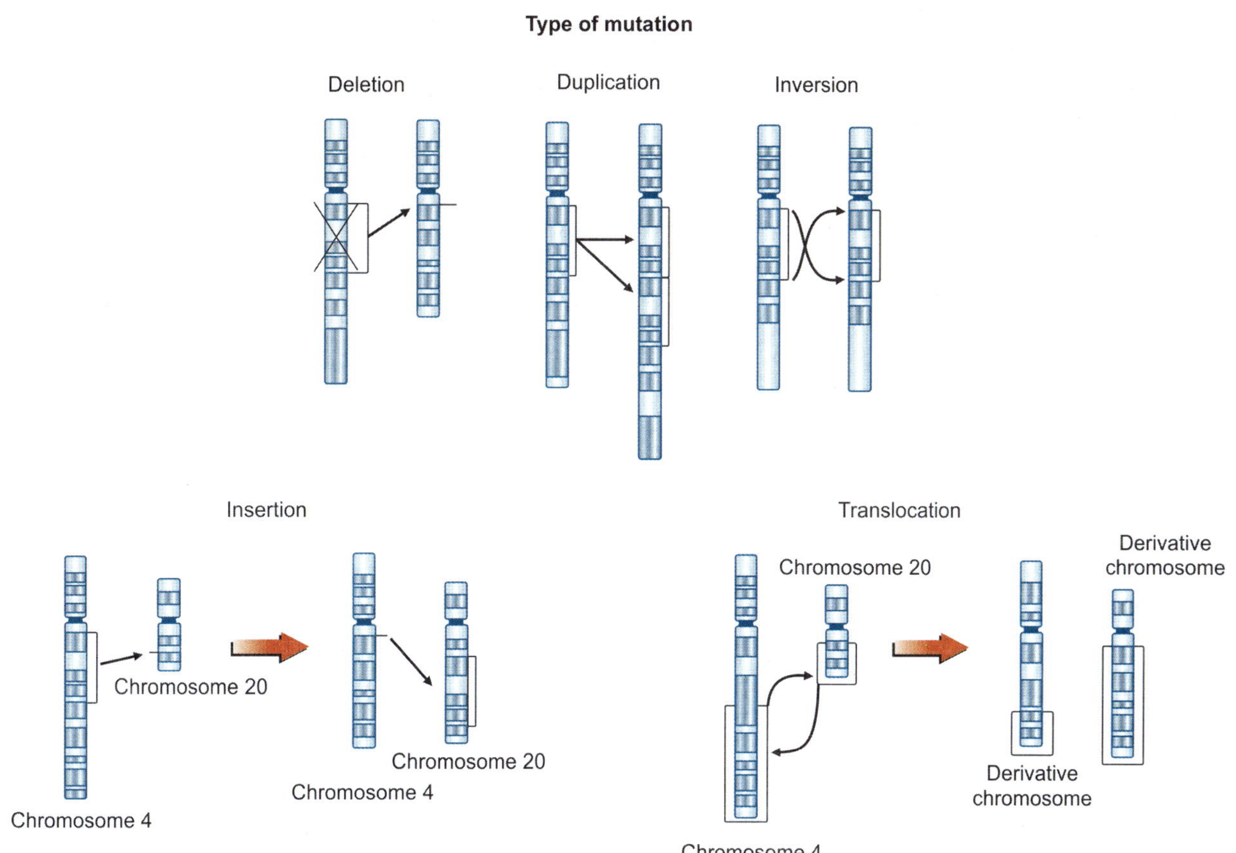

FIG. 4.11: Main types of chromosome mutation

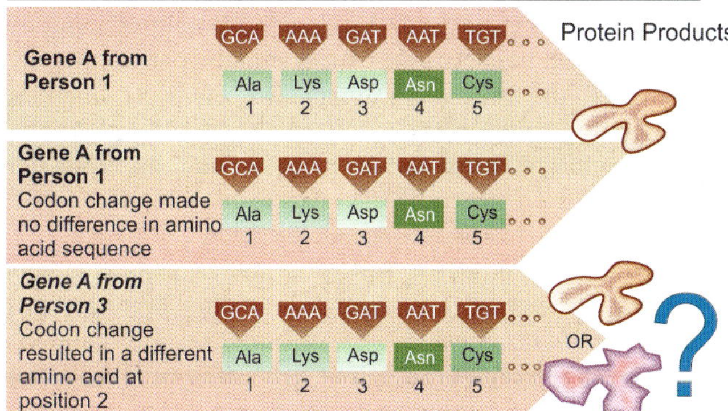

FIG. 4.12: DNA sequence variation. Base pairs include A, adenine, pairs with T, thymine; G, guanine, pairs with C, cytosine. Amino acids illustrated include Ala, alanine; Asp, aspartic acid; Asn, asparagines; Cys, cystenine; Lys, lysine

triplet or trinucleotide repeat, involves expansion to more than the usual number of copies of a triplet repeat sequence within a gene. Myotonic dystrophy, Huntington disease, and fragile X syndrome are examples of conditions caused by this type of gene mutation.

Gene mutations may be inherited or acquired. Inherited or germline gene mutations are present in the DNA of all body cells and are passed on in reproductive cells from parent to child. Germline mutations are passed on to all daughter cells when body cells replicate (Fig. 4.12). The gene that causes Huntington is one example of a germline mutation.

Spontaneous mutations take place in individual oocytes or sperm at the time of conception. These mutations are not inherited in other family members. However, a person who carries the new "spontaneous" mutation may pass on the mutation to his or her children. Achondroplasia, Marfan syndrome, and neurofibroma-tosis type 1 are examples of genetic conditions that may occur in a single family member as a result of spontaneous mutation.

Acquired mutations take place in somatic cells and involve changes in DNA that occur after conception, during a person's lifetime. Acquired mutations develop as a result of cumulative changes in body cells other than reproductive cells (Fig. 4.13). Somatic gene mutations are passed on to the daughter cells derived from that particular cell line.

Gene mutations occur in the human body all the time. Cells have built in mechanisms by which they can recognize mutations

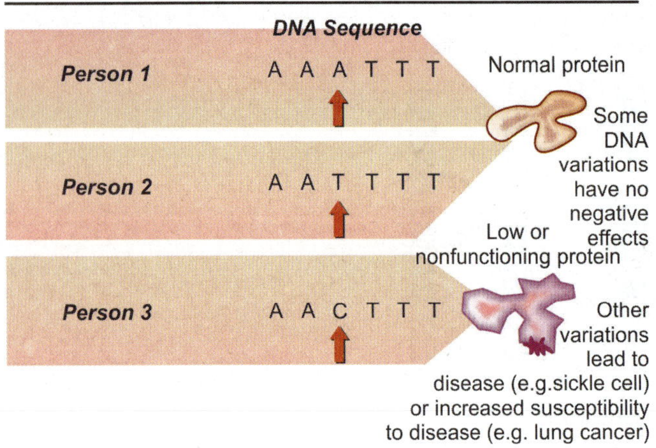

FIG. 4.13: Health or disease. A, adenine, pairs with T, thymine: G, guanine, pairs with C, cytosine. The substitution of one base pair can change the protein produced and lead to disease

in DNA, and in most situations they correct the changes before they are passed on by cell division. However, over time, body cells they may lose their ability to repair damage from gene mutations, causing an accumulation of genetic changes that may ultimately result in diseases such as cancer and possibly other conditions of aging, such as Alzheimer's disease.

Genetic Variation

Research is ongoing to sort out the genetic components of complex conditions (e.g. heart disease, diabetes, common cancers, psychiatric disorders) that result from the interaction of environment, lifestyle, and genetic effects. New studies of genetic variation in humans are underway to develop a map of common DNA variants. Genetic variations occur among people of all populations. *Polymorphisms* and single nucleotide polymorphisms (SNP's, or "snips") are the terms used for common genetic variations that occur most frequently throughout the human genome. Some SNP's may contribute directly to a trait or disease expression by altering function. SNP's are becoming increasingly important for the discovery of DNA sequence allows clinicians to subclassify diseases and adapt therapies to individual patients. For example, a polymorphism or SNP can alter protein or enzyme activity, and thereby affect drug efficacy and safety, if it occurs in proteins that are targets of medication regimens or that are involved in drug transport or drug metabolism.

A number of variables have been observed that explain or modify basic inheritance patterns and the effects of chromosome abnormalities. Some of these variations have been recognized for some time; others are newly discovered phenomena that explain some apparent contradictions in the established patterns of inheritance. Some of the variations involve individual genes, and others involve whole-chromosome behavior but will still affect manifestation of single-gene disorders. Also, some disorders have been reported to follow more than one inheritance pattern in different families (e.g. a classically recessive disorder may occasionally be reported as following a dominant or X-linked pattern in other families).

The most notable of these gene variations is mutation. A **mutation** is any heritable change in the DNA sequence of a gene. Mutations can be a deletion, duplication, or alteration in the base pair sequence. A mutation may cause the protein made by that gene to be produced in an altered, less functional form; to be produced in a decreased amount; or to be entirely absent. A gene mutation may have occurred generations ago and be passed down unchanged until it dies out because an individual does not reproduce, or a new gene mutation can occur spontaneously in an individual. Certain disease-producing gene mutations are known to be "old" mutations, such as the mutation that causes fragile X-syndrome, and new mutations are seldom if ever identified. Other disease known to have a high new mutation rate, such as the 30 to 50% rate for neurofibromatosis and Duchenne muscular dystrophy. This type of definitive determination of a gene mutation is possible only for those single-gene disorders in which the gene site has been located and characterized. Some disorders previously described as exhibiting sporadic occurrence (e.g. Williams syndrome) not attributable to a traditional inheritance pattern may be new mutations with effects such that the individual does not reproduce and the mutation is not passed on to offspring.

Variable expression is an important concept that describes differences in the extent and severity of manifestations of genetic diseases. There is a continuum of expression for any affected person from undetectable (mild) to severe clinical manifestation. Therefore a phenotypically normal person may still possess the mutant gene. This situation most often applies to autosomal dominant disorders; for example, a parent of a child with neurofibromatosis may exhibit only a couple of café-au-lait spots. Genomic imprinting and X-inactivation, discussed later in this section, may account for some variation in expression and penetrance, a term used less often as these new discoveries explain variation in phenotypic manifestation.

The discovery of a new type of mutation in some genetic disorders has helped explain their variation in inheritance patterns and clinical expression. Within genes are sequences **DNA nucleotide repeats**. A normal gene has a certain number of these repeats; for example, in the fragile X syndrome gene there are about 30 to 50 repeats. Some persons, however, have additional repeats of from 50 to 200, which have been termed **permutations**. These permutations in females are unstable and during meiosis can undergo amplification, expanding to hundreds more repeats, thereby becoming a full mutation and causing the offspring to be affected. Because fragile X is an X-linked disorder, females are less likely to be affected because of the tempering effect of the second X chromosome. These expanding repeats have also been found to occur in myotonic dystrophy, Huntington's disease, and spinocerebellar ataxia, which are autosomally transmitted disorders. This expanding-gene discovery exhibits the old concept of **genetic anticipation**, in which certain dominantly inherited disorders tend to worsen or have an earlier age of onset with succeeding generations. It is believed that additional disorders may be discovered to exhibit this type of mutation. In fact, the first recessively inherited disorder to exhibit an expansion mutation is Friedreich ataxia. This disorder usually demonstrates an onset in puberty or early adulthood, depending on the repeat size of the smaller of the two expansion alleles. Recent evidence suggests genetic anticipation may be a factor for the presence of father-son testicular tumors.

Genomic imprinting and uniparental disomy are two genetic phenomena that consider the parental origin of genetic information (i.e. maternally or paternally derived). The concept of *genomic imprinting* refers to modification, in some instances, of genetic material, resulting in phenotypic differences based on whether the genes/chromosomes were from the mother or the father. Genomic imprinting is exhibited during pregnancy, when paternally derived chromosomes seem to positively influence placental development and maternally derived chromosomes seem to positively influence fetal development. It has also been shown to be a factor in some genetic disorders, most classically Prader-Willi and Angelman syndrome. In both of these disorders, about two thirds of affected individuals have a deletion of the same segment of chromosome 15. However, the clinical manifestations of Prader-Willi and Angelman syndromes are markedly different. If the deletion occurs on the paternally derived chromosome 15, the child exhibits Prader-Willi's syndrome; if the deletion occurs on the maternally derived chromosome 15, Angleman's syndrome is manifested.

Prader-Willi syndrome is characterized by central hypotonia, cognitive dysfunction, dysmorphic appearance, behavioral disturbances, hypothalamic hypotonadism, short stature, and obesity, as well as abnormal low body temperature, an increased tolerance to pain, and diminished salivation. In contrast, **Angelman's syndrome** (also called happy puppet syndrome) includes severe mental retardation, characteristic facies, abnormal (puppet like) gait, and paroxysms of inappropriate laughter. Children with Angelman's syndrome are usually nonverbal, although they may vocalize.

In some cases both copies of a chromosome pair are determined to have come from one parent, either the mother or the father, instead of one from each, a phenomenon called uniparental disomy. An other example of **uniparental disomy** has been reported with cystic fibrosis, in which both chromosomes, each with a mutant recessive gene, came from the carrier mother; the father was not a carrier. In cases that appear to be nonpaternity, uniparental disomy may be a factor. One of the several theories about uniparental disomy is that the chromosome pair was originally a trisomy and the father's chromosome was randomly expelled, leaving two copies of the mother's chromosome. Because the chromosomes appear as a normal "pair", diagnosis of this situation is only possible with molecular (DNA) techniques. Uniparental disomy has also been reported with Beckwith-Weidemann syndrome, which is characterized by overgrowth and hypoglycemia at birth.

Mitochondrial Disorders

Mitochondrial DNA mutations also account for nontraditional inheritance patterns. Mitochondria are components of the cell cytoplasm involved in energy production. They perform many different functions in different tissues of the body. They are the only cellular organelles to have their own DNA distinct from nDNA and inheritance is exclusively maternal. A defect in the mtDNA can lead to altered functions of the proteins in some or all of the cells. Because the mitochondria perform so many different functions in the body, when a mutation has occurred, the spectrum of symptoms is enormous. Individuals with the same mtDNA mutation may be symptom free or severely affected with seizures, pancreatitis and metabolic disease. Even within the same family, different manifestations of the mitochondrial condition are seen. Mutations may be inherited or occur spontaneously. It is now believed that mitochondria are responsible not only for diseases occurring in childhood, such as Leigh disease (with symptoms of hypotonia, seizures, and failure to thrive), but they can be responsible for many common diseases associated with aging such as diabetes, parkinsonism, and dementia. Because there is such variability of expression with mitochondrial disorders, it can be very confusing to determine the diagnosis. However, when a child has an unexplained constellation of symptoms, a mitochondrial disorder should be considered.

Diagnosis of a mitochondrial disorder can be very difficult and therefore genetic counseling may be possible only in a small number of cases. Nuclear DNA mutations can also cause disorders of the mitochondria, and, with the advances in the detection of nDNA mutations, accurate diagnosis and therefore accurate information about recurrence risk and prenatal diagnosis is possible. Currently, treatment for these disorders is symptomatic and some patients show benefits from vitamin and cofactor supplementation. Referral to mitochondrial support groups can be very helpful to parents.

All cancers are "genetic". In DNA, cellular maintenance and repair genes inhibit abnormal cell growth that may become malignant. To lose this function, mutations must occur in both alleles of one of these genes. These mutations usually result from exposure to carcinogens, with exposure occurring over a lifetime. Only 5 to 10% of cancer occurs as a single gene abnormality, and in these hereditary cancer syndrome a person is born with a mutation already existing in one of the alleles. For this reason the cancer is much more likely to develop earlier in life. One of the cardinal clues to an inherited cancer syndrome is early onset.

Some of the inherited cancer syndromes for which DNA testing is available and medical surveillance and intervention is indicated in children include retinolblastoma, medullary thyroid carcinoma, familial adenomatous poluposis coli, multiple endocrine neoplasia, and Wilms tumor. Inherited cancer syndromes tend to follow an autosomal dominant inheritance pattern in families.

Testing may help identify family members who could benefit from medical intervention as well as those who do not need the expensive and uncomfortable screening tests. However, the benefits and risks of testing, confidentiality of results, and potential psychologic impact on the child need to be discussed with the parents before testing. Nurses play a key role in identifying and educating families with an increased cancer risk. Available testing can be discussed with these families, and they can be referred for genetic counseling.

CONGENITAL MALFORMATIONS

The development of an organism, especially during embryogenesis, is an intricate process in which all parts must be properly integrated to ensure a coordinated whole. The rate must be such that one part is ready when needed by another part; otherwise, wither part may cease to grow or may deviate from its normal path. **Congenital anomalies**, or **birth defects**, occur in 2 to 4% of all live born children and can arise at any stage of development. There is wide variability in etiologic factors, as well as in type, extent, and frequency of defects. Some defects result when a state present in one phase of development as a normal condition persists into another phase as abnormal. For example, a cleft lip is normal in a young embryo, and a patent ductus arteriosus is essential during fetal life. Any agent that interferes with these complex processes will produce a defect in development ranging in severity from an insignificant local anomaly to complete degeneration.

A few congenital are clearly caused by a single gene mutation, some are associated with chromosome abnormalities, and others are produced by known intrauterine environmental factors. However, many of the more common and severe defects (e.g. pyloric stenosis, central nervous system malformations, cataracts, and congenital heart disease) appear to be consistant with multifactorial inheritance.

The types of malformations that can result from genetic and/or prenatal environmental causes can be **major structural abnormalities** with serious medical, surgical, or quality-of-life consequences, or they can be **minor anomalies** or **normal variants** with no serious consequences, such as a sacral dimple, an extra nipple, or an umbilical hernia. Malformations can occur in isolation, such as congenital heart defect, or multiple anomalies may be present. A recognized pattern of malformations due to a single specific cause is called **syndrome**, such as Down syndrome or fetal alcohol syndrome. A nonrandom pattern of malformations for which an etiology has not been determined is called an **association** such as VATER (vertebral defects, imperforate anus, tracheoesphageal fistula, and radial/renal defects) association. Neural tube defects, cleft lip and/or cleft palate, deafness, congenital heart defects, and mental retardation are examples of anomalies that can occur in isolation or as part of a syndrome or association and can have different etiologies, such as single-gene or chromosome abnormalities, prenatal exposures, or multifactorial causes.

Chromosome (Cytogenetic) Disorders

Chromosome or **cytogenetic disorders** are deviations in either structure or number of a chromosome; the consequences in either situation can be readily observed in the affected individual and are often severe or even lethal. The reason for this is that a numerical or structural chromosome abnormality involves a duplication or loss of at least a few genes, or up to thousands of genes. Although the types of cytogenic disorders are not as varied as those caused by a single gene, the incidence for many of the specific abnormalities is significantly higher than that for any of the single-gene (monogenic) disorders.

A **structural abnormality** involves loss, addition, rearrangement, or exchange of some of the genes of a chromosome. If there is sufficient remaining genetic material to render the organism viable, structural alterations can produce an endless variety of clinical manifestations. These deviations are usually a result of an error in cell division in the sperm or ovum that resulted in that individual, but the parents are chromosomally normal.

Sometimes, however, the chromosome abnormality can be inherited from a parent who is a balanced translocation carrier. Also, fragile, or weak, sites have been identified on both autosomes and on the X-chromosome. An X-chromosome fragile site has been associated with physical and mental abnormalities termed **fragile X-syndrome**.

The normal number of chromosomes in a somatic cell is 23 pairs, or 46 total. Deviations in chromosome number involve the gain or loss of a chromosome and are designated with the suffix **somy**. A cell that contains one fewer than the total number of chromosomes is called a **monosomy** of the loss of one member of a chromosome pair; a cell that contains one more than the total number of chromosomes resulting from the addition of an extra member to a normal pair is called **a trisomy**. A number of deviations compatible with life occur in humans, especially those involving the sex chromosomes; the more serious outcomes are related to abnormalities of the autosomes. Trisomies are the chromosome aberrations encountered most commonly by health care workers. Monosomies may occur as often in concept uses but are usually nonviable. A relatively rare but clinically recognized variation is triploidy, in which there are three chromosomes in every pair, so that the total chromosome number is 69. This condition is lethal in early infancy.

The clinical consequences that attend variations in chromosome number frequently consist of discrete, identifiable syndromes, particularly in regard to the trisomies. The chromosome structural anomalies form a more diverse group of reported physical deviations with few recognized syndromes. Some of the chromosome disorders, such as Down's syndrome, can be identified on the basis of physical characteristics but require chromosome analysis to rule out the less common situation of translocation Down's syndrome.

CAUSES OF CHROMOSOME DEFECTS

There is considerable speculation regarding the precise cause of chromosome errors. Ionizing radiation—especially large doses or from occupational exposure—has been found to be a cause of chromosome breaks, rearrangements, and nondisjunction. Autoimmune diseases appear to have a role in the pathogenesis of nondisjunction during cell division. Viruses have also been implicated, especially in relation to chromosome breakage. However, only germ cell chromosome errors or breaks have the potential to cause chromosome abnormalities in offspring. Somatic errors do not have reproductive consequences.

Most of the information regarding factors that cause chromosome errors is related to parental age. The incidence of trisomic births corresponds strongly with increasing maternal age, regardless of the number of pregnancies. For example, the risk for trisomy 21, or Down's syndrome, increases dramatically for mothers more than 35 years of age. There is no positive explanation for this observation. However, throughout a lifetime the germ cells are vulnerable to a variety of exogenous influences and to the normal effects of the aging process. Increasing paternal age is not associated with most chromosome abnormalities, but it is associated with an increased risk for new mutation cases of autosomal dominant disorders, such as skeletal dysplasias.

Errors in Cell Division

The process by which chromosomes are distributed to the daughter cells during cell division is very complex and therefore prone to error. These errors can occur during **gamete formation (meiosis)** or in early **postzygotic cell division (mitosis)**. The resulting unequal distribution of genetic material may involve the gain or loss of a whole chromosome or part of a chromosome.

The most common cause of numeric chromosome abnormalities is the process of nondisjunction during cell division. **Nondisjunction** is the failure of separation of homologous chromosomes during meiosis I (or of **sister chromosomes** during meiosis II or mitosis. The term sister chromatid refers to the pair of stands that constitute a metaphase (a stage of mitosis) chromosome. This failure to separate can result in one or both members of the pair not passing (segregating) to either daughter cell. Nondisjunction can involve either the autosomes or the sex chromosomes. If nondisjunction takes place at meiosis I, the gamete will contain both the maternally and the paternally derived chromosomes of the pair involved. If it occurs at meiosis II, the gamete will contain a double complement of either the maternal or the paternal chromosome. In either case the resulting gamete will have too many or too few chromosomes. If this gamete is fertilized with a sperm or ovum with a normal chromosome complement, the resulting fetus will be either trisomic (3) or monosomic (1) for the chromosome pair involved. Monomies are usually not viable, with the exception of monosomy X (Turner's syndrome).

Mosaicism is the presence of two or more chromosomally distinct cell lines, usually one normal and one abnormal. This situation occurs when nondisjunction occurs in the later cell division (postzygotic) of a chromosomally normal fertilized egg. The abnormality may be either numeric mosaicism is the most common type seen clinically. Postzygotic mitotic nondisjunction results in a fetus with two or more cell lines. This early cell division error following fertilization is the most common cause of mosaicism and usually results showing a mosaic Turner syndrome (normal and monosomic X-cell line) are seen. The percentage, or level, of mosaicism depends on the stage of embryonic development in which the cell division error occurs. If it occurs at the first cell division after fertilization, the level of mosaicism may be as high as 50%. If the cell division error occurs in later development, the abnormal cells may be localized to one cell type, such as the brain tissue or germ cell line (ovaries or testes). The extent of clinical manifestations is determined by the type of tissues that contain cells with abnormal chromosome numbers and the percentage of affected cells, and may vary from near normal to a fully manifested syndrome.

Placental tissue is commonly found to be mosaic and may determine the variability to term of fetuses with chromosome abnormalities. It is now understood that different percentages of mosaicism; for example, a parents germline cells (which produce the sperm and egg) may be mosaic, but other tissues, (e.g. skin, blood [somatic cells]) may be normal. Therefore, a phenotypically normal parent could test negative for a mutation from the DNA of the lymphocytes yet carry the gene mutation in his or her germ cell line, with all the attendant risks of transmission. Different percentages of mosaicism in different tissues can also explain variable phenotypic expression.

X-inactivation also produces a functional mosaicism. It is also now known that not all of the second X-chromosome is inactivated and that inactivation is not random, which further explains variable phenotypic expression in regard to genes on the X-chromosome.

A **translocation** is a structural abnormality that involves an exchange of genetic material between two or more chromosomes. A simple translocation results when a break occurs in one arm of each of any two nonhomologous (non-paired) chromosomes and the segments below or above the break points change places. A variation of this occurrence, called a **Robertsonian translocation**, occurs between **acrocentric chromosomes**; group D (13, 14, 15) and group G (21, 22). In an acrocentric chromosome, the centromere is near one end, so that one arm is much longer than the other. Translocations between those groups involving the No.21 chromosome can result in an inherited form of Down syndrome, called **translocation Down's syndrome**, which accounts for approximately 4.7 to 6.7% of cases.

If there is essentially no loss or gain of genetic material in the exchange, the translocation is **balanced**, or **reciprocal**. Carriers of a balanced translocation are phenotypically normal and occur with a frequency of about 1 in 600 in the general population. These carrier individuals (either male or female) may pass the translocation to their offspring in a balanced or **unbalanced** form, depending on how the chromosomes segregate to the gametes. If it is passed in the unbalanced form, the combination is often lethal, and an early spontaneous abortion occurs. However, the risk of having a live born offspring with birth defects associated with the unbalanced translocation is 5 to 20%. Approximately 5% of cases of repeated spontaneous abortion (two or more) can be attributed to a balance translocation carrier parent. Unlike nondisjunction, translocations are not related to increasing maternal age. Translocations, balance or unbalanced, can be passed from a carrier parent or be de novo (arising as a new change), which subsequently can be passed to future offspring.

Autosomal Chromosome Abnormalities

Both numeric and structural abnormalities of autosomes account for a variety of syndromes usually characterized by mental deficiencies. A few are associated with a group of characteristics that clearly indicate the precise chromosome anomaly. The first and the most common disorder in which an associated chromosome abnormality was demonstrated is Down syndrome. The most viable trisomies are trisomy 21 (Down syndrome), trisomy 18 (Edward syndrome), and trisomy 13 (Patau). Nurses often note dysmorphic facial features (Table 4.2), behavioral characteristics such as an unusual cry and poor feeding behavior, and other neurologic manifestations such as hypotonia or abnormal reflex responses, which may alert them to these and other chromosome abnormalities.

Partial chromosome abnormalities involve a missing (deletion) or extra (duplication) segment of a chromosome. The features of classic deletion and contiguous gene (microdeletion and microduplication) syndromes are usually less recognizable at birth. Phenotypic effects of these syndromes may include a cluster of known single-gene disorders. The **classic deletion syndromes** can be detected on a routine chromosome analysis and include cri-du-chat (Table 4.2), Wolf-Hirschhorn, and chromosome 18 deletions. **Contiguous gene syndrome** are disorders characterized by a microdeletion or microduplication of smaller chromosome segments, which may require special analysis techniques or molecular testing to detect. Microdeletion syndromes are more common and may have more clinically obvious phenotypic effects than microduplication syndromes. Examples of these syndromes include Prader-Willi, Angelman, DiGeorge, and Beckwith-Wiedemann.

Sex Chromosome Abnormalities

The possible mechanisms by which sex chromosome abnormalities may occur are the same as those previously described (i.e. prefertilization nondisjunction during one of the meiotic divisions of gametogenesis in either parent or in the early postfertilization divisions of the zygote). An alteration in the number of sex chromosomes usually does not produce the profound effects that are associated with the autosomal trisomies. Intelligence may be normal or low-normal, or the child may have some learning disabilities, but moderate or severe mental retardation is less common.

Turner syndrome (45, X) is essentially the only viable monosomy. It is still extremely lethal prenatally, with 99% of these fetuses being spontaneously aborted. Most girls have one +X chromosome missing from all cells (45, X). Some have mosaic cells lines with some cells 45, X and others 46, XX. The syndrome should be suspected in the newborn period by the presence of lymphedema of the hands and feet and a low posterior hairline, in child hood by a webbed neck and short stature, and at puberty by delayed development and primary amenorrhea. The reason for the growth is usually until 3 years of age and then slows, gradually drifting away from the normal

TABLE 4.2: Common autosomal aberrations

Syndrome	Chromosome abnormality and nomenclature	Average incidence (live birth)	Major clinical manifestations
Cri-du-chat	Deletion of short arm of No.5 chromosome – 46, XY, 5p-	1: 50,000	Distinctive weak, high-pitched, mew-like cry resembling the cry of a cat; small head, hyperteloism; failure to thrive; severe mental retardation – profound with age
Trisomy 13 (Patau)	Trisomy of No.13 chromosome – 47, XY, +13	1: 4,000–15,000	Cleft lip and palate (frequently bilateral); ear malformations; microphthalmia; polydactyly; eye defects; cardiac defects; mental retardation; early death
Trisomy 13 (Edward)	Trisomy of No.18 chromosome – 47, XY,+18	1: 3,500–8,000	Deformed and low-set ears; micrognathia; rocker-bottom feet; overlapping (index over third) fingers; retardation; failure to thrive; early death
Trisomy 13 (Down)	Trisomy of No. 21 chromosome – 47, XY,+21 (trisomy); 46, XY, +(14;21) (translocation); 46 ,XY/47, XY, +21 (mosaic)	1: 700+	Brachycephaly with flat occiput; inner epicanthal folds; small ears, nose, and mouth with protruding tongue; muscular hypotonia; broad, short hands with stubby feet with wide space between big and second toes; cardiac defects, mental retardation, variable life expectancy

growth curve. There is no prepubertal growth spurt, and girls with Turner syndrome are generally infertile. These girls may have difficulty with peer relationships and with understanding social cues. They may exhibit behavioral problems, especially in relation to immature, socially isolated behavior. Most, however, lead productive lives and function as independent adults.

Klinefelter syndrome, the most common of all sex chromosome abnormalities, is caused by the presence of one or more additional X-chromosomes. The majority of males with this syndrome have a chromosome complement of 47, XXY, but there are numerous variants in the number of extra sex chromosomes. There are no distinctive physical characteristics that are helpful in detecting Klinefelter syndrome before the advent of puberty. Mental impairment of varying degrees is a frequent finding and appears to have a direct relationship to the number of X-chromosomes in the cells. The severity of retardation increases with the number of X-chromosomes.

The milder physical and mental deficiencies of children with sex chromosome abnormalities compared with children with autosomal abnormalities are due in part to a phenomenon called X inactivation or Lyon hypothesis. In all body cells one X chromosome is biologically active; if more than one X chromosome is present, most (but not all, as previously thought) of the other(s) are in some way "switched off", or inactivated, during the very early divisions of the zygote and remain so throughout life. Because of the milder effects of sex chromosome abnormalities, many individuals are phenotypically normal and may remain undiagnosed. Sex chromosome mosaicism occurs, which also accounts for some variation in phenotype. The aberrant social behavior described as typical of multiple-Y chromosome abnormalities is thought to have been exaggerated and is more limited to poor impulse control, hyperactivity, and learning disability.

Multiples of the X and Y-chromosomes exist, in trisomic or greater numbers (Table 4.3). Regardless of the number of X-chromosomes, the presence of a Y-chromosome appears to be a male determining factor. Therapy of sex chromosome disorders consists primarily of hormone treatment to initiate appropriate pubertal sexual development. Growth hormone therapy may be used in girls with Turner syndrome to increase growth velocity and, hopefully, final height.

Single-Gene (Monogenic) Disorders

Disorders that are the result of a defect or mutation of a single gene, rather than a partial or whole chromosome abnormality, are called **single-gene disorders**. These disorders, which generally follow a simple, definite inheritance pattern, are rare individually, but collectively they constitute a significant portion of health problems seen in infants and children. They can involve any system in the body. They can be of such minor importance that they have little effect on the child or be so severe as to cause serious disability or to be incompatible with life.

The defective or mutated gene cannot be diagnosed by chromosome analysis, because it is at a more basic level of the chromosome, that of the DNA structure. These disease producing mutant genes are usually distributed or transmitted in families according to basic Mendelian principles of dominant or recessive behavior on the autosomes or sex chromosomes (usually the X-chromosome). Some generalizations can be applied to dominant and recessive inheritance patterns of the autosomes or sex chromosomes and the resultant diseases and malformations.

TABLE 4.3: Partial list of few single-gene disorders

Disease	Inheritance	Basic defect	Manifestations	Therapy
Achondroplasia	Autosomal dominant, new mutation	Defect in ossification at epiphyseal plate (growth portion of bones)	Very short limbs; large head; lordosis	Supportive
Albinism (ocular)	Autosomal recessive	Deficiency of tyrosinase: Failure to convert tyrosine to dopa, and, hence, lack of melanin synthesis	Lack of pigment in skin, hair, and eyes, eye defects	Symptomatic, avoid exposure to sunlight, ophthalmologic care
Cystic fibrosis	Autosomal recessive	Defect in pancreatic enzymes	Abnormal secretions, chronic pulmonary disease; malabsorption	Symptomatic, enzyme therapy
Fragile X-syndrome	X-linked dominant	Unknown	Long face; large ears; large testicles; mental retardation	Symptomatic
Galactosemia	Autosomal recessive	Defect in galactose metabolism	Hypotonia, vomiting, hepatosplenomegaly; cataracts	Galactose-free diet
Hemophilia A	X-linked recessive	Defect in factor VII production	Hemorrhage into tissues, joints after injury	Factor VIII replacement therapy

Contd...

Contd...

Disease	Inheritance	Basic defect	Manifestations	Therapy
Hypothyroidism	Autosomal recessive	Deficiency of iodotyrosine deiodinase	Lethargy; stunted growth; mental retardation	Early administration of thyroid hormone
Maple syrup urine disease	Autosomal recessive	Defective metabolism of branched-chain amino acids	Onset in early infance; neurologic disorders; odor of urine similar to that of maple syrup	Diet low in branched-chain amino acids
Marfan syndrome (arachnodactyly)	Autosomal dominant, new mutation	Defect in elastic fibers of connective tissues	Tall and thin, with long tapering fingers; poorly developed musculature; associated defects include aortic aneurysm, dislocation of optic lens, winged scapula	Supportive surgical correction of deformities
Muscular dystrophy (Duchenne)	Autosomal dominant, new mutation	Protein dystrophin is absent	Muscular atrophy; progressive deterioration of motor function and mental development	Symptomatic
Myotonic dystrophy	Autosomal dominant,	Defective calcium metabolism in nerve and muscle cells	Hypotonia; characteristic facial features; respiratory distress; poor feeding; high-arched palate; cataracts; severe neonatal form leads to early death	Symptomatic
Neurofibromatosis (von Reckling Hausen disease)	Autosomal dominant, new mutation	Defect in neural cells – exact mechanism unknown	Café-au-lait spots; multiple fibromas; neurologic and ophthalmologic defects; skeletal anomalies	Symptomatic, surgical removal of tumors
Noonan syndrome	Autosomal dominant	Unknown	Small stature; shield-shaped chest; webbed neck; low posterior hairline; narrow maxilola; low-set ears; ptosis; hypertelorism; cardiac anomalies (pulmonic stenosis)	Correct cardiac anomalies Supportive
Osteogenesis imperfecta	Autosomal dominant, new mutation	Defect in production of type 1 procollagen	Fragile, short, bowed bones; blue sclera; hyperextensible joints; hearing loss	Symptomatic, surgical orthopedic procedures
Phenylketonuria	Autosomal recessive	Defect in phenylalanine metabolism	Eczema; poor feeding; seizures; musty smell to urine; mental retardation	Low-phenylalanine diet
Tay-Sachs disease (amaurotic familial idiocy)	Autosomal recessive	Defect of hexosaminidase; defect in synthesis of gangliosides	Predominantly in Ashkenazi Jews; progressive neurologic deterioriation; blindness, cherry red spot in macula; early death	Supportive
Thalassemias	Autosomal recessive	Defect in synthesis of one or more globin chains of hemoglobin	Anemia; hepatosplenomegaly; thinning of bones	Symptomatic, transfusions
Wilson disease	Autosomal recessive	Failure of biliary excretion of copper, leading to copper toxicity	Liver failure, speech abnor- malities; tremors; psychiatric and behavior problems	Chelation agents, treatment of liver disease

Some examples of single-gene disorders, including the inheritance pattern, basic defect, and manifestations, are outlined in Table 4.3.

A number of variables are observed in many disorders that modify the basic inheritance patterns. In addition, there are genetic phenomena that are not explained by traditional Mendelian inheritance. These variations and concepts are discussed following presentation of traditional autosomal dominant, recessive, and sex chromosomes X-linked patterns.

AUTOSOMAL INHERITANCE PATTERNS

Autosomal Dominant Inheritance. Children with an autosomal dominant disorder have usually inherited it from an affected parent, although the parent's case may have been mild or detected. When a first case in a family appears, it is usually as a result of a new mutation. It is being recognized, however, that in rare cases, especially when a second affected child is

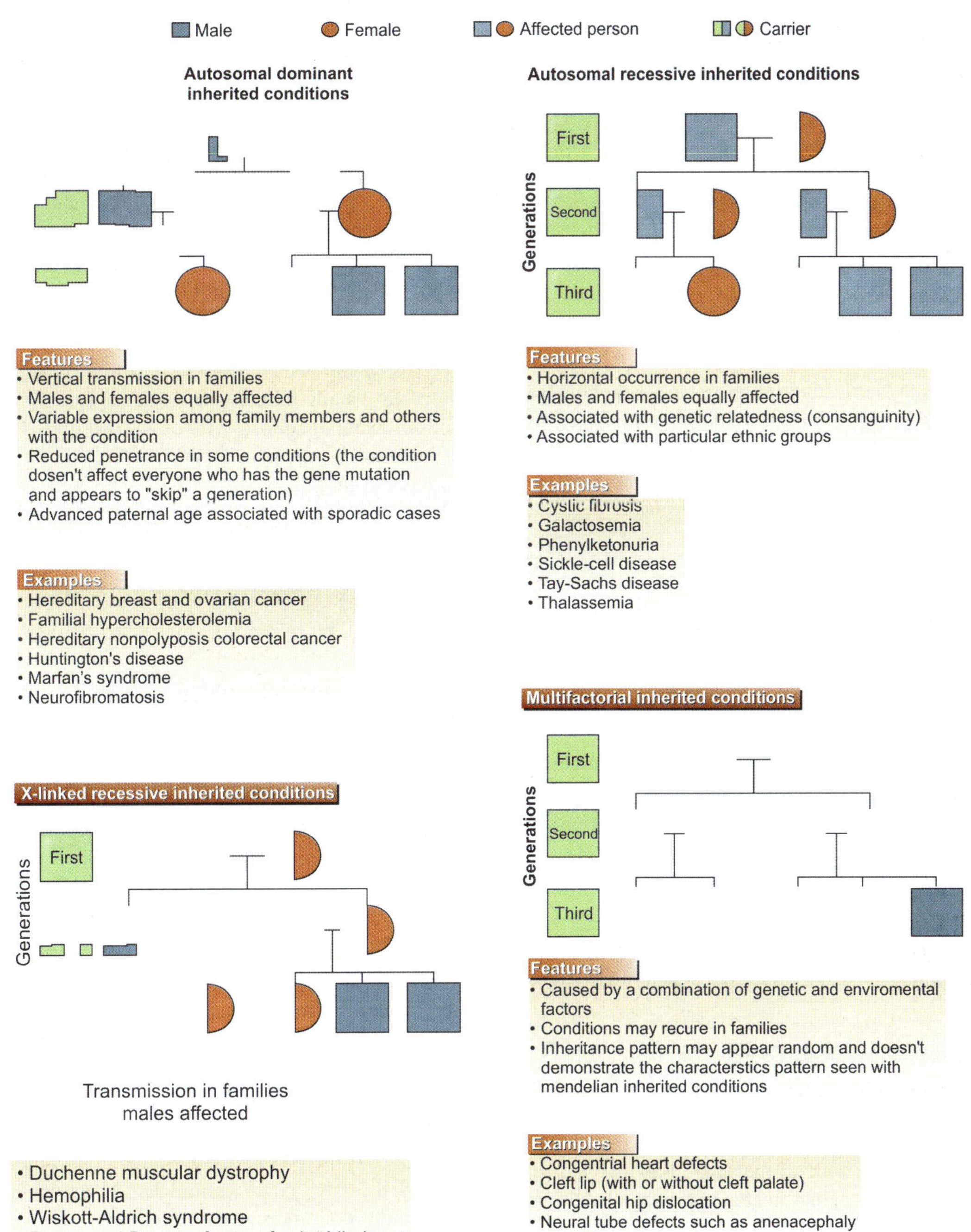

FIG. 4.14: Mapping out hereditary conditions

born, one parent could have germline mosaicism (i.e. the gene mutation for a disorder is only present in the egg or sperm cells). Depending on the degree of disability the condition imposes on the individual and the age of onset, the gene will either die out or continue to be passed on through several generations. For example, Huntington's disease, a progressive incapacitating and fatal neuromuscular disease, is usually not manifested until age 40 or later, after the affected person may have passed on the defective gene to offspring. Incomplete penetrance of autosomal dominant disorders is common, and there is wide variability in expression. Regardless of penetrance or variable expression in the parent, there is a 50% risk of passing on the defective gene to offspring, where it may be fully expressed. Other examples of autosomal dominant disorders include achonodroplasia, neurofibromatosis, and Marfan syndrome (Fig. 4.14).

Characteristics of Autosomal Dominant Inheritance

- Males and females are affected with equal frequency
- Affected individuals will have an affected parent although expression may be variable (unless the condition is caused by a new mutation or germline mosaicism)
- Children of a heterozygous affected parent have a 50% probability of possessing the defective gene, although it may be nonpenetrant
- Children of affected parents who did not receive the affected gene will have unaffected children.
- Traits can be traced vertically through previous generations—a positive family history—unless it is a new mutation, germline mosacism, or nonpenetrant
- Autosomal dominant disorders are more common than recessive disorders and are usually less severe.

Characteristics of Autosomal Recessive Inheritance

- Males and females are affected with equal frequency
- Affected individuals will have unaffected parents who are heterozygous for the trait
- There is a 1 in 4 (25%) chance that any child of two unaffected heterozygous parents will be affected
- Unaffected siblings of an affected person have a 2/3 risk of being a carrier
- Affected individuals mated to normal individuals will have normal children, all of whom will be carriers
- There is usually no evidence of the trait in previous generation —a negative family history—unless consanguinity is a factor.

Characteristics of X-linked Recessive Inheritance

- Affected individuals will have an affected parent
- All the daughters but none of the sons of an affected male have the probability of being affected (although usually more mildly)
- Half the sons and half the daughters of an affected female will be affected
- Normal children of an affected parent will have normal offspring
- There are no carriers (although expression may vary)
- The inheritance pattern shows a positive family history.

Autosomal Recessive Inheritance

Children who display an autosomal recessive disorder will always be homozygous for that trait. The heterozygous person, with only one gene for a rare recessive disorder, remains undetected in the population. It is estimated that each person carries from three to eight genes for a severe genetic disease. For example, 1 in 20 persons in the US and Northern European populations carry the recessive gene for cystic fibrosis. In the African-American population, 1 in 10 persons is a carrier for the sickle rate is 1 in 50. However, the probability of the mating of two persons who carry the same gene is highly unlikely. The chances are increased if the mating occurs in persons who select a mate because of geographic, ethnic, or religious restrictions or blood relationship **(consanguinity)**. For example, 1 in 30 Ashkenazi Jews is a carrier of the Tay-Sachs disease gene. The age of onset for autosomal recessive disorders is early, and, because they are usually biochemical defects, heterozygote detection and prenatal diagnosis are often possible. Other examples of autosomal recessive disorders include the thalassemias, congenital adrenal hyperplasia, galactosemia and cystic fibrosis (Fig. 4.14).

X-Linked Inheritance Patterns

Genes on the X-chromosome differ from those on the Y chromosome; therefore the transmission of traits caused by these genes will vary according to the sex of the individual who carries the gene. The two X-chromosomes in the female are alike in gene constitution, with two genes for each trait. Genes on the X-chromosome have no counterpart on the Y-chromosome; therefore a characteristic determined by a gene on the X-chromosome is always expressed in the male. One of the most significant aspects of X-linked inheritance is the absence of father-to-son transmission. Although it is essential for development of the male phenotype, the Y-chromosome carries no known medically significant characteristics.

X-linked dominant inheritance: Superficially this pattern resembles an autosomal dominant inheritance pattern. This type of inheritance is relatively uncommon. An example of an X-linked dominant disorder is hypophosphatemic vitamin D-resistant rickets. The inheritance pattern of fragile X-syndrome is complex and may not follow the standard X-linked pattern.

X-linked recessive inheritance: The abnormal gene behaves as any recessive gene would; that is, its effect is hidden by a normal dominant gene. Therefore, two recessive genes are usually present if manifestations in the female are seen. This rare situation would require the father to be affected and the mother to be a carrier. However, unequal X inactivation can also produce manifestations in a carrier female. New mutations are not uncommon. Examples of X-linked disorders include hemophilia types A and B and Duchenne muscular dystrophy.

Multifactorial Disorders

A number of diseases and defects that are encountered frequently in the population show an increased incidence in some families but have no clear-cut-affected-unaffected classification. Although the incidence is higher than would be expected by chance, no specific mode of inheritance can be identified. In some, environmental factors, including the prenatal environment, appear to play an important role. These conditions are classified as **multifactorial** disorders, in which a genetic susceptibility and appropriate environmental agents interact to produce a disease state. Diseases considered to be multifactorial (at least an isolation) include neural tube defects, cleft lip and cleft palate, many congenital heart defects, congenital hip dislocation, and pyloric stenosis. Determining risks of recurrence is more difficult than for single-gene disorders, but the risk is usually low, less than 10%. For example, anencephaly and/or spina bifida occur in 0.2 to 5 births per 1000 in the general population. The recurrence risk after the first affected child is 3 to 6%. Advances in genetics are enhancing knowledge of multifactorial inheritance to better understand familial risks (Fig. 4.14).

Disorders of the Intrauterine Environment

The prenatal intrauterine environment can have a profound and permanent effect on a developing fetus, even when chromosome or single-gene abnormalities are not present. Sometimes, however, intrauterine effects occur in tandem with genetic factors. Intrauterine growth retardation (IGUR), for example, can occur with many genetic syndromes, such as Down, Russell-Silver, Prader-Willi, and Turner syndromes, or can occur from nongenetic causes such as maternal alcohol ingestion. Placental abnormalities are increasingly being found to be the etiologic factor in neurodevelopmental disorders (such as cerebral palsy and mental retardation) that were previously attributed to asphyxia during delivery.

Teratogens, agents that cause birth defects when present in the prenatal environment, account for the majority of adverse intrauterine effects not attributable to genetic factors. Types of teratogens include drugs (phenytoin [Dilantin], warfarin [Coumadin], tretinoin [Accutane]): chemicals (ethyl alcohol, cocaine, lead); infectious agents (rubella, cytomegalovirus); physical agents (maternal hyperthermia); and metabolic agents (maternal phenylketonuria). Many of these teratogen exposures and the resulting effects are completely preventable, such as ingestion of alcohol resulting in fetal alcohol syndrome/fetal alcohol effects (FAS/FAE), which causes severe birth defects including mental retardation. The incidence of FAS is estimated at 5.2 per 10,000 live births.

Genetic Testing

Genetic tests provide information leading to the diagnosis of inherited conditions or other conditions with a known genetic contribution. Genetic testing involves the use of specific laboratory analyses of chromosomes, genes, or gene products (e.g. enzymes, proteins) to learn whether a genetic alteration related to a specific disease or condition is present. This testing may be DNA-based, chromosomal, or biochemical.

Genetic testing can be used for a variety of purposes in prenatal, pediatric, and adult populations. Prenatal testing is widely used for **prenatal screening** and diagnosis of such conditions as Down syndrome. Carrier testing is used to determine carrier status - that is, to discover whether a person carries a recessive allele for an inherited condition (e.g. cystic fibrosis, sickle cell anemia, Tay-Sachs disease) and therefore risks passing it on to his or her children. Genetic testing is also used widely in newborn screening. In the United States, it is made available for an increasing number of genetic conditions (e.g. PKU, galactosemia). Diagnostic testing is used to detect the presence or absence of a particular genetic alteration or allele to identify or confirm a diagnosis of a disease or condition (e.g. myotonic dystrophy, fragile X-syndrome). Increasingly, genetic tests are being used to predict drug response and to design specific and individualized treatment and management plans. For example, genetic testing is used to identify specific gene variants that can predict therapeutic success of treatments for human immunodeficiency virus (HIV) infection and the use of tacrine for Alzheimer's disease. Examples of current uses of genetic tests are shown in Table 4.4.

Nurses are increasingly participating in genetic testing, especially in the area of patient education. In addition, they contribute by ensuring informed health choices and consent, advocating for privacy and confidentiality with regard to genetic test results, and helping patients understand the complex issues involved.

Genetic Screening

Genetic screening in contrast to genetic testing, is a broader concept and applies to testing of populations or groups independent of a positive family history or symptom manifestation. Genetic screening has several major aims. The first aim is to improve management—that is, to identify people with treatable genetic conditions that could prove dangerous to their health if left untreated. For example, newborns are screened for an increasing number of conditions, including PKU, congenital hypothyroidism, and galactosemia. The second aim is to provide reproductive options to people with a high probability of having children with severe, untreatable diseases and for whom genetic counseling, prenatal diagnosis, and other reproductive options could be helpful and of interest. The third aim is to screen pregnant women using multiple marker screening to detect birth defects such as neural tube defects and Down syndrome. Genetic screening may also be used for public health purposes to determine the incidence and prevalence of a birth defect or to investigate the feasibility and value of new genetic testing methods.

Most commonly, genetic screening occurs in prenatal and newborn programs that involve nurses in various roles and settings. In the failure, population-based (widespread)

TABLE 4.4: Genetic tests: Examples of current uses

Purpose of genetic test	Type of genetic test
Carrier testing	
Cystic fibrosis	DNA analysis
Tay-Sachs disease	Hexosaminidase A activity testing and DNA analysis
Canavan disease	DNA analysis
Sickle cell anemia	Hemoglobin electrophoresis
Thalassemia	Complete blood count and hemoglobin electrophoresis
Prenatal diagnosis– amniocentesis is often performed when there is a risk for a chromosomal or genetic disorder	
Risk for Down syndrome	Chromosomal analysis
Risk for cystic fibrosis	DNA analysis
Risk for Tay-Sachs disease	Hexosaminidase A activity testing and/or DNA analysis
Risk for open neural tube defect	Protein analysis
Diagnosis	
Down syndrome	Chromosomal analysis
Fragile X-syndrome	DNA analysis
Myotonic dystrophy	DNA analysis
Presymptomatic testing	
Huntington disease	DNA analysis
Myotonic dystrophy	DNA analysis
Susceptibility testing	
Hereditary breast/ovarian cancer	DNA analysis
Hereditary nonpolyposis colorectal cancer	DNA analysis

genetic screening will be used to help identify people who are predisposed to conditions such as breast and colon cancer, diabetes, and heart disease. Nurses will be expected to participate in explaining risk and genetic predisposition, supporting informed health decisions and opportunities for prevention and early intervention, and protecting patients' privacy. Table 4.5 gives examples of genetic screening.

Testing and Screening for Adult-Onset Conditions

Adult-onset conditions are disorders (Table 4.6) with a genetic basis that are manifested in later life. Often clinical signs or symptoms occur only in late adolescence or adulthood, and disease is clearly observed to run in families. Some of these conditions are attributed to specific genetic mutations and follow either an autosomal dominant or an autosomal recessive inheritance pattern. However, the majority of adult-onset condition are considered to be multifactorial (polygenetic); examples include heart disease, diabetes and arthritis. Multifactorial influences involve the interactions among several genes (gene-gene interaction) and between genes and the environment (gene-environment interactions).

Nursing assessment for adult-onset condition is based on family history, personal and medical risk factors, and identification of associated diseases or clinical manifestations. Knowledge of adult-onset conditions and their genetic bases (i.e. Mendelian versus multifactorial conditions) influences the nursing considerations for genetic testing and health promotion.

If a single gene accounts for an adult-onset condition in a symptomatic person, diagnostic testing is used to confirm a diagnosis to assist in the plan of care and management. Diagnostic testing for adult-onset conditions is most frequently used with autosomal dominant conditions. Such as Huntington's disease or factor V Leiden thrombophilia, and with autosomal recessive conditions such as hemochromatosis. In families with known adult-onset conditions or with a confirmed genetic mutation in

TABLE 4.5: Applications for genetic screening

Timing of screening	Purpose	Examples
Preconception screening	For autosomal recessive inherited genetic conditions that occur with greater frequency among individuals of certain ethnic groups	Cystic fibrosis–all couples, but especially Northern European Caucasian, and Ashkenazi Jewish Tay-Sachs disease–Ashkenazi Jewish sickle cell anemia – African American, Puerto Rican, Mediterranean, Middle Eastern alpha-thalassemia – Southeast Asian, African American
Prenatal screening	For genetic conditions that are common and for which prenatal diagnosis is available when a pregnancy is identified at increased risk	Neural tube defects– spina bifida, anencephaly, Down syndrome, other chromosomal abnormalities–trisomy 18
Newborn screening	For genetic conditions for which there is specific treatment	Phenylketonuria (PKU), galactosemia, homocystinuria, biotinidase deficiency

TABLE 4.6: Adult-onset disorders

Medical description	Age of onset (y)	Inheritance	Risk factors
Neurologic conditions			
Early-onset familial Alzheimer disease			
Progressive dementia, memory failure, personality disturbance, loss of intellectual functioning associated with cerebral cortical atrophy, beta-amyloid plague formation, intraneuronal neurofibrillary tangles	<60–65 and often before 55	AD <2% (autosomal dominant)	Mutations on preslin 1, preslin 2 and/or beta-amyloid precursor protein Carriers of apolipoprotein E4
Late-onset familial Alzheimer disease			
Progressive dementia, cognitive decline	>60–65	AD ~25% MF ~75% (Multi-factorious)	Gene-gene interactions Diabetes Hypercholesterolemia Cerebrovascular or cardiovascular disease
Huntington disease			
Widespread degenerative brain change with progressive motor loss, both voluntary and involuntary disability, cognitive decline, cholera (involuntary movements) at later stage, psychiatric disturbances	35–44 (mean)	AD 100%	HD gene
Hematologic conditions			
Hereditary hemochromatosis (HHC)			
High absorption of iron by gastrointestinal mucosa, resulting in excessive iron storage in liver, skin, pancreas, heart, joints, and testes Early symptoms of abdominal pain, weakness, lethargy, weight loss Possible pigmentation, diabetes mellitus, hepatic fibrosis or cirrhosis, heart failure, and arrhythmias or arthritis in untreated people	40–60 in males; after menopause in females	AR ~60-90% (autosomal recessive) MF ~10–30%	Carrier or sibling of carrier of HFE gene mutations Liver disease such as alcoholic liver disease, acute viral hepatitis, or chronic hepatitis C Iron overload resulting from ingested iron in foods, cookware, and medicines, as well as parenteral iron from iron injections or transfusions for a chronic anemia such as beta-thalassemia or sickle cell disease
Factor V Leiden thrombophilia			
Poor anticoagulant response to activated protein C with increased risk for venous thrombosis and risk for increased fetal loss during pregnancy	30s; during pregnancy in females	AD	Carriers or relatives of individuals known to have factor V Leiden mutations Families with high rates of venous thromboembolism, deep venous thrombosis, or pulmonary embolism, especially if age<50y Women with recurrent pregnancy loss or venous thromboembolism during pregnancy or who use oral contraceptives
Diabetes mellitus type 2			
Insulin resistance, impaired glucose tolerance	Variable onset; most often >30	MF	Gene-gene interactions Obesity Hypertension Hyperlipidemia High intake of refined carbohydrates
Cardiovascular disease			
Familial hypercholesterolemia Elevated LDL levels leading to coronary artery disease, xanthomas, and corneal arcus	35–50	AD	Family or personal history of coronary heart disease at <45 years in women or <40 years in men Elevated LDL
Oncology conditions			
Multiple endocrine neoplasia Familial medullary thyroid cancer, pheochromocytoma, and parathyroid abnormalities	Early adulthood; 40–50 y	AD	Carrier or relative of carrier of a RET mutation Family history of medullary thyroid cancer, pheochromocytoma, and parathyroid abnormalities
Breast cancer			
BRCA1 and BRCA2 hereditary breast/ovarian cancer Breast, ovarian, an prostate (BRCA1) Breast, ovarian, and other cancer (BRCA2)	30–70; often <50	AD ~5–10% of breast and ovarian cancers MF >75%	Mutations in BRCA1 BRCA2
Hereditary non-polyposis colorectal cancer (HNPCC)			
Colorectal, ovarian, endometrial, bladder, gastric, biliary, and renal cell cancers	<50	AD ~1–3% of colorectal colon cancer, ~1% of endometrial cancers	Mutations in family of repair genes

an affected family member, **presymptomatic testing** provides asymptomatic people with information about the presence of a genetic mutation and about the likelihood of developing the disease. Huntington disease has served as the model for presymptomatic testing because the presence of the genetic mutation predicts disease onset and progression. Although preventive measures are not yet available for Huntington disease, the genetics information enables health care providers to develop a clinical, supportive, and psychological plan of care. Presymptomatic testing is considered for people in families with a known adult onset condition in which either a positive or a negative test result indicates an increased or reduced risk for developing the disease, affects medical management, or allows earlier treatment of a condition.

The foremost factor that may influence the development and severity of disease is a persons genetic makeup. However, in the absence of a single disease-causing gene, it is thought that multiple genes and other environmental factors are related to the onset of most adult diseases. For some diseases, the interactions among several genes and other environmental or metabolic events affect disease onset and progression. Specific gene-gene interactions or SNPs can confer susceptibility to disease. Most susceptibility testing is conducted in the research setting to identify candidate genes for diseases such as Alzheimer disease, psychiatric conditions, heart disease, hypertension and hypercholesterolemia. Susceptibility testing helps distinguish variations within the same disease or response to treatment. For example, no single gene is associated with osteoporosis. Several polymorphisms on candidate genes related to the vitamin D receptor, estrogen and androgen receptors and cytokine production and its associated stimulation of osteoclasts are under study to predict bone mineral density and fracture risk. Some susceptibility genes may predict treatment response. For example, people may present with similar clinical signs and symptoms of asthma but have different responses to treatment. Susceptibility testing helps classify people with asthma as sensitive or resistant to treatment with corticosteroids.

Population screening, the use of genetic testing for large groups or whole populations, to identify late-onset conditions is under development. For a test to be considered for population screening, there must be (1) sufficient information about gene distribution within populations, (2) accurate prediction about the development and progression of disease, and (3) appropriate medical management for asymptomatic people with a mutation. Currently, population screening is offered in some ethnic groups to identify cancer-predisposing genes. For example, Ashkenazi Jews (Jews of Eastern European origin) have a greater chance of having a specific genetic mutation in the BRCA1 and BRCA2 gene. People with one of these BRCA mutations have approximately an 80% risk for breast cancer, a 40 to 65% risk for ovarian cancer (BRCAI carriers), a 20% risk for ovarian cancer (BRCA2 carriers), and a 16% risk for prostate cancer. The identification of one of these mutations gives patients options for cancer screening as well as chemoprevention or prophylactic mastectomy or oophorectomy in carriers. Population screening is being explored for other adult-onset conditions such as type 2 diabetes and hereditary hemochromatosis (iron overload disorder).

Nurses must be alert for family histories indicating that multiple generations (autosomal dominant inheritance) or multiple siblings (autosomal recessive inheritance) are affected with the same condition or that onset of disease is earlier than expected (e.g. multiple generations with early-onset hyperlipidemia). Possible adult-onset conditions are discussed with other members of the health care team for appropriate resources and referral. When a family history of disease is identified, the nurse must be responsible for making the patient aware that this is a risk factor for disease. Regardless of whether a particular patient pursues a genetic testing workup, risk information for the disease should be explained. For example, if a 45 years old woman presents for her annual gynecology visit and has a family history showing colon cancer in multiple paternal relatives, including her father, the nurse discussed the family history with the gynecologist. In addition, the woman is alerted to the risk for colon cancer based on the family history, and she is given information about possible genetic testing and referral for a colonoscopy.

If the existence of a mutation for an adult-onset condition in a family is identified, at-risk family members can be referred for **predisposition testing**. If the patient is found to be a carrier of the mutation, the nurse provides him or her with information about the risk to other family members. In that discussion, the nurse assures the patient that the test results are private and confidential and will not be shared with others, including family members, without the patients permission. If the patient is an unaffected family member, the nurse discusses inheritance and the risk for developing the disease, provides support for the decision-making process, and offers referral for genetics services.

Management of Genetic Disease

There is no cure for genetic disease at present, although preventive and corrective therapy is helping to reduce the harmful effects in an increasing number of conditions. Genetic research is making progress in the art of altering the genetic material directly. Meanwhile, the major goal of therapy is modification of the internal or external environment to correct or minimize the effects of the genetic defect.

Therapeutic Modalities

The therapeutic modalities available for genetic disorders are few when compared with the infinite variety of conditions afflicting the population, but with increased understanding of the basic defects and the technical advances being made, an increasing number of genetic disorders are becoming amenable to treatment.

Surgical repair: Surgical repair of structural defects has made it possible to prolong life in a number of multifactorial disorders. Numerous facial and limb deformities can be altered by plastic and reconstructive techniques. In cases of familial polyposis coli, surgical removal of the colon eliminates the countless polyps that invariably become cancerous. Splenectomy prevents the trapping of abnormal blood cells in that organ in several hereditary disorders of red blood cells. Early diagnosis and enucleation in retinoblastoma have reduced the mortality from this malignant eye tumor. Fetal surgery may also be performed for some life-threatening anomalies, particularly urinary tract abnormalities.

Diet modification: For disorders in which an enzyme deficiency causes a toxic accumulation of a substance or its by-products, restricting the intake of foods containing the offending substance often prevents irreversible damage from the improper metabolism of these compounds, this dietary control is a life-long recommendation. Examples include the low-phenylalanine diet prescribed for children with phenylketonuria (PKU), elimination of diary products containing lactose for infants and children with hereditary lactase deficiency, avoidance of foods containing or producing galactose for children with galactosemia, and a diet low in branched-chain amino acids for infants and children with maple syrup urine disease. Women with PKU who have not phenylalanine diet before conception and maintain it throughout pregnancy to prevent a high risk of adverse fetal effects. Folic acid supplementation preconceptionally has been shown to reduce the incidence or recurrence of neural tube defects (NTDs).

Folic acid: Folic acid supplementation before conception can have a major impact in the prevention of NTDs. Therefore, in 1992 there was recommendation that all women capable of becoming pregnant should consume 0.4 mg of folic acid per day. It is mandatory that folic acid would be added to enriched grain products. This would add 0.1 mg folic acid to the daily diet of the average person. Since that time there has been a 19% reduction in the incidence of NTDs.

Women who have previously had a pregnancy affected with an NTD are advised to take 4.0 mg of folic acid per day beginning 1 month before conception and continuing throughout the first trimester of pregnancy. The risk of recurrence in another pregnancy affected by an NTD is reduced by 72% in women following this regimen.

Product replacement: In some deficiency diseases, supplying the missing product that cannot be synthesized prevents undesirable effects. For example, thyroid extract is prescribed to prevent the damaging effects of hypothyroidism and providing the missing blood factors prevents life-threatening and debilitating hemorrhages in persons with hemophilia. Other examples are insulin for diabetes mellitus, growth hormone for growth hormone deficiency, and corticosteroids for adrenogenital syndrome.

Avoidance of drugs or other substances: In drug induced disease, such as glucose-6-phosphate dehydrogenase (G-6-PD) deficiency and the porphyries, avoidance of the drugs that precipitate a reaction provides a simple preventive measure.

Removal of toxic substances: Removal of toxic substances that accumulate in vital tissues as a result of a hereditary disease can prevent disabling complications. Some of the deleterious effects of hemochromatosis, a hereditary disorder characterized by an excess accumulation of iron in the liver, heart, and pancreas, can be reduced with the removal of iron by administration of chelating agents or periodic phlebotomies.

Immunologic prevention: The administration of immunoglobulin to Rh-negative mothers following the birth of an Rh-positive infant is effective in preventing Rh-antibody formation that causes hemolytic disease of the newborn in subsequent births.

Transplantation: Replacement of nonfunctioning organs with normal organs is increasing the survival of children with defective organs because the problems of tissue incompatibility are better controlled. Examples of organ transplants include the kidneys in nereditary polycystic kidneys, the heart in severe cardiac myopathy, liver in hepatic atresia, and bone marrow.

Cofactor administration: Diet supplements can be given when the body is unable to synthesize or effectively use some substances needed as cofactors in metabolism, such as vitamin B_{12} in pernicious anemia, in which absorption of this vitamin is absent. Vitamin and cofactor supplementation may be used in the treatment of mitochondrial disease.

Recombinant DNA: The transfer of modified genetic material from one organism (a virus) to another causes the viral DNA to become integrated into the cellular DNA of a recipient cell, often a bacteria cell. This recombinant DNA multiplies, producing the missing substance in the host cell. This technology has been applied in growth hormone therapy and factor VIII synthesis.

Gene transfer: Fragments of DNA from a normal gene can be introduced directly into a recipient cell lacking such a gene. This approach has been attempted in humans with the transfer of normal gene copies of β-hemoglobin into bone marrow cells in an effort to treat a form of β-hemoglobin and has been used in sickle cell disease. Gene transfer has also been successfully used in adenosine deaminase deficiency. Gene therapy is the introduction of healthy genes into patients to replace their own defective genes. This concept of delivering genes to specific target has been widened the field from treatment of single-gene defect (e.g. cystic fibrosis and DMD) to alleviation of multi-gene defects (e.g. neurodegenerative disease cardiac disease). Gene therapy research has suffered a number of setbacks in clinical research, and the search for safer, more effective ways to transfer genes into human cells continues.

Other therapies: Other methods such as enzyme repression and competitive inhibition are providing effective treatment in some metabolic disorders. Growth hormone therapy is used in

Turner and Noonan syndromes. Future therapies include the possibility of replacement or stabilization by infection or oral administration of a substance that the patient lacks.

Environmental Manipulation

Inherited diseases or defects for which there is no therapeutic modality can be modified to enhance the quality of life for the affected individual. Some examples of environmental manipulation include hearing aids for deaf children, glasses or vision enhancers such as enlarged print and books in Braille for the visually impaired, mobilizing devices such as braces and wheelchairs for persons with muscle and bone impair-ment, prosthetic devices for limb deficiencies, and infant stimulation programs to maximize the potential of children who are mentally retarded.

ROLE OF NURSES IN APPLICATIONS OF GENETICS IN HEALTH CARE

Nurses in genetics-related health care blend the principles of human genetics with nursing care in collaborations with other professionals, including genetic specialist, to foster improvement, maintenance, and restoration of patient's health. In all nursing practice setting, nurses have five main tasks:

1. Help collect and interpret relevant family and medical histories
2. Identify patients and families who need further genetics evaluation and counseling and refer them to appropriate genetics services
3. Offer genetics information and resources to patients and families
4. Collaborate with genetics specialists, and
5. Participate in the management and coordination of care of patients with genetic conditions.

Genetics-related nursing practice involves the care of people who have genetic conditions, those who may be predisposed to develop or pass on genetic conditions, and those who are seeking genetics information and referral for additional genetics services.

Nurses support patients and families with genetics-related health concerns by ensuring that their choices are informed ones and by advocating for the privacy and confidentiality of genetics information and for equal access to genetic testing and treatments.

Health Assessment

Assessment of a persons genetics-related health status is an ongoing process. Nurses collect information that can help identify individuals and families who have actual or potential genetics-related health concerns or who may benefit from further genetics information, counseling, testing and treatment. This process can begin before conception and continue throughout the lifespan. Nurses evaluate family and past medical histories, including prenatal history, childhood illnesses, developmental history, adult-onset conditions (in adults), past surgeries, treatments, and medications, this information may relate to the genetic condition at hand or to a condition being considered. Nurses also identify the patient's ethnic background and conduct a physical assessment to gather pertinent genetics information. The assessment also includes information about culture, spiritual beliefs, and ancestry. Genetics-related health assessment always includes determining a patients or family's understanding of actual or potential genetics-related health concerns awareness of how these issues are communicated within a family.

Family History Assessment

Nurses in any practice setting continuously assess families' genetics histories to identify the presence of a genetic trait, inherited condition, or predisposition. Targeted questions are used to identify genetic conditions for which further information, education, testing or treatment can be offered. In consultation and collaboration with other health care providers and specialists, nurses can then determine whether further genetic testing and evaluation should be offered for the trait or condition in question. A well-documented family history is a tool used by the health care team to make a diagnosis, identify testing strategies, and establish a pattern of inheritance. The family history should include at least three generations, as well as information about the current and past health status of all family members, including the age at onset of any illnesses, cause of death, and age at death. Nurses also inquire about medical conditions that are known to have a heritable component and for which genetic testing may be available. Nurses obtain information about the presence of birth defects, mental retardation, familial traits, or similarly affected family members (Box 4.1).

Nurses also consider the presence of genetic relatedness (consanguinity) among family members when assessing the risk for genetic conditions in couples or families. For example, when obtaining a preconception or prenatal family history, the nurse asks if the prospective parents have common ancestors (i.e. are they first cousins?). This is important to know, because people who are related have more genes in common than those who are unrelated, thus increasing their chance for having children with an autosomal recessive inherited conditions such as cystic fibrosis. The number of shared genes depends on the degree of relationship. For example, a parent and child share one half of their genes, whereas first cousins share one eighth of their genes. Ascertaining genetic relatedness gives nurses the opportunity to offer additional genetic counseling and evaluation. It may also serve as an explanation for parents who have a child with a rare autosomal recessive inherited condition or for a person who is similarly affected.

Box 4.1 Genetics family history

A well-documented family history can be used to:
- Assess risk of certain diseases
- Decide on testing strategies, such as what genetic and other diagnostic tests to order
- Establish a pattern of inheritance
- Identify other family members who are at increased risk
- Calculate risks
- Assess risk of passing on conditions to children
- Determine and recommend treatments that modify disease risk making decisions risk
- Making decisions about management or surveillance
- Develop patient rapport
- Educate patients

Key questions to ask about each family member include:
- What the current age or what was the age at death?
- What is the ethnic background (some genetic conditions are more common in certain ethnic groups)?

Is there a history of:
- Multiple pregnancy losses/stillbirths?
- Unexplained infertility?
- Birth defects?
- Mental retardation or developmental delay?
- Learning disabilities?
- Medical problems in children whose parents are closely related (second cousins or closer)?
- Congenital or juvenile blindness, cataracts, hearing loss, or deafness?
- Very short or very tall stature?
- Several close relatives with the same or related conditions (e.g. breast or colon cancer, diabetes, heart disease, asthma, stroke, high blood pressure, kidney disease)?
- Occurrence of a common condition with earlier age of onset than is usual (e.g. breast or colon cancer, hearing loss, dementia, heart disease)?

When the assessment of family history reveals that a patient has been adopted, genetics-based health assessment becomes more challenging. The nurse and the health care team should make all efforts to help the patient obtain as such information as possible about his or her biologic parents, including their ethnic backgrounds.

Questions regarding reproductive history (e.g., history of miscarriage or stillbirth) are included in genetics family history health assessments to identify possible chromosomal conditions. Nurses also inquire about any history of family members with inherited conditions or birth defects; maternal health conditions such as type 1 diabetes, seizure disorders, or PKU, which may increase the risk for birth defects in children, and about exposure to alcohol or other drugs during pregnancy. Maternal age is also noted; women who are 35 years of age or older who are considering pregnancy and childbearing or who are already pregnant should be offered prenatal diagnosis (e.g. testing through amniocentesis) because of the association between advanced maternal age and chromosomal abnormalities such as Down's syndrome.

Physical Assessment

Physical assessment may provide clues that a particular genetic condition is present in a person and family. Family history assessment may offer initial guidance regarding particular area for physical assessment. For example, a family history of familial hypercholesterolemia would alert the nurse to assess family members for symptoms of hyperlipidemias (xanthomas, corneal arcus, abdominal pain of unexplained origin). As another example, a family history of neurofibromatosis type 1, an inherited condition involving tumors of the central nervous system, would prompt the nurse to carry out a detailed assessment of closely related family members. Skin findings such as café-au-lait spots, axillary freckling, or tumors of the skin (neurofibromas) would warrant referral for further evaluation, including genetic evaluation and counseling.

If a genetic condition is suspected as a result of a family history or physical assessment, the nurse, in collaboration with the health care team, may initiate further discussion and evaluation. Providing genetics information, offering and discussing genetic tests, and suggesting a referral to a geneticist are part of the nurse's role. Indications for genetics referral are given in Box 4.2.

Ancestry, Cultural, Social, and Spiritual Assessment

When collecting and discussing genetics information, nurses assess the ancestry of patients and families, as well as their ethnic, cultural, social and spiritual orientation. Assessment of ancestry and ethnicity helps identify individual patients and groups who could benefit from genetic testing for carrier identification, prenatal diagnosis.

The assessment of a client's psychosocial genetic health is based on the nurse's professional responsibility to demonstrate in practice the importance of tailoring genetic and genomic information and services to clients based on their culture, religion, knowledge level, literacy and preferred language.

The nurse assesses:
- Educational level and understanding of the genetic condition or concern in the family
- Desired goals and health outcomes in relation to the genetic condition or concern
- Family rules regarding disclosure of medical information (e.g. some families may not reveal a history of a disease such as cancer or mental illness during the family history assessment)
- Family rules, bounderies, and cultural practices as well as personal preference about knowing genetic information

Box 4.2 Indications for making a genetics referral

Prepregnancy and Prenatal
- Maternal age of 35 years or greater at expected time of delivery
- Previous child with a chromosome problem
- Positive alpha-fetoprotein profile screening test
- Previous child with a birth defect or family history of birth defects
- Pregnancy history of two or more unexplained miscarriages
- Maternal conditions such as diabetes, epilepsy, or alcoholism
- Exposures to certain medications or drugs during pregnancy
- Family history of mental retardation
- Either member of the couple has a birth defect such as cleft lip or palate, spina bifida, or congenital heart defect
- Either member of the couple has a chromosome abnormality

Pediatric
- Positive newborn screening test
- One or more major birth defects
- Unusual (dysmorphic) facial features
- Development delay/mental retardation
- Suspicion of a metabolic disorder
- Unusually tall or short stature, or growth delays
- Known chromosomal abnormality

Adult
- Mental retardation without a known cause
- Unexplained infertility or multiple pregnancy losses
- A personal or family history of thrombotic events
- Adult-onset conditions such as hemochromatosis, hearing loss, visual impairment
- Family history of an adult-onset neurodegenerative disorder (e.g. Huntington disease)
- Features of a genetic condition such as neurofibromatosis (cafe-au-lait spots, neurofibromas on the skin), Marfan syndrome (unusually tall stature, dilation of the aortic root), others
- Personal of family history of cardiovascular disorders known to be associated with genetic factors such as cardiomyopathy or long QT syndrome
- Family history of cancers known to be associated with specific genes such as hereditary breast/ovarian cancer or hereditary nonpolyposis colorectal cancer (HNPCC)
- Family history of early onset cancers and familial clustering of related tumors

- Past coping mechanisms and social support
- Ability to make an informed decision (e.g. is the patient under stress from family situations, acute or chronic illness, or medications that may impair the patient's ability to make an informed decision?).

Genetic Counseling

Genetic counseling is a combination process that deals with human problems associated with the occurrence, or recurrence, of a genetic disorder in a family. There is a specific concern about risk associated with a certain problem or because of the relationship to someone who is affected, the proband. Several steps occur in the genetic evaluation, including obtaining and reviewing the medical history and records of the affected; eliciting the family history, with special attention to factors pertinent to the diagnosis in the proband; evaluating and examining the affected (if available and indicated); ordering appropriate tests and interpreting results; and then meeting with the person seeking the consultation and/or the proband.

Goals of Genetic Counseling

Assist the proband and/or consultant to:

1. Comprehend the medical facts, including the diagnosis, the possible course of the disorder, and the available management.
2. Understand the inheritance of the disorder and the risk of recurrence in specified relatives.
3. Understand the options for dealing with the risk of recurrence.
4. Choose the course of action that seems appropriate to the individuals involved, in view of their risk, family goals, and religious beliefs, and act in accordance with that decision.
5. Make the best possible adjustment to the disorder.

Components of counseling are given in Box 4.3.

Box 4.3 Components of genetic counseling

Information and assessment sources
- Reason for referral
- Family history
- Medical history/records
- Relevant test results and other medical evaluations
- Social and emotional concerns
- Relevant cultural, educational, and financial factors

Analysis of data
- Family history
- Physical examination as needed
- Additional laboratory testing and procedures (e.g. echocardiogram, ophthalmology or neurologic examination)

Communication of genetic finding
- Natural history of disorder
- Pattern of inheritance
- Reproductive and family health issues and options
- Testing options
- Management and treatment issues

Counseling and support
- Identify individual and family question and concerns
- Identify existing support systems
- Provide emotional and social support
- Refer of additional support and counseling as indicated

Follow-up
- Written summary to referring primary care providers and family
- Coordination of care with primary care providers and specialists
- Additional discussion of test results or diagnosis

Identify Persons in Need of Genetic Assessment and Counseling

1. Parents of a child with a birth defects, mental retardation, or known/possible genetic disorder.
2. Any individual with a genetic or potentially genetic disorder.
3. Persons with a family history of mental retardation, birth defects(s), genetic disorder, or condition that tends to run in the family.
4. Pregnant women who will be 35 or older at the time delivery.
5. Couples of ethnic origin known to be at an increased risk for a specific genetic disorder.
6. Couples who have experienced two or more miscarriages.
7. Pregnant women who have an elevated or low maternal serum screening test result, such as alpha-fetoprotein.
8. Women who have been exposed to drugs or infections during pregnancy.
9. Couples who are related to each other.
10. Persons who are concerned about the risk for a genetic disorder.

Genetic Screening, Testing and Research Screening

1. Screening is the level of testing offered to large population (e.g. newborn) or to high-risk segments of the population (such as African-Americans, Ashkenazi Jews, Mediterranean people) to identify individual with a genetic disorder, increased risk for abnormality, or carriers of a genetic disorder.
2. Criteria include that the test itself must be reliable, appropriate to the designated population, and cost-effective and that the condition being tested for must be treatable or that early identification will enhance health.
3. Newborn screening varies among states, testing for disorders such as phenylketonuria (PKU), hypothyroidism, maple syrup urine disease (MSUD), and histidinemia.
4. Prenatal screening-maternal serum alpha-fetoprotein (AFP) or triple screen (includes measurement of maternal serum AFP, beta-human chorionic gonadotropin [bHCG], and estriol) or quad screen. After 14 weeks gestation can identify pregnancies at increased risk for neural tube defects (NTD), Down sydrome, and trisomy 18.

Testing

1. Biochemical testing is done on body tissue or fluid to measure enzyme levels and activity.
2. DNA testing is done on blood or tissue samples to look for a gene mutation or to study DNA linkage.
3. Chromosomal testing is done on nucleated cells (usually blood cells) or other tissue for detection of various conditions, such as extra, missing, deleted, duplicated, or rearranged chromosomes.

Prenatal Testing

1. *Chorionic villus sampling (CVS)*—for chromosomal, biochemical, and DNA testing; done at 9 to 12 weeks gestation.
2. *Amniocentesis*—for chromosomal, biochemical, and DNA testing at 13 weeks (early amniocentesis), AFP can be done at 14 to 18 gestation.
3. *Ultrasound*—for dating pregnancy and assessing fetal structures, placenta, and amniotic fluid; done throughout pregnancy, but fetal structures are best visualized after 12 weeks.
4. *Acetylcholinesterase* (ACH) in amniotic fluid for suspected NTD.
5. *Fetoscopy*—for obtaining fetal blood samples or visualizing details of fetal structures, done during second trimester.
6. *Percutaneous umbilical blood sampling (PUBS)*—for obtaining fetal blood, done during second trimester.

Research

1. Testing done to further understand the genetics of a disorder or biochemical process.
2. Not clinical testing, and may have no clinical value to the patients case.
   a. Some states, such as New Work, mandate that genetic research specimens must be kept anonymous and that results not be provided to an individual for any clinical use.
3. There is ongoing and extensive research on cancer susceptibility genes.

Additional Genetic Testing Consideration

DNA banking—extraction and storage of one's DNA from blood through a qualified genetics laboratory; requires informed consent, proper collection, and prompt handling.

Genetic counseling across the lifespan are given in Box 4.4.

Nursing Roles and Responsibilities

1. Recognize or suspect genetic disorders by their physical characteristics and clinical manifestations.
2. Create a genetic pedigree (diagram of the family history), including cause of death and any genetically linked ailments.

Box 4.4 Genetic counseling across the lifespan

Prenatal issues
- Understanding prenatal screening and diagnosis testing
- Implications of reproductive choices
- Potential for anxiety and emotional distress
- Effects on partnership, family and parental-fetal bonding

Newborn issues
- Understanding newborn screening results
- Potential for disrupted parent-newborn relationship on diagnosis of a genetic condition
- Parental guilt
- Implications for siblings and other family members
- Coordination and continuity of care

Pediatric issues
- Caring for children with complex medical needs
- Coordination of care
- Potential for impaired parent-child relationship
- Potential for social stigmatization

Adolescent issues
- Potential for impaired self-image and decreased self-esteem
- Potential for altered perception of family
- Implication for lifestyle and family planning

Adult issues
- Potential for ambiguous test results
- Identification of a genetic susceptibility or diagnosis without an existing cure
- Effect on marriage reproduction, parenting, and lifestyle
- Potential impact on insurability and employability

3. Explain/review those aspects of diagnosis, prognosis, and treatment that affect the patients growth and development and that parents or caretakers need to know to plan for the care of the patient.
4. Clear up misconceptions and allay feelings of guilt.
5. Assist with the diagnostic process by exploring medical and family history information, by using physical assessment skills, by obtaining blood samples, and/or by assisting with CVS or amniocentesis, as indicated.
6. Enhance and reinforce self-image and self-worth of parents and child.
7. Encourage interaction with family and friends; offer referrals, phone numbers of support groups.
8. Refer and prepare family for genetic counseling
   a. Inform that prenatal testing does not mean termination of pregnancy (e.g. it may confirm that the fetus is not affected, thus eliminating worry throughout pregnancy, although the determination of an abnormality is also a possibility).
   b. Encourage the parents to allow adequate time to deliberate on a course of action (e.g. do not rush into a tubal ligation, because in a few years they may want more children).
   c. Remain nonjudgmental.
9. Check within state (for example, state health department) for information and resources regarding newborn testing required, state regulations on genetic testing and research, etc.
10. Recognize that there are many ethical, legal, psychosocial, and professional issues associated with obtaining, using, and storing genetic information.
    a. Be aware of associated professional responsibilities, including informed consent, documentation in medical records, medical releases, and individual privacy of information.
    b. Refer to state legislation that deals with protection from genetic discrimination in medical insurance; individual state legislation; genetics professional societies and the World Health Organization document on ethical considerations in genetic testing and services.
11. Refer for further information and support to genetic services agencies.

People seek genetic counseling for a variety of reasons and at different stages of life. Some are seeking preconception or prenatal information, others are referred after the birth of a child with a birth defect or suspected genetic condition, and still others are seeking information for themselves or their families because of the presence of, or a family history of, a genetic condition. Regardless of the timing or setting, genetic counseling is offered to all people who have questions about genetics and their health. In collaboration with the health care team, nurses consider referral for genetic counseling for any patient who belongs to a family with a hereditary condition and who asks questions such as, "What are my chances for having this condition? Is there a genetic test that will tell me? Is there gene-based treatment or cure? What are my options?"

As the contribution of genetics to the health-illness continuum is recognized, the process of genetic counseling is expected to become a responsibility of all health care professionals in clinical practice. Nurses are obvious and natural providers of genetics services because they are often aware of the patient's personal and family history. Nurses assess the patient's health and make referrals for specialized diagnosis and treatment. They offer anticipatory guidance by explaining the purpose and goals of a referral. They collaborate with primary healthcare providers and specialists in giving supportive and follow-up counseling. They coordinate follow-up and case management.

Genetic Services

Genetics services provide genetic information, education, and support to patients and families with genetics-related health concerns. Genetics professionals, including medical geneticists, genetics counselors, and advanced practice nurses in genetics, provide specific genetics services to patients and families who are referred by their primary health care providers. A team approach is often used by genetics specialists to obtain and interpret complex family history information, evaluate and diagnose genetic conditions, interpret and discuss complicated genetic test results, support patients throughout the evaluation process, and offer resources for additional professional and family support. Patients participate as team members and decision-makers throughout the process. Overall, genetics services are an evaluation and communication process by which patients and their families come to learn and understand relevant aspects of genetics, to make informed health decisions, and to receive support as they integrate personal and family genetics information into daily living.

Genetic counseling may take place over an extended period and may entail more than one counseling session, which may include other family members. This allows patients and families to learn and understand genetics information, to receive support and guidance in decision-making, and to obtain comprehensive and coordinated care if they have specific genetic conditions or concerns.

Nursing Intervention in Genetic Counseling

The process of genetic counseling and evaluation often involves additional genetic testing and procedures as well as decisions by patients and families with regard to reproduction, fertility, testing of children, and management options such as prophylactic surgery. Nurses have responsibilities in each of these areas for assessment and for providing psychosocial interventions and accurate information as family members consider their genetic testing and treatment options. In all of these areas, nurses consider individual patients in the context of the family.

When patients or family members are considering genetic testing, nurses provide accurate information as patients consider their options. For prenatal testing, this includes information and support for subsequent decisions regarding the pregnancy in the event of diagnosis of a genetic condition in the fetus. When a diagnosis such as Down syndrome or hereditary breast or ovarian cancer is made, families need information about the range and severity of potential problems, the proportion of people with milder aspects of the condition, management options, support organizations, and current understanding of the long-term prognosis.

Decision-making support is an important nursing intervention in many genetic counseling situations. Examples include consideration of pregnancy termination, presymptomatic testing for conditions such as Huntington disease, or predisposition testing for a hereditary cancer. Nurses help patients and families acquire information about options, identify the "pros" and "cons" of each option, and explore their values and beliefs. In addition, nurses help patients respect each persons right to receive or not to receive information an help them explain their decision to others.

Other essential components of nursing care and genetic counseling include teaching and an intervention known as "coping enhancement". For example, teaching is needed when a new genetics diagnosis is made. Patients and families need information about the range of possible health outcomes, treatment options, and, in the case of prenatal diagnosis of a genetic condition, management options regarding continuing or ending the pregnancy. Coping enhancement involves helping people adapt to perceived stressors or changes that interfere with daily living and functioning. Coping enhancement is essential throughout the entire genetic counseling, evaluation, and testing process. Indicators of patient knowledge, decision-making and coping outcomes have been developed, and nurses can use these indicators when documenting nursing care provided to families and its effectiveness.

Specific Nursing Roles in Genetic Counseling

Nurses refer patients, collaborative with genetic specialists, and participate in genetic counseling when they carry out the following activities:

- Provide appropriate genetics information before, during, and in follow-up to genetic counseling
- Help gather relevant family and medical history information
- Offer support to patients and families throughout the genetic counseling process
- Coordinate genetics-related health care with relevant community and national support resources.

These activities are carried out in collaboration with patients and families and help ensure that they receive the most benefit from genetic counseling, which includes the following:

- *Respecting patients' rights:* Respecting the patients' rights to self-determination—that is, supporting decisions that reflect the patient's personal beliefs, values, and interests—is a central principle directing how nurses provide genetics information and counseling. Genetics specialists and nurses participating in genetic counseling make every attempt to respect the patient's ability to make autonomous decisions. A first step in providing such nondirective counseling is recognizing one's own values and how communication of genetics information may be influenced by those values.

  Confidentiality of genetics information and respect for privacy are other essential principles underlying genetic counseling. Patients have the right to have testing without having the results divulged to anyone, including insurers or physicians. Some patients pay for testing themselves so that insurers will not learn of the test, and others use a different name for testing to protect their privacy.

  All genetics specialists, including nurses who participate in the genetic counseling process and those with access to people's genetics information, must honor a patients desire for confidentiality. Genetics information should be kept from family members, insurance companies, employers, and schools if the patient so desires, even if keeping the information confidential is difficult. A nurse may want to disclose genetics information to family members who could experience significant harm if they do not know such information. However, the patient may have other views and may wish to keep this information from the family, resulting in an ethical dilemma for both patient and nurse. The nurse must honor the patient's wishes, while explaining to the patient the potential benefit this information may have for other family members.

- *Providing precounseling informatiin:* Preparing the patient and family, promoting informed decision-making, and obtaining informed consent are essential in genetic counseling. Nurses assess the patient's capacity and ability to give voluntary consent. This includes assessment of factors that may interfere with informed consent, such as hearing loss, language differences, cognitive impairment, and the effects of medication. Nurses make sure that a person's decision to undergo testing is not affected by coercion, persuasion, or manipulation. Because information may need to be repeated over time, nurses offer follow-up discussion as needed.

  The genetics service to which a nurse refers a patient or family for genetic counseling will ask the nurse to provide background information for evaluation. Genetics specialists need to know the reason for referral, the patients or family's reason for seeking genetic counseling, and potential genetics-related health concerns. For example, a nurse may refer a family with a new diagnosis of hereditary breast or ovarian cancer to obtain more information or counseling or to discuss the likelihood of developing the disease and the implications for other family members. The family may have concerns about confidentiality and privacy. Using the nursing assessment, the genetics specialist tailors the genetic counseling to respond to these concerns.

  With the patient's permission, nurses may also provide genetics specialists with the relevant test results and medical evaluations. Nurses need to obtain permission from the patient and, if applicable, from other family members to retriever, review, and transfer medical records that document the genetic condition of concern. In some situations, evaluation of more than one family member may be necessary to establish a diagnosis of a genetic disorder. Nurses can prepare the family for this assessment by explaining that the medical information and evaluation are necessary to ensure that appropriate information and counseling (including risk interpretation) are provided.

  Nurses will be asked to provide information about the emotional and social status of the patient and family. Genetics specialist will want to know the coping skills of patients and families who have recently learned of the diagnosis of a genetic disorder and will want to know what type of genetics information is being sought. Nurses help identify cultural and other issues that may influence how information is provided and by whom. For example, for patients with hearing loss, a sign interpreters services may have to be arranged. For those with vision loss, alternative forms of communication may be necessary. Genetics professionals prepare for the genetic counseling and evaluation with these relevant issues in mind.

- *Preparing patients for genetics evaluation:* Before a genetic counseling appointment, the nurse discusses with the patient and family the type and nature of family history information that will be collected during the consultation. Family history collection and analysis are comprehensive and focus on information that may be relevant to the genetics-related concern in question. Although targeted to each genetic counseling situation, such analysis always includes assessment for any potentially inherited conditions for which testing and preventive and treatment measures may be available.

  A physical examination performed by the medical geneticist may be needed to identify specific clinical features that are diagnostic of a genetic condition. The examination also helps determine whether additional laboratory tests are needed to clarify the diagnosis of a genetic disorder. The detailed physical examination generally involves assessment of all body systems, with a focus on specific physical characteristics considered for diagnosis. The nurse describes the diagnostic evaluations that are part of a genetics consultation and explains their purposes.

- *Communicating genetics information to patients:* After the family history and physical examination are completed, the genetics team reviews the information gathered before beginning genetic counseling with the patient and family. The genetics specialists meet with the patient and family to discuss their findings. If information from family and medical histories and examination confirms the presence of a genetic condition in a family, genetics specialists discuss with the patient the natural history of the condition, the pattern of inheritance, and the implications of the condition for reproductive and general health. When appropriate, the specialists also discuss relevant testing and management options. The nurse assesses the patients understanding of the genetics consultation and clarifies information given by specialists.

- *Providing support:* The genetics team provides support throughout the counseling session and makes every effort to elicit personal and family concerns. Genetics specialists use principles of active listening to interpret patient concerns and emotions, seek and provide feedback, and demonstrate understanding of those concerns. When necessary, genetics specialists suggest referral for additional social and emotional support. Genetics specialists discuss pertinent patient and family concerns and need with nurses regarding primary care and guidance. The nurse assesses the patients understanding of the information given during the counseling session, clarifies information, answers questions, assess patient reactions, and identifies support systems.

- *Follow-up after genetic evaluation:* As follow-up to genetic evaluation and counseling, genetics specialists prepare a written summary of the evaluation and counseling session and, with the patients permission, send this summary to the primary health care provider as well as all other providers and participants in the patients care, as identified by the family. The consultation summary outlines the results of the family history and physical and laboratory assessments, provides a discussion and associated risk of recurrence for the patient and family, presents reproductive and general health options, and make recommendations for further testing and management. The summary is also sent to the patient, and a copy is retained in the patient medical record. The nurse plays an important role in reviewing the summary with the patient and family identifying information, education, and counseling for which follow-up counseling may be useful.

  Follow-up genetic counseling is always offered to patients and families, because some people may need more time to understand and discuss the specifics of a genetic test or diagnosis, or they may wish to review reproductive options again later, when pregnancy is being considered. Follow-up genetic counseling is also offered to patients when further evaluation and counseling of extended family members is recommended. As part of follow-up, nurses can educate patients about where to find information about genetics issues.

To a patient, a family, other care providers, community agencies and organizations, and society as a whole. In addition it provides support for nurses facing clinical situations that involve ethical dilemmas. Principle-based ethics offers moral guidelines that nurses can use to justify their nursing practice. The emphasis is on ethical principles of beneficence (to do good) and nonmaleficence (to do no harm), as well as autonomy, justice, fidelity, and veracity, to help solve ethical dilemmas that may arise in clinical care. Respect for people is the ethical principle underlying all nursing care. Using an ethical foundation based on these principles that incorporates the values of caring, nurses can promote the kind of thoughtful discussions that are useful when patients and families are facing genetics-related health and reproductive decisions and consequences.

CHAPTER

5

Immunological Problems and Nursing

INTRODUCTION

The term immunity refers to the body's specific protective response to an invading foreign agent or organism. In other words, immunity is a state of responsiveness to foreign substance such as microorganisms and tumor proteins. The immune system functions as the body's defense mechanism against invasion and allows a rapid response to foreign substance in a specific manner. Immune response serve three functions.

1. *Defense:* The body protects against invasion by microorganisms and prevents the development of infection by attacking foreign antigen and pathogens.
2. *Homeostasis:* Damaged cellular substances are digested and removed. Through this mechanisms, the body's different cell types remain uniform and unchanged.
3. *Surveillance:* Mutations continually arise in the body but are normally recognized as foreign cells and destroyed.

Immune response occur at genetic and cellular levels. Any qualitative or quantitative change in the components of the immune system can produce profound effect, on the integrity of the human organism. Immune function is affected by a variety of factors such as central nervous system integrity, emotional status, medications, and the stress of illness, trauma or surgery dysfunctions involving the immune system occur across the lifespan. Many are genetically based; others are acquired.

Immune memory is a property of immune system that provides protection against harmful microbial agents despite the timing of re-exposure to the agent. Tolerance is the process by which the immune system is programmed to eliminate foreign substances such as microbes, toxins, and cellular mutations but maintain the ability to accept self-antigens. Some evidence is given to the concept of surveillance in which the immune system is in a perpetual state of vigilance, screening and rejecting any invader that is recognized as foreign to the host.

The term 'immunopathology' refers to the study of diseases than result from dysfunctions within the immune system. Disorders of the immune system may stem from excesses or deficiencies of immune competent cells, alteration in the functions of these cells, immunologic attack on self-antigens, or inappropriate or exaggerated responses to specific antigens.

To gain insight into immunopathology and the growing number of immunologic disorders, and to assess and care of people with immunologic disorders, the nurse needs to understand the immune system and how it functions; to recognize its importance in understanding disease processes, and to apply this knowledge in making appropriate patient care decisions.

REVIEW IMMUNE SYSTEM

The immune system is composed of an integrated collection of various cell types, each with a designated functional role in defending against infection and invasion by other organisms. Supporting this system are molecules that are responsible for the interactions, modulations and regulation of the system. These molecules and cells participate in specific interactions with immunogenic **epitopes** (antigenic determinants) present on foreign materials and initiate a series of actions in a host, including the inflammatory response, the lysis of microbial agents, and the disposal of foreign toxins. The major components of the immune system include the bone marrow and the lymphoid tissues, including the thymus gland, the spleen, the lymph nodes, the tonsils and adenoids, and similar tissues in the gastrointestinal, respiratory and reproductive systems.

Bone marrow: The WBCs involved in immunity are produced in the bone marrow. Like other blood cells, lymphocytes are generated from stem cells, which are undifferentiated cells. Descendants of **stem cells** become lymphocytes—the B-lymphocytes **(B-cells)**, and the T-lymphocytes **(T-cells)**,

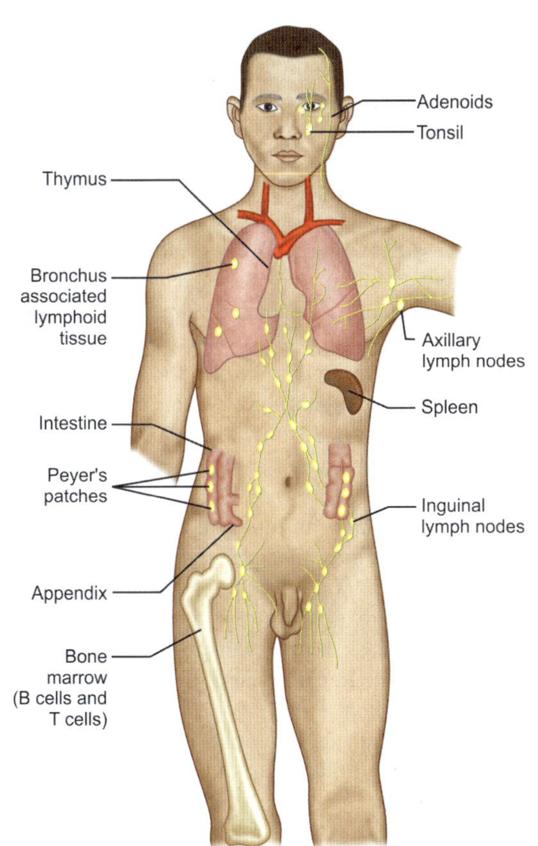

FIG. 5.1: Central and peripheral lymphoid organs and tissues

B-lymphocytes mature in the course bone marrow and then enter the circulation. T-lymphocytes move from the bone marrow to the thymus, where they mature into several kinds of cells with different functions.

Lymphoid tissues: The spleen, composed of red and white pulp, acts somewhat like a filter. The red pulp is the site where old and injured red blood cells (RBCs) are destroyed. The white pulp contains concentrations of lymphocytes. The lymph nodes are distributed throughout the body. They are connected by lymph channels and capillaries, which remove foreign material from the lymph system before it enters the bloodstream. The lymph nodes also serve as centers for immune cell proliferation. The remaining lymphoid tissues contain immune cells that defend the body's mucosal surfaces against microorganisms (Fig. 5.1).

TYPES OF IMMUNITY

There are two general types of immunity—natural (innate) and acquired (adaptive). Natural immunity is a nonspecific immunity that is present at birth. Acquired or specific immunity develops after birth. Natural immune responses to a foreign invader are very similar from one encounter to the next, regardless of the number of times the invader is encountered—in contrast, acquired responses increase in intensity with repeated exposure to the invading agent. Although each type of immunity has a distinct role in defending the body against harmful invaders, the various components usually act in an interdependent manner.

Natural Immunity

The natural (innate) system provides rapid nonspecific immunity and is present at birth. Because of its nonspecificity, it has a broad spectrum of defense against and resistance to infection. Natural (innate) immunity provides a nonspecific response to any foreign invader, regardless of the invader's composition. The basis of this defense mechanism is the ability to distinguish between friend and foe or "self" and "nonself". Natural (innate) immunity coordinates the initial response to pathogens through the production of cytokines and other effector molecules, which either activate cells for control of the pathogen (by elimination) or promote the development of the acquired immune response. The cells involved in this response include macrophages, dendritic cells, and natural killer (NK) cells, which have the ability to recognize and respond to a wide variety of pathogens long before the development of antigen-specific acquired immunity. The early events in this immune response are critical in determining the nature of the adaptive immune response. Innate immune mechanisms can be divided into two stages—immediate (generally occurring within 4 hours) and delayed (occurring between 4 and 96 hours after exposure).

White blood cell action: Cellular response is key to the effective initiation of the immune response. WBCs or leukocytes, participate in both the natural and the acquired immune responses. Granular leukocytes, or granulocytes (so called because of granules in their cytoplasm), fight invasion by foreign bodies or toxins by releasing cell mediators, such as histamine, bradykinin, and prostaglandin's, and engulfing the foreign bodies or toxins. Granulocytes include neutrophils, eosinophils, and basophils.

Neutrophils (also called polymorphonuclear leukocytes, or PMNs, because their nuclei have multiple lobes) are the first cells to arrive at the site where inflammation occurs. Eosinophils and basophils, other types of granulocytes, increase in number during allergic reactions and stress responses. Nongranular leukocytes include monocytes or macrophages (referred to as histocytes when they enter tissue spaces) and lymphocytes. Monocytes also function as **phagocytic cells**, engulfing, ingesting and destroying greater numbers and quantities of foreign bodies or toxins than granulocytes do. Lymphocytes, consisting of B-cells and T-cells, play major roles in humoral and cell-mediated immune responses. About 60 to 70% of lymphocytes in the blood are T-cells, and about 10 to 20% are B-cells.

Inflammatory response: The inflammatory response is a major function of the natural immune system that is elicited in response to tissue injury or invading organisms. Chemical mediators assist this response by minimizing blood loss, walling off the invading organism, activating phagocytes, and promoting formation of fibrous scar tissue and regeneration of injured tissue. The inflammatory response is facilitated by physical and chemical barriers that are part of the human organism.

Physical and chemical barriers: Activation of the natural immunity response is enhanced by processes inherent in physical and chemical barriers. Physical surface barriers include intact skin, mucous membranes, and cilia of the respiratory tract, which prevent pathogens from gaining access to the body. The cilia of the respiratory tract, along with coughing and sneezing responses, filter and clear pathogens from the upper respiratory tract before they can invade the body further. Chemical barriers, such as mucus, acidic gastric secretions, enzymes in tears and saliva, and substances in sebaceous and sweat secretions, act in a nonspecific way to destroy invading bacteria and fungi. Viruses are countered by other means, such as interferon. **Interferon**, one type of biologic response modifier, is a nonspecific viricidal protein that is naturally produced by the body and is capable of activating other components of the immune system.

Immune regulation: Regulation of the immune response involves balance and counterbalance. Dysfunction of the natural immune system can occur when the immune components are inactivated or when they remain active long after their effects are beneficial. A successful immune response eliminated the responsible antigen. Immunodeficiencies are characterized by inactivation (e.g. asthma, allergy, arthritis) are characterized by persistent inflammatory responses. The immune system recognition of one's own tissues as "foreign" rather than as self is the basis for many autoimmune disorders. Despite the fact that the immune response is critical to the prevention of disease, it must be well controlled to curtail immunopathology. Most microbial infections include an inflammatory response mediated by T-cells and cytokines, which in excess, can cause tissue damage. Therefore, regulatory mechanisms must be in place to suppress or halt the immune response. This is mainly achieved by the production of cytokines and transformation of growth factor that inhibits macrophage activation. In some cases, T-cell activation is so overwhelming that these mechanisms fail and pathology results. Research on **immunoregulation** holds the promise of preventing graft rejection and aiding the body in eliminating cancerous or infected cells.

Acquired Immunity

Acquired (adaptive) immunity—immunologic responses acquired during life but not present at birth—usually develops as a result of prior exposure to an antigen through immunization (vaccination) or by contracting a disease, both of which generate a protective immune response. Weeks or months after exposure to the disease or vaccine, the body produces an immune response that is sufficient to defend against the disease on re-exposure. In contrast to the rapid but nonspecific innate immune response, this form of immunity relies on the recognition of specific foreign antigens. The two components of the immune response are strongly interrelated. Events occurring early in injection dictate the direction of the adaptive response and activate the acquired immune effector mechanisms, which have a direct feedback on the cells of the innate (natural) system. The acquired immune response is broadly divided into two mechanisms—the cell-mediated response, involving T-cell activation, and effector mechanisms, involving B-cell maturation and production of antibodies.

The two types of acquired immunity are known as active and passive. In active acquired immunity, the immunologic defenses are developed by the person's own body. This immunity typically lasts many years or even a lifetime. Passive acquired immunity is temporary immunity transmitted from a source outside the body that has developed immunity through previous disease or immunization. For example, immune globulin or antiserum, obtained from the blood plasma of people with acquired immunity, is used in emergencies to provide immunity to diseases when the risk for contracting a specific disease is great (e.g. after exposure to hepatitis) and there is not enough time for a person to develop adequate active immunity. Immunity resulting from the transfer of antibodies from the mother to an infant in utero or through breastfeeding is another example of passive immunity. Active and passive acquired immunity involve humoral and cellular (cell-mediated) immunologic responses.

STAGES OF IMMUNE RESPONSE AND ITS TYPES

When the body is invaded or attacked by bacteria, viruses, or other pathogens, it has three means of defense:

1. The phagocytic immune response.
2. The humoral or antibody immune response.
3. The cellular immune response .

The first line of defense, the *phagocytic immune response*, involves the WBCs (granulocytes and macrophages), which have the ability to ingest foreign particles. These cells move to the point of attack, where they engulf and destroy the invading agents. Phagocytes also remove the body's own dying or dead cells. Cells in necrotic tissue that are dying release substances that trigger an inflammatory response. Apoptosis, or programmed cell death, is the body's way of destroying worn-out cells such as blood or skin cells or cells that need to be renewed. Apoptosis involves the digestion of DNA by endonucleases, which results in targeting of the cells from phagocytosis. Unlike macrophages, eosinophils are only weakly phagocytic. On activation, eosinophils probably kill parasites by releasing specific chemical mediators into the extracellular fluid. Additionally, eosinophils secrete leukotrienes, prostaglandins, and various cytokines.

A second protective response, the **humoral immune** response (sometimes called the **antibody** response), begins with the B-lymphocytes, which can transform themselves into plasma cells that manufacture antibodies. These antibodies are highly specific proteins that are transported in the bloodstream and attempt to disable invaders. The third mechanism of defense, the **cellular immune response**, also involves the T-lymphocytes, which can turn into special cytotoxic (or killer) T-cells that can attack the pathogens.

The structural part of the invading or attacking organism that is responsible for stimulating antibody production is called an **antigen** (or an immunogen). For example, an antigen can be a small patch of proteins on the outer surface of a microorganism. Not all antigens are naturally immunogenic; some must be coupled to other molecules to stimulate the immune response. A single bacterium or large molecule, such as a diphtheria or tetanus toxin, may have several antigens, or markers, on its surface, thus inducing the body to produce a number of different antibodies. Once produced, an antibody is released into the blood stream and carried to the attacking organism. There, it combines with the antigen, binding with it like an interlocking piece of a jigsaw puzzle. There are four well-defined stages in an immune response—recognition, proliferation, response, and effector (Fig. 5.2).

Recognition stage: Recognition of antigens as foreign, or non-self, by the immune system is the initiating event in any immune response. The body must first recognize invaders as foreign before it can react to them. The body accomplishes recognition using lymph nodes and lymphocytes for surveillance. Lymph nodes are widely distributed internally throughout the body and in the circulating blood, as well as externally near the body's surfaces. They continuously discharge small lymphocytes into the bloodstream. These lymphocytes patrol the tissues and vessels that drain the areas served by that node.

Lymphocytes recirculate from the blood to lymph nodes and from the lymph nodes back into the bloodstream, in a never-ending series of patrols. Some circulating lymphocytes can survive for decades. Some of these small, hardy cells maintain their solitary circuits for a person's entire lifetime.

The exact way in which circulating lymphocytes recognize antigens on foreign surfaces is not known: however, recognition is thought to depend on specific receptor sites on the surface of the lymphocytes. Macrophages play an important role in helping the circulating lymphocytes process the antigens. Both macrophages and neutrophils have receptors for antibodies and complement; as a result, they coat microorganisms with antibodies, complement, or both, enhancing phagocytosis. The engulfed microorganisms are then subjected to a wide range of toxic intracellular molecules. When foreign materials enter the body, circulating lymphocytes come into physical contact with the surfaces of these materials. Upon contact with the foreign material, lymphocytes, with the help of macrophages, whether remove the antigen from the surface or obtain an imprint of its structure, which becomes important in subsequent re-exposure to the antigen.

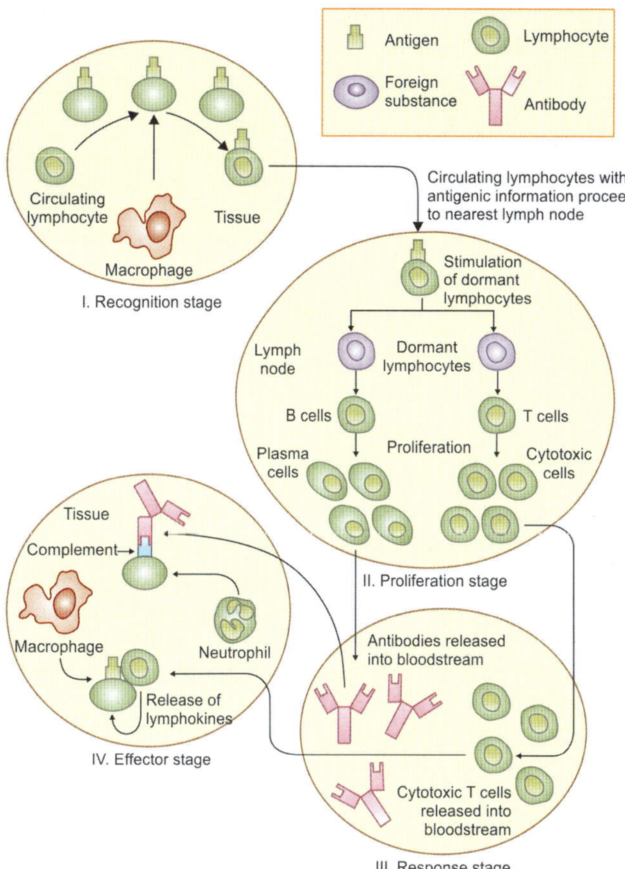

FIG. 5.2: Stages of the immune response **I,** In the recognition stage, antigen are recognized by circulating lymphocyte and macrophages. **II,** In the proliferation stage, the dormat lymphocyte proliferate and differentiate into cytotoxic (killer) T cells or B cells responsible for formation and release of antibodies. **III,** In this response stage, the cytotoxic T cells and the B cells perform cellular and humoral functions, respectively. **IV,** In the effector stage, antigens are destroyed or neutralized through the action of antibodies complement, macrophages, and cytotoxic T-cells

In a streptococcal throat infection, for example, the streptococcal organism gains access to the mucous membranes of the throat. A circulating lymphocyte moving through the tissues of the throat comes in contact with the organism. The lymphocyte, familiar with the surface markers on the cells of its own body, recognizes the antigens on the microbe as different (nonself) and the streptococcal organism as antigenic (foreign). This triggers the second stage of the immune response—proliferation.

Proliferation stage: The circulating lymphocyte containing the antigenic message returns to the nearest lymph node. Once in the node, the sensitized lymphocyte stimulates some of the resident dormant T- and B-lymphocytes to enlarge, divide, and proliferate. T-lymphocytes differentiate into cytotoxic (or killer)

T-cells, whereas B-lymphocytes produce and release antibodies. Enlargement of the lymph nodes in the neck in conjunction with a sore throat is one example of the immune response.

Responses stage: In the response stage, the differentiated lymphocytes function in either a humoral or a cellular capacity. The production of antibodies by the B-lymphocytes in response to a specific antigen begins the humoral response. Humoral refers to the fact that the antibodies are released into the bloodstream and therefore reside in the plasma (fluid fraction of the blood).

With the initial cellular response, the returning sensitized lymphocytes migrate to areas of the lymph node other than those areas containing lymphocytes programmed to become plasma cells. Here, they stimulate the residing lymphocytes to become cells that will attack microbes directly rather than through the action of antibodies. These transformed lymphocytes are known as cytotoxic (killer) T-cells. The T-stands for thymus, signifying that during embryologic development of the immune system, these T-lymphocytes spent time in the thymus of the developing fetus, where they were genetically programmed to become T-lymphocytes rather than the antibody-producing B-lymphocytes. Vital rather than bacterial antigens induce a cellular response. This response is manifested by the increasing number T-lymphocytes (lymphocytosis) seen in the blood tests of people with viral illnesses such as infectious mononucleosis.

Most immune responses to antigens involve both humoral and cellular responses, although one usually predominates. For example, during transplant rejection, the cellular response predominates, whereas in the bacterial pneumonias and sepsis, the humoral response plays the dominant protective role.

Effector stage: In the effector stage, either the antibody of the humoral response or the cytotoxic (killer) T-cell of the cellular response reaches and connects with the antigen on the surface of the foreign invader. The connection initiates a series of events that is most instances results in the total destruction of the invading microbes or the complete neutralization of the toxin. The events involve interplay of antibodies (humoral immunity), complement, and action by the cytotoxic T-cells (cellular immunity).

(i) Humoral Immune Response

The humoral response is characterized by the production of antibodies by B-lymphocytes in responses to a specific antigen. Although the B-lymphocytes is ultimately responsible for the production of antibodies, both the macrophages of natural immunity and the special T-cell lymphocytes of cellular immunity are involved in recognizing the foreign substance and in producing antibodies.

Antigen recognition: Several theories explain the mechanisms by which B-lymphocytes recognize the invading antigen and respond by producing antibodies. It is known that B-lymphocyte recognize and respond to invading antigens in more than one way.

The B-lymphocytes appear to respond to some antigens by directly triggering antibody formation: however, in response to other antigens, they need the assistance of T-cells to trigger antibody formation. The T-lymphocytes are part of a surveillance system that is dispersed throughout the body and recycles through the general circulation, tissues, and lymphatic system. With the assistance of macrophages, the T-lymphocytes are believed to recognize the antigen of a foreign invader. The T-lymphocyte picks up the antigenic message, or "blueprint", of the antigen and returns to the nearest node with that message.

B-lymphocytes stored in the lymph nodes are subdivided into thousands of clones, each responsive to a single group of antigens having almost identical characteristics. When the antigenic message is carried back to the lymph node, specific clones of the B-lymphocyte are stimulated to enlarge, divide, proliferate, and differentiate into plasma cells capable of producing specific antibodies to the antigen. Other B-lymphocytes differentiate into B-lymphocyte clones with a memory for the antigen. These memory cells are responsible for the more exaggerated and rapid immune in a person who is repeatedly exposed to the same antigen.

Role of Antibodies

Antibodies are large proteins called immunoglobulins (because they are found in the globulin fraction of the plasma proteins). All immunoglobulins are glycoproteins and contain a certain amount of carbohydrate. The carbohydrate concentration, which ranges from approximately 3 to 13%, is dependent on the class of the antibody. Each antibody molecule consists of two subunits, each of which contains a light and a heavy peptide chain. The subunits are held together by a chemical link composed of disulfide bonds. Each subunit has a portion, referred to as the Fab fragment, that serves as a binding site for a site for a specific antigen. The Fab fragment (antibody-binding site) binds to the antigenic determinant similar to a lock-and-key mechanism. The Fab fragment provides the "lock" portion that is highly specific for an antigen. An additional portion, known as the Fc fragment, allows the antibody molecular to take part in the complement system.

Antibodies defend against foreign invaders in several ways, and the type of defense employed depends on the structure and composition of both the antigen and the immunoglobulin. The antibody molecule has at least two combining sites or Fab fragments. One antibody can act as a cross-link between two antigens, causing them to bind or clump together. This clumping effect, referred to as **agglutination**, helps clear the body of the invading organism by facilitating phagocytosis. Some antibodies assist in removal of offending organisms through **opsonization**. In this process, the antigen-antibody molecule is coated with a sticky substance that also facilitates phagocytosis.

Antibodies also promote the release of vasoactive substances, such as histamine and slow-reacting substance, two of the chemical mediators of the inflammatory response. Antibodies do not function in isolation; rather, they mobilize other components of the immune system to defend against the invader. The typical role of antibodies is to focus components of the natural immune system on the invader. This includes activation of the complement system and activation of phagocytosis.

The body can produce five different types of immunoglobulins (Ig). Each of the five types, or classes, is identified by a specific letter of the alphabet: IgA, IgD, IgE, IgG, and IgM. Classification is based on the chemical structure and biologic role of the individual immunoglobulin.

Antigen-antibody binding: The portion of the antigen involved in binding with the antibody is referred to as the **antigenic determinant**. The most efficient immunologic responses occur when the antibody and antigen fit like a lock and key. Poor fit can occur with an antibody that was produced in response to a different antigen. This phenomenon is known as cross-reactivity. For example, in acute rheumatic fever, the antibody produced against *Streptococcus pyogenes* in the upper respiratory tract may cross-react with the patients heart tissue, leading to heart valve damage.

Antigen-antibody binding: **Left**—a highly specific antigen-antibody complex. **Middle**—no match and therefore, no immune response. **Right**—poor fit or match with low specificity, antibody reacts to antigen with similar characteristics, producing cross-reactivity.

Major Characteristics of the Immunoglobulins

IgG (75% of Total Immunoglobulin)

- Appears in serum and tissues (interstitial fluid)
- Assumes a major role in bloodborne and tissue infections
- Activates the complement system
- Enhances phagocytosis
- Crosses the placenta.

IgA (15% of Total Immunoglobulin)

- Appears in body fluids (blood, saliva, tears, breast milk, and pulmonary, gastrointestinal, prostatic, and vaginal secretions)
- Protects against respiratory, gastrointestinal, and genitourinary infections
- Prevents absorption of antigens from food
- Passes to neonate in breast milk for protection.

IgM (10% of Total Immunoglobulin)

- Appears mostly in intravascular serum
- Appears as the first immunoglobulin produced in response to bacterial and viral infections
- Activates the complement system.

IgD (0.2% of Total Immunoglobulin)

- Appears in small amounts in serum
- Possibly influences B-lymphocyte differentiation, but role is unclear.

IgE (0.004% of Total Immunoglobulin)

- Appears in serum
- Takes part in allergic and some hypersensitivity reactions
- Combats parasitic infections.

(ii) Cellular Immune Response

The B-lymphocyte are responsible for humoral immunity, and the T-lymphocyte are primarily responsible for cellular immunity. Stem cells continuously migrate from the bone marrow to the thymus gland, where they develop into T-cells. T-cells continue to develop in the thymus gland, despite the partial degeneration of the gland that occurs at puberty. By spending time in the thymus, these cells are programmed to become T-cells rather than antibody-producing B-lymphocytes. Several types of T-cells exist, each with designated roles in the defense against bacteria, viruses, fungi, parasites, and malignant cells. T-cells attack foreign invaders directly rather than by producing antibodies.

Cellular reactions are initiated by the binding of an antigen to an antigen receptor located on the surface of a T-cell. This may occur with or without the assistance of macrophages. The T-cells then carry the antigenic message, or blueprint, to the lymph nodes, where the production of other T-cells is stimulated. Some T-cells remain in the lymph nodes and retain a memory for the antigen. Other T-cells migrate from the lymph nodes into the general circulatory system and ultimately to the tissues, where they remain until they either come in contact with their respective antigens or die.

Role of T-lymphocytes

T-cells include effector T-cells, suppressor T-cells, and memory T-cells. Two major categories of effector T-cells exist—helper T-cells and cytotoxic T-cells. These effector T-cells participate in the destruction of foreign organisms. T-cells interact closely with B-cells, including that humoral and cellular immune responses are not separate, unrelated processes, but rather, branches of the immune response that interact.

Helper T-cells are activated on recognition of antigens and stimulate the rest of the immune system. When activated, helper T-cells secrete **cytokines**, which attract and activate B-cells, cytotoxic T-cells, natural killer (NK) cells, macrophages, and other cells of the immune system. Separate subpopulations of helper T-cells produce different types of cytokines and determine whether the immune response will be the production of antibodies or a cell-mediated immune response. Helper T-cells produce **lymphokines**, one category of cytokines. These lymphokines activate other T-cells (e.g. interleukin-2 [IL-2]), natural cytotoxic T-cells (e.g. interferon-γ), and other inflammatory cells (e.g. tumor necrosis factor). Helper T-cells produce IL-4 and IL-5, lymphokines that activate B-cells to grow and differentiate (Table 5.1).

Cytotoxic T-cells (killer T-cells) attack the antigen directly by altering the cell membrane and causing cell lysis (disintegration)

TABLE 5.1: Cytokines and their biologic activity

Cytokine*	Biologic activity
Interleukin-1 (α and β)	Promotes differentiation of T- and B-lymphocytes, natural killer (NK) cells, and null cells
Interleukin-2	Stimulates growth of T-lymphocytes and special activated killer lymphocytes (known as lymphocyte activated killer cells [LAK cells])
Interleukin-3	Stimulates growth of mast cells and other blood cells
Interleukin-4	Stimulates growth of T- and B-lymphocytes and antibodies
Interleukin-5	Stimulates antibody responses
Interleukin-6	Stimulates growth and function of B-lymphocytes and antibodies
Interleukin-7	Stimulates growth of pre-B, CD4+ and CD8+ T-lymphocytes
Interleukin-8	Promotes chemotaxis and activation of neutrophils
Interleukin-9	Stimulates growth and proliferation of T-lymphocytes
Interleukin-10	Inhibits interferon-gamma and mononuclear cell inflammation
Interleukin-11	Promotes induction of acute phase proteins
Interleukin-12	Introduces helper T-lymphocytes
Interleukin-13	Inhibits mononuclear phagocyte inflammation and promotes differentiation of B-cells
Interleukin-16	Promotes chemotaxis CD4+ T-lymphocytes and eosinophils
Permeability factor	Increases vascular permeability, allowing white cells into area
Interferon-γ	Activates macrophages; increases expression of class I and II MHC** antigen processing and presentation
Interferon – (type 1α and type β)	Exerts antiviral activity in body cells; induces class I antigen expression; activates NK cells
Migration inhibitory factor	Suppress movement of macrophages, keeping macrophages in area of foreign cells
Skin reactive factor	Induces inflammatory response
Cytotoxic factor (lymphotoxin)	Kills certain antigenic cells
Macrophage chemotactic factor	Attracts macrophages into the area
Lymphocyte blastogenic factor	Stimulates more lymphocytes, recruiting additional lymphocytes into the area
Macrophage aggregation factor	Causes clumping to adhere to surfaces more readily
Macrophage activation factor	Allows macrophages to adhere to surfaces more readily
Proliferation inhibitor factor	Inhibits growth of certain antigenic cells
Cytophilic antibody	Binds to an Fc receptor on macrophages, thereby permitting macrophages to bind to antigens
Tumor necrosis factor-alpha	Stimulates inflammation, wound healing, and tissue remodeling
Tumor necrosis factor-beta	Mediates inflammation and graft rejection

*Cytokines are biologically active substances that are released by cells to regulate growth and function of other cells within the immune system.
**Lymphocytes produce lymphokines, and monocytes and macrophages produce monokines. This table lists some of the cytokines that play a role in immune system functioning. MHC = major histocompatibility complex

and by releasing cytolytic enzymes and cytokines. Lymphokines can recruit, activate, and regulate other lymphocytes and WBCs. These cells then assist in destroying the invading organisms. Delayed-type hypersensitivity is an example of an immune reaction that protects the body from antigens through the production and release of lymphokines.

Another type of cell, the **suppressor T-cell**, has the ability to decrease B-cell production, thereby keeping the immune response at a level that is compatible with health (e.g. sufficient to fight infection adequately without attacking the body's healthy tissues). **Memory cells** are responding for recognizing antigens from previous exposure and mounting an immune response (Table 5.2).

Roles of Null Lymphocytes and Natural Killer Cells

Null lymphocytes and NK cells are other lymphocytes that assist in combating organisms. These cells are distinct from B-cells and T-cells and lack the usual characteristics of those cells. **Null lymphocytes**, a subpopulation of lymphocytes, destroy antigens already coated with antibody. These cells have special Fc-receptor sites on their surface that allow them to connect with the Fc-end of antibodies; this is known as antibody-dependent, cell-mediated cytotoxicity.

Natural killer cells, another subpopulation of lymphocytes, defend against microorganisms and some types of malignant cells. NK cells are capable of directly killing invading organisms

TABLE 5.2: Lymphocytes involved in immune responses

Type of immune response	Cell type	Function
Humoral	B-lymphocyte	Produces antibodies or immunoglobulins (IgA, IgD, IgE, IgG, IGM)
Cellular	T-lymphocyte	
	Helper T	Attacks foreign invaders (antigens) directly. Initiates and augments inflammatory response
	Helper T1	Increases activated cytotoxic T-cells
	Helper T2	Increases B-cell antibody production
	Suppressor T	Suppresses the immune response
	Memory T	Remembers contact with an antigen and on subsequent exposures mounts an immune response
	Cytotoxic T (killer T)	Lyses cells infected with virus; plays a role in graft rejection
Nonspecific	Non-T or non-B lymphocyte	
	Null cell	Destroys antigens already coated with antibody
	Natural killer (NK) cell (granular lymphocyte)	Defends against microorganisms and some type of malignant cells; produces cytokines

TABLE 5.3: Complement-mediated immune responses

Response	Complement products	Effects
Cytolysis	C5b-C9	Lysis and destruction of cell membranes of body's cells or pathogens
Opsonization	C3b, C5b	Targeting of the antigen so that it can be easily engulfed and digested by macrophages and other phagocytic cells
Chemotaxis	C3a, C5a	Chemical attraction of neutrophils and phagocytic cells to the antigen
Anaphylaxis	C3a, C5a	Activation of mast cells and basophils with release of inflammatory mediators that produce smooth muscle contraction and increased vascular permeability

and producing cytokines. The helper T-cells contribute to the differentiation of null and NK cells.

Complement System

Circulating plasma proteins, known as **complement**, are made in the liver and activated when an antibody connects with its antigen. Complement plays an important role in the immune response. Destruction of an invading or attacking organism or toxin is not achieved merely by the binding of the antibody and antigens; it also requires activation of complement, the arrival of killer T-cells, or the attraction of macrophages. Complement has three major physiologic functions—defending the body against bacterial infection, bridging natural and acquired immunity, and disposing of immune complexes and the byproducts associated with inflammation. Complement-mediated immune responses are summarized in Table 5.3.

The proteins that comprise complement interact sequentially with one another in a cascading or "falling domino" effect. The complement cascade is important to modifying the effector arm of the immune system. Activation of complement allows important events, such as removal of infectious agents and initiation of the inflammatory response, to take place. These events involve active parts of the pathway that enhance chemotaxis of macrophages and granulocytes, alter blood vessel permeability, change blood vessels diameters, cause cells to lyse, alter blood clotting, and cause other points of modification. These macrophages and granulocytes continue the body's defense by devouring the antibody-coated microbes and by releasing bacterial products.

There are several ways to activate the complement system—the classic pathway, the alternative pathway, and the lectin pathway.

Classic Pathway of Complement Activation

The classic pathway (the first method discovered) is activated by antigen-antibody complexes; it begins when antibody binds to a cell surface and ends with lysis of the cell. This involves the reaction of the first of the circulating complement proteins (C1) with the receptor site of the Fc portion of an antibody molecule after formation of an antigen-antibody complex. The activation of the first complement component then activates all the other components, in the following sequence: C4, C2, C3, C5, C6, C7, C8 and C9 (the components are named in the sequence in which they were discovered).

Alternative and Lectin Pathways

The alternative and lectin pathways of complement are activated without the formation of antigen-antibody complexes. These pathways can be initiated by the release of bacterial products, such as endotoxins. When complement is activated without the formation of antigen-antibody complexes, the process bypasses the first three components (C1, C4 and C2) and begins with C3. Regardless of the method, once activated, the complement system destroys cells by altering or damaging the cell membrane of the antigen, by chemically attracting phagocytes to the antigen (chemotaxis), and by rendering the antigen more vulnerable to phagocytosis (opsonization). The complement system enhances the inflammatory response by releasing vasoactive substances. The alternative and lectin pathways of complement are activated without the formation of antigen-antibody complexes. These pathways can be initiated by the release of bacterial products, such as endotoxins. When complement is activated without the formation of antigen-antibody complexes, the process bypasses the first three components (C1, C4 and C2) and begins with C3. Regardless of the method, once activated, the complement system destroys cells by altering or damaging the cell membrane of the antigen, by chemically attracting phagocytes to the antigen (chemotaxis), and by rendering the antigen more vulnerable to phagocytosis (opsonization). The complement system enhances the inflammatory response by releasing vasoactive substances.

Complement components, prostaglandins, leukotrienes and other inflammatory mediators all contribute to the recruitment of inflammatory cells, as do chemokines, a group of cytokines. The activated neutrophils pass through the vessel walls to accumulate at the site of infection, where they phagocytose complement-coated microbes. This response is usually therapeutic and can be lifesaving if the cell attacked, by the complement system is a true foreign invader, such as streptococcal or staphylococcal organism. However, if that cell is actually part of the person—for example, a cell of the brain or liver, the tissue lining the blood vessels, or the cells of a transplanted organ or skin graft—the result can be devastating disease and even death. This vigorous and deadly attack on the material identified as foreign is underscored by the resulting purulent material (the remains of microbes, granulocytes, macrophages, T-cells, plasma proteins, complement, and antibodies) that accumulates in wound infections and abscesses. In addition, many autoimmune diseases (e.g. systemic lupus erythematosus) and disorders characterized by chronic infection (e.g. myocardial infarction, stroke) are thought to be caused in part by continued or chronic activation of complement, which in turn results in chronic inflammation.

The RBCs (erythrocytes) and platelets (thrombocytes) also have a role in the immune response. RBCs and platelets have complement receptors and, as a result, play an important role in the clearance of immune complexes that consist of antigen, antibody and components of the complement system.

Role of Interferons

Biologic response modifiers, such as the interferons, continue to be investigated to determine their roles in the immune system and their potential therapeutic effects in disorders characterized by disturbed immune responses (Korholz and Kiess, 2003). Interferons have antiviral and anti-tumor properties. In addition to responding to viral infection, interferons are produced by T-lymphocytes, B-lymphocytes, and macrophages in response to antigens. They are thought to modify the immune response by suppressing antibody production and cellular immunity. They also facilitate the cytotytic role of macrophages and NK cells. Interferons are undergoing extensive testing to evaluating their effectiveness in treating tumors and acquired immunodeficiency syndrome (AIDS). Some interferons are already used to treat immune-related disorders (e.g. multiple sclerosis) and chronic inflammatory conditions (e.g. chronic hepatitis).

Genetic Engineering

One of the more remarkable evolving technologies is **genetics engineering**, which uses recombinant DNA technology. Two facets exist with this technology. The first permits scientists to combine genes from one type of organisms with genes of a second organisms. This type of technology allows cells and microorganisms to manufacture proteins, monokines and lymphokines, which can alter and enhance immune system function. The second facet of recombinant DNA technology involves gene therapy. If a particular gene is abnormal or missing, experimental recombinant DNA technology may be capable of restoring normal gene function. For example, a recombinant gene is inserted onto a virus particle. When the virus particle splices its gene, the virus automatically inserts the missing gene, and theoretically corrects the genetic anomaly. Extensive research into recombinant DNA technology and gene therapy is ongoing.

Stem Cells

Stem cells are potentially immortal cells that are capable of self-renewal and differentiation; they continually replenish the body's entire supply of both RBCs and WBCs. Some stem cells, described as totipotent cells, have tremendous capacity to self-renew and differentiate. Embryonic stem cells, described as pluripotent, give rise to numerous cell types that are able to form tissues (Porth, 2005). Research has shown that stem cells can restore an immune system that has been destroyed. Stem cell transplantation has been carried out in humans with certain types of immune dysfunction, such as severe combined immunodeficiency (SCID); clinical trials using stem cells are underway in patients with a variety of disorders having an autoimmune component, including systemic lupus erythematosus, rheumatoid arthritis, scleroderma, and multiple sclerosis. Research with embryonic stem cells has enabled investigators to make substantial gains in developmental biology, gene therapy, therapeutic tissue engineering, and the treatment of a variety of diseases. However, along with these remarkable opportunities, many ethical challenges arise, which are largely based on concerns about safety, efficacy, resource allocation, and human cloning.

PRIMARY IMMUNE ABERRATIONS AND DISEASE

The immune response is protective in healthy individuals; however, that protection depends on an intact immune system. Four primary immune aberrations can lead to disease:

1. A deficiency of one or more immune components **(immunodeficiency)**
2. An abnormal production of antibodies **(gammopathy)**
3. An exaggerated or inappropriate immune response **(hypersensitivity)**, and
4. Immunologic attacks on host cells **(autoimmunity)**.

(1) IMMUNODEFICIENCIES

The four components of the immuno system—humoral (B cell mediated) immunity, cellular (T-cell) immunity, phagocytosis, and complement—act together and independently to protect the host from infection and disease. Both primary (congenital) and secondary (acquired) immunodeficiencies produce chronic or recurring infections that can, without effective treatment, lead to death.

(a) Primary Immunodeficiences

Primary immunodeficiencies (PIs) are a group of disorders that occur from congenital genetic defects that block or prevent the maturation or function of immune cells. Most PIs are autosomal, or X-linked, and have both dominant and recessive inheritance patterns. They commonly occur in persons under the age of 20 and, because of inheritance patterns, affect males in 70% of cases. The most common immunodeficiencies are secondary or acquired. Most people are born with a normal immune response, but secondary factors or occurrences affect the immune system, causing dysfunction. Immunosuppressive agents; malignancies; chronic diseases; nutritional deficits; age; and some viral infections, such as human immunodeficiency virus (HIV), can cause secondary immunodeficiency.

Pathophysiology of Primary Immunodeficiencies

The PI disorders are characterized by defects in immunologic cell development or function that result in B-lymphocyte (also known as B cell) T cell, complement, or phagocytic cell deficiency. Recurrent infections or repeated infection treatment failures generally prompt the clinician to suspect the presence of immunodeficiency. Without treatment, most individuals suffering from these deficiencies die of overwhelming infectious early in life.

Immunodeficiencies produce a variety of clinical manifestation based on the type of deficiency. Not all patients experience all manifestations listed. Common manifestations include:

- Frequent bacterial and viral infections
- Infection with unusual or opportunistic organisms
- Associated autoimmune disease
- Painful, swollen, wrist, elbow, ankle, or knee joints
- Digestive problems, nausea, or vomiting
- Chronic skin or mucous membrane infections
- Blood disorders
- Diarrhea
- Fever
- Fatigue
- Weakness
- Enlarged lymph noses or spleen.

Antibody Deficiencies

Selective immunoglobulin A (IgA) deficiency is the most common PI and has both autosomal dominant and recessive inheritance traits. The exact defect that leads to low serum IgA levels is unknown, but may be related to impaired B cell differentiation and subsequent loss of immunoglobulin secreting ability. The disorder is associated with increased incidence of infections, autoimmunity, allergies, gastrointestinal disorders, and cancer. B-lymphocytes produce *antibodies* that recognize mark foreign antigens so that other immune components will react and destroy them. X-linked agammaglobulinemia is an example of an inherited, B cell immunodeficiency that results from failure of pre-B cells to differentiate into mature B cells. This disorder occurs exclusively in males and is usually diagnosed within the first 3 years of life. Individuals with agammaglobulinemia are particularly susceptible to infections from pyrogenic bacteria such as streptococci, staphylococci, *Pseudomonas* organisms, and *Haemophilus influenzae*; infections of the eyes, sinuses, ears, nose, and lungs, and viruses such as hepatitis and polio.

Combined B and T Cell Deficiencies

Stem cell immunodeficiency (severe combined immuno-deficiency, or SCID) refers to the complete absence of both T cell (cellular) and B cell (humoral) immunity. This disorder has many variants. In the most severe form the common stem cell for white blood cells is absent, resulting is subsequent loss of B cells, T cells, and phagocytic cells. Infants with this condition generally die in utero or soon after birth. A less severe form of SCID results from impaired stem cell maturation, which interferes with T and B cell development. T and B cells are significantly reduced or absent even though other white blood cells are present in normal numbers. People with SCID are at high risk for developing nearly every type of infection because of pancytopenia. Thymic hypoplasia (DiGeorge syndrome) is a cellular immunodeficiency resulting from thymus gland hypoplasia and inability to assist in the maturation of T cells. Even though B cells are normal, children with total loss of thymic function are at increased risk for infection and may not live more than 5 to 6 years without treatment.

Phagocytic Defects

Phagocytes (neutrophis and macrophages) are white blood cells that engulf and destroy antibody-coated antigens. Phagocytic defects may interfere with their ability to move to the site of an infection or destroy pathogens. Chronic granulomatous disease is the most severe form of phagocytic cell deficiency. It involves a deficiency in the molecules needed by neutrophils to destroy foreign antigens. Individuals with phagocytic disorders are at risk for developing mild to severe bacterial infections. Signs and symptoms depend on the site of infection and type of infecting organism.

Complement System Defects

The complement system is composed of proteins that attach themselves to antibody-coated antigens and facilitate destruction of the antigen. Persons with complement deficiency have a diminished ability to destroy invading pathogens and are at increased risk for infection. A common complement deficiency. C2 deficiency, is associated with an increased incidence of autoimmune disease, such as glomerulonephritis or rheumatoid arthritis, and severe infection such as meningitis.

(b) Secondary Immunodeficiencies

Secondary immunodeficiencies result from numerous factors. Generalized **immunosuppression** is often induced therapeutically to decrease unwanted immune reactions, such as hypersensitivity reactions, autoimmune diseases, neoplasia, or organ rejection.

Immunosuppressive Therapies

Corticosteroids have both anti-inflammatory and immunosuppressive properties. They inhibit movement of leukocytes and alter cellular and humoral immunity. When infection is present in a person receiving corticosteroids, the severity of the infection may increase despite the induced minimization of symptoms. Cyclosporine, a primary immunosuppressant drug used after organ transplantation, acts by inhibiting helper T cells and facilitating development of suppressor T cells.

Cytotoxic drugs and other cancer chemotherapeutic agents (alkylating agents, antifolates, and antimetabolites) destroy replicating cells. Consequently, they produce immunosuppression by destroying rapidly dividing immunologically stimulated cells. They also interfere with basic cellular metabolic processes in which B and T cell numbers are reduced.

Specific immunosuppression may be induced in people with hypersensitivities by administration of antigens in small amounts over time. This antigenic stimulation forms circulating immunoglobulin G (IgG) antibodies (immunoglobulins) that combine with the offending antigen to block contact with immunocompetent cells or immunoglobulin E (IgE)—coated mast cells, thus suppressing the immune response and preventing hypersensitivity reactions. Allergists use an adaptation of this method to desensitize persons who are allergic to antigens such as pollens or dust mites. A slightly different method of immunosuppression involves administration of a specific antibody, which then combines with the antigen to block contact with the immunocompetent cell. This method is used successfully in obstetrics in preventing the sensitive Rh-negative mother from reacting to an Rh-positive fetus during pregnancy.

Antilymphocytic globulin and antithymocytic globulin are antisera prepared by isolating the active globulin fraction from the serum of horses, goats, or rabbits that have been immunized with human lymphocytes or thymocytes. These antisera produce immunosuppression by decreasing all lymphocytes, although T cells are more affected than B cells. Because these globulins are xenogeneic (from another species), serum sickness may occur, and this limits their use to short-term therapy.

Monoclonal antibodies (MoAbs) are also used to suppress immunity because they are derived from a single cell line (monoclonal). They are very specific and can be targeted against subpopulations of lymphocytes, such as helper T cells. Monoclonal antibodies are useful in treating cancers, autoimmune disorders, and renal allograft rejection.

Many chemicals have immunosuppressive effects in exposed humans. T lymphocytes seem to be affected more severely than other immune cells. Examples of potentially damaging environmental chemicals are asbestos, dioxin, insecticides, and heavy metals. Irradiation also suppresses immunity by suppressing both primary and secondary immune responses, although primary suppression is more effective. Irradiation destroys lymphocytes either directly or through depletion of precursor stem cells.

Other factors: Prolonged physical and psychosocial stress stimulates the production of corticosteroids, which suppress immunity and increase the risk for infections and tumors. T and B cells are reduced for up to a month after surgery, most likely because of stress. Chronic conditions such as diabetes mellitus are common causes of secondary immunodeficiency. Malnutrition and subsequent protein and calorie deficiencies result in reduced T cell numbers. The immune systems of older adults are less efficient, with decreased Y cell function, variable ability to respond to antigenic stimulation, and decreased proliferation of immune cells. HIV causes a serious secondary immunodeficiency, acquired immunodeficiency syndrome (AIDS).

Complications: Frequent acute and chronic bacterial, viral and fungal infections and repeated infection treatment failures are the complications of primary and secondary immunodeficiencies. Without adequate treatment, these complications can lead to weight loss, fatigue, poor quality of life, sepsis, septic shock, and death.

Management of Immunodeficiency Disorder

The primary goals of collaborative management for patients with suspected immunodeficiency disorders are to:

- Identify those at risk for the disorder
- Prevent infection or effectively treat existing infections
- Replace missing humoral or cellular immunologic factors as possible.

Diagnosis is based on patient history, physical examination, and laboratory findings; however, there is no one specific test for all diseases.

Antimicrobial agents to treat existing and prevent new infections are key to the successful management of both primary and secondary immunodeficiencies. Immmunoglobulin replacement therapy, which contains intravenous immunoglobulin (IVIG), is accepted treatment for patients with antibody deficiencies. The optimal dose of immunoglobulin, which is usually between 400 and 500 mg/dL, is maintained by monitoring the trough of immunoglobulin levels in the blood. Immunoglobulin are usually given intramuscularly or intravenously on a monthly basis. Reactions to immunoglobulins can include back or abdominal pain, nausea and vomiting, chills and fever, headache, myalgia, or fatigue. Fortunately, anaphylactic reactions to immunoglobulins are rare.

Other chemotherapeutic treatments for immunodeficiency include:

- Injections of interferon gamma, a cytokine that activates phagocytes
- Injections of growth factors,, which increase neutrophil production; and
- Granulocyte-macrophage colony stimulating factor or granulocyte colony-stimulating factor, both of which stimulate the production of granulocytes (white blood cells).

Bone marrow transplantation may be used for patients with T cell deficiencies. The major risk of this therapy is graft-versus-host disease. Bone marrow cells from family members with identical human leukocyte antigens have been used successfully in treating patients with combined immunodeficiencies.

Patients with immunodeficiency diseases have no specific dietary restrictions. A well-balanced, nutritious diet that includes all food groups and has adequate calories and protein to support tissue healing and growth is recommended, since it helps support immunity. Efforts should be made to prevent the transfer of food-borne microbes that may be potential sources of infection by thoroughly washing or cooking fruits and vegetables, thoroughly cooking meat products, and avoiding placing cooked foods on surfaces where raw meat was prepared and also be alert for the following signs and symptoms for assessing immune dysfunction.

Respiratory System

- Changes in respiratory rate
- Cough (dry or productive)
- Abnormal lung sounds (wheezing, crackles, rhonchi)
- Rhinitis
- Hyperventilation
- Bronchospasm.

Cardiovascular System

- Hypotension
- Tachycardia
- Dysrhythmia
- Vasculitis
- Anemia.

Gastrointestinal System

- Hepatosplenomegaly
- Colitis
- Vomiting
- Diarrhea.

Genitourinary System

- Frequency and burning on urination
- Hematuria
- Discharge.

Musculoskeletal System

- Joint mobility, edema, and pain.

Skin

- Rashes
- Lesions
- Dermatitis
- Hematomas or purpura
- Edema or urticarial
- Inflammation
- Discharge.

Neurosensory System

- Cognitive dysfunction
- Hearing loss
- Visual changes
- Headaches and migraines
- Ataxia
- Tetany.

Nursing Management

The nurses has to assess for:
- Frequency and length of any chronic bacterial or viral infections
- Bacterial infections of the ears, sinuses, lungs, bronchi
- Painful joints of the wrist, elbows, ankles, or knees
- Digestive problems, nausea, or vomiting
- Frequent bouts of diarrhea
- Chronic skin infections
- Blood disorders
- Enlarged lymph nodes or spleen
- Fever
- Poor skin turgor, bruising, lesions on the skin or mucous membranes
- Swollen joints
- Decreased weight for height.

Problems usually associated with immunodeficiency disorder includes the following:

Risk for Infection

Common nursing objective for the patient with a diagnosis of risk for infection are:

Patient will:

- Recognize signs of new infections and report for treatment early
- Use precautions to prevent new infections
- Maintain treatment regimens for treatment or prevention of infections.

For which the nurse consistently monitors patients who have immunodeficiencies or are undergoing immunosuppression therapy for indications of systemic infection, such as fever, changes in vital sign pattern, irritability, fatigue, or cough. Meticulous skin an perineal care and a clean environment reduce the patients potential for contact with infectious organisms. Injections are avoided and invasive lines kept to a minimum to prevent a portal of entry for microbes. When invasive lines are necessary, the nurse carefully monitors insertion sites for signs of localized infection. The nurse cultures suspicious drainage and monitors laboratory data to detect new infections and to determine the effectiveness of medications and other treatments. Live immunizations and oral polio vaccines are avoided in immunocompromised patients because of the risk of contracting infections via the immunization (Box 5.1).

Immunodeficient or immunosuppresed patients and their families need to know the nature of the immunodeficiency and how to avoid infection. Many patients do not require hospitalization, but they do need to be taught about infection control measures to follow at home. They need to be able to recognize the signs and symptoms of infection and which symptoms to report to the health care provider. Teaching includes information about the use of protective strategies such as hand washing techniques and asking people with infections such as colds or chickenpox not to visit. Frequent turning and deep breathing exercises are encouraged to prevent atelectasis and pneumonia. Careful attention should be given to older adults because of their increased risk for infection resulting from a decline in T cell function and immune response efficiency.

There are no specific activity restrictions; however, the nurse counsels patients about the need to avoid becoming overly fatigued. Patients with immunodeficiency disorders need to understand the importance of ongoing follow-up care. Referrals to community or home health nurses for continued assessment and treatment of infections may be necessary. Hospice care may be appropriate for patients with terminal primary or secondary immunodeficiency disorders.

Patient teaching should include information about the nature of immunodeficiency and prescribed medications, as

Box 5.1 Assessing for infection

Be alert for the following signs and symptoms:
- Fever with or without chills
- Cough with or without sputum
- Shortness of breath
- Difficulty breathing
- Difficulty swallowing
- White patches in the oral cavity
- Swollen lymph nodes
- Nausea with or without vomiting
- Persistent diarrhea
- Frequency, urgency, or pain on urination
- Change in the character of the urine
- Lesions on the face, lips or perianal area
- Redness, swelling, or drainage from skin lesions
- Persistent vaginal discharge with or without perianal itching
- Persistent abdominal pain

well as the following instructions regarding the preventions and management of the infection:

- Avoid persons with infections (especially colds)
- Inspect skin daily for lesions or breaks
- Avoid bumping, breaking, or tearing skin
- Eat a well-balanced diet with sufficient calories to maintain ideal weight
- Drink at least six glasses of fluid daily
- Avoid becoming overly fatigued
- Try to get sufficient sleep every night
- Decrease environmental contaminants:
  - Take prophylactic antibiotics before any manipulative or invasive procedures (dental procedures, biopsies, endoscopies, arteriograms)
  - Keep scheduled follow-up appointments with health care provider
  - Report signs of infection immediately (increased temperature, redness of swelling of skin or mucous membranes, change in color of sputum, unusual drainage, diarrhea).

(2) GAMMOPATHIES

Gammopathies, also known as hypergammaglobulinemias, refer to elevated levels of serum gamma globulin resulting from overproduction. The blood normally contains a large number of different proteins collectively called plasma proteins. One type of protein, gamma globulin, combines to make varying types of antibodies for fighting different infections. When the majority of protein produced is an identical type of gamma globulin, the abnormally produced protein is called *monoclonal gammopathy or plasma* cell dyscrasia. Multiple myeloma and macroglobulinemia are plasma cell dyscrasias that have distinctive clinical patterns.

Polyclonal gammopathies involve the overproduction of virtually all classes of immunoglobulins in response to inappropriate antigenic stimulation. High levels of dysfunctional immmunoglobulins depress the synthesis of normal immunoglobulins, leaving the patient susceptible to infection. IgG and IgM are most commonly involved. The immunoglobulin levels reflect the severity of disease produced. Polyclonal gammopathies are associated with chronic bacterial infections and connective tissue diseases such as lupus erythematosus and rheumatoid arthritis.

Multiple Myeloma

Multiple myeloma, which is plasma cell cancer, is the most serious and prevalent of the monoclonal gammopathies. The cause of multiple myeloma is unknown, but studies have shown possible associations with genetic factors, a decline in immune function, exposure to chemicals or radiation, and more recently a viral origin.

Pathophysiology

Multiple myeloma is a type of bone marrow cancer, which occurs from uncontrolled growth of plasma cells. Normally the bone marrow contains less than 5% plasma cells. Patients with multiple myeloma have bone marrow that contains between 10 to 90% plasma cells. The malignant plasma cells are most often monoclonal, originating from one single defective cell. The cancerous plasma cells collect in many bones, where they may form tumors, weaken bones, and cause pain and fractures. Calcium is released from damaged bones, causing hypocalcemia and resultant fatigue, muscle weakness, or confusion. The increased numbers of myeloma cells within bone marrow prevent the formation of white blood cells, erythrocytes, and normal plasma cells, leading to anemia and increased susceptibility to infections. The kidneys are also affected and at increased risk for damage because of the excretion of excess antibodies and calcium.

Patients with multiple myeloma are staged to determine treatment options and prognosis. Staging is based on the estimated number of myeloma cells calculated from the amount of abnormal monoclonal immunoglobulin in the urine and blood; the amount of calcium in the blood; the degree of bone destruction noted on X-ray examination; and the amount of hemoglobin in the blood.

Early in the disease process patients may be symptom free. When manifestations do occur, they may consist of back or rib pain, weight loss, fatigue, weakness, or repeated infections. Later stages of the diseases are associated with nausea, vomiting, anemia, renal damage, or extremity weakness. By the time of diagnosis, bone lesions are typically present in the skull, spine, and pelvis. The major problems encountered by patients with multiple myeloma are related to the complication of pathologic fractures, renal failure, and infection.

Clinical Manifestations

- *Pain (an early symptom):* Plasma cells accumulate within the bone marrow, causing destruction of bone, which results in fractures.
- *Renal compromise:* Excessive amounts of protein excreted in the urine and hypercalcemia adversely affect renal function.
- *Infections:* Abnormal plasma cells accumulate in the bone marrow, decreasing the production of normal white blood cells (WBCs). Decreased WBCs result in increased bacterial infections.
- *Weakness:* The accumulation of abnormal plasma cells in the bone marrow prevents red blood cells production and results in anemia.

Management

Collaborative management of multiple myeloma is directed at improving the quality of the patients life by controlling symptoms, reducing tumor cell burden, and preventing complications. Chemotherapy prolongs the survival for patients with stage I disease for 40 to 46 months, stage II disease for 35 to 40 months, and stage III disease for 24 to 30 months.

Various laboratory and other diagnostic tests are completed when patients are symptomatic. Summation of common diagnostic tests for multiple myeloma include the following:

- Urine and serum protein electrophoresis to determine the presence of abnormal proteins and number of normal immunoglobulins
- Bone marrow biopsy to determine the presence and number of cancerous plasma cells
- Computed tomography scans and radiography that show a "punched-out" type of bone lesion or generalized osteoporosis of the axial skeleton
- Complete blood count to determine the presence of anemia, leukopenia or thrombocytopenia
- Magnetic resonance imaging to detect the presence of bone abnormalities and fractures
- Blood chemistries to detect the presence of hypercalcemia and elevated uric acid levels
- Estimated myeloma cell mass to estimate the tumor burden.

Combination drug therapy has proven to be a more effective treatment for multiple myeloma than single chemotherapeutic agents. Oral melphalan combined with prednisone is the treatment of choice to reduce tumor load. Other chemotherapy combinations are:

- Vincristine sulfate, doxorubicin, cyclophosphamide, and carmustine
- Vincristine, doxorubicin and dexamethasone; and
- Thalidomide and dexamethasone.

Interferon-alpha therapy has been shown to prolong the duration of initial remission once achieved. Glucocorticoids and calcitonin reduce the lytic bone destruction of hypercalcemia. Erythropoietin stimulates the production of red blood cells and helps correct anemia.

The type of combination therapy or other agents used depends on several factors, including the patients age, the stage of the disease, and the patients kidney function. If cell transplantation is being considered, drugs with increased risk for bone marrow damage are avoided.

For patients who have a solitary skeletal lesion (plasmacytoma) but are otherwise asymptomatic and have fewer than 50% plasma cells in their bone marrow, radiotherapy has been shown to increase survival rates. When bone damage to the spine is extensive, orthopedic fixation devices may be used for stabilization and to prevent cord compression. For patients in renal failure, dialysis may be necessary to correct azotemia and hypercalcemia. Plasmapheresis, a process that filters the blood, may be useful in removing accumulated myeloma proteins that thicken blood and impede circulation to the brain.

Adequate hydration is necessary to prevent renal complications related to the excretion of increased amounts of urates and calcium in the urine. Fluid intake needs to be sufficient to ensure a minimal urinary output of 1500 mL/day to maintain renal function. If the patient is unable to maintain adequate fluid intake orally or requires nothing-by-mouth status for diagnostic or surgical procedures, intravenous fluids need to be administered. The nurse weighs the patient daily to assess for fluid retention, and monitors the patients blood urea nitrogen and serum creatinine levels to evaluate renal function. A well-balanced diet is encouraged, but there are no specific dietary restrictions unless renal failure occurs.

Nursing Management

The nurses to assess for:

- Back or rib pain
- Excessive fatigue or weakness
- Increased incidence of bacterial infections, urinary tract infections, or shingles
- Changes in urinary pattern or output
- Recent or frequent fractures
- Increased thirst, nausea, loss of appetite.

And also assess for:

- Weight gain and edema
- Pale skin or mucous membranes
- Cough
- Abnormal lung sounds.

The main problem associated with multiplex is pain (acute or chronic).

Common examples of nursing objective for the patient with a diagnosis of pain are:

Patient will:

- Use nonanalgesic measures to control pain (e.g. relaxation)
- Rate pain as 3 or less on a scale of 1 (no pain) to 10 (severe pain)
- Verbalize satisfactory control of pain.

For pain in the early stages of multiple myeloma, patients may experience little pain or discomfort. During the advanced stage of disease, pain is likely due to fragile bones and fractures. General comfort measures, such as back care, fresh linens, or a quiet environment, may reduce the patients discomfort. Analgesic medications may include nonsteroidal anti-inflammatory agents or narcotic analgesics. Ambulation is encouraged to prevent further bone demineralization associated with immobility, but skeletal pain may be a deterrent to ambulation. A light-weight spinal brace, analgesics, local radiotherapy, and nonanalgesic pain control methods such as distraction may be of benefit.

Safety is of vital importance because of the risk of fractures. Area rugs should be removed from the home to eliminate a potential source of falls. If the patient is completely immobile, careful turning is important. Even a tug on the arm or a turn toward the bed rail can cause a fracture. A lift sheet and the assistance of several people are necessary to facilitate moving the patient gently and safely without causing extensive pain.

(3) HYPERSENSITIVITIES

The immune system is always ready to respond to foreign antigens. Under certain circumstances, however, this response may bring harm as well as protection. Hypersensitivity diseases may be related to two abnormalities: the immune response to antigens may be unrestrained, producing tissue injury; or the immune response may be directed toward self-antigens because of a loss of self-tolerance, which is known as autoimmunity.

Hypersensitivity diseases are broadly divided into five categories based on the immunologic mechanisms involved in the reaction. Immediate hypersensitivity (type I) is mediated by IgE and causes injury from the release of histamine from mast cells. Antibody-mediated (type II) hypersensitivity exists when antibodies are directed against self-antigens. When antigen-antibody complexes collect in blood vessels or other tissues, immune complex disease (type III) hypersensitivity disease exists. T cell mediated hypersensitivity (type IV or delayed) exists when T cells are directed against self-antigens in tissues. Another relatively new hypersensitivity, known as stimulatory (type V), involves the binding the autoantibodies to hormone receptors that mimic the hormone itself, which stimulates target cells (Fig. 5.3).

Immediate Hypersensitivity

Immediate or type I hypersensitivity is an exaggerated immune response occurring in persons who have been previously sensitized to the specific antigen. The antigen producing the reaction is referred to as an *allergen*, and the reaction itself is called allergy or atopy. Immediate hypersensitivities are characterized by inappropriate, rapid and exaggerated responses mediated by IgE antibodies and mast cells. People who tend to produce IgE in response to antigens such as pollen or dust mites are said to be atopic. A severe, potentially lethal systemic form of immediate hypersensitivity reaction is known as systemic anaphylaxis or *anaphylactic shock*.

The onset of allergic diseases generally occurs between the ages of 2 and 15 years, although they can begin at any age. Atopic dermatitis is the most common skin disease, but allergic rhinitis accounts for the majority of visits to health care providers each year. It is estimated that 8% of children under the age of 6 and 1 to 2% of adults have food allergies. Allergic reactions account for 5 to 10% of all above drug reactions.

The tendency to become hypersensitive and produce IgE antibodies in response to inhaled or ingested substances is inherited as a dominant trait. If both parents have allergies, their children have a 50% probability of also having allergies. The specific substances that an individual develops hypersensitivity to, however, are determined by the allergens to which that individual is exposed. A person does not inherit a specific allergy, only the predisposition to develop allergies. No association has been found between gender, race, or geographic area and an increased risk of anaphylaxis.

Allergens are primarily characterized by their route of exposure. Inhaled allergens such as pollens, dust mite fecal matter, fungal hyphae or spores, animal dander are main casual agents of hay fever, chronic rhinitis, and asthma. Common food allergens, such as peanuts, eggs, milk, soy, chicken and shellfish, are thought to trigger mast cell degranulation in the gut after entering the circulation. Whether an allergic response occurs and to what degree depends on a combination of interrelated factors.

Pathophysiology

Immediate hypersensitivities are medicated by the IgE class of immunoglobulins. In generally predisposed people, initial exposure to an allergen prompts the activation of TH2 cells, which are not produced by normal individuals. TH2 cells stimulate the production of IgE antibodies that sensitize the person to the allergen. This initial contact with the allergen is known as the *sensitizing dose*. In some cases it may take several doses of allergen before the persons immune system is fully sensitized. Once sensitization is complete, subsequent exposure (termed the *challenging dose*) results in the allergen combining with IgE and binding to receptor sites on mast cells and basophils. This antigen-antibody reaction results in a rapid release of potent vasoactive mediators such as histamine, kinins, chemotactic factors, and active products of arachidonic acid metabolism (leukotrienes, prostaglandins, and thromboxanes).

Vasoactive mediators produce the clinical manifestations associated with immediate hypersensitivity, which includes smooth muscle contraction, increased vascular permeability and increased mucus gland secretion. These changes may occur locally or at the site of the antigen-antibody reaction. Atopic allergens generally produce localized tissue reactions that remain confined to a specific area such as the skin, nasal passages, or lungs. Hives (urticaria) are pruritic lesions characterized by a pale pink elevated edge (wheal) on an erythematous background. Skin exposed to latex can precipitate contact urticaria. Chronic urticaria that occurs in response to heat, cold, or various light waves is not an IgE-mediated hypersensitivity. Angioedema is a form of urticaria that involves the subcutaneous tissue rather than the skin. It can affect an entire anatomic part, such as the eyelid, thumb, or lip. Swelling is present, but not pruritus. Atopic diseases are not usually life threatening, but the symptoms can be uncomfortable and may cause the individual to miss school or work. A mosquito bite is a classic example of this type of reaction; the intradermal injection of the mosquito anticoagulants produces a wheal-flare type of reaction within minutes.

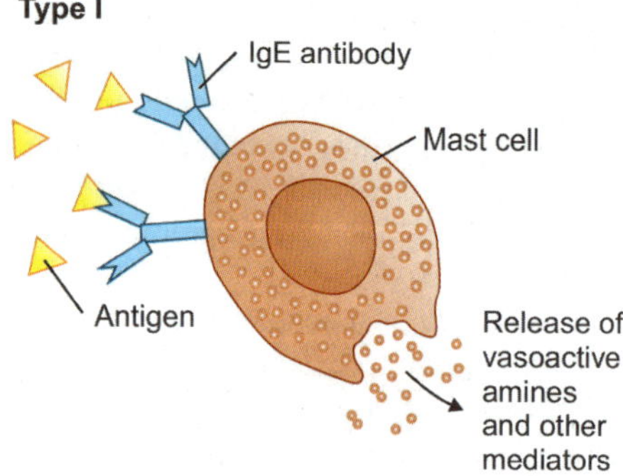

Type I. An anaphylactic reaction is characterized by vasodilation, increased capillary permeability, smooth muscle contraction, and eosinophilia. Systemic reactions may involve laryngeal stridor, angioedema, hypotension, and bronchial, GI, or uterine spasm; local reactions are characterized by hives. Examples to types I reactions include extrinsic asthma, allergic rhinitis, systemic anaphylaxis, and reactions to insect stings

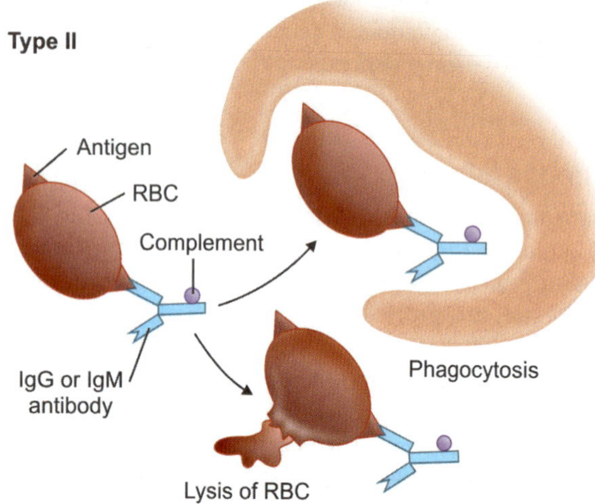

Type II. A cytotoxic reaction, which involves binding either the IgG or IgM antibody to a cell-bound antigen, may lead to eventual cell and tissue damage. The reaction is the result of mistaken identity when the system identifies a normal constituent of the body as foreign and activates the complement cascade. Examples of type II reactions are myasthenia gravis, Goodpasture's syndrome, pernicious anemia, hemolytic disease of the newborn, transfusion reaction, and thrombocytopenia

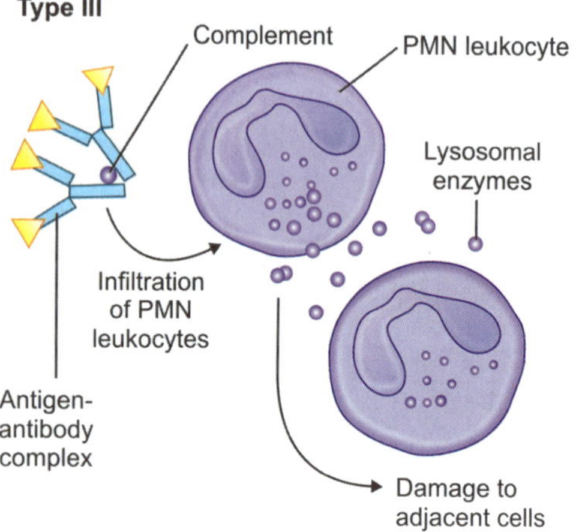

Type III. An immune complex reaction is marked by acute inflammation resulting from formation and deposition of immune complexes. The joints and kidneys are particularly susceptible to this kind of reaction, which is associated with systemic lupus erythematosus, serum sickness, nephritis, and rheumatoid arthritis. Some signs and symptoms include uritcaria, joint pain, fever, rash, and adenopathy (swollen glands)

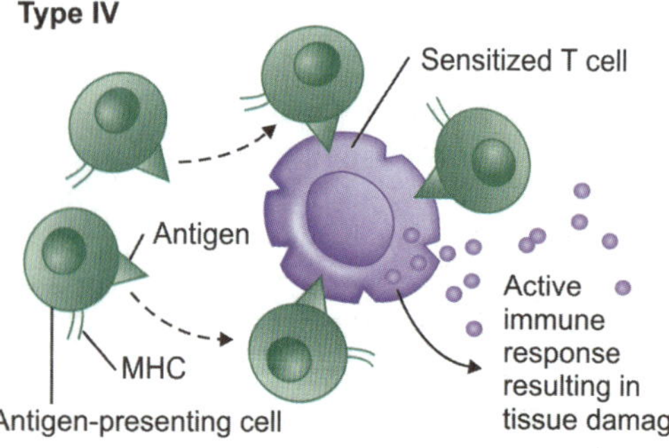

Type IV. A delayed, or cellular, reaction occurs 1 to 3 days after exposure to an antigen. The reaction, which results in tissue damage, involves activity by lymphokines, macrophages, and lysozymes. Erythema and itching are common; a few examples include contact dermatitis, graft-versus-host disease, Hashimoto's thyroiditis, and sarcoidosis

FIG. 5.3: Four types of hypersensitivity reactions (Ig, immunoglobulin; PMN, polymorphonuclear; RBC, red blood cell)

Clinical manifestations immediate (Type I) hypersensitivity include the following:

Respiratory
- Rhinorrhea
- Watery, itching eyes
- Obstruction of eustachian tubes
- Sneezing
- Sinusitis
- Headache
- Facial pain
- Bronchospasm
- Dyspnea
- Stridor
- Tachypnea
- Wheezing
- Cyanosis
- Use of accessory muscles for breathing
- Flaring of nare

Dermal
- Hives
- Rash
- Angioedema

Abdominal
- Nausea
- Vomiting
- Cramping
- Diarrhea

General
- Fever
- Diaphoresis
- Malaise
- Joint pain
- Hematopoietic suppression
- Anxiety
- Anaphylaxis

Anaphylaxis

Anaphylaxis is a severe, life-threatening allergic response to an immunologic reaction (type I hypersensitivity) between a specific antigen and an immunoglobulin E (IgE) antibody. Type I hypersensitivity requires previous exposure to the specific antigen through inhalation, injection, ingestion, or skin contact (Fig. 5.4). An anaphylactoid (anaphylaxis-like) reaction is clinically similar to anaphylaxis. Anaphylaxis may occur with medications, food, latex, insect sting, and cytotoxic antibody transfusion. Reactions may be local or systemic. Local anaphylactic reactions usually involve urticaria (hives) and angioedema (swelling) at the exposure site. The reaction can be severe but is rarely fatal. Systemic reactions occur in major organ systems within minutes of exposure.

Anaphylaxis may be localized or widespread. Localized anaphylaxis produces hives and angioedema. If widespread mast cell degranulation occurs, producing systemic effects such as decreased blood pressure, bronchial obstruction, and edema in many tissues, systemic anaphylaxis or anaphylactic

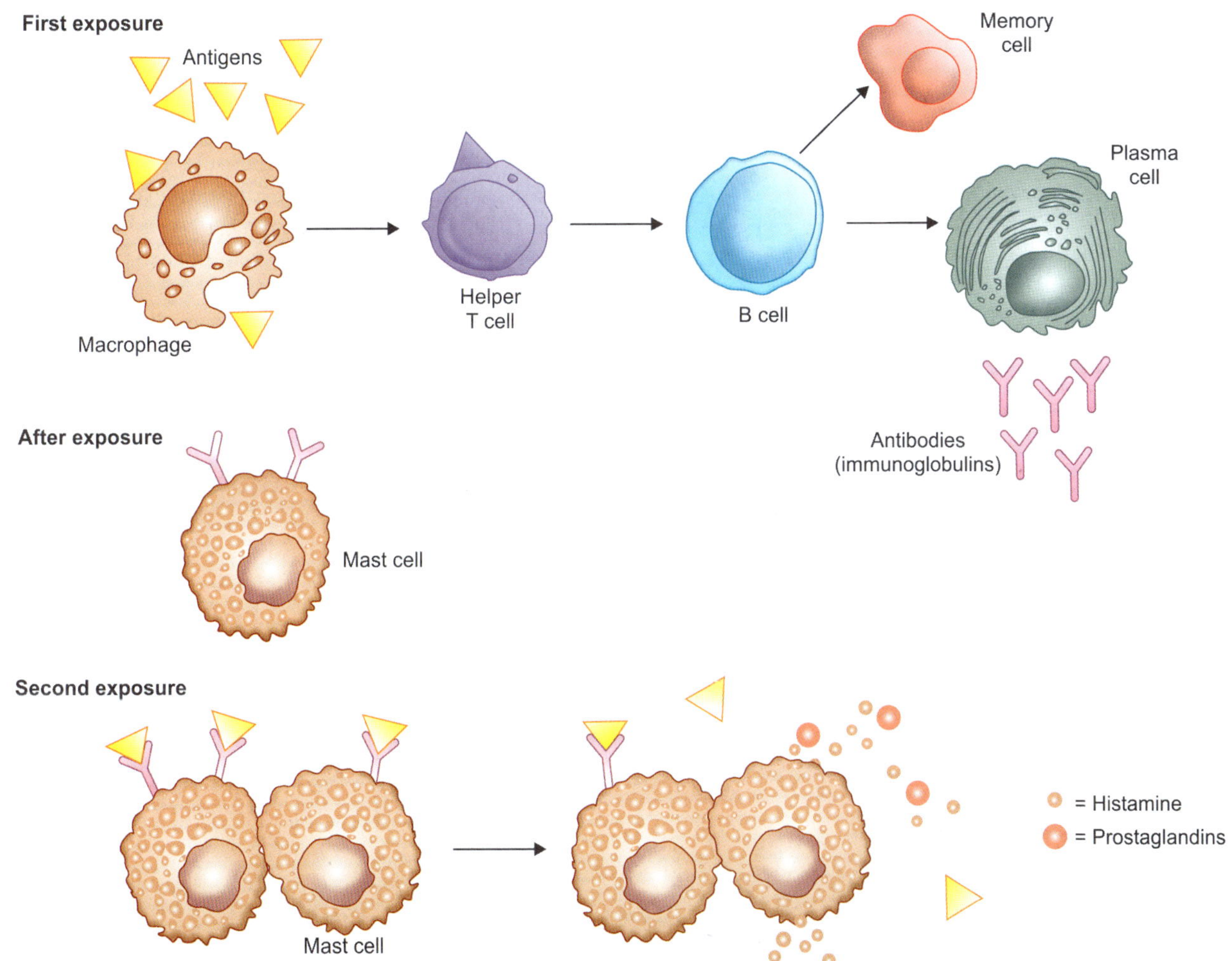

FIG. 5.4: Type I hypersensitivity

shock is said to exist. It is the most severe form of immediate hypersentivity in humans. Apprehension and sneezing are two of the earliest symptoms of systemic anaphylaxis. Edema and itching may also occur at the site of antigen entrance. These mild reactions are rapidly followed, sometimes in a matter of seconds or minutes, by severe manifestations that lead to vascular collapse shock, and death unless rapid action is taken. Insect or snake venoms; foods; and drugs such as penicillin, streptokinase, or amphotericin B are most often associated with anaphylaxis, although almost any antigen to which a person is hypersensitive has the potential for producing a systemic reaction. The causes of anaphylaxis are given in Box 5.2.

Box 5.2 Causes of anaphylaxis

Antibiotics	Aminoglycosides Amphotericin B Cephalosporins Penicillins Sulfonamides Tetracyclines
Anesthetics	Lidocaine
Antiarrhythmics	Procaine
Hormones	Adrenocorticotropic hormone Estradiol Insulin Vasopressin
Other medications	Barbiturates Diazepam (Valium) Phenytoin (Dilantin) Protamine Salicylates
Diagnostic agents	Contrast dyes
Medical products	Latex rubber
Foods	Beans Chocolate Eggs Fruits (e.g. strawberries) Grains (e.g. wheat) Nuts Shellfish
Food additives	Bisulfites Monosodium glutamate (MG)
Proteins	Horse serum Rabbit serum
Venoms	Bees, wasps, hornets Fire ants Snakes
Pollens	Grass Ragweed

Clinical Manifestations

Clinical symptoms are determined by the amount of the allergen, the amount of mediator released, the sensitivity of the target organ, and the route of allergen entry. Type I hypersensitivity reactions may include both local and systemic anaphylaxis.

Mild: Symptoms include peripheral tingling; a warm sensation; fullness in the mouth and throat; nasal congestion; periorbital swelling, pruritus, sneezing, and tearing eyes. Symptoms begin within 2 hours of exposure.

Moderate: May include nay of the mild symptoms plus anxiety, bronchospasm, and edema of the airways or larynx with dyspnea, cough, and wheezing. Symptom onset is the same as that of a mild reaction.

Severe: An abrupt onset with the same signs and symptoms described above, progressing rapidly to bronchospasm, laryngeal edema, sever dyspnea, cyanosis and hypotension. Dysphagia, abdominal cramping, vomiting, diarrhea, and seizures are additional symptoms, with cardiac arrest and coma occurring rarely.

If the second antigen exposure is localized, the reaction is mild and remains local. However, if the exposure is systemic, the reaction is massive and widespread. Respiratory allergies, such as allergic rhinitis and allergic asthma, with associated disorders of atopic dermatitis, tend to be reaction of a larger scale. Anaphylaxis, urticarial, and angioedema are the severest forms of types I reactions.

A type I reaction occurs when the patient has a positive reaction to a scratch test. A scratch test is done to identify specific allergens to which a patient is reactive. Tiny amounts of a variety of common allergens are scratched onto the skin, which is then observed for indication of a reaction—redness, edema, and pruritus. If these indications occur, it is considered to be a local reaction.

Localized

- Hives
- Angioedema

Systemic

- Apprehension
- Edema of the face, hands, or other parts of the body
- Wheezing
- Dyspnea
- Respiratory collapse
- Vascular collapse with shock
  - Rapid, weak pulse
  - Falling blood pressure
  - Cyanosis
  - Death.

The factors that determine a hypersensitivity response will include the following:

- *Responsiveness of the host to the allergens:* If the host is highly sensitive to the antigen, a greater than normal chance exists that a tissue-damaging reaction will occur.
- *Amount of allergen:* Generally the greater the amount of allergen contracted, the more severe the reaction.
- *Nature of the allergen:* Any foreign protein or protein-containing component can serve as an allergen when coupled with a normal tissue protein carrier. Examples include pollens, foods, animal dander, house dust, and feathers.
- *Route of entrance of the allergen:* Allergens may gain host entry via the respiratory tract, through epidermal or mucosal surfaces, by injection, or through the digestive tract.
- *Timing of exposure to the allergens:* If the host's contacts with the allergen are widely separated by time, the immunologic mediators may be so dilute that little responses occurs. Conversely, if frequent contact is made with the allergen, reactions are more likely to occur.
- *Site of the allergen immune mediator reaction:* A reaction can occur in the tissues with little consequence; however, the same reaction occurring in the bloodstream can lead to a severe reaction.
- *Host's threshold of reactivity:* The host's immune system can be changed by factors such as stress, fatigue, or infection, all of which can decrease the immune system's responsiveness to potential allergens.

Latex hypersensitivity, which has a high potential for producing anaphylaxis, has become a universal concern among health care workers, since numerous medical products such as gloves, catheters, and tubes contain latex. The prevalence of latex allergy is estimated at about 6% for the general population. Signs of latex allergy depend largely on the route of exposure. When latex particles are aerosolized, wheezing, rhinitis, and conjunctivitis may occur. Mucosal exposure frequently results in angioedema. There is no cure for latex hypersensitivity, and avoidance is the principal treatment. To sum up anaphlaxis see Box 5.3.

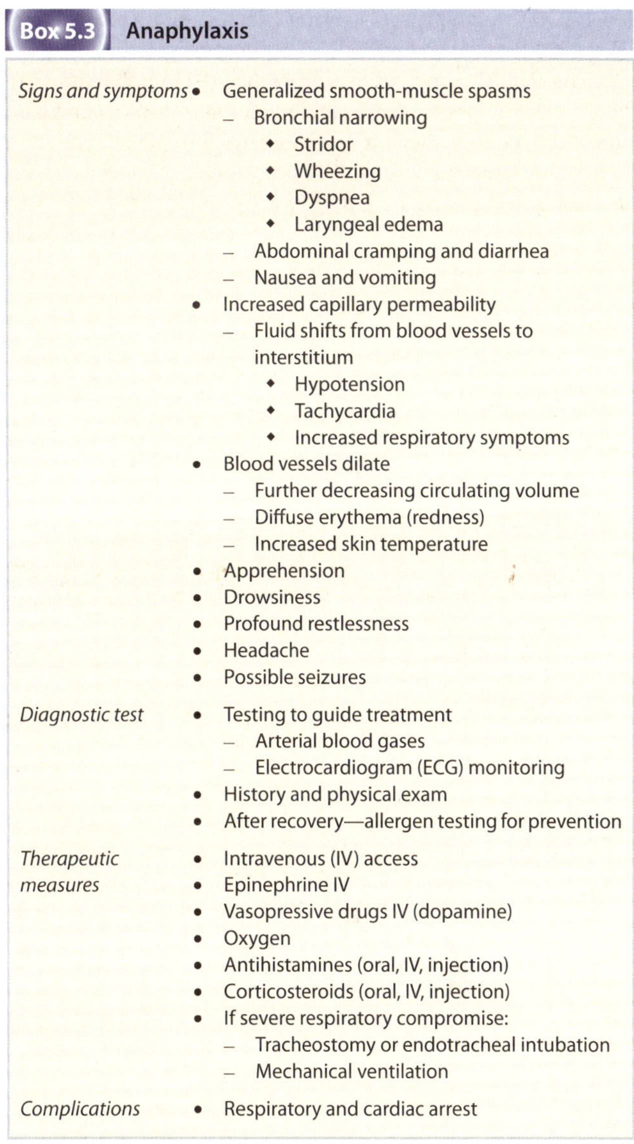

Box 5.3 Anaphylaxis

Signs and symptoms

- Generalized smooth-muscle spasms
  - Bronchial narrowing
    - Stridor
    - Wheezing
    - Dyspnea
    - Laryngeal edema
  - Abdominal cramping and diarrhea
  - Nausea and vomiting
- Increased capillary permeability
  - Fluid shifts from blood vessels to interstitium
    - Hypotension
    - Tachycardia
    - Increased respiratory symptoms
- Blood vessels dilate
  - Further decreasing circulating volume
  - Diffuse erythema (redness)
  - Increased skin temperature
- Apprehension
- Drowsiness
- Profound restlessness
- Headache
- Possible seizures

Diagnostic test

- Testing to guide treatment
  - Arterial blood gases
  - Electrocardiogram (ECG) monitoring
- History and physical exam
- After recovery—allergen testing for prevention

Therapeutic measures

- Intravenous (IV) access
- Epinephrine IV
- Vasopressive drugs IV (dopamine)
- Oxygen
- Antihistamines (oral, IV, injection)
- Corticosteroids (oral, IV, injection)
- If severe respiratory compromise:
  - Tracheostomy or endotracheal intubation
  - Mechanical ventilation

Complications

- Respiratory and cardiac arrest

Management of Hypersensitivity

Diagnostic evaluation of the patient with allergic disorders commonly includes blood tests (CBC with differential, high total serum IgE levels), smears of body secretions, skin tests, and the radioallergosorbent test (RAST).

The health history, including an environmental assessment, is one of the most valuable diagnostic tools for the health care provider evaluating the patient for immediate hypersensitivities. Intradermal skin testing and the radioallergosorbent test (RAST) may be helpful in identifying antigens and determining therapy for persons with allergens. Eosinophilia (increased eosinophil count) is associated with antigen-antibody reactions and occurs in persons with allergies, and drug hypersensitivity.

Medications

Respiratory and cardiovascular functions are evaluated and cardiopulmonary resuscitation (CPR) is initiated in cases of cardiac arrest. Oxygen is administered in high concentrations during CPR or when the patient is cyanotic, dyspneic, or wheezing. Patients with mild reactions need to be educated about the risk for recurrences. Patients with severe reactions need to be observed for 12 to 14 hours.

Symptom relief is the primary aim of drug therapy for allergies. Urticaria and angioedema are usually self-limiting; therefore treatment is often not required. Anaphylaxis is treated with epinephrine to shorten its duration and prevent relapse. When intravenous access is not available, epinephrine is administered by intramuscular injection to provide the highest level of absorption. Antihistamines, such as diphenhydramine (Benadryl), are given to block histamine receptors. Short-term corticosteroid therapy, either oral or inhaled (cromolyn sodium), may be useful for decreasing the inflammation associated with allergic responses. Leukotriene-mediated bronchoconstriction is treated with leukotriene receptor blocking agents such as montelukast (singulair) or zafirlukast (accolate). Aminophylline or inhalants such as isoproterenol (terbutaline, albuterol) may also provide symptomatic relief from bronchoconstriction. Common medications used for type 1 hypersensitivities are given in Table 5.4.

Prevention by avoidance of allergens is of utmost importance. Health care providers should always obtain a careful history of any sensitivities before administering medications. Venom immunotherapy may be given to people who are allergic to insect venom. Insulin-allergic diabetic patients or penicillin-sensitive patients may require desensitization as well.

Avoidance therapy, in which the patient is taught to reduce exposure to triggering antigens, is the most effective treatment to decrease allergic attacks, especially for food, drug, and animal dander, but it can be useful in treating seasonal allergies. For instance, limiting outdoor activities and staying in air-conditioned settings when the pollen counts are high decrease seasonal allergy symptoms.

Immunotherapy is often useful in reducing symptoms in patients who cannot avoid antigens such as dust mites or pollen. The health care provider injects an extract of the allergen subcutaneously starting with the dose at which the person was found to be sensitive by skin testing. Over time, serum IgE-specific antibody levels fall, IgG blocking antibodies increase,

TABLE 5.4: Common medications for type I hypersensitivities

Drug	Action	Nursing intervention
Antihistamines		
Diphenhydramine (Benadryl)	Antihistamine; compete with histamine for effector cell H1-receptor sites, thus preventing action of histamine	May produce significant drowsiness (Benadryl) or central nervous system stimulation (Chlor-Trimeton); causes dry mouth; may produce blurred vision Do not use for patients with hypersensitivity narrow-angle glaucoma, lower respiratory tract disease, or acute asthma attacks; patient who are pregnant or breastfeeding; or patients who took monoamine oxidase inhibitors within past 14 days Advise patient to take 1 hour before or 1 hour after meals to facilitate drug absorption
Chlorpheniramine (Chlor-Trimeton)		
Brompheniramine (Dimetane)		
Astemizole (Hismanal)		
Loratadine (Tavist)		
Fexofenadine hydrochloride (Allergra)		
Decongestants	Stimulate alpha-adrenergic receptors to shrink respiratory mucous membranes	May produce nausea, vomiting, headache, anxiety, tremors, dizziness, seizures, tachycardia, hypertension, dysrhythmias, mucous membrane irritation, or dry mouth Monitor blood pressure and pulse; give several hours before bedtime if drug produces sleeplessness Do not use for patients with hypertension. Teach patient to stop drug if tremors or restlessness occurs Phenylephrine (Neo-Synephrine) Pseudoephedrine (Sudafed)
Mast cell degranulator Inhibitor		
Cromolyn sodium inhaler (Intal)	Inhibit mast cell release of histamine and slow-reacting substance of anaphylaxis, thus preventing allergic response	Give for prophylactic use only. May produce nasal irritation and burning, sneezing, cough, or throat irritation; dry mouth; nausea and vomiting; angioedema; or bronchospasm. Do not give to patients with hypertensitivity, acute asthma, or history of coronary artery disease or dysrhythmias. Teach effective use of inhaler for accurate dosing.

Contd...

Contd...

Drug	Action	Nursing intervention
Cromolyn sodium nasal spray (Nasalcrom)		
Corticosteroids		
Prednisone	Suppress migration of polymorphonuclear leukocytes and fibroblasts, thereby reducing inflammation	Do not give to patients with hypersensitivity, psychoses, fungal, acquired immunodeficiency syndrome, tuberculosis Monitor for thrombocytopenia, increased intraocular pressure, poor wound healing, nausea, diarrhea, headache, mood changes Monitor daily weight, serum potassium levels, blood glucose levels, blood pressure, signs of infection, mood changes Tell patients to take with food or milk to decrease gastrointestinal irritation Caution patient not to stop taking drug abruptly and to notify health care provider if infection develops
Methyprednisone		
Dexamethasone (Decadron)		
Beclomethasone (Vancenase, Beconase)		
Adrenalin		
Epinephrine	Opposes action of histamine through vasoconstriction to raise blood pressure; promotes bronchiole relaxation of facilitate breathing; stimulates both alpha and beta receptors to reproduce effects of sympathetic nervous system	Use for temporary relief from anaphylaxis, hypersensitivity reactions, bronchospasm, and acute asthma attacks Do not use for patients with hypersensitivity, narrow-angle glaucoma, dysrhythmias Monitor for anxiety, tremors, palpitations, tachydysrhythmias, hypertension, pulmonary edema Use intramuscular route when intravenous access is not available, since it provides highest level of absorption during systemic anaphylaxis
Aminophylline		
Theophylline (Theo-Dur)	Xanthine blocks phosphodiesterase, thus increasing cyclic adenosine monophosphate, which alters intracellular calcium and ion movement, produces respiratory tract relaxation and bronchodilation, and increases pulmonary blood flow	Monitor for central nervous system stimulation, dizziness, anxiety, restlessness, seizures, tachycardia, dysrhythmias, nausea, vomiting, insomnia Do not give a patients with hypersensitivity to xanthine or history of tachydysrhythmias Instruct patient to avoid intake of stimulant foods such as coffee, tea, and colas Monitor theophylline blood levels. Instruct patient to avoid smoking because it interferes with absorption

and lymphocyte responsiveness to the antigen is reduced. Increasing amounts of allergen are injected at weekly intervals. If large local reactions occur during therapy, the dose is lowered until better tolerated. Systemic reactions, although uncommon, may occur within 30 minutes of injection of the allergen extract. Treatment includes placing the person in a supine position and administering epinephrine. If the nurse notes signs and symptoms of systemic anaphylactic shock, oxygen is administered and intravenous fluids infused rapidly to support blood pressure. Because of its potential for anaphylaxis and death, the patient and primary caregiver must be certain that the symptoms warrant the risk, expense, and inconvenience of immunotherapy.

Clinical manifestations of immunotherapy reactions include the following:

Localized

- Redness
- Pruritus
- Edema
- Tenderness

Systemic

- Nasal stuffiness
- Reddening of conjunctiva
- Wheezing
- Apprehension
- Sneezing
- Chest tightness
- Fainting
- Anaphylactic shock

The future of immediate hypersensitivity treatment appears to lie in learning how to more effectively modulate the immune response. Possible therapies include manipulating IgE response by using IgE-specific suppressor T cells; using antibodies against IgE idiotopes; or using cytokines to suppress IgE synthesis.

Diet: The diet may be altered in patients with food allergies to avoid those foods precipitating the response. Suspected foods fare eliminated to see if allergy symptoms disappear. They may be reintroduced to see if they again cause symptoms. Foods suspected of causing systemic anaphylaxis are not reintroduced or only reintroduced under supervision in a hospital setting.

Nursing Management

- Teach people who are sensitive to insect bites and stings, certain medications, or foods, and people who have idiopathic or exercise-induced anaphylactic reactions to avoid exposure to allergens
- Instruct patient always to carry an emergency kit that contains injectable epinephrine
- Provide verbal and written instruction about the emergency kit
- Ensure that patient can perform correct self-injection
- Encourage patient always to wear or carry medical identification.

Nursing Management of the Patient with Immediate Hypersensitivity (Type 1)

Assess for:

- History of allergic reactions (type, frequency, or perceived causes)
- Familial history of allergies
- Recent exposure to sensitizing substances (chemicals, drugs)
- Changes in living, working, or environmental conditions
- Characteristics of present environment (house, clothing, plants, trees or animals)
- Symptoms experienced: Respiratory, dermal, gastrointestinal, or general
- Alleviating factors, either prescribed, herbal or over the counter.

And also assess for:

- Rashes (location, color)
- Mouth breathing (nasal obstruction)
- Flaring nares
- Difficulty hearing (plugged Eustachian tubes)
- Pale bluish turbinates that are edematous with clear secretions
- Tearing or dark areas under eyes (venous dilation of skin).
- Scleral or conjunctival infections
- Increased respiratory rate
- Use of accessory muscles for breathing
- Audible wheezing
- Anxious expression.

Problem Associated with Hypersensitivity

Risk for Latex Allergy Responses

Common nursing objectives for the patient with a diagnosis of risk for latex allergy response (or other allergy responses) are:

Patient will:

- Verbalize understanding of approaches for avoiding allergen (all latex-containing products)
- Plan to alter habits or environment to reduce exposure to antigens
- Verbalize understanding of prescribed and alternative approaches to symptom relief.

Here, an important aspect of nursing care for the patient with allergies is helping the patient identify and adjust to lifestyle changes to reduce exposure to allergens and maintain health. In many cases this involves few lifestyle changes, and the patient and family readily adjust. In other cases the patient may need to adjust to a complex medication schedule, give up a beloved pet, or move to another climate. Patients may have a change employment to avoid allergens such as chemicals, molds, or fibers. These changes may place emotional or financial burdens on the patient and family, especially if the job market or patients skills are limited. The nurses role is to help the patient explore alternative solutions and make the best choices possible to maintain health.

Teaching the patient and family about the disorder and methods to avoid the allergen is another important nursing interventions for the patient with allergies. The nurse reviews results of allergy testing, assessment findings, and patient history so the patient and family understand which allergens need to be controlled or avoided. The nurse teaches patients the importance of controlling their living and working environments to reduce exposure to antigens and, hence, the risk of reactions. If animal dander is a source of allergy and removal of a family pet is unacceptable to the patient or family, they may explore ways to decrease the pets impact on the allergic patient, such as keeping the pet outdoors or away from the room where the patient sleeps or spends large amounts of time.

The nurse emphasizes the need for total avoidance for patients who are latex sensitive. Patients are taught about prescribed medications, including desired actions, dosage schedules, and potential side effects. The nurse stresses the importance of maintaining drug schedules for prophylactic drugs, such as cromolyn, and reminds the patient and family that these drugs are of no value during an acute allergic attack.

Anaphylaxis can occur after exposure to offending antigens or from immunotherapy; consequently, the nurse teaches the patient and family about symptoms that need to be reported, potential reactions that necessitate emergency measures, and use of emergency care kit. If the patient chooses to undergo immunotherapy, the nurse discusses the risks and benefits, schedules, and costs. The nurse informs the patient that immunotherapy can be reinstituted if symptoms recur.

Patients with immediate hypersensitivities need to be aware of situations in which their specific allergens are likely to be present. The nurse gives those with insect sting sensitivity information about where to obtain and how to use emergency kits for insect stings. The nurse teaches both the patient and family how to use the self-injecting syringe to administer epinephrine. If the patient is unable to use the syringe, an inhalation of high-dose epinephrine may be taken from a metered dose aerosol, which is found in some emergency kits.

Ineffective Airway Clearance

Common nursing objective for the patient with a diagnosis of *ineffective airway clearance* are:

Patient will:

- Maintain a patent airway
- Correctly demonstrate the use of emergency anaphylactic equipment
- Verbalize the need to have emergency anaphylactic equipment available at all times
- Verbalize the need to inform all health care providers regarding his or her latex sensitivity.

Death from anaphylaxis occurs from asphyxiation because of upper airway edema and congestion, irreversible shock, or a combination of these factors (see the section on clinical manifestation of systemic anaphylaxis). The primary concern during an anaphylactic reaction is ensuring that the patient's airway is patent. The nurse positions the patient in a high Fowler's position to maximize ventilation; inserts an oral airway if necessary; and removes secretions by suction or by encouraging the patient to cough. Oxygen therapy is initiated in accordance with facility protocols. The nurse encourages slow, deep breathing to facilitate the intake of oxygen and decrease anxiety. The administration of epinephrine or bronchodilators such as aminophylline may be necessary to decrease bronchospasm. In severe cases, tracheostomy may be necessary to maintain a patent airway. The nurse closely monitors the patient both during and after anaphylaxis, since recurrence is possible.

Respiratory compromise can lead to impaired cardiac function and death within minutes. At the first sign of anaphylaxis, the nurse gives the patient epinephrine, 1:1000 solution, 0.3 to 0.5 mL subcutaneously or intramuscularly. If shock continues, the nurse may administer albuterol (Ventolin) or epinephrine through aerosol treatments. Vasopressors such as dopamine may be prescribed for severe shock to assist in maintaining blood pressure and cardiac output.

Since drug allergies are a significant cause of anaphylaxis, the nurse questions all patients about allergies and drug sensitivities before initiating drug therapy. High-risk persons are instructed to wear an identification bracelet or necklace at all times that indicates the known allergy. Such devices may be obtained from Guinine or other commercial sources. Persons with known drug allergies are advised to alert health care workers of their allergies when animal sera, allergenic extracts, or contrast media containing iodide need to be given for any reason, so that epinephrine can be readily available. The nurse monitors the patient for at least 30 minutes after administration of such substances. Any reaction that occurs within a few minutes forewarns of an impending emergency.

Nurses need to recognize the potential for drug cross-sensitivity what administering alternative drugs to allergic patients. For example, cephalosporins are frequently administered to patients who are sensitive to penicillin. A small percentage of patients will, however, also be sensitive to cephalosporin because it has a cross-sensitivity with penicillin. The yellow dye contained in some tablets has cross-sensitivity with aspirin and may cause anaphylaxis in aspirin-sensitive patients.

Health Education for Patient with Allergies

Patient teaching should include information about the allergy and prescribed medication, as well as the following instructions on avoiding allergens.

Animal Dander

- Avoid fur-bearing pets if possible, or keep pets outdoors
- Avoid furniture stuffed with horsehair or feathers.

Pollen Spores

- Use air conditioning if possible; keep windows closed at night; if using air condition in car, start car, roll down windows, and allow air conditioner to run for 10 to 15 minutes before entering car
- Limit time outdoors between sunset and sunrise, especially when windy
- Do not hang wash outside to dry (pollen and molds stick to wet wash)
- Avoid gardening, raking leaves, mowing lawn, or being near freshly cut grass
- Keep car windows closed when driving
- Minimize number of indoor plants
- Vacation in selected geographic areas, such as beach or sea, that are free of specific allergen during seasonal height, if possible.

House Dust

- Use synthetic materials; avoid wool and cotton
- Use a minimum of lint-producing articles
- Put away items that are difficult to dust
- Dust with damp cloth daily
- Use air conditioner if possible
- Change furnace filter every month when in use.

The Patient with Immediate Hypersensitivity: Sting

Patient teaching should include:

- Emergency care for the specific allergy
- Availability and use of commercially prepared emergency kit
- Concentration and route of emergency use epinephrine (1:1000 epinephrine injection)
- Use of self-injection syringe of epinephrine supplied with kit (spring loaded; can be given through clothing).

Also include the following instructions about the emergency procedure if sting occurs:

- Immediately swallow the uncoated antihistamine tablet
- Inject the epinephrine
- If unable to self-inject, inhale high-dose epinephrine from metered-dose aerosol (if included in kit).

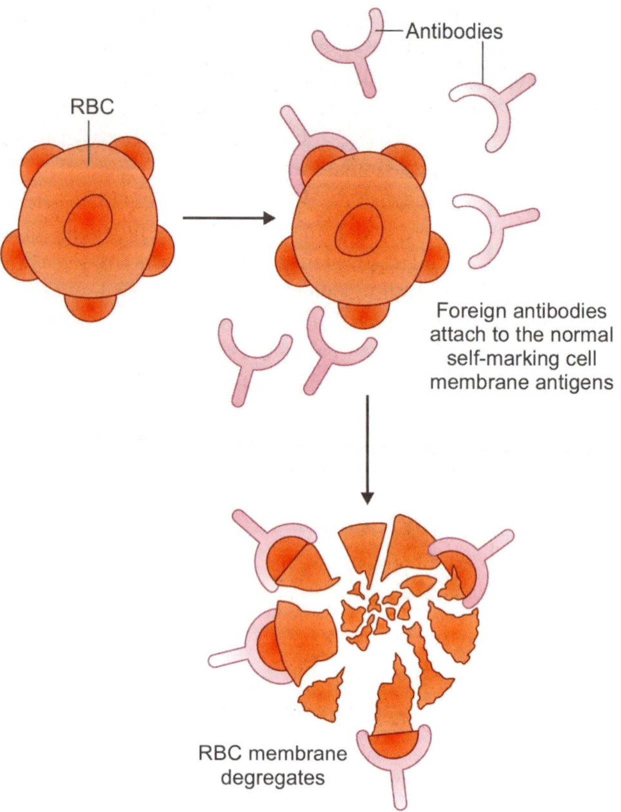

FIG. 5.5: Type II hypersensitivity

Tissue-specific Antibody Hypersensitivities

In antibody-mediated hypersensitivity, also known as cytotoxic hypersensitivity, antibodies are directed against specific target cells or tissues; thus the damage is restricted to those cells or tissues that bear the specific antigen, such as platelets. These reactions differ from immune-complex (type III) reactions in that type III reactions involve circulating antigen-antibody complexes.

A classic example of a specific antibody-mediated (type II) hypersensitivity reaction occurs with the infusion of mismatched blood (Fig. 5.5). *Acute hemolytic transfusion reaction* (ABO incompatibility) is the most serious adverse reaction to blood transfusions and results in approximately 1 death per 1,00,000 units of blood infused. The reaction occurs within the first 30 minutes of blood administration. Studies of **hemolytic** reactions have shown that mistakes in specimen collection and labeling or inadequate patient identification are the primary errors responsible.

Another type of antibody-mediated hypersensitivity occurs when the mother is sensitized to antigens on the infant's erythrocytes and makes antibodies against those antigens. This condition is known as *hemolytic disease of the newborn*. The Rhesus D (RhD) factor is the most commonly involved antigen of the antigen RhD is present; the term Rh-negative means that the RhD antigen is absent. Approximately, 85% of the population has Rh-positive blood. Between 10 and 15% of Caucasian infants and approximately 5% of African-American infants experience Rh incompatibility.

Tissue-specific hypersensitivities injure host cells by binding IgG or IgM to an antigen on the surface of a target cell, such as a platelet. Once binding occurs, the cell is destroyed by phagocytic attack, nonspecific lymphocytic attack or lysis of the cell through the activation of the full complement cascade.

Immunologic Transfusion Reactions

Acute hemolytic reactions are caused by antigen-antibody complexes on the erythrocyte membrane. These complexes activate Hageman factor (coagulation factor XII) and the complement cascade. The Hageman factor initiates the kinin system, causing increased capillary permeability, arteriole vasodilation, and hypotension. The complement system initiates intravascular hemolysis, as well as histamine and serotonin release from the mast cells. Hageman factor also combines with free compatible erythrocytes, activating the intrinsic clotting cascade, which causes disseminated intravascular coagulation (DIC) (Table 5.5).

Febrile nonhemolytic reactions are among the most common transfusion reactions. They occur when the recipient becomes sensitized to the donor's white blood cells, platelets, or plasma.

TABLE 5.5: Immunologic reactions to blood transfusion

Reaction	Clinical manifestations	Management	Prevention
Acute hemolytic	Chills, fever, lower back pain, flushing, tachycardia, tachypnea, hypotension, vascular collapse, hemoglobinuria, hemoglobinemia, bleeding, acute renal failure, shock, cardiac arrest, death	Treat shock. Draw blood samples for serologic testing. To avoid hemolysis from procedure, use new venipuncture (not existing central line) and avoid small-gauge needles. Send urine specimen to laboratory Maintain blood pressure with intravenous (IV) colloid solutions Insert indwelling as prescribed to maintain urine flow Insert indwelling catheter or measure voided amounts to monitor hourly urine output Dialysis may be required if renal failure occurs Do not transfuse additional red blood cell-containing components until transfusion service has provided newly cross-matched units	Meticulously verify and document patient identification from sample collection to component infusion Transfuse blood slowly for first 15–20 minutes with nurse at patients side
Febrile, nonhemolytic (most common)	Sudden chills and fever (rise in temperature of greater than 2°F [1°C]), headache, flushing, anxiety, muscle pain	Give antipyretics as prescribed. Do not give aspirin to thrombocytopenic patients. Do not restart transfusion	Consider leukocyte-poor blood products (filtered, washed or frozen)
Mild allergic	Flushing, itching, urticaria (hives)	Give antihistamines as directed If symptoms are mild and transient, restart transfusion slowly Do not restart transfusion if fever or pulmonary symptoms develop	Treat prophylactically with glucocorticosteriods or antihistamines (dexamethasone), [Decadron], diphenhydramine [Benadryl]) given 30–60 minutes before transfusion
Anaphylactic	Anxiety, urticaria, wheezing, tightness and pain in chest, difficulty swallowing, progressing to cyanosis, shock and possible cardiac arrest	Initiate cardiopulmonary resuscitation if indicated. Have epinephrine ready for injection (0.4 mL of a 1:1000 solution diluted to 10 mL with saline for IV use) Do not restart transfusion	Transfuse extensively washed red blood cell products from which all plasma has been removed. Alternatively, use blood from IgA-deficient donor
Delayed hemolytic	Fever, chills, back pain, hemoglobinuria	Monitor adequacy of urinary Treat fever with acetaminophen (Tylenol) May need further blood transfusion.	Do more specific type and cross-match jaundice, anemia, output and degree of anemia. When giving patient blood
Posttransfusion graft-versus-host disease	Anorexia, nausea, diarrhea, high fever, rash, stomatitis, liver dysfunction	No effective treatment Administer steroids	Give irradiated blood products
Noncardiac pulmonary edema	Fever, chills, hypotension, cough, orthopnea, cyanosis	Shock stop transfusion Continue IV saline Give oxygen prn Administer steroids as directed	Give furosemide (Lasix) and epinephrine as ordered

Symptoms usually begin 30 minutes after the start of the infusion. Although this reaction is not usually serious, it is uncomfortable.

Allergic transfusion reactions are due to the recipient's sensitivity to foreign plasma proteins. Common symptoms include hives, rash, and urticaria. If the symptoms are mild, the patient is treated with antihistamines and the transfusion is restarted slowly. Anaphylaxis can occur but fortunately is rare.

Delayed hemolytic reactions occur 7 to 14 days after the transfusion and are thought to be the result of sensitization of the recipient's immune system to the transfused erythrocyte antigens. The recipient may also have been previously sensitized but have antibody titers that are undetectable at the time of transfusion.

Post-transfusion graft-versus-host disease, which was once relatively rare, is occurring more frequently because of increased use of purposeful immunosuppression as treatment (e.g. bone marrow transplantation). The donor lymphocytes begin to reject the patient's host cells 4 to 30 days after the infusion of blood.

Noncardiac pulmonary edema is thought to be caused by a high titer of leukocyte antibodies in either the donor or recipient plasma. These antibody-to-granulocyte reactions cause granulocyte aggregates that are filtered out by the lung. The antibodies attached to initiate the complement cascade and promote histamine release, causing an influx of inflammatory cells into the lung (Table 5.5).

Hemolytic Disease

Hemolytic disease, most commonly seen in newborns, occurs when the Rh-negative mother is first exposed to the fetus's Rh-positive blood. Rh antibodies are formed against the Rh-positive blood. On subsequent exposures to Rh-positive blood, such as a second pregnancy, the Rh antibody binds to its corresponding antigen on the surface of the erythrocyte containing Rh factor. The Rh-antibodies do not usually fix complement; therefore hemolysis does not occur immediately as it does in the ABO system. Instead, the Rh-factor erythrocytes are rapidly broken down by macrophages in the spleen, with conversion of hemoglobin to bilirubin, resulting in jaundice.

Nonimmunogenic transfusion reactions: The administration of blood can cause reactions that are not immunologic. These include circulatory overload, sepsis, and transmission of disease. The clinical manifestations of nonimmunogenic transfusion reactions (Box 5.4).

Box 5.4 Hemolytic transfusion reaction

Signs and symptoms	Low back or chest pain Hypotension Fever rising more than 1.8°F (1°C) Chills Tachycardia Tachypnea, wheezing, dyspnea Urticaria Anxiety Headache Nausea
Diagnostic test	Direct Coomb's test • Small amount of patient's RBCs are washed • Antihuman globulin is added • If agglutination (clumping) occurs, an immune reaction is occurring
Therapeutic measures	Depends on severity of reaction and organs affected Antihistamins Corticosteroids Epinephrine Diuretics, to assist kidneys
Complications	If severe: shock, acute renal failure

- *Circulation overload:* This can occur when blood is given to rapidly or in large quantities. Older adults are particularly vulnerable. Patients develop signs of fluid overload and pulmonary congestion. The transfusion is stopped and oxygen and diuretics may be administered.
- *Sepsis:* Bacterial contamination can occur at time during the collection or handling of blood. Signs of sepsis being almost immediately. The transfusion is stopped, and the patient receives antibiotics and treatment for shock if it occurs.
- *Disease transmission:* Hepatits, cytomegalovirus, and human immunodeficiency virus are the most common diseases transmitted by blood transfusions. Hepatitis A and B are effectively identified with current screening capabilities, but hepatitis C is still readily transmissible.

Management: Prevention is the key to management of transfusion reactions. Blood received from volunteer donors through the blood banks is carefully screened and labeled. Most of the serious reactions that occur from transfusions are the result of human error. Typing, screening and cross-matching of blood in the laboratory must be accurate. Typing is established by testing the recipients serum against commercial A and B cells to detect isoaglutinins. The recipient's serum is then screened for all antibodies that were not found in the typing. The goal of cross-matching is to ensure the recipient's blood does not contain antibodies that will attack and destroy the transfused erythrocytes.

One method for preventing immunologic blood transfusion reactions and disease transmission is planned autologous transfusion, which involves using the persons own blood for replacement. Health care providers collect blood at regular intervals before anticipated use, such as forthcoming surgery, and store and freeze the blood until needed. This method is especially useful for persons with rare blood types, for those whose religious beliefs preclude receiving donor blood, or for those expected to need several units of blood during surgery (e.g. selected heart surgeries or joint replacements).

Auto transfusion, which consists of collecting, filtering, and immediately reinfusing the persons own blood, may be performed in the emergency department, the operating room suite during surgery, the post anesthesia care unit, or the critical care unit. Blood draining from the surgical site is suctioned into a bag and passes through a filter to remove microaggregates. When the bag is full, it is disconnected from the system and the blood is infused into the patient with an administration set, using a standard or microembolic filter.

Blood components are often administered rather than whole blood. Blood can be fractionated into red blood cells, platelets, and plasma either by centrifuge or automated cell separators. Blood can also be withdrawn from a donor, a portion separated out, and the remainder returned to the donor (apheresis). Using blood components rather than whole blood is a more efficient use of a scarce commodity for more recipients, prevents fluid overload, and decreases the risk of adverse effects.

The nurse administering blood or blood products carefully monitors it and follows strict institutional protocols. If a patient reports any of the symptoms associated with transfusion reaction, the nurse stops the transfusion immediately, maintains venous patency by administering normal saline, and notifies the primary care provider immediately. Patients who exhibit any sign of anaphylaxis or hemolytic reaction receive frequent vital sign monitoring and are assessed for signs of impending shock, renal failure, or DIC. The blood and tubing are returned to the laboratory for analysis, and a first-voided urine specimen is collected to analyze for signs of hemolysis. The patients hemoglobin and hematocrit levels are carefully monitored to determine the extent of the reaction. Patients who experience mild allergic reactions to blood may receive premedication with an antihistamine if they should need transfusion in the future.

Persons with any of the following are not permitted to donate blood:

- History of infectious diseases such as hepatitis, human immunodeficiency virus infection, acquired immuno-deficiency syndrome (AIDS), tuberculosis, or malaria
- Malignant diseases
- Allergies of asthma
- Polycythemia vera
- Abnormal bleeding tendencies
- Hypotension (current)
- Anemia (current)
- Recent pregency or major surgery
- Men with at least one homosexual or bisexual contact since 1975 (concern for AIDS)
- International travel to malarial areas or high-risk countries (concern for AIDS)
- Blood transfusion during past 6 months
- History of jaundice
- Disease of the heart, lung, or liver
- Immunizations or vaccinations with attenuated viral vaccine rubella or rabies vaccine
- Hemoglobin level below 13.5 g/dL for men or 12.4 g/dL for women
- Abnormalities in vital signs, particularly fever.

Treatment for hemolytic disease of the newborn involves the administration of Rh-immunoglobulin (RhoGAM) to mothers who have not been sensitized by a former pregnancy. The immunoglobulin is given by injection at about 28 weeks of pregnancy or within 72 hours after birth, amniocentesis, or interrupted pregnancy because of miscarriage or abortion. The immunoglobulin contains antibodies that destroy any of the fetus's red blood cells that have entered the mother's blood, preventing sensitization and Rh incompatibility during the next pregnancy.

Antigen-Antibody Complex Hypersensitivities

Antigen-antibody complex (type III) (also known as immune-complex) hypersensitivities are caused by the formation or deposition of antigen-antibody complexes in various tissues, which results in complement activation and inflammation. These reactions generally occur several hours after exposure to the antigen. Unlike antibody mediated (type II) responses, these reactions tend to be systemic and characterized by widespread vasculitis, arthritis, or nephritis. Systemic lupus erythematosus, post-streptococcal immune complex glomerulonephritis and serum sickness are examples of antigen-antibody hypersensitivity diseases (Fig. 5.6).

Guidelines for Safe Practice of Blood Transfusion

Patient Receiving Blood Transfusion

Carefully check all of the following:

1. Obtain baseline vital signs and check at frequent intervals throughout the procedure.
2. Administer all blood products through micron mesh filters.
3. Assess patient for any unusual sensations felt throughout the transfusion. (This information may help with early identification of any reactions).
4. Infuse blood within 4 hours after it is taken from the blood bank (to prevent bacterial growth).
5. If blood cannot be infused within 4 hours, return it to the blood bank for proper refrigeration.
6. Follow facility guidelines for proper disposal of empty blood bag and tubing.
7. Record patients response to the infusion.
8. Report any adverse effect to the primary care provider immediately.
9. Return the blood bag and tubing to the laboratory for testing if a reaction occurs.

Serum Sickness

Serum sickness develops within 1 to 3 weeks after administration of a foreign serum, such as horse or rabbit serum. It may also occur after administration of certain drugs (e.g. antimicrobials such as penicillin and sulfonamides). Classic serum sickness is rarely encountered today because large doses of foreign sera are rarely administered.

The pathogenesis of serum sickness involves the attachment of foreign serum proteins to IgM and IgG. These antigen-antibody complexes bind to complement, initiating the complement cascade and resulting in chemotaxis, vasodilation, and cell lysis. These chemotactic factors lead to an influx of phagocytes, which tend to intensify the inflammatory response.

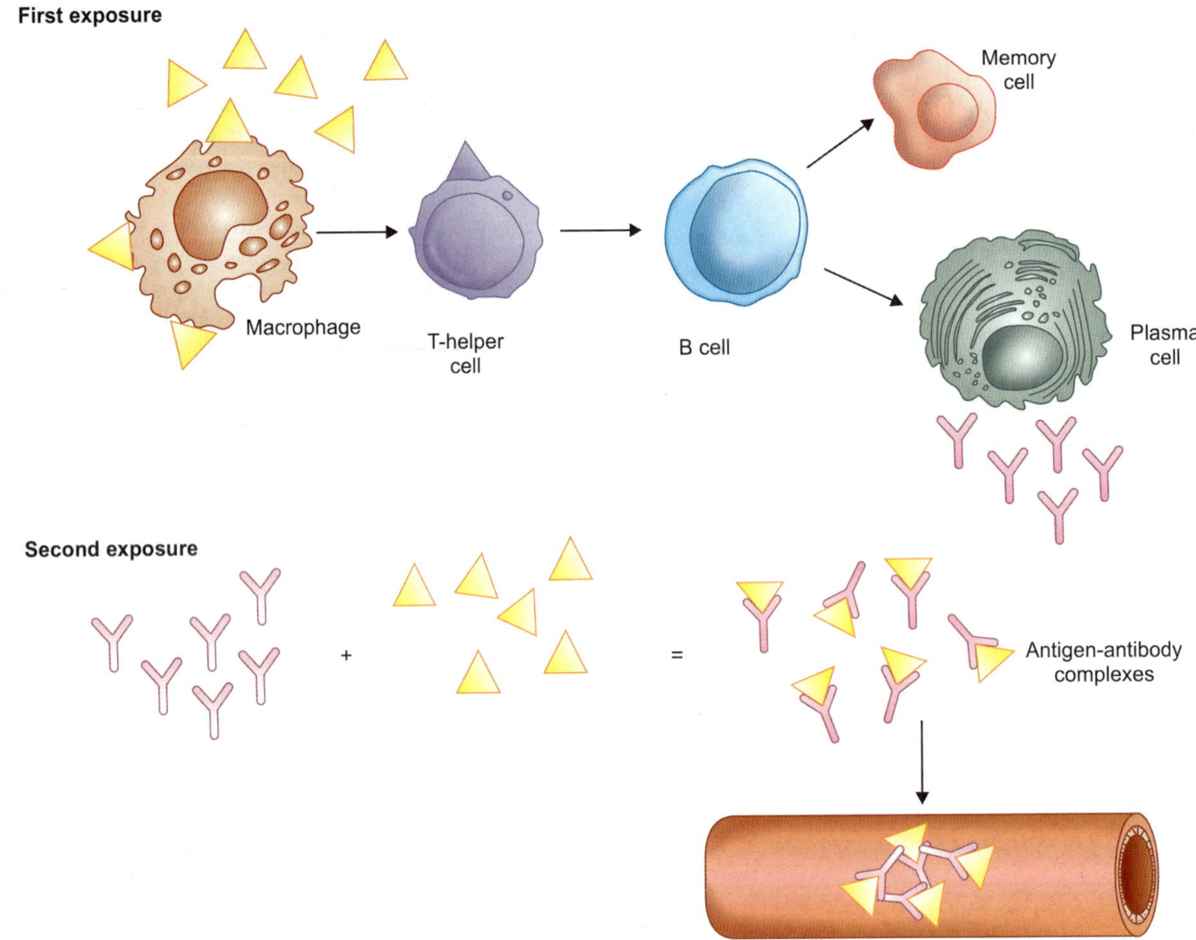

FIG. 5.6: Type III hypersensitivity

The antigen-antibody reactions of serum sickness occur in many organs, but the kidneys, choroids plexus, joints, skin and lungs are primarily affected. Itching and discomfort at the injection site are usually the first symptoms, followed by lymphadenopathy, fever, urticaria or erythematous rash, angioedema of the face, and joint pain. Splenomegaly, abdominal pain, headache, nausea, and vomiting may also occur.

Treatment of antigen-antibody hypersensitivity depends on the cause. Serum sickness is a self-limiting disease. Mild symptoms respond well to antihistamines salicylates. More sever symptoms are treated with steroids such as prednisone, and symptom relief is often achieved within hours. Epinephrine is given if an anaphylactic reaction occurs.

T cell-Mediated Hypersensitivity

T cell-mediated (type IV) hypersensitivity, also known as delayed hypersensitivity, is mediated by T cells rather than antibodies. Graft rejection, contact dermatitis, and hypersensitivity induced by chronic infection (e.g. tuberculosis) are examples of T cell-mediated hypersensitivity reactions.

T cell-mediated hypersensitivity generally occurs within 12 to 72 hours after a sensitized individual comes in contact with the offending antigen. The reaction occurring from an inactivated or purified protein derivative (PPD) tuberculin test is a classic example. People who have undergone sufficient exposure to *Mycobacterium tuberculosis* to be sensitized to the organism, whether or not they have the disease, develop redness and in duration in response to the injection within 8 to 12 hours.

Allergic contact dermatitis is an inflammatory response confined to the skin that results from repeated exposure of a sensitized person to an allergen. Environmental substances such as cosmetics, hair dyes, detergents, poison ivy or oak, or latex may serve as the offending antigen in these reactions.

Another important T-cell mediated hypersensitivity reaction occurs when organs or tissues are transferred from one person to another. Transplantations have been performed for many years, but they remain limited because of the rejection process resulting from this type of hypersensitivity.

Pathophysiology

T cell-mediated hypersensitivities do not involve antibodies such as IgE. Rather, macrophages identify the antigen as foreign, encode it, and present it to T cell lymphocytes, which become sensitized lymphocyte forms cytotoxic T cells or activates nonspecific phagocytic cells (macrophages and polymorphonuclear leukocytes) through release of lymphokines. The cytotoxic T cell lymphocytes destroy the antigen directly by breaking down the cell membrane, causing lysis and cell death (Fig. 5.7).

Allergic contact dermatitis is one of the most commonly encountered T cell-mediated hypersensitivities and type of allergic disease. Dermal contact with the antigen produces sensitization and the clinical manifestations associated with the reaction. The allergen attaches to skin proteins, which function as haptens to stimulate the proliferation of a T cell population sensitized to the allergen. After sensitization, subsequent exposure to the contact allergen leads to formation of an erythematous, vesiculated (blistered) lesion. The inflamed area is red, swollen, and warm and may itch, burn or sting. The location of the lesions often provides data but the causative allergic agent.

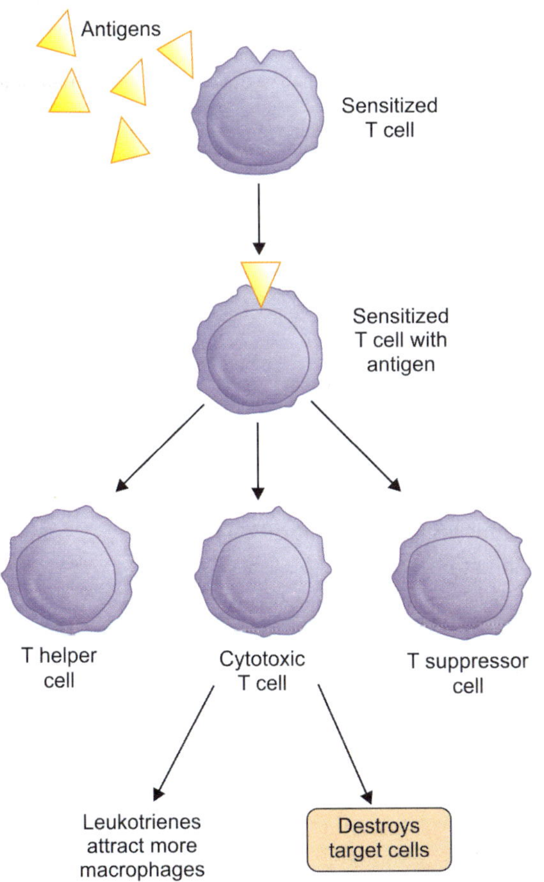

FIG. 5.7: Type IV hypersensitivity

The tubercle bacillus *(M. tuberculosis)* itself is not directly toxic to human cells or tissues. The organism invades the tissues of a nonsensitized host and establishes residence in the host tissues, causing virtually no damage. However, in time, as the organism sheds antigenic material, the T cell-mediated response is triggered. The sensitized lymphocytes and activated macrophages attack not only the organism but also the tissues surrounding the organism. This process is aimed at destroying the foreign organism, but tissue destruction may result. The lesions associated with tuberculosis (such as caseation necrosis cavitations) and general toxemia are results of the hypersensitivity. After the initial sensitization with the infectious organism, subsequent contact with the tuberculosis organism or an extract of a purified protein from the organism elicits a hypersensitivity reaction. This is the basis of the Mantoux tuberculin skin test. The skin rashes of smallpox and measles and the lesions of herpes simplex virus are all examples of microbially induced T cell hypersensitivities.

In organ transplantation the foreign tissue or organ serves as the allergen against which the cell-mediated response is directed. Cytotoxic T lymphocytes attack and destroy the tissues directly, resulting in destruction of transplanted tissues. Discussions of specific types of transplants are found in chapters dealing with the disorders for which they are used as treatment.

Management

Treatment for contact dermatitis includes elimination of known allergens, decreased exposure, or both. Topical anti-inflammatory agents such as corticosteroid creams may be useful in reducing the discomfort associated with itching and in decreasing healing time. For severe reactions, systemic corticosteroids and antihistamines may be necessary. There is no specific treatment, other than treatment of the underlying infection, for hypersensitivity reactions to infective agents. If secondary infection develops as a result of the patient scratching the area, antibodies may be prescribed. Immunosuppression therapy is used to control transplant rejection.

Stimulatory Hypersensitivity

Stimulatory hypersensitivity is a B cell-mediated response that occurs when auto-antibodies bind to target cell surface receptors and cause inappropriate stimulation of the cell, such as the thyroid gland. The usual feedback mechanism is lost; consequently the cell continuously secretes its hormone in an uncontrolled manner. Thyrotoxicosis (Grave's disease) is thought to be induced by this mechanism. It is believed that thyroid-stimulating immunoglobulin and thyrotoxicosis (Grave's disease) is thought to be induced by this mechanism. It is believed that thyroid-stimulating immunoglobulin and thyroid-stimulating hormone-binding inhibitory immunoglobulin stimulate the secretion of thyroid hormone. Signs and symptoms of hyperthyroidism are produced even though the actual condition is not present and the thyroid gland itself is completely normal.

The causes of stimulatory reactions are unknown but may be related to loss of self-tolerance. Treatment of stimulatory hypersensitivity involves removing the focus of the abnormal secretion when only one organ is involved, such as the thyroid gland. If multiple tissues are involved, immunosuppression is used in an attempt to suppress the production of autoantibodies, halt over secretion of the hormone, and prevent associated symptoms.

(4) AUTOIMMUNITY

The cause of autoimmunity, or the loss of self-tolerance, is not clearly understood. Autoimmune diseases occur more frequently in women, especially during the childbearing years, than in men. Some autoimmune diseases affect certain populations more than others. For example, rheumatoid arthritis and scleroderma are more common among Native Americans than in the general population. Lupus erythematosus affects African-American and Hispanic women more than Caucasian women.

Pathophysiology: Autoimmunity refers to the formation of antibodies against self-cells. The principal factors in the development of autoimmunity are genetic predisposition, environment, and viral infections. Antibodies produced against one's own cells are referred to as *autoantibodies*. When produced against deoxyribonucleic acid (DNA), they are called anti-DNA antibodies. These self-reactive immunoglobulins are often associated with pathologic states in the body; however, they can also be isolated from the serum of disease-free individuals and are present in about half of adults over the age of 70 years.

Several theories exist about the mechanism of autoimmunity:

- *Release of sequestered antigens:* If an antigen does not come into contact with the immune system during fetal development when self-tolerance normally develops, the antigen remains antigenic. Later, as a result of trauma or infection, the antigen may be exposed to the immune system, eliciting an autoimmune response (e.g. autoantibodies against heart muscle after acute myocardial infarction).
- *Defective suppressor T cells:* Suppressor T cell function may be lost or altered so that autoantibodies are allowed to proliferate without control.
- *Synthesis of cross reactive antibodies:* Antibodies synthesized in response to certain foreign antigens may have cross-reactivity with similar antigenic components within human tissues.
- *Alteration of self-antigens:* Normal body proteins may be altered by chemicals, infectious organisms, or therapeutic drugs and present new antigenically active groups to the immune system. Autoimmune hemolytic anemia may result from alteration of the Rh antigens of the red blood cells, rendering it antigenic. Certain antibodies can have a similar effect.

Autoimmune disorders are grouped into categories according to the body part or tissues involved. *Organ-specific* diseases produce chronic inflammatory changes in a specific organ, such as the kidney or heart. *Nonorgan-specific* autoimmune disorders are characterized by chronic inflammatory changes in many different organs and tissues throughout the body.

Classifications of autoimmune disorders

Organ specific

Blood

- Autoimmune hemolytic anemia
- Idiopathic thrombocytopenic purpura

Heart

- Rheumatic fever

Central nervous system

- Multiple sclerosis
- Guillain-Barre' syndrome

Muscles

- Myasthenia gravis

Endocrine System

- Addison's disease
- Autoimmune thyroiditis (Hashimoto's disease)
- Graves disease
- Hypothyroidism

Eye

- Uveitis

Gastrointestinal system

- Pernicious anemia
- Ulcerative colitis

Kidneys

- Glomerulonephritis
- Goodpasture's syndrome

Skin

- Pemphigus vulgaris

Nonorganspecific

- Systemic lupus erythematosus
- Rheumatoid arthritis
- Progressive systemic sclerosis

Treatment for autoimmune disorders consists of immunosuppression and control of clinical manifestations, primarily through systemic corticosteroid therapy. Initial doses of 60 mg of oral prednisone often bring about a noticeable decrease in symptoms. Once symptoms are controlled, dosages are slowly decreased and then discontinued until the next exacerbation. Cytotoxic drugs such as cyclophosphamide, azathioprine, and methotrexate are sometimes prescribed for patients with severe or persistent manifestations. Treatment of specific autoimmune disorders is discussed elsewhere in this textbook.

Patients with autoimmune disorders are encouraged to eat well-balanced diets, maintain daily exercise patterns without becoming excessively fatigued, and get adequate rest and sleep. The nurse explains the anticipated benefit of prescribed medications, dosage schedules, and adverse effects, especially when patient are taking corticosteroids or other immunosuppressive drugs. The nurse cautions patients against abruptly withdrawing steroid medications, since abrupt cessation can result in adrenal insufficiency or crisis. Close follow-up care is emphasized for all patients taking immunosuppressive agents.

Chronic Fatigue Syndrome

Chronic fatigue syndrome (CFS) is a condition of unexplained fatigue that lasts 6 months or longer and eventually leads to disability. CFS may follow a cold, influenza, bronchitis, or mononucleosis. In other instances CFS develops gradually, with no clear initiating event. Accompanying manifestations, such as muscle and joint discomfort, headache, loss of concentration, weakness and tender lymph nodes, may go unnoticed because they are similar to the flu. Unlike the flu, however, the fatigue and other symptoms remain or reappear frequently. CFS is now recognized in people of all ages, races, and socioeconomic groups. The primary clinical manifestations of CFS is prolonged, debilitrating fatigue accompanied by any or all of the symptoms listed below.

1. Clinically evaluated, unexplained, persistent or relapsing chronic fatigue that is of new or definite onset (i.e. not lifelong), is not the result of ongoing exertion, is not substantially alleviated by rest, and results in substantial reduction in previous levels of occupational, educational, social, or personal activities.
2. The concurrent occurrence of four or more of the following symptoms:
   - Substantial impairment in short-term memory or concentration
   - Sore throat
   - Tender lymph nodes
   - Muscle pain
   - Multijoint pain without swelling or redness
   - Headaches of a new type, pattern, or severity
   - Unrefreshing sleep
   - Postexertional malaise lasting more than 24 hours

These symptoms must have persisted or recurred during 6 or more consecutive months of illness and must not have predated the fatigue.

Conditions that Exclude a Diagnosis of Chronic Fatigue Syndrome

1. Any active medical condition that may explain the presence of chronic fatigue, such as untreated hypothyroidism, sleep apnea and narcolepsy, and iatrogenic conditions such as side effects of medication.
2. Some diagnosable illnesses that may relapse or may not have completely resolved during treatment. If the persistence of such a condition could explain the presence of chronic fatigue, and if it cannot be clearly established that the original condition has completely resolved with treatment, the such patients should not be classified as having chronic fatigue syndrome. Examples of illnesses that can present such a picture include some types of malignancies and chronic cases of hepatitis B or C virus infection.
3. Any past or current diagnosis of a major depressive disorder with psychotic or melancholic features; bipolar affective disorders; schizophrenia of any subtype; delusional disorders of any subtype; dementias of any subtype; anorexia nervosa; or bulimia nervosa.
4. Alcohol or other substance abuse, occurring within 2 years of the onset of chronic fatigue and any time afterward.
5. Severe obesity as defined by a body mass index [body mass index = weight (kg)/height (m)^2] equal to or greater than 45. (*Note:* Body mass index values vary considerably among different age groups and populations. No "normal" or "average" range of values is meaningful. The range of 45 or greater was selected because it clearly falls within the range of severe obesity.)

The exact cause of CFS remains unknown. Conditions that may trigger its development are genetic and environmental factors, viral infection, transient traumatic conditions, toxins, or stress. The clinical course of CFS varies considerably among patients, and it is difficult to diagnose because the same symptoms occur with many other conditions and diseases. CFS often follows a cyclic course, alternating between illness and relatively symptom-free intervals, which is similar to that of autoimmune disorders such as lupus erythematosus or multiple sclerosis. About 50% of patients recover within the first 5 years after onset. No characteristics of the disease or persons with the disease have been identified to show that one person is more likely to recover than another.

Management

Treatments for CFS have included antiviral agents, antidepressants, and immune modulators, but none have proven effective. Consequently, treatments are aimed at controlling symptoms and helping patients return to a normal or near-normal lifestyle. Non-steroidal anti-inflammatory drugs may be beneficial in reducing body aches or fever, and nonsedating antihistamines have been useful for relieving allergy symptoms. No cure for this disease exists at this time.

Patient care focuses on self-management of fatigue to improve function and quality of life. The nurse helps the patient identify potential triggers to fatigue and encourages them to avoid situation or activities adversely affect their energy levels. Periods of activity are scheduled at times when patients feel better and are alternated with rest periods. Exercise may seem contradictory in the presence of fatigue, but exercise improves conditioning and can restore energy. Patients are assisted with developing individualized exercise programs that incorporate a gradual increase in exercise intensity and duration. Exercise beds to be incorporated in a manner that does not exacerbate fatigue, yet promotes regular participations.

A well-balanced diet is essential to promote adequate energy stores. Nighttime sleep should be as free of interruption as possible, and daytime naps are avoided if they interfere with night-time sleep. The patient may also benefit from relaxation, meditation, massage, imagery, therapeutic touch, music, or biofeedback.

Chronic fatigue syndrome is disease with overwhelming subjective symptoms, and health care providers commonly treat patients experiencing persistent debilitating fatigue with over skepticism, if not direct accusations of malingering. Symptoms of CFS may be attributed to life stress, unhappiness, female hormone imbalances, or simply psychosomaticism. The nurse plays an important role in reassuring the patient about the validity and severity of the symptoms. Family members should be included in discussions and teaching sessions about disease etiology and management. Family support is critical to the patient because many occupational and family roles may have to be reduced or eliminated in the face of overwhelming fatigue. Patient and families may be encouraged to contact local or national CFS support groups to establish networks of information and support for dealing with this debilitating chronic disease.

HUMAN IMMUNODEFICIENCY VIRUS INFECTION (HIV)

Human immunodeficiency virus (HIV) infection is an acquired infection in which the HIV integrates itself into CD4 (helper T4) cells, causing severe immune dysfunction. HIV infection renders the person unusually susceptible to other life-threatening infections and malignancies. In its most serious form, HIV results in acquired immunodeficiency syndrome (AIDS).

Etiology

The origin of HIV is still largely unknown. Evidence suggests an African origin, since an AIDS-like illness in Central Africa has been known to exist the early 1960s. Some researches hypothesize that the most likely source of human infection was from nonhuman primates. The causative agent of HIV infection is HIV, a **retrovirus** belonging to the *Lentivirus* subfamily (Fig. 5.8). Several human retroviruses have been identified. Two of them, HIV-1 and HIV-2 are associated with depletion of helper T4 cells and subsequent loss of cellular immunity.

HIV is a blood borne, sexually transmitted disease (STD). The routes of viral transmission are well documented: (1) direct transmission from person to person by sexual contact, (2) direct inoculation with contaminated blood products, needles, or syringe, and (3) infection from mother to her fetus or newborn.

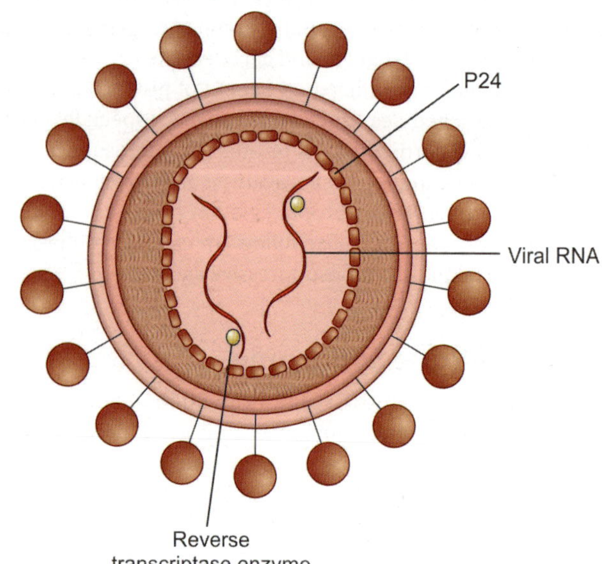

FIG. 5.8: HIV is surrounded by an envelope made up of proteins (including gp 120) and contains a core of viral RNA and proteins

Sexual practices, including vaginal or anal penetration without a condom and oral sexual practices, are associated with a high risk for infection. The use of contaminated needles for subcutaneous, intramuscular, or IV injection is another source of infection. Women who are HIV infected may pass the virus onto their newborns via three potential routes: gestation, delivery, and rarely, breast milk.

Blood, semen and vaginal secretions are primary sources for infection, and epidemiologic studies indicate that transmission via saliva, tears, and breast milk is sufficient and unlikely to produce infection. HIV is not transmitted by casual contact, including sneezing; coughing; spitting; hand shaking; and contacting potential secretions in toilet seats, bathtubs, showers, swimming pools, utensils, dishes, or linens used by infected persons. HIV is not transmitted by biting or blood-sucking insects.

Blood transfusions are not a significant source of HIV infection today. In each unit of donated blood is tested of HIV infection, as well as several other blood borne infections, such as hepatitis B. HIV screening of blood products has been conducted since 1985, only recipients of transfusions before that time were at significant risk for infection via the blood supply. It is possible for a contaminated unit of blood to test negative for HIV if the donor has not yet formed antibodies to the virus at the time of donation. As a result, the risk of exposure to HIV via blood supply is estimated to be 1 in 1.4 to 1.8 million units of blood. Since 1985, seven cases have been reported of organ transplant recipients contracting HIV. In all cases, problems prevented the identification of the donor's HIV status before harvesting of organs.

The risk for HIV transmission to health care workers prompted the CDC to implement Universal Precautions. Those precautions, now known as Standard Precautions, apply to all patients regardless of their medical diagnosis. The Standard Precaution protocol acknowledges that recognized and unrecognized microorganisms can exist in any body fluid, and the use of appropriate precautions reduces the risk for transmission within the hospital environment.

Risk Factors of HIV

- Sexual practices
  - Unprotected sex
  - Multiple sexual partners
  - Anal or oral sexual activity
  - Improper condom use or condom breakage
  - Open sores, lesions, or irritation in the genital area
- Contaminated blood
- Contaminated needles
- Occupational exposure
  - All health care workers—acute care, long-term care and home care
  - Dental workers
  - Corrections officers and law enforcement personnel
- Perinatal exposure (during pregnancy, birth, or breast-feeding).

HIV is transmitted through bodily fluids by high-risk behaviors such as heterosexual intercourse with an HIV-infected partner, injection drug use, and male homosexual relations. Also at risk are people who received transfusions of blood or blood products contaminated with HIV, children born to mothers with HIV infection, breastfed infants of HIV-infected mothers, and health care workers exposed to needle-stick injury associated with an infected patient.

Transmission of HIV

HIV is a fragile virus. It can only be transmitted under specific conditions that allow contact with infected body fluids, including blood, semen, vaginal secretions, and breast milk. Transmission of HIV occurs through sexual intercourse with an infected partner, exposure to HIV infected blood or blood produces, and perinatal transmission during pregnancy, at the time of delivery, or through breastfeeding.

HIV infected individuals can transmit HIV to others within a few days after becoming infected. After that, the ability to transmit HIV is lifelong. Transmission of HIV is subject to the same requirements as other microorganisms (i.e. a large enough amount of the virus must enter the body of a susceptible host). Duration and frequency of contact, volume of fluid, virulence and concentration of the organism, and host immune status all affect whether infection is established after an exposure. The viral load (or the number of viruses) in the blood, semen, vaginal secretions, or breast milk of the "donor" is an important variable. Large amounts of HIV can be found in the blood during the first 6 months of infection and again during the late stages of the diseases. Unprotected sexual or blood exposure to an infected individual is more risky during these periods, although HIV can be transmitted during all phases of the disease.

HIV is not spread casually. The virus cannot be transmitted through hugging, dry kissing, shaking hands, sharing eating utensils, using toilet seats, or attending school or working with an HIV infected person. It is not transmitted through tears, saliva, urine, emesis, sputum, feces, or sweat. Repeated studies have failed to demonstrate transmission of the virus by respiratory droplets, enteric routes, or casual encounters in any setting. Health care workers have a very low risk of acquiring HIV at work, even after a needle-stick injury.

Sexual Transmission

Unprotected sexual contact with an HIV-infected partner is the most common mode of transmission. Sexual activity provides an opportunity for contact with semen, vaginal secretions, and/or blood, all of which have lymphocytes that may contain HIV.

Although men who have sex with men (MSM) still account for most cases of HIV in the United States and Canada, heterosexual transmission has become more prevalent and is now the most common method of infection for women. The riskiest sexual activity is unprotected anal intercourse. During any form of sexual intercourse (anal, vaginal, or oral), the risk of infection is greater for the partner who receives the semen, although infection can also be transmitted to an inserting partner. This occurs because the receiver has prolonged contact with infected fluids, and helps explain why women are more easily infected than men during heterosexual intercourse. Sexual activities that involve blood, such as during menstruation or as a result of trauma to local tissues, also increase the risk of transmission. In addition, the presence of genital lesions caused by other sexually transmitted disease (e.g. herpes, syphilis) significantly increases the likelihood of infection.

Contact with Blood and Blood Products

HIV can be transmitted during exposure to blood through drug-using equipment. Used equipment may be contaminated with HIV and other blood-borne organisms, and sharing that equipment can result in disease transmission.

It has been reported that transfusion of infected blood and blood products has caused only 1% of adult AIDS cases. In 1985, routine screening of blood donors to identify at-risk individuals and testing donated blood for the presence of HIV were implemented, thereby improving the safety of the blood supply. HIV infection as a result of blood transfusions is now unlikely, but still possible because blood donated during the first few months of infection may not test positive for HIV antibodies.

Clotting factors used by people with hemophilia are now treated with heat or chemicals that kill HIV and other blood-borne viruses, thus eliminating that risk.

Puncture wounds are the most common means of work-related transmission. The risk of infection after a needle-stick exposure to HIV-infected blood is 0.3 to 0.4% (or 3 to 4 out of 1000). The risk is higher if the exposure involves blood from a patient with a high viral load, a deep puncture wound, a needle with a hollow bore and visible blood, a device used for venous or arterial access, or a patient who dies within 60 days. Splash exposures of blood on skin with an open lesion present some risk, but it is much lower than from a puncture wound.

Perinatal Transmission

Perinatal transmission is the most common route of infection for children. Transmission from an HIV-infected mother to her infant can occur during pregnancy, at the time of delivery, or after birth through breastfeeding. On average, 25% of infants born to untreated HIV-infected women will be born with HIV. This means that 75% of these infants would not have been infected even without treatment.

Pathophysiology

The **human immunodeficiency virus (HIV)**, a ribonucleic acid (RNA) virus, was discovered in 1983. RNA viruses are called **retroviruses** because they replicate in a "backward" manner (going from RNA to deoxyribonucleic acid [DNA]). Like all viruses, HIV cannot replicate unless it is inside a living cell. The life cycle of HIV is given in Figure 5.9.

The natural history of HIV infection is associated with an unpredictable course of disease progression. Patients may undergo a prolonged period of clinically silent infection, often lasting more than 10 years, during which the virus remains dormant. Although the virus is consistently detected throughout this time, patients may exhibit only subtle immunologic alterations. Once viral replication begins, which can occur rapidly, **CD4 lymphocytes** are destroyed and the patient becomes symptomatic.

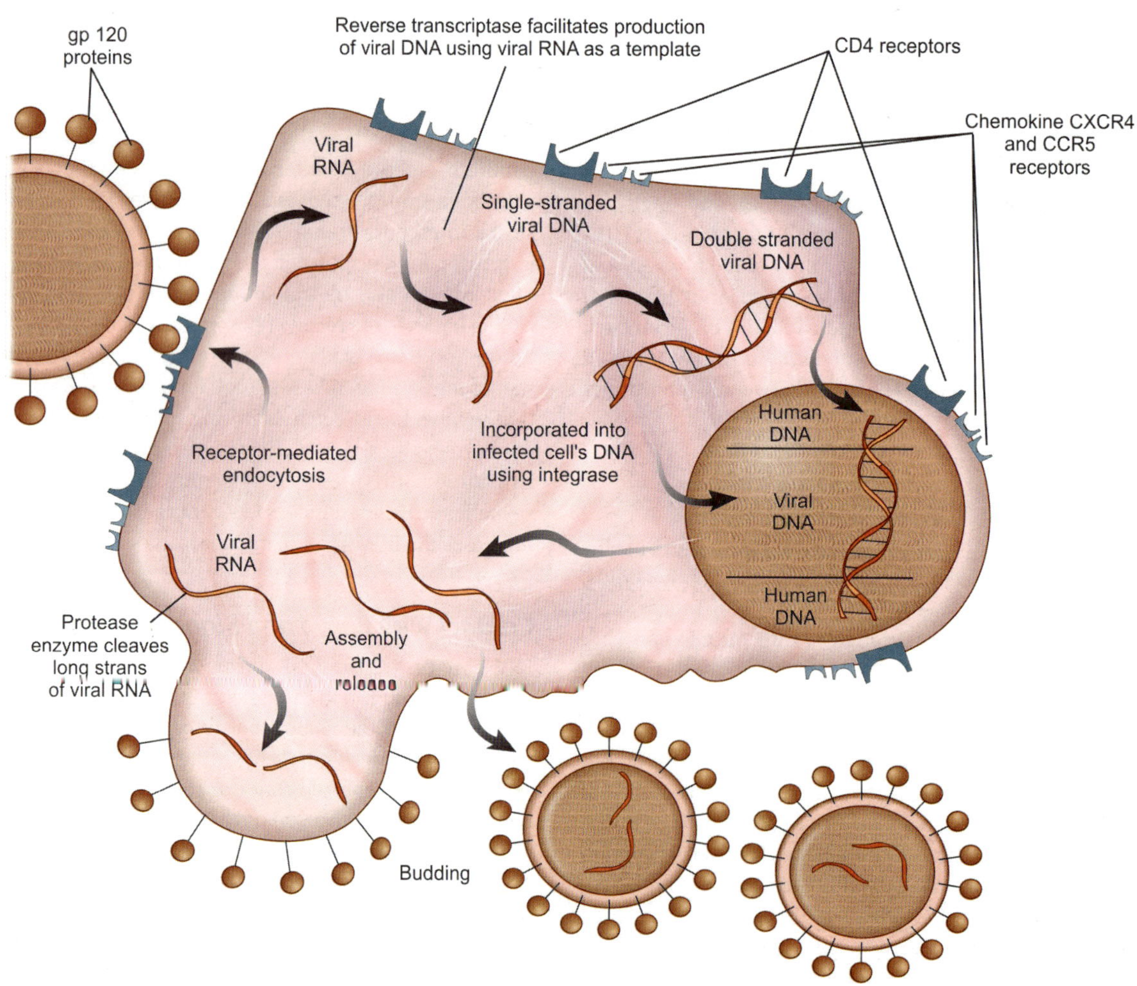

FIG. 5.9: Life cycle of HIV

The life cycle of HIV is similar to that of the other retroviruses. HIV interacts with a CD4 glycoprotein found on the membrane of CD4 lymphocytes. CD4 refers to the particular protein expressed on the surface of the helper T4 lymphocyte. The CD4 glycoprotein is also found on the surface of several other cells, including some monocytes, macrophages, glial cells, and gastrointestinal (GI) cells. Presence of the CD4 glycoprotein allows the virus to fuse to the host cell. Once fused, the virus is infected into the cell cytoplasm, where it sheds its two outer coats, releasing two ribonucleic acid (RNA) copies, which are subsequently transcribed into proviral deoxyribonucleic acids (DNA). The proviral DNA is then integrated into the CD4 cell by the retroviral enzyme reverse transcriptase (Fig. 5.10).

HIV has gp 120 glycoprotiens that attach to CD4 and chemokine CXCR4 and CCR5 receptors on the surface of Cd4 T cells. Viral RNA then enters the cell, produces viral DNA in the presence of reverse transcriptase, and incorporates itself into the cellular genome in the presence of integrase, causing permanent cellular infection and the production of new virions. New viral RNA develops initially in long strands that are cut in the presence of protease and leave the cell through a budding process that ultimately contributes to cellular destruction.

The virus may remain dormant in the CD4 cells, or replicate by using the host cell's genetic machinery to assemble and release new viral particles. Viral replication eventually depletes the host's CD4 cells, resulting in a dramatic loss of immune protection. Infections that were once disarmed by the healthy immune system, are eventually able to cause serious and potentially life-threatening disease. HIV escapes the host's immune system may be thought that viral entry into host cells occurs before the host's virus-specific immune response is initiated. Once HIV gains entry into T cells, the virus reshapes the host's immune system, impairing antigen-processing function, humoral neutralizing response, the production of new CD4 cells, and HIV-specific CD8 cells.

Several potential cofactors, which may be viral, host, or environmental, are thought to directly influence the replication of HIV or the severity of its pathogenic effects. Viral cofactors may include herpes simplex virus, cytomegalovirus (CMV), and Epstein-Barr virus. Host cofactors may include a variety of cytokines and intracellular mediators. Environmental cofactors may include repeated exposure to HIV, which may induce hyper activation of the immune system, resulting in an expansion of the pool of HIV-replicating cells.

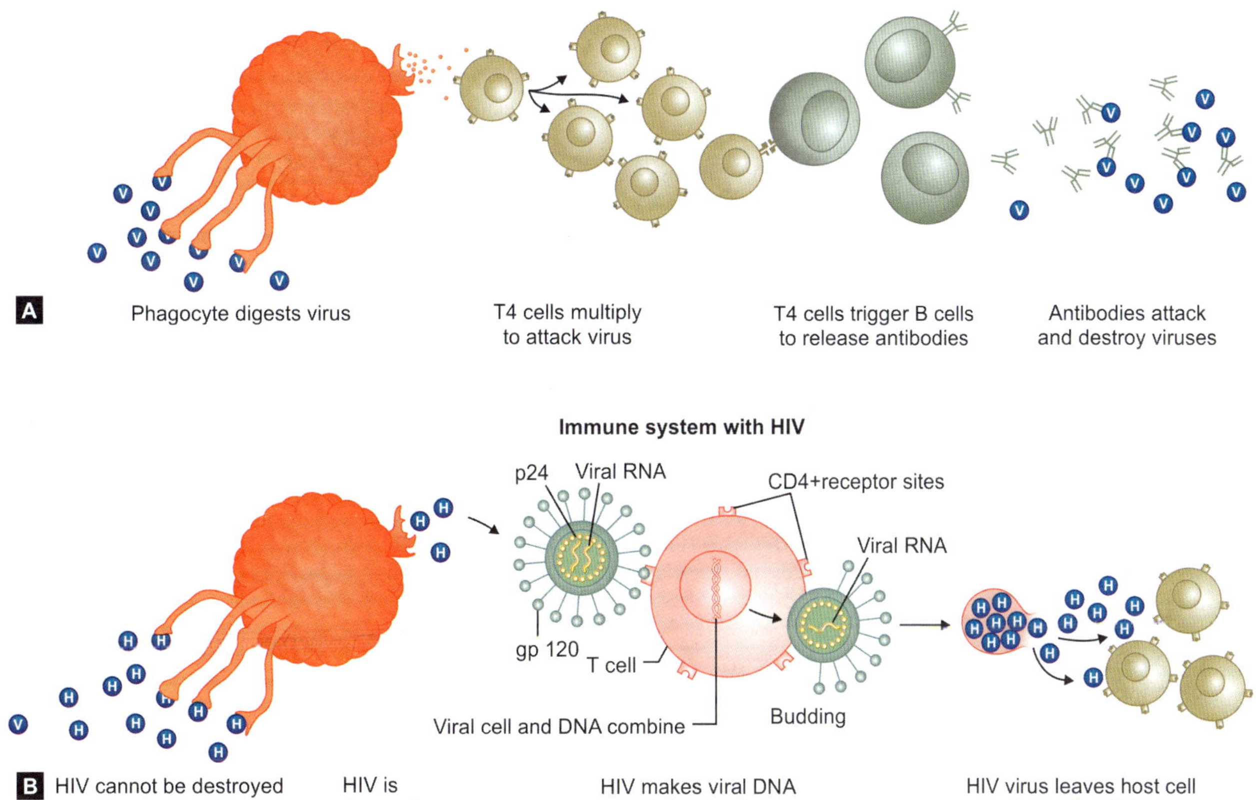

FIGS 5.10A AND B: (A) Normal immune system; (B) HIV contains several proteins: gp 120 protein around it and viral RNA and p24 protein inside. The gp 120 protiens attach to CD4+ receptors to T lymphocytes; HIV enters the cell and makes viral DNA; the enslaved host cell produces new viruses that bud, which destroys the host cell's membrane, causing cellular death and allowing the virus to leave the attack other CD4+ T-lymphocyte cells

The spectrum of HIV infection ranges from asymptomatic primary infection to overt AIDS, which is characterized by potentially life-threatening opportunistic infections. Early in the AIDS epidemic, it was believed that HIV infection could be divided into four separate processes: acute HIV infection, latent infection, AIDS-related complex, and AIDS. It is now known that the infection is one continuous disease process with three stages: primary HIV infection, chronic asymptomatic disease, and AIDS. The CDC uses a case definition for AIDS surveillance and reporting, which has evolved over time and incorporates both laboratory and clinical stages. However, it is more useful to discuss the disease in terms of staging.

Primary HIV-1 infection: Symptoms of primary HIV infection generally occur within 2 to 4 weeks after HIV exposure and last between 2 and 10 weeks. Symptoms are similar to the flu or mononucleosis, consisting of fever, sore throat, fatigue, nausea, vomiting, headache, rash or lymphadenopathy. Most of these manifestation go away without intervention; however, the lymphadenopathy usually persists throughout the course of the disease. During this time there is a corresponding rapid rise in serum HIV RNA copies, which may reach 1 million copies/mL or more; a decrease in CD4 cell numbers; and a large increase in CD8 cell numbers. The decline in viral copies coincides with the resolution of clinical manifestations. Antibodies to HIV-1 are usually negative during the primary HIV-1 phase of infection.

Clinical Manifestations

Symptoms are widespread and may affect any organ system. Manifestations range from mild abnormalities in immune response without overt signs and symptoms to profound immunosuppression, life-threatening infection, malignancy, and the direct effect of HIV on body tissues.

Respiratory

- Shortness of breath, dyspnea, cough, chest pain, and fever are associated with opportunistic infections, including *Pneumocystis jiroveci* pneumonia (PCP), the most common infection, and the immune reconstitution syndromes, such as *Mycobacterium avium complex* (MAC)/*Mycobacterium avium intracellulare* (MAI), which is a leading bacterial infection in AIDS patients. Legionella and CMV are other opportunistic organisms
- HIV-associated tuberculosis occurs early in the course of HIV infection, often preceding a diagnosis of AIDS.

Gastrointestinal

- Loss of appetite
- Nausea and vomiting
- Oral and esophageal candidiasis (white patches, painful swallowing, retrosternal pain, and possibly oral lesions)
- Chronic diarrhea, possible with devastating effects (e.g. weight loss, fluid and electrolyte imbalances, perianal skin excoriation, weakness and inability to perform activities of daily living).

Wasting Syndrome (Cachexia)

- Multifactorial protein-energy malnutrition
- Profound involuntary weight loss exceeding 10% of baseline body weight
- Chronic diarrhea, chronic weakness and documented intermittent of constant fever with no concurrent illness
- Anorexia, diarrhea, gastrointestinal malabsorption, lack of nutrition, and for some patients a hypermetabolic state.

Neurologic

Neurologic complications involve central, peripheral and autonomic functions.

- HIV encephalopathy (AIDS dementia complex [ADC]) occurs in two thirds of patients with AIDS. Symptoms include memory deficits, headache, lack of concentration, progressive confusion, psychomotor slowing, apathy and ataxia, and in later stages global cognitive impairments, delayed verbal responses, spastic paraparesis, hyperreflexia, psychosis, seizures, incontinence, mutism, and death
- HIV-related peripheral neuropathy is thought to be a demyelinating disorder; it is associated with pain and numbness in the extremities, weakness, diminished deep tendon reflexes, orthostatic hypotension, and impotence.
- *Cryptococcus neoformans*, a fungal infection (fever, stiff neck, nausea and vomiting seizures)
- Central and peripheral neuropathies, including vascular myelopathy (spastic paraparesis, ataxia, and incontinence)
- Progressive multifocal leukoencephalopathy (PML), a central nervous system demyelinating disorder, can occur
- Other neurologic disorders include *Toxoplasma gondii,* CMV, and *Mycobacterium tuberculosis* infection, with symptoms ranging from confusion to blindness, aphasia, paresis, and death.

Integumentary

- Kaposi's sarcoma (KS), herpes simplex and herpes zoster viruses, and various forms of dermatitis associated with painful vesicles
- Folliculitis, associated with dry flaking skin or atopic dermatitis (eczema or psoriasis).

Reproductive (Female)

- Persistent recurrent vaginal candidiasis may be the first sign of HIV infectioin

- Ulcerative sexually transmitted diseases, such as chancroid, syphilis, and herpes, are more severe in women with HIV
- Venereal warts and cervical cancer/cervical intraepithelial neoplasia (CIN) may be noted
- Women with HIV have a higher incidence of pelvic inflammatory disease (PID) and menstrual abnormalities (amenorrhea or bleeding between periods).

Hematologic/Lymphatic

B-cell lymphomas, such as non-Hodgkin's lymphoma, are the second most common AIDS-related cancer (the first is KS). These lymphomas usually differ from those in the general population because they develop outside the lymph nodes (mostly in the brain, bone marrow, and GI tract), grow aggressively, affect multiple organs, and exhibit resistance to treatment, which may be complicated by severe hemotologic toxicity.

Other: Chronic Illness and Cancers

Early diagnosis and treatment of opportunistic diseases and antiviral therapy have brough HIV infection into the chronic illness category. Additional clinical manifestations follow:

- Fatigue, headanche, profuse night sweats, unexplained weight loss, dry cough, shortness of breath, extreme weakness, diarrhea, decreased endurance, edema, blindness swallowing difficulties, and possible neurologic involvement resulting in dementia, hemiplegia, spastic paraparesis, painful neuropatheis, proximal and distal muscle weakness, and presistent lymphadenopathy
- Higher than usual incidence of cancer, including KS, B-cell lymphomas, and carcinomas of cervix, skin stomach, pancreas, rectum, and bladder
- Depressive symptoms from multiple causes, including preexisting mental illness, neuropsychiatric disturbances, and psychosocial factors
- Irrational guilt, shame, loss of self-esteem, helplessness, worthlessness, and suicidal ideation.

Chronic Asymptomatic Infection

The initial phase of infection may be followed by a period of latency that can last from several months to 10 years or more. During this time the person may be completely **asymptomatic** or experience only mild symptoms such as fatigue, headache, or lymphadenopathy. Over time, however, active viral replication begins. As viral load increases, CD4 cell counts gradually decline. The actual rate of decline varies among individuals and can be altered by antiretroviral therapy. Generally, by 12 weeks after infection, anti- HIV antibodies have been produced and can be detected by immunoassay even when the patient is asymptomatic. An overviw of HIV/AIDS are given in Box 5.5.

Box 5.5 Overview of HIV/AIDS

Signs and symptoms	• Initially vary; none or acute retroviral syndrome • Asymptomatic phase • Immune system impairment: Dyspnea, fever, weight loss, fatigue, night sweats, persistent diarrhea, oral or vaginal candidiasis ulcers, dry skin, skin lesions, peripheral neuropathy, shingles, or dementia
Diagnostic test	• HIV antibody tests • Complete blood cell count/lymphocyte count • CD4 +/CD8 + T-lymphocyte count • Viral load testing • Genotyping
Therapeutic measures	• Non-nucleoside reverse transcriptase inhibitors (NRTIs) • Nucleoside/nucleotide reverse transcriptase inhibitors (NNRTs) • Protease inhibitors (PIs) • Fusion inhibitors • Integrase inhibitors
Complications	• AIDS wasting syndrome • Opportunistic infections and cancer • AIDS dementia complex

AIDS

As viral replication continues and more CD4 cells are destroyed, the immune system becomes further compromised. Clinical manifestations associated with AIDS are primarily those of opportunistic infections, which are discussed later in this chapter. The clinical manifestations box summarizes other manifestations. AIDS is the end stage of HIV infection. Without treatment death occurs within 3 to 5 years. Acquired immunodeficiency syndrome (AIDS) is defined as the most severe form of a continuum of illnesses associated with human immunodeficiency virus (HIV) infection. HIV belongs to a group of viruses known as retroviruses. These viruses carry their genetic material in the form of ribonucleic acid (RNA) rather than deoxyribonucleic acid (DNA). Infection with HIV occurs when it enters the host CD4 (T) cell and causes this cell to replicate viral RNA and viral proteins, which in turn invade other CD4 cells.

The stage of HIV disease is based on clinical history, physical examination, laboratory evidence of immune dysfunction, signs and symptoms, and infections and malignancies. The stage of primary infection is acute and spans the time from infection to antibody development. Four categories of infected states have been denoted:

- Primary infection (part of CDC Category A: Dramatic drop in CD4 T-cell counts from normal level between 500 and 1500 cells/mm^3)
- HIV asymptomatic (CDC Category A: More than 500 CD4+ T lymphocytes/mm^3)

- HIV symptomatic (CDC Category B: 200–499 CD4+ T lymphocytes/mm^3)
- AIDS (CDC Category C: Fewer than 200 CD4+ T lymphocytes/mm^3).

Clinical Manifestations of HIV/AIDS

- Chills and fever
- Night sweats
- Dry, productive cough
- Dyspnea
- Lethargy
- Confusion
- Stiff neck
- Seizures
- Headache
- Malaise
- Fatigue
- Oral lesions
- Skin rash
- Abdominal discomfort
- Diarrhea
- Weight loss
- Lymphadenopathy
- Progressive generalized edema.

Complications: AIDS and its associated opportunistic infections can affect every organ and body system. *Opportunistic* infectious are those pathogens that take advantage of decreased immunity to produce disease. Pulmonary infection from a variety of organism is a constant threat and is often the first manifestation of AIDS. Such infections can rapidly lead to severe hypoxemia. Numerous GI problems are associated with opportunistic infections or antiretroviral therapy. Other common problems include granulomatous hepatitis, drug toxicity hepatitis, or coinfection with a hepatitis virus; masses or lesions from lymphomas and Kaposi's sarcoma; cholangitis eating or swallowing or may experience dyspepsia, diarrhea, and weight loss. Loss of lean muscle mass is common.

HIV crosses the blood HIV-brain and blood-cerebrospinal fluid (CSF) barriers and infects microglia and possibly other cells, resulting in encephalopathy. This process results in loss of cognitive and motor function. Many of the opportunistic infections also can affect the central nervous system. Peripheral neuropathy with loss of motor function often occurs. The eyes are vulnerable to CMV, which can result in blurred vision and decreased acuity. The lesions are progressive and may lead to total blindness unless early and aggressive treatment is instituted.

Thrombocytopenia, anemia, and neutropenia may be present with AIDS. The causes of these problems are not precisely known, but it is thought that HIV decreases red blood cell production. Drug side effects also affect the hematologic system and can cause impaired production and increased destruction of red blood cells.

Opportunistic infections can affect the heart by producing pericarditis or myocarditis. Severe pulmonary hypertension associated with multiple episodes of *Pneumocystis carinii* pneumonia can cause right ventricular failure.

Although not as common as other system dysfunctions, all endocrine glands can be infiltrated with HIV. The adrenal gland is most commonly affected. Adrenal insufficiency may result from invasion by infective organism, tumor growth, or drug therapy.

Musculoskeletal manifestations of HIV are common and may be mild or severe. Arthralgia is seen with acute infection and may also result from drug therapy. Myalgia, weakness, and wasting may also occur secondary to decreased appetite.

Fluid and electrolyte and acid-base imbalances occur from a variety of causes, including renal, GI, or endocrine changes or drug therapy. Renal dysfunction may occur from acute kidney failure secondary to hypovolemia, interstitial nephritis caused by invasion of renal tissue by tumors or infective organisms, or glomerulosclerosis from HIV-associated nephropathy. Specific opportunistic infections are discussed later in the chapter (Table 5.6).

Management of HIV

Diagnostic Tests of HIV AIDS includes the following:

Antibody Assays

Antibody assays measure the immune system's response from exposure to a specific antigen. When an antigen enters the host, the immune system recognizes the antigen and produces specific antibodies against it. Antibody assay tests depend on antibody formation, but a patient's serum may not have detectable levels of antibody during the initial stage of infection. Approximately 90% of the population forms antibodies in response to HIV and the production of detectable antibodies is known as the "window period". Newborns maintain maternal antibodies for as long as 18 months; therefore antibody testing is unreliable until the infant is 18 months of age.

Enzyme-linked Immunosorbent Assay (ELISA)

The ELISA is a highly specific test that is close to 99.6% sensitive for HIV-1 antibodies. If the patients serum is reactive, the patient is considered seropositive for HIV antibodies. False-positive tests are possible and may occur from recent influenza or hepatitis B vaccines; in multiparous women; after multiple blood transfusion; or with multiple myeloma, alcoholic hepatitis, or biliary cirrhosis.

TABLE 5.6: Manifestations and treatment of common opportunities diseases associated with HIV infection.

Organism/disease	Clinical manifestations	Prophylaxis and treatment
Candida albicans	Thrush, esophagitis, vaginitis; whitish yellow patches in mouth, esophagus, GI tract, vagina	Treatment—fluconazole (Diflucan), clotrimazole (Lotrimin), nystatin (Mycostatin), itraconazole (Sporanox); if fluconazole refractory; amphotericin B (Fungizone) 2°Prophylaxis—only if subsequent episodes are frequent or severe recurrences: fluconazole (Diflucan), itraconazole (Sporanox)
Coccidioides immitis	Pneumonia/fever, weight loss, cough	Treatment—amphotericin B (Fungizone), fluconazole (Diflucan), itraconazole (Sporanox) 2°Prophylaxis—to prevent recurrence of documented disease—fluconazole (Diflucan), amphotericin B (Fungizone), itraconazole (Sporanox)
CNS lymphoma	Cognitive dysfunction, motor impairment, aphasia, seizures, personality changes, headache	Treatment—radiation, chemotherapy
Cryptococcus neoformans	Meningitis, cognitive impairment, motor dysfunction, fever, seizures, headache	Treatment—amphotericin B (Fungizone), fluconazole (Diflucan), itraconazole (Sporanox) 2°Prophylaxis—to prevent recurrence of documented disease: fluconazole (Diflucan), amphotericin (Fungizone), itraconazole (Sporanox)
Cryptosporidium muris	Gastroenteritis, watery diarrhea, abdominal pain, weight loss	Treatment—antidiarrheals, nitazoxanide (Alinia), paromomycin (Humatin)
Cytomegalovirus (CMV)	Retinitis–retinal lesions, blurred vision, loss of vision Esophagitis/stomatitis – difficulty swallowing; colitis/gastritis – bloody diarrhea, pain, weight loss Pneumonitis – respiratory symptoms Neurologic disease – CNS manifestations	Treatment—ganciclovir (Cytovene), foscarnet (Forcavir), cidofovir (Vistide), valganciclovir (Valcyte) 2°Prophylaxis—to prevent recurrence of documented disease: ganciclovir (Cytovene), foscarnet (Foscavir), cidofovir (Vistide), valganciclovir (Valcyte)
Hepatitis B virus (HBV)	Jaundice, fatigue, abdominal pain, loss of appetite, nausea, vomiting, dark urine; 30% may have no signs or symptoms	1°Prevention—hepatitis B vaccine series; screen and vaccinate those with no evidence of previous HBV infection; encourage for IDU, sexually active MSM, sexual partners or household contacts of HBV-infected individuals, and those with hepatitis C virus; hepatitis A vaccine series should be given to prevent additive effects and advanced liver damage; screen and vaccinate those without evidence of previous HAV infection Treatment—adefovir dipivoxil (Hepsera), α-interferon, lamivudine (Epivir), entecavir (Baraclude)
Hepatitis C virus (HCV)	Jaundice, fatigue, abdominal pain, loss of appetite, nausea, vomiting, dark urine; 80% may have no signs or symptoms	Prophylaxis—none for HCV. Hepatitis A and B vaccine series should be given to prevent additive affects and advanced liver damage; screen and vaccinate those without evidence of previous HAV/HBV infection Treatment—α-interferon, ribavirin (Virazole)
Herpes simplex	HSV1 (type 1): orolabial and mucocutaneous vesicular and ulcerative lesion; keratitis – visual disturbances; encephalitis – CNS manifestations HSV2 (type 2): gential and perianal vesicular an ulcerative lesions	Treatment—acyclovir (Zovirax), famciclovir (Famvir), valacyclovir (Valtrex), foscarnet (Foscavir), cidofovir (Vistide) 2°Prophylaxis—only if subsequent episodes are frequent or severe: acyclovir (Zovirax), famciclovir (Famvir), valacyclovir (Valtrex)
Histoplasma capsulatum	Pneumonia –fever, cough, weight loss Meningitis – CNS manifestations; disseminated disease	Treatment—amphotericin B (Fungizone), itraconazole (Sporanox), fluconazole (Diflucan) 2°Prophylaxis—to prevent recurrence of documented disease: itraconazole (Sporanox), amphotericin B (Fungizone)
Influenza virus	Fever (usually high), headache, extreme tiredness, dry cough, sore throat, runny or stuffy nose, muscle aches; nausea, vomiting, if initial vaccine was given when CD4 +T cell count was and diarrhea can occur	1°Prevention—inactivated trivalent influenza virus vaccine; provide annually, before influenza virus season; revaccinate <200 µL; treatment: supportive therapy

Western Blot

If a patient has a positive ELISA, as it confirmed by the Western blot technique, another more sensitive test for HIV-1 antibodies. The Western blot test for antibodies to four major HIV antigens, two of which must be present for a positive result. Like the ELISA, the Western blot test relies on the production of antibodies and, therefore, may not detect antibodies during the early stages of infection.

Rapid Tests

The ELISA and Western blot tests have been the most widely used tests to determine the presence of antibodies to HIV-1. However, these tests are technically demanding and require sophisticated equipment. Rapid HIV antibody tests are being more widely used today because of ease of use and convenience. Many have comparable sensitivities to the ELISA and Western blot.

Viral Load

Plasma HIV RNA levels indicate the amount of virus in the persons serum, which is a reflection of active viral replication, or viral load. The steeper the rate of increase in plasma HIV RNA, the greater the risk of disease progression unless antiretroviral therapy is started. HIV RNA viral load is measured by one of three assays—quantitative RNA-PCR, branched DNA(bDNA) assay, or nucleic acid sequence-based amplification (NASBA). These tests are greater than 98% sensitive and can detect as few as 40 HIV RNA copies/mL. Another test, the p24 antigen assay, detects the viral protein p24 in the blood of HIV-infected patients. Since the assay is only about 50% sensitive, it is used less often than the quantitative tests for HIV RNA.

Viral load is measured periodically in HIV-positive persons to assess their disease progression and to monitor the effectiveness of antiretroviral therapy. Therapy is aimed at reducing plasma HIV RNA levels of below the limit of detection by assay. For accuracy, two HIV RNA assays are completed within 1 to 2 weeks, and both values are used to establish a baseline for the infected person. It is important for nurses to understand that suppression of HIV RNA levels to below the limits of detection does not mean that HIV infection has been eliminated or that viral replication has been halted completely. It simple means that HIV levels have been reduced to such a degree that they cannot be measured by present methods.

CD4 Cell Counts

CD4 cell counts are used to measure the extent of immune damage that has occurred as a result of HIV infection and its complications, and to monitor the immunologic benefit of antiretroviral therapy. CD4 cell counts are obtained on all newly diagnosed patients to establish a baseline and every 3 to 4 months thereafter if counts are above 350/mm^3 and the patient is asymptomatic and not receiving drug therapy. Once drug therapy is initiated, counts are monitored every 2 to 4 weeks initially and then every 3 to 4 months if the patient stabilizes.

CD4 cell counts are used in conjunction with viral load to predict the possibility of disease progression, determine when to start antiretroviral therapy, and monitor the effectiveness of treatment. Patients with plasma HIV RNA levels of less than 7000 copies/mL and Cd4 counts of greater than 350/mm^3 have less than a 2% likelihood of progressing to AIDS within 3 years without treatment. Conversely, those with viral loads greater than 55,000 copies/mL and CD4 counts of less than 200/mm^3 have an 85% likelihood of progressing to AIDS within 3 years.

Other Tests

Other diagnostic studies are obtained to establish baselines, monitor patient progress, and identify possible coinfections.

Medications for HIV/AIDS

Recent drug developments have decreased the speed of disease progression in many HIV-infected individuals and increased the life span of those living with AIDS. In 1995, the US food and Drug administration approved a class of drugs named protease inhibitors. When a protease inhibitor is combined with two other drugs (reverse transcriptase inhibitors), a highly active antiretroviral therapy (HAART) "cocktail" is created that reduces HIV viral load to undetectable levels. Those drug combinations are the mainstay of HIV treatment.

HAART works by disrupting HIV at different stages during its replication process. The nucleoside and nucleotide reverse transcriptase inhibitors (NRTIs), abacavir (ABC), zidovudine (AZT), didanosine (ddl), stavudine (d4T), lamivudine (3TC), zalcitabine (ddC), and tenofovir, act through two mechanisms. They competitively bind to reverse transcriptase, and they block the elongation of the DNA chain, both of which interfere with the early stages of HIV viral replication. The nonnucleoside reverse transcriptase, and they block the elongatin of the DNA chain, both of which interfere with the early stages of HIV viral replication. The nonnucleoside reverse transcriptase inhibitors (NNRTIs, or nucleoside analogs), nevirapine (NVP), efavirenz(EFV), and delavirdine (DLV), prevent viral replication through competitive binding of reverse transcriptase, but they do not terminate DNA chains.

The protease inhibitors (PIs) indinavir (IDV), ritonavir (RTV), amprenavir (APV), saquinavir (SAQ), lopinavir (LPV), and nelfinavir (NFV) prevent HIV from making the long protein molecules necessary to create new viruses, thus halting replication toward the end of viral replication. Enfuvirtide is a class of drugs known as a fusion inhibitor. It is the first agent of its class to be approved for treatment of HIV. It binds the glucoprotein region of the HIV envelope and prevents viral fusion with the CD4 target cell membrane.

The goals of HAART treatment are to maximally suppress plasma HIV RNA levels of below detectable levels on assay, restore or preserve immunologic function by preventing the destruction of CD4 cells for as long as possible, improve the quality of life, and reduce mortality. Clinical trials are ongoing to find more effective drug therapies with fever side effects.

In 2004, the CDC revised their guidelines for use of antiretroviral agents in HIV-infected adults and adolescents. The guidelines include recommendations for initiating antiretroviral therapy in persons who are asymptomatic, as well as those with established disease. The recommendations were derived from studies designed to identify the risks versus benefits of treatment. Clinical trials indicated that patients whose Cd4 T cell counts fell below 200 cells/mm^3 were at significantly increased risk for opportunistic infections and should be offered antiretroviral therapy.

Medical Management

Currently there is no cure for HIV or AIDS, although researchers continue to work on developing a vaccine. Treatment decisions for an individual patient are based on three factors: HIV RNA (viral load), CD4 T-cell counts, and the clinical condition of the patient (severity of symptoms and patient's commitment to participate in lifelong therapy). The goals of tratment are maximal and durable suppression of viral load, restoration and/or preservation of immunologic function, improvement of quality of life, and reduction of HIV-related morbidity and mortality. To determine and evaluate the treatment plan, viral load testing is recommended at diagnosis and then every 3 to 4 months thereafter in the untreated person. CD4+ T-cell counts should be measured at diagnosis and generally every 3 to 6 months thereafter.

Combination therapy is defined as a regimen containing at least two antiretroviral agents; highly active antiretroviral therapy (HAART) includes at least one nucleoside reverse transcriptase inhibitor plus various other drug combinations. As new medications are developed, the number of combinations continues to increase. Highcost of medications, difficulties with adherence to the regimen, drug resistance, and drug toxicities present problems in drug therapy. Intermittent therapy is under investigation as an alternative regimen.

Pharmacologic Therapy

Antiretroviral Therapy (ART)

(For combination regimens with at least three medications)

- Nucleoside/nucleotide reverse transcriptase inhibitors (NRTI)
- Non-nucleoside reverse transcriptase inhibitors (NNRTI)
- Protease inhibitors (PI)
- Fusion inhibitors (FI).

Drug Resistance Testing

Helps determine which antiretroviral agents to eliminate from the antiretroviral regimen (rather than which agents should be used).

Treatment Interruption and Reinstitution

Depending on the patient and CD4 cell count, ART may be temporarily discontinued when immune competence recurs and stabilizes (e.g. sustained CD4 count between 500 and 800 cells/mm^3). Then, when CD4 counts fall between 350 and 400 cells/mm^3, ART should restart.

Medications for HIV-related Infections

- *PCP:* Trimethoprim-sulfamethoxazole (TMP-SMZ) and antibacterial agents, such as dapsone; alternatively, pentamidine, an antiprotozoal agent
- *MAC:* Treatment for MAC infections involves use of either clarithromycin (Biaxin) or azithromycin (Zithromax). The combination of azithromycin with rifabutin (Mycobutin) is more effective but costly, with more adverse effects and interactions
- *Cryptococcal meningitis:* Intravenous amphotericin B with or without antifungal agents, such as fluconazole (Diflucan) or flucytosine (Ancobon)
- *CMV retinitis:* Ganciclovir, foscarnet, or cidofovir
- *Encephalitis:* Pyrimethamine (Daraprim) and sulfadiazine or clindamycin (Cleocin)
- *Candidiasis:* Clotrimazole (Mycelex), ketoconazole, or fluconazole

Anticancer Agents

- *KS:* Alpha-interferon, surgical excision of lesions, liquid nitrogen to lesions, vinblastine injected into intraoral lesions, interferon; chemotherapy with doxorubicin (adriamycin), bleomycin, and vincristine (ABV); radiation
- *Lymphomas:* Limited successful treatment; chemotherapy and radiation therapy may be used.

Immunomodulators

- Alpha-interferon
- Other substances under evaluation (interleukin-2 interleukin-12, and other cytokines and lymphokines).

Antidepressants

Psychotherapy is integrated with pharmacology (imipramine [Tofranil], desipramine [Norpramin], fluoxetine [Prozac], methylphenidate [Ritalin]; electroconvulsive therapy if depression is severe).

Antidiarrheal Agents and Appetite Stimulants

Octreotide acetate (Sandostatin) is given to treat diarrhea and megestrol acetate (Megace) or dronabinol (Marinol) to stimulate appetite.

No optimal time to initiate anteretroviral therapy has been identified for HIV-infected patients with CD4 cell counts greater than 200 cells/mm^3 who are asymptomatic, although many clinicians offer therapy when CD4 counts are less than 350 cells/mm^3. The available drug regimen are potent, complex, and challenging for adherence. Thus the decision to initiate therapy must be a joint decision between the patient and practitioner.

Patients are likely to experience drug toxicity and numerous side effects. They must be compliant with large pill burdens and tightly prescribed administration regimens; be able to financially withstand the cost of therapy; and be prepared for the possibility of drug resistance, which may limit future therapy options. Drug resistance can develop if viral replication is not sufficiently suppressed or the person is already infected with a resistant strain of HIV. On the other hand, patient who delay therapy run the risk of permanent immune system damage, inability to effectively inhibit vital replication at a later stage in the disease, and increased risk of HIV transmission.

At present HIV infection and AIDS have no vaccine or cure, although the number of potential HIV vaccines in clinical trails supported by the International AIDS Vaccine Initiative and other agencies has doubled since 2000. Although many trials show promise, more research and funding are needed. In addition, ethical questions regarding testing of potential vaccines on healthy subjects must be addressed as trials go forward.

No special treatments exist for the early stages of HIV infection. Respiratory treatments may become necessary as the patients disease progresses. Standard precautions are necessary during hospitalization and at home. Treatments associated with maintenance and improvement of nutritional status usually become necessary. Specific treatments related to opportunistic infections are discussed in Table 5.6.

Surgery does not play a role in the standard management of HIV. Patients may undergo surgical biopsy of skin lesions, surgical treatment of internal Kaposi's sarcoma lesions that do not respond to chemotherapy, or drainage of abscesses or other sites of infection. Those all represent management of AIDS complications, however, and are not primary therapies for HIV disease.

Supportive Care and Alternative Therapies

- Spiritual: Laughter, hypnosis, faith healing, guided imagery, positive affirmations
- Nutrituional: Goal is to attain or maintain ideal weight and decrease risk for infections. Appetite stimulants (megestrol [Megacel]) have been successful; dronabinol (Marinol), which contains synthetic tetrahydrocannabinol (THC), the active ingredient in marijuana, has been effective when used to relieve nausea and vomiting. Alternative nutritional measures include oral supplements, such as Advera, and parenteral nutrition as well as vegetarian and macrobiotic diets, vitamin C or beta-carotene supplements, turmeric (curcumin), and Chinese herbs
- Administraiton of intravenous fluid and electrolyte replacement may treat imbalances
- Drug and biologic medicines not approved by the FDA; oxygen, ozone, and urine therapy
- Physical forces and devices: Acupuncure, acupressure, massage therapy, yoga, therapeutic touch, reflexology crystals.

Diet: Although no particular diet is indicated for persons with HIV, nutritional deficits commonly develop from both the disease itself and the opportunistic infections associated with the disease. Anorexia, nausea, and diarrhea are commonly associated with antiretroviral therapy, further contributing to nutritional alterations. Many persons with AIDS develop wasting syndrome, especially late in the disease. Wasting syndrome involve involuntary weight loss in excess of 10 to 15% of normal baseline weight. It is related to decreased nutrient intake, decreased nutrient absorption, and metabolic disturbances.

Patients must be carefully monitored to evaluate the adequacy of intake and food intolerances. A high-protein diet is encouraged to prevent weight loss and potential cachexia. In the later stages of disease, when infections and muscle wasting prevent adequate food intake, IV nutritional support may be necessary.

Nursing Management of HIV Infection

Nursing assessment for individuals not known to be infected with HIV should focus on behaviors that could put the person at risk for HIV infection and other sexually transmitted and blood-borne diseases. All patients should be assessed for risky behaviors on a regular basis. The assumption should not be made that someone is without risk because he is too young or because she is married or sings in the church choir. Nurses can help individuals assess risk by asking four basic questions: (1) Have you ever had a blood transfusion or used clotting factors? If so, was it before 1985? (2) Have you ever shared drug-using equipment with another person? (3) Have you ever had a sexual experience in which your penis, vagina, rectum, or mouth? And (4) Have you ever had a sexually transmitted disease (STD)? These questions provide the minimum data needed to initiate a risk assessment. A positive response to any of these questions requires an in-depth exploration of issues related to the identified risk.

Specific assessments are needed when an individual has been diagnosed with HIV infection. Repeated nursing assessments over time are essential because people's circumstances change. Early recognition and treatment of problems can decrease the progression of HIV infection and prevent new infections.

A complete history and thorough systems review can help the nurse identify and address problems in a timely manner. Identify potential risk factors, including sexual practices and IV/ injection drug use history. Assess physical and psychological status. Thoroughly explore factors affecting immune system functioning.

Nutritional Status

- Obtain dietary history
- Identify factors that may interfere with oral intake, such as anorexia, nausea, vomiting, oral pain, or difficulty swallowing
- Assess patient's ability to purchase and prepare food
- Measure nutritional status by weight, anthropometric measurements (triceps skin-fold measurement), and blood urea nitrogen, serum protein, albumin, and transferrin levels.

Skin and Mucous Membranes

- Inspect daily for breakdown, ulceration, and infection
- Monitor oral cavity for redness, ulcerations, and creamy-white patches (candidiasis)
- Assess perianal area for excoriation and infection
- Obtain wound cultures to identify infectious organisms.

Respiratory Status

- Monitor for cough, sputum production, shortness of breath, orthopnea, tachypnea, and chest pain; assess breath sounds
- Assess other parameters of pulmonary function (chest X-rays, arterial blood gases, pulmonary function tests).

Neurologic Status

- Assess mental status as early as possible to provide a baseline. Note level of consciousness and orientation to person, place, and time and the occurrence of memory lapses
- Observe for sensory deficits, such as visual changes, headache, and numbness and tingling in the extremities
- Observe for motor impairments, such as altered gait and paresis
- Observe for seizure activity.

Fluid and Electrolyte Status

- Examine skin and mucous membranes for turgor and dryness
- Assess for dehydration by observing for increased thirst, decreased urine output, low blood pressure, weak rapid pulse, or urine specific gravity
- Monitor electrolyte imbalances (laboratory studies show low serum sodium, potassium, calcium, magnesium, and chloride)
- Assess for signs and symptoms of electrolyte depletion, including decreased mental status, muscle twitching, muscle cramps, irregular pulse, nausea and vomiting, and shallow respirations.

Level of Knowledge

- Evaluate patient's knowledge of disease and transmission
- Assess level of knowledge of family and friends
- Explore patient's reaction to the diagnosis of HIV infection or AIDS
- Explore how patient has dealt with illness and major life-stressors in the past
- Identify patient's resources for support.

Use of Alternative Therapies

- Question patient about use of alternative therapies
- Encourage patient to report any use of alternative therapies to primary health care provider
- Become familiar with potential side effects of alternative therapies; if side effect is suspected to result from alternative therapies, discuss with patient and primary and alternative health care providers
- View alternative therapies with an open mind, and try to understand the importance of the treatment to patient.

Nursing Diagnoses

Nursing diagnoses related to HIV infection are indicated by several variables: the stage (e.g. Is prevention of HIV infection the issue? Are there concerns related to ongoing infection? Is the patient dying?); the presence of specific etiologic problems (e.g. respiratory distress, depression, pain); and psychosocial factors (e.g. issues related to self-esteem, sexuality, family interaction, finances). Because HIV infection is a complex and individually experienced disease, a broad spectrum of nursing diagnoses may include, but are not limited to, those presented below:

- Acute pain
- Anxiety
- Caregiver role strain
- Chronic low self-esteem
- Decisional conflict
- Diarrhea
- Disturbed body image
- Disturbed thought processes
- Fatigue
- Fear
- Grieving
- Hyperthermia
- Imbalanced nutrition—less than body requirements

- Impaired oral mucous membrane
- Ineffective coping
- Ineffective denial
- Ineffective therapeutic regimen management
- Insomnia
- Interrupted family processes
- Noncompliance
- Powerlessness
- Relocation stress syndrome
- Risk for disuse syndrome
- Self-care deficit
- Situational low self-esteem
- Social isolation
- Spiritual distress.

Nursing Diagnoses of HIV Includes

- Impaired skin integrity related to cutaneous manifestations of HIV infection, excoriation, and diarrhea
- Risk for infection related to immunodefciency
- Activity intolerance related to weakness, fatigue, malnutrition, impaired fluid and electrolyte balance, and hypoxia associated with pulmonary infections
- Disturbed thought processes related to shortened attention span, impaired memory, confusion, and disorientation, (HIV encephalopathy)
- Ineffective airway clearance related to PCP, increased bronchial secretions, and decreased ability to cough related to weakness and fatigue
- Imbalanced nutrition: Less than body requirements related to decreased oral intake
- Diarrhea related to enteric pathogens or HIV infection
- Pain related to impaired perianal skin integrity secondary to diarrhea, KS, and peripheral neuropathy
- Social isolation related to stigma of the disease, withdrawal of support systems, isolation procedures, and fear of infecting others
- Anticipatory grieving related to changes in lifestyle and roles and unfavorable prognosis
- Deficient knowledge related to self-care and preventing HIV transmission.

Collaborative Problems/Potential Complications

- Opportunistic infections
- Impaired breathing or respiratory failure
- Wasting syndrome and fluid and electrolyte imbalance
- Adverse reaction to medications.

Planning

Prevention of HIV infection presents a number of challenges for the patient, many of which are related to the difficulties of behavior change. Nurses can be instrumental in this process. Nursing interventions to prevent disease transmission depend on assessment of the patients individual risk behaviors, knowledge, and skills. Nursing orders based on these assessments can encourage the patient to adopt, healthier, and less risky behaviors.

Infection with HIV affects the entire of a person's life from physical health to social, economic, and spiritual well-being. Once infected, no known treatment can eliminate HIV from the body. Therefore the overriding goals of therapy are to keep the viral load as low as possible for a long time to maintain or restore a functioning immune system, improve the patients quality of life, prevent opportunistic disease, reduce HIV-related disability and death, and prevent new infections. Nursing interventions can assist the patient to (1) adhere to drug regimens; (2) promote a healthy lifestyle that includes avoiding exposure to additional sexual and blood-borne disease; (3) protect others from HIV; (4) maintain or develop healthy and supportive relationships; (5) maintain activities and productivity; (6) explore spiritual issues; (7) come to terms with issues related to disease, disability, and death; and (8) cope with the frequent symptoms caused by HIV and its treatments. Goals are individualized and change as new treatment protocols develop and/or as HIV disease progresses. Goals include improved airway clearance, achievement and maintenance of skin integrity, resumption of usual bowel patterns, absence of infection, relief of pain and discomfort, improved nutritional status, activity tolerance, improved thought processes, increased socialization, expression of grief, absence of complications, and increased knowledge of disease prevention and self-care.

The objective of nursing care will be:

- Maintains skin integrity
- Resumes usual bowel habits
- Experiences no infections
- Maintains adequate level of activity tolerance
- Maintains usual level of thought processes
- Maintains effective airway clearance
- Experiences increased sense of comfort, less pain
- Maintains adequate nutritional status
- Experiences decreased sense of social isolation
- Progresses through grieving process
- Reports increased understanding of AIDS and participates in self-care activities as possible
- Remains free of complication.

Implementation

The complexity of HIV disease is related to its chronic nature. As with most chronic and infectious diseases, primary prevention and health promotion are the most effective health care strategies. When prevention fails, disease results. HIV has no cure, continues for life, causes increasing physical disability, contributes to impaired health and ultimately leads to death.

Nursing interventions at every stage of HIV disease can be instrumental in improving the quality and quantity of the patients life. Nurses who emphasize a holistic and individualized approach to care as well-suited to provide optimal care to these patients. Table 5.7 presents a synopsis of nursing goals, assessments, and interventions at each stage of HIV infection.

Nursing Interventions includes

Improving Airway Clearance

- At least daily, assess respiratory status, mental status and skin color
- Note and document presence of cough and quantity and characteristics of sputum; send specimen for analysis as ordered
- Encourage adequate rest to minimize energy expenditure and prevent fatigue

TABLE 5.7: Nursing intervention in HIV disease

Levels of nursing care/goals	Assessment	Nursing interventions
i. **Prevent HIV infection**		
Detect HIV infection early	*Risk factors:* What behaviors or social, physical, emotional, pathologic, and immune factors place the patient at risk? Does the patient need to be tested for HIV?	• Education, including knowledge, attitudes, and behaviors, with an emphasis on risk reduction to • *General population:* Cover general information and information specific to HIV infection and pregnancy • *Individual patient:* Specific to assessed need • Empower patients to take control of prevention measures • Provide HIV antibody testing with pretest and posttest counseling
ii. Acute intervention		
1. Promote health and limit disability 2. Manage problems caused by HIV infection	*Physical health:* Is patient experiencing problems? *Mental health status:* How is the patient coping? *Resources:* Does the patient have family/social support? Is patient accessing community services? Is money/insurance a problem? Does the patient have access to spiritual support?	• Provide case management • Educate regarding HIV, the spectrum of infection, options for care, signs and symptoms to report, treatment options, immune enhancement, risk reduction, and ways to adhere to treatment regimens • Refer to needed resources • Establish long-term, trusting relationship with patient, family and significant others
		• Provide emotional and spiritual support • Provide care during acute exacerbations: Recognition of life-threatening developments, life support, rapid intervention with treatments and drugs, patient and family emotional support during crisis, comfort and hygiene needs • Develop resources for legal needs: Discrimination prevention, wills and powers of attorney, child care wishes • Empower patient to identify needs, direct care, seek services
iii. Ambulatory and home care		
1. Maximize quality of life 2. Resolve life and death issues developing? Is the patient experiencing	*Physical health:* Are new symptoms drug side effects or interaction? *Mental health:* How is the patient coping? What adjustments have been made? *Finances:* Can the patient maintain health care and basic standards of living? *Family/social/community supports:* Are these available? Is the patient using supports in an effective manner? Do family/significant others need education, encouragement, or stress relief? *Spirituality issues:* Does the patient desire support from a religious organization? Are spirituality issues private and personal? What assistance does the patient need?	• Continue case management • Educate about changing treatment options and continued adherence • Empower patient to continue to direct

- Provide pulmonary therapy, such as coughing, deep breathing, postural drainage, percussion, and vibration, every 2 hours to prevent stasis of secretions and promote airway clearance
- Assist patient into a position (high- or-semi-Fowler's) that facilitates breathing and airway clearance
- Evaluate fluid volume status; encourage intake of 3 liters daily
- Provide humidified oxygen, suctioning, intubation, and mechanical ventilation as necessary.

Promoting Skin Integrity

- Assess skin and oral mucosa for changes in appearance, location and size of lesions, and evidence of infection and breakdown; encourage regular oral care
- Encourage patient to balance rest and mobility whenever possible; assist immobile patients to change position every 2 hours
- Use devices such as alternating-pressure mattresses and low-air-loss beds
- Encourage patient to avoid scratching, to use nonabrasive and nondrying soaps, and to use nonperfumed skin moisturizers on dry skin; administer antipruritic agents, antibiotic medication, analgesic agents, medicated lotions, ointments, and dressings as prescribed; avoid excessive use of tape
- Keep bed linen free of wrinkles, and avoid tight or restrictive clothing to reduce friction to skin
- Advise patient with foot lesions to wear white cotton socks and shoes that do not cause feet to perspire.

Maintaining Perianal Skin Integrity

- Asses perianal region for impaired skin integrity and infection
- Instruct patient to keep the area as clean as possible, to cleanse after each bowel movement, to use sitz bath or irrigation, and to dry the area thoroughly after cleaning
- Assist debilitated patient in maintaining hygiene practices
- Promote healing with prescribed topical ointments and lotions
- Culture wounds if infection is suspected.

Promoting Usual Bowel Habits

- Assess bowel patterns for diarrhea (frequency and consistency of stool, pain or cramping with bowel movements)
- Assess factors that increase frequency of diarrhe
- Assess self-care strategies patient uses to control diarrhea
- Measure and document volume of liquid stool as fluid volume loss; obtain stool cultures
- Counsel patient about ways to decrease diarrhea (rest bowel, avoid foods that act as bowel irritants, including raw fruits and vegetables); encourage small, frequent meals
- Administer prescribed medications, such as anticholinergic antispasmodic medications or opiates, antibiotic medications, and antifungal agents.

Preventing Infection

- Instruct patient and caregivers to monitor for signs and symptoms of infection. Recommend strategies to avoid infection (upper respiratory infections)
- Monitor laboratory values that indicate the presence of infection, such as white blood cell count and differential; assist in obtaining culture specimens as ordered
- Strongly urge patients and sexual partners to avoid exposure to body fluids and to use condoms for any sexual activities
- Strongly discourage IV/injection drug use because of risk to patient of other infections and transmission of HIV infection
- Maintain strict aseptic technique for invasive procedures.

Observe universal precautions in all patient care. Teach colleagues and other health care workers to apply precautions to blood and all body fluids, secretions, and excretions except sweat (e.g. cerebrospinal fluid; synovial, pleural, peritoneal, pericardial, amniotic, and vaginal fluid; semen). Consider all body fluids to be potentially hazardous in emergency circumstances when differentiating between fluid types is difficult.

A major goal of health promotion is to prevent disease. Even with recent successes in the treatment of HIV, prevention is crucial for control of the epidemic. In addition, health promotion encourages early detection of disease so that, if primary prevention has failed, early intervention can be implemented. HIV infection is preventable. Avoiding and/or modifying risky behaviors are the most effective prevention tools. All patients should be provided with education and behavior change counseling that is specific to the patient's need, culturally sensitive, language appropriate, and age specific. Nurses are excellent resources for this type of education, but they must be comfortable with and know how to talk about sensitive topics such as sexuality and drug use.

Prevention behaviors have been known and recommended since the mid-1980s. It is important to remember that a range of activities can reduce the risk of HIV infection and that individuals will choose methods that best fit their life circumstances. The goal is for the person to develop safer, healthier, and less risky behaviors. These techniques can be divided into *safe activities* (those that eliminate risk) and *risk-reducing* activities (those that decrease risk, but do not eliminate it). The more consistently and correctly prevention methods are used, the more effective they are in preventing HIV infection.

Relieving Pain and Discomfort

- Assess patient for quality and severity of pain associated with impaired parianal skin integrity, KS lesions, and peripheral neuropathy

- Explore effects of pain on elimination, nutrition, sleep, affect, and communication, along with exacerbating and relieving factors
- Encourage patient to use soft cushions or foam pads while sitting and topical anesthetic or ointments as prescribed
- Instruct patient to avoid irritating foods and to use antispasmodic agents and antidiarrheal preparations if necessary
- Administer non-steroidal anti-inflammatory agents and opiates, and use nonpharmacologic approaches, such as relaxation techniques
- Administer tricyclic antidepressants and recommend elastic stockings as prescribed to help alleviate neuropathic pain.

Improving Nutritional Status

- Assess weight, dietary intake, anthropometric measurements, serum albumin, blood urea nitrogen, protein, and transferrin levels
- Instruct patient about ways to supplement nutritional value of meals (e.g. add eggs, butter milk)
- Based on assessment of factors interfering with oral intake, implement specific measures to facilitate oral intake; consult dietitian to determine nutritional requirements
- Control nausea and vomiting; encourage patient to eat easy-to-swallow foods; encourage oral hygiene before and after meals
- Encourage rest before meals; do not schedule meals after painful or unpleasant procedures
- Provide enteral or parenteral feeding to maintain nutritional status, as indicated.

Improving Activity Tolerance

- Monitor ability to ambulate and perform daily activities
- Assist in planning daily routines to maintain balance between activity and rest
- Instruct patient in energy conservation techniques (e.g. sitting while washing or preparing a meal)
- Decrease anxiety that contributes to weakness and fatigue by using measures such as relaxation and guided imagery
- Strategize with other health care team members to uncover and address factors associated with fatigue (e.g. epoetin alfa [Epogen] for fatigue related to anemia).

Maintaining Thought Processes

- Asses for alterations in mental status
- Reorient to person, place, and time as necessary; maintain and post a regular daily schedule
- Give instructions, and instruct family to speak to patient, in a slow, simple and clear manner
- Provide night lights for bedroom and bathroom. Plan safe leisure activities that patient previously enjoyed
- Provide around-the-clock supervision as necessary for patients with HIV encephalopathy (Box 5.6).

Box 5.6 Care of the patient with HIV encephalopathy

Disturbed thought processes
- Assess mental status and neurologic functioning
- Monitor for medication interactions, infections, electrolyte imbalance, and depression
- Frequently orient the patient to time, place, person reality, and the environment
- Use simple explanations
- Teach the patient to perform tasks in incremental steps
- Provide memory aids (clocks and calendars)
- Provide memory aids for medications administration
- Post activity schedule
- Give positive feedback for appropriate behavior
- Teach caretakers how to orient patient to time, place, person, reality, and the environment
- Encourage the patient to designate a responsible person to assume power of attorney

Disturbed sensory perception
- Assess sensory impairment
- Decrease amount of stimuli in the patient's environment
- Correct inaccurate perceptions
- Provide reassurance and safety if the patient displays fear
- Provide a secure and stable environment
- Teach caregivers how to recognize inaccurate sensory perceptions
- Teach the patient and caregivers to report any changes in the patient's vision to the patient's health care provider

Risk for injury
- Assess the patient's level of anxiety, confusion, or disorientation
- Assess the patient for delusions or hallucinations
- Remove potentially dangerous objects from the patient's environment
- Structure the environment for safety (ensure adequate lighting, avoid clutter, provide bed rails if needed)
- Supervise smoking
- Do not let the patient drive a car if confusion is present
- Instruct the patient and caregiver in home safety
- Provide assistance as needed for ambulation and getting in and out of bed
- Pad headboard and side rails if the patient has seizures

Self-care seficits
- Encourage activities of daily living within the patient's level of ability
- Encourage independence but assist if the patient cannot perform an activity
- Demonstrate any activity that patient is having difficulty accomplishing
- Monitor food and fluid intake
- Weight patient weekly
- Encourage the patient to eat, and offer nutritious meals, snacks, and adequate fluids
- If patient is incontinent, establish a routine toileting schedule
- Teach caregivers how to meet the patients self-care needs

Decreasing Sense of Social Isolation

- Provide an atmosphere of acceptance and understanding of AIDS patients, their families, and partners
- Assess patient's usual level of social interaction early to provide a baseline for monitoring changes in behavior
- Encourage patient to express feeling of isolation and aloneness; assure patient that these feelings are not unique or abnormal
- Assure patients, family and friends that AIDS is not spread through casual contact.

Coping with Grief

- Help patients explore and identify resources for support and mechanisms for coping
- Encourage patient to maintain contant with family, friends, and coworkers and to continue usual activities whenever possible
- Encourage patient to use local or national AIDS support groups and hotlines and to identify losses and deal with them when possible.

Research shows that the majority of new HIV infections were transmitted by individuals who were not aware that they were infected. CDC develop four strategies in the *Advancing HIV Prevention (AHP)* initiative: (1) HIV testing should be a part of routine health care based on risk assessment and clinical need; (2) rapid HIV testing should also be used to diagnose HIV outside of traditional care settings (e.g. in community-based organizations and at health fairs), (3) providers should work with HIV-infected patients and their partners to change risky behaviors and decrease the risks of HIV transmission, and (4) perinatal transmission should be further reduced by universally offering HIV tests to pregnant women and appropriate treatment to those found to be infected.

Monitoring and Managing Complications

- Respiratory failure and impaired breathing; monitor arterial blood gas values, oxygen saturation, respiratory rate and pattern, and breath sounds; provide suctioning and oxygen therapy; assist patient on mechnical ventilation to cope with associated stress
- Inform patient that signs and symptoms of opportunistic infections include fever, malaise, difficulty breathing, nausea or vomiting diarrhea, difficulty swallowing, and any occurrences of swelling or discharge. These symptoms should be reported to the health care provider immediately
- Wasting syndrom and fluid and electrolyte disturbances: Monitor weight gain or loss, skin turgor and dryness, ferritin levels, hemoglobin and hematocrit, and electrolytes. Assist in selecting foods that replenish electrolytes. Initiate measure to control diarrhea. Provide intravenous fluids and electrolytes as prescribed
- Side effects of medications: Provide information about purpose, administration, side effects (those reportable to physician), and strategies to manage or prevent side effects of medications. Monitor laboratory test values.

Promoting Home and Community-based Care

Teaching Patients Self-Care

- Thoroughly discuss the disease and all fears and misconceptions; instruct patient, family, and friends about the transmission of AIDS
- Discuss precautions to prevent transmission of HIV: Use of condoms during vaginal or anal intercourse; using dental dam or avoiding oral contact with the penis, vagina, or rectum; avoiding sexual practices that might cut or tear the lining of the rectum, vagina, or penis; and avoiding sexual contact with multiple partners, those known to be HIV positive, those who use illict injectable drugs, and those who are sexual partners of people who inject drugs
- Teach patient and family how to prevent disease transmission, including hand hygiene and methods of safely handling items soiled with bodily fluids
- Instruct patient not to donate blood
- Emphasize importance to taking medication as prescribed. Assist patient and caregivers in fitting the medication regimen into their lives
- Teach medication administration, including intravenous preparations
- Teach guidelines about infection, follow-up care, diet, rest, and activities
- Instruct patient and family how to administer enteral or parenteral feedings, if applicable
- Offer support and guidance in coping with this disease.

Continuing Care

- Refer patient and family for home care nursing or hospice for physical and emotional support
- Assist family and caregivers in providing supporitve care
- Assist in administration of parenteral antibiotics, chemotherapy, nutrition, complicated wound care, and respiratory care
- Provide emotional support to patient and family
- Refer patient to community programs, housekeeping assistance, meals, transportation, shopping, individual and group therapy, support for caregivers, telephone networks for the homebound, and legal and financial assistance
- Encourage patient and family to discuss end-of-life decisions.

Decreasing Risks Related to Sexual Intercourse

Safe sexual activities eliminate the risk of exposure to HIV in semen and vaginal secretions. Abstaining from all sexual activity is the most effective way to accomplish this goal, but there are safe options for those who cannot or do not wish to obtain. Limiting sexual behavior to activities in which the mouth, penis, vagina or rectum does not come into contact with a partners mouth, penis, vagina or rectum is safe because there is no contact with blood, semen or vaginal secretions. Safe activities include massage, masturbation, mutual masturbation (hand job), telephone sex, and other activities that meet the "no contact" requirements. *Insertive sex* between partners who are not infected with HIV or not at risk of becoming infected with HIV is also considered to be safe.

Risk-reducing sexual activities decrease the risk of contact with HIV through the use of barriers. Barriers should be used when engaging in insertive sexual activity (oral, vaginal or anal) with a partner whose HIV status is not known or with a partner who is known to have HIV. The most commonly used barrier is the male condom. The efficacy (protection provided under ideal circumstances) of male condom is essentially 100%; their effectiveness (protection provided in actual or "real life" circumstances) is 80 to 90%. Correct use of male condoms, increased effectiveness. Female condoms provide an excellent alternative to male condoms (Fig. 5.12). Female condom efficacy is also close to 100% and effectiveness is 94 to 97% against HIV and STD transmission. Use can be complicated, so careful instruction and practice are required. In addition, squares of latex (known as dental dams) or plastic food wrap can be used to cover the external female genitalia during oral sexual activity (Box 5.7).

Proper Use of the Male Condom

1. Use only condoms that are made with latex or polyurethane. "Natural skin" condoms have pores that are large enough for HIV to penetrate.
2. Store condoms in a cool, dry place and protect them from trauma. The friction caused by carrying them in a back pocket, for instance, can damage the latex.
3. Do not use a condom if the expiration date has passed or if the package looks worn or punctured.
4. Lubricants used in conjunction with condoms must be water soluble. Oil-based lubricants can weaken latex and increase the risk of tearing or breaking.
5. Nonlubricated, flavored, or unflavored condoms can provide protection during oral intercourse.
6. The condom must be placed on the erect penis before any contact is made with the partner's mouth, vagina, or rectum to prevent exposure to preejaculatory secretions that may contain HIV.
7. See Figures 5.11A to C for proper steps in male condom placement.
8. Remove the penis and condom from the partner's body immediately after ejaculation and before the erection is lost. Hold the condom at the base of the penis and remove both from the partner's body at the same time. This keeps semen from leaking around the condom as the penis becomes flaccid.
9. Remove the condom after use, wrap in tissue, and discard. Do not dispose in the toilet, as this can cause plumbing problems.
10. Condoms are not reusable! A new condom must be used for every act of intercourse (Box 5.8).

Box 5.7 Condom use to prevent HIV transmission

Condoms should be:
- New for each sex act
- Made of latex (polyurethane if allergic to latex) because other material's have large pores that allow HIV to pass
- Nondamaged and within expiration date
- Applied before partner is touched (tip of condom is held while unrolling over erect penis, allowing room at tip for semen collection)
- Used with adequate amount of only water-soluble lubricant (petroleum or oil-based lubricants such as petroleum jelly, cooking oil, shortening, or lotions can damage latex condoms)
- Replaced if broken (if ejaculation occurs before replacement, immediate use of a spermicide may give some protection)
- Withdrawn from partner by holding condom against base of erect penis to avoid semen leakage

Box 5.8 Safer sexual behaviors

- Advise patients to abstain from sharing sexual fluids
- Advise patients to reduce the number of sexual partners to one
- Advise patients to always use latex condoms. If the patient is allergic to latex, nonlatex condoms should be used
- Advise patients to avoid reusing condoms
- Advise patients to avoid using cervical caps or diaphragms without using a condom as well
- Advise patients to always use dental dams for oral-genital or anal stimulation
- Advise patients to avoid anal intercourse because this practice may injure tissues
- Advise patients to avoid manual-anal intercourse (fisting)
- Advise patients not to ingest urine or semen
- Educate patients about nonpenetrative sexual activities, such as body massage, social kissing (dry), mutual masturbation, fantasy, and sex films
- Advise patients to avoid sharing needles, razors, toothbrushes, sex toys, or blood-contaminated articles
- Advise HIV-seropositive patients to inform previous, present and prospective sexual and drug-using partners of their HIV positive status. If the patient is concerned for his or her safety, advise the patient that many states have established mechanisms through the public health department in which professionals are available to notify exposed people
- Advise HIV seropositive patients to avoid having unprotected sex with another HIV seropositive person. Cross-infection with that person's HIV can increase the severity of infection
- Advise HIV seropositive patients to avoid donating blood, plasma, body organs, or sperm

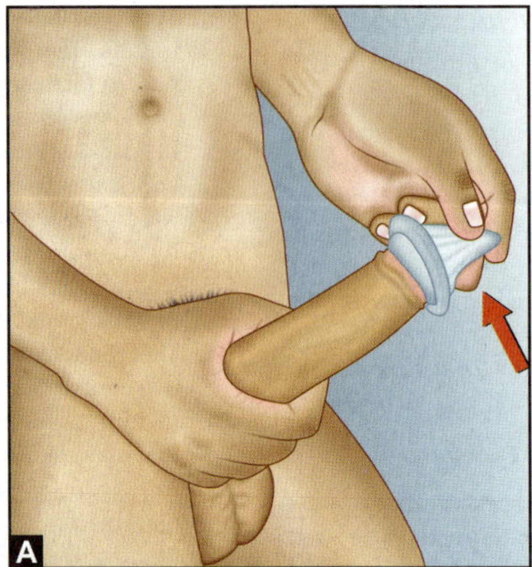

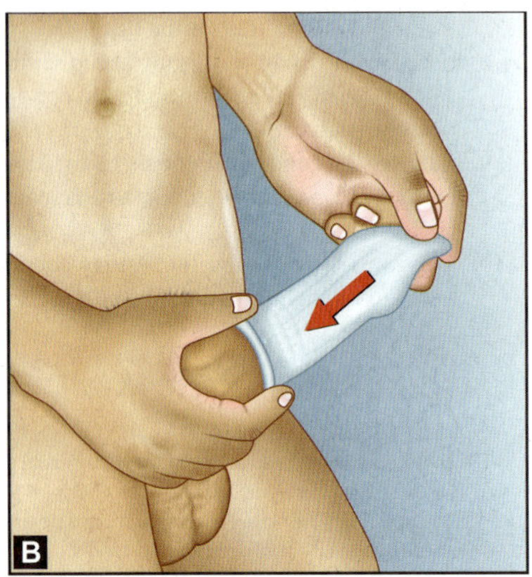

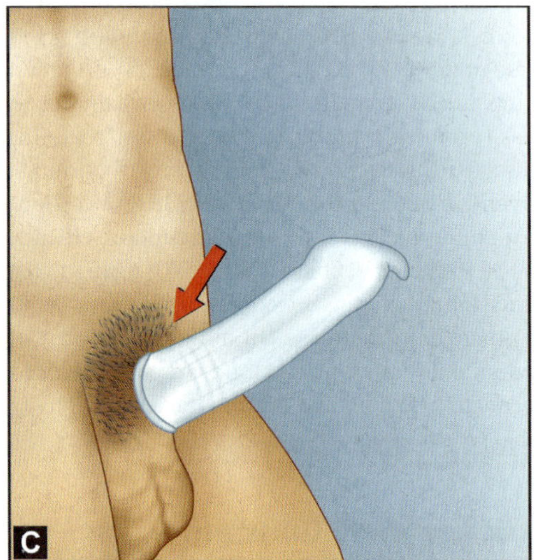

FIGS 5.11A TO C: Proper placement of the male condom. (A) The condom is placed over the glans of the effect penis, being careful to squeeze air out of the reservoir (tip); (B and C). The condom is then rolled down the shaft of the penis to the hairline

Decreasing Risks Related to Drug Use

Drug use, including alcohol, is harmful. It can cause immune suppression and malnutrition, as well as a host of psychological problems. However, drug use in and of itself does not cause HIV infection. The major risk for HIV infection is related to sharing equipment and/or having unsafe sexual experiences while under the influence of drugs. Basic risk reduction rules are: (1) do not use drugs; (2) if you use drugs, do not share equipment; and (3) do not have sexual intercourse when under the influence of any drug (including alcohol) that impairs decision-making ability.

The safest mechanism is to abstain from drugs. Although this is the best option for those who do not currently use drugs, it may not be a viable option for users who are not prepared to quit or for those who have no access to drug treatment services. The risk of HIV for these individuals can be eliminated if they do not share equipment. Injecting equipment (works) includes needles, syringes, cookers (spoons or bottle caps used to mix the drug), cotton and rinse water. Equipment used to snort (straws) or smoke (pipes) drugs can also be contaminated with blood. None of this equipment should be shared. Access to sterile equipment is an important risk elimination tactic. Some communities have needle and syringe exchange programs (NSEPs) that provide sterile equipment to users in exchange for used equipment. Opposition to these programs is supported by the fear that ready access to injecting supplies will increase drug use. However, studies have shown that, in communities where exchange programs have been established, drug use does not increase, rates of HIV and other blood-borne infections are controlled, and an overall cost benefit results.

are the clinicians who work most closely with patients who are trying to cope with these issues. Interventions include education about (1) the advantages and disadvantages of new treatments, (2) the dangers of nonadherence to therapeutic regimens, (3) how and when to take each drug, (4) drug interaction to avoid, and (5) side effects that must be reported to the health care provider.

Health Teaching Guide Use of Antiretroviral Drugs

Resistance to antiretroviral drugs is a major problem in treating HIV infection. To decrease the risk of developing resistance:

1. Take at least three different antiretroviral drugs from at least two different drug classes; discuss options with your health care provider to find the best regimen for you.
2. Know what you are taking and how to take them (some have to be taken with food, some must be taken on an empty stomach, some cannot be taken together). If you do not understand, ask. Get your nurse to write the instructions clearly for you.
3. Take the full dose prescribed and take it on schedule. If you cannot take the drug because of side effects or other problems, report it to your health care provider immediately.
4. Take all of the drugs as prescribed. Do not quit taking one drug while continuing the others. If you cannot tolerate one of your drugs, talk to your health care provider, who will recommend a new set of drugs.
5. Many of the antiretroviral drugs interact with other drugs, including a number of common drugs you can buy without a prescription. Be sure your health care provider and pharmacist know all of the drugs that you are taking, and do not take any new drugs without checking for possible interactions.
6. The goal of antiretroviral therapy is to decrease the amount of virus in your blood. This is called your *viral load*. The best result is to get your viral load below detectable levels. Most health care providers will check for possible interactions.
7. Two to four weeks after you start on drug therapy (or change your therapy), your health care provider will test your viral load to find out if the drugs are working. These results are reported in absolute numbers or in logarithms (a mathematical concept). All you need to know is that you want to see the viral load drop. If reports are in logarithms, you want to see a drop of at least 1 unit, which means that 90% of your viral load has been eliminated. If your viral load drops by 2 units, your viral load will have decreased by 95%. If your viral load drops by 3 units, your viral load will have decreased by 99%.
8. An undetectable viral load means that the amount of virus is extremely low and viruses cannot be found in the blood using the current technology. It does not mean that the virus is gone because much of the virus will be in lymph nodes and organs that the tests cannot detect. It also does not mean that you are no longer able to transmit HIV to others; you will need to continue protecting call of your sexual and drug-using partners from HIV.

When to start antiretroviral therapy: ART has evolved continuously since the first antiretroviral drug was released in 1987. When new drugs were developed, clinicians had the ability to combine and substitute medications. For a while, the preferred treatment strategy was known as "hit it early, hit it hard". This was thought to be appropriate because decreasing the viral load provides for better health outcomes. However, side effects and treatment "burnout" often led to non-adherence, which increased the risk of developing resistance to medications. For this reason, federal guidelines now suggest that treatment can be delayed until greater immune suppression is observed. The most important consideration for initiating therapy is patient readiness. Nurses can provide in-depth education and counseling for patients as they struggle to make this decision.

Adherence: Adherence is the accurate and consistent fidelity to a treatment regimen. Adherence to drug regimens is a critical component of drug therapy for people with HIV infection and an area when nurses are uniquely well prepared to provide assistance. Taking drugs as ordered (right dose and time) every day is important for all drug therapy. The difference with HIV is that missing even a few doses can lead to viral mutations that allow HIV to become resistant to the drug.

The difficulty of adhering consistently is probably clear to anyone who has tried to take a 10-day course of antibiotics. Patients with HIV infection to take anywhere from 2 to 20 pills a day, at precise times during the day. This process must be repeated every day for the rest of their lives even though they often suffer uncomfortable side effects. Nurses have learned that helping people adhere to difficult treatment regimens requires a number of things. The most important is to remember that each patient is a unique individual with unique ways of dealing with therapy. Patients may be helped with technologies such as electronic reminders, beepers, or timers on pillboxes. Group support and individual counseling can also help, but the best approach is to learn about the patient's life and assist with problem solving within the confines of that life. The strategies proven to assist with adherence to antiretroviral.

Antiretroviral therapy includes the following:

- Establish the patients readiness to start therapy
- Provide education on dosing of medication
- Review potential side effects of drugs
- Anticipate and treat side effects
- Use educational aids, including pictures, pillboxes, and calendars
- Engage family and friends in the education process
- Simplify regimens, dosing, and food requirements
- Use team approach with nurses, pharmacists, and peer counselors

- Provide accessible and trusting health care team
- Integrate medication doses into patients life and work schedules.

Health promotion: HIV disease progression may be delayed by promoting a healthy immune system whether the patient choosers to use ART or not. Useful interventions for HIV-infected patients include (1) nutritional support to maintain lean body mass and ensure appropriate levels of vitamins and micronutrients; (2) moderation or elimination of alcohol, tobacco, and drug use; (3) keeping recommended vaccines up to date; (4) adequate rest, exercise, and stress reduction; (5) avoiding exposure to new infectious agents; (6) mental health counseling; and (7) getting involved in support groups and community activities.

Patients should be taught to recognize symptoms that may indicate disease progression and/or drug side effects so that prompt medical care can be initiated. Nurse provides an overview of symptoms that patients should report. In general, patients should have as much information as needed to make the informed decisions that guide appropriate nursing intervention.

Acute exacerbations: Chronic diseases are characterized by acute exacerbation of recurring problems. This is especially true in HIV disease where infections, cancers, debility and psychosocial/economic issues may interact to overwhelm the patients ability to cope. Nursing care becomes more complex as the patients immune system deteriorates and new problems arise to compound existing difficulties. When opportunistic diseases or difficult side effects of treatment develop, symptom management, education, and emotional support are necessary.

Nursing care assumes primary importance in helping patients prevent the many opportunistic diseases associated with HIV infection. The best prevention of opportunistic disease is adequate treatment of the underlying HIV infection. In addition to assisting the patient with the medication prescribed for these diseases, the nurse will need to provide appropriate supportive care. If the patient has *Pneumocystis jiroveci* pneumonia, for example, nursing interventions will be required to assure adequate oxygenation. If the patient has cryptococcal meningitis, an important nursing concern will be to maintain a safe environment for a confused patient.

Ambulatory and Home Care

Ongoing care: HIV-infected patients share problems experienced by all individuals with chronic diseases, but these problems are exacerbated by negative social constructs surrounding HIV. In HIV, the stigma of illness is compounded by several factors. HIV-infected people may be seen as lacking control over urges to have sex or use drugs. It is then easy to jump to the conclusion that they brought the disease on themselves and therefore deserve to be sick. Behaviors associated with HIV infection may be viewed as immoral (e.g. homosexuality, having many sexual partners) and are sometimes illegal (e.g. using drugs, sex work). The fact that infected individuals can transmit HIV to others increases stigma, and stigma leads to discrimination in all facets of life. For example, HIV-infected people have lost jobs, homes and insurance, even though these forms of discrimination are illegal according to the Disabilities Act. Unfortunately, this problem occurs all over the world and is often more severe for women.

Discrimination related to HIV infection can lead to social isolation, dependence, frustration, lowered self-image, loss of control, and economic pressures. It is of interest that all of these variables may have contributed to the patients infection in the first place. Low self-esteem, searching for social contact, frustration, and economic difficulties can all contribute to drug use and risky sexual behaviors.

Disease and drug side effects: Physical problems related to HIV and/or the treatment of HIV can interrupt the patients ability to maintain a desired lifestyle. HIV-infected patients frequently experience anxiety, fear, depression, diarrhea, peripheral neuropathy, pain, nausea, vomiting, and fatigue. These are symptoms that nurses deal with routinely. Interventions for these symptoms do not change significantly based on the primary diagnosis. Individual considerations will, of course, influence the way that the nurse approaches each patient. Nursing management of diarrhea, for instance, still includes helping patients collect specimens, recommending dietary changes, encouraging fluid and electrolyte replacement, instructing the patient about skin care, and managing skin breakdown around the perineal area. Nursing approaches for fatigue in HIV include teaching patients to assess fatigue patterns, determine contributing factors, set activity priorities, converse energy, schedule rest periods, exercise and avoid substances such as caffeine, nicotine, alcohol, and other drugs that may disturb sleep.

Report the following signs and symptoms immediately to health care provider:

- Any change in level of consciousness: Lethargy, hard to arouse, unable to arouse, unresponsive, unconscious
- Headache accompanied by nausea and vomiting, changes in vision, changes in ability to perform coordinated activities, or after any head trauma
- Vision changes: Blurry or black areas in vision field, new floaters, double vision
- Persistent shortness of breath related to activity and not relieved by a short rest period
- Nausea and vomiting accompanied by abdominal pain
- Vomiting blood
- Dehydration: Unable to eat or drink because of nausea, diarrhea, or mouth lesions; severe diarrhea or vomiting; dizziness when standing
- Yellow discoloration of the skin
- Any bleeding from the rectum that is not related to hemorrhoids or trauma (from anal sexual intercourse)

- Pain in the flank with fever and unable to urinate for more than 6 hours
- Blood in the urine
- New onset of weakness in any part of the body, new onset of numbness that is not obviously related to pressure, new onset of difficulty speaking
- Chest pain not obviously related to cough
- Seizures
- New rash accompanied by fever
- New oral lesions accompanied by fever
- Severe depression, anxiety, hallucinations, delusions, or thoughts of causing danger to self or others.

Report the following signs and symptoms within 24 hours:

- New or different headache; constant headache not relieved by aspirin or acetaminophen
- Headache accompanied by fever, nasal congestion, or cough
- Burning, itching, or discharge from the eyes
- New or productive cough
- Vomiting 2–3 times a day
- Vomiting accompanied by fever
- New, significant, or watery diarrhea (more than 6 times a day)
- Painful urination, bloody urine, urethral discharge
- New, significant rash (widespread, painful, itchy, or following a path down the leg or arm, around the chest, or on the face)
- Difficulty eating or drinking because of mouth lesions
- Vaginal discharge, pain or itching.

Some HIV-infected patients, especially those who have been infected for a long time and who have been on ART, develop a set of metabolic disorders that include changes in body shape (fat deposits in the abdomen, upper back, and breasts along with fat loss in the arms, legs, and face) due to lipodystrophy, hyperlipidemia (elevated triglycerides and decreases in high-density lipoproteins), insulin resistance and hyperglycemia, bone disease (osteoporosis, osteopenia, avascular necrosis), lactic acidosis, and cardiovascular disease. It is still not clear why these disorders develop, but it is probably a combination of factors such as long-term infection with HIV, side effects of ART, genetic predisposition, and chronic stress.

Management of metabolic disorders currently focuses on detecting problems early, dealing with the symptoms, and helping the patient cope with new problems and changes to treatment regimens. It is important to recognize and treat these problems early, especially since cardiovascular disease and lactic acidosis are potentially fatal complications. A frequent first intervention is to change ART medications because some drugs are more often associated with these problems. Lipid abnormalities are generally treated with lipid-lowering drugs, dietary changes, and exercise. Insulin resistance is treated with hypoglycemic drugs and weight loss. Bone disease may be improved with exercise, dietary changes, and calcium and vitamin D supplements.

Body changes that combine fat accumulation and wasting are major problems for patients with this syndrome. There is little evidence that exercise or dietary changes make any difference. Human growth hormone, testosterone, and anabolic steroids have been used to help resolve these changes, but they frequently are not effective or even available. Some patients have had plastic surgery to reduce areas of fat and to build up sunken areas of the face, but access to these procedures is limited. Nursing interventions can focus on helping the patient to make treatment decisions and cope with negative changes in body image.

Terminal care: Despite exciting new developments in the treatment of HIV infection, many patients eventually experience disease progression, disability and death. Sometimes these occur because treatments do not work for the patient. Sometimes the patients HIV becomes resistant to all available drug therapies. In other cases, a patient may make a calculated decision to forego further treatment, allowing the disease to progress toward death. Nursing care during the terminal phase of any disease needs to focus on keeping the patient comfortable, facilitating emotional and spiritual acceptance of the finite nature of life, helping the patients significant others deal with grief and loss, and maintaining a safe environment. Nurses become pivotal care providers during the terminal phase of illness, especially when patients and families choose terminal care at home.

CHAPTER

6

Perioperative Nursing

INTRODUCTION

The word 'surgery' comes from the '*kheirurgos*', which means working by hand. Surgery is defined as "the branch of medicine dealing with manual and operative procedures for correction of deformities and defects, repair of injuries.

Surgery has always been practiced; what has changed over the years is the extent of surgery and its complexity, from Homer's reference to battlefield surgery in 800 BC, to bladder and plastic surgery operations in India in 650 AD, with the first manual of surgery produced by Paracelsus, 'Die Kleine Chirurgia' in 1528. Today's surgery has developed from the days of the barber to advanced techniques including the use of lasers, endoscopes and microscopes. Surgical techniques now allow 'free tissue transfer' due to advances in microsurgical techniques and cardiac surgery to the 'beating heart' rather than utilizing bypass techniques. These techniques and others allow surgery to benefit individuals, who may previously not have been offered this option.

The advance in perioperative care and the use of evidence-based practice ensure that care throughout the perioperative period is optimal. Also appreciation of the morbid events that affect the outcome of surgery, specifically inadvertent hypothermia and pressure injuries, improve the quality of care.

Throughout surgery, there has been the presence of an assistant to the surgeon. This is currently a surgical practitioner, either a nurse of operating department practitioner. Their role is multifunctional, to provide quality care for individual patients, manage resources related to surgical episodes, act as the patient's advocate, all the time ensuring that teamworking is practised.

Surgery long back became a medical speciality, because often the treatment of a wide variety of illness and injuries include some types of surgical intervention. Surgery is an invasive method of treatment that may be planned or unplanned, major or minor, and that may involve any body part or system. Care for the client during all phases of the surgical experience needs to be continuous, and integrated surgical procedures require physical and psychosocial adaptations and are stressors for both the client and the family. The client's recovery from a surgical procedure requires skillful and knowledgeable nursing care whether the surgery is of outpatient or in the hospital setting. Nurses working in both settings must understand the principles of caring for surgical clients.

As stated earlier, a client faces variety of stressors when confronting surgery. Anticipatory surgery leads to fear and anxiety for clients who associate surgery with pain, possible disfigurement, dependence, and perhaps even loss of life. Family members often fear a disruption in life-style and experience a sense of powerlessness as the surgery approaches. The trauma sustained during surgery creates physical needs requiring close supervision and skilled intervention by the nurse and surgeon. Nurses use all phases of nursing process used perioperatively to make assessment and provide interventions necessary to promote the recovery of health, prevent further injury or illness, and facilitate coping with alterations in physical structure and function.

DEFINITION OF PERIOPERATIVE NURSING AND NURSE

Perioperative nursing refers to the role of nurse during the perioperative, intraoperative and postoperative phases of a clients surgical experience. The concept of perioperative nursing stresses the importance of providing continuity of care.

- Perioperative nursing refers to the role of the nurse during the preoperative, intraoperative and postoperative phases of a client's surgical experience. The concept of perioperative nursing stresses the importance of providing continuity of care

- A perioperative nurse is defined as the registered nurse, who, using the nursing process, designs, coordinates and delivers care to meet the identified needs of the clients whose protective reflexes or self-care abilities are potentially compromised because they are under the influence of anesthesia during operative or other invasive procedures
- Perioperative nurse, possesses and applies knowledge of the procedure and the client's intraoperative experience throughout the client-care continuum. And also they assess, diagnose, plan, intervene and evaluate the outcome of interventions based on criteria and support of a standard care targeted towards the population
- The perioperative nurse addresses the changing physiological, pathophysiological, sociocultural and spiritual responses of the client that have been initiated by the prospect of performance of the invasive procedure.

SCOPE OF THE PERIOPERATIVE NURSING

The scope of perioperative nursing practice consists of three phases:

1. Preoperative;
2. Intraoperative; and
3. Postoperative.

Preoperative Phase

It begins where the decision for surgical intervention is made and ends with transference of the client to the operative site. Nursing activities range from a baseline assessment of the client during the preoperative interview and continues with assessment in the pre-admission unit, client room, holding area, or induction room on the day of surgery. Before surgery, the nurse prepares the client and family for the surgery, performs diagnostic tests, and assesses the client in preparation for the operation.

Intraoperative Phase

It begins where the client is transferred to the operating room bed and ends when the client is transferred to an area of recovery from anesthesia. In this phase, nursing interventions range from communicating the client's plan of care, identifying nursing activities, necessary for expected outcome and establishing priorities for nursing actions. During surgery, the nurse assists surgeons and other operating room nurses to ensure that the client receives optimal care. The nurse also coordinates client needs with team members and personnel's from other disciplines, coordinates the use of the supplies and equipment, controls the environment, prepares for potential emergencies, and communicates and documents the client's plan of care.

Postoperative Phase

It begins with the client's transfer to an area for recovery and ends with client's recovery from surgery. Nursing activities range from communicating pertinent information about the client's surgery, to assist the client to be physical stability and wakefulness and institute measures to help the client achieve maximum recovery. See Box 6.1 for an overview of perioperative care.

Box 6.1 An overview of the perioperative phases of care

Preoperative phase

Preadmission testing
- Initiates initial preoperative assessment
- Initiates teaching appropriate to patient's needs
- Involves family in interview
- Verifies completion of preoperative diagnostic testing
- Verifies understanding of surgeon-specific preoperative orders (e.g. bowel preparation, preoperative shower)
- Discusses and reviews advanced directive document
- Begins discharge planning by assessing patient's need for postoperative transportation and care

Admission to surgical procedure
- Completes preoperative assessment
- Assesses for risks for postoperative complications
- Reports unexpected findings or any deviations from normal
- Verifies that operative consent has been signed
- Coordinates patient teaching and plan of care with nursing staff and other health team members
- Reinforces previous teaching
- Explains phases in perioperative period and expectations
- Answers patient's and family's questions.

In the holding area
- Assesses patient's status, baseline pain, and nutritional status
- Reviews chart

Contd...

Contd...

- Identifies patient
- Verifies surgical site and marks site per institutional policy
- Establishes intravenous line
- Administers medications if prescribed
- Takes measures to ensure patient's comfort
- Provides psychological support
- Communicates patient's emotional status to other appropriate members of the health care team

Intraoperative phase

Maintenance of safety

- Maintains aseptic, controlled environment
- Effectively manages human resources, equipment, and supplies for individualized patient care
- Transfers patient to operating room bed or table
- Positions patient based on functional alignment and exposure of surgical site
- Applies grounding device to patient
- Ensures that the sponge, needle, and instrument counts are correct
- Completes intraoperative documentation

Physiologic monitoring

- Calculates effects on patient of excessive fluid loss or gain
- Distinguishes normal from abnormal cardiopulmonary data
- Reports changes in patient's vital signs
- Institutes measures to promote normothermia

Psychological support (before induction and when patient is conscious)

- Provides emotional support to patient
- Stands near or touches patient during procedure and induction
- Continues to assess patient's emotional status

Postoperative phase

Transfer of patient to postanesthesia care unit

- Communicates intraoperative information:
  - Identifies patient by name
  - States type of surgery performed
  - Identifies type and amounts of anesthetic and analgesic agents used
  - Reports patient's vital signs and response to surgical procedure and anesthesia
  - Describes intraoperatiye factors (e.g. insertion of drains or catheters, administration of blood, medications during surgery, or occurrence of unexpected events)
  - Describes physical limitations
  - Reports patient's preoperative level of consciousness
  - Gommunicates necessary equipment needs
  - Communicates presence of family or significant others

Postoperative assessment recovery area

- Determines patient's immediate response to surgical intervention
- Monitors patient's vital signs and physiologic status
- Assesses patient's pain level and administers appropriate pain relief measures
- Maintains patient's safety (airway, circulation, prevention of injury)
- Administers medications, fluid, and blood component therapy, if prescribed
- Provides oral fluids if prescribed for ambulatory surgery patient
- Assesses patient's readiness for transfer to in-hospital unit or for discharge home based on institutional policy (e.g. Alderete score)

Surgical nursing unit

- Continues close monitoring of patient's physical and psychological response to surgical intervention
- Assesses patient's pain level and administers appropriate pain relief measures
- Provides teaching to patient during immediate recovery period
- Assists patient in recovery and preparation for discharge home
- Determines patient's psychological status
- Assists with discharge planning

Home or clinic

- Provides follow-up care during office or clinic visit or by telephone contact
- Reinforces previous teaching and answers patient's and family's questions about surgery and follow-up care
- Assesses patient's response to surgery and anesthesia and their effects on body image and function
- Determines family's perception of surgery and its outcome

CLASSIFICATION OF SURGICAL PROCEDURE

Surgery can be defined as the art and science of treating diseases, injuries and deformities by operation and instrumentation. The surgical procedure involves the interaction of the patient, the surgeon, and the nurse. Surgical procedures usually are classified on the basis of urgency degree of risk, and purposes.

Based on Urgency

Surgery may be classified as elective surgery, urgent surgery and emergency surgery.

Elective surgery: It is preplanned and performed on the basis of client's choice. It is not essential and may not be necessary for health and delay in surgery has no ill effects, can be scheduled in advance based on the choice of client.

The purposes of elective surgery are as follows:

- To remove or repair a body part
- To restore function
- To improve health
- To improve self-concept.

For example, tonsillectomy, hernia repair, cataract extraction and lens implant, hip prosthesis, hemorrhoidectomy, etc.

Urgent surgery: In which the surgery is the necessity for the client's health, but not an emergency. This is performed for the purposes as in elective surgery and to prevent further tissue damage. For example, removal of gallbladder, coronary artery, removal of tumor, etc.

Emergency surgery: When surgery must be done immediately to preserve the client's life, remove or repair body part, restore function, improve health and self concept. For example, perforated ulcer, intestinal obstruction, tracheostomy, Cesarean section etc.

Based on Degree of Risk or Seriousness

Surgery has been classified as major or minor on the basis of risk for the client:

Major surgery: It involves extensive reconstruction or alteration in body parts poses great risks to well-being. It requires hospitalization usually belonged to well-being; has a high degree of risk; involves major body organs, life-threatening situations and potential postoperative complications. Major surgery may be elective, urgent, or emergency. For example, nephrectomy, cholecystectomy, colostomy, hysterectomy.

Minor surgery: It is primarily elective; it is usually a brief, carries low risk and results in few complications. It can be performed in clinics, outpatient clinic and minor operation theaters. For example, teeth extraction, removal of warts, skin biopsy, laparoscopy, dilatations and curettage.

Based on Purpose

Surgical procedures based on purpose include diagnostic, ablative, palliative, reconstructive, transplant, constructive.

Diagnostic: It is surgical exploration that allows physician to make or to confirm diagnosis, may involve removal of tissue for further diagnostic testing. For example, breast biopsy, laparoscopy, bronchoscopy, exploratory laparotomy (incision in peritoneal cavity to inspect abdominal organs).

Ablative: It is excision or removal of diseased body part. For example, appendicectomy, subtotal thyroidectomy, partial gastrectomy, colon resection, amputation, cholecystectomy, etc.

Palliative surgery: It is performed to relieve or reduce intensity of an illness or disease symptoms will not produce cure. For example, colostomy, nerve root resection (rhizotomy) debridement of necrotic tissue, balloon angioplasty, arthroscopy, etc.

Reconstructive surgery: It is performed to restore function to traumatized or malfunctioning tissues and to improve self-concept. For example, scar revision, plastic surgery, skin graft, internal fixation of fractures, breast reconstruction.

Transplant: It is performed to replace organs or structures that are diseased or malfunctioning. For example, kidney, cornea, liver, heart, joints, total hip replacement.

Constructive surgery: It is performed to restore function lost or reduced as a result of congenital anomalies. For example, repair of cleft palate, closure of a trial defect in heart.

Sometimes combination of several surgery explained above also are performed as and when needed.

The common prefixes and suffixes used to explain the types of surgical procedures are described in Table 6.1.

ROLE OF NURSE IN PERIOPERATIVE CARE

General Care

Each surgical client responds differently in surgery, when he/she enters the healthcare setting in different stages of health. Many variables influence a person's physiologic and psychological responses to the surgical experience. These include physical and mental status, extent of disease, magnitude of the surgery, social and financial resources, and psychological and physiological preparation for surgery. When considered effectively, these variables reveal the degree of risk for a client undergoing surgery.

While making physiological assessment before surgery, nurse elicits information about age; presence of pain; nutritional status; fluid and electrolyte balance; presence of

TABLE 6.1: Common prefixes and suffixes in surgery

Prefixes		Suffixes	
Terms	**Definitions**	**Terms**	**Definitions**
Supra-	Above, beyond	-oma	Tumor, swelling
Artho-	Joint	-ectomy	Removal of organ
Chole-	Bile or gall	-rrhaphy	The suturing or stitching of part of an organ
Cysto-	Bladder	-scopy	Looking into
Endocephalo-	Brain	-ostomy	Making an opening or stoma
Hystero-	Uterus	-otomy	Cutting into
Mast-	Breast	-plasty	To repair or restore
Meningo-	Membrane	-cele	Tumor, hernia, swelling
Myo-	Muscle	-itis	Inflammation of
Nephro-	Kidney		
Oophor-	Ovary		
Pneumo-	Lung		
Pyelo-	Pelvis, kidney		
Salpingo-	Fallopian tube		
Thoraco-	Chest		
Viscero-	Organ especially abdomen		

Box 6.2 Purposes of preoperative diagnostic tests

Diagnostic test	**Purpose**
Chest X-ray	Detect pulmonary and cardiac abnormalities
Oxygen saturation	Obtain baseline level and detect abnormality
Serum tests	
Arterial blood gases	Obtain baseline levels and detect pH and oxygenation abnormalities
Bleeding time	Detect prolonged bleeding problem
Blood urea nitrogen	Detect kidney problem
Creatinine	Detect kidney problem
Complete blood cell count	Detect anemia, infection, clotting problems
Electrolytes	Detect potassium, sodium, chloride imbalances
Fasting blood glucose	Detect abnormalities, monitor diabetes control
Pregnancy	Detect early, unknown pregnancy
Partial thromboplastin time	Detect clotting problem
International normalized ratio (INR) prothrombin time	Detect clotting problem, monitor warfarin therapy
Type and crossmatch	Identify blood type to match blood for possible transfusion
Urine tests	
Pregnancy	Detect early, unknown pregnancy
Urinalysis	Detect infection, abnormalities

infections; physical mobility, skin integrity, cardiovascular; pulmonary, renal, gastrointestinal, liver, endocrine, neurologic and hematologic function; sensory medication history, abnormalities, injuries and previous surgeries, health habits, and sociocultural history and note any abnormalities and report to the concerned and take suitable measures to correct and sending the client to operating room.

The possible preoperative tests include the following purposes/reasons for those tests and normal ranges stated are as follows (Box 6.2):

- Complete blood count and picture should be tested
- Serum potassium (normal 3.5–5 mEq/L) to identify hyperkalemia or hypokalemia
- Serum sodium (normal 136 to 145 mEq/L) to identify hypernatremia, dehydration or overhydration
- Serum chloride (normal 96–100 mEq/L) to identify hyperchloremia, hypochloremia, or metabolic disorder
- Glucose (normal 60–100 mg/dL) to identify hypoglycemia or hyperglycemia
- Creatinine (normal 0.7–1.4 mg/dL) to identify acute or chronic renal disease
- Blood urea nitrogen (BUN) (10–20 mg/dL) to identify impaired liver or kidney function or excessive protein or tissue catabolism
- Hemoglobin (Hb) (Female) (12 to 15 g/dL; Male 13–17 g) to identify the presence and extent of anemia
- Hematocrit (Hct) (Female 36%; Male 39–51%) to identify the presence and extent of anemia
- Prothrombin time (PT) or clotting time (CT) (11 18 seconds) to identify dysfunction of blood clotting (prothrombin level)
- Partial thromboplastin time (PTT) to identify deficiencies of coagulation factors
- Chest X-ray (no abnormal heart of lung lesion) to determine size and contour of heart, lungs, and major vessels
- Electrocardiogram (ECG) (normal rate and rhythm) to determine the electrical activity of the heart
- Urine analysis to identify abnormalities.

Any deviations from the normal, should be noted and reported to take precautions during surgery. And the common medical conditions that increase the high risk in surgery will include bleeding disorders, diabetes mellitus, heart diseases, upper respiratory infection, liver diseases, fever, chronic respiratory diseases, and immunological disorders. A special precaution should be taken on these cases before, during and after surgery.

PREOPERATIVE NURSING

Persons who require surgical intervention and nursing care enter the health care settings in a variety of situations, ranging from essentially healthy people who have planned elective procedure to emergency admissions for treatment of trauma. Surgical client may be of any age and at any point on the health-illness continuum. It is the nurse's responsibility to identify factors that affect risk from a surgical procedure, assess physical and psychosocial needs of the client and family and establish a plan of care, based on appropriate nursing diagnoses, that includes interventions to meet needs and facilitate recovery as the client progresses through the perioperative period. Nurse has to perform preoperative assessment and teaching as discussed below:

Preoperative Assessment

The nurses make preoperative assessment by taking history, conducting physical examination, performing diagnostic tests as required preoperatively according to client's status/requirements, and takes informed consent in preoperative phase. Informed consent is very essential for anyone is undergoing any invasive procedure like surgery. A consent form is the legal document which signifies the client's informed consent for the procedure. The consent form guards the client against unwanted invasive procedure. It also protects the healthcare facility and healthcare professional (use consent form as per Policy of Hospital).

In addition, preoperative teaching is an important component in the client's operative experience. Teaching about postoperative phase is the nurse's responsibility. Clients and families need to know about surgical events, and sensations, how to perform physical activities necessary to decrease postoperative complications and facilitate recovery. The teaching-learning process is individualized to meet both specific and common client needs. Preoperative teaching allays anxiety and encourages clients to participate actively in their own care.

Preoperative nursing interventions are derived from the nursing assessment and must reflect each individual patients specific needs. Physical preparations will be determined by the pending surgery and the routines of the surgery setting. Preoperative teaching may be minimal or extensive. General information for surgery should be given. Nursing assessment includes following:

Cardiovascular System

- Identify acute or chronic problems; focus on presence of angina, hypertension, heart failure, recent history of myocardial infarction
- Auscultate and palpate baseline pulses; apical, radial, and pedal for rate and characteristics (compare one side to the other)
- Inspect and palpate for presence of edema (including dependent areas) noting location and severity
- Inspect and palpate neck veins for distention
- Take baseline blood pressure in both arms
- Identify any drug or herbal product that may affect coagulation (e.g. aspirin, ginkgo, ginger)
- Review laboratory and diagnostic tests for cardiovascular function
- Identify patients with pacemakers and/or implantable defibrillators.

Respiratory System

- Identify acute or chronic problems; note the presence of infection or chronic obstructive pulmonary disease (COPD), asthma
- Assess history of smoking, including the time interval since the last cigarette and the number of pack-years (remember that although smoking should be discouraged preoperatively, it may be difficult for patients to stop during this time of anxiety)
- Auscultate lungs for normal and adventitious breath sounds
- Determine baseline respiratory rate and rhythm, and regularity of pattern
- Observe for cough, dyspnea and use of accessory muscles of respiration.

Neurologic System

- Determine orientation to time, place, and person
- Identify presence of confusion, disorderly thinking, or inability to follow commands
- Identify past history of strokes, transient ischemic attacks or nervous system diseases (e.g. Parkinson's disease, multiple sclerosis).

Urinary System

- Identify any pre-existing disease
- Determine ability to void. Prostate enlargement may affect catheterization during surgery and ability to void postoperatively
- If necessary, note color, amount, and characteristics of urine
- Review laboratory and diagnostic tests for renal function.

Hepatic System

- Inspect skin color and sclera of eyes for any signs of jaundice
- Review past history of substance abuse, especially alcohol and IV drug use
- Review laboratory and diagnostic tests for liver function

Integumentary System

- Assess mucous membranes for dryness and intactness
- Determine skin status; note drying, bruising, or breaks in surface
- Inspect skin for rashes, boils or infection, especially around the planned surgical site
- Assess skin moisture and temperature
- Inspect the mucous membranes and skin turgor for dehydration.

Musculoskeletal System

- Examine skin/bone pressure points
- Assess for presence of any pressure ulcers
- Assess for limitations in joint range of motion and muscle weakness
- Assess mobility, gait, and balance
- Assess for presence of joint pain.

Gastrointestinal System

- Determine food and fluid intake patterns and any recent weight loss
- Weigh and measure patient
- Assess for the presence of dentures and bridges (loose dentures or teeth may be dislodged during intubation).

Immune System

- Identify any immunodeficiency or autoimmune disorders
- Assess for use of corticosteroids or other immuno suppressant drugs.

For common preoperative diagnostic test see Table 6.2.

TABLE 6.2: Common preoperative diagnostic tests

Test	Assessment
Urinalysis infection	Renal status, hydration, urinary tract and disease
Chest X-ray	Pulmonary disorders, cardiac enlargement
Blood studies	Anemia, immune status, infection
(RBC, Hb, Hct, WBC, WBC differential)	
Electrolytes	Metabolic status, renal function, diuretic side effects
ABGs, oximetry	Pulmonary and metabolic function
PT, PTT, INR, platelet count	Bleeding tendencies
Blood glucose	Metabolic status, diabetes mellitus
Creatinine	Renal function
Blood urea nitrogen	Renal function
Serum albumin	Nutritional status
Electrocardiogram	Cardiac disease, electrolyte abnormalities
Pulmonary function studies	Pulmonary status
Liver function tests	Liver function
Type and crossmatch	Blood availability for replacement (elective surgery patients may have own blood available)
hCG	Pregnancy

Preoperative Teaching

The patient has a right to know what to expect and how to participate effectively during the surgical experience. Preoperative teaching increases patient satisfaction and may reduce postoperative fear, anxiety, and stress. Teaching may also decrease complication, the duration of hospitalization and the recovery time following discharge. In most surgical settings, patients often arrive only a short time before surgery is scheduled. This includes patients arriving for ambulatory surgery and patient who will be hospitalized postoperatively. Preoperative teaching for these patients is generally done in the surgeon's office or preadmission surgical clinic and reinforced on the day of surgery. The patient usually goes home several hours after ambulatory surgery, the patient usually goes home several hours after recovery depending on the patient's progress and procedure-specific needs. If ambulatory patients have not had preoperative teaching in an outpatient setting before surgery, teaching must address needs of the highest priority and include information that focuses on the safety of the patient. Written materials must be provided for patient to use for review and reinforcement at home. When providing preoperative teaching for a patient several days before surgery, the nurse must provide a balance between telling so little that the patient is unprepared and explaining so much that the patient is overwhelmed. The nurse who observes carefully and listen sensitively to the patient can usually determine how much information is enough in each instance, remembering that anxiety and fear may decrease leaning ability. The nurse must also assess what the patient wants to know right away and give priority to his or her concerns.

Generally, preoperative teaching concerns three types of information: sensory, process and procedural. Different patients, with varying cultures, backgrounds, and experience may want different types of information. With *sensory information*, patients want to know what they will see, hear, smell and feel during the surgery. For example, the nurse may tell them that the OT (operation theater) will be cold, but they can ask the OT nurse for a warm blanket; the lights in the OT are very bright; or there will be lots of sounds that are unfamiliar and there may be specific smells present. Patients wanting *process information* may not want specific details but desire the general flow of what is going to happen. This information would include the patient's transfer to the OT, and waking up in the POCU (postoperative care unit). Patients may also be informed that as soon as they are awake, their family may come in to visit them. With *procedural information*, desired details are more specific. For example, this information would include that an IV line will be started while patients are in the holding area and the surgeon may mark the operative site with an indelible marker to verify site and side. Other procedural information includes that when patients are transferred to the OR (operating room), they will be asked to move onto the narrow bed and a safety strap will be put over their thighs.

Preoperative teaching provided to the patient must be communicated to the nurses providing postoperative care so that learning can be evaluated and duplication of teaching can be prevented. Because the nurse has limited time for teaching, the team approach is usually used. Nurses in offices, homes, or clinics may initiate the teaching. The perioperative nurses continue teaching and evaluate the patients understanding of the content. The discharge nurse provides written instructions and additional information for reinforcement. Community nurses may also be involved if the patient has continuing learning needs that these nurses can address during home visits after patients are discharged.

All teaching should be documented in the patient's medical record. A patient and family teaching guide for preoperative preparation is presented as follows:

Sensory Information

- Holding area may be noisy
- Drugs and cleaning solutions may be smelled
- Operation theater (OT) can be cold; warm blankets are available
- Talking may be heard in the OT but may be distorted because of masks. Questions should be asked if something is not understood
- OT bed will be narrow. A safety strap will be applied over the knees
- Lights in the OT may be very bright
- Monitoring machines (ticking and pinging noises) may be heard when awake. Their purpose is to monitor and ensure safety.

Procedural Information

- What to bring and what type of clothing to wear to the ambulatory surgery center
- Any changes in time of surgery
- Fluid and food restrictions
- Physical preparation required (e.g. bowel of skin preparation)
- Purpose of frequent vital signs assessment
- Pain control and other comfort measures
- Why turning, coughing, and deep breathing postoperatively is important; practice sessions need to be done preoperatively
- Insertion of intravenous lines
- Procedure for anesthesia administration
- Expected surgical site and/or side to be marked with indelible ink or marker.

Incentive spirometry may also be ordered postoperatively to prevent atelectasis by increasing lung volume, alveoli expansion, and venous return. All patients can benefit from incentive spirometry, especially the elderly and those at increased risk for lung complications. The spirometer stays at the patient's bedside for hourly use while awake (not on the window sill or in a drawer where it cannot be reached by the patient!). Offer the spirometer to the patient each hour to ensure that it is used. Teach patients to do the following:

- Sit upright, at 45 degrees minimum, if possible
- Take two normal breaths. Place mouthpiece of spirometer in mouth
- Inhale until target, designated by spirometer light or rising ball, is reached, and hold breath for 3 to 5 seconds
- Exhale completely
- Perform 10 sets of breaths each hour.

Coughing moves secretions to prevent pneumonia. Teach patients how to cough effectively if not contraindicated by the patient's condition (such as hernia repair or head injury) (Box 6.3). Give pain medication before asking the patient to cough and offer reassurance that coughing should not harm the incision. Splinting the incision with a pillow may be comforting. Several sets of coughing are performed every 1 to 2 hours while the patient is awake.

Leg exercises, if not contraindicated, improve circulation and help prevent complications related to stasis of blood, such

Box 6.3 Teaching coughing technique

Procedure	Rationale
Have patient sit up and lean forward	Promotes lung expansion and ability to generate forceful cough
Show patient how to splint incision with hand, pillow, or blanket	Reduces incision pressure so it does not feel as if incision is opening
Have patient inhale and exhale deeply three times through mouth	Helps expand lungs
Have patient take in deep breath and cough out the breath forcefully with three short coughs using diaphragmatic muscles. Take in quick deep breath through mouth, cough deeply, and deep breathe	Generates forceful cough and expands lunges to help move secretions

as emboli formation. Instructions are to lie down, raise the leg, bend it at the knee, flex the foot, extend the leg, and lower it to the bed. Each leg is exercised in sets of five. Foot circles are also done every hour while awake. Teach the patient to raise a leg slightly off the bed with toes pointed. Draw a circle in the air with the great toe, rotating to the right four times, then to the left. Repeat this five time and then do the same with the other foot.

Patients are taught that turning from side to side in bed is aided by bending the leg that is to be on top and placing a pillow between the legs to support the top leg. They are told, unless contraindicated, to use the bed's side rail to pull themselves over to the side. To promote comfort, patients are encouraged to deep breathe while turning instead of holding their breath (see preoperative instruction in Box 6.4).

Box 6.4 Preoperative instructions to prevent complications

Diaphragmatic breathing

Diaphragmatic breathing refers to a flattening of the dome of the diaphragm during inspiration, with resultant enlargement at the upper abdomen as air rushes in. During expiration, the abdominal muscles contract.

- Practice in the same position you would assume in bed after surgery: a semi-Fowler's position, propped in bed with the back and shoulders well supported with pillows
- With your hands resting lightly on the front of the lower ribs, and fingertips against lower chest to feel the movement

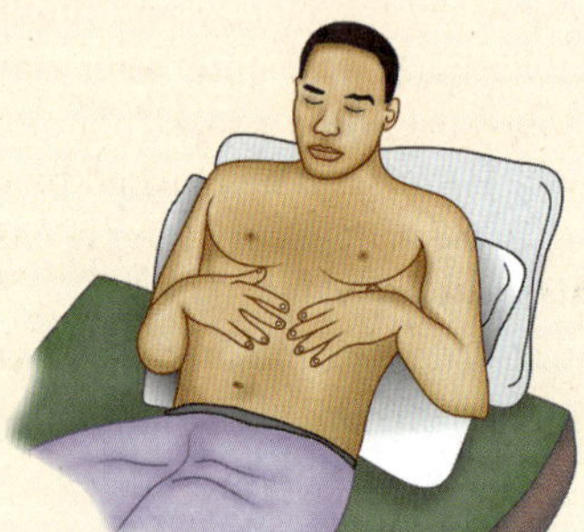

Diaphragmatic breathing

- Breath out gently and fully as the ribs sink down and inward toward midline
- Then take a deep breath through your nose and mouth, letting the abdomen rise as the lungs fill with air
- Hold this breath for a count of five
- Exhale and let out all the air through your nose and mouth
- Repeat this exercise 15 times with a short rest after each group of five
- Practice this twice a day preoperatively

Coughing

- Lean forward slightly from a sitting position in bed, interlace your fingers together, and place your hands across the incisional site to act as a splint like support when coughing

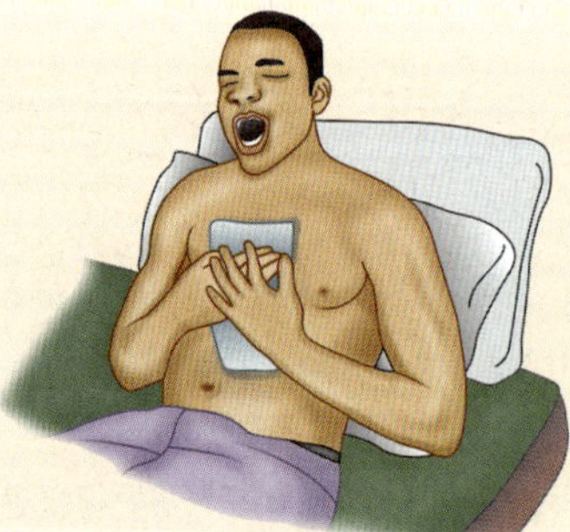

Splinting of chest when coughing

- Breathe with the diaphragm as described under "diaphragmatic breathing"
- With your mouth slightly open, breathe in fully
- "Hack" out sharply for three short breaths
- Then, keeping your mouth open, take in a quick deep breath and immediately give a strong cough once or twice. This helps clear secretions from your chest. It may cause some discomfort but will not harm your incision

Leg exercises

- Lie in a semi-Fowler's position and perform the following simple exercises to improve circulation
- Bend your knee and raise your foot—hold it a few seconds, then exted the leg and lower it to the bed

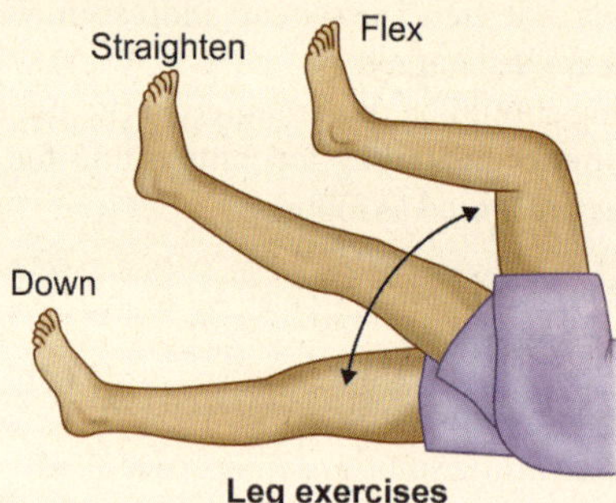

Leg exercises

- Do this five times with one leg, then repeat with the other leg
- Then trace circles with the feet by bending them down, in toward each other, up, and then out
- Repeat these movements five times

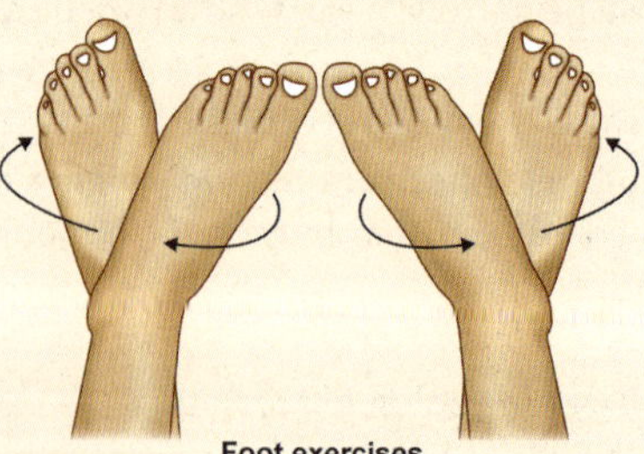

Foot exercises

Turning to the side

- Turn on your side with the uppermost leg flexed most and supported on a pillow
- Grasp the side rail as an aid to maneuver to the side
- Practice diaphragmatic breathing and coughing while one your side

Getting out of bed

- Turn on your side.
- Push yourself up with one hand as you swing your legs out of bed

To make it easier for patients to get out of bed and to reduce strain on the incision, patients are instructed to turn to their side without pillows between their knees. Then they should place their hands flat against the bed and push up while swinging their legs out of bed and into a sitting position. Patients should be told to sit for a few minutes after changing position to avoid dizziness and falling. They should also deep breathe while sitting to promote lung expansion.

Process Information

Information about General Flow of Surgery

- Admission area
- Preoperative holding area, OR, and recovery area
- Families can usually stay in holding area until surgery
- Families may be able to enter recovery area as soon as patient is awake
- Identification of any technology that may be present on awakening, such as monitors and central lines.

Where Families can Wait during Surgery

- Patients and family members need to be encouraged to verbalize concerns
- OR staff will notify family when surgery is completed
- Surgeon will usually talk with family following surgery.

All patients should receive instruction about deep breathing, coughing, and moving postoperatively. This is essential because patients may not want to do these activities postoperatively unless they are taught the rationale for them and practice them preoperatively. Patients and families should be told if there will be tubes, drains, monitoring devices, or special equipment after surgery, and that these devices enable the nurse to safely care for the patient. Examples of individualized teaching may include how to use incentive spirometers or postoperative patient-controlled analgesia pumps. The patient should also receive accurate surgery-specific information, such as a patient having an immobilizer following a total joint replacement, a patient having an epidural catheter for postoperative pain control, or the patient being told about waking up in the intensive care unit following extensive surgery.

The ambulatory surgery patient or the patient admitted to the hospital the day of surgery will need to receive information before admission. Some ambulatory surgical centers have the staff to telephone the patients in the evening before surgery to answer last-minute questions and to reinforce teaching. Each surgical center has policies and procedures that direct and enable this communication in a timely manner.

The patient will need basic information such as time to arrive at the surgery center and the time of surgery. Arrival time is usually 1 to 2 hours before the scheduled time of surgery to allow for the completion of the preoperative assessment and paperwork preparation. Information can also include the day-of-surgery events such as patient registration, parking, what to wear, what to bring, and the need to have a responsible adult present for transportation home after surgery. To provide for general hygiene and preparation of surgical areas the surgeon may order a preoperative shower, an enema, and food and fluid restrictions. Historically, patients having elective surgery were usually instructed by the anesthesia care provider (ACP) to have nothing by mouth (NPO) starting at midnight on the night before surgery. Protocols may vary if the patient is having local anesthesia or the surgery is scheduled for late in the day. The NPO protocol of each surgical facility should be followed because varying NPO protocols exist. Providing the patient with the rationale for adhering to NPO orders can significantly increase the patient's perception of their importance. Restriction of fluids and food is designed to minimize the potential risk of aspiration and to decrease the risk of postoperative nausea and vomiting. The patient who has not followed this instruction may have surgery delayed or cancelled, so it is critical that the surgical patient understands and adheres to these restrictions.

Legal Preparation

Legal preparation for the client undergoing surgery consists of checking that all required forms have been correctly signed and are present on the chart, and that the patient and family clearly understand what is going to happen. Standard consent forms include those for the surgical procedure and blood transfusions. Other forms may include those that have been completed for advance directives and power of attorney. Before nonemergency surgery can be legally performed, the patient must voluntarily sign an **informed consent** form in the presence of a witness. Informed consent is an active, shared decision-making process between the provider and the recipient of care. Three conditions must be met for consent to be valid. First, there must be *adequate disclosure* of the diagnosis; the nature and purpose of the proposed treatment; the risks and consequences of the proposed treatment; the probability of a successful outcome; the availability, benefits, and risks of alternative treatments, and the prognosis if treatment is not instituted. Second, the patient must demonstrate clear *understanding and comprehension* of the information being provided before receiving sedating preoperative medications. Third, the recipient of care must *give consent voluntarily*. The patient must not be persuaded or coerced in any way by anyone to undergo the procedure.

Although the surgeon is ultimately responsible for obtaining the patient's consent for surgical treatment, the nurse may be responsible for witnessing the patient's signature on the consent form. At this time the nurse can be patient advocate, verifying that consent for surgery is truly voluntary. If the patient is unclear about operative plans, the nurse should contact the surgeon about the patients need for additional information. The patient also should be aware the consent, even when signed, can be withdrawn at any time if the desire to give permission for the procedure changes. If the patient is a minor, is unconscious, or is mentally incompetent to sign the permit, the written permission may be given by a legally appointed representative or responsible family member. Procedures for obtaining consent, especially from minors and patients who are mentally incompetent, vary among states and institutions. Therefore the nurse should follow specifics required by the states nurse practice act and the institutional or agency policies that apply to an individual situation.

A true medical emergency may override the need to obtain consent. When immediate medical treatment is needed to preserve life or to prevent serious impairment to life and the individual patient is incapable of giving consent, the next of kin may give consent. If reaching the next of kin is not possible, the physician may institute treatment without written consent. A note is written in the chart documenting the medical necessity of the procedure. In the case of emergency where consent cannot be obtained, the intraoperative nurse will usually need to complete an incident report because it is an occurrence that is inconsistent with routine facility operations.

The motive of any OT nurse should be to make the operating room a safe place for patient as well as the staff.

1. Safe for the *patient* who must be protected from infection and other harm.
2. Safe for the *staff* from the risk of needle-stick and other injuries. These can spread hepatitis, HIV and other infections.
3. Safe for the *community* by careful and safe disposal of soiled materials, especially sharp instruments and needles.

Great importance is being given to prevention of harm to the patient with considerable success. However, even the staff working in the OT should be protected from risks, infections and the law. Theater procedures depend on many different factors—the work-load; the equipment available; the choice of the surgeon; etc. The staff should be aware of the legal responsibilities in order to safeguard themselves from legal lawsuits. Now-a-days nursing has developed its all functional activities in accordance with technological, political or socioeconomical rapid charge. From the legal, ethical or professional perspective nursing within the perioperative environment has become a new challenges. Some of the legal issues include:

1. *Consent:* It is the prime responsibility of the nurse to check that informed consent has been taken from the patient. During checking the consent, she should also re-establish the identity of the patient by matching all the particulars from the patient's record as well as from the patient. Special care should be taken regarding site of the surgery, patients with similar names and psychiatric patients.

   The signed consent form is placed in a prominent place on the patient chart and accompanies the patients to operation theater.
2. *Lack of consensus between surgeon and the nurse:* At time there may be lack of consensus between the nurse and any other member of the team. Sometimes the surgeon may do wrong thing in regarding to very crucial issues. It is the nurse's responsibility in such a situation to either achieve consensus or confront to the OT policies in the regard.
3. *Nurse as a link between the patient and the surgical team:* It is also true that the patient has the right to know who assists in performing his or her treatment. So it is required to introduce them to the doctor and the nurse from the accountability and legal perspective.
4. *Gauze counting:* As discussed earlier (safety issues) that foreign articles such as gauze or surgical instruments may be left inside the patient during surgery, which may place the patient under harm. So nurses should be very cautious in counting all the sponges and instruments during the surgery and just before the closure of the incision.

The nurse discusses a patient's impending surgery in the preoperative holding area. It becomes obvious that this competent adult patient was not fully informed of the alternatives to this surgery. She has signed the consent form but clearly was not fully informed about her treatment options. An important points to be considered here are as given below:

- Informed consent requires that patients have complete information about the proposed treatment and its possible consequences, as well as alternative treatments and possible consequences
- Risks and benefits of each treatment option must also be explained in order for patients to weigh treatment options
- An opportunity to have questions answered about the various treatment options and their possible outcomes is also an important element of informed consent
- Informed consent is an ongoing process that needs periodic assessment and discussion, not an event where a person signs a document
- Paternalism results when health care providers do not provide complete information for patients to make fully informed decisions or when they decide what is best for patients.

Nursing Responsibilities in the day-of-surgery

Day-of-surgery preparation will vary a great deal depending on whether the patient is an inpatient or an outpatient. The nursing responsibilities immediately before surgery include final preoperative teaching, assessment and communication of pertinent findings, ensuring that all preoperative preparation orders have been completed, and ensuring that records and reports are present and complete to accompany the patient to the OR. It is especially important to verify the presence of a signed operative consent, laboratory data, a history and physical examination report, a record of any consultations, baseline vital signs, and nurses notes complete to that point. In addition, the site and side of the anticipated surgery may be marked with an indelible marker and documented to indicate agreement with the patient.

If the patient is an inpatient, the hospital nurse is responsible to ensure that the patients is ready and appropriately prepared for surgery. If the patient is an outpatient, the patient or family member will share the responsibility for preoperative preparation. Hospitals may require that a patient wear a hospital gown with no underclothes, whereas surgery centers may allow the patient to wear underwear, depending on the surgical procedure to be performed. The patient should not wear cosmetics because observation of skin color will be important. Nail polish and artificial nails should be removed so that capillary refill and pulse oximetry can be assessed. An identification band is put on the patient and, if applicable, an allergy band. All patient valuables are returned to a family member or secured according to institutional protocol. If the patient prefers not to remove a wedding ring, the ring can be taped securely to the finger to prevent loss. All prostheses, including dentures, contact lenses, and glasses, are generally removed to prevent loss or damage to them. Hearing aids may be left in place to allow the patient to better follow instructions. Glasses and hearing aids must be returned to the patient as soon as possible following surgery.

The patient should be encouraged to void before preoperative medications are administered if the medications will interfere with maintaining balance and increase the risk for a fall when ambulating to the bathroom. The patient should have an empty bladder on transfer to the OT to prevent involuntary elimination under anesthesia and reduce the possibility of urinary retention during early postoperative recovery. The use of preoperative checklist ensures that all preoperative preparations have been completed before the patient is given any sedating medications (Table 6.3).

TABLE 6.3: Preoperative checklist

Preoperative requirements	Initials	Day of surgery	Initials
Height _____ Weight ______		Surgical site marked Y N NA	
Isolation? ______ Type _____		ID band on patient	
Allergies noted on chart		Allergy band on patient Y NA	
Vital signs (initial)			
T ___ P ____ R ____ BP ____		Vital signs time _______	
		T ____ P ____ R _____ BP ____	
		Procedures	
Chart review		NPO since ________	
H and P on chart		Capillary blood glucose Y NA	
H and P within 30 days? Y N		Preoperative skin prep Y NA	
		Shower scrub shave	
Signed and witnessed informed consent form on chart		Makeup, nail polish, false fingernails, and false eyelashes removed Y NA	
Signed consent for blood administration Y NA		Hospital gown applied Y NA	
Blood type and cross match Y NA		**Valuables** Y or N	
Name plate on chart		Dentures ________	
Old chart requested and sent Y NA		Wig or hairpiece ______	
Diagnostic results		Eyeglasses _________	
Hb/Hct ______/ _____ NA		Contact lenses _________	
PT/INR/PTT ____/____/_____ NA		Hearing aid _________	
CXR _________ NA		Prosthesis __________	
ECG _________ NA		Jewelry __________	
Other laboratories		Clothing __________	
		Disposition of valuables:	
		Family rings taped safe	
Final chart review:		Voided/catheter Time:	
New forms added			
Signed off		Preoperative medications given	
		Time ________ NA	
		Preoperative antibiotics given	
		Time ________ NA	
Time to OT _________________ Date ___________			
Transported to OT by ____________________________			
Final check by ______________________________ RN			

Preoperative Medications

Preoperative medications are used for a variety of reasons. A patient may receive a single drug or a combination of drugs. Benzodiazepines and barbiturates are used for their sedative and amnesic properties. Anticholinergics are given to reduce secretions. Opioids may be given to decrease intraoperative anesthetic requirements and to decrease pain. Antiemetics may be given to decrease nausea and vomiting. It identifies common preoperative medications and the purposes of their use preoperatively (Table 6.4).

The nurse must assess and document the patient's use of prescription medication (because of possible adverse effects). If any, nurse must clearly communicate to anesthetists.

Other medications that may be administered preoperatively include antibiotics, eye drops, and routine prescription drugs. Antibiotics may be administered throughout the perioperative period for a patient with a history of congenital or valvular heart disease to prevent the development of infective endocarditis. Antibiotics may also be ordered for the patient undergoing surgery where wound contamination is either a potential risk (e.g. gastrointestinal surgery) or where wound infection could have serious postoperative consequences (e.g. cardiac and joint replacement surgery). Antibiotics are most commonly administered intravenously (IV) and may be started either preoperatively or in the OT (operation theater).

Eye drops commonly ordered and administered preoperatively for the patient undergoing cataract and other eye surgery. Many times the patient will require multiple sets of eye drops administered at 5-minute intervals. It is important to administer these drugs as ordered and on time to adequately prepare the eye for surgery.

TABLE 6.4: Commonly used preoperative medications

Class	Drug	Purpose and effects
Benzodiazepines	Midazolam (Versed) Diazepam (Valium) Lorazepam (Ativan)	Reduce anxiety, amnesic effects Induce sedation Induce amnesia
Opiodis	Morphine Meperidine (Demerol) Fentanyl (Sublimaze)	Relieve discomfort during preoperative procedures
Histamine (H2)–receptor antagonists	Cimetidine (Tagamet) Famotidine (Pepcid) Ranitidine (Zantac)	Decrease HCl acid secretion Increase gastric pH Decrease gastric volume
Antiemetics	Metoclopramide (Reglan) Droperidol (Inapsine) Ondansetron (Zofran)	Increase gastric emptying Decrease nausea and vomiting Prevent nausea and vomiting
Anticholinergics	Atropine Glycopyrrolate (Robinul) Scopolamine	Decrease oral and respiratory secretions Prevent bradycardia

Medications that patients routinely use for health maintenance or disease management may or may not be used on the day of surgery. To facilitate patient teaching and eliminate confusion about which medications should be taken, the nurse should carefully check written preoperative orders and clarify the orders with the surgeon and/or ACP if there is any question.

Premedications may be administered orally (PO), IV, subcutaneously (SC), or intramuscularly, (IM). Oral medications are given 60 to 90 minutes before the patient goes to the OR unless otherwise ordered. Because patients are fluid restricted before surgery, the patient should swallow these medications with a minimal amount of water. IM and SC injections are usually to be given 30 to 60 minutes before arrival at the OT (minimally 20 minutes). Intravenous medication are usually administered to the patient after arrival in the preoperative holding area or operating room. The patient should be informed about the expected effects of the medications, such as relaxation, drowsiness, and dryness of the mouth.

Transportation to the Operation Theater

If the patient is an inpatient, the OT staff sends transport personnel to the patient's room with a cart or trolley to transport the patient to surgery. The nurse assists the patient in transferring from the hospital bed to the OR cart, and the side rails of the cart are raised and secured. The nurse should ensure that the completed chart goes with the patient, as well as any ordered preoperative equipment, such as antiembolism devices or the patient's inhaler. In many institutions, the family may accompany the patient to the holding area.

In an ambulatory surgical center, the patient may be transported to the OT by cart or wheelchair, or, if no sedatives have been administered, the patient may even walk accompanied to the OT. In all cases it is important for the nurse to ensure patient safety during transport. The method of transportation and the person who transported the patient should be documented by the nurse responsible for the transfer.

The family should be instructed where to wait for the patient during surgery. Many hospitals have a surgical waiting room where OT personnel communicate the status of the patient to the family. It is in this waiting room that the surgeon can locate the family after surgery and where families can be notified that the surgery is complete. Some hospitals provide pagers to waiting family members so that they may eat or do errands during the surgery.

While the patient is in surgery the inpatient nurse should have the patients room prepared for the postoperative arrival. Any additional necessary equipment, including IV poles, oxygen, suction, and additional pillows for positioning, should also be placed in the room. The room also is organized to facilitate entry of the transport cart.

In addition, preoperative teaching is an important component in the client's operative experience. Teaching about postoperative phase is the nurse's responsibility. Clients and families need to know about surgical events, and sensations, how to perform physical activities necessary to decrease postoperative complications and facilitate recovery. The teaching-learning process is individualized to meet both specific and common client needs. Preoperative teaching allays anxiety and encourages clients to participate actively in their own care. The basic areas that must be covered in preoperative teaching are the following:

Deep breathing exercises and coughing exercises: These help expand collapsed lung and prevent postoperative pneumonia atelectasis. Coughing exercise help to guard the suture.

Turning exercises: These help prevent venous stasis, thrombophlebitis, decubitus ulcer formation, and respiratory complications.

Extremity exercises: These help prevent circulatory problems, such as thrombophlebitis, by facilitating venous return to the heart.

Ambulation: Early ambulation when appropriate, helps prevent postoperative complications.

Pain control: Regarding medication (IV or IM) or NPO (nothing per oral), relaxation technique are advisable. In addition, TENS and PCA are taught for pain control measure.

Postoperative equipments: Client may be instructed about equipments that may be used postoperatively. Depending upon the surgery, various tubes, drains, and IV lines are used.

Physical preparation: The physical preparation of the client for surgery may vary, depending on the client's physical status and special needs, type of surgery to be done and surgeon's order. Certain nursing interventions are appropriate for all surgical clients in the areas of hygiene and skin preparation, elimination, nutrition, and fluids and rest and sleep. The nurse is responsible for the preparation and safety of the client on the day of surgery.

i. *Skin preparation:* The skin is cleaned by scrubbing the operative site one or more times with an antiseptic soap or solution to remove bacteria. This can be done by the client while taking a bath or shower. Ideally, a shower is taken in the evening before the morning of surgery. Shampooing the hair and the cleaning of the fingernails also help to reduce number of organism present. The incisional area usually is shaved before surgery because hair serves as a reservoir of bacteria. Usually the operative area is washed before surgery with an antiseptic such as povidone-iodine (Betadine) to clean and disinfect the skin.

ii. *Elimination:* The gastrointestinal tract needs special preparation on the evening before surgery to:
   - Reduce the possibility of vomiting and aspiration during anesthesia
   - Reduce the possibility of a bowel obstruction, and
   - Prevent contamination from fecal material during intestinal tract or bowel surgery.

   Emptying the bowel of feces in no longer routine procedure before surgery, but the nurse should use preoperative assessment to determine the need for an order of bowel elimination. If the client is scheduled for surgery of the GI tract, cleansing enema usually ordered.

   Insertion of an indwelling urinary catheter may be ordered before surgery, especially in clients having pelvic surgery, to prevent bladder distention or accidental injury. If an indwelling catheter is not in place, the client should void immediately before receiving premedication to ensure an empty bladder during surgery.

iii. *Nutrition and fluids:* Preparation involves restricting food and fluid. If a client undergoing surgery is to receive a general anesthesia, foods and fluids are restricted 8 to 10 hours before the operation. This restriction significantly reduces the possibility of aspirations of gastric contents, which can cause aspiration pneumonia. Most clients have an NPO status after midnight.

iv. *Rest and sleep:* These are important components in reducing stress before surgery and in healing and recovery after surgery. The nurse can facilitate rest and sleep in the immediate preoperative period by meeting psychological needs, carrying out teaching, providing a quiet environment, and administering prescribed bedtime sedative medication.

To sum up immediate preoperative preparations begin at least 1 to 2 hours before surgery in the hospital. The nurse's responsibility on the day of surgery will include the following:

- Note allergies according to institutional policy
- Take and record the vital signs, assess and report the abnormalities for elevated temperature
- Check the identification band to make sure it is legible, accurate and securely fastened to the client
- Be sure that informed consent has been obtained and is clearly documented
- If a skin preparation has been ordered, check that it has been completed accurately and thoroughly
- Check for the carry out any special orders, such as administering enema or starting on IV line, recurred previous records, inserting nasogastric tube, giving medications
- Verify that the client has not eaten for the last 8 hours. Check that fluids have been restricted although sometimes the physician will order clients to take their usual oral medication with a small sip of water
- Ask the client to void, measure and record the amount of urine (if indicated)
- Assist the client with oral hygiene, if necessary
- Help the client to remove jewelery to prevent loss or injury from swelling, during or after surgery. Many facilities allow the client to keep wedding band or Mangalasutra (Tali) on as long as they are taped securely. If jewelery is removed, it

should be stored according to policy or given to authorized member of their family

- Remove all hairpins or hairpieces. This prevents injury to the client during surgery as well as possible loss or hairpieces or wigs
- Remove colored nail polish from at least one nail for the pulse oximeter to allow intraoperative and postoperative assessment of skin and nailbeds for circulation and oxygenation of tissues
- If the client is wearing hearing aid, notify the operating room nurse. Leave it in place so that operating room personnel know it is there and can communicate with the client
- Remove all prosthesis, such as dentures, or partial plates, eye glasses, contact lenses and artificial limbs and store them safely (dentures may cause respiratory, distress)
- Give the preoperative medications that are prescribed, either at a scheduled time or "on call". The commonly ordered medications are:
  - Sedatives and tranquilizers to alleviate anxiety and facilitate anesthesia induction, e.g. nembutal, chlorpromazine, or diazepam
  - Anticholenesterase to decrease pulmonary and oral secretions to prevent laryngospasm, e.g. atropine
  - Narcotic analgesics to facilitate client's sedation and relaxation and to decrease the amount of anesthetic agent need, e.g. morphine
  - Neurolephanalegiscs agents to cause a general state of calmness and sleepness.

To prevent omissions and preoperative nursing intervention, most facilities supply nurses with a preoperative checklist. As each intervention on the list is completed, the nurse initials it. Documents through checklists and narrative charting, the nursing intervention carried out.

Assist in moving client from the bed to the operating room stretcher when it is time to transport the client to surgery, ensuring accurate identification.

INTRAOPERATIVE NURSING

Intraoperative phase begins when the client enters the surgical suite and ends with admission to the recovery area. Nursing care during this phase focuses on the client's emotional well-being, as well as on physical factors such as safety positioning, maintaining asepsis and controlling the surgical environment. The nurses are the client's advocates upon induction of anesthesia.

It is imperative that the correct patient identity, surgical procedure and surgical site be verified prior to surgery.

In the surgical holding area, the nurse is responsible for reviewing the record for completeness, ensuring proper identification of the client, client's safety and providing emotional support. It is important to deal with the fears and concerns of a frightened or agitated client. A relaxed client undergoes anesthetic induction easier than who is anxious. If the client still seems anxious despite sedation and reassurance, notify the surgeon or anesthesia personnel. Here the anesthesiologist sees the client, IV fluids starts by him or her or nurse-anesthetist. Nurse-anesthetist also can administer medication needed during surgery. The procedures vary among institutions of health care. Nurse has to perform following activities during intraoperative phase.

The preoperative assessment of the surgical patient establishes baseline data for intraoperative and post-anesthesia care. Assessment data provided by the patient and family in the holding area and data from the inpatient-nursing units are verified and used to develop a plan of care for the patient.

Psychosocial Assessment

The perioperative nurse who cares for the patient in the OT is knowledgeable about the activities that occur when a patient is transferred into the surgical suite. This knowledge allows for informative and reassuring explanations, especially to the anxious patient. General questions regarding surgery or anesthesia can usually be answered by the perioperative nurse. Examples of these questions include, "When will I go to sleep?" "Who will be in the room?" "When will doctor arrive?" "How much of my body will be exposed and to whom?" "Will I be cold?" "When will I wake up?" Specific questions relating to details of the surgical procedure and anesthesia may be referred to the surgeon or ACP.

Cultural assessment is essential to understanding the patient's response to the surgical experience. For example, members of the Jehovan's Witness community may refuse blood transfusions. For Muslims, the left hand is considered unclean, so the nurse should use the right hand to administer forms, drugs, and treatments. Some patients may request that surgically removed body tissue be preserved so that it may be ritually buried. Some body piercings may also have cultural meaning. An interpreter may be necessary if the patient does not speak local language or English. Spiritual considerations, attitudes, and expression regarding pain and health beliefs and practices should individualize the plan of care.

Physical Assessment

A thorough physical assessment should be made during the preoperative preparation of the patient. Physical assessment data that are specifically important to intraoperative nursing care include baseline data such as vital signs, height, weight, and age; allergic reactions to food, drugs and latex; condition and cleanliness of skin; skeletal and muscle impairments; perceptual difficulties; level of consciousness; nothing-by-mouth (NPO) status; and any sources of pain or discomfort. Vital signs are important as baseline data to evaluate the effects of intraoperative medications and body positioning. Height and weight of the patient guide the nurse regarding the width and length of the OR bed. The need for extra warmth is indicated by the patient's age, metabolic problems, and planned surgical procedures.

Some allergic reactions may be avoided with such simple measures as a change in "pepping" solutions or the type of tape used with dressings. Catastrophic reactions can possibly be avoided if latex sensitivity is determined before the procedure begins. The condition and cleanliness of the skin determine the amount and type of intraoperative skin preparation solutions, and will alert the team to the potential for infection as a result of open or closed skin lesions. Knowledge of skeletal and muscle impairments helps prevent injury during positioning. Knowledge of the presence of piercings will allow jewelery to be removed to prevent site burns when using electrosurgery. Perceptual difficulty, such as vision or hearing impairment, will guide the nurse in adapting communication techniques to individual needs. An altered level of consciousness necessitates increased safety and protection techniques. Communicating identified sources of pain to other health team members prevents subjecting the patient to unnecessary discomfort.

Transferring the Patient

Before transferring the patient into the scheduled OT, the nurse spends significant time preparing the room to ensure privacy, safety, and prevention of infection. Surgical attire (pants and shirts, masks, protective eyewear, and caps or hoods) is worn by all persons entering the OT suite. All electrical and mechanical equipment is checked for proper functioning. Aseptic technique is practiced as each surgical item is opened and placed systematically on the instrument table. Sponges, needles, and instruments are counted to ensure accurate retrieval at the close of the procedure.

During room preparation and during the procedure the functions of the team members are delineated. The scrub person will scrub hands and arms, don sterile gown and gloves, and touch only those items in the sterile field. The circulating nurse remains in the unsterile field and implements those activities that permit touching all unsterile items and the patient. Every person on the surgical team must share the responsibility for monitoring aseptic practice and initiating corrective action when a sterile field is compromised.

Once the patient has been properly identified and the OT has been adequately prepared, the patient is transported into the room for the surgery. Each time a patient is transferred from one bed to another, the wheels of the stretcher should be locked, and a sufficient number of personnel should be available to lift, guide, and prevent accidental falling. Once the patient is on the OT bed, safety straps should be snugly placed across the patients thighs. At this time the monitor leads (e.g. ECG leads), blood pressure cuff, and pulse oximeter are usually applied and an IV catheter is inserted if it was not in place when the patient arrived from the holding area.

Scrubbing, Gowning and Gloving

Scrubbing: All sterile team members should perform the hand and arm scrub before entering the surgical suite. The basic principle of the scrub is to wash the hands thoroughly, and then to wash from a clean area (the hand) to a less clean area (the arm). A systematic approach to the scrub is an efficient way to ensure proper technique. There are two methods of scrub procedure (Fig. 6.1).

1. Numbered stroke method: In this method each finger, palm, back of hand, and arm is assigned a certain number of brush strokes.
2. Timed scrub method: This method designates specified time for washing hands. Generally each scrub should last from 3 to 5 minutes, depending on organizational protocols. This is the commonly used method.

The procedure for the timed 5 minutes scrub consists for following steps:

- Remove all jewelery (rings, watches, bracelets)
- Wash hands and arms to two inches above the elbow and clean finger nails under running water. Avoid using too hot water as it may dry the skin, and could be uncomfortable to wash for the recommended amount of time. However, because cold water prevents soap from lathering properly, soil and germs may not be washed away
- Start timing
- Begin scrubbing palm, other and inner aspect of each finger, finger nails, the dorsum of the hand and circumferentially work up to the elbow
- Scrub each side of each finger, between the fingers, and the back and front of the hand for 2 minutes
- Proceed to scrub the arms, keeping the hand higher than the arm at all times. This prevents bacteria-laden soap and water from contaminating the hand
- Wash each side of the arm to three inches above the elbow for 1 minute
- Repeat the process on the other hand and arm, keeping hands above elbows at all times. If the hand touches anything except the brush at any time, the scrub must be lengthened by 1 minute for the area that has been contaminated
- Rinse hands and arms by passing them through the water in one direction only, from fingertips to elbow. Do not move the arm back and forth through the water
- The hands should be held above elbows once the procedure is completed
- If the hands and arms are grossly soiled, the scrub time should be lengthened
- At all times during the scrub procedure, care should be taken not to splash water onto surgical attire
- Once in the operating room suite, hands and arms should be dried using a sterile towel and aseptic technique.

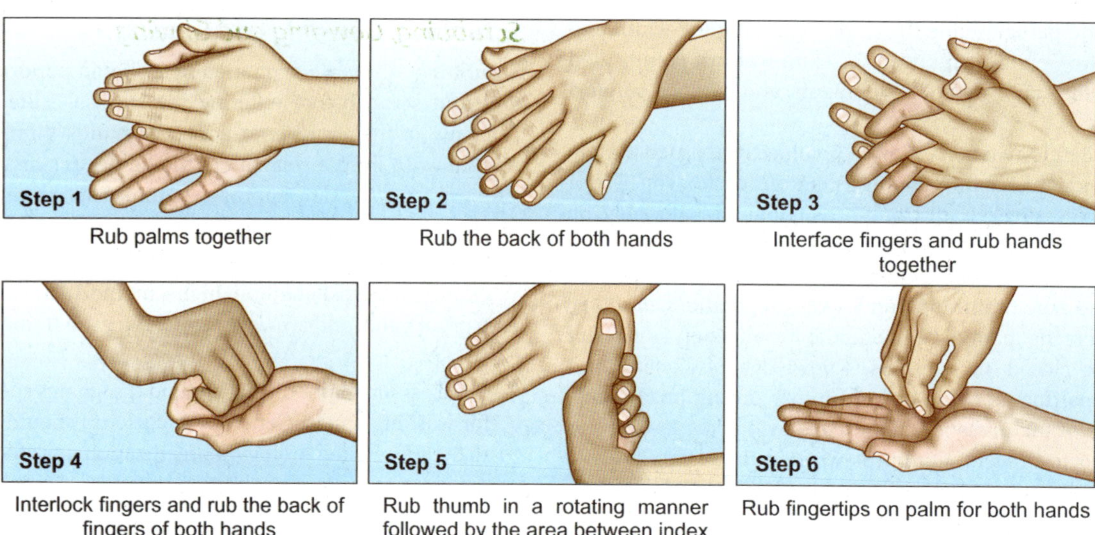

Rub palms together

Rub the back of both hands

Interface fingers and rub hands together

Interlock fingers and rub the back of fingers of both hands

Rub thumb in a rotating manner followed by the area between index finger and thumb for both hands

Rub fingertips on palm for both hands

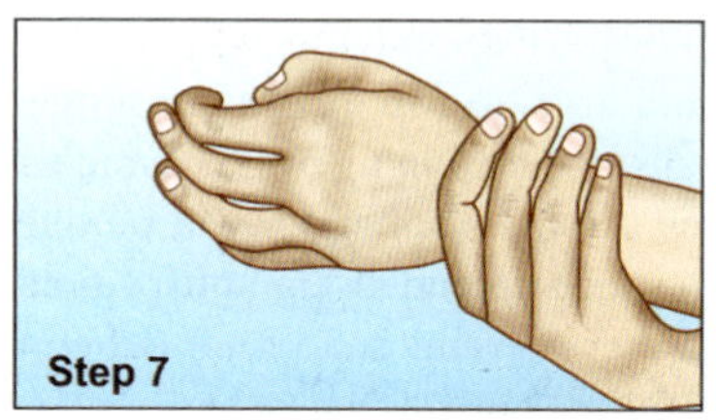

Rub both wrists in a rotating manner, rinse and dry thoroughly

FIG. 6.1: Scrubbing of hands

Surgical hand antiseptics is required of all sterile members of the surgical team (scrub assistant, surgeon, and assistant). This is done to eliminate dirt, skin oil, and transient microorganisms, to decrease the microbial count as much as possible; and to inhibit rapid rebound growth of microorganisms. The agent used for antisepsis should be an effective antimicrobial agent. It should significantly reduce microorganisms on the skin; contain a nonirritating; antimicrobial preparation; be broad spectrum and fast acting; and have a persistent effect. The procedure should be standardized for all personnel. When the procedure of scrubbing is the chosen method for surgical hand antisepsis, the team members fingers and hands should be scrubbed first with progression to the forearms and elbows. The hands should be held away from surgical attire and higher than the elbows at all times to prevent contamination from clothing or detergent suds and water from draining from the unclean area above the elbows to the clean and previously scrubbed areas of the hands and fingers. Waterless, alcohol-based agents are replacing traditional soap and water in many facilities. When a waterless hand rub product is chosen, the team member should first wash and dry hands and forearms with soap and water.

Gowning: Gowning is an important procedure of the scrubbing process. In order to minimize the risk of contaminating the sterile operative set up during the process of gowning and gloving a separate table should be used. Only the scrub nurse should gown and glove herself, the rest should avoid self gowning and gloving. Members of the team should be gowned and gloved as soon as they enter the room. Once gowned and gloved, they should remain in the sterile end of the room until the patient is draped and the sterile setup is moved into place. During any waiting period, the sterile gowned and gloved members of the team must keep their hands as above waist level in front of them during this time. They should never sit, place their hands on lap or fold their hands. During the surgery if the gown is contaminated with blood or fluids, it should be changed immediately.

Steps of gowning (Fig. 6.2)

- The first step in wearing gown is to select the appropriate type and size of gown
- The gown is then opened in the pack
- Unfold the gown. Hold the gown so that the opening faces you
- Then pull up the arms through the sleeves one at a time and then over the shoulders
- Once the gown is on the shoulders secure at the neck and waist
- Tie the neck strings so that the gown overlaps
- Tie the waist strings so that the gown ends overlap.

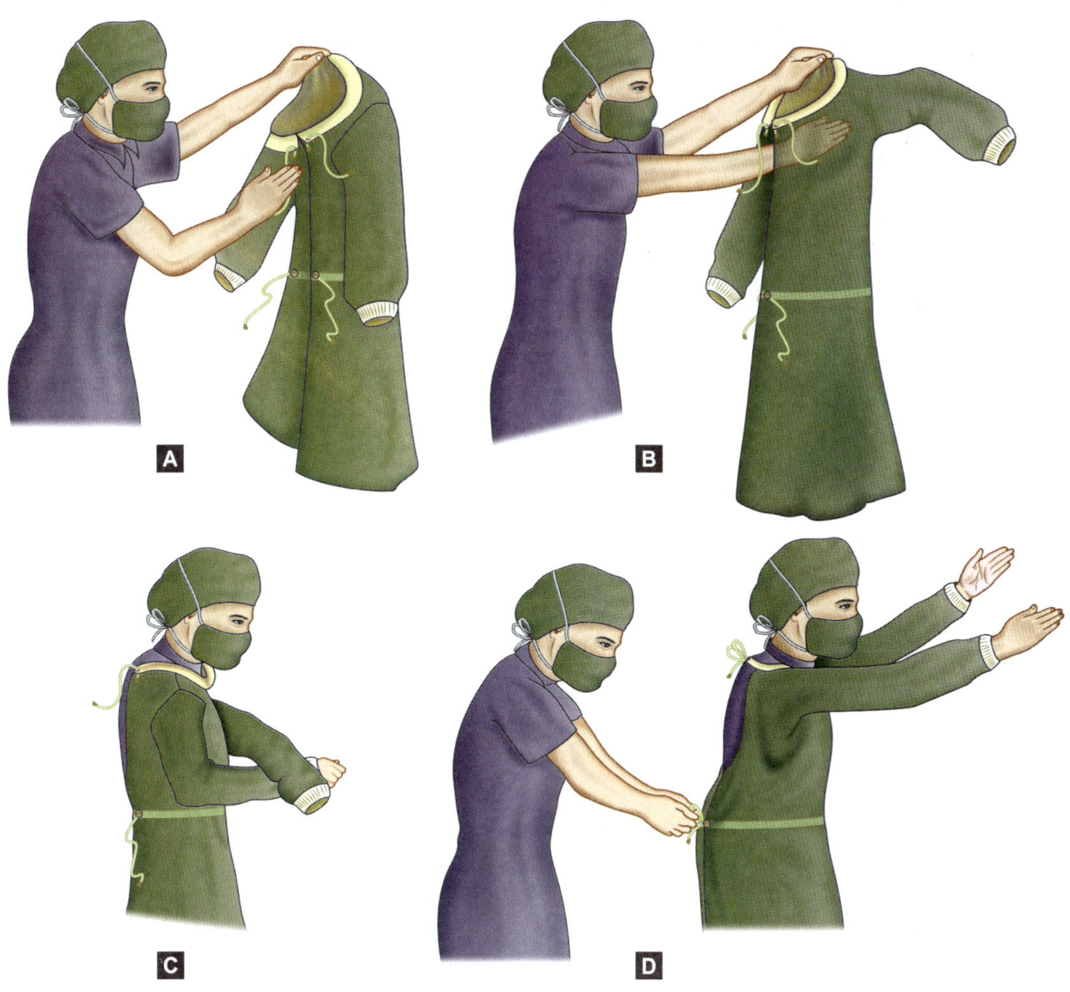

FIGS 6.2A TO D: Putting on a sterile gown
(*Note*: All shaded areas are considered as contaminated)

Removing the gown

- If the gown is disposable and designed to be removed quickly, the gloves may be removed with the gown and rolled together to prevent contamination
- If not using a breakaway gown, it is important to untie the waist tie before removing the gloves
- If not using a breakaway gown, untie the gown at the neck and pull it away from the shoulders with ungloved hands
- Then roll gown into a bundle with ungloved hands, it is important to avoid contact with outside of the gown.

Gloving: Gloves provide a barrier against potentially infectious microorganisms that can be found in blood, other body fluids, and waste. Gloves act as a barrier that protects health care workers and clients. Several recent studies have shown that "double gloving" (wearing two surgical gloves of each hand) may reduce the risk of contamination of the provider's hands with blood and other matter during major surgical procedures.

Steps for putting on surgical gloves (Fig. 6.3)

- The first step in gloving is to determine the appropriate glove size
- Prepare a large, clean, dry area for opening the package of gloves
- Scrub the and for surgery and ask someone (e.g. circulating nurse) to open the package of gloves
- Open the inner glove wrapper, exposing the cuffed gloves with the palms up
- Pick up the first glove by the cuff, touching only the inside portion of the cuff (the inside is the side that will be touching your skin when the glove is on)
- While holding the cuff in one hand, slip your other hand into the glove (pointing the fingers of the glove toward the floor will keep the fingers open). Be careful not to touch anything, and hold the gloves above your waist level

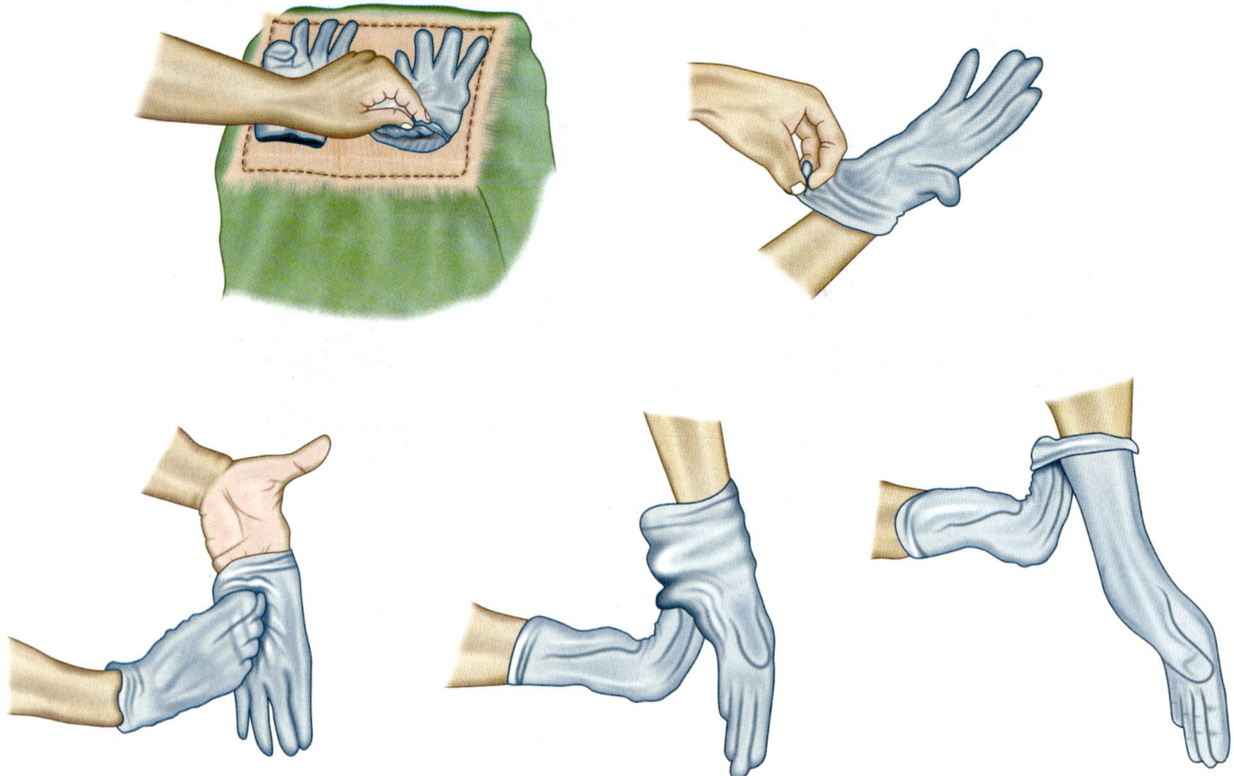

FIG. 6.3: Wearing gloves

- Pick up the second glove by sliding the fingers of the gloved hand under the cuff of the second glove. Be careful not to contaminate the gloved hand with the ungloved hand
- Put the second glove on the ungloved hand by maintain a steady pull through the cuff. Adjust the glove fingers and cuffs until the gloves fit comfortably.

Steps for removing surgical gloves

- Grasp on glove near the cuff and pull it partway off. The glove will turn inside out
- Keep the first glove partially on before removing the second one the protect from touching the outside of a glove with bare hand
- Leaving the first glove over the fingers, grasp the second glove near the cuff and pull it partway off. Keep the second glove partially on
- Pull of the two gloves at the same time, being careful to touch only the inside surface of the gloves with bare hand and make sure not to result in splashes in the environment
- Dispose off the gloves immediately and wash hands immediately after gloves are removed.

Once surgical hand antisepsis is completed, the team members enter the OT to put the surgical gowns and gloves. Because the gowns and gloves are sterile, it is permissible for the scrubbed people to manipulate and organize all sterile items for use during the procedure.

Basic Aseptic Technique

To prevent infections, aseptic technique is practiced in the OT. This is implemented through the creation and maintenance of a sterile field. The center of the sterile field is the site of the surgical incision.

There are specific principles that the team members should understand to practice aseptic technique. Unless these principles are followed, the safety of the patient is compromised, and the potential for postoperative infection is increased. It presents basic principles of aseptic technique.

- All materials that enter the sterile field must be sterile
- If a sterile item comes in contact with an unsterile item, it is contaminated
- Contaminated items should be removed immediately from the sterile field
- Sterile team members must wear only sterile gowns and gloves; once dressed for the procedure, they should recognize that the only parts of the gown considered sterile are the front from chest to table level and the sleeves to 2 inches above the elbow

- A wide margin of safety must be maintained between the sterile and unsterile fields
- Tables are considered sterile only at tabletop level; items extending beneath this level are considered contaminated
- The edges of a sterile package are considered contaminated once the package has been opened
- Bacteria travel on airborne particles and will enter the sterile field with excessive air movements and currents
- Bacteria travel by capillary action through moist fabrics and contamination occurs
- Bacteria harbor on the patients and the team members hair, skin, and respiratory tracts and must be confined by appropriate attire.

In addition to following the principles of aseptic technique, the surgical team is responsible for following the guidelines to protect the patient and the team from exposure to blood-borne pathogens. These guidelines emphasize standard and transmission-based precautions; engineering and work practice controls; and the use of personal protective equipment such as gloves, gowns, aprons, caps, face shields, masks, and protective eyewear. This is especially important in the OT environment because of the high potential for exposure to blood-borne pathogens.

Assisting the Anesthesia Care Provider

While the perioperative nurse checks the OT to complete its preparation, the anesthesia care provider (ACP) prepares the patient for the administration of the anesthetic. The nurse must understand the mechanism of anesthetic administration and the pharmacologic effects of the agents. The nurse should know the location of all emergency drugs and equipment in the OT area.

The circulating nonsterile perioperative nurse may be involved in placing monitoring devices to be used during the surgical procedure (e.g. urinary catheter, ECG leads). If the patient is to have a general anesthetic, the nurse remains at the patient's side to ensure safety and to assist the ACP. These responsibilities may include obtaining blood pressure measurements and assisting in the maintenance of the patient's airway. During the surgical procedure, the circulating nonsterile perioperative nurse also provides a vital communication link for the ACP to ancillary departments such as the laboratory or blood bank.

Maintenance of Safety

All surgical procedures, regardless of where they take place, can put the patient at risk for injury. These injuries can be infectious, physical trauma from positioning or equipment used, or physiologic effects of surgery itself. The perioperative nurse must be alert to all safety issues as the patient in the OT is often compromised from the effects of anesthesia. Smoke particles produced during laser procedures may contain trace hydrocarbons, including acetone, isopropanol, toluene, formaldehyde, and cyanide. These airborne contaminates can cause respiratory irritation and have mutagenic and carcinogenic potential. Smoke evacuators may be used to minimize this exposure. Care must be taken with correct placement of the grounding pad and all aspects of the electrosurgical equipment to prevent injury from burns of fire. All members of the surgical team stop what they are doing during a *surgical time-out* just before the procedure is started to verify patient identification, surgical procedure, and surgical site.

It is the responsibility of the nurses to be aware of latex allergies, necessary precautions and products that are latex free. Nursing staff also at risk for development of latex allergy secondary to repeated exposure to latex products.

Positioning the Patient

Positioning the patient is a critical part of every procedure and usually follows administration of the anesthetic. The ACP will indicate when to begin the positioning. The position of the patient should allow for accessibility to the operative site, administration and monitoring of anesthetic agents, and maintenance of the patients airway. When positioning for the surgical procedure, care must be used to (1) provide correct skeletal alignment; (2) prevent undue pressure on nerves; (3) provide for adequate thoracic excursion; (4) prevent occlusion of arteries and veins; (5) provide modesty in exposure; and (6) recognize and respect individual needs such as previously assessed aches, pains, or deformities. It is a nursing responsibility to secure the extremities, provide adequate padding and support, and obtain sufficient physical or mechanical help to avoid unnecessary straining of self or patient.

Various positions in which the patient may be placed include supine, prone, Trendelenburg, lateral, kidney, lithotomy, jackknife, and sitting. The supine is the most common used. It is suited for surgery involving the abdomen, heart, and breast. The prone position allows easy access for back surgeries (e.g. laminectomies). The lithotomy position is used for some types of pelvic organ surgery (e.g. vaginal hysterectomy) (Fig. 6.4).

Whatever position is required for the procedure, great care is taken to prevent injury to the patient. Because anesthesia has blocked the nerve impulses, the patient will not feel pain or discomfort, or stress being placed on the nerves, muscles, bones, and skin. Improper positioning could potentially result in muscle strain, joint damage, pressure ulcers, nerve damage, and other untoward effects.

General anesthesia causes peripheral vessels to dilate. Position changes affect where the pooling of blood occurs. If the head of the OT bed is raised, the lower torso will have increased blood volume and the upper torso may become compromised. Hypovolemia and cardiovascular disease can

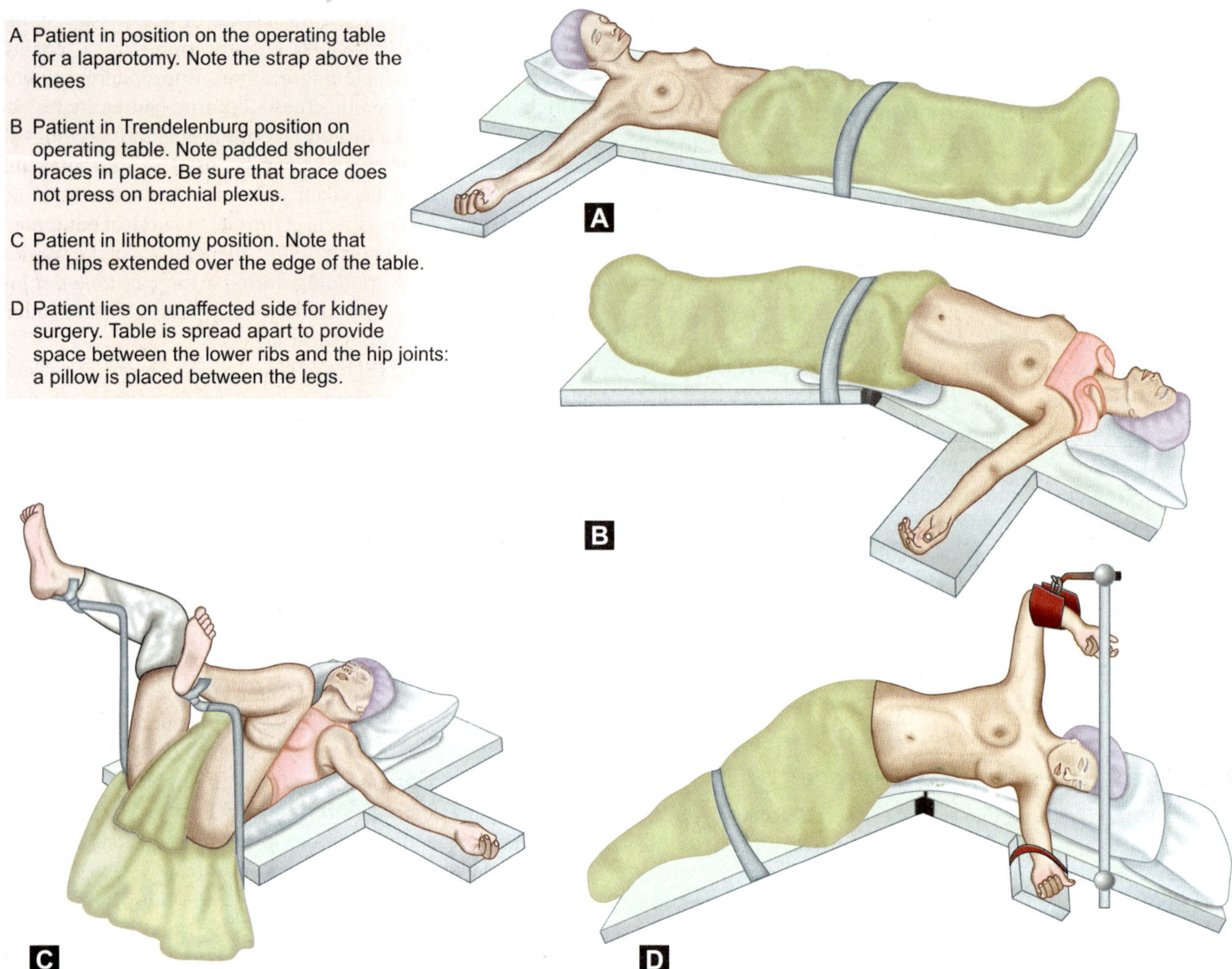

FIGS 6.4A TO D: Positions on the operating table. All surgical patients wear caps to cover the hair completely

further compromise the patient's status. Consequently the perioperative nurse, working with the entire surgical team, carefully plans and implements the patients positioning, and then closely monitors the patient throughout the surgical procedure.

Preparing the Surgical Site

The purpose of skin preparation, or "prepping", is to reduce the number of organisms available to migrate to the surgical wound. The task of prepping is usually the responsibility of the circulating nurse.

The skin is prepared by mechanically scrubbing or cleansing around the surgical site with antimicrobial agents identified as being nonallergic to the patient. Hair that will interfere with the surgical procedure is removed. The area is then scrubbed in a circular motion. The principle of scrubbing from the clean area (site of the incision) to the dirty area (periphery) is observed at all times. A liberal area is cleansed to allow for added protection and unexpected occurrences during the procedure.

Patient After Surgery

Through constant observation of the surgical progress, the ACP anticipates the end of the surgical procedure and uses appropriate types and doses of anesthetic agents so that their effects will be minimal at the end of the surgical procedure. This also allows greater physiologic control of the patient during the transfer to the Post Anesthesia Care Unit (PACU) or Post Operative Care Unit (POCU). The patient's response to nursing care is evaluated by the OR nurse based on outcome criteria established during the development of the patients plan of care. The ACP and the perioperative nurse or another member of the surgical team accompany the patient to the PACU. A report of the patient's status and the procedure is communicated to the nurse receiving the patient in the PACU to promote safe, continuing care.

ANESTHESIA

Anesthesia is derived from Greek word "*anaisthesis*" which means "not sensation". This term was listed in Bailey's dictionary in 1721. The word anesthesia was used to describe the namely discovered effect of ether. Werr kitchel called it as Death of pain. The word anesthesia was first suggested by Oliver Wendell Holmes. It is defined as the absence or abolition of sensation.

Criteria for choosing anesthesia

- Type, duration and extent of surgery
- Patient's hemodynamic stability
- Presence and severity of co-existing diseases
- Patient mental and emotional status
- The postoperative recovery from various kinds of anesthesia
- Options for management of postoperative pan
- Surgeon preference and any particular requirements of the surgeon.

General anesthesia is a reversible, unconscious state characterized by amnesia (sleep, hypnosis), analgesia (freedom from pain) depression of reflexes and muscle relaxation.

Anesthesia is a mandatory component of the surgical department. Anesthesia in some or the other form is required for every surgery. Thus, nurses must understand this field to an extent that they utilize this information in supporting the patient and the health care team.

Anesthesia Administration

Anesthesia means the absence of pain (Greek: an = without + aisthesis = feeling). Anesthesia is an artificially-induced state of partial or total loss of sensation, with or without loss of consciousness. Anesthesia produces muscle relaxation, blocks transmission of nerve impulses and suppresses reflexes.

There are two types of anesthesia, i.e. general anesthesia and regional anesthesia.

Types of Anesthesia

Anesthesia can be dividing into various catagories on the basis of method of administration and the parts involved in its effect.

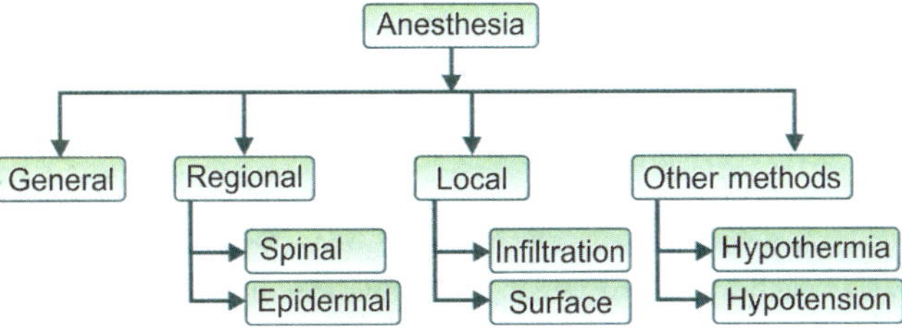

General Anesthesia

This type of anesthesia is required for extensive surgeries. It involves sensual loss in the overall body. Since general anesthesia involves the whole body and may disturb some physiological balances, suitability of the client for anesthesia must be assessed. This is generally referred to as pre-anesthetic checkup (PAC). This assessment involves a thorough examination of body for its ability to literate the stress of anesthesias intubation.

Any signs of infection, hyperthermia altered blood pressure and respiratory compromise may render the patient insuitable for general anesthesia. In suitable clients, some medication may be given prior to surgery. These medicators are called pre-medicationis. These medications facilitate anesthesia administration, relaxes the patient, keeps his anxiety level low. In addition, pre-medications also reduces the respiratory tract secretions and cardiac activity.

Types of pre-medications

1. **Anticholenergics:** These drugs act to diminish the respiratory tract secretions which may interfere with intubation and administration of inhalation anesthesia. These drugs also reduces heart rate suppresses severe reflexes. Examples of this group of drugs are atropine and scopolamine.
2. **Opiates:** These drugs help in causing relaxation and thus contributes to reduction of anxiety. However, patient should not be left attended as the patient becomes drowsy. These drugs include morphine and meperidine.
3. **Barbiturates and tranquilizers:** They are generally given in the night before the surgery to facilitate sound sleep as surgery associated anxiety may induce sleeplessness. Examples of this group of drugs include phenobarbital.

Antibiotics: Since surgery exposes the body tissues to external environment, part operative infections may be expected. Thus antibiotics may be given prophylactically preferably just before the incision is made.

Once pre-medication is done, patient is taken for general anesthesia. The two modes of general anesthesia are:

1. **Intravenous:** When anesthetic drugs are administered intravenously to achieve anesthetic effect, it is called intravenous anesthesia. This is a rapid mode of achieving unconsciousness and may take less than 1 minute. Although this mode may be an initiating phase for inhalation anesthesia, it can also be used alone for some minor surgical procedures like dental extraction, some painful examinations.
2. **Inhalation anesthesia:** When the anesthetic drugs are administered as volatile liquids and gases in the form of inhalation, this is referred to as inhalation anesthesia. The mixture of drugs can be given through a mask or through endotracheal intubation. Commonly used inhalation drugs are halothane and nitrous oxide.

General anesthesia is a drug-induced depression of the central nervous system (CNS) that is reverted either by metabolic elimination in the body or by pharmocologic means. General anesthetic agents produces analgesia, amnesia and unconsciousness, characterized by loss of reflexes and muscle tone.

There are four stages of anesthesia. Brief explanation and nursing intervention in these stages are as follows:

Onset: Starts from anesthetic administration to loss of consciousness. In this stage, client may be drowsy or dizzy and may experience auditory or visual hallucinations. Nursing action in this stage will include, close operating room doors, keeping room quiet, and standby to assist client.

Excitement: Starts from loss of consciousness to loss of eyelid reflexes. Here there will be increase in automatic activity, irregular breathing, client may struggle. In this stage, nurse has to remain quietly at client's side, assist anesthetists if needed.

Surgical anesthesia: This stage starts with loss of eyelid reflexes, to lose of motor reflexes and depression of vital function. Here client is unconscious, muscles are relaxed and no blink or gag reflexes. In this stage, begin preparation (if indicated) only when anesthetists indicate stage III has been reached and client is under good control.

Danger (death) stage experiences: Vital functions too depressed may lead to respiratory and circulatory failure. In this stage, client is not breathing and he may or may not have a heartbeat. If arrest occurs, nurse responds immediately to assist establishing airway, provide cardiac arrest tray, drugs, syringes, long needles, assist surgeon with closed or open cardiac massage.

General anesthesia can be administered by inhalation or intravenously. An inhalation agent will include nitrous oxide, halothane (fluothane) enflurane (ethrane) and isoflurane (forane) and the intravenous drugs are thiopental sodium (pentothal), fentanyl citrate droperidol (innovar) and ketamine hydrochloride. The selections of anesthetic agents are according to decision of the anesthesiologist. But continuous monitoring of side effects of the drugs, vital signs are essential.

Regional Anesthesia

Regional anesthesia blocks the pain stimulus at the origin and along afferent neurons of along the spinal cord. Regional anesthesia produces a loss of painful sensation in only one region of the body and does not result in unconsciousness. The client may receive sedative that produces drowsiness. The Regional anesthetic agents block the conduction of impulses in nerve fiber without depolarizing the cell membrane are: Local agents and topical agents. An example of local agents are Bupivacaine HCl (Marcaine HCl) (xylocaine) and examples of topical agents will include benzocaine, ethylchloride spray, tetracaine HCl. All these agents have their own side effects. Contraindication for children, test dose can be given prior to use of these agents to know any allergies to these agents.

The types of regional anesthesia are:

- Topical anesthesia
- Local infiltration anesthesia
- Field block anesthesia
- Peripheral nerve block anesthesia
- Spinal anesthesia
- Epidural anesthesia
- Caudal anesthesia.

The other types of anesthesia are used in modern drugs acupuncture, cryothermia and hypnoanesthesia. The type of anesthesia chosen depends on the surgery performed and level of unconscious desired.

These anesthetic agents work by blocking the impulse conduction through the nerve fibers without cell membrane depolarization. This type of anesthesia can be given in a number of different ways. It is often divided into two categories, i.e.

1. **Major conduction anesthesia (or central):** This type of anesthesia allows the patient to control his own respiration. Less medication is required to achieve the effect and their enhancement of postoperative analgesic affect. Moreover, there may be beneficial effects on cardiopulmonary function coagulation and less blood loss. This mode includes spinal and epidural anesthesia. Both these anesthesia disrupt afferent neural impulse by depositing the drug close to the spinal cord.

   The common types are explained here:

   a. **Spinal anesthesia:** This anesthesia is very suitable for surgeries involving lower parts of the body. Since this type of anesthesia does not cause unconsciousness, it is highly preferred in surgeries of lower half of the body and for the clients unsuitable for inhalation of general anesthesia. This method is comparatively safe and requires minimal preoperative preparation such as empty stomach. Spinal anesthesia is also referred to as subarachnoid block. On the basis of site of insertion of anesthetic agent spinal anesthesia may be categorised as low, mid or high spinal (Fig. 6.5).

      i. **Low spinal anesthesia:** This is also called saddle or caudal block and is used for surgeries of perineal and rectal areas.

      ii. **Mid spinals:** This type of anesthesia is generally given below the level of umbilicus at T_{10}. Hernial repair, appendectomy are the surgeries which can be performed using this level of spinal anesthesia

      iii. **High spinals:** This type of anesthesia is given higher on the spine generally at the middle line at T_4 level. This level is used for obstratical surgeries such as cesarian section.

   b. **Epidural anesthesia:** This is also a major conduction anesthesia involving epidural space. This is the space in the spinal cord which is outside the dura mater. Effects

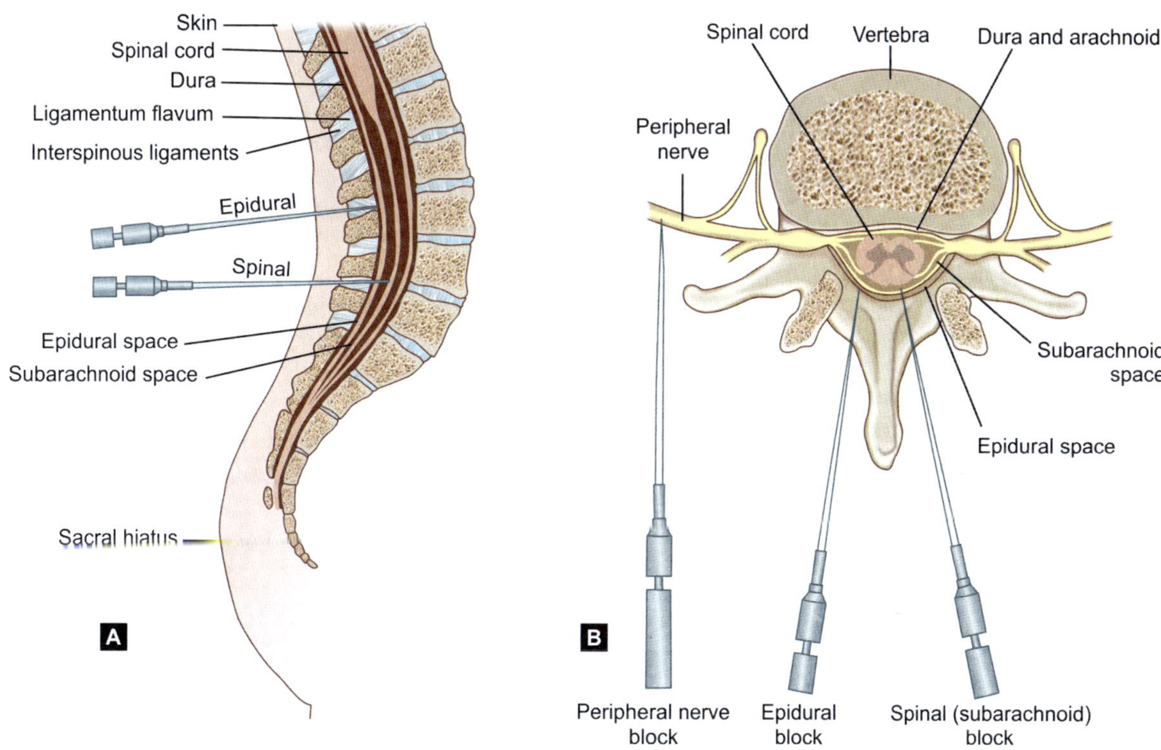

FIGS 6.5A AND B: (A) Injection sites for spinal and epidural anesthesia; (B) Cross-section of injection sites for peripheral nerve, epidural, and spinal blocks

similar to spinal anesthesia are achieved with an injection of anesthetic age into the epidural space. This anesthesia has emerged as the most popular means of pain relief during lobar and has received recognition for the painless deficiency. The benefit of this type of anesthesia is it provides analgesia and pain relief rather than complete lack of feelings. These are two basic modes of giving epidurals:

i. Regular epidurals: As the name indicates regular epidural involves continuous slow infusion of anesthetic agent (general narcotics such as fentanyl or morphine) by using a pump or periodic injections into the epidural space.
ii. Combined spinal epidural: This combined mode of anesthetization is also called as walking epidural because of freedom it provides in the movements own during anesthesia. In this technique first an epidural needle is positioned followed by a spinal needle is placed a quick acting narcotic is given through it to achieve the analgesic effect.

2. **Nerve blockage:** This is also a form of regional anesthesia as it involves anesthetic effect only on a selected portion of the body. This mode of anesthesia offer the benefits of providing intensive anesthetic effect and muscle relaxation to a limited portion of the body. Thus maintaining other vital functions irrespective of the generalized effects of anesthesia. In addition the post-surgical analgesic effect is also prolonged. Commonly used modes of major nerve block are as follows:
   i. **Peripheral nerve block:** This form anesthetize individual nerves or nerve plexus. Commonly used drugs used for nerve block are lidocaine, bupivacaine, etc. The drug is injected along the nerve and not the nerve. This minimizes the risk of nerve damage. This peripheral nerve block coma be used for individual nerves such as digital nerve block for a finger commonly used plexus block are:
      a. Brachial plexus block: This block is used for surgeries on arm or shoulder. It may be given as intercalene, supraclavicular and axillary.
      b. Cervical plexus block: This block is used for neck and carotid artery procedures.
      c. Femoral-sciatic nerve block is used for upper and lower leg surgeries.
      d. Para-vertebral block may be used for upper abdominal and thoracic procedures.
      e. Other blocks: Some other blocks are popliteal fossa block for lower leg procedures, retrobulbar blocks for eye procedures, 3 in one nerve (femoral, obturator and lateral femoral cutaneous nerves) blocks for upper leg procedures.

ii. **Field block anesthesia:** This type of anesthesia is used to create a barrier between the area to be operated and the nervous system by injecting and infilterating the area proximal to the incision with a local anesthetic agent. In this block, all the local nerves are anesthetized contrary to nerve plexus block where individual plexus or major nerve is anesthetized.

3. **Intravenous regional extremity block ansthesia (Bieri block):** As the name indicates it is the use of intravenous anesthetic agent such as lidocaine to achieve the anesthetic effect in an extremity. Since the vein is used for injecting the agent, the desired limb has to be applied with a dual ruff tourniquet for 2 hours so that the drug does not circulate beyond the area in which anesthesia is desired.
4. **Local anesthesia (infilteration):** This is the most common form of anesthesia used in day-to-day hospital procedures. This method interferes with neural transmission to produce its effect. Local anesthetic agents such as lidocain (xylocaine) is infilteratd into the skin and the subcutaneous tissue of the site where anesthetic effect is to be achieved. However, care should be taken, not to inject the agent into the vein by aspirating before the membrane of the nerve and inhibit transmission of nerve impulses by reducing the membrane permeability for sodium and displacement of calcium ions. Thus the threshold potential for the activation of depolarization is not achieved making it unable to conduct the action potential. This duration of action depends on the time the anesthetic agent is in contact with the nerve fibers. These drugs can be used to produce both sensory and motor block. Local anesthetic agents are weak bases and are poorly soluble in water. They are thus available as their water soluble, hydrocholoride salts.

   Local anesthesia can also be given as a spray or topical application. Such technique is generally used as a spray lignocain jelly for pain control in minor nasal procedures, nasogastric tube insertion, etc.

Other Methods of Anesthesia

In addition to the methods discussed above some less common methods are also used in certain surgeries. At times a combination of two or more methods may be used to achieve better effect and acceptability. For example, epidural anesthesia may be obtained with a general anesthetic for a repeat hip replacement.

Some other methods include acupuncture, cryothermia, and normovalemic hypotension. These methods prevent hematocrit blood loss. However, their usge is limited only to some rare situations such as unsuitability of the patient for other forms of anesthesia.

Nursing care during surgery will include providing emotional care, assessing the client with positioning (as required for type of surgery) maintaining safety, maintaining surgical asepsis, prevent client heat loss, monitoring malignant hyperthermia, assisting with surgeon to perform surgery by providing proper equipments and supplies, assisting with wound closure, assessing drainage, and transferring client to recovery room.

Anesthetists and anesthesiologists use the physical (P) status classification system to describe the patients general status and identify potential risks surgery. There are six classes of physical status:

- P1. A normal healthy patient .

  Example: No systemic abnormality, localized infection without fever, benign tumor, hernia.
- P2. A patient with mild systemic disease, without functional limitations.

  Example: Well-controlled hypertension, well-controlled diabetes mellitus, chronic bronchitis, obesity, age over 80 years.
- P3. A patient with severe systemic disease associated with functional limitations.

  Example: Severe disease, compensated heart failure, myocardial infraction more than 6 months ago, angina pectoris, severe dysrhythmia, cirrhosis, poorly controlled diabetes or hypertension, ileus.
- P4. A patient with an incapacitating systemic disease that is a constant threat to life.

  Example: Sever heart failure, myocardial infarction less than 6 months ago, severe respiratory failure, advanced liver or renal failure.
- P5. A moribund patient who is not expected to survive for 24 hours with or without operation.

  Example: Unconscious patient with traumatic head injury and agonal respirations.
- P6. Patient is brain dead and is being prepared as an organ donor.

Stage of Anesthesia

There are four stages of delivering anesthesia. Although these four stages were categorized on the basis of ether as the agent for anesthesia, which is no more in use because of its explosive nature, they can be applied to any form of modern general anesthesia. Since the mode of action of present day anesthetic drugs is comparatively quite rapid, these stages may not be readily identifiable.

Different anesthetic agent may have distinctive stages. For example, nitrous oxide has a highly analgesic effect while thiopental does not show stage 1 at all. The four stages described here are based upon patients body movements, respiratory rhythm, oculomotor reflexes and muscle tone. As nurses it is important to remember than hearing is the last sense to be depressed during anesthesia, so a quite atmosphere should be maintained during anesthesia induction, as well as reversal as hearing is also the first sense to be returned.

The four stages of anesthesia were given by Arthur Guedel in 1937, which were framed on the basis of the use of diethyl ether for general anesthesia. Yet they are applicable to modern agent as well with some variations.

1. **Stage 1 (Analgesia):** This stage is also referred as the stage of amnesia. It extends from induction till there is loss of eyelid reflex. The speed with a patient progresses depends upon the amount and charactersitcis of the anesthetic agent being used. This stage has been considered as a period of altered consciousness. During this stage, the patient may become drowsy or dizy and may have hallucinations. A nurse, is important to maintain silence in the room and assist the client. Although patient can communicate when induction to initiate, he may feel the transition very fast.
2. **Stage 2:** This stage was called as "delirium by Guedel". Commonly stage is referred to as the stage of excitement. This stage is marked by the patient becoming unconscious but the body may respond to some stimuli irrationally and reflexually. This stage may not occur with some ultra short acting drugs such as barbiturates. This stage extends from loss of consciousness to the onset of automatic respiration. During this stage pupils may become dilated and some untoward signs such as breath holding, hypoxia, hypertension, tachycardia, laryngospasm and vomiting may occur. The nurses must always anesthetize the patient and be ready to support and assist the patient.
3. **Stage 3:** This stage is known as the surgical anesthesia stage. This stage extends from the onset of automatic respiration to respiratory paralysis and it characterized by increased muscular relaxation, absence of protective pharyngotracheal, eyelid and conjunctival reflexes. The patients reaction to surgical manipulation should be continously observed. This is the actual stage, during which the surgery is performed. On the initiation of surgical manipulations such as incision if there is no response by the patient, if the respirations are mouth, if eyelid reflex is absent and the patient's color is good, it is justified to proceed with the surgery.
4. **Stage 4:** This stage is called as overdose stage. As the name suggest, it generally means that too much anesthetic has been given to the patient which has led him to move from respiratory paralysis to death. All the reflex activities are lost and pupils may be widely dilated. As a nurse, it is important to observe the patient and monitor carefully. If cardiac arrest occurs immediate assistance in establishing airway, CPR, cardiac arrest tray and required drugs must be provided to save the patient's life. Without ventilatory support and cardic support, the patient may die at this point.

Guedel also described various planes within the surgical anesthesia stage (stage 3). These planes are based on progressive suppression of ocular signs and respiratory activity.

1. **Plane 1:** This is the period from return of regular respiration to the cessation rapid eye movement. This plane generally considered as light anesthesia.
2. **Plane 2:** This is the plane of medium anesthesia characterized by increasing intercostal paralysis. This plane is from cessation of eyeball movement to the beginning of intercostal muscles. Although there is respiratory reflex, irritability is increased, there is loss of laryngeal reflex, corneal reflex may also be lost. Respiration is automatic, regular and deep.
3. **Plane 3:** This is the plane of deep anesthesia characterized by diaphragmatic respiration. This plane is from beginning to completion of intercostal muscle paralysis. Pupils are dilated and light reflex is abolished. This plane used to be the most suitable plane for surgeon before the introduction of muscle relaxant in anesthesiology.
4. **Plane 4:** This plane is considered to be from complete intercostal paralysis till diaphragmatic paralysis and may be characterized by presence of apnea.

In 1954, Artusio divided the first stage of Guedel's classification into further 3 planes

1. First Plane: No amnesia or analgesia.
2. Second Plane: Complete amnesia but parital analgesia.
3. Third Plane: Complete amnesia as well as analgesia.

This classification into four stages was basically designated for sole inhalation anesthetic agent 'ether' with patients given morphine and atrophine as pre-medication. During that time muscle relaxants and intravenous anesthetics were not used. However, with the advent of modern modes of anesthesia, some of the signs typical of each stage may not be detectable making Guedel's classification obsolete. Although controversial 'BIS monitor' may be better estimate of depth of anesthesia in the light of modern anesthesiology.

Bispectral index (BIS) is a modern technology in monitoring the depth of anesthesia which purports to replace or supplement Guedel's classification system, under the light of usage of modern nodes of general anesthesia. Use of this index allows better adjustment of anesthesia agents and thus facilitates more rapid emergence from anesthesia. This system was introduced by Aspect Medical system, Inc in `994. It is statistically based, empirically derived complex parameter. It is weighted sum of EEG subparameters including a time and frequency domain and high order spectral subparameters. This monitors utilizes a gradation scale from O (EEG silence) to 100 (awake/alert EEG). BIS value of 40 to 60 is considered as the appropriate level for general anesthesia (manufacturer recommendation). On the basis of plotting of the patient on this scale, the depth of anesthesia could be estimated. The value on 0–100 scale is generated through the complex EEG signal analysis which is processed into a single member. This single member is used as a guide to identify, the depth of anesthesia and any alterations needed in the anesthesia delivery. The major disadvantage of BIS is that in some cases this scale may underestimate the depth of anesthesia, leading to administration of higher than necessary dose of anesthetic agents.

Instruments Used for Anesthesia

As with any procedure, anesthesia administration requires some important instruments to be gathered and checked before anesthesia is to be administered. The instruments for a local anesthesia generally are available in all health care facilities and may not require any specific preparation. However, for general anesthesia highly specialized machines and equipments would be required. The most commonly used instruments are:

- Continuous flow anesthetic machine
- Anesthetic vaporizers
- Oxygen masks
- Nasal oxygen set
- Guedel airways.

For anesthetic delivery method see Figure 6.6.

Surgical Asepsis Maintenance

Surgical asepsis prevents the contamination of surgical wounds. The patients natural skin flora or a previously existing infection may cause postoperative wound infection. Rigorous adherence to the principles of surgical asepsis by OT personnel is basic to preventing surgical site infections. All surgical supplies, instruments, needles, sutures, dressings, gloves, covers and solutions that may come in contact with the surgical wound or exposed tissues must be sterilized before use. Traditionally, the surgeon, surgical assistants, and nurses prepared themselves by scrubbing their hands and arms with antiseptic soap and water, but this traditional practice is being challenged by research investigating the optimal length of time of scrub and the best preparation to use. In some institutions, an alcohol based product or scrubless soap is used to prepare for surgery.

Surgical team members wear long-sleeved, sterile gowns and gloves. Head and hair are covered with a cap, and a mask is worn over the nose and mouth to minimize the possibility that bacteria from the upper respiratory tract will enter the wound. During surgery, only personnel who have scrubbed, gloved, and gowned touch sterilized objects. Nonscrubbed personnel refrain from touching or contaminating anything sterile. An area of the patients skin considerably larger than that requiring exposure during the surgery is meticulously cleansed, and an antiseptic solution is applied. If hair needs to be removed, this is done immediately before the procedure to minimize the risk of wound infection. The remainder of the patient's body is covered with sterile drapes.

In addition to the protocols described previously, surgical asepsis requires meticulous cleaning and maintenance of the OT environment. Floors and horizontal surfaces are cleaned frequently with detergent, soap, and water or a detergent germicide. Sterilizing equipment is inspected regularly to ensure optimal operation and performance. All equipments that come into direct contact with the patient must be sterile. Sterilized linens, drapes, and solutions are used. Instruments are cleaned and sterilized in a unit near the OT. Individually wrapped sterile items are used when additional individual items are needed.

To decrease the amount of bacteria in the air, standard OT ventilation provides 15 air exchanges per hour, at least 3 of which are fresh air. A temperature of 20° to 24° C (68° to 73°F), humidity between 30 to 60%, and positive pressure relative to adjacent areas are maintained. Staff members shed skin scales, resulting in about 1000 bacteria-carrying particles (or colony-forming units [CFUs]) per cubic foot per minute. With the standard air exchanges, air counts of bacteria are reduced to 50 to 150 CFUs per cubic foot per minute. Systems with high-efficiency particulate air (HEPA) filters are needed to remove particles larger than 0.3 μm. Unnecessary personnel and physical movement may be restricted to minimize bacteria in the air and achieve an OT infection rate no greater than 3 to 5% in clean, infection-prone surgery. Some OTs have laminar airflow units. These units provide 400 to 500 air exchanges per hour. When used appropriately, laminar airflow units result in fewer than 10 CFUs per cubic foot per minute during surgery. The goal for a laminar airflow-equipped OT is an infection rate of less than 1%. An OR equipped with this unit is frequently used for total joint replacement or organ transplant surgery.

Despite these precautions, wound contamination may occur during surgery but may only become apparent days or weeks later in the form of a surgical site infection that results in a longer hospital stay. Constant surveillance and conscientious technique in carrying out aseptic practices are necessary to reduce the risk of contamination and infection.

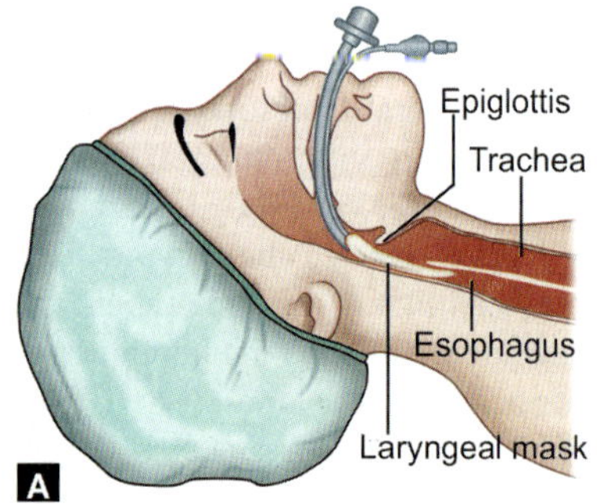

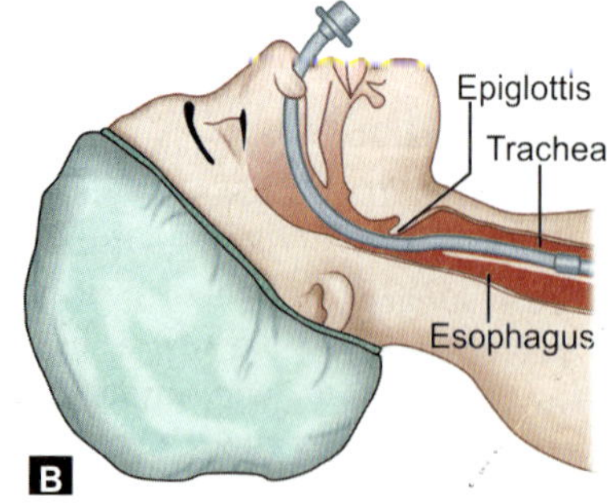

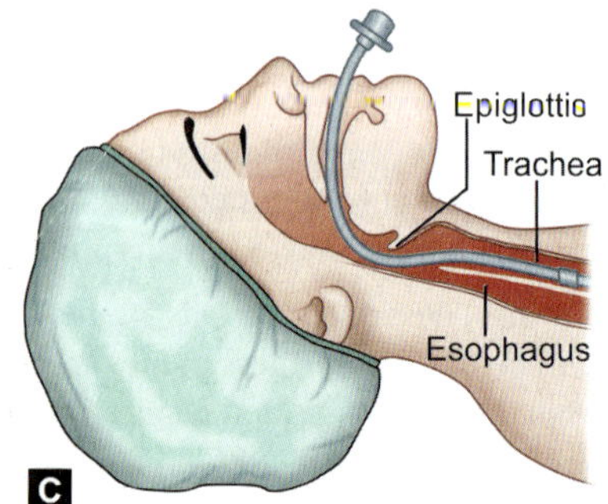

FIGS 6.6A TO C: Anesthetic delivery methods. (A) Laryngeal mask airway (LMA); (B) Nasal endotracheal catheter (in position with cuff inflated); (C) Oral endotracheal intubation (tube is in position with cuff inflated)

All practitioners involved in the intraoperative phase have a responsibility to provide and maintain a safe environment. Adherence to aseptic practice is part of this responsibility. The basic principles of aseptic technique follow:

- All materials in contact with the surgical wound or used within the sterile field must be sterile. Sterile surfaces or articles may touch other sterile surfaces or articles and remain sterile; contact with unsterile objects at any point renders a sterile area contaminated
- Gowns of the surgical team are considered sterile in front from the chest to the level of the sterile field. The sleeves are also considered sterile from 2 inches above the elbow to the stockinette cuff
- Sterile drapes are used to create a sterile field. Only the top surface of a draped table is considered sterile. During draping of a table or patient, the sterile drape is held well above the surface to be covered and is positioned from front to back
- Items are dispensed to a sterile field by methods that preserve the sterility of the items and the integrity of the sterile field. After a sterile package is opened, the edges are considered unsterile. Sterile supplies, including solutions, are delivered to a sterile field or handed to a scrubbed person in such a way that the sterility of the object or fluid remains intact
- The movements of the surgical team are from sterile to sterile and from unsterile to unsterile areas. Scrubbed persons and sterile items contact only unsterile areas
- Movement around a sterile field must not cause contamination of the field. Sterile areas must be kept in view during movement around the area. At least a 1-foot distance from the sterile field must be maintained to prevent inadvertent contamination
- Whenever a sterile barrier is breached, the area must be considered contaminated. A tear or puncture of the drape permitting access to an unsterile surface underneath renders the area unsterile. Such a drape must be replaced
- Every sterile field is constantly monitored and maintained. Items of doubtful sterility are considered unsterile. Sterile fields are prepared as close as possible to the time of use
- The routine administration of hyperoxia (high levels of oxygen) is not recommended to reduce surgical site infections. In a study of 165 patients undergoing general surgery, the rate of surgical site infection was higher in patients who received 80% oxygen during surgery than in those who received 35% oxygen.

Nursing Intervention of Intraoperative Patient

Nursing assessment of the intraoperative patient involves obtaining data from the patient and the patients record to identify variables that can affect care and serve as guidelines for developing an individualized plan of patient care. The intraoperative nurse uses the focused preoperative nursing assessment documented on the patient record. This includes assessment of physiologic status (e.g. health-illness level, level of consciousness), psychological status (e.g. anxiety level, verbal communication problems, coping mechanisms), and physical status (e.g. surgical site, skin condition, and effectiveness of preparation; immobile joints), and ethical concerns.

Based on the assessment data, some major nursing diagnoses may include the following:

- Anxiety related to expressed concerns due to surgery or OR environment
- Risk for perioperative positioning injury related to positioning in the OR (operating room)
- Risk for injury related to anesthesia and surgery
- Disturbed sensory perception (global) related to general anesthesia or sedation.

Based on the assessment data, potential complications may include the following:

- Nausea and vomiting
- Anaphylaxis
- Hypoxia
- Unintentional hypothermia
- Malignant hyperthermia
- DIC
- Infection.

Goals for care of the patient during surgery include reducing anxiety, preventing positioning injuries, maintaining safety, maintaining the patient's dignity and avoiding complications. To achieve goals of care following nursing intervention are performed.

Reducing Anxiety

The OT environment can seem cold, stark, and frightening to the patient, who may be feeling isolated and apprehensive. Introducing yourself, addressing the patient by name warmly and frequently, verifying details, providing explanations, and encouraging and answering questions provide a sense of professionalism and friendliness that can help the patient feel secure. When discussing what the patient can expect in surgery, the nurse uses basic communication skills, such as touch and eye contact, to reduce anxiety.

Attention to physical comfort (warm blankets, position changes) helps the patient feel more comfortable. Telling the patient who else will be present in the OR, how long the procedure is expected to take, and other details helps the patient prepare for the experience and gain a sense of control.

Preventing Intraoperative Positioning Injury

The patient's position on the operating table depends on the surgical procedure to be performed as well as on the patients physical condition. The potential for transient discomfort or permanent injury is present, because many positions are awkward. Hyperextending joints, compressing arteries, or pressing on nerves and bony prominences usually results in discomfort simply because the position must be sustained for a long period of time. Factors to consider include the following:

- The patient should be in as comfortable a position as possible, whether conscious or unconscious
- The operative field must be adequately exposed
- An awkward position, undue pressure on a body part, or use of stirrups or traction should not obstruct the vascular supply
- Respiration should not be impeded by pressure of arms on the chest or by a gown that constricts the neck or chest
- Nerves must be protected from undue pressure. Improper positioning of the arms, hands, legs, or feet can cause serious injury or paralysis. Shoulder braces must be well padded to prevent irreparable nerve injury, especially when the Trendelenburg position is necessary
- Precautions for patient safety must be observed, particularly with thin, elderly, or obese patients and those with a physical deformity
- The patient may need light restraint before induction in case of excitement.

The usual position for surgery, called the dorsal recumbent position, is flat on the back. One arm is positioned at the side of the table, with the hand placed palm down; the other is carefully positioned on an armboard to facilitate IV infusion of fluids, blood, or medications. This position is used for most abdominal surgeries except for surgery of the gallbladder or pelvis.

The Trendelenburg position usually is used for surgery on the lower abdomen and pelvis to obtain good exposure by displacing the intestines into the upper abdomen. In this position, the head and body are lowered. The patient is held in position by padded shoulder braces (Fig. 6.4).

The lithotomy position is used for nearly all perineal, rectal, and vaginal surgical procedures. The patient is positioned on the back with the legs and thighs flexed. The position is maintained by placing the feet in stirrups.

The Sims or lateral position is used for renal surgery. The patient on the nonoperative side with an air pillow 12.5 to 15 cm (5 to 6 inches) thick under the loin, or on a table with a kidney or back lift.

Other procedures, such as neurosurgery or abdominothoracic surgery, may require unique positioning and supplemental apparatus, depending on the operative approach.

Protecting the Patient from Injury

A variety of activities are used to address the diverse patient safety issues that arise in the OR. The nurse protects the patient from injury by providing a safe environment. Verifying information, checking the chart for completeness, and maintaining surgical asepsis and an optimal environment are critical nursing responsibilities. Verifying that all required documentation is completed is one of the first functions of the intraoperative nurse. The patient is identified, and the planned surgical procedure, correct surgical site, and type of anesthesia are verified. It is important to review the patients record for the following:

- Correct informed surgical consent, with patients signature
- Completed records for health history and physical examination
- Results of diagnostic studies
- Allergies (including latex).

In addition to checking that all necessary patient data are complete, the perioperative nurse obtains the necessary equipment specific to the procedure. The need for nonroutine medications, blood components, instruments, and other equipment and supplies is assessed, and the readiness of the room, completeness of physical setup and completeness of instrument, suture and dressing setups are determined. Any aspects of the OT environment that may negatively affect the patient are identified. These include physical features, such as room temperature and humidity; electrical hazards; potential contaminants (dust, blood, and discharge on floor or surfaces, uncovered hair, faculty attire of personnel, jewelry worn by personnel); and unnecessary traffic. The circulating nurse also sets up and maintains suction equipment in working order, sets up invasive monitoring equipment, assists with insertion of vascular access and monitoring devices (arterial, Swan-Granz, central venous pressure, IV lines), and initiates appropriate physical comfort measures for the patient.

Preventing physical injury includes using safety straps and side rails and not leaving the sedated patient unattended. Transferring the patient from the stretcher to the OR table requires safe transferring practices. Other safety measures include properly positioning the grounding pad under the patient to prevent electrical burns and shock, removing excess antiseptic solution from the patient's skin, and promptly and completely draping exposed areas after the sterile field has been created to decrease the risk for hypothermia.

Nursing measures to prevent injury from excessive blood loss include blood conservation using equipment such as a cell-saver (a device for recirculating the patient's own blood cells) and administration of blood products. Few patients undergoing an elective procedure require blood transfusion, but those undergoing higher-risk procedures (such as orthopedic or cardiac surgeries) may require an intraoperative transfusion. The circulating nurse anticipates this need, checks that blood has been cross-matched and held in reserve, and is prepared to administer blood.

Serving as Patient Advocate

Because the patient undergoing general anesthesia or moderate sedation experiences temporary sensory/perceptual alteration or loss, he or she has an increased need for protection and advocacy. Patient advocacy in the OR entails maintaining the patient's physical and emotional comfort, privacy, rights, and dignity. Patients, whether conscious or unconscious, should not be subjected to excess noise, inappropriate conversation, or, most of all, derogatory comments. As surprising as this sounds, banter in the OR occasionally includes jokes about the patient's physical appearance, job, personal history, and so forth. Cases have been reported in which seemingly deeply anesthetized patients recalled the entire surgical experience, including disparaging personal remarks made by OR personnel. As an advocate, the nurse never engages in this conversation and discourages others from doing so. Other advocacy activities include minimizing the clinical, dehumanizing aspects of being a surgical patient by making sure the patient is treated as a person, respecting cultural and spiritual values, providing physical privacy, and maintaining confidentiality.

Monitoring and Managing Potential Complications

It is the responsibility of the surgeon and the anesthesiologist or anesthetist to monitor and manage complications. However, intraoperative nurses also play an important role. Being alert to and reporting changes in vital signs and symptoms of nausea and vomiting, anaphylaxis, hypoxia, hypothermia, malignant hyperthermia, or DIC and assisting with their management are important nursing functions. Each of these complication was discussed earlier. Maintaining asepsis and preventing infection are responsibilities of all members of the surgical team.

The surgical team consists of the patient, the anesthesiologist or anesthetist, the surgeon, nurses, and the surgical technologists (or assistants). The anesthesiologist or anesthetist (often a nurse anesthetist) administers the anesthetic agent and monitors the patient's physical status throughout the surgery. The surgeon, nurses, and assistants scrub and perform the surgery. The person in the scrub role, either a nurse or a surgical technologist, provides sterile instruments and supplies to the surgeon during the procedure. The circulating nurse coordinates the care of the patient in the OR. Care provided by the circulating nurse includes assisting with patient positioning, preparing the patient's skin for surgery, managing surgical specimens, anticipating the needs of the surgical team, and documenting intraoperative events. Collaboration of the surgical team using evidence-based practice tailored to the specific case results in optimum patient care and improved outcomes.

Expected patient outcomes may include the following:

1. Exhibits low level of anxiety while awake during the intraoperative phase of care.
2. Remains free of perioperative positioning injury.
3. Experiences no unexpected threats to safety.
4. Has dignity preserved throughout OR experience.
5. Is free of complications (nausea and vomiting, anaphylaxis, hypoxia, hypothermia, malignant hyperthermia, or DIC) or experiences successful management of adverse effects of surgery and anesthesia should they occur (Box 6.5).

Box 6.5 Potential adverse effects of surgery and anesthesia

Anesthesia and surgery disrupt all major body systems. Although most patients can compensate for surgical trauma and the effects of anesthesia, all patients are at risk during the operative procedure. These risks include the following:

- Allergic reactions
- Cardiac dysrhythmia from electrolyte imblance or adverse effect of anesthetic agents
- Myocardial depression, bradycardia, and circulatory collapse
- Central nervous system agitation seizures, and respiratory arrest
- Oversedation or undersedation
- Agitation or disorientation, especially in elderly patients
- Hypoxemia or hypercarbia from hypoventilation and inadequate respiratory support during anesthesia
- Laryngeal trauma, oral trauma and broken teeth from difficult intubation
- Hypothermia from cool operating room temperatures, exposure of body cavities, and impaired thermoregulation secondary to anesthetic agents
- Hypotension from blood loss or adverse effect of anesthesia
- Infection
- Thrombosis from compression of blood vessels or stasis
- Malignat hyperthermia secondry to adverse effect of anesthesia
- Nerve damage and skin breakdown from prolonged or inappropriate positioning
- Electrical shock or burns
- Laser burns
- Drug toxicity, faulty equipment, and human error.

POSTOPERATIVE NURSING

The postoperative phase of surgery is final phase of the surgical experience. Nursing plays a critical role in returning the client to an optimal level of functioning. The postoperative period can be divided into two phases, i.e. immediate postanesthesia and postoperative period, and later in postoperative phase.

Immediate Postoperative Phase

Immediate postoperative phase is the first few hours after surgery when the client is recovering from the effect of anesthesia. Here the nurse has to keep all emergency equipment and drugs, etc. for the use of patient's recovery from anesthesia and on admission to postoperative unit, the nurse performs the following:

- Assess airway patency and support as needed, cramp, strider, wheezes or decreased breath sounds
- Applies humidified oxygen via nasal cannula or facemask (unless otherwise ordered)
- Records vital signs (blood pressure, heart rate, strength and regularity, respiratory rate and depth, oxygen saturation, skin color, and temperature)
- Assess the client's level of consciousness, muscle strength and ability to follow commands

- Observe the client's IV infusions, dressings, drains and special equipment
- Remain at the client's bedside, continuing close observations of the client's conditions.

After the client has been positioned safely and baseline vital signs status has been ascertained, the nurse receives verbal report regarding surgery in detail, i.e. type of surgery, time of incision, patient's condition during surgery, type of anesthesia, sedative, all untoward incident happened and everything about surgery and documents the reliable and retainable information for further care that follow surgeon's and anesthetist's instructions for patient's recovery.

It is very important that nursing intervention associated with immediate recovery (ABCs) are as follows:

Airway (A)

- Maintain patency, keep head tilted up and back may position on side with the face down and neck slightly extended
- Note presence or absence of gag / swallowing reflex
- Suction until awake and alert
- Provide oxygen if necessary.

Breathing (B)

- Evaluate depth, rate, sounds, rhythm and chest movement
- Assess color of mucous membrane
- Place hand above nose to detect respirations if shallow
- Initiate coughing and deep breathing as soon as able to respond
- Chart time oxygen is discontinued.

Consciousness (C)

- Able to extubate airway
- Responds to commands
- Verbalizes responses
- Reacts to stimuli.

Circulation (C)

- Monitor TPR every 15 minutes, to take axillary or rectal temperature, if necessary
- Assess rate, rhythm, quality of pulse
- Evaluate color and warmth of skin and nailbeds
- Check peripheral pulse if indicated
- Monitor IVS solution, rate, site.

System Review (S)

- Assess neurological functions
- Monitor drains, tubes, color and amount of output
- Evaluate pain response, may need to give analgesics
- Observe for allergic reactions
- Assess urinary output, if Foley's catheter is in place.

For remaining postoperative period, nurse has to take following measures to:

- Continuous assessment of respiratory and circulatory assessment
- Ensure optimal respiratory function—deep breath and coughing exercises
- Relieving postoperative discomforts by relieving pain, restlessness nausea and vomiting, abdominal distention, hiccups, etc.
- Maintaining normal body temperature
- Avoid injury by providing proper positioning in bed
- Maintaining normal nutritional status by IV fluids, total parenteral nutrition
- Promoting normal urinary functions
- Promoting bowel elimination—preventing paralytic ileus, and constipation
- Restoring mobility by proper positioning
- Early ambulation—bed exercises
- Prevent and treatment of complication like shock, hemorrhage, deep venous thrombosis (DVT), pulmonary embolism, respiratory complication like undetected hypoxemia, atelectasis, bronchitis, bronchopneumonia and lobar pneumonia, hypostatic pulmonary congestion, pleuracy, etc. and gastric complication like nutritional anemia, intestinal obstruction and postoperative psychosis

Potential Postoperative Problems and Their Management

Respiratory Problems and Their Management

In the immediate postanesthetic period, the most common causes of airway compromise include obstruction, hypoxemia, and hypoventilation. Patients at risk include those who have had general anesthesia, are older, smoke heavily, have lung disease, are obese, or have undergone airway, thoracic, or abdominal surgery. However, respiratory problems may occur with any patient who has been anesthetized.

Airway obstruction is most commonly caused by blockage of the airway by the patient's tongue. The base of the tongue falls backward against the soft palate and occludes the pharynx. It is most pronounced in the supine position and in the patient who is extremely sleepy after surgery. Less common causes of airway obstruction include laryngospasm, retained secretions, and laryngeal edema.

The treatment of hypopharyngeal obstruction involves tilting the head back and pushing forward on the angle of the lower jaw, as if to push the lower teeth in front of the upper teeth. This maneuver pulls the tongue forward to open the air passage.

Hypoxemia, specifically a partial pressure of arterial oxygen (PaO_2) of less than 60 mm Hg, is characterized by a variety of nonspecific clinical signs and symptoms, ranging from agitation to somnolence, hypertension to hypotension, and tachycardia to bradycardia. Pulse oximetry will indicate a low oxygen saturation (less than 90 to 92%). Arterial blood gas analysis should be used to confirm hypoxemia if the pulse oximetry indicates a low oxygen saturation.

The most common cause of postoperative hypoxemia is atelectasis. **Atelectasis** (alveolar collapse) may be the result of bronchial obstruction caused by retained secretions or decreased respiratory excursion. Atelectasis occurs when mucus blocks bronchioles or when the amount of alveolar surfactant (the substance that holds the alveoli open) is reduced). As air becomes trapped beyond the plug and is eventually absorbed, the alveoli collapse. Atelectasis may affect a portion or an entire lobe of the lungs. Hypotension and low cardiac output states can also contribute to the development of atelectasis.

Other causes of hypoxemia that may occur include pulmonary edema, aspiration, and bronchospasm. *Pulmonary edema* is caused by an accumulation of fluid in the alveoli and may be the result of fluid overload; left ventricular failure; or prolonged airway obstruction, sepsis, or aspiration. Pulmonary edema is characterized by hypoxemia, crackles on auscultation, decreased pulmonary compliance, and the presence of infiltrates on chest X-ray.

Aspiration of gastric contents into the lungs is a potentially serious airway emergency. Symptoms include bronchospasm, hypoxemia, atelectasis, interstitial edema, alveolar hemorrhage, and respiratory failure. Gastric aspiration may also cause laryngospasm, infection, and pulmonary edema. Because of the serious consequences of gastric aspiration, prevention, as opposed to treatment, is the goal.

Bronchospasm is the result of an increase in bronchial smooth muscle tone with resultant closure of small airways. Airway edema develops, causing secretions to build up in the airway. The patient sured that these activities will not cause the incision to separate. Adequate hydration, either parenteral or oral, is essential to maintain the integrity of mucous membranes and to keep secretions thin and loose for easy expectoration.

Common immediate postoperative problems, and their mechanism, manifestation and nursing intervention are listed in Table 6.5.

Cardiovascular Problems and Their Management

In the immediate postanesthetic period, the most common cardiovascular problems include hypotension, hypertension, and dysrhythmias. Patients at greatest risk for alterations in cardiovascular function include those with alterations in respiratory function, those with a history of cardiovascular disease, the elderly, the debilitated, and the critically ill.

Hypotension is evidenced by signs of hypoperfusion to the vital organs, especially the brain, heart, and kidneys. Clinical signs of disorientation, loss of consciousness, chest pain, oliguria, and anuria reflect hypoxemia and the loss of physiologic compensation. Intervention must be timely to prevent the devastating complications of cardiac ischemia or infarction, cerebral ischemia, renal ischemia, and bowel infarction.

A systolic blood pressure less than 90 mm Hg is usually considered immediately reportable. However, the patients preoperative or baseline blood pressure used to make informed postopereative comparison. Any deviation should be reported.

The most common cause of hypotension in the POCU is unreplaced fluid and blood loss, which may lead to hypovolemic shock. Hemorrhage is always a risk of surgery, and marked blood loss is possible when cauterization or ligatures fail. Hemorrhage most often occurs internally, requiring assessment for changes in level of consciousness and vital signs. If changes are detected, treatment will be directed toward restoring circulating volume. If there is no response to fluid administration, cardiac dysfunction should be considered to be the cause of hypotension.

Primary cardiac dysfunction, as may occur in the case of myocardial infarction, cardiac tamponade, or pulmonary embolism, results in an acute fall in cardiac output. Secondary myocardial dysfunction occurs as a result of the negative chronotropic (rate of cardiac contraction) and negative inotropic (force of cardiac contraction) effects of drugs, such as β-adrenergic blockers, digoxin, or opioids. Other causes of hypotension include decreased systemic vascular resistance, dysrhythmias, and measurement errors that may occur if a blood pressure cuff is incorrectly sized.

Hypertension, a common finding in the POCU is most frequently the result of sympathetic nervous system stimulation that may be result of pain, anxiety, bladder distention, or respiratory compromise. Hypertension may also be the result of hypothermia and pre-existing hypertension. It may be seen after vascular and cardiac surgery as a result of revascularization.

In the POCU, *dysrhythmias* are often the result of an identifiable cause other than myocardial injury. The leading causes include hypokalemia, hypoxemia, hypercarbia, alterations in acid-base status, circulatory instability, and preexisting heart disease. Hypothermia, pain, surgical stress, and many anesthetic agents are also capable of causing dysrhythmias.

In the clinical unit, postoperative fluid and electrolyte imbalances are contributing factors to cardiovascular problems. Such imbalances may develop as a result of a combination of the body's normal response to the stress of surgery, excessive fluid losses, and improper IV fluid replacement. The body's fluid status directly affects cardiac output. Fluid retention during the first 2 to 5 postoperative days can be the result of the stress response. This response serves to maintain both blood volume and blood pressure. Fluid retention results from the secretion and release of two hormones by the pituitary—antidiuretic hormone (ADH) and adrenocorticotropic hormone (ACTH)—and activation of the rennin-angiotensin-aldosterone system. ADH release leads to increased water reabsorption and decreased urinary output, increasing blood volume. ACTH stimulates the adrenal

TABLE 6.5: Common immediate postoperative respiratory complications care

Complications and causes	Mechanisms	Manifestations	Nursing interventions
Airway Obstruction			
Tongue falling back	Muscular flaccidity associated with ↓ consciousness and muscle relaxants	Use of accessory muscles Snoring respiration ↓ Air movement	Patient stimulation Jaw thrust Chin lift Artificial airway
Retained thick secretions	Secretion stimulation by anesthetic agents Dehydration of secretions	Noisy respirations Coarse crackles	Suctioning Deep breathing and coughing IV hydration Chest physical therapy
Laryngospasm	Irritation from endotracheal tube or anesthetic gases Most likely to occur after removal of endotracheal tube	Inspiratory stridor (crowing respiration) Sternal retraction Acute respiratory distress	O_2 Positive pressure ventilation IV muscle relaxant Lidocaine Corticosteroids
Laryngeal edema	Allergic drug reaction Mechanical irritation from intubation Fluid overload	Similar to laryngospasm	O_2 Antihistamines Corticosteroids Sedatives Possible intubation
Hypoxemia			
Atelectasis	Bronchial obstruction caused by secretions or ↓ lung volume	↓ Breath sounds ↓ O_2 saturation	Humidified O_2 Deep breathing Incentive spirometry Early mobilization
Pulmonary edema	↑Hydrostatic pressure ↓ Interstitial pressure ↑ Capillary permeability	Crackles Infiltrates on chest X-ray Fluid overload ↓ O_2 saturation	O_2 therapy Diuretics Fluid restriction
Pulmonary embolism	Thrombus dislodged from peripheral venous system; lodged in pulmonary arterial system	Acute tachypnea Dyspnea Tachycardia Hypotension ↓ O_2 saturation	O_2 therapy Cardiopulmonary support Anticoagulant therapy
Aspiration	Inhalation of gastric contents	Wheezing Dyspnea Tachypnea ↓ O_2 saturation	O_2 therapy Cardiac support Antibiotics
Bronchospasm	↑ Smooth muscle tone with closure of small airways	Wheezing Dyspnea ¯ O_2 saturation	O_2 therapy Bronchodilators
Hyperventilation			
Depression of central respiratory drive	Medullary depression from anesthetics/ opioids/sedatives	Shallow respirations ↓ Respiratory rate/apnea ↓ PaO_2 ↑ $PaCO_2$	Stimulation Reversal of opioids/benzodiazepines Mechanical ventilation
Poor respiratory muscle tone	Neuromuscular blockade Neuromuscular disease	As above	Reversal of paralysis Mechanical ventilation
Mechanical restriction	Tight casts, dressings, positioning, and obesity preventing lung expansion	As above	Elevate head of bed Repositioning Loosen dressings
Pain	Shallow breathing to prevent incisional pain	As above Complaints of pain Guarding behavior	Opioid analgesic therapy in reduced dose

cortex to secrete cortisol and, to a lesser degree, aldosterone. Fluid losses resulting from surgery decrease kidney perfusion, stimulating the rennin-angiotensin-aldosterone system and causing marked release of aldosterone. Both of the mechanisms that increase aldosterone lead to significant sodium and fluid retention, increasing blood volume.

Fluid overload may occur during this period of fluid retention when IV fluids are administered too rapidly, when chronic (e.g. cardiac, renal) disease exists, or when the patient is an older adult. Conversely, fluid deficit may be related to slow or inadequate fluid replacement, which leads to decreases in cardiac output and tissue perfusion. Untreated preoperative dehydration or intraoperative or postoperative losses from vomiting, bleeding, wound drainage, or suctioning may be contributing factors to fluid deficits.

Hypokalemia can be a consequence of urinary and gastrointestinal (GI) tract losses, and it results when potassium is not replaced in IV fluids. Low serum potassium levels directly affect the contractility of the heart and this may also contribute to decreases in cardiac output and in overall body tissue perfusion. Adequate replacement of potassium is usually 40 mEq/day. However, potassium should not be given if adequate renal function has been established. Urine output of at least 0.5 mL/kg/h is generally considered indicative of adequate renal function.

Cardiovascular status is also affected by the state of tissue perfusion or blood flow. The stress response contributed to an increase in clotting tendencies in the postoperative patient by increasing platelet production. Deep vein thrombosis (DVT) may form in leg veins as a result of inactivity, body position, and pressure, all of which lead to venous stasis and decreased perfusion. DVT, especially common in the order adult, obese individual, and immobilized patient, is a potentially life-threatening complication because it may lead to pulmonary embolism. Patients with a history of DVT have a greater risk for pulmonary embolism. Pulmonary embolism should be suspected in any patient complaining of tachypnea, dyspnea, and tachycaradia, particularly when the patient is already receiving oxygen therapy. Other manifestations may include chest pain, hypotension, hemoptyis, dysrhythmias, and heart failure. Superficial thrombophlebitis is an uncomfortable but less ominous complication that may develop in a leg vein as a result of venous stasis or in the arm veins as a result of irritation from IV catheters or solutions. If a piece of a clot becomes dislodged and travels to the lung, it can cause a pulmonary infarction of a size proportionate to the vessel in which it lodges.

Nursing Management of Cardiovascular Problems

The most important aspect of the cardiovascular assessment is frequent monitoring of vital signs. They are usually monitored every 15 minutes in Phase I, or more often until stabilized, and then at less frequent intervals. Postoperative vital signs should be compared with preoperative and intraoperative readings to determine when the signs are stabilizing at a level that is normal for the patient's condition. The ACP or surgeon should be notified if the following occur:

1. Systolic BP is less than 90 mm Hg or greater than 160 mm Hg.
2. Pulse rate is less than 60 beats per minute or greater than 120 beats per minute.
3. Pulse pressure (difference between systolic and diastolic pressures) narrows.
4. BP gradually decreases during several consecutive readings.
5. There is a change in cardiac rhythm.
6. There is a significant variation from preoperative readings.

Cardiac monitoring is recommended for patients who have a history of cardiac disease and for all older adult patients who have undergone major surgery, regardless of whether they have cardiac problems. The apical-radial pulse should be assessed carefully, and any irregularities should be reported.

Assessment of skin color, temperature, and moisture provides valuable information in detecting cardiovascular problems. Hypotension accompanied by a normal pulse and warm, dry, pink skin usually represents the residual vasodilating effects of anesthesia and suggests only a need for continued observation. Hypotension accompanied by a rapid pulse and cold, clammy, pale skin may be caused by impending hypovolemic shock and requires immediate treatment.

Nursing diagnoses and collaborative problems related to potential cardiovascular problems for the postoperative patient include, but are not limited to, the following:

- Decreased cardiac output
- Deficient fluid volume
- Excess fluid volume
- Ineffective tissue perfusion
- Activity intolerance
- Potential complication—hypovolemic shock
- Potential complication—thromboembolism.

Nursing interventions in the POCU are designed to prevent and treat cardiovascular problems. Treatment of hypotension should always begin with oxygen therapy to promote oxygenation of hypoperfused organs. Volume status should be assessed as described, and errors of BP measurement should be ruled out. Because the most common cause of hypotension is fluid loss, IV fluid boluses will be given to normalize BP. Primary cardiac dysfunction may require drug intervention. Peripheral vasodilation and hypotension may require vasoconstrictive agents to normalize systemic vascular resistance.

Treatment of hypertension will center on addressing the cause of sympathetic nervous system stimulation and eliminating the precipitating cause. Treatment may include the use of analgesics, assistance in voiding, and correction of respiratory problems. Rewarming will correct hypothermia-induced hypertension. If the patient has preexisting hypertension or has undergone cardiac or vascular surgery, drug therapy designed to reduce BP will usually be required.

An accurate intake and output record should be kept during the postoperative period, and laboratory findings (e.g. electrolytes, hematocrit) should be monitored. Nursing responsibilities relating to IV management are critical during this period. In particular, the nurse should be alert for symptoms of too slow or too rapid a rate of fluid replacement. Assessment should also be made of the hazards associated with the IV administration of potassium, such as cardiac dysrhythmias and pain at the infusion site.

Leg exercises should be encouraged 10 to 12 times every 1 to 2 hours while awake. The muscular contraction produced by these exercises and by ambulation facilitates venous return from the lower extremities. When confined to bed, the patient should alternately flex and extend the legs. When the patient is sitting in a chair or lying in bed, there should be no pressure to impede venous flow through the popliteal space. Crossed legs, pillows behind the knees, and extreme elevation of the knee gatch of the bed must be avoided.

Early ambulation is the most significant general nursing measure to prevent postoperative complications. The exercise associated with walking (1) increases muscle tone; (2) improved GI and urinary tract function; (3) stimulates circulation, which prevents venous stasis and speeds wound healing; and (4) increases vital capacity and maintains normal respiratory function.

Currently the most effective means of preventing DVT and pulmonary emboli in surgical patients is use of subcutaneous heparin (or low-molecular-weight heparin [LMWH] in combination with antiembolism stockings. One recent study indicated that the combination LMWH and thigh-length stockings was the best method to decrease the risk for developing a DVT.

The nurse may prevent syncope by making changes slowly in the patient's position. Progression to ambulation can be achieved by first raising the head of the patient's bed for 1 to 2 minutes and then by assisting the patient to sit on the side of the bed while monitoring the radial pulse for rate and quality. If no changes or complaints are noted, ambulation can be started. If faintness occurs, the nurse can help the patient sit on the edge of the bed while continuing of feeling faint during ambulation, the nurse should provide assistance to a nearby chair or ease the patient to the floor. The patient should remain in either location until recovery is evidenced by BP stability, and then be helped back to the bed. If faintness occurs, it is often frightening for the patient and for the unprepared nurse, but syncope poses no real physiologic danger, although injury can result from a fall.

Syncope (fainting) is another factor that reflects the cardiovascular status. It may indicate decreased cardiac output, fluid deficits, or defects in cerebral perfusion. Syncope frequently occurs as a result of postural hypotension when the patient ambulates. It is more common in the older adult or in the patient who has been immobile for long periods of time. Normally when the patient quickly moves to a standing position, the arterial press receptors respond to the accompanying fall in blood pressure with sympathetic nervous system stimulation, which produces vasoconstriction and thereby maintains blood pressure. These sympathetic and vasomotor functions may be diminished in the older adult and the immobile or postanesthetic patient.

Neurologic Problems

Postoperatively, emergence delirium is the neurologic **alteration** that causes the most concern. **Emergence** delirium, or *waking up wild*, can include behaviors such as restlessness, agitation, disorientation, thrashing, and shouting. This condition may be caused by anesthetic agents, hypoxia, bladder distention, pain, electrolyte abnormalities, or the patient's state of anxiety preoperatively. Hypoxia should be suspected first.

Delayed emergence may also be a problem postoperatively. Fortunately, the most common cause of delayed emergence is prolonged drug action, particularly of opioids, sedatives, and inhalational anesthetics, as opposed to neurologic injury. Normal awakening can be predicted by the ACP based on the drugs used in surgery.

Two types of postoperative cognitive impairment are seen in surgical patients—delirium and postoperative cognitive dysfunction (POCD). POCD is almost exclusively seen in the older surgical patient. While postoperative confusion and delirium are also more commonly seen in the older patient, they may occur in patients of any age. Confusion or delirium may arise from a variety of psychologic and physiologic sources, including fluid and electrolyte imbalances, hypoxemia, drug effects, sleep deprivation, and sensory deprivation or overload.

Anxiety and depression may also occur in postoperative patients. Any patient may experience these responses as part of grieving for lost body parts or function or for decreased independence during the recovery and rehabilitation process. Radical surgeries leading to changes in body function or surgical findings that suggest a poor prognosis may cause more pronounced psychologic reactions.

Alcohol withdrawal delirium may also occur as a result of alcohol withdrawal in a postoperative patient. Alcohol withdrawal delirium is a reaction characterized by restlessness, insomnia and nightmares, irritability, and authority or visual hallucinations.

The nurses in the POCU, should assess the patients level of consciousness, orientation, and memory and his or her ability to follow commands should be assessed. The size, reactivity, and equality of the pupils should be determined. The patients sleep/wake cycle and sensory and motor status should also be assessed. If the neurologic status is altered, possible causes should be determined. If the patient was mentally alert before surgery and becomes cognitively impaired postoperatively, the nurse should suspect delirium.

Nursing diagnoses related to potential neurologic or psychologic problems for the postoperative patient include, but are not limited to the following:

- Disturbed sensory perception
- Risk for injury
- Disturbed thought processes
- Impaired verbal communication
- Anxiety
- Ineffective coping
- Disturbed body image
- Fear.

The most common cause of postoperative agitation in the POCU is hypoxemia. As a result, attention must focus on evaluating respiratory function. Once hypoxemia has been ruled out as the cause of postoperative delirium and all potentially known causes have been addressed, sedation may prove beneficial in controlling the agitation and providing for patient and staff safety. Emergence delirium is usually time limited and will resolve before the patient is discharged from the POCU. Because the most common cause of delayed emergence is prolonged drug action, delays in awakening usually spontaneously resolve with time. If necessary, benzodiazepines and opioids may be pharmacologically reversed with antagonists.

Until the patient is awake and able to communicate effectively, it is the responsibility of the POCU nurse to act as a patient advocate and to maintain patient safety at all times. This includes having the side rails up, securing IV lines and artificial airways, verifying the presence of identification and allergy bands, and monitoring physiologic status.

To prevent or manage postoperative delirium, the nurse should address factors that are known to contribute to the condition. Maintenance of normal physiologic function is important and includes fluid and electrolyte balance, adequate nutrition, pain management, proper bowel and bladder function, and early mobilization. The nurse can also use environmental aids, such as clocks, calendars, and photographs, to help orient the patient.

The nurse should attempt to prevent psychologic problems in the postoperative period by providing adequate support for the patient. Supportive measures include taking time to listen to and talk with the patient, offering explanations and genuine reassurance, and encouraging the presence and assistance of significant others. The nurse must observe and evaluate the patients behavior to distinguish a normal reaction to the stress situation from one that becoming abnormal or excessive.

The nurse should discuss the patient's expectations regarding activity and assistance needed following discharge. The patient must be included in discharge planning and should be provided with the information and support to make informed decisions about continuing care.

The recognition of alcohol withdrawal delirium in a patient not previously known to be an alcoholic presents a particular challenge. Any unusual or disturbed behavior should be reported immediately so that diagnosis and treatment may be instituted.

Pain and Discomfort and Their Management

Despite the availability of analgesic drugs and pain-relieving techniques, pain remains a common problem and a significant fear for the patient in the POCU and during the postoperative period. Postoperative pain is caused by the interaction of a number of physiologic and psychologic factors. The skin and underlying tissues have been traumatized by the incision and retraction during surgery. In addition, there may be reflex muscle spasms around the incision. Anxiety and fear, sometimes related to the anticipation of pain, create tension and further increase muscle tone and spasm. Positioning during surgery or the use of internal devices such as an endotracheal tube or catheters may also result in pain. The effort and movement associated with deep breathing, coughing, and ambulating may aggravate pain by creating tension on the incision area. Pain can contribute to complications such as dysfunction of the immune system and blood clotting, and delayed return of normal gastric and bowel function. It also increases the risk of atelectasis and impaired respiratory function. When the internal viscera are cut, no pain is felt. However, pressure in the internal viscera elicits pain. Therefore, deep visceral pain may signal the presence of a signal the presence of a complication such as intestinal distention, bleeding, or abscess formation.

The patient's self-report is the single most reliable indicator of pain. Since this is not always possible in the POCU, the patient should be observed for other indications of pain (e.g. restlessness, increased heart rate, diaphoresis). Identifying the location of the pain is important. Incisional pain is to be expected, but other causes of pain, such as a full bladder, may be present.

Nursing diagnoses for the patient experiencing pain and discomfort include, but are limited to the following:

- Acute pain
- Anxiety.

The most effective interventions for postoperative pain management include using a variety of analgesics. Intravenous opioids provide the most rapid relief. Drugs are administered slowly and titrated to allow for optimal pain management with minimal to no adverse drug side effects. More sustained relief may be obtained through the use of epidural catheters, patient-controlled analgesia, or regional anesthetic blockade.

Postoperative pain relief is a nursing responsibility because the surgeons orders for analgesic medication and other comfort measures are usually written on an as-needed as basis. During the first 48 hours or longer, opioid analgesics (e.g. morphine) are required to relieve moderate to severe pain. After that time, nonopioid analgesics, such as nonsteroidal anti-inflammatory agents, may be sufficient as pain intensity decreases.

Analgesic administration should be timed to ensure that it is in effect during activities that may be painful for the patient, such as ambulating. Although opioid analgesics are often essential for the postoperative patients comfort, there are undesirable side effects. Side effects such as constipation, nausea and vomiting, respiratory and cough depression, and hypotension are most common with the opioids. Before administering any analgesic, the nurse should first assess the nature of the patients pain, including location, quality, and intensity. If it is incisional pain, analgesic administration is appropriate. If it is chest or leg pain, medication may simply mask a complication that must be reported and documented. If it is gas pain, opioids can aggravate it. The nurse should notify the physician and request a change in the order if the analgesic either fails to relieve the pain or makes the patient excessively lethargic or somnolent.

Patient-controlled analgesia (PCA) and epidural analgesia are two alternative approaches for pain control. The goals of PCA are to provide immediate analgesia and to maintain a constant, steady blood level of the analgesia agent. PCA involves self-administration of predetermined doses of analgesia by the patient. The route of delivery may be IV, oral, or epidural. Some advantages of PCA are early ambulation, improved wound healing, and earlier hospital discharge.

Epidural analgesia is the infusion of opioid analgesics through a catheter placed into the epidural space surrounding the spinal cord. The goal of epidural analgesia is delivery of medication directly to opiate receptors in the spinal cord. Administration methods include intermittent bolus dosing, continuous infusion, and patient-controlled epidural analgesia (PCEA). The overall effectiveness and the technique of administration result in a constant circulating level and a reduced total dose of medication. The use of epidural analgesia for postoperative pain is increasing based on research that has demonstrated superior pain relief and improved functional outcomes after major surgery in patients who receive epidural analgesia compared with patients receiving IV PCA.

The acute pain of surgery almost always requires the use of analgesics. However, nonpharmacologic approaches such as repositioning, massage, distraction, relaxation, and deep breathing can enhance pain management. Music and educational interventions have also been shown to be effective adjuncts to pain medication.

Alterations in Temperature and Their Management

Hypothermia, a core temperature of less than 96.8°F (36°C), occurs when heat loss exceeds heat production. In addition to the usual heat loss mechanisms of radiation, convection, conduction, and evaporation, heat loss may occur in the perioperative setting because of infusion of cool IV fluids and ventilation with dry gases.

Although all patients are at risk for hypothermia, the older, debilitated, or intoxicated patient is at an increased risk. Long surgical procedures and prolonged anesthetic administration lead to redistribution of body heat from the core to the periphery. This places the patient at increased risk for hypothermia. Complications from hypothermia may include compromised immune function, postoperative pain, bleeding, myocardial ischemia, impaired wound healing, and delayed drug metabolism.

Another complication of hypothermia is shivering. Shivering can increase oxygen consumption, carbon dioxide production, and cardiac output, as well as significantly affect the patient's comfort level.

Temperature variation in the postoperative period provides valuable information about the patient's status. Fever may occur at anytime during the postoperative period. A mild elevation (up to 100.4°F [38°C]) during the first 48 hours usually reflects the surgical stress response. A moderate elevation (higher than up to 100.4°F [38°C]) is caused more frequently by respiratory congestion or atelectasis and less frequently by dehydration. After the first 48 hours, a moderate to marked elevation (higher than 99.9°F [37.7°C]) is usually caused by infection.

Wound infection, particularly from aerobic organisms, is often accompanied by a fever that spikes in the afternoon or evening and returns to near-normal levels in the morning. The respiratory tract may be infected secondary to stasis of secretions in areas of atelectasis. The urinary tract may be infected secondary to catheterization. Superficial thrombophlebitis in the leg veins may produce a temperature elevation between 7 and 10 days after surgery.

Nosocomial infectious diarrhea caused by *Clostridium difficile* may be signaled by fever, diarrhea, and abdominal pain. Surgical patients who receive antibiotics for a period of time are at risk.

Intermittent high fever accompanied by shaking chills and diaphoresis suggests septicemia. This may occur at any time during the postoperative period because microorganism may have been introduced into the blood stream during surgery, especially in GI or genitourinary (GU) procedures, or picked up later from the site of a wound or from a urinary tract or vein infection.

The nurses in POCU, should perform frequent assessment of the patient's temperature is important to detect patterns of hypothermia and/or fever that may be present in the postoperative period. Temperature may be taken orally, or via the tympanic membrane or axilla. The color and temperature of the skin should also be assessed. The nurse should observe the patient for early signs of inflammation and infection that may precede a fever so that any complications that arise may be treated in a timely manner.

Nursing diagnoses for the patient with an altered temperature include, but are not limited to, the following:

- Hyperthermia
- Hypothermia
- Risk for imbalanced body temperature.

The nursing intervention for altered temperature will include the following:

Passive rewarming in a patient with hypothermia (i.e. shivering) raises basal body metabolism. *Active rewarming* requires the application of external warming devices, including warm blankets, heated aerosols, radiant warmers, forced air warmers, and heated water mattresses. When using any external warming device, body temperature should be monitored at

15-minute intervals, and care should be taken to prevent skin injuries. In addition, oxygen therapy via nasal prongs or mask is used to treat the increased demand for oxygen accompanying the increase in body temperature. Shivering is usually quickly suppressed by opioids.

The nurse's role with respect to postoperative fever may be preventive, diagnostic, and therapeutic. The patient's temperature is usually measured every 4 hours for the first 48 hours postoperatively and then less frequently if no problems develop. Meticulous asepsis is maintained with regard to the wound and the IV site, and airway clearance is encouraged. If fever develops, chest X-rays may be taken, and depending on the suspected cause, cultures of the wound, urine, or blood are obtained. If infection is the source of the fever, antibiotics are started as soon as cultures have been obtained. If the fever rises above 103° F (39.4°C), antipyretic drugs and body-cooling measures may be employed.

Gastrointestinal Problems and Their Management

Postoperative nausea and vomiting occur in 20 to 30% of adult patients. These problems are responsible for unanticipated hospital admission of day-surgery patients, increased patient discomfort, delays in discharge, and patient's dissatisfaction with the surgical experience. Numerous factors have been identified as contributing to the development of nausea and vomiting, including gender (female), history of motion sickness or previous postoperative nausea and vomiting, and action of anesthetics or opioids, as well as duration and type of surgery. At the slightest indication of nausea, the patient is turned completely to one side to promote mouth drainage and prevent aspiration of vomitus, which causes asphyxia and death. Delayed gastric emptying and slowed peristalsis that result from handling of the bowel during abdominal surgery also contribute to nausea and vomiting, as does the assumption of oral intake too soon after surgery.

Abdominal distention is another common problem caused by decreased peristalsis as a result of handling of the intestine during surgery and limited dietary intake before and after surgery. Following abdominal surgery, motility in the large intestine may be reduced for 3 to 5 days, although motility in the small intestine resumes within 24 hours. Swallowed air and GI secretions may accumulate in the colon, producing distention and gas pains.

Hiccups (singultus) are intermittent spasms of the diaphragm caused by irritation of the phrenic nerve, which innervates the diaphragm. Postoperative sources of direct irritation of the phrenic nerve may be gastric distention, intestinal obstruction, intra-abdominal bleeding, and a subphrenic abscess. Indirect irritation of the phrenic nerve may be produced by acid-base and electrolyte imbalances. Reflex irritation may come from drinking hot or cold liquids or from the presence of a nasogastric tube. Hiccups usually last a short time and subside spontaneously; occasionally they may be persistent, but they are rarely debilitating.

The nurses in POCU should perform following activitations. The patient should be questioned about feelings of nausea. If vomiting occurs, it is important to determine the quantity, characteristics, and color of the vomitus. The abdomen should be assessed for distention and the presence of bowel sounds. Because bowel sounds are frequently absent or diminished in the immediate postoperative period, all four quadrants should be auscultated to determine the presence, frequency, and characteristics of the sounds. The return of normal bowel motility is usually accompanied by the passage of flatus in addition to normal bowel sounds and the absence of distention.

Nursing diagnoses for the patient experiencing GI problems include, but are not limited to, the following:

- Nausea
- Risk for aspiration
- Risk for deficient fluid volume
- Imbalanced nutrition—less than body requirements
- Potential complication—fluid and electrolyte imbalance
- Potential complication—hiccups.

Postoperative nausea and nausea are treated with the use of antiemetic or prokinetic drugs. Other methods of decreasing nausea and vomiting are being tested, such as giving carbohydrate-rich fluid to patients before laparoscopic cholecystectomy. In the POCU, oral fluids should be given only as indicated and tolerated. Intravenous fluids will provide hydration until the patient is able to tolerate oral fluids. Care should be also be taken to prevent aspiration if the patient vomits while still sleepy from anesthesia. Having suction equipment readily available at the bedside and turning the patients head to the side will help protect the patient from aspiration. Other nonpharmacologic nursing interventions that may be effective include biofeedback, hypnosis, relaxation, guided imagery, music therapy, distraction, and acupressure.

Depending on the nature of the surgery, the patient may resume oral intake as soon as the gag reflex returns. The patient who had abdominal surgery is usually allowed nothing by mouth (NPO) until the presence of bowel sounds indicates the return of peristalsis. When the patient is NPO, IV infusions are given to maintain fluid and electrolyte balance. A nasogastric tube may be used to decompress the stomach to prevent nausea, vomiting, and abdominal distention. Regular mouth care is essential for comfort and stimulation of salivary glands when the patient is NPO or has a nasogastric tube. When oral intake is allowed, clear liquids are offered first and the IV infusion is continued, usually at a reduced rate. If oral intake is well tolerated by the patient, the IV infusion is discontinued, and the diet is advanced until a regular diet is tolerated.

Abdominal distention may be prevented or minimized by early and frequent ambulation, which stimulates intestinal motility. The nurse should assess the patient regularly to detect the resumption of normal intestinal peristalsis as evidenced by the return of bowel sounds and the passage of flatus. The nasogastric tube must be clamped. Resumption of a normal diet after bowel sounds have returned will also enhance the return of normal peristalsis.

The patient may need to be encouraged to expel flatus and assured that expulsion is necessary and desirable. Gas pains, which tend to become pronounced on the second or third postoperative day, may be relieved by ambulation and frequent repositioning. Positioning the patient on the right side permits gas to rise along the transverse colon and facilitates its release. Bisacodyl (Dulcolax) suppositories may be ordered to stimulate colonic peristalsis and expulsion of flatus and feces.

Urinary Problems and Their Management

Low urine output (800 to 1500 mL) in the first 24 hours after surgery may be expected, regardless of fluid intake. This low output is caused by increased aldosterone and ADH secretion resulting from the stress of surgery, fluid restriction before surgery, and fluid loss through surgery, drainage, and diaphoresis. By the second or third day, the patient will begin to have increasing urinary output after fluid has been mobilized and the immediate stress reaction subsides.

Acute urinary retention can occur in the postoperative period for a variety of reasons. Anesthesia depresses the nervous system, including the micturition reflex arc and the higher centers that influence it. This allows the bladder to fill more completely than normal before the urge to void is felt. Anesthesia also impedes voluntary micturition. Anticholinergic and opioid drugs may also interfere with the ability to initiate voiding or to empty the bladder completely.

Retention is more likely to occur after lower abdominal or pelvic surgery because spasms or guarding of the abdominal and pelvic muscles interferes with their normal function in micturition. Pain may alter perception and interfere with the patient's awareness of bladder filling. Voiding ability is probably impaired to the greatest extent by immobility and the recumbent position in bed. The supine position reduces the ability to relax the perineal muscles and external sphincter.

Oliguria (the diminished output of urine) can be a manifestation of renal failure and is a less common, although more serious problem after surgery. It may result from renal ischemia caused by inadequate renal perfusion or altered cardiovascular function.

The nurses in the POCU should monitor the following:

The urine of the postoperative patient should be examined for both quantity and quality. The color, amount, consistency, and odor of the urine should be noted. Indwelling catheters should be assessed for patency, and urine output should be at least 0.5 mL/kg/h. Most patients urinate within 6 to 8 hours after surgery. If no voiding occurs, the abdominal contour should be inspected and the bladder assessed for distention.

Nursing diagnoses and collaborative problems related to potential urinary problems for the postoperative patient include, but are not limited to, the following:

- Impaired urinary elimination
- Potential complication: acute urinary retention.

The nurse may facilitate voiding by normal positioning of the patient—sitting for women and standing for men. Providing reassurance to the patient regarding the ability to void and the use of techniques such as providing privacy, running water, having the patient drink water, or pouring warm water over the perineum may also be of assistance. Ambulation, preferably to the bathroom, and the use of a bedside commode are additional helpful measures to assist in voiding.

The surgeon often leaves an order to catheterize the patient in 6 to 8 hours if voiding has not occurred. Because of the possibility of infection associated with catheterization, the nurse should first try other measures to induce voiding and validate that the bladder is actually full. In assessing the need for catheterization, the nurse should consider fluid intake during and after surgery and determine bladder fullness (e.g. palpable fullness above the symphysis pubis, discomfort when pressure is applied over the bladder, or the presence of the urge to void). Straight catheterization is preferred because of the possibility of infection associated with an indwelling catheter.

Integumentary Problems and Their Management

Surgery generally involves an incision through the skin and underlying tissues. An incision disrupts the protective skin barrier. Therefore, wound healing is one of the major concerns during the postoperative period.

An adequate nutritional state is essential for wound healing. Amino acids are readily available for the healing process because of the catabolic effects of the stress-related hormones (e.g. cortisol). The patient who was well nourished preoperatively can tolerate the postoperative delay in nutritional deficits that occur with chronic disease (e.g. diabetes, ulcerative colitis, alcoholism) is more prone to problems of wound healing. Abdominal wound healing is affected by obesity. Wound healing is also a concern for the older adult. The patient who is unable to meet nutritional needs postoperatively may be provided with enteral nutrition or parenteral nutrition to promote healing (Box 6.6).

Wound infection may result from contamination of the wound from three major sources: (1) exogenous flora present in the environment and on the skin; (2) oral flora and (3) intestinal flora. The incidence of wound sepsis is higher in patients who are malnourished, immunosuppressed, or older, who have had a prolonged hospital stay or a lengthy surgical procedure (lasting more than 3 hours). Patients undergoing bowel surgery, particularly following a traumatic injury, are at particularly high risk. Infection may involve the entire incision and may extend downward through the deeper tissue layers. An abscess may form locally, or the infection may spread throughout entire body cavities, as in peritonitis. Evidence of wound infection usually does not become apparent before the third to the fifth postoperative day. Local manifestations include redness,

Box 6.6 Nutrients important for wound healing

Nutrient	Rationale for increased need	Possible deficieny outcome
Protein	To allow collagen deposition and wound healing to occur	Collagen deposition leading to impaired/delayed wound healing Decreased skin and wound strength Increased wound infection rates
Arginine (amino acid)	To provide necessary substrate for collagen synthesis and nitric oxide (crucial for wound healing) at wound site To increase wound strength and collagen deposition To stimulate T-cell response Associated with a variety of essential reactions of intermediary metabolism	Impaired wound healing
Carbohydrates and fats	Primary source of energy in the body and consequently in the wound healing process To meet the demand for increased essential fatty acids needed for cellular function after an injury To spare protein To restore normal weight	Signs and symptoms of protein deficiency due to use of protein to meet energy requirement Extensive weight loss
Water	To restore normal weight To replace fluid lost through vomiting, hemorrhage, exudates, fever, drainage, diuresis To maintain homeostasis	Signs, symptoms, and complications of dehydration, such as poor skin turgor, dry mucous membranes, oliguria, anuria, weight loss, increased pulse rate, decreased central venous pressure
Vitamin C	Important for capillary formation, tissue synthesis, and wound healing through collagen formation Needed for antibody formation	Impaired/delayed wound healing related to impaired collagen formation and increased capillary fragility and permeability Increased risk for infection related to decreased antibodies
Vitamin B complex	Indirect role in wound healing through their influence on host resistance	Decreased enzymes available for energy metabolism
Vitamin A	Increases inflammatory response in wounds, reduces anti-inflammatory effects of corticosteroids on wound healing	Impaired/delayed wound healing related to decreased collagen synthesis; impaired immune function Increased risk for infection
Vitamin K	Important for normal blood clotting Impaired intestinal synthesis associated with the use of antibiotics	Prolonged prothrombin time Hematomas contributing to impaired healing and predisposition to wound infections
Magnesium	Essential cofactor for many enymes that are involved in the process for protein synthesis and wound repair	Impaired/delayed wound healing (impaired collagen production)
Copper	Required cofactor in the development of connective tissue	Impaired wound healing
Zinc	Involved in DNA synthesis, protein synthesis, cellular proliferation needed for wound healing Essential to immune function	Impaired immune response

swelling and increasing pain and tenderness at the site. Systemic manifestations are fever and leukocytosis.

An accumulation of fluid in a wound may create pressure, impair circulation and wound healing, and predispose to infection. For these reasons, the surgeon may place a drain in the incision or make a stab wound adjacent to the incision to allow for drainage. These drains may be firm catheters attached to a Hemovac or other source of gentle suction.

Nursing assessment of the wound and dressing requires knowledge of the type of wound, the drains inserted, and expected drainage related to the specific type of surgery. A small amount of serous drainage is common from any type of wound. If a drain is in place, a moderate to large amount of drainage may be expected. For example, an abdominal incision with an accompanying drain is expected to have a moderate amount of serosanguineous drainage in the first 24 hours. In contrast, an inguinal herniorrhaphy should have only minimal serous drainage during the postoperative period.

In general, drainage is expected to change from sanguineous (red) to serosanguineous (pink) to serous (clear yellow).

The drainage output should decrease over hours or days, depending on the type of surgery. Wound infection may be accompanied by purulent, wound edges) and preceded by a sudden discharge of brown, pink, or clear drainage.

Nursing diagnoses related to surgical wounds of the postoperative patient include, but are not limited to, the following:

- Risk for infection
- Potential complication—impaired wound healing.

When drainage occurs on the dressing, the type, amount, color, consistency, and odor of drainage should be noted and recorded. The effect of position changes on drainage should also be assessed. The surgeon should be notified of any excessive or abnormal drainage and significant changes in vital signs.

The incision may be covered with a dressing immediately after surgery. If there is no drainage after 24 to 48 hours, the dressing may be removed and the incision left open to the air. If the initial operative dressing is saturated, institutional policy determines whether the nurse may change the dressing or simply reinforce it.

When a dressing is changed, the number and type of drains present should be noted. Care should be taken to avoid dislodging drains during dressing removal. When the dressing is changed, the incision site should be examined carefully. The area around the sutures may be slightly reddened and swollen, which is an expected inflammatory response. However, skin around the incision should be of normal color and temperature. Clinical manifestations of infection include redness, swelling, pain, fever, and increased white blood cell count. If healing is by primary intention, little or no drainage is present, and no drains are in place, a single-layer dressing or no dressing is sufficient. When drains are in place, when moderate to heavy drainage is occurring, or when healing occurs other than by primary intention, a multiple-layer dressing is needed.

DISCHARGE FROM THE POCU

The choice of discharge site is based on patient acuity, access to follow-up care, and the potential for postoperative complications. The decision to discharge the patient from the POCU is based on written discharge criteria. Examples of discharge criteria are provided in as given below:

Postanesthesia Discharge Criteria (Phase I)

- Patient awake (or baseline)
- Vital signs stable
- No excess bleeding or drainage
- No respiratory depression
- Oxygen saturation >90%
- Report given.

Ambulatory Surgery Discharge Criteria (Phase II/III)

- All POCU discharge criteria met
- No IV opioid drugs for last 30 minutes
- Minimal nausea and vomiting
- Voided (if appropriate to surgical procedure/orders)
- Able to ambulate if age appropriate and not contraindicated
- Responsible adult present to accompany patient
- Discharge instructions given and understood.

Discharge to the Clinical Unit

Before discharging the patient from the POCU to the clinical unit, the POCU nurse provides a verbal report about the patient to the receiving nurse. The report summarizes the operative and postanesthetic period.

The nurse who receives the patient on the clinical unit assists POCU transport in transferring the patient from the POCU cart onto the bed. Care must be taken to protect IV lines, wound drains, dressings, and traction devices. The use of a draw sheet or transfer board and sufficient personnel facilitates transfer of the patient.

Vital signs should be obtained, and patient status should be compared with the report provided by the POCU. Documentation of the transfer is then completed, followed by a more in-depth assessment. Postoperative orders and appropriate nursing care are then initiated.

Nursing Assessment and Care of Patient on Admission to Clinical Unit

- Record time of patients return to unit
- Take baseline vital signs
- Assess pain and discomfort
  - Note last dose and type of pain control
  - Note current pain intensity
- Assess airway and breath sounds
- Assess neurologic status, including level of consciousness and movement of extremities
- Assess wound, dressing, and drainage tubes:
  - Type and amount of drainage
  - Connect tubing to gravity or suction drainage (per orders)
- Assess color and appearance of skin
  - Time of voiding
  - Presence of catheter, patency, and total output
  - Bladder distention or urge to void
- Assess urinary status
- Position for airway maintenance, comfort, and safety (bed in low position, side rails up)

- Check IV infusion:
  - Type of solution
  - Amount of fluid remaining
  - Flow rate
  - Integrity of insertion site and size of catheter
- Attach call light within reach, and orient patient to use of call light
- Ensure that emesis basin and tissues are available
- Determine emotional condition and support
- Check for presence of family member or significant other:
  - Orient patient and family to immediate environment
- Check and carry out postoperative orders
- Give wound care instructions:

Until sutures are removed

a. Keep the wound dry and clean.
   - If there is no dressing, ask your nurse or physician if you can bathe or shower
   - If a dressing or splint is in place, do not remove it unless it is wet or soiled
   - If wet or soiled, change dressing yourself if you have been taught to do so; otherwise, call your nurse or physician for guidance
   - If you have been taught, instruction might be as follows:
     - Cleanse area gently with sterile normal saline once or twice daily
     - Cover with a sterile Telfa pad or gauze square large enough to cover wound
     - Apply hypoallergenic tape (Dermacel or paper). Adhesive is not recommended because it is difficult to remove without possible injury to the incisional site.

b. Immediately report any of the these signs of infection:
   - Redness, marked swelling exceeding 1/2 inch (2.5 cm) from incision site; tenderness; or increased warmth around wound
   - Red streaks in skin near wound
   - Pus or discharge, foul odor
   - Chills or temperature higher than 37.7°C (100°F)

3. If soreness or pain causes discomfort, apply a dry cool pack (containing ice or cold water) or take prescribed acetaminophen tablets (2) every 4-6 hours. Avoid using aspirin without direction or instruction because bleeding can occur with its use.
4. Swelling after surgery is common. To help reduce swelling, elevate the affected part to the level of the heart.
   - Hand or arm
     - Sleelp—elevate arm on pillow at side
     - Sitting—place arm on pillow on adjacent table
     - Standing—rest affected hand on opposite shoulder; support elbow with unaffected hand
   - Leg or foot
     - Sitting—place a pillow on a facing chair; provide support underneath the knee
     - Lying—place a pillow under affected leg

After sutures are removed

Although the wound appears to be healed when sutures are removed, it is still tender and will continue to heal and strengthen for several weeks.

a. Follow recommendations or physician or nurse regarding extent of activity.
b. Keep suture line clean; do not rub vigorously; pat dry. Wound edges may look red and may be slightly raised. This is normal.
c. If the site continues to be red, thick and painful to pressure after 8 weeks, consult the health care provider. (This may be due to excessive collagen formation and should be checked.)

Common Trays used in Preoperative Nursing

1. Preoperative skin preparation tray (Fig. 6.7)
   - A bowl of hot water
   - A bowl with cotton wool and gauze swabs
   - A receiver with a razor and a pair of scissors
   - A small bowl with warm ether soap
   - A receiver or disposal bag for soiled swabs
   - A protection for the bed
   - A disposable drape.

   When a skin disinfectant and sterile dressing is to be applied add:
   - A bottle with the ordered disinfectant, e.g. hibitane
   - A gallipot for the lotion
   - A receiver or suitable container with set of dressing forceps
   - A small packet containing the necessary sterile dressings and towels.
2. Local anesthetic tray (Fig. 6.8)
   - Small packet containing sterile towel and swabs
   - A bottle with cetavlon (1%)

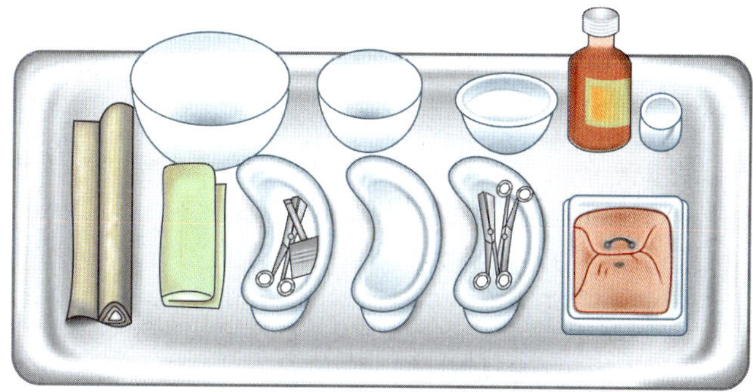

FIG. 6.7: Tray for preoperative skin preparation

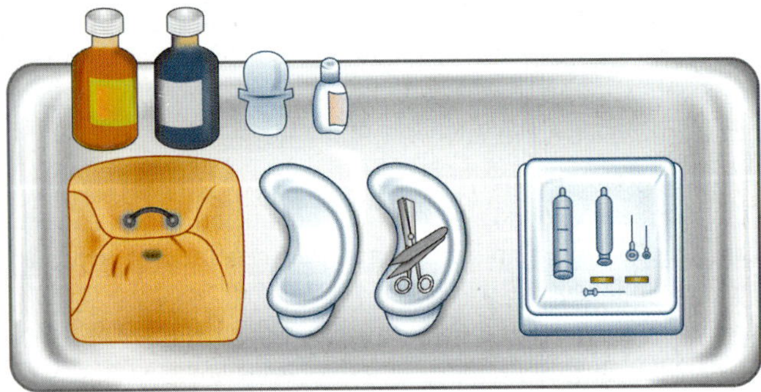

FIG. 6.8: Tray for local anesthetic by injection

- A bottle of methylated spirit
- Two sterile gallipots
- Bottle containing the local anesthetic, e.g. xylocaine (0.5%)
- Packet or box with 5 and 2 mL dry sterile syringes and assorted suitable-sized needles
- A receiver or suitable container with three pairs of sterile dressing forceps
- A receiver or disposal bag for soiled swabs (local anesthesia may also be produced using, e.g. a spray or drops):
  - A bowl of gauze swabs
  - A jar with dressed wooden probes
  - A bottle with the local anesthetic, e.g. cocaine (10 %)
  - A suitable measure for the anesthetic
  - De Vilbiss spray
  - A small tray with laryngoscope(s)
  - A receiver with angled tongue depressor and grasping forceps.
  - Sickness basin
  - Denture jar
  - A receiver or disposal bag for soiled swabs
  - A disposable drape.

c. Direct laryngoscopy tray (Fig. 6.9)

(*Note:* Patient premedicated. Several sizes of laryngoscope available. Extra-electric bulbs at hand. Suction apparatus in readiness.)

(It may be necessary to have tracheotomy instruments also in readiness.)

For bronchoscopy: Requirements are similar with the addition of a bronchoscope.

d. Lumbar puncture trolley (Fig. 6.10)

- A jar with Cheatle's forceps
- A small tray with a packet containing sterile towels and dressings
- A bottle of cetavlon (1%)
- A bottle of methylated spirit

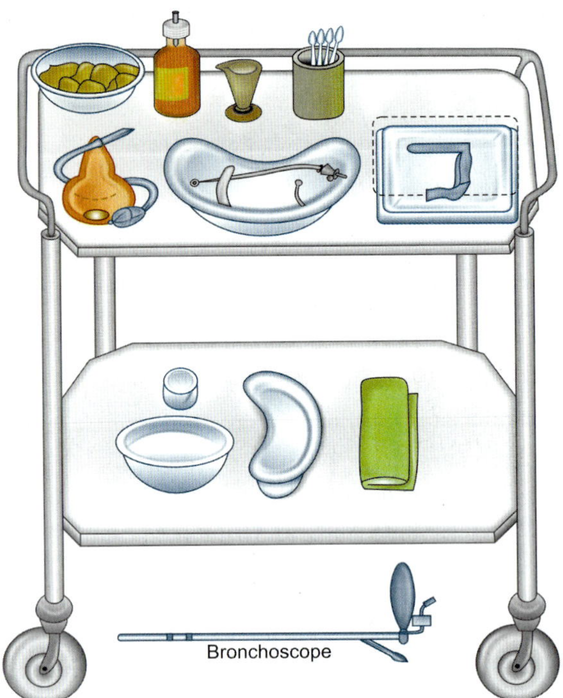

FIG. 6.9: Trolley for direct laryngoscopy

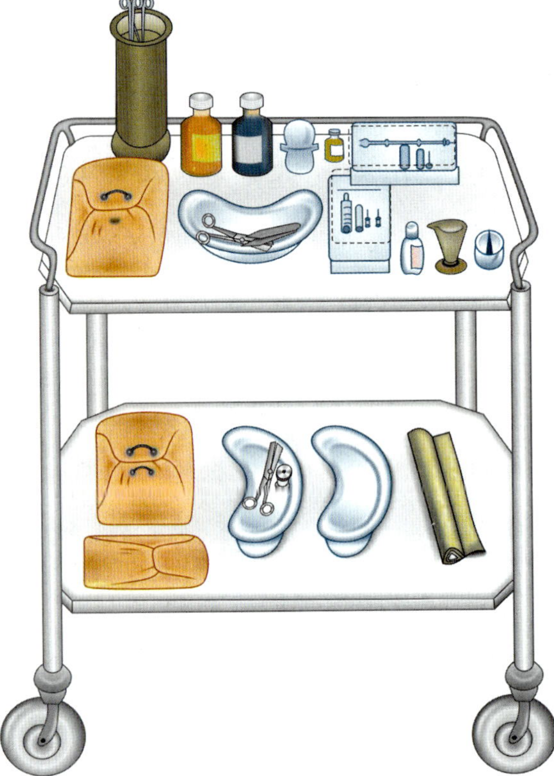

FIG. 6.10: Trolley for lumbar puncture

- Two sterile gallipots
- A covered receiver or suitable container with three pairs of sterile dressing forceps
- Hypodermic syringe and needles in syringe box or packet
- A bottle with local anesthetic, e.g. novocaine (2%) or xylocaine (0.5%)
- Two lumbar puncture needles, a spinal manometer, 10 or 20 mL syringe and cannula; these may be autoclaved in a packet or a special covered tray. A tenotomy knife may also be required
- A sterile specimen bottle
- A small glass measure for the fluid
- When a drug is being introduced intrathecally, the ampoule may be standing in a bowl of warm water to heat it to body temperature
- A receiver with adhesive strapping and scissors
- A receiver or disposal bag for soiled swabs
- A protection for the bed
- Packets containing sterile gowns, masks and gloves
- A stimulant should be at hand

5. Spinal anesthesia trolley: (Fig. 6.11)

For cisternal puncture or ventricular puncture: Requirements are similar, but the appropriate needle is substituted for the lumbar puncture needle. (Omit: Cheatle's forceps and make necessary modification when equipment is available from Central Sterile Supply Department).

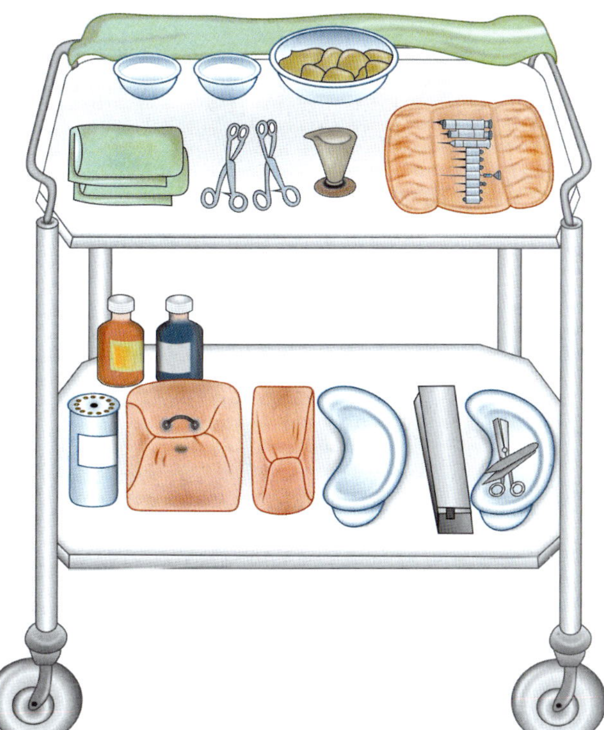

FIG. 6.11: Trolley for spinal anesthesia

Sterile towel on trolley—

i. A gallipot with hibitane and cetavlon
ii. A gallipot with skin hibitane
iii. A bowl with sterile gauze swabs
iv. Two swab-holding forceps
v. Sterile towels
vi. A small measure or gallipot for cerebrospinal fluid.
vii. A spinal bundle containing:
    a. 120 mL syringe
    b. 110 mL syringe
    c. 12 mL syringe
    d. 1 ampoule of heavy spinal nupercaine
    e. 1 ampoule of light spinal nupercaine
    f. 1 ampoule of 0.5 percent, xylocaine
    g. 2 lumbar puncture needles
    h. 2 large wide-bore needles for emptying ampoules
    i. 2 hypodermic needles
    j. An ampoule file
    (This bundle is autoclaved at 20 lb pressure at a temperature of 260° F (126.6°C) for 20 minutes)
    (All ampoules must be discarded and renewed before resterilizing as the drug must be autoclaved once only)
viii. Bottles with lotions for skin
ix. Small drum from which spinal set is removed
x. Gowns, caps, masks and gloves for anesthetists
xi. Receiver for discarded equipment
xii. Sphygmomanometer
xiii. Adhesive strapping and scissors
xiv. Disposal bag for soiled dressings

(A sterile spinal manometer should be at hand. Trolley covered with a sterile towel).

OPERATION THEATER INSTRUMENTS

It must be understood that lists of instruments for different operations vary with different surgeons and circumstances, but the following have been found generally satisfactory:

General (Fig. 6.12)
Bone set (Fig. 6.13)
Bone sharps (Fig. 6.14)
Gastrectomy and resection of gut (Fig. 6.15)
Tonsillectomy (Fig. 6.16)
Gynecological work (Fig. 6.17)
Ophthalmic work (Fig. 6.18)

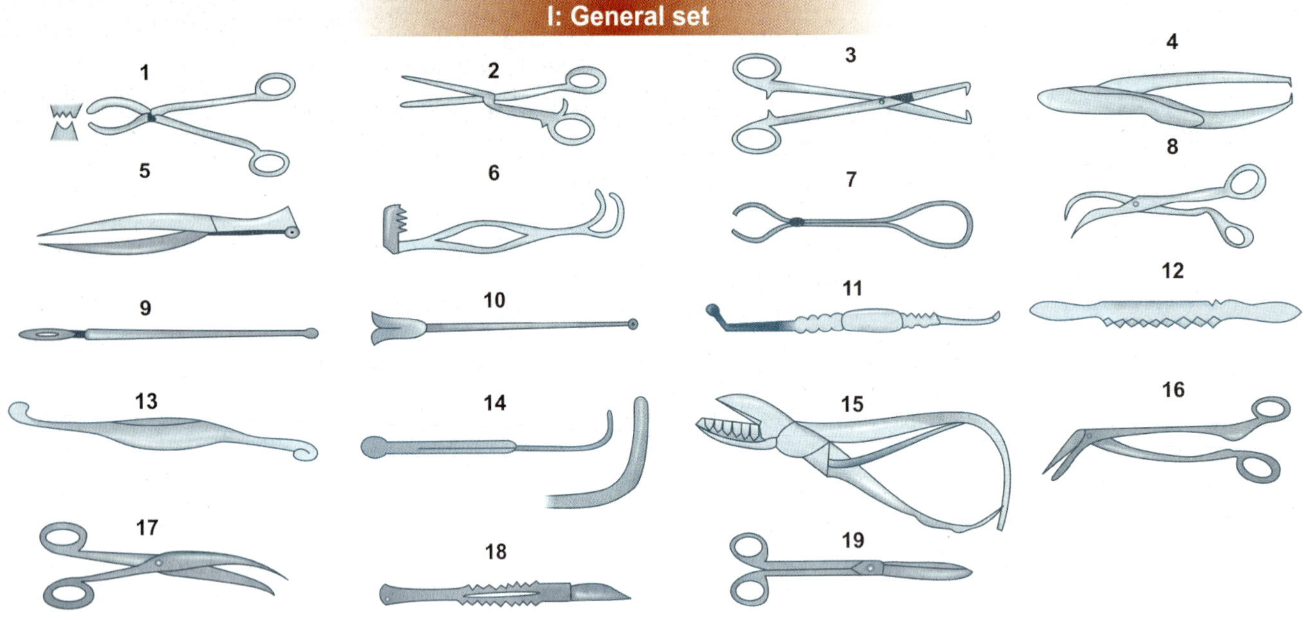

FIG. 6.12: General set (plate I)

15 Lane's tissue forceps (I, 1).
9 Spencer Wells artery forceps (I, 2).
9 Mayo Ochsner's forceps (I, 3).
4 Toothed dissecting forceps (I, 4).
2 Non-toothed dissecting forceps (I, 5).
2 Retractors (I, 6).
2 Sponge-holding forceps (I, 7).
4 Towel clips (I, 8).
1 Small probe (I, 9).
1 Long probe (I, 9).
1 Grooved director (I, 10). 9 extras
1 Blunt dissector (I, 11).
1 Raspatory (I, 12).
1 Sharp spoon (I, 13).
1 Aneurysm needle (I, 14). 9 extras
1 Needle holder (I, 15).
1 Suture holder (I, 16).
1 Pair curved scissors (I, 17).
2 Scalpels (I, 18).
2 Pairs straight scissors (I, 19).

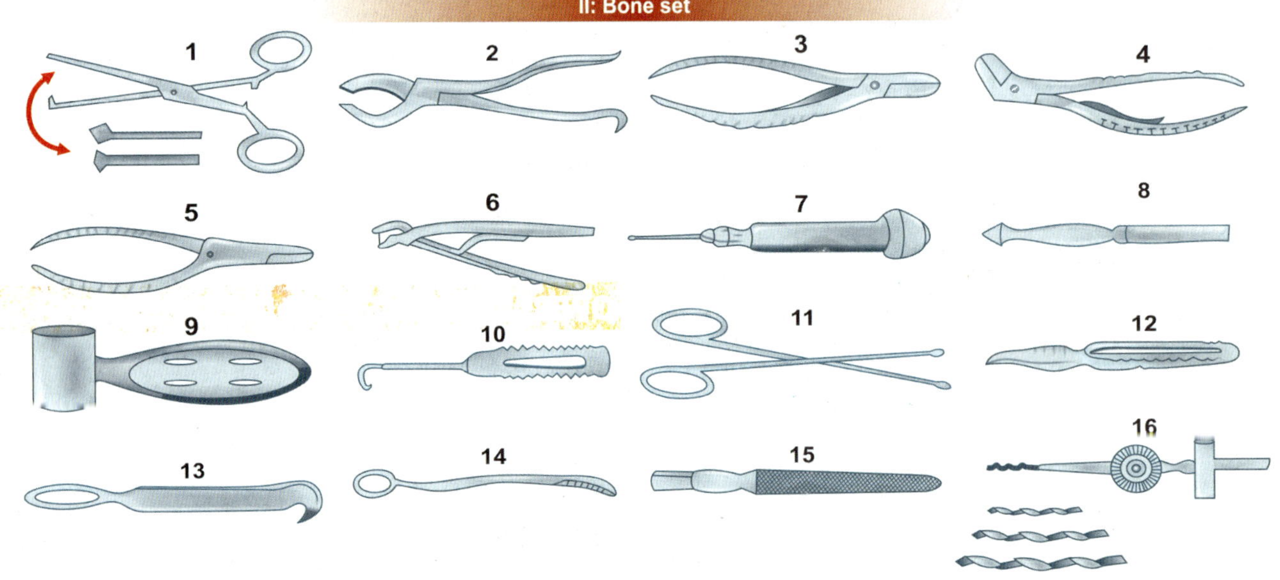

FIG. 6.13: Bone set (plate II)

9 Skin clips (II, 1).
2 Lion bone-holding forceps (II, 2).
2 Small lion-holding forceps (II, 2).
1 Large straight bone cutting forceps (II, 3).
1 Large curved bone cutting forceps (II, 4).
1 Small straight bone cutting forceps.
1 Small curved bone cutting forceps (II, 4).
2 Pairs necrosis forceps (II, 5).
1 Pair sequestrum forceps (II, 6).
1 Awl (II, 7).
1 Grooved awl (II, 8).
1 Mallet (II, 9).
Langenbeck retractors (II, 10).
1 Pair sinus forceps (II, 11).
2 Rugines (II, 12)
1 Pair large bone levers or spikes (II, 13).
1 Pair medium bone levers (grooved) (II, 14).
1 Pair small bone levers (or more according to operation)
1 File (II, 15).
1 Mechanical drill and drill points (II, 16).

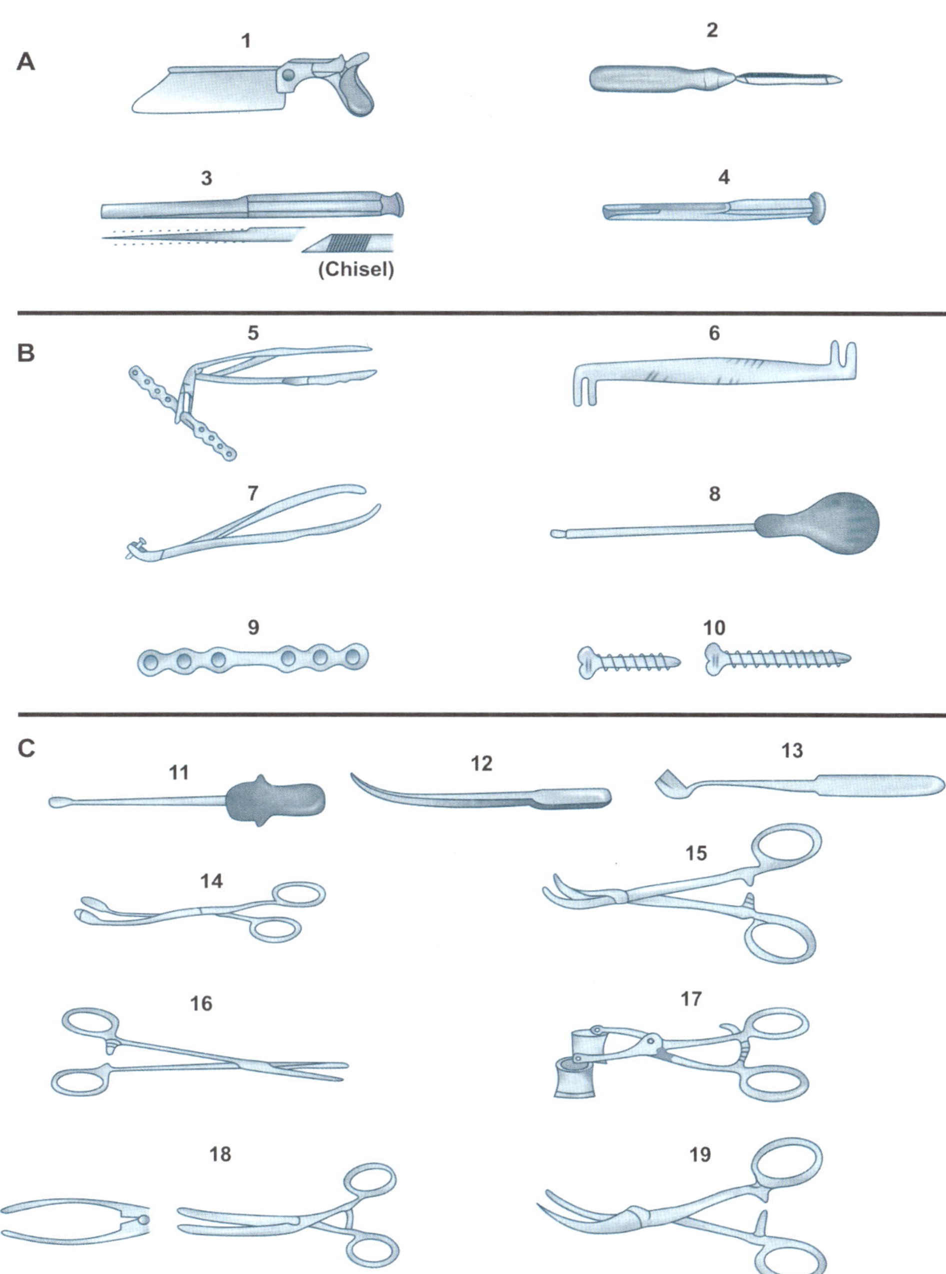

FIG. 6.14: Bone sharps (plate IIIA to C)

Bone plating set (plate IIIA)

1 Large saw (III, 1).
1 Small saw.
Osteotomes varying sizes (III, 2).
Chisels of varying sizes (III, 3).
Gouges varying sizes (III, 4).
Drill points varying sizes (II, 16).

Bone plating set (plate IIIB)

General set and bone set, plus—
2 Plate-holding forceps (III, 5).
2 Plate benders (III, 6).
2 Screw-holding forceps (III, 7).
2 Screwdrivers (III, 8).
Plates (III, 9) and screws (III, 10).

Extra laparotomy instruments (plate IIIC)

General set, plus.—
1 Malleable probe (III, 11).
1 Pliable probe (III, 12). 4 gallbladder extras
1 Malleable spoon or scoop (III, 13).
1 Gallstone forceps (Desjardin's) (III, 14).
2 Moynihan's pedicle forceps (III, 15).
2 Straight compression forceps (III, 16).
2 Abdominal retractors (III, 17).
2 Pairs curved intestinal clamps (III, 18).
2 Curved compression forceps (III, 19).

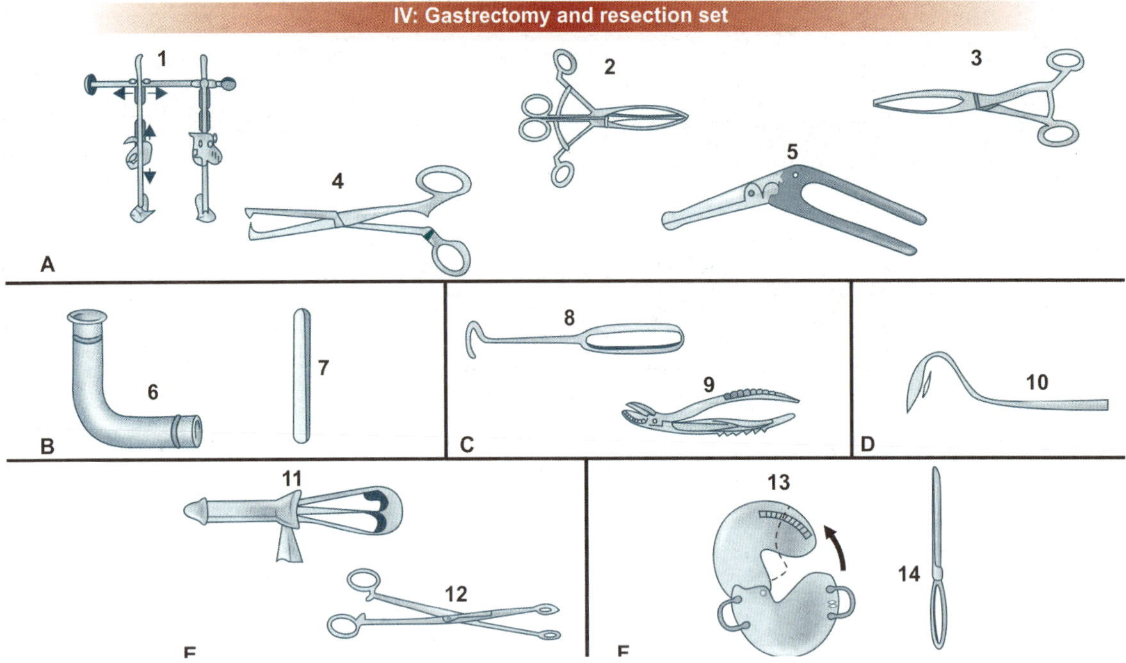

FIG. 6.15: Gastrectomy and resection of gut (plate IVA to F)

Gastrectomy and resection of gut (plate IVA)

General set, plus.—

2 Abdominal retractors (III, 17).
1 Self-retaining retractor (IV, 1).
2 Straight compression forceps (III, 16).
2 Curved compression forceps (III, 19).
2 Moynihan's pedicle forceps (III, 15).
1 Double intestinal clamp (IV, 2).
2 Large straight intestinal clamps (IV, 3).
2 Small straight intestinal clamps (IV, 3).
2 Curved intestinal clamps (III, 18).
4 Ludd's or Allis's basting forceps (IV, 4).
1 Large Payr's clamp (IV, 5).
1 Small Payr's clamp (IV, 5).

Colostomy (plate IVB)

General set, plus—
Abdominal retractors (III, 17).
2 Small intestinal clamps (III, 18).
Paul's tube (IV, 6) and colostomy rod (IV, 7).

Empyema (plate IVC)

Herniotomy (plate IVD)

General Set, plus-
Rugine (II, 12).
Hernia needle (IV, 10).
2 Rib raspatories (IV, 8).
Rib cutting forceps (II, 3, 4).
Rib shears (IV, 9).
Necrosis forceps (II, 5).

Hemorrhoids (plate IVE)

General set, plus—
Proctoscope (IV, 11).
4 Hemorrhoid clamps (IV, 12).

Amputation (plate IVF)

General set, plus—
Extra artery forceps (I, 2).
Bone set (II).
Bone sharps (IIIA).
Flat retractor (IV, 13).
Amputation knife (IV, 14).

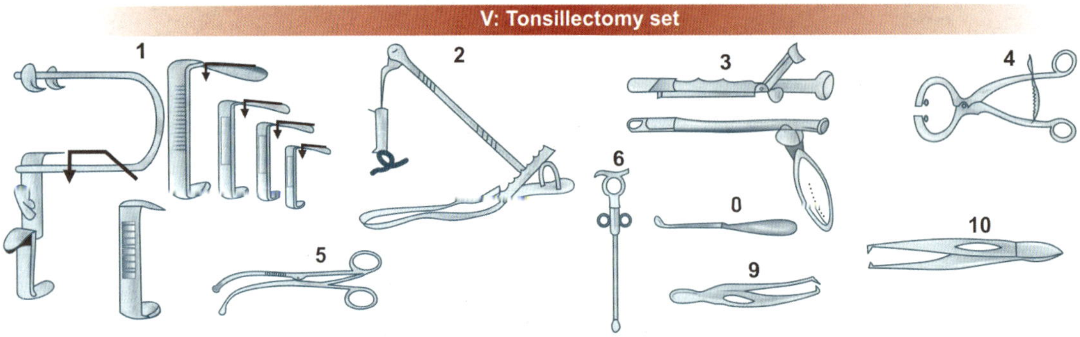

V: Tonsillectomy set

FIG. 6.16: Tonsillectomy set (plate V)

1 Towel clip (I, 8).
4 Tongue depressors (V, 1).
1 Davis gag (V, 1).
Suspension apparatus for gag (V, 2).
2 Tonsil guillotines (V, 3).
2 Doyen's gags (V, 4).
2 Mayo Ochsner's artery forceps (I, 3).
1 Tracheotomy dilator (V, 5).
2 Tonsil snares (V, 6).
1 Tonsil dissector.
2 Adenoid curettes (V, 8).
2 Pairs toothed dissecting forceps (I, 4).
2 Curved tonsil forceps (V, 9).
1 Toothed tonsil forceps (V, 10).
4 Straight artery forceps (I, 2).
4 Curved artery forceps (I, 1).

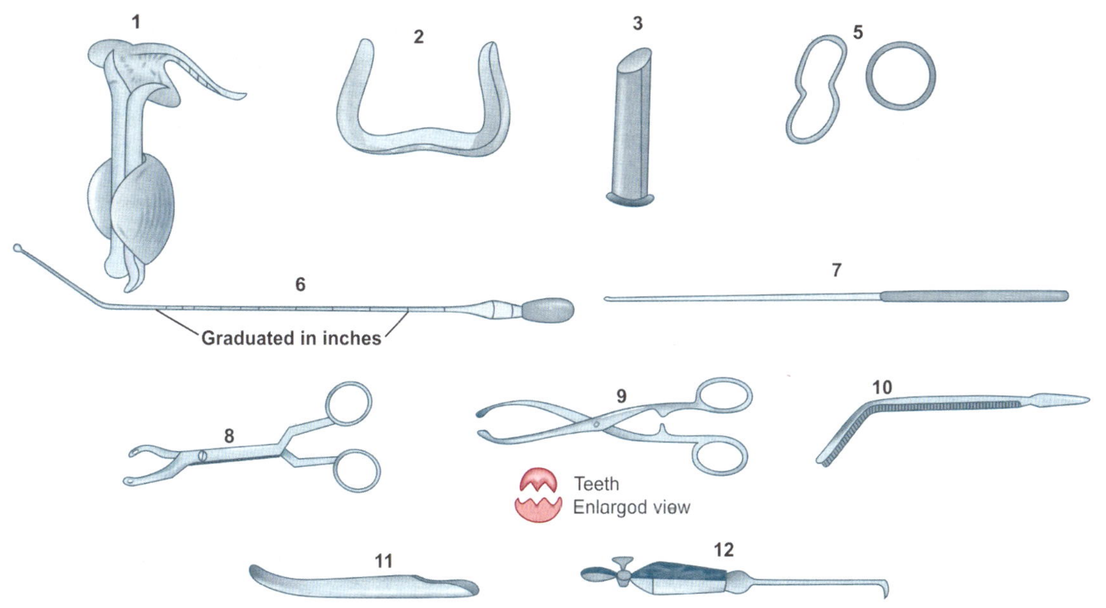

FIG. 6.17: Some special instruments for gynecological work (plate VI)

Vaginal speculae, Auvard's (VI, 1).
Vaginal speculae, Sims' (VI, 2).
Vaginal speculae, Fergusson's (VI, 3).
Pessaries (VI, 5).
Uterine sound (VI, 6).
Playfair's probe (VI, 7).
Ovum forceps (VI, 8).
Vulsellum forceps (VI, 9).
Intrauterine douche nozzle (VI, 10).
Dilators for cervix (VI, 11).
Intrauterine flushing curette (VI, 12).

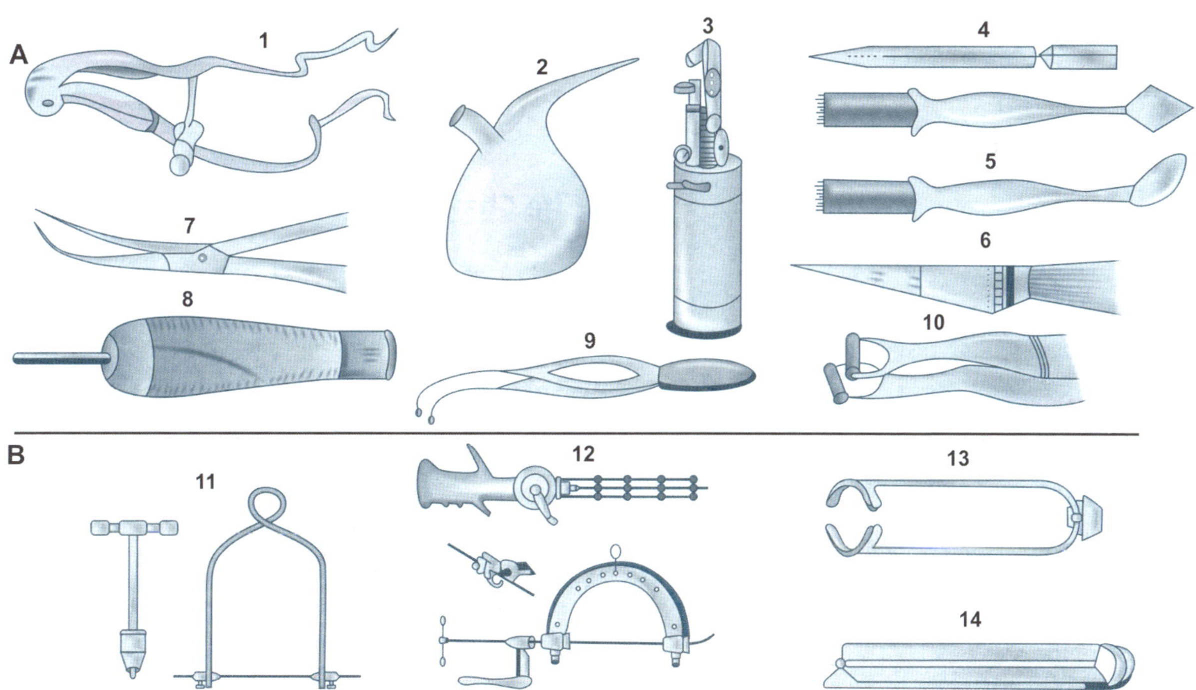

FIG. 6.18: Some special instruments for ophthalmic work (plate VIIA and VIIB)

Some special instruments for ophthalmic work (plate VIIA)

Retractor (VII, 1).
Undine (VII, 2).
Ophthalmoscope (VII, 3).
Graefe's knife (VII, 4).
Keratome (VII, 5).
Beer's knife (VII, 6).
Iris scissors (VII, 7).
Elliott's trephine (VII, 8).
Iris forceps (VII, 9).
Roller forceps for trachoma (VII, 10).

Operative Treatment of Fractures (Plate VIIB)

Steinmann's pin, introducer, stirrup (VII, 11).
Apparatus for the insertion of Kirschner's wire (VII, 12).
A Bohler's iron (VII, 13).
A Smith-Petersen nail (VII, 14).

(This plate is much reduced from the actual size.)

INFECTION CONTROL IN OPERATION THEATER

This chapter intends to explore further some of the principles that aid in enabling the success of surgery and without which would result in an increase in the morbidity or mortality of surgical patients.

INFECTION CONTROL

Infection control within the theater environment covers a vast area. This section intends to review basic infection control issues within the environment, explore infection transmission and examine how the obtaining and maintaining of a sterile field reduces the risk of transmission. Finally sterilization and disinfection methods in current use will be discussed.

Management of infection control is the responsibility of all staff under health and safety guidelines (Health and Safety Executive 1999); therefore it is essential that everyone has a good understanding of the rationale behind practice and takes individual responsibility of implementing policies. Policies and guideline should be in place to guide individuals, minimizing the risk of infection transmission to both staff and patients.

Design of the operating theater has an impact on the ability of the environment to prevent the transmission of infection. Ventilation, humidity and baseline temperature all affect the presence and spread of microorganisms within the operating environment. Assuming that these factors are externally controlled, what actions could surgical, practitioners take to affect the incidence of surgical infections?

In the 1500s, Fracastorius stated that disease was spread via three methods: direct contact; handling articles that infected patients had handled; and distance transmission. Today the focus remains the same; it is recognizd that there is a chain of events that needs to be broken to prevent transmision (Fig. 6.19). Transmission of infecting requires: the presence of a pathogenic organism; a reservoir; method of exit-transmission; portal of entry; plus susceptibility of the host . Only by breaking this chain can infection be prevented.

Application of the principles of infection control is a fundamental part of effective health care. In order to manage infection control effectively, all practitioners need knowledge, in relation to key micro-organisms, their mode of transmission, methods of control and how to apply these in practice. The general principles of infection control are based on the use of practices and procedures that prevent or reduce the likelihood of infection being transmitted from a source (e.g. person, contaminated fluids, equipment) to a susceptible individual. This is commonly referred to as the chain of infection.

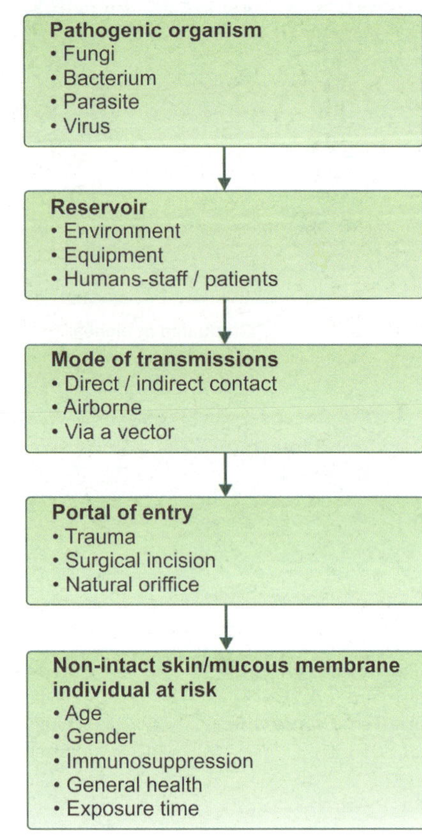

FIG. 6.19: Chain of infection

The Chain of Infection

The chain of infection is often described as having six links that represent the chain of events leading to the transmission of infection:

1. **A source of infectious agents** (bacteria, viruses, fungi).
2. Reservoirs in which the organisms may survive to multiply (e.g. people, animals, food, water, equipment). The most common reservoir and source of microorganisms in clinical areas are the patients themselves, particularly their exertions (such as blood, urine, feces, and vomit), secretions (such as pus, wound exudates) and skin lesions. Since it is impossible to eliminate exposure to all body fluids, it is important that all practitioners should follow standard (universal) precautions at all times and hence remove one or more of the other links in the chain of infection.
3. Portals of exit are where these microorganisms leave the body of the infected or colonized individual (e.g. droplets, excreta, secretions, skin).

4. Methods of transmitting these microorganisms from person to person by the following routes:
   - Direct contact: With body surfaces or fluids of an infected person
   - Indirect contact: Involves the transfer of microorganisms indirectly from one body site to another) via contaminated hands, equipment (e.g. urine measuring jugs, laryngoscope blade), surfaces, animals, food or water
   - Airborne spread: Contaminated skin scales, aerosols of contaminated skin scales, aerosols of contaminated droplets from patient sneezing and coughing
   - Vectors: Such as files, fleas, cockroaches, mosquitoes and other insects that harbor infectious agents
   - Ingestion: Microorganisms enter the gastrointestinal tract with contaminated food and water (e.g. *Salmonella*)
   - Inoculation: Microorganisms may be introduced via skin and mucous membranes by accidental injury, injection, bites or during surgical incision.
5. Portals of entry are ways through which the microorganisms are able to enter the body of another individual. This can be via the genitorurinary tract, the alimentary tract through the ingestion of contaminated food, the skin, mucous membranes and the respiratory tract via inhalation of organism such a tuberculosis.
6. **Susceptible individuals** have variable resistance to infection depending on their age, underlying disease and other factors that may compromise their immune status such as medical treatment with immunosuppressive drugs or irradiation. The risk of transmission of infection is higher for patients undergoing invasive procedures, and for patients who stay in hospital for a long time. Indwelling devices like catheters may also increase the risk of infection, particularly when used over long periods. Glynn, et al. (1997) found that invasive devices increase a patient's risk of infection sevenfold.

A complete chain of events is necessary for infection to occur. Figure 6.20 illustrates the elements of the chain and identifies points where nurses can intervene to interrupt the chain. Six elements are necessary for infection to occur. These essentials are (1) a causative organism, (2) a reservoir of available organisms, (3) a portal or mode of exit from the reservoir,

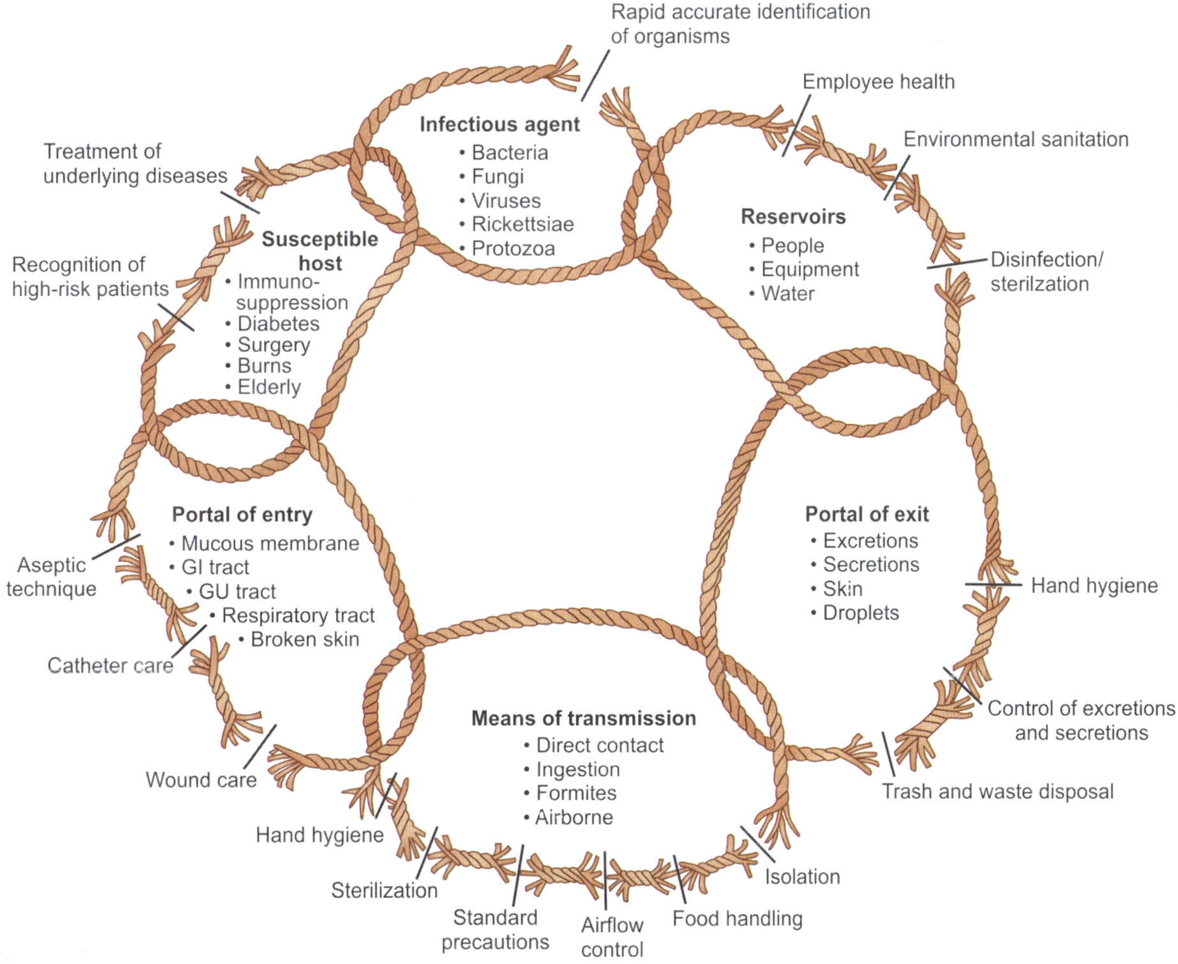

FIG. 6.20: Nurses interventions used to break the chain of infection transmission

(4) a mode of transmission from reservoir to host, (5) a susceptible host, and (6) a mode of entry to the host.

An infection will not be able to develop if one of the links in the chain is removed or controlled. However, it would be impossible to eradicate the second and sixth links, namely the reservoirs of infection and the susceptible individuals. For that reason, infection control practice tries to eliminate the third and fourth links, i.e. the means of transmission so as to prevent pathogenic organisms from gaining access via the portals of entry. The single most effective means of achieving this is through effective handwashing.

HOST-SPECIFIC DEFENSE MECHANISMS AGAINST INFECTION

All infections need a route of some sort by which to gain access to the body and the body in turn has developed defence mechanisms to reduce its vulnerability.

First Lines of Defense

- **Skin**: The first line of defense that an invading microorganism meets is the physical barrier provided by intact skin. Skin has a low pH and pathogenic bacteria fail to survive for long in this acid environment, but it allows the growth of harmless bacteria such as *Staphylococcus epidermidis*, micrococci and diptheroids (normal skin flora organisms). However, this balance is easily disrupted by the use of broad-spectrum antibiotics. These wipe out the normal flora which is replaced by potentially more harmful organisms, particularly if the individual is hospitalized. When the integrity of the skin is broken, for example, by a surgical incision or inflammation, it provides an obvious portal of entry for infection.
- **Respiratory tract:** The majority of microorganisms are prevented from entering the bronchial tree by hairs in the nose, which filter particles, and the cough reflex, which prevents their aspiration. However, procedures such as intubations and tracheotomy bypass the normal respiratory defence mechanism.
- **Conjunctiva:** The surface of the eyeball is constantly irrigated with tears from the lachrymal glands. Tears remove microorganisms by mechanical action (with eyelids). The enzyme lysozyme in tears has antibacterial properties that form an effective barrier against infection.
- **Genitourinary tract:** The constant downward flow of urine through the ureter and bladder helps avoid ascending infections. However, this is bypassed when a urinary catheter is inserted.
- **Gastrointestinal tract:** Gastric juices are highly acidic and a pH of between 2 and 3 destroys most ingested bacteria.

Second Lines of Defense

If invading microorganisms get through the first line of defense and enter the tissues, further non-specific host responses are stimulated. These include the inflammatory response, phagocytic cells, eosinophils, complement proteins, interferon and natural killer cells.

BLOOD-BORNE VIRUSES AND THE PERIOPERATIVE ENVIRONMENT

Theater practitioners on a daily basis are exposed to blood and body fluids, aerosols from power tools, splashes and risk of percutaneous injury from instruments, blades and needles. For this reason alone, it is essential that practitioners working in the high-risk environment of an operating theater are aware of the potential risks and incorporate safe systems of practice to avoid occupational exposure to blood-borne pathogens.

Conversely, patients can be at risk of acquiring blood-borne viruses from healthcare workers (HCWs). The three most important blood-borne viruses from an occupational exposure point of view are hepatits B, hepatitis C and HIV.

While environmental design is out of the practitioner's control, the management of reservoirs is certainly within their domain. Surgical practitioners can ensure that zoning for unrestricted semi-restricted and restricted access is fully maintained. They must ensure that within all these areas adequate cleaning of the environment occurs; this is essential to break the reservoir link of the chain. This requires the removal of obvious surface dirt and the thorough disinfection of floors. Additionally, in restricted areas the scrubbing of floors daily and disinfection of all equipment and surfaces is required.

There should be liaison with the hospital infection control team and an evidence-based use of competencies ensures their understanding of the environmental cleaning requirements, plus the impact of their non-compliance with policies. In addition to routine cleaning, there should be local polices on the management of spillages that prevent these from acting as a reservoir of infection.

Equipment is a reservoir that potentially places patients at risk and practitioners have the responsibility for ensuring that all equipment used during surgery is sterile. Methods of sterilization will be examined later. Besides ensuring equipment is sterile prior to use, practitioners need to maintain its sterility when handing to a sterile area, additionally ensuring that they retain appropriate information to ensure traceability of the equipment at a later date. For such equipment this requires the retention of the adhesive label supplied by their sterile service provider. Where departmental equipment is used for sterilization , this may entail noting date and time of activation, length of immersion and staff members involved. However, equipment has been sterilized prior to use, this information should be made available within each individual patient's notes. This demonstrates good practice, ensures standards are maintained and provides a resource for identifying equipment used on individuals should recall of equipment of patients be required.

Following use equipment still remains a reservoir, having the potential to place other patients and staff at risk. All equipment once finished with should be removed from the surgical site, handled with gloves and returned to the sterile service supplier as soon as possible to allow decontamination to occur. Supplementary sharps such as blades, needles, etc. should be handled with care, placed in a neutral zone on the practioner's trolley, and a solid disposal case used.

Practitioners, patients and other staff within the perioperative environment are potential reservoirs of infection. It is each practitioner's responsibility to recognize and report any infection or open lesion that may place susceptible individuals at risk. They should also recognize that infection or open lesions place themselves in the position of being the susceptible recipient of pathogenic organisms.

Transmission

Contact, be it direct or indirect, is essential to manage when attempting to break the infection chain. The wearing of gloves is good practice but only if worn appropriately, i.e. when at risk of being in contact with blood or body fluids. Once gloves have been in contact they should be discarded and hands washed before commencing other activities. Good quality hand hygiene is regarded as the single most important factor and essential in combating spread of infection . It is recognized that it is the quality of washing and sufficient drying rather than the cleaning product used that reduces the potential of spreading infection (Davey and Ince 2000). All staff should remember that good hand hygiene not only protects patients but also individuals and their work colleagues.

Other methods of transmission that specifically affect staff are splashes and aerosolizalion during surgery; this could be from irrigation, drills or the transfer of specimens. To protect themselves all staff should be routinely wearing facemasks and goggles and local policies should be in place.

Airborne

The dispersion of microbes is increased with movement, the majority of these microbes from staff. Practical aspects to reduce dissemination require the reduction of movement. During surgery doors should remain closed preventing the ingress of corridor air plus utilizing only the required number of staff for surgery and restricting the number and movement of visitors.

While it is recognized that practitioners cannot affect the ventilation system in place, they should ensure it is working on the day of surgery. Those practicing in areas with laminar flow have additional responsibilities to ensure they utilize it effectively and contain all trolleys and equipment within the laminar flow area.

Vector

A vector may be any mechanical agent that picks up an infectious agent and then carries it to a susceptible host. Glove powder is considered a vector, though powdered gloves are now not used. In surgery, practitioners need to be aware of the principles of vector contamination.

Portal of Entry

Patients undergoing a surgical incision all have a potential entry site for infection. Those who arrive for surgery following a trumatic accident will have increased their opportunity for infection development due to contamination of the wound. Additionally patients with multiple injuries develop the risk of contamination from one site to another. With multiple operation sites, the scrub practitioner can influence and reduce the risk of cross-site contamination by preparing wound sites in a logical sequence starting with the least contaminated or from a non-open surgical site.

Natural orifices are also an entry site for infection; therefore staff should ensure they remain vigilant during procedures that involve any natural body opening. Opportunities remain frequent with endotracheal tubes inserted nasally/orally, urinary catheters and cystoscopes used urethrally, and gastroscopes used via the esophagus, to name a few opportunities for the introduction of infection. Alongside the protection of patients, staff must remain vigilant for their own wellbeing, protecting open wounds that may act as an entry gate.

Individuals at Risk

Those who may be at risk from infection are wide and varied, an individual's general health and nutritional state playing a large part. Those whose risk is increased are young children due to their immature immune system, the elderly who have a diminished immune response so cannot respond appropriately to infection, and those whose immune system has been damaged or compromised. Additionally others whose immune system may be affected and thus susceptible to infection are those who have undergone a large emotional or physical stress. This would include those undergoing extensive surgery. Patients considered not be at risk initially may become at risk due to local factors affecting blood supply to a wound, such as edema or ischemia. The longer the length of surgery the more there is an increased risk of infection due to the opportunities from exposure to the environment, the invasive use of equipment and handling of body tissue.

Combined with the principles of infection control is the need to obtain and maintain a sterile field for surgical procedures. Actions to this effect will enable a break in the transmission of infection.

OBTAINING AND MAINTAINING A STERILE FIELD

The obtaining and maintaining of a sterile field is designed to reduce the risk of infection transmission to individual patients and at the same time to protect staff from infection. This is achieved by combining a number of practices: staff dress and preparation; patient preparation; utilization of sterile equipment; and etiquette during surgery. The key infection control procedures in two phases—pre- and perioperative that all practitioners should use in the care of all patients undergoing a surgical procedure to minimize the transmission of infection to staff and between patients.

Preoperative Phase

Admission

Pre-admission assessment and an increase in day-case surgery have reduced the length of time patients have to be in hospital prior to surgery. In demonstrated that shorter stays are associated with lower infection rates. The relationship between the numbers of preoperative days and the likelihood of infection are—after 1 day, the wound infection rate is 1.2%; after 7 days this increases to 3.1% and after 14 days or more the wound infection rate increases to 3.4%.

Preoperative Preparation of the Patient's Showering

The benefit of preoperative bathing, with or without antiseptic soaps to reduce skin flora, remains unclear. A number of studies demonstrated that showering using an antimicrobial product reduced the bacterial load on the skin.

Shaving

A number of studies have demonstrated that shaving the skin before an operation increases the risk of wound infections. The criteria to shave should be based on the need to view or access the surgical site and should be carried out close to the time of surgery. This avoids the risk of traumatizing the skin and providing an opportunity for the skin to become heavily colonized with bacteria at the surgical site.

Patients' Clothing

The routine removal of patients' underwear was first introduced when nylon underwear could potentially cause static electricity. Today the removal of the patient's underwear should only occur if it is going to interfere, with the operation site or there is a risk of the patient's own underwear being soiled by the use of skin preparations in theaters. In both cases, disposable underwear should be made available in order to maintain the patient's dignity. Brown (1993), described this ritual of removing patients' underwear as the "most illogical of rituals'. However, in respect of removing all other times of the patient's own clothing prior to some surgery is required to confirm whether this is necessary.

Transport of the patient to theater: Prior to the patient going to theater they should be dressed in a freshly laundered theater gown. If being transported on a bed then it should be made up with fresh bed linen to minimize the shedding of particles into the air when the bedding is disturbed. Moreover, the patient can be transferred to the anesthetic room or to the operating theater on their bed, without additional risk of infection, providing the bed linen pack (i.e. the upper layers rather than under sheet) is not brought into the operating theater itself.

Provision of Overshoes

The issue of hand contamination by donning and removal of overshoes was highlighted as a potential risk to patients. It has been suggested that overshoes could be worn to avoid shoes being overly contaminated by blood and body fluids. The patient preparation incorporates skin preparing and draping. Shaving of skin prior to surgery has been shown to cause injury and increase infection risk. Studies demonstrate that where possible patients who require hair removal to provide access to the incision site should (where possible) use a depilatory cream on the day prior to surgery, otherwise clippers should be used to remove hair.

Skin preparation at the time of surgery is performed to prevent bacteria entering the incision site. Solutions used vary widely but they should all be rapidly effective, broad spectrum and effective against both Gram-negative and Gram-positive bacteria plus fungi and viruses. They need to remain active when in contact with blood or body fluids/secretions/excretions. No known toxic or allergic solutions should be used on an individual. Solutions should ideally be available in single-use containers. Ideally only one solution should be applied to prevent inactivation. Current recommendation is that alcoholic solutions are the most effective, though care must be taken to prevent pooling and time allowed to ensure the solution is dry prior to application of the drapes or the use of electrocautery - due to the risk of combustion. Additionally pooling under pneumatic tourniquets, around ECG electrodes and diathermy plates can result in chemical burn injury to the patient.

Preparation should not commence until all non-scrubbed staff have completed all care requirements for the individual. Prior to commencing the scrub, the practitioner needs to have ensured, the patient has no allergy to the solution to be applied.

Cleansing commences with the cleanest area moving to less clean areas, working from the incision site outwards unless this is a contaminated area. Where open wounds or areas such as anus or vagina, are to be prepared, these areas are prepared last, the sponges used once and immediately discarded. Following skin preparation, all sponges and holders are discarded and never returned to the instrument trolley. Care must be taken to ensure spongeholder tips are protected, solutions are not allowed to pool and any wet linen/protection is removed prior to draping.

The use of adhesive sheets with the or without antiseptic impregnation and wound guards to prevent postoperative wound infection and intraoperative contamination have been shown to provide no clear benefits to patients in either the prevention of postoperative infection or in reduction of contamination; therefore their use can be questioned.

Theater Footwear

Well-fitting footwear with impervious soles should be worn. These need to be cleaned after every use to remove splashes of blood and body fluid. Procedures need to be in place to ensure that this is undertaken at the end of every session.

Removal of Jewelery

In recommend that jewelery (i.e. necklaces, ear-rings and rings with stones) be removed. However on the issue of wedding rings that theater practitioner (scrub and non-scrub) may continue to wear these. But in the case of surgeons they may be advised to remove a wedding ring when working with metal prostheses.

Scrubbing

Preoperative hand scrubbing is used to reduce the bacteria count on the hands of scrub staff and is the first defence for preventing transmission of pathogens. Prior to scrubbing all jewelery with the exception of a single plain band should be removed as they may be a source of microorganisms. The wearing of false nails should be prohibited due to evidence supporting the presence of pathogens. For the same reason, the wearing of nail polish should also be prohibited. The recommended length of scrub of the day must include cleaning beneath the nail.

Methodology of scrubbing should ensure that hands and arms are scrubbed effectively from fingertips to elbows and that hands are held higher than elbows. Subsequent hand cleaning can utilize an alcoholic hand rub.

Finger nails: Finger nails should be kept short, clean and free of artificial nails demonstrated that artificial nails harbor more pathogens such as Gram-negative bacilli and yeast bacteria, even after handwashing, than nurses with natural nails.

Theater Caps

Theater caps are principally worn to reduce the dispersal of hair and skin scales and protect the wearer from contamination such as blood and body fluid. It have been recommended that all theater staff keep their hair covered as a matter of routine at all times including non-scrubbed staff members of the operating team to wear disposable headgear; however common sense dictates that hair should be kept clean and out of the way.

Hand Hygiene

The single most important factor in prevention of infection in hospitals is hand hygiene. Infection control required to have a policy an hand hygiene and provide education and training in this area and pointed out that the recent national evidence-based guidelines included seven recommendations on hand hygiene.

The aim of hand decontamination is to significantly reduce the carriage of potential pathogens on the hands. Gould (2002) suggests that the terminology surrounding hand washing should be changed to hand 'decontamination' so that all health care staff view hand hygiene as a priority when they have direct patient contact. All theater practitioners are aware of the importance of a diligent scrub technique, but may fail to remember to wash their hands when carrying out other activities in the operating department. One of the seven recommendations on hand hygiene is that all health care workers' hands must be decontaminated immediately before each and every episode of direct patient contact or care and in hands becoming contaminated.

The aim of hand decontamination is to significantly reduce the carriage of potential pathogens on the hands. Gould (2002); suggests that the terminology surrounding hand washing should be changed to hand 'decontamination' so that all health care staff view hand hygiene as a priority when they have direct patient contact. All theater practitioners are aware of the importance of a diligent scrub 'technique, but may fail to remember to wash their hands when carrying out other activities in the operating department. One of the seven recommendations on hand hygiene is that all health care workers' hands must be decontaminated immediately before each and every episode of direct patient contact or care and in hands becoming contaminated.

Choice of cleansing agents commonly found in operating departments are as follows:

- *Liquid soap and water*: It is used to remove transient microorganisms acquired on the hands before they can be transferred commonly referred to as a 'social' hand wash. Unlike antiseptics they do not kill microorganisms or inhibit their growth, so their effectiveness is limited. In the operating department, it can be used in areas such as changing facilities, toiled areas and all other areas where a higher level of skin disinfection is not required.
- *Chlorhexidine, iodophors (e.g. povidone iodine) and triclosan:* These are products used either for hygienic hands disinfection where the transient microorganisms are largely destroyed or for a surgical scrub where the transient microorganisms and readily detachable residents are removed or destroyed.
- *Alcohol-based products:* These can be used for both hygiene hand disinfection and surgical scrub. However, it is important to highlight that alcohol-based products do not remove microorganisms but rapidly destroy them on skin surfaces, so they are therefore only suitable to be used for

clean hands. All visible contaminates must be first removed with soap and water or a detergent-based solution. Ethyl alcohol and isopropanyl or n-propyl alcohol are the two main alcohols that are combined with other antimicrobials, e.g. chlorhexidine or triclosan, plus the addition of an emollient to reduce the drying effect on skin. They have a rapid broad-spectrum antimicrobial activity but have limited effect on spores.

Skin Care

Skin damage is generally associated with the detergent base of the preparation and possibly poor handwashing technique. Common errors seem to be; not wetting the hands before applying soap or antiseptic detergent; not rinsing thoroughly to remove residual soap; and not drying the hands carefully. The epic guidelines recommend that a hand cream should be applied regularly to the hands to protect the skin from the drying effects of regular hand decontamination. Also, should a particular product currently used in the workplace cause skin irritation, occupational health advice should be sought.

PERSONAL PROTECTIVE EQUIPMENT (PPE)

Select protective equipment on the basis of an assessment of the risk of transmission of microorganisms in the patient, and the risk of contamination of health care practitioners' clothing and skin by the patient' blood, body fluids, secretions and excretions.

Plastic aprons: Single use fluid repellent aprons will protect the practitioner from contamination with blood, body fluids and microorganisms and must be discarded after each task or epidosode of care.

Examples of use are:

- Prior to handling contaminated swabs and specimens
- Cleaning in between cases and at the end of theater lists
- Dealing with spillages
- When cleaning contaminated equipment
- Whenever there is a risk of contamination to theater attire.

A full-body, fluid repellent gown should be worn where there is a risk of extensive splashing of blood, body fluids, secretions and excretions, with the exception of sweat, on the skin of health care practitioners.

Theater, Gowns and Drapes

Traditionally, the sole purpose of theater gowns and drapes was to reduce wound infection by providing a barrier to prevent the transfer of microorganisms from the patient's 'own skin flora and the skin of operating staff, into the surgical wound.

Gowns

Gowns are worn during sterile procedures to prevent bacteria from the scrubbed practitioner passing through the fabric to the environment or the operation site. When wet the fabric needs to prevent the transfer of bacteria through the fabric. Gowns currently supplied are made from polyimpermeable material. Best practice suggests that only gowns that are waterproof and disposable should be used; where material gowns are used they should be checked for faults and aprons underneath to protect the wearer from contamination. Microfilament gowns should be checked for faults, observed for strike-through and monitored to ensure appropriate disposal following the maximum number of uses. Gowns may be back-fastening or wrap around. Back-fastening gowns should never be exposed to the operation site as the area is unprotected. Wrap around gowns should only be considered sterile at the commencement of 4 procedure; after this they are at risk of contamination and are not visible to the wearer all gowns are supplied sterile and donned following the scrubbing of hands. They should be handled with dry hands, by the inside only, then assistance given to secure by a circulator. Hands do not protrude from the cuffs until gloves have been donned.

While the main rationale for gowns wearing is to protect the patient, they have the additional benefit of providing protection to the wearer from contamination from blood or body fluids. Theater gowns are considered as medical devices and in the future will have to comply with legal minimum standards. These standards will include wet and dry microbial penetration and a requirement to meet performance standards in relation to wet and dry sterile and resistance to penetration and linting. The same regulation will apply to drapes as these are also considered to be medical devices.

Draping

As with gowns, theater drapes should prevent bacteria from the scrubbed practitioner or from non-sterile areas of the patient passing through the fabric to the environment or the operation site. Should the fabric become wet it needs to prevent the transfer of bacteria through the fabric. Drapes are supplied currently made from cotton fabric, microfilament or a disposable impermeable material. Best practice would suggest that only drapes that are waterproof and disposable should be used (Woodhead, et al. 2002). Where material; drapes are used they should be checked for faults and protection applied underneath to protect the patient from self contamination and to protect the skin from excess moisture. With microfilament owns these should be check ked for faults, observed for strike-through and monitored to ensure that following 1he maximum number of uses they are disposed of.

Before applying drapes, skin preparation solutions should have been allowed to dry. Care must be taken with adhesive drapes to ensure patients have no allergies. Where drapes have no adhesive, they should be secured using towel clips that do not perforate the fabric. Additional care should be taken to ensure that the patient's skin is not injured by the used of towel clips.

When applying drapes practitioners should ensure they have sufficient drapes folded and prepared. These need to be held at waist height until placed on the patient with controlled movements that minimally disturb the air, ideally by two people to reduce the risk of contaminating the drapes or practitioners involved. Practitioners need to protect their hands by folding the drape over them to prevent contamination. Draping commences from the incision site working out towards the peripheries. Once in place drapes should not be moved; any drape below the edge of the operating table is considered unsterile (Meeker and Rothrock 1999).

Drapes should not be 'removed until the completion of surgery and until after the application of the wound dressings. Drapes should then be removed and disposed appropriately by the scrub practitioner; this prevents contamination of others and ensures that all equipment has been removed prior to drape removal. Health care workers require protection from splashes of potentially infected blood and bodily fluids onto the mucous membranes of the eyes and mouth.

Masks

Masks are donned prior to scrubbing and while their benefit in preventing infection is questionable they do prevent bacterial shedding onto the wound sire though an alternative view is that wearing of masks causes rubbing and the release of potentially harmful skin flakes. Currently there is insufficient research to prove or disprove either theory. Recommendations indicate that all staff involved in prosthetic implant surgery under laminar flow should wear masks to protect the patient. Where masks are worn they should be changed at the end of each case.

Mask provide the wearer with prevention from the body fluid and blood splashes also providing protection from in handling smoke and laser plume. The wearing of mask by scrub staff following risk assessment of invasive procedures is that mask should be worn at all times by all scrub staff.

Eye Protection

Eye protection is donned prior to scrubbing and may be in the form of a visor, spectacle or goggle. Though not worn to protect the patient they protect the scrubbed individual from penetration injury, conjunctiva contact with blood or body fluid splashes, or aerosolization. The increasing usage of power tools and lavage would suggest following risk assessment that for the majority of surgical cases scrubbed staff should wear eye protection.

Utilization of Sterile Equipment

Prior to the commencement of surgery all required and anticipated equipment for surgery is collected and checked for sterility. The scrub practioner prepares the equipment. If any set is found to contain moisture on opening it is discarded, as its sterility cannot be guaranteed. Any equipment found to be contaminated is discarded; if this is a part of a tray the whole tray is discarded. The circulating practitioner ensures that they maintain a wide berth around the sterile trolley and provide all supplementary equipment to the scrub practioner in a manner that maintains sterility. Preparation of equipment should only occur immediately prior to commencement of surgery; this reduces the risk of contamination of equipment to be used. All equipment should be laid out in a manner that facilitates ease of recognition and availability for immediate use.

Once at the operating table all trolleys and tables should be positioned adjacent to the operating table ensuring access to the surgeon. Positioning also needs to ensure there is sufficient space around the trolleys to reduce the risk of contamination of equipment or practitioners. When positioning, care must be taken to ensure no pressure is placed on any part of the patient. During use, all equipment should be replaced on trolleys or tables to reduce the risk of equipment falling to the floor or becoming contaminated in error.

Equipment used to remove tumors or used on 'dirty' areas, for example open bowel, should be used for these areas only and contained on separate trolleys or separate demarcated areas of a trolley. They must be user on these areas and not moved to potentially contaminate other surgical areas.

Following completion of surgery, once all equipment is accounted for. It is immediately sent for decontamination following hospital policy.

Causes of Needle Stick Injuries

It includes that were recapping of needles, transfer of used sharps to point of disposal, sharps not discarded after used, or overfilled sharp containers. Resheathing of needles has been proven to be, by and large, a dangerous practice, because if the needle misses the sheath, it will puncture the hand holding. In order to reduce the risk of percutaneous exposure at the operating table, the following actions required which includes.

- Avoid hand to hand passing of sharp instruments during an operation
- Establish a 'neutral zone'; this can be tray, kidney basin or an identified area in the operative field, which ensures the safe passage of sharps
- Ensure scalpels and sharp needles are placed in the designated neutral zone and removed promptly away from the operative field when not in use.

Safe Management of Spillages

All blood and body fluid spillages should be removed promptly, using 1% hypochlorite solution (10,000 parts per million [ppm] of available chlorine) or chlorine-releasing granules; this is necessary to neutralize and make safe the spillage prior to disposal. In situations, where there are minor contaminations of surfaces, a dilution of 0.1 % hypochlorite (1000 ppm available) can be used. If chlorine disinfectants cannot be used then spills should be removed using detergent and hot water. It should be noted that in the case of urine spillages, chlorine-based products should not be used as they may react with urine to produce a chlorine vapor. Consult local infection control policy for further information on the products used and the procedure for dealing with body fluids spills in your workplace.

Safe Management of Linen

Linen should be separated into used linen (soiled or fouled) and infected linen and then re-processed according to local infection control policy in your workplace.

Safe Disposal of Waste

All waste must be properly segregated, labeled, stored, transported and disposed of in accordance with expert guidance and the local infection control policies in your work area for further information. A surgical client is at a high risk of getting hospital acquired infection because of exposure of internal body tissue to the exterior environment. Thus, it is mandatory to practice standard safety measures.

Infection Control

This discipline is concerned with preventing nosocomial or healthcare-associated infections. Infection control practices focus at prevention of infection transmission. Since transmission of infection follows a chain of events involving pathogen, portal of entry and exit, transmission and host susceptibility. Infection control practices in OT perspective would include:

- *Personal methods:* These measures are used by an individual to prevent infection transmission. These measures include skin disinfection such as hand washing, scrubbing, skin decontamination, surgical site preparation, other personal measures may include maintaining health, avoiding infections, avoiding cuts, bruises on skin, wearing sterilized/disinfected clothing before entering the OT area. The principle of confine and confirm should be followed by the staff working in OT.
- *Administrative measures:* These measures are taken by the organization in an effort to minimize patients contact with any contaminated area surface of vehicle. The organization should formulate, and implement rules and regulations related infection control policies, provision of a adequate facilities for sterilization and disinfection surgical supplies and operative instruments.

Infection control considers factors related to spread of infection between various sources such as from patient to patient, patient to staff, from staff to patient or among the staff members. Since infection continues to be major source of morbidity in surgical patients, a conscious effort is necessary to control this infection in any possible way.

Infection control measures necessitates use of aseptic techniques in all invasive procedures and use universal precautions as it is excepted that undiagnosed infections are prevalent. The measures which can be taken to ensure infection control include:

Hand Washing

Hands of the hospital staff is a common source of bacterial contamination and most of these bacteria are multi-drug resistant. Thus, they act as an important source of nosocomial infection. The best way to control infection from this source is to wash hands frequently, and before and after every patient contact. However, health care worker's compliance with hand washing is poor and various reasons have been attributed to this such as lack of time, poor availability of soap and sinks, etc. Yet good amount of literature exist to justify hand washing. The center for disease control and prevention has stated that it is well documented that the most important measure for preventing the spread of pathogens is hand washing.

Hand washing is a procedure of washing hands with soap and water or an antiseptic solution in an attempt to reduce the number of microorganisms in an attempt to minimize risk of transferring infection from one individual to the other. The main medical purpose of hand washing is to remove pathogens and other harmful contents from the hands which may be harmful for the patients.

Environmental Cleaning in the Theater Suite

Floors of the operating room should be disinfected at the end of each session and scrubbed daily. Wall washing is recommended twice yearly. Specific spillages of blood or body fluids should be dealt with immediately. Mop buckets for spillage should be emptied after each use and kept dry until the next occasion when they are required. Lint-free cloth is recommended for all operating theater cleaning.

Sterilization and Disinfection

Patients admitted for surgery expect to find a clean, safe environment and to be protected from preventable infections. All practitioners have a professional responsibility to ensure that where possible practices in relation to sterlization and disinfection are carried out and monitored.

Decontamination

Cleaning, disinfection and sterilization are all forms of decontamination. Decontamination is the process that removes organic matter and removes or destroys microorganisms, allowing equipment to then be safe for handling or for use on patients. Methods used for decontamination on equipment are dependent upon the equipment's susceptibility to heat, chemicals, moisture and corrosion. Equipment design is also relevant, if it is fine-bored or porous. Other factors that may affect the process instigated are time, cost and safety.

Cleaning

Cleaning is a process that physically removes contamination, namely dirt, grease, tissue, etc. and does not necessarily destroy microorganisms. It is essential to perform before disinfection or sterilization of equipment as physical contamination reduces the ability of disinfectants or sterilants to achieve contact with the equipment. Failure to perform cleaning prior to disinfection and sterilization places patients at risk of infection and thus potentially an increased hospital stay, an increased risk of mortality plus increased costs to the hospital and risk of acquiring infections. Further consequences to equipment will result if cleaning is not performed, resulting in blockage of fine-bore equipment or malfunction. Cleaning may be performed manually; here appropriate protection should be worn; gloves, aprons and goggles. Cleaning may also be carried out with automated washers utilizing water, detergent and heat, or ultrasonic cleaners where cavitations agitates the liquid and results in cleaning. Cleaning as a final process is appropriate for use where there is low risk, items do not come into contact with patients, or with healthy skin. Therefore, the process is suitable for items such as furniture, walls and floors. In some instances disinfection may be preferable.

Cleaning and Mopping in Operation Theater before Starting in the Morning (everyday)

1. Clean using vacuum cleaner (using broom increases bacterial counts in air which is highly undesirable).
2. After 10 minutes of cleaning, mopping should be done using plain water with 10 grams of bleaching powder per liter.
3. Let the floor dry after the first mop, second round of mopping is done using 2–5% phenol (carbolic acid 20–50 mL per liter of water) or a good quality disinfectant like Lysol can be used as per the manufacturer's instructions.
4. Lower concentration of phenol acts as a perfume rather than a disinfectant.
5. Clean the operation theater (OT) table, instruments coming in intimate contact with patient and door handles with 70% alcohol solution.
6. Do not enter OT till the floor is completely dry.
7. After mopping, mops must be kept dry by exposure to sunlight. Continuous use of mops without intermittent drying leads to contamination more than disinfection.

Between Two Procedures in the Same Session

1. Clean the operation theater table and instruments coming in intimate contact with patient with 70% alcohol solution.
2. Discard waste immediately into respective plastic bags.

After Concluding in the Evening (Everyday)

1. Wait for at least 30 minutes after all the OT personnel are out of the room.
2. Mopping is to be done using 2% phenol solution.
3. Bathrooms and toilets should be disinfected with bleaching powder (10 grams per liter).

Disinfection

Disinfection results in the reduction of viable microorganisms to the extent they are not harmful to health. Disinfection does not achieve the same microbial reduction as sterilization and does not inactivate some 'slow' viruses or bacterial spores. The main methods of disinfection are boiling; washer disinfectors; chemical disinfection; and low-temperature steam.

Disinfection is suitable where there is an intermediate risk, i.e. contact with mucous membranes during endoscopy or for respiratory equipment, though in some instances sterilization may be preferable.

Physical Disinfectants

1. *Boiling water:* Minimum boiling of water for 30 minutes ensures disinfection of steel articles. Boiling water cannot kill spores.
2. *Pasteurization:* It can be used for disinfection of reusable respiratory devices and anesthesia breathing circuits (e.g. anesthesia hoses, masks and fluted breathing bags).
3. *Ultraviolet radiations:* UV radiations kill selective vegetative bacteria, fungi, lipoprotein virus on contact in air or water. UV lights are used in operative rooms to decrease air borne microorganisms to low levels.

Boiling should occur in soft water at 100°C for 5 minutes; items should then be allowed to dry and cool. This lack of rigour, the time allowing for recontamination, and risk of injury from boiling water renders this method inappropriate within the surgical setting. Washer disinfectors achieve physical cleaning with heat disinfection of equipment. All microorganisms bar some heat-resistant viruses and bacterial spores are inactivated.

- Chemical disinfection may be achieved via a washer disinfector that utilizes chemicals:
  - Chlorine dioxide (Tristel®): Rapidly bacteriocidal, veridical and mycobactericidal; high level disinfection is achieved in 5 minutes and sporicidal in 10 minutes.
  - Electrolyzed water (Sterilox™): Freshly generated solutions are sporicidal and mycobactericidal. The solution is produced by electrolyzing a salt solution .
  - Glutaraldehyde 2% (Cide™): Most bacteria and viruses are inactivated in 10 minutes. Mycobacteria require

20 minutes and spores 3 hours. Potential harm to practitioners is well-recognized and use is being curtailed within most surgical areas and alternatives used.
- Peracetic acid (Nu Cidex®): Bacteriocidal, virucidal and mycobactericidal within 5 minutes and sporicidal within 10 minutes.

Chemical disinfectants: Disinfectants are effective against *Staphylococcus aureus, Salmonella choleraesuis* and *Pseudomonas aeruginosa.* These are following disinfectants used in OT:

1. Alcohol (ethyl alcohol, isopropyl): It is bactericidal agent, kills some virus, fungi.
2. Aldehyde (aqueous acidic 2%, glutaraldehyde): It kills virus, bacteria but not spermicidal but kills fungi.
3. Phenol compound (64% with 0.95% glutaraldehyde): It kills virus, bacteria, fungi and spores.
4. Halogens (chlorine and chlorine compounds such as sodium chlorite): It kills virus, fungi, bacteria but limited spermicidal.

For all chemical disinfectants practitioners should be aware of COSHH (Control of Substances Hazardous to Health) implications for staff. They should also be aware whether his chemical disinfectant of choice is corrosive to the equipment to be immersed and that all equipment should be rinsed to remove toxic residues prior to use. The advantage of chemical disinfectants is that they can be used at the point of use, although practitioners should be able to apply traceability principles in case an infection develops requiring patient in case an infection develops requiring patient or equipment recall. When using chemically disinfected equipment on patients, equality of care should be practiced. If some patients have sterilized equipment while others receive similar equipment that has been disinfected, this demonstrates that patients are receiving differing standards of care.

Further chemical disinfectants available are hypochlorites. Different concentrations achieve differing outcomes, for example when used for blood spillages and environmental disinfection. Alcohol is bactericidal and mycobactericidal, but is not active against spores and has the advantage of leaving surfaces dry. Solutions of 60% and 70% (isopropanolol and ethanol) are more effective than absolute alcohol. Care is required due to flammability (Steer 2002)

Sterilization

Sterilization achieves inactivation of microorganisms including viruses and bacteria spores. Sterilization is required where there is a high risk to individuals, i.e. where equipment is introduced into a normally closed body cavity or is in contact with broken skin/membranes. Therefore, surgical equipment and sundries require sterilizing. It can be achieved via a number of methods including.

Sterilization is the process by which an article or a solution or surface is made free of microbes as well as their spores. According to Miller "Sterilization is a process intended to kill all microorganisms and is the highest level of microbial kill that is possible". Heat, steam or liquid chemicals may be used to achieve this. A properly performed sterilization is an effective way of preventing bacteria from spreading. All the instruments used for any invasive procedure or surgery must be adequately sterilized. The action of agents used for sterilization depends upon a variety of factors including inmate characteristics of the involved organism as well as the agents used for sterilization. An understanding of these factors helps in achieving a better sterilization.

- *Dry heat sterilization:* Here temperatures need to reach 160°C for 2 hours, 170°C for 1 hour or 180°C for 30 minutes. This method is used for the sterilization of solids, non-aqueous liquids and item damaged by steam. The main disadvantage of the method is the length of cycle time and the temperature that may affect items containing some rubbers and plastics .
  - Dry heat penetrates certain substances that cannot be sterilized by steam sterilization or another method. Dry heat given in the form of hot air mainly at temperature of 320° to 340°F (160°C to 171°C) for the period of 1–2 hours. Dry heat method is a protective method of sterilizing some delicate, sharp or cutting edge instruments (like scissors) as steam may erode or corrode cutting eges.
- *Chemical sterilization:* Ethylene oxide gas sterilization—EO gas is used to sterilize items that is sensitive to heat or moisture. EO gas kills microorganisms including spores. All plastic and rubber items (e.g. disposable syringes and needles, dialysis set, endotracheal tubes, internal pacemakers, gloves, all type of catheters, RT tubes, etc.) are sterilized by EO gas. Oil and talc are not sterilized through EO gas.
  - Ethylene oxide: This is active against bacteria, viruses and spores though it is toxic, irritant, explosive and expensive. Microbiological monitoring is required to ensure efficacy of the process, therefore use is generally limited to industrial use with single-use plastic items frequently sterilized by this method.
- *Irradiation:* Used industrially to sterilize single-use items. Gamma rays or electron beam are used to achieve sterilization.
- *Low temperature steam and formaldehyde:* Dry saturated steam and formaldehyde are used together at sub-atmospheric pressures to kill bacteria, spores and most viruses. Hollow items may be damaged due to the pressure, and formaldehyde is corrosive to some materials. A process that is toxic and irritant, and expensive.
- *Hydrogen peroxide plasma sterilization:* This method is used for sterilization of metal and non-metal surgical devices at low temperature in a dry environment (e.g. box locks on clamps, instruments with lumens). Hydrogen peroxide can be activated to create reactive plasma. The cloud of plasma created plasma consists of ions, electrons and neutral atomic particles that produce visible pink glow. Free radicals of hydrogen peroxide in cloud interact with cell membrane,

enzymes or nucleic acids to destruct the life functions of microorganisms.

- *Ozon gas sterilization:* Ozone sterilizes by oxidation. Oxidation is a process that destroys organic and inorganic matter. It penetrates into the membrane of cells and causing them to explode. Ozone gas sterilization provides alternative to EO gas sterilization.
- *Steam:* This is effective, non-toxic and non-corrosive. This form of sterilization is achieved within an autoclave where steam is placed under pressure and air removed. Air may be removed by displacement or vacuum. Direct contact needs to occur between the steam and the items for sterilization. Autoclaves reach 134°C for three minutes or 121°C for 15 minutes to achieve sterilization. Equipment that is wrapped is managed within porous load autoclaves where air is removed by vacuum, so allowing steam to penetrate wrapping and also hollow items. Performance testing monitors the effectiveness of autoclaving with visual evidence available to end-users via indicators/tape that changes color on completion of effective processing.
- *Autoclave:* This is one of most safe and reliable methods of sterilization. Moreover in certain commodities such as dressings, drapes etc., it is the only effective way of sterilization. Autoclave kills both pathogens and their spores to achieve high efficient sterilization. Thus it is considered as the best to sterilize surgical instruments. Autoclave works on the principle of pressure cooker utilizing the specific heat of steam (water vapors) to kill the pathogens. Since the temperature achieved under pressure is as high as 140°C, it is capable of killing even the spores which generally survive at lower temperatures. A coordination of the temperature and time required for achieving optimum sterilization is very important in autoclaving. The table below shows the variation in time according to the temperature inside the autoclave.

Temperature in degrees	Duration of autoclaving
134–138	3 minutes
126–129	10 minutes
121–123	15 minutes
115–116	30 minutes

The time given in the above table is the duration after the requisite temperature has been achieved. Thus the total time required for a set of articles to be sterilized can be calculated as per the following equation :

Let T= Time required for achieving the requisite temperature.
t = Time needed for sterilization (after reaching the required temperature)
Then,

Tat = T + t (i)

Where Tat =Total time to be spent by a nurse for sterilizing an equipment.

For example, if T = 15 minutes to reach 126°C
T = 10 minutes (refer above table)

Thus, the total time required for sterilizing an equipment or article will be:

T = 15 + 10
T = 25 minutes (as per equation)

- Spermicidal chemicals (discussed previously), though considered disinfectants can act as sterilizing agents if used for an extended period of time. Spermicidal chemicals that may be used include: Chlorine dioxide—spermicidal in 10 minutes; glutaraldehyde 2%—spermicidal in 3-10 hours; and per acetic acid—spermicidal in 3-10 hours; and per acetic acid—spermicidal in 10 minutes.
- Chemical sterility in solutions: Articles are immersed in solutions of chemical as recommended by manufacturer's instructions. If EO gas sterilization is not available these; chemical can be used.
  a. Acetic acid: It takes 20 minutes at room temperature of 77°F for sterilization.
  b. Formaldehyde: 37% aqueous solution (formalin) or 8% formaldehyde in 70% isopropyl alcohol kills microorganisms by coagulating protein in cells.
  c. Glutaraldehyde: 2.4%, 2.5% or 3.4% aqueous solution of activated, buffered alkaline glutaraldehyde kills microorganisms by the denaturation of protein in cells.
  d. Para acetic acid-STERIS: Chemical form of 35% para acetic acid, hydrogen peroxide and water (inactivates critical microbial cell system and cause cell death. The solution is heated 122°-310°C for 20-30 minute in self processing chamber and all items are submerged in the heated sterialnt.
  e. Hypochlorous acid: It is derived from electrochemical activation of chlorine solution. It is high level disinfectant, kills many spores on well cleaned endoscopes and other heat sensitive items.

A large bin with a perforated inner tray and lid is used with chemical sterilant solutions at room temperature. The outside of bin should be labeled with product name, date of activation, date of expiration and initials of person who mixed the solution. The inside of lid and inner side should be kept sterile throughout the duration of exposure. After completion of exposure period all items should be rinsed thoroughly in sterile distilled water before use.

When any form of sterilization has been used on surgical equipment and sundries all practitioners need to be aware of observing indicators and expiry dates of equipment and ensure these are monitored prior to use of equipment to reduce the potential risk to patients . Where tracing is applicable, local policies should be followed to ensure patients or equipment can be recalled in the future. Practitioners additionally have a responsibility to ensure that all single-use items are used for their original purpose and disposed of, not returned to sterile service departments for resterilization (MDA 2000).

EQUIPMENT

Equipment required, during surgery is wide and varied; this section intends to examine suture and instrument design that caters for a wide variety of surgical requirements. Individuals need to be aware of the physical properties of the variety of suture materials available for use and alternatives that may be available, plus the body's response to the various materials used. With regard to instruments, practitioners need to be aware of what an instrument is designed for to avoid inappropriate use and thus injury to patients or damage to the instrument resulting in costly repair replacement bills. The use of electro surgery and laser equipment will also be explored, highlighting the need for practitioner knowledge in order to prevent injury to patients when using these pieces of equipment.

Sutures

The use of sutures enables wound closure and allows for the removal of dead space, realignment of tissue planes and the securing of tissue edges until healing by first intention has occurred. This section will examine suture use in more detail, though practitioners should also be aware of other closure methods available, i.e. tissue adhesive, staples and adhesive strips. Whatever the choice of closure material, practitioners should be knowledgeable as to the properties of the option of choice and of the alternatives, should the first choice be unavailable. Thought should be given to any tissue action, the final cosmetic result and removal. The age of the patient may be a significant factor; pediatric patients require a smaller suture size than adults, and dependent upon age the method of removal should be considered. Older patients require consideration, as their skin may be less elastic, more friable and prone to bruising or damage; these changes are dependent upon age, concurrent disease or pharmacological agents.

Suture Categories

Sutures are divided into two categories—absorbable and non-absorbable.

Absorbable sutures are designed to hold the wound together and withhold normal stresses until healing has occurred. Presentation is as a synthetic material, which is hydrolyzed by body fluids; it may be a braided or monofilament suture. Length of time taken to be hydrolyzed will vary; dependent upon the suture of choice the minimal time varies from 40 to 90 days, with complete absorption varying from 60 to 210 days.

Non-absorbable sutures are not affected by body fluids and once within a body cavity become encapsulated. Presentation may be as a natural or synthetic material and either twisted, braided or monofilament.

Gauge of suture ranges from 1 mm to as line as 15 microns (7–11/0); best practice indicates that the finest gauge that will hold tissues securely should be used. Castile (1998) recommends 5/0 fan faces, scalp and upper limbs; 4/0 and 3/0 for trunk and lower limbs.

Needles

In addition to decisions about suture type, there is the choice of needle; these again are varied.

The shape of needle used is restricted by the surgeon's degree of access to the site to be sutured (Fig. 6.21). Besides shape there is also the bore description to be considered. This may be round-bodied to separate tissues rather than cut them, cutting to address dense tissue, or speculated as in the case of needles for ophthalmic use.

Having identified the appropriate suture material and size plus needle shape, errors can still occur that will reduce the effectiveness of the suturing or cause damage to wounds. The most common errors include: (i) pulling sutures too tight, so causing swelling and reducing vascularity to the wound edges; (ii) allowing sutures to be too loose resulting in the wound gaping and not haling by first intention; (iii) placing sutures too near the wound edge, so that they may pull out; (iv) overlapping of the wound egos, which can result in wound dehiscence. These aspects can be, identified easily on final skin closure, but may cause irreparable damage or complications if involving internal sutures. The type of suturing technique used is the choice of the surgeon and may include interrupted, continuous, subcuticular and endoscopic sutures.

All practitioners involved with suturing have a responsibility to have a working knowledge of sutures in use within their practice area plus knowledge of alternative materials available. They also must ensure that all sutures within the surgical field are accounted for and added to the visible swab count. On closure of each layer, a further count should be undertaken to ensure all sutures and their packaging are accounted for. On completion of surgery this count should be documented within the patient's care plan/surgical record.

Instruments

Instrumentation within all surgical specialities is wide and varied, but the role of practitioners taken with their management is the same. All practitioners need to be competent to use the

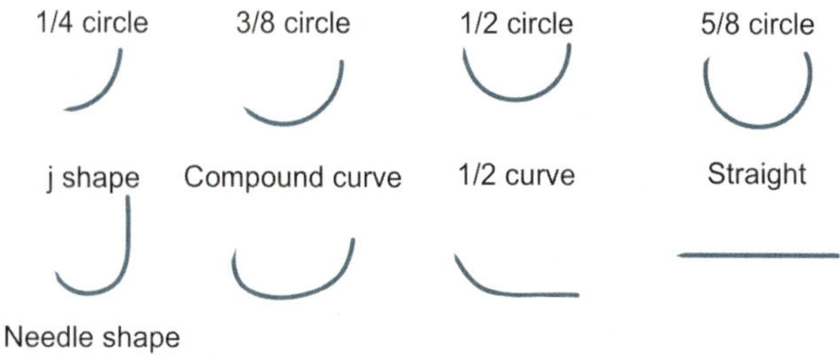

FIG. 6.21: Needle shape

equipment, be able to recognize their instruments, be aware of their uses and understand the principles of how to care for them. Misuse of instrumentation can place the patient and practitioners at risk of injury and may become costly if instruments become damaged or broken when used incorrectly or inappropriately. Practitioners involved in the buying of equipment need to ensure that any equipment bought/supplied to their department conforms to current Medical Devices Agency guidelines.

Presentation of instruments may come in a variety of forms from preset instrument and drape packs, Edinburgh pre-set trays or via a container system. Whatever the format of presentation all practitioners should be aware of how they identify that their equipment is sterile and within its usable date. They should also know how they identify the traceability of the set, should there be a need to track and identify equipment used on a specific patient at a later date. Prior to use the practitioner must ensure that they have checked which instruments are present against the set checklist and also that all components of instruments are accounted for. Any supplementary instruments should be recorded and checked prior to use. Items identified as faulty should be removed and replaced where possible. Faulty items should then be tagged to identify them to sterile service staff as requiring repair or replacement. Prior to commencing surgery, practitioners should ensure they have all the instrumentation they need, along with any additional instrumentation that may be required in the event of unanticipated extension of planned surgery or emergency.

Instruments can be broadly discussed under five categories: cutting instruments; artery forceps; clamps; tissue forceps; and retractors. Instrumentation additional to these can be considered as accessory equipment.

Cutting Instruments

Cutting instrumentation includes both scalpel handles (BP handles/Barron handles) and scissors. Scalpel handles come in a variety of sizes and require blades to be attached. To reduce the risk of sharps injury, blades should be attached and removed using appropriate tools/aids and not by hand. Prior to use the blade should be checked for security to ensure no injuries occur due to blade slippage.

Scissors vary from extremely fine to large and heavy, being angled, straight or curved. All scissors are designed for a specific use and should only be used for that purpose. Misuse could result in damage to the patient and to instrumentation . Prior to use these should be checked for smooth action and sharpness; blunt scissors must be identified for repair/resharpening.

Artery Forceps

Artery forceps (hemostats/hemostatic forceps) are utilized for clamping blood vessels, blunt dissection, handing or holding supplementary items, i.e. ties/pledges. These come in a variety of sizes and may be curved or straight, giving the user the ability to vary the pressure applied via the ratchet lock. Prior to use the tips should be inspected to ensure they meet.

Clamps

A variety of claps are available and those used are dependent upon the surgery to be undertaken. Vascular clamps are designed to be traumatic and, as with artery forceps, may have a ratchet lock to allow variable degrees of pressure to be applied. Bowel clamps are designed to be crushing for application to distal and proximal ends, or non-crushing for application at the site of anastomosis. In use, crushing and non-crushing must be clearly identified by practitioners to ensure accurate identification and usage.

Tissue Forceps

Tissue forceps may be for tissue dissection or holding. Dissecting forceps are supplied in a variety of lengths and weights and may be toothed or non-toothed. The former are presented as interlocking grooves or teeth. Heavy teeth allow for the holding of heavier tissues such as muscle, while finer teeth are utilized on finer tissues . Plain, non-toothed forceps are for holding very delicate tissue such as vessels. Prior to use all dissection forceps should be checked for approximation of the tips.

Holding forceps are of various sizes and weights from the finer Allis to the heavy Lanes, again for use on various weights of tissue. Again inspection of alignment is required. Within this category are included needle holders and sponge-holders. Needleholders are provided in different weights and lengths to balance the depth of suturing and the weight of the needle in use. Care should be taken to use an appropriate weight of needleholder for each needle used; too heavy a needle with a fine needleholder will result in strain on the joint and tips leading to costly damage of the needleholder. Passing of loaded needleholders should ideally occur via a 'safe transfer zone to reduce the risk of accidental injury to scrubbed practitioners or the patient.

Retractors

Retractors may be hand-held or self-retaining, allowing access to the site of surgery, Where self-retaining retractors are used any screws should be confirmed as present prior to and on commencement of surgery. Retractors are provided in a variety of lengths and widths to allow for accurate retraction and with those that contain teeth, additional care should be taken to ensure that no accidental injury is caused to the patient or to scrubbed personnel.

This has provided an insight into types of instrumentation in use; a wide variety are available and their use will be dependent upon the surgical speciality undertaken. During use instruments should be maintained in an organized manner to allow for immediate identification and allow for prompt retrieval. Any question as to the sterility of an item should result in its being removed from use and returned for sterilization at the end of surgery with the remainder of the set. Throughout surgery, the practitioner should ensure that all instruments are handled carefully and passed to users in a safe manner, sharp instruments ideally via a 'safe transfer zone' such as a recover. Instruments other than blades and needles should be considered as sharps as many scissors and retractors have aspects that can inflict injury to receiving personnel. Items found to be blunt should be identified and notified to the sterile service department; the items should then be sent for sharpening,

Following completion of surgery, instruments should be counted against the initial set list along with supplementary items to confirm all instruments are present and accounted for following surgical closure. Instruments should then be returned to the sterile service departments following local policy guidelines and utilizing the systems and processes in place to identify the location of equipment sets. The patient's individual care plan/documentation should be completed to indicate who has accounted the instrumentation used.

Practitioners need to be aware of their professional accountability with regard to surgical counts. While no legal requirement exists to perform a surgical count, practitioners have a duty of care to their patient to ensure that they come to no harm, For this reason the National Association or theater Nurses has provided a number of documents that indicate what can be considered best practice when performing a surgical count. Within these they indicate the necessity to ensure the following :

- All swabs, instruments and sharps are accounted for prior to the commencement of surgery and as they are added to the surgical field
- Counts should be performed by two staff members who can identify and recognize all items to be counted; one of these must be a qualified staff member
- Counts to be audible
- No items to be removed from theater until the final count has been completed and confirmed as correct
- Counts to be performed at the commencement of any cavity closure
- On completion a verbal acknowledgement that the count was correct is made
- At the end of surgery the count is documented and signed for by the scrub and circulating staff performing the count.

During use, equipment that is sharp has the potential to injure patients and staff; therefore appropriate handling is essential. Practitioners need to ensure that sharp prongs, scissor tips, etc. are maintained within a 'safe transfer' area away from the patient and staff when not required, but convenient to access safely. Should injury occur to the patient or staff member this should be documented and appropriate action taken under hospital policy.

Education on the use and handling of equipment is essential. Practitioners new to theater practice can benefit from handling and passing clean instrumentation away from the surgical field. This is an opportune time to consider equipment against set lists with discussion from experienced practitioners.

FUMIGATION OF OPERATION THEATER

To sterilize the operation theater formaldehyde gas (bactericidal and sporicidal) is widely employed (cost effective) for fumigation. Formaldehyde kills the microbes by alkylating the amino acids and sulfhydryl group of proteins and urine bases.

Step 1: Preparation for fumigation

1. Thoroughly clean windows, doors , floor, walls and all washable equipments with soap and water.
2. Close windows and ventilators tightly. If any openings found in the room, seal it with cellophane tape or other material.
3. Switch off all lights, A/C and other electrical and electronical items.
4. Calculate the room size in cubic feet (L × B × H) and calculate the required amount of formaldehyde as given in Step 3.

Step 2 : Precaution

1. Adequate care must be taken by wearing cap, mask, foot cover, spectacle, etc.
2. Formaldehyde is irritant to eye and nose; and it has been recognized as a potential carcinogen.
3. So the fumigating employee must be provided with the personal protective equipments (PPE).

Step 3: Fumigation

1. Electric boiler fumigation method: For each 1000 cu.ft, 500 mL of formaldehyde (40% solution) added in 1000 mL of water in an electric boiler. Switch on the boiler, leave the room and seal the door. After 45 minutes (variable depending to volume present in the boils apparatus) switch off the boiler without entering in to the room (switch off the main from outside).
2. Potassium permanganate method: For every 1000 cubic feet and 450 g of potassium permanganate ($KMnO_4$) to 500 mL of formaldehyde (40% solution). Take about 5 to 8 bowels (heat resistant; place it in various locations) with equally divided parts of formaldehyde and add equally divided $KMnO_4$ to each bowl. This will cause auto boiling and generate fume.
3. After the initiation of formaldehyde vapor, immediately leave the room and seal it for at least 48 hour.

Step 4: Neutralization

1. After the fumigation process neutralize the formaldehyde vapor with ammonia solution. On inspection (or surgery) day enter the operation theater at 7 AM with 150 mL of 10% ammonia (for 500 mL of formaldehyde used, i.e. for 100 cu feet.

2. Place the ammonia solution in the center of the room and leave it for 3 hours to neutralize the formalin vapor.

Example:

Operation theater volume = L × B × H = 20 × 15 × 10 = 3000 cubic feet

Formaldehyde required for fumigation = 500 mL for 1000 cubic feet. So, 1500 mL of formaldehyde required.

Ammonia required for neutralization = 150mL of 10% ammonia for 500 mL of formaldehyde. So, 450 mL of 10% ammonia, required.

Guidelines to be considered for operation theater sterility check:

1. Construction carpentry, plumbing, electrical, cleaning and other works should be completed before (the initiation of fumigation procedure.
2. If exhaust fan is used (instead of A/C) its exterior level fins should be closed.
3. Rooms allotted for operation should not be used for other purposes.
4. The construction must have
   a. Separate dressing room for medical officer and staff nurses
   b. Patient waiting room
   c. Operation room
   d. Veranda
5. The entire block should be cleaned and fumigated.
6. Entry should be restricted to OT staff only.
7. All apparatus such as boils apparatus, suction machine, OT table, cautery, focus lights, A/C units, exhaust fans should be cleaned completely as per the manufacturer instructions.
8. Theater dress (includes head cap, mask, apron, chapel, ect.) should be made available for all persons who are entering into the operation theater (surgeons, anesthetist, microbiologist team, nurses, theater assistants and helper).
9. Surroundings should be clean and free from garbage, open drainage, bushes, shrubs, wastes, etc.
10. Operation theater should be cleaned and fumigated once a month periodically.
11. Walls should be disinfected only once in 6 months and roof/ceiling is to be disinfected only once a year unless obvious fungal growth/dampness is noticed. In such case, report immediately to the concerned authorities.

Bacillocid Rasant spray or Virkon disinfectant are excellent alternatives for fumigation, which should be considered if feasible as fumigation has certain major health concerns.

CHAPTER

7

Critical Care Nursing

EVOLUTION OF CRITICAL CARE NURSING

Since the earliest days of nursing, the sickest patients have been placed near the nurse's station, underlining the importance of frequent assessment and rapid intervention. From the development of postoperative wards and polio centers to triage centers during various wars, to the evolution of the coronary care unit, this concentration of highly specialized caregivers with access to unique technology has remained the guiding principle for the evolution of critical care environment.

The delivery of critical care as we know it today originated from the need to centralize specially trained personnel and equipment in a separate area of the hospital to optimize the care of critically ill and injured patients. Nurses began to group their most unstable patients closer to the nurse's station, so they provide "watchful vigilance" or intensive observation. The concept of gathering patients together for care can be traced back to Florence Nightingale.

It is common in small country hospitals, to have a recess or small room leading from the operating theater in which the patients remain until they have recovered, or at least recovered from the immediate effects of the operation.

Critical care units have evolved over the last four decades in response to medical advances. During 1970's the term critical care unit came into existence which covered all types of special care units. The American Association of Critical Care Nurses was a response to the demands placed on nurses for safe knowledgeable patient care and it played an important role as vehicle for nurses and physicians, in supporting education and standard formation.

As the medical technology advanced more subspecialities such as cardiothoracic, renal, coronary, respiratory and neurosurgical units were established. No hospital is complete without establishment or critical care unit. A critical care unit is defined as the unit in which comprehensive care of a critically ill patient, which is deemed to recoverable stage is carried out. Critical care unit is specially designed and equipped facility staffed by skilled personnel to provide effective and safe care for dependent patient with life threatening or potentially life threatening problems.

Critical care units or intensive care units were designed to meet the special needs of acutely and critically ill patients. The concept of clustering the most acutely ill is not new. Florence Nightingale recommended grouping acutely ill patients together. During poliomyelitis and tuberculosis pandemics earlier in 20th century, special units were established, equipped with technical apparatus to manage the airway and ventilate the patient and staffed by specialized care providers. During World War II and Vietnam War, trauma units were developed for battle casualties.

In the 1960s, technical developments allowed for more accessible monitoring of electrocardiogram (ECG), arterial and central venous pressures, and arterial blood gases. Coronary care units were developed for patients with acute myocardial infarction. In these units patients were continually monitored for cardiac dysrhythmias and nurses were trained to identify and aggressively manage dysrhythmias. By the 1970s, the intensive care unit (ICU) was a standard component of most general hospitals. Since that time, technologic advances have continued at a rapid pace, bringing improved monitoring capabilities and new strategies to manage life-threatening problems.

The term critical care nursing is often used interchangeably with the term ICU nursing. The critical care nurse is responsible for diagnosing life-threatening conditions and instituting appropriate treatment. Today the technology and equipment available in the ICU are extensive and continually evolving. In ICUs the capability exists to continuously monitor ECG, blood pressure, oxygenation, and temperature. More advanced monitoring devices allow for the measurement of stroke volume, ejection fraction, end tidal carbon dioxide, and oxygen consumption. Patients may be receiving continual support from the ventilator, cardiac assist devices, or dialysis machines.

Now *critical care unit* continues to be a unique, high-paced environment in which the most sophisticated medical, nursing, and technical interventions are integrated to combat life-threatening illness. These units are referred to as intensive care units, critical care units, coronary care units, and other names that identify the type and intensity of patient care. The one constant is that the role of nursing is critical to success. Through vigilant observation of a patients ever-changing condition, the critical care, nurse monitors the complex treatment regimen, quickly identifies problems and initiates appropriate therapies, and intervenes to prevent or correct life-threatening situations. However, the focus of critical care nursing practice is no longer only on the patients critical illness or injury. Critical care nurses have broadened their focus to include preventive care and risk modification to decrease future patient hospitalizations.

Critical care nursing is the field of nursing, in which the focus is on the care of the critically ill or unstable patients. Critical care nurses can be found working in a wide variety of environments and specialities, such as emergency departments and the intensive care units.

Critical care nurses work in a variety of different areas, with a diverse patient population. There are many critical care nurses working in hospitals in intensive care units, postoperative care and high dependency units. They also work on medical evacuation and transport teams.

Critical care nurse and critical care nursing offers challenge and excitement to the role of the nurse. Physicians have relied heavily on the skills of critical care nurses and respect them for their expertise. Aside from job satisfaction, salaries are highly rewarding in some parts of the country.

CLASSIFICATION OF CRITICAL CARE UNITS

Critical care units may be classified into three levels depending on the staffing and support facilities of the hospital. A three level classification consist of:

Level 1: It is a high dependency unit which could be either separate or attached to a general ward patient nursed in these units is those who require special observation following an uncomplicated myocardial infarction or surgical procedures. These units undertake only immediate resuscitation, short-term ventilation and cardiac monitoring. The nurse patient is 1:3 and the medical staffs are not present in the unit all the time.

Level 2: This level of critical care unit is capable of providing prolonged mechanical ventilation but does not have access to comprehensive support facilities. The nurse patient ratio is 1:2 and junior medical staff is available in the unit all the time and consultant medical staff is available if needed.

Level 3: This level of critical care unit is capable of providing prolonged mechanical ventilation and has access to comprehensive support facilities. The nurse : patient ratio is 1:1 and consultant medical staff is available in the unit all the time.

TYPES OF CRITICAL CARE UNIT/ICU

Specialized types of ICUs include:

1. Neonatal intensive care unit (NICU)
2. Special care nursery (SCN)
3. Pediatric intensive care unit (PICU)
4. Psychiatric intensive care unit (PICU)
5. Coronary care unit (CCU) for heart disease
6. Cardiac surgery intensive care unit (CSICU)
7. Cardiovascular intensive care unit (CVICU)
8. Medical intensive care unit (MICU)
9. Medical surgical intensive care unit (MSICU)
10. Surgical intensive care unit (SICU)
11. Overnight intensive recovery (OIR)
12. Neuroscience/neurotrauma intensive care unit (NICU)
13. Neurointensive care unit (NICU)
14. Burn intensive care unit (BICU)
15. Trauma intensive care unit (TICU)
16. Shock trauma intensive care unit (STICU)
17. Trauma-neuro critical care unit (TNCC)
18. Respiratory intensive care unit (RICU)
19. Geriatric intensive care unit (GICU).

Critical care units should be staffed by highly trained and skilled nurses. Specialized critical care units have been developed to meet the needs of individual patients. The size and number of critical care units vary from one institution to another. Categories of some of these specialized units are listed:

- ICU: Intensive care unit
- CCU: Coronary care unit
- MICU: Medical intensive care unit
- SICU: Surgical intensive care unit
- PICU: Pediatric intensive care unit
- NICU: Neonatal intensive care unit
- PMU: Progressive medical care unit
- PSU: Progressive surgical care unit
- BU: Burn unit.

Some of the functions of skilled critical care nurses include:

- Performing basic bedside care-meeting bio-psychosocial needs
- Identifying cardiac arrhythmias
- Administering and adjusting medications
- Initiating and maintaining intravenous therapy
- Performing cardiopulmonary resuscitation
- Performing defibrillation
- Completing physical assessment
- Taking health histories

- Interpreting 12-lead electrocardiograms
- Monitoring hemodynamic Swan-Ganz catheter
- Maintaining arterial lines and pressure interpretation
- Monitoring intra-aortic ballon pumps
- Providing patient/family teaching
- Interpret and order diagnostic laboratory tests
- Make nursing diagnoses
- Identify community resources
- Collaborate with the physician regarding treatment
- Prescribe symptomatic treatment in select situations.

Roles and functions of critical care nurses vary from state to state depending on the Nurse Practice Act. In some states, Licences laws dictate, in part, the level of nurse eligible for employment in critical care units. The nursing administration office of the institution establishes the job description and qualification based on the Nurse Practice Act of the state.

Job opportunities are abundant because there are not enough qualifed nurses to meet the job openings in all parts of the country. Salaries depend on the geographic location but are usually higher than those for RNs on a general medical/ surgical unit.

The critical care nurse cares for patients and the families of patients with acute and unstable physiologic problems in an environment equipped for technically advanced methods of assessing and managing patient problems. Critical care nursing as that specialty dealing with human responses to life-threatening problems. The specialty requires knowledge of physiology, pathophysiology, pharmacology, and the ability to use advanced technology to accurately measure physiologic parameters. It is important that the nurse understand the assumptions on which measurements depend and determine if those assumptions are correct for each specific patient. The nurse provides ongoing assessment and early recognition and management of complications while fostering healing and recovery. Appropriate actions by an astute nurse can prevent complications. The nurse must be able to provide psychologic support to the patient and the family. To be effective the critical care nurse must be able to communicate clearly and work as a team member.

PRINCIPLES OF CRITICAL CARE NURSING

Critical care unit is a specially designed and equipped facility staffed by skilled personnel to provide effective and safe care for dependent patients with life threatening or potentially life threatening problems. There are following principles of critical care nursing:

1. Anticipation
2. Early detection and prompt action
3. Collaborative practice
4. Communication
5. Prevention of infection
6. Crisis intervention and stress reduction.

1. *Anticipation*: The first principle in critical care is anticipation. One has to recognize the high-risk patients and anticipate the requirements, complication and be prepared to meet any emergency. Unit properly organized which all necessary equipment and supplies are mandatory for smooth running of the unit.
2. *Early detection and prompt action*: The prognosis of the patient depends on the early detection of variation, prompt and appropriate action to prevent or combat complication. Monitoring of cardiac respiratory function is of prime importance in assessment.
3. *Collaborative practice*: Critical care, which has originated as technical subspecialized body of knowledge, has evolved into a comprehensive discipline requiring a very specialized body of knowledge for the physicians and nurses working in the unit. Collaborative practice between the physicians and nurses working in the critical care unit fosters a partnerships for decision making and ensures quality and compassionate patient care. Collaborative practice is more and more than warranted for critical care more than in any other field.
4. *Communication*: Intraprofessional, interdepartmental and interpersonal communication has a significant importance in the smooth running of unit. Collaborative practice of communication model unlike the traditional practice model enhances better outcome as far as patient, nurse, physician and hospital are concerned. This model centers around the patient, fosters individual clinical decision making, uses integrated medical records and joint review of care.
5. *Prevention of infection*: Nosocomial infection cost a lot in the health care services. Critically ill patients requiring intensive care are at a greater risk than other patients due to the immunocompromised state with the antibiotic usage and stress, invasive lines, mechanical and stress, mechanical ventilators, prolonged stay and severity of illness and environment of the critical care unit itself.
6. *Crisis intervention and stress reduction*: Partnerships are formulated during crisis. Bonds between nurses, patients and families are stronger during hospitalization. As patient advocates, nurse assist the patient to express fear and identify their grieving pattern and provide avenues for positive coping.

Critical care nursing is concerned with human responses to life-threatening problems, such as major surgery, trauma, infection, and shock, as well as prevention of potential life-threatening conditions. The critical care nurse is a patient advocate responsible for ensuring that all critically ill patients and families receive optimal care through a process of establishing goals for patient care and providing mechanisms to assess the patients progress toward the goals. Clinical competencies for critical care nurses include clinical judgment and reasoning skills coupled with the ability to think critically and make decisions. The critical care nurse relies on specialized skills and knowledge to monitor and support the patient's physiologic stability of patients and provides an interface between the patient and technology. The nurse tailors clinical practices to the needs of each individual patient and family through collaboration with the health care team members to meet desired patient outcomes. Today's critical care is provided by a multidisciplinary team of health care professionals, including physicians, respiratory therapists, social workers, and clergy. The critical care nurse is an integral part of this team in coordinating care activities for patients and families.

Nursing practice in the ICU often follows a primary care model with the patient cared for by a limited group of nurses who become intensely familiar with the patient's condition and needs and needs of the patient's family. That primary care nurse spends most working hours near the patients bedside. Specialization in ICU nursing usually requires formal training and mentored clinical practice, followed by an internship. Training takes place in a variety of settings. Only a small percentage of baccalaureate nursing programs include critical care as a separate course, often with a minimal clinical component. The number of associate degree programs offering critical care content is unknown. Many clinical institutions offer ICU preparation, as do continuing education agencies.

Advanced practice critical care nurses generally have a graduate (master's or doctorate) degree. These nurses are employed as patient and staff educators, consultants, administrators, researchers, or practitioners. The critical care clinical nurse specialist role traditionally includes aspects of each of these role components. An important emerging role is the acute care nurse practitioner. These master's prepared nurses provide advanced, comprehensive, risk-appropriate care to selected critically ill patients and their families. The acute care nurse practitioner is prepared to conduct comprehensive health assessments, order and interpret diagnostic tests, diagnose and treat health problems and disease-related symptoms, prescribe and evaluate drugs and treatments, and coordinate care during transitions in settings. They may practice independently (e.g. providing comprehensive care to the chronically critically ill), or collaboratively (e.g. providing symptom management in conjunction with physician specialists).

CRITICAL CARE UNIT/ICU

Establishment of care requires intelligent planning. One must keep the need of the hospital and its location. One ICU may not cater to all needs. An institute may plan beds into multiple units under separate management by single discipline specialist viz. medical ICU, surgical ICU, CCU, burns ICU, trauma ICU, etc. It may be useful but experience in Australia has favored multi-disciplinary ICUs, which are managed by specialist intensive lists. Duplication of services and equipment is to be avoided. Critically ill patients develop the same pathophysiological process no matter whether they are classified as medical or surgical. They require the same approaches to support the organs. The problems of critically ill patients do not confine to their primary disease and the single discipline doctor lacks the experience and expertise to deal with the complexities of the multi-organ failure.

The number of ICU beds in hospital ranges from 1 to 10 per 100 total hospital beds. Multidisciplinary requires more beds than single speciality. ICUs with fewer that 4 beds are not cost effective and over 20 beds are unmanageable. ICU should be sited in close proximity to relevant areas viz. operating rooms, imageology, acute wards, emergency department. There should be sufficient number of lifts available to carry these critically ill patients to different areas.

Design of ICU

There should be a single entry and exit. There should not be any through traffic of goods or hospital staff. ICU must have areas and rooms for public reception, patient management and support services. Full commitment must be given from administration and a designated team to work on various tasks. Patient areas each patient requires a floor space 18.5 cm^2 (200 sq ft) with single room being larger about 26–30 m^2 to accommodate patient, staff, equipment without overcrowding. There should be at least 3 to 3.67 meters between the bed centers. Single rooms are essential for isolation and privacy. The ratio of single room beds to open ward beds depends on the role and type of ICU. Service outlets could conform to local standards (electrical safety, and emergency supply). Three oxygen, two air, four suction and 16 power outlets and bedside lamp are optimum for level III ICU. They can be either wall mounted, or bed pendants. Many of the charts, syringes, sampling tubes pillows should be kept in bed dividers. Lead lining these dividers will help minimize X-ray radiation risk to staff and patients. There should be source of natural light coming from the windows. Lack of natural light has shown to cause patient disorientation and increased stress to the staff. A central station will have central monitor, drug cupboard, telephone, refrigerator and patient records. Nursing in ICU is always at the bedside. Sufficient hand wash areas should be provided. X-ray views are needed in multi-bed wards. Proper facilities for hemodialysis such as filtered water should be incorporated at the time of ICU planning.

Storage Areas/Service Areas

Most ICUs lack storage space. They should have a total of 25–30% of all patient and central station areas for storage. Clean and dirty utility rooms should be separate each with its own access. Disposal of soiled linen and waste must be catered for. A laboratory, which estimates blood gases, electrolytes, hemoglobin, is a must. Good communication systems, staff lounge, food areas must be marked out. There should be an area to teach and train students. This completes the design.

Equipment

Use of equipment depends upon the type of ICU. Level II ICUs requirements are necessarily less, may require a two-channel monitor, whereas level III ICU will require multichannel invasive monitors. Inappropriate or unsuitable equipment is brought by inept or less knowledgeable people. Ventilators, infusion pumps, portable X-ray unit, fluid and bed warmers, portable light, defibrillators, anesthesia machine and difficult airway management equipment are necessary. Dialysis unit is essential. An echo, ultrasound machines are necessary but can be commanded from the respective departments when necessary.

Staffing

Large hospital requires bigger team.

Medical staff: Carrier intensivists are the best senior medical staff to be appointed to the CCU. He/she will be the Director. Less preferred are other specialists' viz. from anesthesia, medicine who has clinical commitment elsewhere. Junior staffs are intensive care trainees and trainess on deputation from other disciplines.

Nursing staff: The major teaching tertiary care ICU will require trained nurses in critical care. In our setups it may be ideal to have an in-house training program for critical care nursing. The number of nurses ideally required for such units is 1:1 ratio, however, it may not be possible to have such numbers in our setup. One nurse for two patients is acceptable. In complex situations they may require two nurses per patient. The number of trained nurses should be also worked out by the type of ICU, the workload and work statistics and type of patient load.

Allied services: Physiotherapy, social workers, dieticians, radiology services, respiratory therapists are a useful work force responsible for patient management and equipment maintenance. Biomedical department services are required on a regular basis to service and repair and develop equipment. Adequate secretarial assistance and reception category makes the functioning smooth. For transport of patients, it is ideal if one can have separate teams to lift critically ill patients and transport them to different areas. Trained staff in this area would be very valuable contribution.

In earlier days, critical care units were small carved out of existing recovery rooms or other areas in the hospital. Soon, however, the ICU emerged as a distinct area for care of complex patients, different from the recovery room in that patients were also admitted from outside the hospital and from other units. The units were staffed 24 hours a day, 7 days a week.

Today's critical care unit is designed, equipped, and staffed to meet the anticipated needs of patients in life-threatening situations. The physical layout is frequently a modified circle that allows for direct visualization of all patients at all times. Patients may be separated into cubicles with glass windows or situated in a large open area with curtains for partitions. The advantage of direct nurse-patient visualization is accompanied by the disadvantages of limited privacy and patient exposure to frequent crisis interventions.

Although direct visualization of patients facilitates patient monitoring, maximizes the use of available staff, and is required by some hospital accrediting organizations, the cost to the patient in terms of sensory overload and loss of control can be significant. Optimal patient care requires maintaining a sensitive balance between the needs of patients and those of caregivers.

The central nurse's station contains sophisticated monitoring and even video equipment that enables nurses to continuously monitor vital data for each patient. Certain technologies are available for constant use at each bedside (e.g. cardiac monitor, oxygen, hemodynamic monitoring equipment, and suction equipment), whereas others must be available within seconds (e.g. defibrillator, ventilator, 12-lead electrocardiogram [ECG] machine, emergency medications). Still other technologies must be available for constant or intermittent use with certain patient populations (e.g. intra-aortic balloon pumps, continuous venovenous hemofiltration or hemodialysis, extracorporeal membrane oxygenator, temporary or permanent pacemakers, ventricular assist devices, intermittent conventional hemodialysis, and a variety of pumps for infusion of intravenous fluids or enteral feedings) (Fig. 7.1).

The concentration of complex technologic equipment creates a unique hazard in the critical care environment: the risk of electrical microshock. The invasive monitoring and therapeutic interventions used with critically ill patients (e.g. central venous pressure lines, pulmonary artery catheters, and temporary pacemakers) often create a direct pathway to the heart. Direct contact with stray or leaked current could prove fatal, particularly to critically ill patients whose resistance may be further decreased by other breaks in skin integrity or electrolyte imbalances. Critical care nurses are responsible for using electrical equipment properly and safely.

As the need for more specialized and sophisticated critical care equipment grows, the patient often becomes surrounded by a sea of machinery for monitoring and care delivery. A popular feature of newer or remodeled critical care environments is the centralized or headwall power needs for monitoring equipment, oxygen, suction equipment, and electrical outlets; to store equipment; and to provide a workspace at each patient's bedside. With the advent of microprocessing and digital processing, continued research and development of critical care equipment focus on how to provide the most service in the smallest available space.

Critical Care Patient

A patient is generally admitted to the ICU for one of three reasons. First, the patient may be physiologically unstable, requiring advanced and sophisticated clinical judgments by

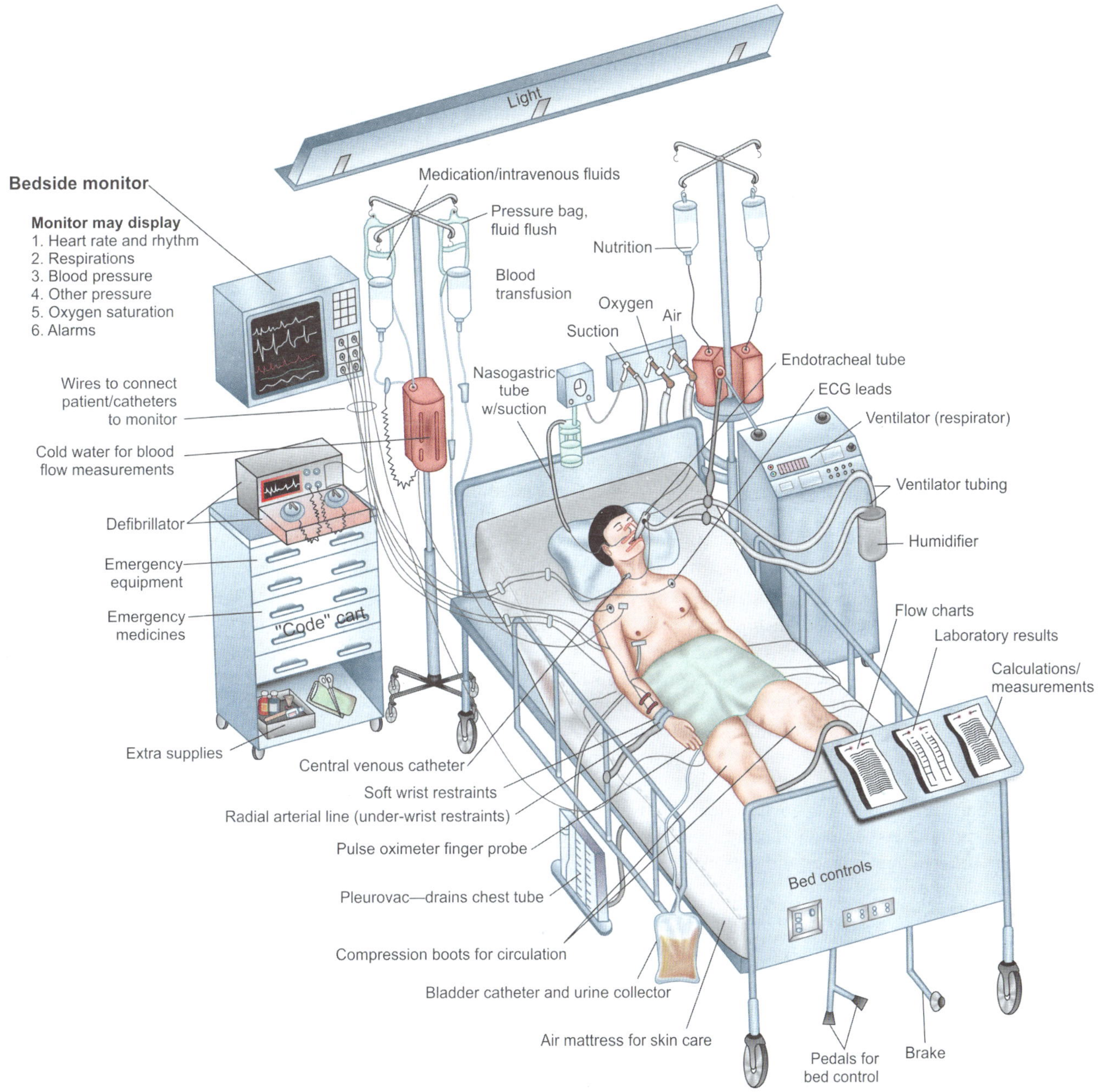

FIG. 7.1: Critical care unit room and equipment

the nurse or physician. Second, the patient may be at risk for serious complications and require frequent and often invasive physical assessment. Third, the patient may be stable but require intensive and complicated nursing support, including ventilation, hemodynamic monitoring, feeding, turning, wound care, and hygiene.

ICUs may serve a variety of patients or specialize in a disease condition (e.g. neurology) or age group (e.g. pediatrics). ICU patients are sometimes clustered by acuity (e.g. acute and unstable versus technology dependent but stable). The patient with myocardial ischemia or infarction or respiratory distress is commonly treated in the ICU, as is the patient with acute neurologic impairment, after cardiac surgery, or after major organ transplantation. Trauma ICUs treat the critically injured. The patient with a medical emergency (e.g. sepsis; diabetic ketoacidosis; drug overdoses; poisonings; thyroid, adrenal, or hematologic crises) is often treated in a medical ICU. The patient with a serious underlying condition may be monitored in the ICU while receiving care for unrelated conditions. The patient who is not expected to recover is not treated in an ICU. The ICU should not be used to treat the patient in a persistent vegetative state, nor should ICU care be used to prolong the natural process of death.

The critical care environment confronts patients with advanced forms of medical and nursing therapies. Although the patient and family are partially aware of the dynamics of critical care, their attention primarily focuses on the confusing and frightening environment: flashing lights, buzzing machines, painful procedures, bright lights, noise, and hyperactivity. The stressors on the patient and family are immense. The recovery period from psychologic stressors experienced in critical care may extend well past discharge from the hospital.

The patient admitted into the ICU is at risk for complications and special problems. Invasive devices carry a risk of infection, particularly in the patient with a compromised immunologic status. Sepsis and multiple organ dysfunction syndrome may follow. Other special problems for ICU patients include anxiety, dependency, impaired communication, sensory-perceptual problems, and sleep difficulties These complications are discussed as follows:

Anxiety: Patients commonly find the ICU frightening. Frequently patients are at risk of dying and fear death. Many patients and families feel uncomfortable in the ICU environment with its equipment, high noise and light levels, and intense pace of activity. The nurse can assist the patient and family with their feelings of anxiety by encouraging them to express concerns, ask questions, and state their needs. The nurse should explain equipment and procedures. The nurse may be able to structure the patients surrounding environment in a way that may decrease anxiety. For example, family members can be encouraged to bring in photographs and personal items.

Dependency: Patients in the ICU commonly are unable to perform self-care activities such as eating, bathing and oral hygiene. The patient may lack control over bodily functions such as elimination and breathing. The patient is frequently dependent on the nursing staff for access to food, liquids, the bedpan and other needed items. In addition, the ICU patient is frequently connected equipment and placed on bed rest. The degree of dependency experienced by an ICU patient can be distressing. Although the highest priority is the safety of the patient, the nurse should provide as much autonomy as the patients condition allows. Family members can be taught to assist the patient with activities of daily living.

Impaired communication: Inability to communicate can be a distressing problem for the patient who may be unable to speak because of the use of paralyzing drugs or an endotracheal tube. As part of any procedure the nurse should explain what will happen or is happening to the patient. When the patient cannot speak, the nurse should explore alternative methods of communication, including the use of devices such as picture boards, magic slates, or computer keyboards. When speaking with the patient, the nurse should look directly at the patient and use hand gestures when appropriate. Nonverbal communication is important. The ICU is characterized by high levels of procedure-related touch and decreased affection-related or comfort-related touch. Patients have different levels of tolerance for being touched, possibly related to cultural background and personal history. It may be appropriate to provide comforting touch with ongoing evaluation of the patients response.

Sensory-perceptual problems: Transient sensory-perceptual changes are common in ICU patients. Approximately 50% of patients treated in the ICU experience decreased orientation and impaired cognition. The combination of changes in mentation (e.g. hallucinations, delusions) and behavior (e.g. shouting, hitting) has been called ICU psychosis. Patients with ICU psychosis or delirium may demonstrate confusion, irritability, an inappropriate behavior. Factors predisposing the patient to sensory-perceptual changes include sleep deprivation, anxiety, sensory overload, stress and many drugs. Physical conditions such as hypoxemia and electrolyte disturbances can produce similar symptoms, including confusion and irritability. Potassium, calcium, and magnesium imbalances are common in the critically ill patient, and each can result in altered cognition.

The task of the ICU nurse is to identify predisposing factors, whether they be physiologic, psychologic, or environmental, and attempt to improve the patients mental clarity and cooperation with therapy. The use of clocks and calendars may help the patient remain oriented. Although symptoms may be managed pharmacologically with a sedative, hypnotic, or a psychotropic (e.g. haloperidol, [Haldol]) medication, these drugs may decrease the patient's ability to interact with family members. This may deprive patients and families of what may be the short and precious time remaining to discuss intimate and important issues.

Sensory deprivation and overload: To interact optimally with the environment, an individual requires the stimulation of all five senses. The optimal level and variety of this stimulation vary significantly among individuals. Patients in a critical care unit have little or no control over the amount or frequency of stimuli they receive. Too much stimuli can be as undesirable as too little. Critical care environments rarely contain the type of sensory stimuli that are familiar or understandable to patients. Unfamiliar voices, equipment noise, continuous bright lights, and frequent assessment interventions all add to the patients stress level. This level of stimulation does not disappear during the night and is in fact minimally diminished. Years of research indicate that sensory overload and sensory deprivation in the critical care environment frequently result in perceptual distortion, hallucinations, and paranoia.

Staff members may not realize the impact of this level of stimuli and frequently perpetuate it. Staff, of course, is also able to leave the high-energy critical care environment at the end of their shift, whereas the patient is unable to escape it. The nurse needs to be constantly aware of the type and amount of stimuli directed toward the patient and must help maintain the level of stimulation within tolerable limits. Research has found that a concentrated effort by staff to reduce environmental stimuli increases the likelihood of patients being able to sleep. Staff should make every effort to reduce noise and other controllable variables and to help the patient understand this complex environment, thereby reducing the stress of the unknown.

Sensory overload can also result in patient distress and anxiety. Noise levels are particularly high in the ICU. The "meaning" of a noise may determine its stressfulness. For example, meaningful noise is less stressful. The nurse can limit noise and assist the patient in understanding noises that cannot be prevented. Conversation is a particularly stressful noise, especially when the discussion concerns the patient and is conducted in the presence of, but without participation from, the patient. The nurse can restructure the environment to eliminate this source of stress by identifying better places for discussing the patient or by including the patient in the discussion. The nurse can also limit noise levels directly by muting phones, setting alarms appropriate to the patients condition, and eliminating unnecessary alarms. For example, the nurse should silence the blood pressure alarms while balancing, calibrating, and flushing lines and reactivate the alarms when the procedures are complete. Similarly, ventilator alarms should be transiently silenced during endotracheal suctioning procedures. Over-head paging should be limited in patient care areas. Music should be played only if it comforts the patient.

Sleep problems: Nearly all ICU patients experience serious sleep disturbances. Patients may have difficulty falling asleep or have disrupted sleep because of frequent monitoring or treatment procedures. Drugs such as sedatives and hypnotics result in disturbed sleep patterns, including reductions in slow wave and rapid eye movement (REM) sleep. Sleep disturbance is a significant stressor in the ICU, contributing to impaired cognition and possibly affecting recovery. The ICU nurse can structure the environment to promote patient sleep. Strategies include clustering activities, scheduling rest, making physiologic measurements without changing the patients position (when appropriate), limiting noise, and promoting comfort and relaxation.

Sleep deprivation: An essential part of the 24-hour cycle, sleep accounts for approximately one third of a person's life. An adequate amount of uninterrupted sleep is essential to prevent exhaustion or illness and maintain physiologic and psychologic well-being. Rapid eye movement (REM) sleep, important for mental restoration, occurs primarily in the last cycles of uninterrupted sleep and is the likely form of sleep to be affected by sleep deprivation in the ICU.

Hourly intervention is frequently necessary in the critical care unit to maintain physiologic homeostasis. This recurrent disruption in the sleep cycle quickly leads to a lack of REM sleep. Adverse effects of REM sleep deprivation include irritability, anxiety, physical exhaustion, disruption of metabolic functions, and respiratory distress.

The critical care nurse must assess the patient and determine whether adequate periods of uninterrupted time have been provided to promote all stages of sleep. Sleep periods should be included in the care plan and adhered to as such much as possible. Consideration must be given to the importance of interventions versus the necessity of uninterrupted sleep periods. Health care personnel should not subject patients to activity or stressful procedures during the early morning hours unless they are imperative. Visiting times should balance the needs of the patient and family while supporting adequate rest. Recent studies suggest that longer but less frequent visits may be more desirable than the traditional plan of a few minutes each hour.

Acute confusion: The risk of developing acute confusion is high in the critical care setting. The high-technology environment is overwhelming and can be frightening for the patient. The presence of serious or traumatic illness adds additional psychologic and physiologic stress. Confusion is common among all patients in ICUs but especially older patients. It has a rapid onset and is generally reversible but can be distressing for both patient and family. Symptoms of acute confusion include hallucinations (both visual and auditory), restlessness, memory impairment, and fluctuations in the patient's level of awareness.

Initial patient assessment should include information about the patient's mental status before admission. If the patient was able to adequately perform activities of daily living, it is reasonable to expect that he or she can return to that level of function once the acute confusion resolves.

Overwhelming stress is a frequent contributor to acute confusion, and the nurse must try to make the critical care environment therapeutic rather than stressful. In the past patients were physically restrained to protect them from harm. This type of intervention controls the patient's behavior but frequently increases confusion and leads to combativeness, which may necessitate chemical sedation. Interventions ideally focus on removing stressors rather than adding to the problem. Current thinking focuses on alternative to physical restraints. Fostering reality orientation by spending time with the patient and encouraging interaction with family and significant others should be priority with the confused patient. Reality orientation is an ongoing regimen of providing information to the patient at regular intervals as needed. This intervention is initiated immediately after admission to the ICU and is maintained until the patient can repeat the information on request.

Problem Related to Family Members of ICU Patient

The experience of having a friend or family member in the ICU is physically and emotionally difficult. Families of the critically ill are usually anxious about the patient's condition and prognosis. They have concerns regarding the patient's pain and other discomforts. They may question the quality of care that the patient is receiving. In addition, it is common for families to experience anxiety regarding the financial problems related to planning and providing care in the next phases of the illness. The family will typically be experiencing disruption of their daily routines in order to support the patient. They may be far from their own home, routines, and supportive friends and family members. During these difficult times, they are often asked to make critical decisions.

Lack of information is a source of anxiety for families. The nurse should assess the family's understanding of the patient's status, goals, treatments, and prognosis and provide information as appropriate. The first time the family member visits it is important for the nurse to prepare the visitor for the experience by briefly describing the patients appearance, condition, treatments, tubes, and equipment. Families should be told what to expect regarding the environment (sounds, noise, odors). It is helpful if the nurse can accompany the family members as they enter the room. They should be encouraged to touch, hug, and speak with the patient. Chairs should be provided whenever possible. The nurse should observe the responses of both patient and family to the visit. The patient may be fatigued by the visitors yet unwilling to ask them to leave. The visitors might have a difficult time dealing with a sick loved one and may need help and support. Rather than a rigid open or closed visiting policy, each patient should have a plan tailored to the patient's and family's needs.

The family needs information about the way in which the patient's care is managed and decisions are made. They should have the opportunity to affect decision-making. The family should be invited to meet the health care team members, including physicians, dietitian, respiratory therapist, social worker, and physical therapist. The nurse should evaluate the appropriateness of including family members to accept and cope with problems if they observe that providers are caring and competent, that decisions are deliberate, and that they themselves have the opportunity to help shape the course of care.

The nurse should assess the family to determine the appropriate extent of their involvement in care. In some cases this might be limited to sitting with the patient and holding the patients hand during quiet periods. Other family members might welcome the opportunity to participate in physical care such as shaving or oral hygiene. The nurse should encourage such activity. Other contributions include assisting with procedures, ambulation and feeding. Family involvement should be included in the plan of care.

While working with families, the ICU nurse should assess the response of the family to the stress. Their feelings should be acknowledged and accepted. They should be supported in their decisions. Institutional support systems such as chaplains, social workers, and psychologists may be helpful in assisting the family and patient to adjust. The extent to which the family is involved and supported will in turn affect the patient's clinical course in the ICU.

Stressors in ICU

The ICU environment is exceptionally stressful for the nursing staff. The nurses stress stems partially from high expectations: advanced knowledge of physiology related to all body systems, astute observational and physical assessment skills, ability to quickly prioritize and make decisions regarding patient care, and technical proficiency in operating the highly sophisticated equipment. Nurses also increasingly face complex ethical issues that consume their time and emotional energy. In addition, the constant vigilance and emergency-ready atmosphere may promote an uneasy sense of impending crisis. Critical care nurses must be able to remain and communicate effectively with the patient and family during crisis situations.

Most critical care nurses select this area of practice at least in part because they feel stimulated by a fast-paced environment that requires them to effectively integrate a detailed knowledge base, excellent assessment skills, and significant technologic proficiency. Manageable stress levels can promote creativity and productivity. However, continuous high-level stress can be as detrimental to the nurse as to the patient in the critical care environment or ICU includes the following:

Patients and Family Stressors

- Unfamiliar environment, new faces
- Noise, light levels
- Sensory deprivation or overload
- Interruption of sleep-wake cycles
- Inaccessibility of family, friends
- Lack of privacy
- Lack of information or understanding of prognosis and care plan
- Lack of information or understanding of policies and procedures
- Anticipation of painful interventions
- Confusion or disorientation related to physiologic factors
- Impaired communication related to intubation
- Observation of crisis interventions in other patients
- Fear related to diagnosis
- Fear of death
- Conflict between patient or family goals and staff goals
- Pain.

Staff Stressors

- Expectations of self
- Expectations of peers, clinical supervisors, other health care team members, hospital administrators
- Intricate machinery and techniques
- Closed, crowded work area

- Constant contact with seriously ill or dying patients
- Continual vigilance over multiple patients
- Constant emergency readiness
- Sustained high activity level
- Limited breaks from high-stress unit
- Limited communication with many patients because of intubation or altered level of consciousness
- Limited opportunity to communicate with families
- Isolation from other nurses in hospital
- Ethical conflicts related to resuscitation and use of life-support equipment
- Legal issues
- Exposure to infectious diseases.

In addition to understanding how stressors affect the patient and family, critical care nurses must guard their own physical and psychologic health by recognizing and decreasing their own stress levels. They must develop in ability to understand and respond appropriately to their own needs for support in the daily work environment, as well as the needs of their colleagues. Failure to develop self-care strategies may hamper the nurse's ability to respond appropriately to patient needs and ultimately leads to nurse burnout and exit from the health care field.

Long-term involvement with patients in a critical care environment is a relatively new phenomenon and is accompanied by significant new stressors. Technology currently enables medical science to extend the life of some critically ill patients, such as those awaiting organ transplantation, who may have critical care hospitalizations that extend weeks to months. Consistent nurse caregivers can develop a strong therapeutic relationship with the patient and family and help them cope with the stressors of the critical care environment. Nurses caring for patients on an ongoing basis may even be able to more quickly assess and respond to changes in the patients' condition. However, they may become so close to the circumstances of the patient's illness that their own psychologic health suffers. It is important for clinicians to recognize when ongoing care of a patient results in undue stress and to develop strategies for protecting their mental health. Strategies include:

- Development of support networks among nursing peers
- Use of employee assistance personnel (counselors, social services personnel, and chaplains: critical stress debriefing) tto cope with stressful circumstances
- Development of interests outside the critical care environment to help keep personal and professional worlds separate
- Careful self-evaluation of the values, beliefs, and feelings associated with the critical care milieu
- Use of a multidisciplinary team approach to nursing care, in collaboration with direct caregivers such as physicians; respiratory, speech, and physical therapists; and other care providers such as nutritionists, pharmacists, clergy, social workers, radiology technicians, clerical assistants, and hospital volunteers
- Acknowledgment of the need to occasionally change assignments to provide respite for the clinician
- Scheduling of regular clinical care conferences with the patient, significant others, and other multidisciplinary team members to help the patient feel less dependent on the nursing staff. Conferences allow the patient and family to provide important input into the overall care plan and to feel the tangible involvement of various members of the multidisciplinary team. This approach is particularly important for the long-term critical care patient. Care goals can be reevaluated, modifications agreed on, or new goals established.

The death of a critically ill patient can be the source of tremendous emotional stress to the nurse. To help protect against overwhelming stress, when caring for a dying patient the nurse should:

- Examine his or her own feelings about death
- Listen attentively to the expressed needs of the patient and family
- Remain available to the patient and family both physically and emotionally
- Use touch, if culturally acceptable, in caring for the patient and family
- Reassure the patient and family that the patient will continue to receive skilled and compassionate care even if a do-not-resuscitate decision has been made
- Attempt to remain nonjudgmental about family or hospital issues
- Respect the strengths and limitations of the patient-family relationship, which existed long before the patient-hospital relationship
- Include the family in care
- Provide for patient and family privacy
- Provide the opportunity for the family to exercise religious or cultural traditions.

Providing comprehensive care to critically ill patients and their families is a challenging opportunity. The critical care nurse combines the technologic sophistication of this unique setting with a personal, individualized care approach to maximize the positive potential outcomes for the patient.

Ethical Decision Making in Critical Care Nursing

In many ways technologic advances in health care have evolved faster than society's ability to understand the associated ethical dilemmas. Life can be prolonged in ways that were previously impossible, sometimes beyond all known hope of recovery. Tremendous emotional, financial, legal, and social ramifications exist as patients are stabilized in conditions for which long-term health care options are limited. For example, few families and even fewer skilled care facilities have the resources to care for a patient who requires continuous mechanical ventilation.

With the advent of advance directives, nurses frequently assume responsibility for gathering information about the patient's wishes concerning the extent of their care or treatment. Patients frequently have not prepared advance directives or are incompetent to render such a decision, leaving the family and significant others to determine the type and extent of medical care the patient would or would not want in this situation. Critical care nurses frequently assist families with highly emotional decisions such as forgoing resuscitation or withdrawing life support systems. Assisting families with these decisions is painfully complex.

All health care professionals must examine their own beliefs about life and death, termination of life, organ and tissue donation, and use of limited resources. Education and support for the nurse are available from formal classes, support groups, peers and hospital ethics committees. Ethics committees are also available to patients, families, and staff members who wish consultation and support in difficult or divisive situations.

Biomedical advances at times seem to challenge the compassionate aspects of care giving. The critical care nurse is the professional caregiver best qualified to play a pivotal role in identifying and supporting the patient's wishes.

Management of the Patient in Critical Care Unit/ICU

Management of critically ill patients requires establishment of a database, identification of actual and potential nursing diagnoses and collaborative problems, delineation of priorities, definition of outcome criteria, execution of planned interventions, and modification of future interventions and plans on the basis of current outcomes.

The assessment process for the critically ill patient differs from the assessment of other patients only in terms of the technologies used. The cardiac monitor, hemodynamic monitoring lines, and laboratory analyses provide data that the nurse must incorporate into the total patient assessment. Technologies provide adjuncts to the data the nurse gathers through observation, history taking, and physical examination. Monitored data are useless unless correlated with physical findings and integrated into meaningful analysis by the critical care nurse.

The importance of accurate, thorough initial information cannot be overemphasized. However, the multiple sources of data and fluctuating condition of critically ill patients make constant priority reorganization a necessity. The critical care nurse continually updates the database to reformulate short-term goals and interventions.

Patient assessment must be thorough, yet rapid. The nurse must consider the physical and psychologic reactions of an entire organism under stress, while remaining open to the unusual or unexpected. Patient assessment also must be organized and repetitive so that small alterations or deviations from previous findings will be apparent. Finally, the assessment must be individualized, with time and attention given to significant aspects.

The patient may be admitted to critical care as either a direct admission (usually through the emergency department), as a transfer from another patient care division in the same or a different hospital, or as a postoperative admission after certain operations. The critical care nurse integrates data from the patient and family, written history, and the transfer report of other nurses into the patient's initial treatment plan. Consultation between transferring and receiving nursing unit staffs is essential to accomplish this process effectively. These data sources help ensure continuity of care and communication of all issues important to the patient or family. The nurse carefully explores the patient's and family's response to the need for critical care placement. A full patient profile may be deferred until later in the hospitalization, as hemodynamic stabilization is always the first priority of care. The initial contact with the critical care personnel sets the tone for all future interactions and is an invaluable opportunity for the nurse to demonstrate competence and caring and begin to establish a foundation of trust.

The physical assessment of the patient, while augmented by the technology of the intensive care unit, still uses the skills of inspection, palpation, percussion, and auscultation to determine the patients care needs and evaluate responses to interventions. The critical care nurse combines these physical assessment may take place hourly or even more frequently as patient status dictates. All disciplines involved in the patient's care participate in the ongoing assessment process. The dynamic and collaborative nature of critical care assessment allows for rapid responses to any changes in patient status, but it may also contribute to the patient's sensory overload. The need to evaluate status changes frequently may leave the patient with little time for rest and privacy. Significant nursing skill is required to balance information gathering and patient rest. It may take years of experience for the nurse to gather and synthesize several pieces of data simultaneously, thoroughly, and rapidly, with the least disruption to the patient.

Monitored data: Nurses in all clinical settings use tools such as stethoscopes, sphygmomanometers, thermometers, and scales to collect patient data. Critical care nurses also have access to tools that are capable of continuous data collection, such as cardiac monitors, hemodynamic pressure lines, intracranial pressure and monitoring devices, and airway pressure monitoring devices. The explosion in critical care technology since the 1970s provides the critical care nurse with amazing quantities of objective data. Digital computerized monitoring systems occupy less space and provide more capabilities than ever before. The most sophisticated patient data management systems take information from all the monitored parameters

(ECG, respirations, intra-arterial pressure, pulmonary artery pressure, venous oxygen saturation, central venous pressure, intracranial pressure, and body temperature), combine it with manually entered data (such as weight, height, intake and output, and times of drug administration), and produce a wide array of hemodynamic and pulmonary calculations and patient response trends for analysis by critical care practitioners.

Technologic adjuncts to critical care assessment are continuously changing, combining older and well-tested monitoring systems with newer advances. Certain types of monitoring equipment are used in all critical care environments. Waveforms and other data produced by these devices may be viewed continuously on a video screen or be graphed for a permanent record.

Many monitoring systems involve use of fluid, tubing, and transducer equipment, which acts as portals of entry for microorganisms. Strict aseptic technique is essential to prevent complications associated with nosocomial infections.

i. *Cardiac monitoring* is a noninvasive procedure that poses minimal risk to the patient. It consists of placing conductive electrodes on the patient's chest that recognize the electrical activity of the heart and relay it to a video display screen. Depending on the sophistication of the monitoring equipment, the clinician may be able to view the patients ECG and heart rate at the bedside and at remote locations in the critical care unit, monitor changes during activity (with mobile equipment), and set flexible monitoring parameters as changes in cardiac status occur. Parameters may include changes in heart rate and rhythm; in respiratory rate and rhythm; in analysis of dysrhythmias; and in specific ECG segments, such as the ST segment for ischemia recognition. Alarms notify the clinician when preset limits have been reached. Most monitors default to preset limits if the clinician does not set specific alarm parameters and only allow clinicians to silence the alarms for a limited time.

ii. *Hemodynamic monitoring* refers to invasive monitoring of the arterial or venous system. Monitoring is accomplished through catheters that measure changes in air and fluid pressures and can also be used to administer intravenous fluids and obtain arterial or venous blood for laboratory analysis. Transducers connected to the system interpret the air and fluid pressure readings and display the results as waveforms on cardiac monitoring equipment. The two most commonly used hemodynamic monitoring systems are intra-arterial monitoring and pulmonary artery monitoring.

It is important for the nurse to verify the digital display of waveform values with a manual sphygmomanometer, regularly calibrate the transducer equipment with the transducer positioned at specific landmarks on the patients body, and assess the entire system for patency and accuracy. The nurse can obtain measurements with the patient in an up to 30° lateral or supine position if the patient is hemodynamically stable. The nurse requires a thorough knowledge of waveform interpretation to appropriately interpret and respond to the values displayed on the screen or on a manual printout. Even minor errors in reading and interpreting values or small problems in the patency of the system, such as a tiny air bubble in the transducer system, can result in inaccurate data and may cause profound complications for the patient.

Aseptic technique is critical to the maintenance of these systems with the least possible risk to the patient. Ongoing assessment of the patient's response to the equipment is also critical to avoid dangerous complications such as air emboli, bleeding, malposition of catheters, tissue damage, or hemodynamic compromise as a result of foreign body insertion or malposition.

iii. *Intra-arterial monitoring* involves inserting a catheter into an artery, usually the radial or femoral artery, and connecting the catheter to a high-pressure flush system filled with either a heparinized or nonheparinized saline solution. The high-pressure flush counterbalances arterial resistance to maintain patency of the system. Intra-arterial systems display a continuous reading of the patient's blood pressure and provide ready access to obtain arterial blood gas or other laboratory specimens.

iv. *Pulmonary artery monitoring* involves inserting a catheter through the subclavian or internal jugular vein and advancing it into the pulmonary artery, usually under fluoroscopic guidance. These catheters have several lumens encased within a larger lumen, and each opens at a different point along the length of the catheter. Each lumen may be used to attach monitoring and transducer equipment. The large bore of the lumens and placement of the catheter in large arteries permit administration of caustic intravenous solutions that could damage peripheral veins.

A balloon at the distal tip of the catheter if filled with approximately 1 mL of air the natural flow of blood through the patient's heart pulls the balloon into place in the pulmonary artery. When the catheter is correctly placed, the balloon is deflated. Monitoring and transducer equipment is attached to the catheter.

The catheter and monitoring equipment are used to obtain significant data about the patient's hemodynamic and cardiac function. Available data include pulmonary artery and central venous pressure recordings and cardiac output measurements. Combining these values with parameters such as blood pressure and body surface area, it is possible to calculate additional information that is not directly available from catheter readings. Newer monitoring equipment calculates these values automatically when data are entered into the database, decreasing the chance for error from manual calculation. The pulmonary artery catheter rapidly provides valuable information to evaluate the patient's response to vasoactive drugs by providing data about left- and right-sided heart function. It is also significant tool for managing severe cardiac failure and cardiogenic shock.

v. *A central venous pressure (CVP)* catheter may be used in lieu of a pulmonary artery catheter when evaluation of pulmonary artery pressure and left-sided heart function are not required. CVP catheters may be connected to a transducer and used to measure right-sided heart pressures and deliver intravenous fluids, but they are more limited than pulmonary artery catheters in the scope of data they provide. A newer type of central line is called a peripherally inserted central venous catheter (PICC). The nurse assess and maintains the external portion of the PICC and may instruct patients and families in these techniques for home use. PICC lines are long-dwell catheters that require the same aseptic care as other central lines. They can be used for long-term fluid and medication administration but at present have no monitoring capabilities.

vi. *Monitoring intracranial pressure (ICP)* involves placing a catheter through the skull into either the subarachnoid space or the cerebral ventricle to monitor changes in pressure within the cranial cavity. A transducer and tubing system gather the data, which are displayed on monitoring screens. Newer monitoring systems have the capacity to sense changes in intracranial pressure and display pressure readings on a bedside monitor without the use of fluid-filled pressure tubing and transducer systems. Although insertion through the skull into the cranial cavity is still required, these newer systems reduce the risk of contamination by microorganisms.

   Patients with unstable intracranial pressure may be sensitive to routine nursing interventions such as turning, suctioning, and changing bed position. Continuous display of ICP readings allows the nurse to constantly evaluate the patient's response to all interventions and take prompt action if the patient's pressure reaches unsafe levels. The catheter also can be used to aspirate cerebrospinal fluid for analysis or culture and to relieve elevated ICP. The nurse is responsible for identifying changes in pressure readings, analyzing trends, evaluating patient responses to interventions or therapies, and preventing complications.

vii. *Continuous airway pressure monitoring (CAPM)* is a simple, noninvasive technique that uses a transducer cable, high-pressure tubing (as used for measuring pulmonary and arterial pressures), and a display monitor. The monitoring equipment is connected to a ventilator circuit at the Y connector near the airway. Standard calibration procedures are used, but the monitoring tubing is filled with air, not fluid, and the transducer can be at any level while calibration is performed. The absence of fluid in the transducer system minimizes the risk of infection. The waveforms produced by CAPM may be continuously displayed, graphed, and compared with hemodynamic waveforms.

The waveforms produced by the system enable the clinician to continuously monitor the patient's response to various modes of mechanical ventilation and therapeutic interventions. CAPM is also useful in identifying one of the most common complications of mechanical ventilation: patient-ventilator asynchrony or intolerance. Asynchrony can result from mechanical malfunction, inappropriate ventilator mode selection and inadequate inspiratory flow rate, airway obstruction from excessive secretions, or patient anxiety or agitation. Asynchrony increases the work of breathing and can result in inadequate gas exchange. When a patient experiences asynchrony, the CAPM waveforms deviate from the expected patterns, altering the nurse to the need for prompt intervention. CAPM can be especially helpful in monitoring sedated, very ill, or chemically relaxed patients who may be unable to communicate patient-ventilator intolerance. CAPM provides the bedside nurse with continuous visual assurance that the patient is receiving adequate ventilation and that chemical relaxation is being delivered at an appropriate dose. Any interruption of ventilation is immediately apparent by waveform absence.

Analysis of the patient's waveforms and comparison with expected waveforms allow the care team to evaluate the patient's response to mechanical ventilation and modify the plan if necessary. Hemodynamic pressure data frequently serve as the foundation of treatment for critically ill patients. However, both real and artificial changes in the hemodynamic waveforms occur in response to pressure in the hemodynamic waveforms occur in response to pressure gradients produced by the pulmonary and systemic circulation. True pressures can be further obscured by tachypnea and underlying cardiac pathologic conditions. CAPM may be used in these situations to help standardize measurements. Simultaneous graphing of CAPM and pulmonary artery pressures provides a clear visual picture of end expiration. CAPM has thus been shown to be a simple, cost-efficient and effective adjunct to critical care monitoring.

In using any invasive or noninvasive tools, the nurse must be knowledgeable about the proper use and maintenance of the equipment, including the appearance of the waveform associated with each line, standard interventions used to prevent complications, signs and symptoms of complications, and troubleshooting techniques for when problem develop. The patient risk associated with invasive monitoring lines is significantly reduced when knowledgeable personnel manage the lines. In addition to the various invasive lines used for monitoring, critical care nurses also must be skillful in using central lines for medication, fluid, and nutrition administration.

As monitoring techniques become increasingly sophisticated, the health care provider may be tempted to treat solely based on the numbers and waveforms produced by the equipment. It is essential for the clinician to remember that these data must always be combined with data from routine physical assessment, including the patient's general appearance and subjective response to all therapeutic measures. A flat line on a waveform may be the result of a disconnected wire to tubing rather than a change in the patient's condition. The nurse must remain vigilant and keep one eye on the monitor and one eye on the patient to avoid treating the equipment instead of the patient. The nurse must also tailor the use of each monitoring technique to each unique patient situation.

Nursing Problems of Patient and Their Interventions in ICU

Impaired Gas Exchange

Common nursing objectives for the patient with a diagnosis of impaired gas exchange are:

Patient will:

- Demonstrate satisfactory pulmonary function: Adequate blood oxygenation, hemoglobin saturation, and forced expiratory volume in 1 second
- Maintain a satisfactory respiratory rate and pattern.

For which nurse in a critical care setting, the immediate goal of ensuring a patients survival determines the priorities for intervention; physiologic problems must be addressed first. Once the critical care team has alleviated life-threatening stressors, they can re-evaluate priorities and address other problems. Physiologic priorities are determined by the degree of threat to the person's survival. Certain body systems are more prone to disorders requiring intensive therapeutic interventions that are frequently encountered in the critical care unit. At the most basic level, these priorities can be organized in the same "ABC" framework as basic cardiac life support. Establishment of airway, breathing, and circulation remains the foundation for therapeutic management of the critical care patient. By applying the ABCs of basic life support, the critical care nurse is able to move from the most parsing to least pressing patient problems. When a patients physiologic status begins to deteriorate, clinicians take immediate actions to reverse the problem. Correct positioning of the endotracheal tube with suctioning as needed ensues airway patency. The nurse then assess the patients ability to breathe and the effect of physical restraints or physiologic conditions such as acute respiratory failure. The patients pulse oximetry and blood gases are also monitored for normalcy and early signs of distress.

Decreased Cardiac Output

Common nursing objectives for the patient with a diagnosis of decreased cardiac output are:

Patient will:

- Maintain systolic blood pressure above 100 mm Hg, urine output greater than 30 mL/h, and cardiac rate and rhythm within acceptable limits
- Maintain good tissue perfusion
- Maintain stable vital signs.

For which after initially focusing on airway and breathing management, the nurse addresses circulatory needs, such as the establishment of normal cardiac rhythm, intravenous access for administration of medications, and adequate cardiopulmonary perfusion of vital organs. The critical care clinician may continue to use this basic ABC principle in ongoing assessments to ensure that problems are recognized before complication develop. The nurse improves cardiac output by reducing workload on the heart and increasing venous return. The patient is placed in the Semi-Fowler's position. Rest and quiet are important. The nurse continues to assess the blood pressure, capillary refill, urine output, presence of edema, and laboratory values. Maintaining intravenous accesses is important, since most medications and fluids are delivered intravenously.

Anxiety

Common nursing objectives for the patient with a diagnosis of anxiety are:

Patient will:

- Report an increase in psychologic comfort
- Report a decrease in restless and other behavioral manifestations of anxiety.

For which the initial step in preventing or alleviating psychologic stress is to identify the patients and family's perception of the critical event. Their perceptions will be affected by their individual personalities, current psychologic health, general understanding of the situation and its projected outcome, tolerance for an ambiguity, and normal pattern of coping. Initial perceptions are often significantly affected by previous exposure to similar events, either positive or negative, and general level of familiarity with medical interventions and the hospital environment. The critically ill person, separated from familiar surroundings and dependent on others to meet the most basic needs, becomes partially or totally isolated from usual support systems. Feelings of helplessness, loneliness, and depersonalization, as well as disturbances in body image, are common. Modes of expressing and thereby relieving frustration, anger, hostility, fear or depression are limited by the physical constraints of the critical care environment. Anger and hostility are often indications of fear and anxiety. Depression and withdrawal may be normal signs of hopelessness, loneliness, powerlessness, or loss.

Consistently assigned caregivers can be an effective way to establish a therapeutic relationship with the patient and family. An atmosphere of openness and acceptance that encourages expression of feelings can help patients cope. The nurse talks openly and honestly with the patient to decrease feelings of depersonalization, isolation and alienation. The nurse encourages the patient and family to express their feelings and assists the patient in identifying the fears and concerns that may be causing unusual or inappropriate behavior. The nurse or other health care team members who help patients talk about feelings must be to accept whatever emotionally laden information might be expressed. Nonjudgmental recognition and acceptance of the patient's feelings help reinforce the patient's right to the feelings.

Intubated patients are unable to express their feelings freely even when alert and oriented and are therefore particularly vulnerable to psychologic stressors. The nurse must guard against the normal inclination to communicate less with persons who cannot talk easily. Strategies such as keeping a letter board, paper and pencil, or "magic slate" within the patient's reach and providing assistance to the patient help reduces the sense of isolation. However, such methods do not allow the patient to truly express feelings and concerns. The nurse carefully assesses the patient for cures concerning his or her emotional state and anticipates common concerns among critically ill patients. The nurse can verbalize the potential concerns and allow the patient to validate them as appropriate. The direct expression of empathy for the patient and family conveys acceptance and understanding.

Interrupted Family Processes

Common nursing objectives for the patient with a diagnosis of interrupted family processes are:

Patient and family will:

- Identify the stress of having a family member admitted to a critical care unit
- State community and personal resources available to enhance coping abilities.

The essence of crisis intervention is helping persons cope with a major life crisis that a critical illness may precipitate. Critical care nursing is far broader in scope and more future oriented than crisis intervention alone, but specific situations frequently require the immediacy and limited focus of crisis intervention. At the time of crisis the nurse helps the patient and family establish short-term goals and minimize the number and scope of decisions they must make. As the crisis situation stabilizes, the nurse provides the patient and family with more information and helps them accept additional responsibility for decision-making and goal setting. When the patient and family are knowledgeable about the goals of therapy and understand the patient's diagnosis, current status, and prognosis, they can be involved in many aspects of care planning and can make decisions consistent with the treatment regimen.

Involvement of significant others decreases the patient's feelings of powerlessness, frustration, and anxiety. The family is likely to be involved in care giving at some point in the patient's recovery, and the maldisciplinary team must begin including them in care planning soon as possible. The patient is reassured by having a loving advocate represent his or her wishes and concerns. Even when a patient is unconscious, visits by key support figures who talk to and touch the patient may have positive, if immeasurable, effects on the patient while ameliorating the family's feelings of helplessness.

The nurse actively involves all alert patients in goal setting and care planning. The nurse seeks to increase the patient's feeling of personal control in structuring the daily schedule of activities. The knowledge that nursing staff values the patient's preferences and views the patient as capable of making decisions reinforces the importance of the patient's role in recovery.

The environment of the critical care unit presents multiple stresses to the patient and family. Narcotics and sedatives, anxiety, hypoxia, sleep deprivation, and multiple metabolic derangements all contribute to acute confusion, disturbed thought processes, and perceptual distortions. The nurse uses reality orientation on an ongoing basis to help patients regain their mental stability. Although some environmental factors cannot be altered, the nurse can use a variety of strategies to control the sensory level of the critical care unit.

Critical care units increasingly recognize the importance of visits by the patients significant others in minimizing psychologic stressors. The practice of restrictive and minimal visitation is being policies range from longer and more frequent visitation hours to true open visitation, where the patient and family participate fully in care activities and care team rounds. Although these policies appear to improve the patient's and family's trust and therapeutic relationship with the care team, the nurse must be careful to avoid overwhelming the family with the daily stress and sensory overload of the critical care unit. The nurse should encourage significant others to meet their own needs for rest, nutrition, psychosocial support, relaxation, and spiritual renewal. Many significant others need support in their decision to leave the critical care environment at regular intervals, even when visitation policies would allow them to remain.

In the critical care setting, the patients psychologic needs often assume priority, and care providers may ignore the patient's needs as a social being. Limited visiting hours, the strange technical environment, and the aura of danger in the critical care unit isolate patients from their usual social roles. For the most part, staff members view a person who is critically ill primarily in the patient role. The more significant roles of spouse, parent, child, lover, sibling, friend, or provider may go virtually unrecognized unless staff members initiate interventions to provide continuity in these relationships.

The nurse can foster continuity in social roles through the same types of interventions used to reduce psychologic stress; increasing visits between patient and family; including the family in discussions of disease process, prognosis, and care plans; and encouraging the family to report events and activities occurring in other significant spheres of the patients life. Relaying telephone messages between the patient and distant friends is another way the nurse can help the patient maintain contact with his or her broader external world.

One effective way to prevent disruption in relationship is for the nurse to carefully explain the patients physical appearance and the critical care environment to family or friends before their first visit with the patient in the critical care unit. Visitors need to understand the patient's level of consciousness, ability to communicate, and comprehension. They need to understand the importance of their presence to the patient and the patients need for their support. When visitors approach the bedside, the nurse remains with them if possible to facilitate their initial interaction with the patient. Family frequently needs to be encouraged to touch the patient and offer other physical expressions of their love and support. Fear of hurting the patient or disrupting the multiple monitoring devices can virtually immobilize the family member. The nurse can help family members find safe places to stand and explain the basic purpose of the various lines and tubes. The nurse also encourages the family to speak with the patient, especially unconscious or intubated patients. At each subsequent visit the nurse caring for the patient meets with the family to answer the questions and apprise them of the patients progress.

The critical care nurse also must recognize the inevitability of role changes for some patients and families during a critical illness. Roles of provider, decision maker, employer, and employee may be altered, reversed, or eliminated. Family and friends may need to assume some or all of the patient's responsibilities at this time.

During the critical phase of illness, family members trying to cope with significant role change and additional responsibilities may need help in working through problems. The nurse needs to be sensitive to these problems and provide the family with professional guidance, such as from a social worker, to assist in reorganizing themselves and their resources. The nurse may help the family appoint a temporary family representative, someone who knows and is able to represent the wishes of a family as a whole and who can be contracted in an emergency. The nurse also may help the family plan visiting schedules that meet the patient's needs without preventing family members from fulfilling their own responsibilities. This is a period of great emotional stress for both patient and family.

Patient and family teaching is an integral part of nursing care for the patient in the critical care unit.

PATIENT MONITORING IN CRITICAL CARE UNIT

Critical care unit (CCU) equipment includes patient monitoring, respiratory and cardiac support, pain management, emergency resuscitation devices, and other life support equipment designed to care for patients who are seriously injured, have a critical or life-threatening illness, or have undergone a major surgical procedure, thereby requiring 24-hour care and monitoring.

A CCU may be designed and equipped to provide care to patients with a range of conditions, or it may be designed and equipped to provide specialized care to patients with specific conditions. For example, a neuromedical CCU cares for patients with acute conditions involving the nervous system or patients who have just had neurosurgical procedures and require equipment for monitoring and assessing the brain and spinal cord. A neonatal CCU is designed and equipped to care for infants who are ill, born prematurely, or have a condition requiring constant monitoring. A trauma/burn CCU provides specialized injury and wound care for patients involved in auto accidents and patients who have gunshot injuries or burns.

Intensive care unit equipment includes patient monitoring, life support and emergency resuscitation devices, and diagnostic devices.

Patient monitoring equipment includes the following:

- Acute care physiologic monitoring system—comprehensive patient monitoring systems that can be configured to continuously measure and display a number of parameters via electrodes and sensors that are connected to the patient. These may include the electrical activity of the heart via an ECG, respiration rate (breathing), blood pressure, body temperature, cardiac output, and amount of oxygen and carbon dioxide in the blood. Each patient bed in an CCU has a physiological monitor that measure these body activities. All monitors are networked to a central nurses' station.
- Pulse oximeter—monitors the arterial hemoglobin oxygen saturation (oxygen level) of the patient's blood with a sensor clipped over the finger or toe.
- Intracranial pressure monitor—measures the pressure of fluid in the brain in patients with head trauma or other conditions affecting the brain (such as tumors, edema; or hemorrhage). These devices warn of elevated pressure and record or display pressure trends. Intracranial pressure monitoring may be a capability included in a physiologic monitor.
- Apnea monitor—continuously monitors breathing via electrodes or sensors placed on the patient. An apnea monitor detects cessation of breathing in infants and adults at risk of respiratory failure, displays respiration parameters, and triggers an alarm if a certain amount of time passes without a patient's breath being detected. Apnea monitoring may be a capability including a physiologic monitor.

Intensive care equipment for life support and emergency resuscitation includes the following:

- Ventilator (also called a respirator)—assists with or controls pulmonary ventilation in patients who cannot breathe on their own. Ventilators consist of a flexible breathing circuit, gas supply, heating/humidification mechanism, monitors and alarms. They are microprocessor-controlled and programmable, and regulate the volume, pressure, and flow of patient respiration. Ventilator monitors and alarms may interface with central monitoring system or information system.
- Infusion pump—device that delivers fluids intravenously or epidural through a catheter. Infusion pumps employ automatic, programmable pumping mechanisms to deliver continuous anesthesia, drugs, and blood infusions to the patient. The pump is hung on an intravenous pole placed next to the patient's bed.

- Crash cart—also called a resuscitation or code cart. This is portable dart containing emergency resuscitation equipment for patients who are "coding". That is, their vital signs are in a dangerous range. The emergency equipment includes a defibrillator, airway intubation devices, a resuscitation bag/mask, and medication obs. Crash carts are strategically located in the CCU for immediate availability for when a patient experiences cardiorespiratory failure.
- Intra-aortic, balloon pump—a device that helps reduce the heart's workload and helps blood flow to the coronary arteries for patients with unstable angina, myocardial, infarction (heart attack), or patients awaiting organ transplants. Intraaortic balloon pumps use a balloon placed in the patient's aorta. The balloon is on the end of a catheter that is connected to the pump's console, which displays heart rate, pressure, and electrocardiogram (ECG) readings. The patient's ECG is used to time the inflation and deflation of the balloon.

Diagnostic Equipment

The use of diagnostic equipment is also required in the CCU. Mobile X-ray units are used for bedside radiography, particularly of the chest. Mobile X-ray units use a battery operated generator that powers an X-ray tube. Handheld, portable clinical laboratory devices, or point-of-care analyzers, and blood chemistry parameters can be provided much faster than if samples were sent to the central laboratory.

Other CCU Equipment for Monitoring

Disposable CCU equipment includes urinary (Foley) catheters, catheters used for arterial and central venous lines, Swan-Ganz catheters, chest and endotracheal tubes, gastrointestinal and nasogastric feeding tubes, and monitoring electrodes. Some patients may be wearing a pose vest, also called a Houdini Jacket for safety; the purpose is to keep the patient stationary. Spenco boots are padded support devices made of lamb's wool to position the feet and ankles of the patient. Support hose may be placed on the patient's legs to support the leg muscles and aid circulation.

Operation

The CCU is a demanding environment due to the critical condition of patients and the variety of equipment necessary to support and monitor patients. Therefore, when operating CCU equipment, staff should pay attention to the types of devices and the variations between different models of the same type of device, so they do not make an error in operation or adjustment. Although many hospitals make an effort to standardize equipment, for example, using the same manufacturer's infusion pumps or patient monitoring systems, older devices and nonstandardized equipment may still be used, particularly when the CCU is busy. Clinical staff should be sure to check all devices and settings to ensure patient safety.

Maintenance

Since CCU equipment is used continuously on critically ill patients. It is essential that equipment be properly maintained particularly devices that are used for life support and resuscitation. Staff in the CCU should perform daily checks on equipment and inform biomedical engineering, staff when equipment needs maintenance, repair or replacement. For mechanically complex devices, service and preventive maintenance contracts are available from the manufacturer or third-party servicing companies, and should be kept current at all times.

Health Care Team Roles

Equipment in the CCU:, is used by a team specialized in their use. The team usually comprises a critical care attending physician (also called an intensives), critical care nurses, and an infectious disease team; critical care respiratory therapists, pharmacologists, physical therapis, and dietitians. Physicians trained in other specialties, such as anesthesiology, cardiology, radiology, surgery, neurology, pediatrics, and other orthopedics may be consulted to perform mobile X-ray examination (beside radiography). Either, nurses or clinical laboratory personnel perform point-of-care blood analysis. Equipment in the CCU is maintained and repaired by hospital biomedical engineering staff and/or the equipment manufacturer.

CHAPTER

8

Oncological Nursing

INTRODUCTION

The word 'onco' originated from Greek word '*onkos*' means 'mass' relating to tumors. Oncogene, a gene which in certain circumstances can transform a cell into a tumor cell, oncology is the study and treatment of tumors, may be benign or malignant. If it is malignant, people used to call it as cancer. Cancer was recognized in ancient times by skilled observers who gave it the name "Cancer" (Latin word *Cancer-crab*) because it stretched out in many directions like the legs of a crab. The term cancer is an "umbrella" word used to describe a group of more than 270 diseases in which cells multiply without restraint, destroy healthy tissue endangering life. The psychological and physiological impact on cancer patients and their families results in profound changes in their lifestyles. Cancer may result in death for some and mutilation for others. The legends, surroundings, malignant diseases often focusing on its incurability help foster feelings of hopelessness and dread. Yet, much progress has been made in prevention, early detection and treatment of cancer and research continue in these areas.

Cancer is not a single disease with a single cause; rather, it is a group of distinct diseases with different causes, manifestations treatments, and prognoses. Cancer nursing practice cover all age groups and nursing specialties and is carried out in variety of health care setting, including the home, community acute care institutions, outpatient centers, rehabilitations and long-term care facilities. The scope, responsibilities and goals of cancer nursing, also called oncology nursing, are adverse and complex as those of any nursing specialty. Because many people associate cancer with pain and death, nurse need to identify their own reactions to cancer and set realist goals to meet the challenges inherent in caring for patient with cancer. In addition, cancer nurses must be prepare to support patients and families through a wide range of physical emotional, social, cultural, and spiritual crises.

Oncology nurses must have a broad base of knowledge in both pathophysiology and psychosocial arena. They care for patients of all ages, both gender and in a variety of settings. The oncology nurse feels and fills the role of care provider, manager, researcher, teacher and consultant. To provide comprehensive care, the nurse must have accurate knowledge about prevention, control and treatment of cancer. Nurse has to teach about cancer in all settings. In addition to teaching, the nurse has an active role in treatment and control programs of cancer. To be effective as a helping person, the nurse must be aware of the emotional impact that the diagnosis of cancer has on the patient and family, because this emotional response affects every aspect of nursing care. Cancer nursing challenges the creativity, skill and commitment of the nurses.

CANCER

The word cancer, often abbreviated Ca, as a term that frightens most people. Cancer is synonymous with the term "malignant neoplasma". Other terms suggest malignant neoplasm includes tumor, malignancy, carcinoma and aberrant cell growth. Strictly speaking, these words are not interchangeable.

Cancer is a disease of the cell in which the normal mechanisms of control of growth and proliferation are disturbed. This results in distinctive morphological alteration of the cells and aberration in tissue pattern. Cancer is a collective term describing a large group of diseases characterized by uncontrolled growth and spread of abnormal cells. This group of diseases:

- Arise from any tissue or organ
- Differ greatly from one another in appearance and growth
- May follow very different courses of developments in their host
- Respond differently to the variety of therapies applied to them.

The word 'neoplasm' is derived from Greek words *neos*: new, and *plasis*: molding. Thus, neoplasm is defined as an abnormal new growth or formation of tissue that serves no useful purpose and may harm the host organism.

A neoplasm may be either benign or malignant:

- Benign is defined as a usually harmless growth that does not spread or invade other tissues
- Malignant is defined as a harmful tumor, capable of spread and invasion of other tissues far removed from the site of origin.

In addition, some other important terms used in cancer are:

- Anaplastic refers to those tumor cells that are completely undifferentiated and bear no resemblance to cells of tissues of their origin
- Hyperplasia refers to an increase in the number of normal cells in a normal arrangement in a tissue or organ, usually leads to an increase in the size or part and an increase in functional activity
- Metaplasia refers to the replacement of one type of fully differentiated cell by another fully differentiated cell in another part of the body where the second cell type does not normally occur
- Dysplasia refers to an alteration in the size, shape, and organization of differentiated cells; cells lose their regularity and show variability in size and shape, usually in response to an irritant; cells may revert to normal when the irritant is removed, but may transform to neoplasia
- Metastasis refers to the ability of neoplastic cells to spread from the original site of the tumor to distant organs, spreading as the same cell type as the original neoplastic tissue
- Carcinoma refers to a form of cancer that is composed of epithelial cells that tend to infiltrate surrounding tissues and may eventually spread to distant sites
- Oncogenes refer to cancer genes that are altered versions of normal genes
- Proto-oncogenes refer to repressed oncogenes existing in normal which can be activated by many different factors and cause the host cell to become malignant
- Tumor refers to usually synonymous with neoplasm.

PATHOPHYSIOLOGY OF CANCER

Cancer is a disease process that begins when an abnormal cell is transformed by the genetic mutation of the cellular DNA.

The exact cause and method of the development of cancer are unknown. Cancer is a group of many diseases of multiple causes that can arise in any cell of the body capable of evading regulatory control over proliferations and differentiation. The two major dysfunctions present in the process of cancer of "defective cellular proliferation (growth)" and "defective cellular differentiation".

The mutant cell forms a clone and begins to proliferate abnormally, ignoring growth-regulating signals in the environment surrounding the cell. The cells acquire invasive characteristics, and changes occur in surrounding tissues. The cells infiltrate these tissues and gain access to lymph and blood vessels, which carry the cells to other areas of the body. This phenomenon is called metastasis (cancer spread to other parts of the body).

Cancer cells are described as malignant neoplasms and are classified and named by tissue of origin. The failure of the immune system to promptly destroy abnormal cells permits these cells to grow too large to be managed by normal immune mechanisms. Certain categories of agents of factors implicated in carcinogenesis (malignant transformation) include viruses, physical agents, chemical agents, genetic or familial factors, dietary factors, and hormonal agents.

Cancer is one of the second leading cause of death, with most cancers occurring in men and in people older than age 65. Cancer also has a higher incidence in industrialized sectors and nations.

Defective Cellular Proliferation

Cancer cells usually proliferate in the manner and at the same rate of the normal cells of the tissue from which they arise. However, cancer cells respond differently than normal cells to the intracellular signals that regulate the state of dynamic equilibrium. Cancer cells divide indiscriminately and haphazardly. Sometime, they produce more than two cells at the time of mitosis. The loss of intracellular control of proliferations may be result of a mutation of the stem cells. The stem cells are viewed as the target or the origin of cancer developed. The DNA of the stem cell is substituted or permanently rearranged. When this happens the stem cell is mutuated and has the potential to become malignant. It will usually proliferate at the rate of the tissue origin, and some subpopulation can promote tumor progression to generate malignant cells. The malignant cells can differentiate to form normal tissue cells (Table 8.1).

Defective Cellular Differentiation

Cellular differentiation is normally and orderly a process that progresses from a state of immaturity to a state of maturity. Because all body cells are derived from the fertilized ova, all cells have the potential to perform all body functions. As cell differentiates, this potential is repressed and the mature cell is capable of performing only specific functions. Genes that are important regulators of these normal cellular processes are the "cellular oncogenes or proto-oncogenes. Mutations that alter the expression of genes or their products can activate proto-oncogenes to function as 'oncogenes' (tumor-inducing genes) by inducing mitosis but inhibiting differentiation of the cell.

The proto-oncogene has been described as the genetic lock that keeps the cell in its mature functioning state. When this lock is 'unlocked' it may occur through exposure to carcinogens or

TABLE 8.1: Characteristics of normal and malignant cells

Normal cells	Malignant cells
A. Mitotic cell division – Mitotic cell division leads to two daughter cells	– Mitosis leads to multiple cell that may or may not resemble the parent, multiple mitotic spindles
B. Appearance – Cells of same type homogeneous in size, shape – Cells cohesive, form regugular – Uniform size to nucleus – Have characteristics pattern of organization – Mixture of stem cells (precursors) and well-differentiated cells	– Cells larger and grow more rapidly than normal, i.e. pleomorphic and heterogeneous growth heterogeneous in size and shape – Cells not as cohesive, irregular pattern or expansion – Larger, more prominent nucleus – Lack of characteristic pattern of organization of host cell – Anaplastic, lack of differentiated cell characteristic, specific functions
C. Growth pattern – Do not invade adjacent tissue – Proliferate in response to specific stimuli – Growth in ideal conditions (e.g. nutrients, oxygen, space, correct biochemical environments) – Exhibit contact inhibition – Cell birth equals or in less than cell death – Stable cell membrane – Constant and predictable cell growth rate – Cannot grow outside specific environment, e.g. breast or lymphatics or seed to distant sites and grow in other sites	– Invade adjacent tissues – Proliferate in response to abnormal stimuli – Growth in adverse conditions such as lack of nutrients – Do not exhibit contact inhibition – Cell birth exceeds cell death – Loss of cell control as a result of cell membrane charges – Erratic cell growth rate – Able to break off cells that migrate through blood stream cell growth and only in breast
D. Function – Have specific and designated purpose – Contribute to the overall being of the host, parasitic – Cells function in specific pre-determined manner (e.g. cells in thyroid secrete thyroxine)	– Serve no useful purpose – Do not contribute to the well-being of the host – If cells function at all, do not function normally or they may actually cause damage (e.g. malignant lung cancer cells secrete ACTH, causing excessive stimulated...cortex)
E. Others – Develop specific antigens, characteristic of particular cell formed – Chromosomes remain constant throughout cell division – Complex metabolic and enzyme pattern – Cannot invade, erode or spread – Cannot grow in the cells and inflammation	– Develop antigens completely different from normal cell – Chromosomal aberrations occur as cell matures – Have more primitive and simplified metabolic and enzyme pattern – Invade, erode and spread – Grow in presence of necrosis presence of necrosis or inflammation – Exhibit periods of latency that vary from tumor to tumor – Have own blood supply and supporting stroma

oncogenic viruses, genetic alterations and mutations occur. The abilities and properties that the cell had in fetal development are again expressed. Although oncogens and oncogenic products, contribute to normal cell function, oncogenes intefere with normal cell expression under some conditions, causing cell to become malignant. The comparison of the characteristics of normal and malignant cells (Table 8.1) are as follows:

The cause and development of each type of cancer are likely to be multifactorial. It is not known how many tumors have chemical, environmental, genetic, immunologic, or viral origin. It is common belief that the development of cancer is rapid, haphazard event. Although scientists have learned a great deal about the causes of cancer, the exact mechanism by which these agents transform healthy cells into neoplastic cells remains obscure. One accepted perception is that cancer develops as a result of genetic alteration from one or more causes, resulting in uncontrolled cellular reproduction and growth. When a defective cell divides, the new cells contain defective genetic code within the DNA. Overtime defective cells divide and multiply and the malignancy grows.

Carcinogens are substances that when introduced into the cell cause changes in the structure and function of the cells that lead to cancer. It is not a simple cause and effect mechanism. However, the natural history of cancer is an orderly process causing several stages and occurring over a period of time. There are three identified stages of carcinogenesis, i.e. initiation, promotion and progression.

Initiation

The first stage, initiation, is an irreversible alteration in the cells' genetic structure resulting from the action of a chemical, physical or biologic agent. This altered cell has the potential for developing into a clone of neoplastic cells. Most carcinogens (see etiology) are detoxified by protective a enzymes and are harmlessly excreted. If this protective mechanism fails, carcinogens enter the cells' nucleus and may irreversibly bind to DNA. DNA repair is possible. However, if repair does not occur before all divisions, the cell will replicate into daughter cells, each with the same genetic alterations. After this damage of DNA cells are more susceptible to progression into malignancies. Irreversibly initiated cells do not display their changes and are not detectable until exposed to a promoting agent.

Promotion

Promotion is usually the result of a second factor acting on the initiated cell. A single alteration of the genetic structure of the cell is not sufficient to result in cancer. At least one or more mutation must occur in cells in which a mutation already occurred. The chances of this occurring, given the billions of cells in the human body, seem highly unlikely. However, the odds of cancer development are increased with the presence of promoting agents.

Promotion—the second stage in the development of cancer is characterized by the reversible proliferation of the altered initiated cells and consequently, with an increase in the initiated cell population likelihood of second cell mutation is increased. Some agents are called complete carcinogens because they produce both initiation and promotion. However, promotion may occur after very long periods of latency, which varies with the type of agent, dose, and characteristics of the target cell. Promoting agents work by changing the expression of genetic information within the cell, increasing DNA synthesis, increasing the number of copies of a particular gene, and altering cellular communication. Often exposure to the promoting agent is under the control of the client as with the tobacco, alcohol and dietary.

An important distinction between initiation and promotion is that the activity of promoters is reversible. This is a key concept in cancer prevention. Promoting factors include such agent as dietary fat, obesity, cigarette smoking, and alcohol consumption. Prolonged stress may also be a promoter. The withdrawal of these factors can reduce the risk of neoplastic formation.

Progression

Progression is the final stage in the nature/history of a cancer; it involves the morphologic and phenotypic changes in cells, which are associated with increasingly malignant behavior leading to invasion of surrounding tissue and metastasis to distant body parts. In other words, this stage is characterized by increased growth rate of the tumor, as well as by increased invasiveness and metastasis.

Metastasis can occur via the vascular system, lymphatic system and the process of implantations. Metastasis via the vascular system occurs in a variety of ways, which includes:

- Proliferating cancer cells in draining lymph nodes may enter a large collecting lymph vessel, such as thoracic duct, that empties into the larger veins leading to the heart
- Surrounding tissue may be invaded from the primary site of the cancer cells. The cancer cells penetrate the blood vessels and are released into bloodstream
- Cancer cells aggregates are trapped in the small capillaries of the tissues and organs
- Through the segregation of proteolytic enzymes, cancer cells penetrate the walls of the capillary and enter the adjacent tissue where they begin to proliferate.

The lymphatic spread occurs in a manner similar to vascular spaces in the body, conducting particles and fluid into lymph nodes. Cancer cells that break free from tissue or invade a lymph vessel almost always become trapped in the meshwork in the draining lymph node. If these cancer cells proliferate, the result is lymphadenopathy. Continued proliferation may result in the release of cancer cells into the lymph vessels leading from the lymph node to the next lymph node up the chain.

Implantation may occur when cancer cells become embedded along the serosal surfaces of body organs, such as the peritoneal cavity or the pleural cavity. During the surgical procedure, implantations may also occur in the primary organ or in the regional area if the environment is suitable.

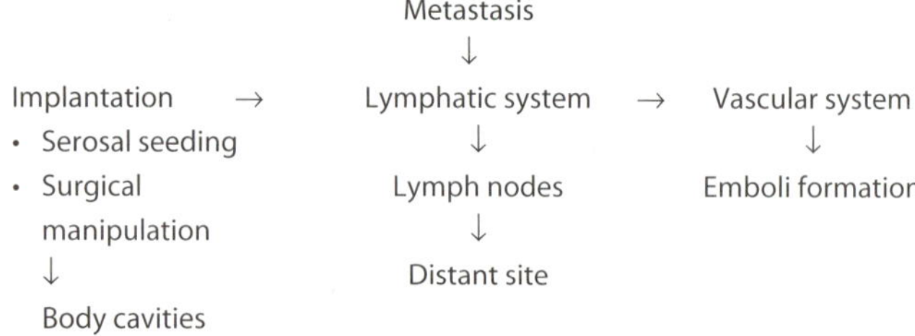

ETIOLOGY OF CANCER

There are approximately 150 types of cancers found in human beings and there are probably at least 500 different cancer-causing agents. Some of the causes on the basis of several studies are as follows:

Viruses

The study of viruses in tumors has lead investigators to discover oncogenes. Oncogenes are small segments of genetic DNA that can transform normal cells into malignant cells, independently or incorporated into a virus. Viruses probably do not, as a single agent cause cancer. However, viruses may be one of multiple agents acting to initiate carcinogenesis. Certain DNA and RNA viruses termed 'oncogenic' can transform the cells they infect and induce malignant transformations. It has been found that viruses have been associated with hepato-cellular carcinoma (hepatitis G Virus) T-cell lymphoma, T-cell leukemia, Burkitt's lymphoma (Epstein-Barr virus), nasopharyngeal carcinoma and cervical cancer.

Chemical Carcinogens

The chemical carcinogens thought to cause cancer in human beings due to close and prolonged contact and persons who are affected usually are workers in industries where these chemicals are used as by-products. The chemical carcinogens and associated neoplasm are as follows (Box 8.1).

Physical Carcinogens

Physical carcinogens cause cellular damage just as chemical carcinogens. The classification of physical carcinogen exists:

- Ionizing radiation
- Ultraviolet radiation, and
- Foreign bodies.

Excessive exposure to ionizing radiation can cause permanent DNA mutation and transformation into a malignant growth. Most radiation from natural resources (radon, cosmic, terrestrial and internal radiation). Certain malignants have been correlated with radiation as carcinogenic agents are leukemia, lymphonce, thyroid cancer, childhood cancer (if exposed) bone cancer (exposed persons include radiologists, radiation chemises, uranium miners).

Ultraviolet radiation from the sun can cause changes in DNA structure that can lead to malignant transformation if it is not repaired. Basal and squamous cell carcinomas of the skin as well as melanoma are linked to ultraviolet exposure.

Foreign bodies that are not biodegradable, such as asbestos fibers and bakelite disk and cellophane implants can induce the development of cancer by stimulating reactions to constant tissue damage such as scar formations, thus increasing the probability of neoplastic formations.

Drugs and Hormones

Certain drugs and hormones have also been identified as carcinogens (Box 8.2). Drugs that are capable of interacting with DNA (e.g. alkylating agents) as immunosuppressive agents, have the potential cause neoplasm in human beings. In addition, certain hormones administered to women has also been linked to the development of cancer. Certain cancers related to drug and hormone exposure in human beings are listed in Box 8.2.

Box 8.1 Chemical carcinogens and affecting organ

Carcinogen	Affecting organ
• Cigarette smoking	Lungs, upper respiratory tract, bladder, cervix, etc.
• Asbestos	Mesothelioma, lung
• Acrylonitrile	Lung, colon, prostate
• Arsenic	Skin, lung, liver
• Benzene	Leukemia
• Cadmium	Prostate, kidney
• Chromium compound	Lung
• Nickel	Lung, nasal sinuses
• Uranium	Lung
• Aflatoxin	Liver
• Nitrates	Stomach
• Chloromethyl ethers	Lung
• Isopropyl oil	Nasal sinuses
• Benzidene	Bladder
• Vinyl chloride	Angiosarcoma of liver
• Radiation	Numerous locations
• Polycyclic hydrocarbons	Lung, skin
• Mustard gas	Lung

Box 8.2 Carcinogen drugs and associated cancer

Carcinogen	Affecting organ
a. *Radioisotopes*	
– Phosphorus (^{32}p)	Acute leukemia
– Radium, mesothorium	Osteosarcoma, sinus carcinoma
– Thorotrast	Hemangioendothelioma of liver
b. *Immunosuppressive agent*	
– Antilymphocyte serum	Reticulum-cell sarcoma,
– Antimetabolites	epithelial cancer of skin and
– Alkylating agents	viscera, acute myelogenous
– Corticosteroids	leukemia
c. *Cytotoxic drugs*	Bladder cancer
– Phenylalanine mustard	Acute myelogenous leukemia
– Cyclophosphamide	
d. *Hormones*	
– Synthetic estrogen-prenatal	Vaginal and cervical
– Synthetic estrogen-	Endometrial carcinoma postnatal (adenosquamous type)
– Androgenic-anabolic steroids	Hepatocellular carcinoma
– Diethylstilbestrol (DES)	Vaginal cancer
e. *Others*	
– Arsenic	Skin, liver cancer
– Phenacetin containing drug	Renal pelvis carcinoma
– Coal tar ointments	Skin cancer
– Diphenyl hydantoin	Skin cancer
– Chloramphenicol	Leukemia
– Amphetamine	Hodgkin's disease

In addition to the carcinogen described above, there are also certain predisposing factors that influence the host susceptibility to various etiologic agents.

i. *Age:* There is an increasing incidence of cancer in the young and in persons more than 55 years of age. Many cancers such as prostate, and colon cancer and some chronic leukemia occur in older people. Testicular cancer is found in men between 20 and 40 years of age. Ovarian cancer is most common in women over 55 years of age. Many cancers occur mainly in childhood, e.g. Ewing's sarcoma, certain acute leukemias, Wilms' tumor and retinoblastoma.

ii. *Sex:* Women are most susceptible to certain types of cancer than men, i.e. cancer cervix, cancer breast, etc.

iii. *Occupation:* People in certain occupations are more susceptible to certain cancers because of their greater contact with specific carcinogens. For example, industrial workers, who expose to certain physical and chemical carcinogens.

iv. *Heredity:* Actually, none of the specific types of cancer are considered heredity. But there are a number of cancers that provide evidence of inheritable predisposed... to cancer. Fanconi anemia, telangiectasia, and xeroderma pigmentosum are examples of autosomal recessive conditions that predisposes persons to a variety of malignancies. Familial polyposis, coli retinoblastoma, Wilms' tumor, and neurofibromatosis are examples of autosomal dominant disorders that follow classic Mendelian patterns of inheritance. Breast, overian and colon cancers may also show a familial pattern.

v. *Diet and nutrition:* A diet high in fat may be a factor in the development of breast, colon and prostate cancer. Excessive alcohol, especially when accompanied by cigarette smoking, increases the risk of cancers of mouth larynx, throat, esophagus and stomach has been noted as area of world where salt-cured smoked, and nitrate cured goods are eaten frequently. People who have more weight have an increased risk of colon breas prostate, gallbladder, ovary and uterine cancer.

   Studies have shown that daily consumptions of vegetables and fresh fruits is associated with decreased risk of lung, prostate bladder, esophagus, colorectal, and stomach cancers. High fiber diet may reduce the risk of colon cancer.

vi. *Stress:* Studies suggest that stress may increase the risk of cancer. Chronic physical and emotional stress preys on the hypothalamus, the portion of the pituitary gland that regulates hormone and immune systems. Increased stress causes hormonal and immunologic changes or both, which may in turn may spur the growth and proliferation of cancer cells.

vii. *Precancerous lesions:* Common precancerous lesions include pigmented moles, burn scars, senile keratoses, leukoplakia, and benign adenomas or polyps of the colon or stomach. These lesions need to be periodically assessed for malignant changes.

Clinical Manifestations

- Cancerous cells spread from one organ or body part to another by invasion and metastasis; therefore, manifestations are related to the system affected and degree of disruption (see the specific type of cancer)
- Generally, cancer causes anemia, weakness, weight loss (dysphagia, anorexia, blockage), and pain (often in late stages)
- Symptoms are from tissue destruction and replacement with non-functional cancer tissue or overproductive cancer tissue (e.g. bone marrow disruption and anemia or excess adrenal steroid production); pressure on surrounding structures; increased metabolic demands; and distruption of production of blood cells.

CLASSIFICATION OF CANCER

Neoplastic tumors classified according to behavior of tumor (benign or malignant) anatomic site, histologic analysis (grading) and extent of disease (staging). This classification systems are intended to provide a standardized way:

- To communicate the status of cancer to all members of health team
- To assist in determining the most effective treatment plan
- To serve as a factor in determining the prognosis, and
- To compare like groups for statistical purposes.

Benign and Malignant

Tumors can be classified on the basis of behavior as benign or malignant. In general, benign neoplasm, are well differentiated and malignant neoplasms range from well-differentiated to undifferentiated. The differences between benign and malignant tumors on the basis of their characteristics given in Box 8.3.

Anatomic Site Classification

In the anatomic classifications of tumors, the tumor is identified by the tissue origin, the anatomic site and the behavior of the tumor, i.e. benign or malignant. Carcinoma originates from embryonical ectoderm (skin and glands) and endoderm (mucous membrane linings of the respiratory tract, GI tract and genitourinary tract). Sarcoma originates from embryonal mesoderm (connective tissue, muscle, bone and fat).

Box 8.3 Differences between benign and malignant tumor

Benign tumor	Malignant tumor
a. Speed of growth:	
• They grow slowly usually continue to grow throughout life unless surgically removed; may have periods of remission	• They usually grow rapidly, tend to grow relentlessly through life, rarely, neoplasm regress spontaneously
b. Mode of growth:	
• Growth by enlarging and expanding, always remaining localized, never infiltrates surrounding tissues	• Grows by infiltrating surrounding tissues; may remain localized (in situ) but usually infiltrates other tissues
c. Cell characteristics:	
• Usually well-differentiated; mitotic figure absent or scanty mature cells; an aplastic cells absent, cell function poorer in comparison with normal cells from which they arise, if neoplasm arises in glandular tissue, cell may secrete hormones	• Usually poorly differentiated large number of normal and abnormal mitotic figures present, cells tend to be anaplastic, i.e. young embryonic type; cells too abnormal to perform any physiologic functions; occasionally a malignant tumor arising in glandular tissue secretes hormones
d. Recurrence:	
• Recurrence extremely unusual when surgically removed	• Recurrence common following surgery because tumor cells spread into surrounding tissues
e. Metastasis:	
• Metastasis never occurs	• Metastasis very common
f. Effect of neoplasm:	
• Not harmful to host unless located in area where it causes compression of tissues or obstruction of vital organs, does not produce cachexia (weight loss, debilitation, anemia, weakness, wasting)	• Always harmful to host. Results in death unless removed surgically or destroyed by radiation or chemotherapy, causes disfigurement, disrupted organ function, nutritional imbalance may result in ulceration, sepsis, perforations, hemorrhage, tissue slough, almost always produces cachexia which leaves person prone to pneumonia anemia, etc.
g. Prognosis:	
• Prognosis is very good speed of diagnosis, poor are poorly differentiated and spread exists; good prognosis indicated when cells still resemble normal cells and there is no evidence of metastasis	• Depends on cell type and tumor generally removed surgically prognosis indicated if cells evidence of metastatic

Symphomas and leukemias originate from the hematopoietic system. The classification of tumor by tissue origin is given in Box 8.4.

Histologic Analytic Classification

The histologic grading of tumors, the appearance of the cells and the degree of differentiation are evaluated. For many tumors, four grades are used.

Grading refers to the classification of the tumor cells. Grading systems seek to define the type of tissue from which the tumor originated and the degree to which the tumor cells retain the functional and histologic characteristics of the tissue of origin (differentiation). Samples of cells used to establish the grade of a tumor may be obtained from tissue scrapings, body fluids, secretions, or washing, biopsy, or surgical excision. This information helps the health care team predict the behavior and prognosis of various tumors. The tumor is assigned a numeric value ranging from I to IV. Grade I tumors, also known as well-differentiated tumors, closely resemble the tissue of origin in structure and function. Tumors that do not clearly resemble the tissue of origin in structure or function are described as poorly differentiated or undifferentiated and are assigned grade IV. These tumors tend to be more aggressive and less responsive to treatment than well-differentiated tumors.

Grade I: Cells differ slightly from normal cells (mils displasia) and are well differentiated.

Grade II: Cells are more abnormal (moderate displasia) and moderately differentiated.

Grade III: Cells are very abnormal (severe dysplasia) and poorly differentiated.

Grade IV: Cells are immature and primitive (anaplasia) and undifferentiated, cell of origin difficult to determine.

Extent of Disease Classification

Staging

Tumors are staged depending on size, lymph node involvement, and metastasis. Staging is also expressed in TNM symbols; T indicated primary tumor; N, lymph node involvement; and M, metastasis (Box 8.5).

Box 8.4 Classification of tumor by tissue origin

Tissue origin	Benign	Malignant
a. Connective tissue		
• Embryonic	...	Sarcoma
fibrous tissue	Myxoma	Myxosarcoma
• Fibrous tissue	Fibroma	Fibrosarcoma
• Adipose tissue	Lipoma	Liposarcoma
• Cartilage	Chondroma	Chondrosarcoma
• Bone	Osteoma	Osteogenic sarcoma
b. Epithelium tissue		
• Skin and mucous	...	Carcinoma
membrane	Papilloma	Squamous cell carcinoma
• Glands	...	Basal cell carcinoma
	...	Transitional cell carcinoma
	Adenoma	Adenocarcinoma
	Cystadenoma	Cystadenocarcinoma
• Pigmented cells (melanocytes)	Nevus	Malignant melanoma
c. Endothelium		
	...	Endothelioma
• Blood vessels	Hemangioma	Hemangioendothelioma
		Hemangiosarcoma
		Kaposi's sarcoma
• Lymph vessels	Lymphangioma	Lymphangiosarcoma
		Lymphangioendothelioma
• Bone marrow	...	Multiple myeloma
		Ewing's sarcoma
		Leukemia
• Lymphoid tissue		Malignant lymphoma
		Lymphosarcoma
		Reticulum cell sarcoma
d. Muscles tissue		
• Smooth muscle	Leiomyoma	Leiomyosarcoma
• Straited muscle	Rhabdomyoma	Rhabdomyosarcoma
e. Nerve tissue		
• Nerve fibers and	Neuroma	Neurogenic sarcoma
sheath	Neurinoma	
	Neurofibroma	Neurofibrosarcoma
• Ganglion cells	Ganglioneuroma	Neuroblastoma
• Glial cells	Glioma	Glioblastoma
• Meninges	Meningioma	Malignant meningioma
f. Gonads	Dermoid cyst	Embryonal carcinoma
		Embryonal sarcoma
		Terato carcinoma

Stage I: Tumor less than 2 cm, negative lymph node involvement, no detectable metastases.

Stage II: Tumor greater than 2 cm but less than 5 cm, negative or positive unfixed lymph node involvement, no detectable metastases.

Stage III: Large tumor greater than 5 cm, or a tumor of any size with invasion of the skin or chest wall or positive fixed lymph node involvement in the clavicular area without evidence of metastases.

Stage IV: Tumor of any size, positive or negative lymph node involvement, and distant metastases.

Box 8.5 TNM staging classification system

Tumor	
T0	No evidence of primary tumor
TS	Carcinoma in situ
T1, T2, T3, T4	Ascending degrees of tumor size and involvement
Nodes	
N0	No evidence of disease in lymph node
N1a, N2a	Disease found in regional lymph nodes, metastasis not suspected
NX	Regional lymph nodes cannot be assessed clinically
Metastasis	
M0	No evidence of distant metastasis
M1, M2, M3	Ascending degrees of metastatic involvement of the host, including distant nodes

The extent of disease classification is often called 'staging'. The clinical staging classification determines the extent of the disease process of cancer by stages:

Stage '0': Cancer in situ. It is defined as a neoplasm of epithelial tissue that remains confined to the site of origin.

Stage I: Tumor linked to the tissue of origin, localized tumor growth.

Stage II: Limited local spread.

Stage III: Extensive local and regional spread.

Stage IV: Metastasis.

This type of classification is used as a basis for staging in cancer of cervix and Hodgkin's disease.

The TNM classification system represents the standardization of the clinical staging of cancer. It is used to determine the extent of disease process of cancer according to three parameters. Tumor size (T), degree of regional spread to the lymph nodes (N) and presence of metastasis (M). TNM system has been used in cancer of breast (Box 8.6).

Prevention of Cancer

The nurse plays a prominent role in all the levels of prevention of cancer. Cancer nursing is directed towards the prevention and early detection of neoplasm as well as the care of the patient in treatment, recovery or advanced stage of cancer. At present, it is not possible to prevent all types of cancer, but some cancers can be prevented by avoidance of recognized carcinogens and by altering health behaviors.

Primary Prevention

Primary prevention of cancer is activity taken to prevent the occurrence or reduce the risk of cancer in healthy persons. Activities in this area of health promotion include identifying

Box 8.6 TNM classification system

T The extent of the primary tumor
N The absence or presence and extent of regional lymph node metastasis
M The absence or presence of distant metastasis
The use of numerical subsets of the TNM components indicates the progressive extent of the malignant disease

Primary tumor (T)
Tx Primary tumor cannot be assessed
T0 No evidence of primary tumor
Tis Carcinoma in situ
T1, T2, T3, T4 increasing size and/or local extent of the primary tumor

Regional lymph nodes (N)
Nx Regional lymph nodes cannot be assessed
N0 No regional lymph node metastasis
N1, N2, N3 Increasing involvement of regional lymph nodes

Distant metastasis (M)
Mx Distant metastasis cannot be assessed
M0 No distant metastasis
M1 Distant metastasis

risk factors, reduction and cancer prevention programs. For example, the dietary changes to reduce cancer which include:

a. Increased intake of high-fiber foods such as fruits and vegetables and whole grain cereals. Dark green and deep yellow fruits and vegetable rich in vitamin A and C (cabbage, broccoli, cauliflower, Brussels sprouts, and kohlrabi).
b. Reduced intake of salt-cured, smoked and nitrite-cured foods, fats and oils especially from animal sources; alcoholic beverages and excess calories leading to obesity.

So, one important aspect of the nurse and other health care provider is to educate the public to do the following:

- Reduce or avoid exposure to known or suspected carcinogens and cancer-promoting agents
- Eat balanced diet that includes vegetables (green, yellow and orange), fresh fruits, whole grains, adequate amount of fiber, and low level of facts and preservatives
- Participate in regular exercise regimens
- Obtain adequate, consistent, periods of rest (at least 6 to 8 hours per night)
- Have a health examination on consistent basis that includes health history physical examination and specific diagnostic tests for common cancers, i.e. lung cancer, colon and rectal cancer, prostate cancer, cervical cancer and breast cancer, etc.
- Eliminate, reduce or change the perceptions of stressors and enhance the ability to positively cope with stressors
- Enjoy consistent periods of relaxation and leisure
- Know the seven warning signals of cancer, which include "CAUTION" as follows:
  1. **C**hange in bowel or bladder habits
  2. **A** sore that does not heal
  3. **U**nusual bleeding or discharge
  4. **T**hickening or lump in the breast or elsewhere
  5. **I**ndigestion or difficulty in swallowing
  6. **O**bvious change in a wart or more
  7. **N**agging cough or hoarseness.
- Learn and practice self-examination of breast and testicles
- Seek immediate medical care if cancer is suspected.

In some occupations, the employees may have contact with carcinogenic substances such as asbestos, chromium, ether, vinyl chloride and benzyprene, etc. In such industries, proper regulation and protective measures can be taken accordingly to reduce the risk of cancer.

The nurses can have a definite impact in convincing people that a change in the lifestyle pattern will have a positive influence on health.

Secondary Prevention

Secondary prevention of cancer is focused on the early diagnosis of which early detection and screening are the major components. Screening and detection programs are concentrated on some of the most common cancers including cancers of the breast, cervix, colon/rectum, prostate, skin and oropharynx.

The screening for specific cancer sites which have high risk profile are as follows:

Lung: The risk of lung cancer can occur with a person of:

- History of 20 pack-years of smoking (1 pack a day for 20 years)
- Exposure to air-borne carcinogens especially asbestos, uranium, hydrocarbon
- Age range 40–80 years
- Chronic lung disease.

The method of screening for any such case will depend on the observation of patient for change in respiratory status, increased frequency of infections and change in cough, sputum, breathing, and voice. Some doctors advise annual chest X-rays.

Colon and rectum: The risk of colon and rectal cancer occurs with a person's:

- History of familial polyposis, ulcerative colitis, Crohn's disease
- Personal or family history of colon or rectal cancer
- Taking diet high in fat and low in fiber
- Age range 40–75 years.

The method of screening will be:

- Blood test on stools every year after age of 50 years
- Digital rectal examination annually after age of 40 years
- Sigmoidoscopic examination (preferably flexible) every 3–5 years after 50 years
- Observations by patients for change in bowel pattern, i.e. diarrhea, constipation, pain, flatus, black tarry stools, bleeding.

Prostate: The risk of prostatic cancer occurs with presence of prostatic hyperplasia and presence of prostatic infection. The methods of screening of such case will be:

- Digital rectal examination of age 40 years and annually thereafter
- Prostate specific antigens blood test every year
- Observation on men aged 50 and older, for dysuria, blood in urine, difficulty in producing stream of urine.

Cervix: The risk of cervical cancer occurs with a person:

- Who has a history of early intercourse (before the age of 20 years) with multiple partners
- Who maintains poor personal hygiene including poor menstrual hygiene
- Who has history of herpes virus type II infections and cervical dysplasia.

For such cases screening measures will include:

- Pap test and pelvic examination every year for those who are or have been sexually active or who have attained the age of 18 years
- Calposcopy if suspicious area is noted
- Observation by patient for abnormal vaginal bleeding or discharge, pain, or bleeding with sexual intercourse.

Endometrium: The risk of endometrial cancer occurs with a person's having infertility, ovarian dysfunction, obesity, uterine bleeding, estrogen therapy over long period of time, diabetes and age range 30–80 years.

By such cases, screening measures will include:

- Pap test every year
- Pelvic examination every year
- Endometrial biopsy every year for women of menopause and
- Observation by patient for abnormal uterine bleeding, pain, change in menstrual pattern.

Skin: The risk of skin cancer occurs with person, having prolonged exposure to sun, and previous radiation exposure; fair, thin skin and positive family history of dysplasia nevus syndrome.

For such cases, screening measures include, self examination monthly with suspicious lesions evaluated promptly, physical examination every year, and observation by patient for sore that does not heal, change in wart or mole.

Breast: The risk of breast cancer occurs with persons who are caucasian, who has early menarche, late menopause, fibrocystic disease, and infertility, more than age of 30 years for first pregnancy, and who has a personal history of breast cancer mother or sister with history of breast cancer, obesity, and whose age range is 35–65 years.

The screening measure will be:

- Monthly breast self-examination
- Breast examination by health professional every 3 years for women aged 20–40 and every year after the age of 40
- Baseline mammogram of age 40 and every 1–2 years between ages 40–49 and every year after the age of 50
- Observation by patient for lungs or thickening discharge from nipple, pain in the breast.

In order to assume the expected role in cancer prevention and early detection programs, the nurse must keep informed about the trends in the incidence of cancer and advances being made. If the nurse is to have a significant impact, the challenge needs to be recognized and strategies must be developed to teach cancer control effectively.

To sum up, the early detection of cancer in asymptomatic population according to American Society Guidelines (1995) are as follows:

1. *Chest X-ray:* It is no longer recommended for smokers to screen for lung cancer, but can be done.
2. *Sputum cytology:* -do-
3. *Physical examination:* For both male and females, after the age of 40 years, yearly including examination of skin, lymph nodes, mouth, thyroid, breast, testes, rectum and prostate.
4. *Health teaching:* For both male and females, who attained the age of 20 years. It has to be done every 3 years to teach about proper diet, exercise, healthy habits, breast and testicular self-examinations, avoidance of sunlight, and smoking cessation.
5. *Breast self examination:* For females who have attained menarchy or 20 years and above, every month after menses before menopause; after menopause, monthly on any specified day such as the first or last of the month.
6. *Mammography:* For women who are between 35 and 40 years of age, baseline mammogram; between 40 and 49 years mammogram should be done every 1–2 years and yearly after 50 years; high risk women should check with their physicians.
7. *Pap smear:* For females who are above 18 years of age, and sexually active women should have pap smears regardless of age, should be performed yearly until there are three negative examinations in a row; at this point, they can be performed yearly or as physician advises.
8. *Pelvic examination:* For females who are between 20–40 and 40 and above, every 3 years, earlier if sexually active, yearly after 40 years.
9. *Endometrial tissue sample:* For female at menopause, high-risk women (obese, abnormal uterine bleeding, estrogen therapy, history of infertility, diabetes, hypertension, failure to ovulate) should have this test performed at menopause.
10. *Testicular self-examination:* For males, monthly, on a set date such as the first of the month following a shower.
11. *Breast physical examination:* For females every 3 years for those who are between 20 and 39 years and annually for those who are above 40.

12. *Digital rectal examination:* For both male and females who are above 40, annually rectal cancer and prostate in men.
13. *Fecal occult blood:* For both males and females those who are above 20 years, done on advice of physician.
14. *Proctoscopy, flexible sigmoidoscopy:* For both men and women who are above 50 years every 3–5 years.

DIAGNOSIS OF CANCER

A diagnostic plan for the person in whom cancer is suspected, includes health history, identification of risk factors, physical examination and specific diagnostic studies.

Screening to detect early cancer usually focuses on cancers with the highest incidence or those that have improved survival rates if diagnosed early. Examples of these cancers include breast, colorectal, cervical, endometrial, testicular, skin and oropharyngeal cancers. Patients with suspected cancer undergo extensive testing for the following reasons:

- To determine the presence of tumor and its extent
- To identify possible spread (metastasis) of disease or invasion of other body tissues
- To evaluate the function of involved and uninvolved body systems and organs
- To obtain tissue and cells for analysis, including tumor stage (tumor size, degree of metastasis, and grade [classification, e.g. TNM stage])

Diagnostic tests may include imaging (magnetic resonance imaging [MRI], computed tomography [CT] scan, endoscopy, fluoroscopy, positron emission tomography [PET] scan, radioimmunoconjugates, ultrasonography) and biopsy.

Laboratory Values

- Tumor marker identification may be beneficial for some cancers
- Complete blood count, electrolytes, hormone levels, liver enzyme studies, as well as other chemistry studies may help to identify secondary effects of tumor (e.g. anemia, neutropenia).

Health History

The health history includes particular emphasis on risk factors, such as family history of cancer, exposure to or use of known carcinogen (e.g. cigarette smoking and exposure to occupational pollutants or chemicals, disease characterised by chronic inflammation (e.g. ulceration colitis) and drug ingestions (e.g. hormone therapy). Other important information related to dietary habits, ingestion of alcohol, lifestyle and patterns and degree of coping with perceived stressors.

Physical Examination

The physical examination should be thorough and particular attention should be given to the respiratory system, the gastrointestinal systems, including colon, rectum, and liver, the lymphatic system (including spleen), the breast, the skin, the reproductive system of the male (testicles, prostate) and of the female (cervix, uterus, ovary and the musculoskeletal and neurologic systems).

When a malignant tumor is in the early stages, there are often few manifestations. Clinical manifestations usually appear once the tumor has grown to a sufficiently large size to cause one or more of the following problems:

- Pressure on surrounding organs or nerves
- Distortion of surrounding tissue
- Obstruction of lumen of tubes
- Interference with the blood supply of surrounding tissues
- Interference with the organ function
- Disturbance of body metabolism
- Parasitic use of the body's nutritional supplies
- Mobilization of the body's defensive responses, resulting in inflammatory changes.

Common clinical manifestations that may arise secondary to cancer include weight loss, weakness or fatigue, CNS alterations, pain and hematologic and metabolic alterations. Close assessment of such manifestations may reveal that they are directly or indirectly related to the tumor growth.

Anorexia, weight loss, weakness and fatigue are related to the body's inability to consume and use nutrients appropriately. Mechanical interference by tumors, malabsorption, paraneoplastic endocrine secretions (such as excessive secretions of thyroid hormone) and tumor, use of nutrient, may all contribute to a cycle that must be interrupted to avoid general physical debilitation.

Pain may occur as a result of obstruction or destruction of a vital organ, pressure on sensitive tissues or bone, or involvement of nerves. If it occurs and is not adequately treated, it may become constraint and progressively severe.

The client who has difficulty with vision, speech, co-ordination or memory may be experiencing primary or metastatic CNS disease. Increased intracranial pressure caused by tumor growth may cause headache, lethargy, nausea and vomiting.

Unexplained anemia often indicates a malignancy. Hematologic changes also include leukopenia, leukocytosis, and bleeding disorders, which in some diseases may occur before local manifestations. Metabolic manifestations also signify the possibility of malignant disease.

A localized tumor usually produces manifestations related to increased pressure or obstruction in a single region. Metastatic disease and extensive tumors of major organs may display a variety of local and systemic manifestations.

Diagnostic Studies

Diagnostic studies to be performed will depend on the suspected primary or metastatic site (s) of the cancer. The common diagnostic studies that may be included in the process of diagnosing cancer include the following:

- Cystologic examination, e.g. pap smear
- Basic X-ray studies for identifying the destructive tumors of the GI, respiratory and renal tracts
- Complete blood count
- Proctoscopic examination
- Liver function studies
- Radiographic studies, e.g. mammogram, (in breast cancer)
- Radioisotopic scans (for liver, brain, bone, lung cancer)
- Computed tomography (CT) scan
- Magnetic resonance imaging (MRI)
- Antigen skin testing (to know the presence of oncofetal antigens)
- Bone marrow examination
- Lymphangiography
- Biopsy (surgical excision of a small piece of tissue for microscopic examination, i.e. needle biopsy, incisional biopsy, excisional biopsy).

MANAGEMENT OF CANCER

Treatment options offered to cancer patients should be based on treatment goals for each specific type of cancer. The range of possible treatment goals may include complete eradication of malignant disease (cure), prolonged survival and containment of cancer cell growth (control), or relief of symptoms associated with the disease (palliation).

The health care team, the patient, and the patient's family must have a clear understanding of the treatment options and goals. Open communication and support are vital as the patient and family periodically reassess treatment plans and goals when complications of therapy develop or disease progresses.

Multiple modalities are commonly used in cancer treatment. A variety of approaches, including surgery, radiation therapy, chemotherapy, and targeted therapies, may be used at various times throughout treatment. Understanding the principles of each and how they interrelate is important in understanding the rational and goals treatment.

Treatment of Cancer

The range of possible treatment goals may include complete eradication of malignant disease (cure), prolonged survival and containment of cancer cell growth (control), or relief of symptoms associated with the disease (palliation).

- A variety of therapies may be used, including surgery (e.g. video-assisted endoscopic surgery, salvage surgery, electrosurgery, cryosurgery, chemosurgery, or laser surgery). Surgery could be for prophylactic, palliative, or reconstructive purposes. The goal of surgery is to remove the tumor as much as is feasible
- Radiation therapy and chemotherapy may be used individually or in combination.
- Biologic response modifier (BRM) therapy may be used at various times throughout treatment.

When caring for the patient with cancer, the nurse should know the goals of the treatment plan to appropriately communicate with and support the patient. The goal of cancer treatment is 'cure', 'control' or palliation.

The major objective of cancer therapy is to treat the client effectively with appropriate therapy for sufficient duration, so that cure results with minimal functional and structural impairment. When cure is the goal, it is expected that after treatment the patient will be free of disease and will have a normal life. Many kinds of cancer have the potential to go into permanent remission with an initial course of treatment or with treatment extending for several weeks, months or years (e.g. basal cell carcinoma of skin is usually cured by surgical removal of lesion or radiation therapy).

When cure is not possible, important alternative goals are:

i. To prevent metastasis
ii. To relieve manifestations, and
iii. To maintain a high quality of life for as long as possible.

Here, the control is the goal of the treatment plan for many cancers considered to be chronic. The patient undergoes the initial course of therapy and is contineud on maintenance therapy for a period of time or is followed closely so that early signs and symptoms of recurrence can be detected. These cancers are usually, not cured, but they are controlled by therapy for long periods of time (e.g. chronic lymphocytic leukemia).

Palliation can also be a goal of the cancer treatment plan. With this treatment, goal, relief of symptoms and the maintenance of a satisfactory quality of life are the primary objective rather than cure or control of the disease process. For example, radiatioan therapy given to relieve the pain of bone metastasis.

The goals of cure, control and palliation are achieved through the use of four treatment modalities for cancer, which includes;

1. Surgery
2. Radiation therapy
3. Chemotherapy
4. Biologic response modifiers.

SURGERY

Surgical removal of the entire cancer remains the ideal and most frequently used treatment method. However, the specific surgical approach may vary for several reasons. Diagnostic surgery is the definitive method of identifying the cellular characteristics that influence all treatment decision. Surgery may be the primary method of treatment, of it may be prophylactic, palliative, or reconstructive.

Surgery is the oldest form of cancer treatment and for many years it was the only effective method of cancer diagnosis and treatment. It is also an integral part of the rehabilitation and palliation of patients with cancer. The types of surgical procedures used in surgical management of cancer are as follows:

i. *Biopsy* is the surgical removal of a piece of tissue from the questionable area, and the tissue sample is sent to the pathology laboratory for diagnostic verification. The sample of tissues can be obtained through the needle biopsy or incisional biopsy or excisional biopsy.

 Diagnostic surgery, such as a biopsy, is usually performed to obtain a tissue sample for analysis of cells suspected to be malignant. In most instances, the biopsy is taken from the actual tumor, but in some situations, it is necessary to biopsy lymph nodes near the suspicious tumor. Many cancers can metastasize from the primary site to other areas of the body through the lymphatic circulation. Knowing whether adjacent lymph nodes contain tumor cells helps physicians plan for systemic therapies instead of or in addition to surgery or radiation, to combat tumor cells that have gone beyond the primary tumor site. The sue of injectable dyes and nuclear medicine imaging can help the surgeon identify the sentinel lymph node or the initial lymph node to which the primary tumor and surrounding tissue drains. Sentinel lymph node biopsy (SLNB), also known as sentinel lymph node mapping, is a minimally invasive surgical approach that in some instances has replaced more invasive lymph node dissections (lymphadenectomy) and their associated complications such as lymphedema and delayed healing. SLNB has been widely adopted for regional lymph node staging in selected cases of melanoma and breast cancer.

 Biopsy types

 The three most common biopsy methods are the excisional, incisional, and needle methods (Szopa, 2005). The choice of biopsy is determined by the size and location of the tumor, the type of treatment anticipated if the cancer diagnosis is confirmed, and the need for surgery and general anesthesia. The biopsy method that allows for the least invasive approach while permitting the most representative tissue sample is chosen. Occasionally, diagnostic imaging techniques are used to assist in locating the suspicious lesion and to facilitate accurate tissue sampling. The patient and family are given the opportunity and time to discuss the option before definitive plans are made. The nurse serves as the patient's advocate and liaison between the patient and physician to facilitate this process.

 Excisional biopsy is most frequently used for easily accessible tumors of the skin, breast, and upper or lower gastrointestinal and upper respiratory tracts. In many cases, the surgeon can remove the entire tumor as well as the surrounding marginal tissues. The removal of normal tissue beyond the tumor area decreases the possibility that residual microscopic disease cells may lead to a recurrence of the tumor. This approach not only provides the pathologist, who stages and grades the cells, with the entire tissue specimen but also decreases the chance of seeding the tumor (disseminating cancer cells throughout surrounding tissues).

 Incisional biopsy is performed if the tumor mass is too large to be removed. In this case, a wedge of tissue from the tumor is removed for analysis. The cells of the tissue wedge must be representative of the tumor mass so that the pathologist can provide an accurate diagnosis. If the specimen does not contain representative tissue and cells, negative biopsy results do not guarantee the absence of cancer.

 Excisional and incisional approaches are often performed through endoscopy. However, surgical incision may be required to determine the anatomic extent or stage of the tumor. For example, a diagnostic or staging laparotomy (the surgical opening of the abdomen to assess malignant abdominal disease) may be necessary to assess malignancies such as gastric cancer.

 Needle biopsies are performed to sample suspicious masses that are easily accessible, such as some growths in the breasts, thyroid, lung, liver, and kidney. Needle biopsies are most often performed on an outpatient basis. They are fast, relatively inexpensive, easy to perform, and usually require only local anesthesia. In general, the patient experiences slight and temporary physical discomfort. In addition, the surrounding tissues are disturbed only minimally, thus decreasing the likelihood of seeding cancer cells. Needle aspiration biopsy involves aspirating tissue fragments through a needle guided into an area suspected of bearing disease. Occasionally, X-ray, computed tomography (CT) scanning, ultrasonography, or magnetic resonance imaging (MRI) is used to help locate the suspicious area and guide the placement of the needle. In some instances, the aspiration biopsy does not yield enough tissue to permit accurate diagnosis. A needle core biopsy uses an especially designed needle to obtain a small core of tissue. Most often, this specimen is sufficient to permit accurate diagnosis.

ii. *Reconstruction/rehabilitative surgery:* Advances in reconstructive surgery offer a different perspective on rehabilitation to the patient who has experienced curative surgery. Here, performing the repair of defects from previous radical surgical resection, it can be performed early (as in head and neck surgery). Restoration of form and function is possible in varying degrees depending on the site and extent of surgery. Reconstructive surgery may be performed concurrently with the radical procedure or delayed for optimal outcome. The major goal of reconstructive surgery is to improve the patient's quality of life by restoring maximal function and appearance.

iii. *Palliative surgery* refers to a surgery that attempts to relieve the complications of cancer. Because of surgical procedures carry an inherent potential for morbidity, use of surgery in palliative care is carefully considered and used only if the risk-benefit ratio is favorable. Palliative surgery can benefit the clients with cancer and improve quality of life include the procedure than reduce pain; relieve airway obstruction, relieve obstructions in the GI and GU tract; relieve pressures on the brain and spinal cord; prevent hemorrhage remove infected and ulcerating tumors and drain abscess. Example of palliative surgical procedure are cordotomy, colostomy, laminectomy, etc.

iv. *Adjuvant surgery* refers to the use of various surgical techniques to facilitate the overall management. These procedures are used to provide supportive care throughout the disease process of cancer. These procedures include:
   - Insertion of feeding tubes in the esophagus or stomach
   - Creation of a colostomy to allow a rectal abscess to heal
   - Suprapubic cystotomy for the patient with advanced prostatic cancer
   - Vascular access devices
   - Radiotherapy implants
   - Peritoneal access
   - Ventricular access
   - Drainage of peritoneal or pleural effusions.

v. *Surgery for primary lesions* is the removal of the primary site of malignancy. The goal of therapy is cure. This depends on the biology of that particular cancer. For example, basal cell carcinoma of skin, early tumor of the rectum or colon.

vi. *Surgery for metastatic lesion* or resection of metastatis is used in selected case where a cure can be obtained or reasonable prolongation of survival is possible. The primary cancer must be under control. The decision to proceed is influenced by the type of histology, number of lesions, their locations and whether they are bilateral, solitary metastatic lesions that appear in the lungs, liver or brain can be removed to effect a surgical cure.

vii. *Preventive/prophylactic surgery* is the removal of lesion, that if left in the body are apt to develop into cancer. Certain conditions or diseases increase the risk of cancer occurrence so significantly that removal of the target organ is justified to prevent cancer development. For example, polyps in the rectum. Clients with high risk factors may consider prophylactic surgery (e.g. prophylactic mastectomy, or oophorectomy).

viii. *Curative surgery* is the removal of the primary site of malignancy and any lymph nodes to which the neoplasm has extended. Such surgery may be all that is required. For example, radical neck dissection, lumpectomy, mastectomy, pneumonectomy, orchiectomy, thyroidectomy and bowel resection.

ix. *Debulking surgery* is the removal of bulk of the tumor; should be performed before the start of chemotherapy whenever possible. This procedure may be used if the tumor cannot be completely removed (e.g. attached to a vital organ). This type of procedure makes the adjuvant therapy more effective.

Assisting in the Grieving Process

Nurses assess the patient's psychological and mental status as the patient and family face this life-threatening experience, unpleasant diagnostic tests and treatment modalities, and progression of disease. The nurse assesses the patient's mood and emotional reaction to the results of diagnostic testing and prognosis and looks for evidence that the patient is progressing through the stages of grief and can talk about the diagnosis and prognosis with family members.

A cancer diagnosis need not indicate a fatal outcome. Many forms of cancer are curable, while others may be cured or controlled for long periods of time if treated early. Despite these facts, many patients and their families view cancer as a fatal disease that is inevitable accompanied by pain, suffering, debilitation, and emaciation. Grieving is a normal response to these fears and actual or potential losses: loss of health, normal sensations, body image, social interaction, sexuality, and intimacy. Patients, families, and friends may grieve for the loss of quality time to spend with other, the loss of future and unfulfilled plans, and the loss of control over the patient's body and emotional reactions.

Patients and their families who have just been informed of a cancer diagnosis frequently respond with shock, numbness, and disbelief. It is often during this stage that patient and family are called on to make important initial decisions about treatment. They require the support of physicians, nurses, and all members of the health care team to make these decisions. The nurse plays an important role in answering any questions the patient and family have and clarifying information provided by physicians. The plan of nursing care addresses anticipatory grieving and nursing strategies for promoting appropriate progression through the grieving process.

If the patient enters the terminal phase of disease, the nurse may realize that the patient and family members are at different stage of grief. In such cases, the nurse helps the patient and family to acknowledge and cope with their reactions and feelings. The nurse also helps the patient and family to explore preferences for issues related to end-of-life care such as withdrawal of active disease treatment, desire for the use of life-support measures, and symptom management. Support, which can be as simple as holding a patient's hand or just being with a patient at home or at the bedside, often contributes to peace of mind. After the death of a patient with cancer, maintain contact with surviving family members may help them work through their feelings of loss and grief.

Nursing Management of Cancer Surgery

- Complete a thorough preoperative assessment for all factors that may affect patients undergoing surgery
- Assist patient and family in dealing with the possible changes and outcomes resulting from surgery; provide education and emotional support by assessing patient and family needs and exploring with them their fear and coping mechanisms. Encourage them to take an active role in decision making when possible
- Explain and clarify information the physician has provided about the results of diagnostic testing and surgical procedures, if asked
- Communicate frequently with the physician and other health care team members to ensure that the information provided is consistent
- After surgery, assess patient's responses to the surgery and monitor for complications such as infection, bleeding thrombophlebitis, wound dehiscence, fluid and electrolyte imbalance, and organ dysfunction
- Provide for patient comfort
- Provide postoperative teaching that addresses wound care, activity, nutrition and medications
- Initiate plans for discharge, follow-up care and treatment as early as possible to ensure continuity of care
- Encourage patient and family to use community resources for support and information.

RADIATION THERAPY

Radiation therapy (RT) is a local treatment modality for cancer. RT is the use of high energy ionizing rays to treat a variety of cancer. Ionizing radiation destroys the cell's ability to reproduce by damaging the cells DNA. Rapidly dividing cells, such as some cancer cells are more vulnerable to radiation than more slowly dividing cells. Furthermore, normal cells have greater ability than cancer cells to repair the DNA damage from radiation. In addition to the DNA effects, a complex chain of chemical reactions occurs in the extracellular fluid resulting in the formation of free radicals. Well oxygenated tumor show a much greater response to radiation than poorly oxygenated tumors. Oxygen free radicals formed during ionization interact readily with nearby molecules causing cellular damage including genetic material.

Radiation is the emission and distribution of energy through space or a material medium. The energy produced by radiation, when absorbed into tissue, produces ionization and excitation. This local energy is sufficient to break chemical bonds in DNA, which leads to biologic effect. The major target of radiation effect is DNA. The ionization that occurs eventually causes damage to DNA, which renders cells incapable of surviving mitosis. Loss of proliferative capacity yields cellular death at the time of division. Cellular death is dependent on the cell going through its mitotic cycle. Thus, death occurs at different rates for different cell types. This is true for both normal cells and cancer cells. However, cancer cells are more likely to be dividing because of the loss of control of cellular divisions. Furthermore, these cells are unable to repair the radiation damage to DNA. Therefore, cancer cells are more likely to be permanently damaged by the cumulative doses of radiation. Normal tissues are usually able to recover from radiation damage of therapeutic doses are kept within certain ranges.

Goals of radiation therapy: The goals of radiation therapy are cure, control and palliation. To accomplish these treatment goals, radiation therapy can be used alone or as an adjuvant treatment modality in combination with surgery chemotherapy and biologic response modifiers.

- Cure is the goal when radiation therapy is used alone as a curative modality for treating patients with basal cell carcinoma of the skin, tumors confined to the vocal cord, and Stage I or II A Hodgkin's disease. Radiation therapy can be combined with surgery and chemotherapy to cure certain cancers such as Stage II B, III A and III B, Hodgkin's disease, Ewing's sarcoma, head and neck cancer and Stage I and II breast cancer
- Control of the disease process of cancer for a period of time is considered to be a reasonable goal in some situations. Initial treatment is offered at the time of diagnosis, and additional treatment is given each time symptoms of disease recur. Most of the patients enjoy a satisfactory quality of life during symptom-free period. It can be combined with surgery to further enhance the local control of cancer. It can be given preoperatively, intraoperatively and also postoperatively as assessed accordingly
- Palliation is often the goal of RT. The patient can be treated to control the distressing symptoms that are occurring as a result of disease process. Tumors can be reduced in size to relieve symptoms more as pain and obstruction. Example of the use of RT for palliatives include the relief of:
  - Pain associated with bone metastasis
  - Pain and neurologic symptoms associated with brain metastasis
  - Spinal cord compression
  - Intestinal obstruction
  - Superior vena cava obstruction
  - Bronchial or tracheal obstruction
  - Bleeding (e.g. bladder and intrabronchial).

Types of radiation therapy: Radiation therapy can be administered from a variety of sources. Sources can be classified into those used outside (i.e. external RT) and those used close to the surface of the body or inside the body (Internal RT).

External radiation: Radiation treatment can be given by external beam radiation delivered from a source placed at some distance from the target site. It is usually administered by high energy X-ray machine (e.g. the betatron and linear accelerator) or machine containing a radioisotope (cobalt 60).

The main advantage of high-energy radiations is its skin-sparing effect. This means that the maximum effect of radiation occurs within the tumor deep in the body and not on the skin surface. Neutron beam therapy is delivered from a cyclotron particle accelerator is currently used to treat many types of cancer (tumor in salivary gland, prostate, lung).

Internal radiation: Internal RT involves the placement of specially prepared radioisotopes, which directly enter near the tumor itself. This is known as brachytherapy in which the implantation or insertion or radioactive materials directly into the tumor or in close proximity of the tumor. An implant may be temporary with the source placed into a catheter or tube inserted into the tumor area and left in place for several days. This method is commonly used for tumors of the head and neck, and gynecologic malignancies.

There are two types of internal RT:

i. Sealed-source in which the radioactive material is enclosed in a sealed container. Sealed source RT includes intracavity and interstitial therapy. In intracavity therapy, the radioiostopes, usually cesium 137 or radium 226, is placed into an applicator, then placed in body cavity for a carefully calculated time usually 24 to 72 hours (e.g. used to treat cancer of uterus or cervix).

   In interstitial therapy, the radioisotope of choice (iridium 192, iodine 125, cesium 137, gold 198 or radon 222) is placed in needles, beads, seeds, ribbons or catheters and then implanted directly into the tumors (e.g. as used in prostate cancer).

ii. Unsealed-sources RT are used in systemic therapy. Radioisotopes may be administered intravenously into a body cavity or orally. For example, sodium phosphate P32 is administered intravenously to treat polycythemia vera.

Iodine 131 is given orally in very low doses to treat Graves' disease.

Measurement of radiation: There are different units which are used to measure radiation as follows:

i. Curie (ci): A measure of the number of atoms of a particular radioisotope that disintegrate in one second.
ii. Rontgen (R): A measure of the radiation required to produce a standard number of ions in air; a unit of exposure to radiation.
iii. Rad: Measurement of radiation dosage absorbed by the tissue.
iv. Rem: Measurement of the biologic effectiveness of various forms of radiation on the human cell (1 Rem = 1 Rad).
v. Gray (Gy): 100 rads - 1 Gy.

The grays and centigrays are the units currently used in clinical practice.

Safety precautions in radiation therapy: There are three key principles to follow to protect nurses and others from excessive radiation exposure, viz. distance, time and shielding.

i. *Distance:* The greater distance from the radiation source, the less exposure dose of ionizing rays. The intensity of radiation decreases inversely to the square of the distance from the source. For example, if a person stands 4 ft from a source of radiation, the person is exposed to approximately 1/4 the amount of radiation the person would receive at 2 ft.
ii. *Time:* Minimal exposure time should be promoted, although patient care needs must still be met. A nurses exposure is generally limited to 30 minutes of direct care per 8 hours shift.
iii. *Shielding:* The dose of X-rays and gamma rays is reduced as the thickness of the lead shield is increased. In practice, nurses have found that leadshielding can be cumbersome to work with. So, it is better to maintain maximum distance from the radioactive source and limiting duration of exposure as safety measure.

The following guidelines will help protecting staff and others from radiation:

1. Place the client in a private room: It prevents undue exposure to other clients and to nurses caring for these clients.
2. Plan care well so that minimal time is spent in direct contact with the client. Do not spend more than 30 minutes per shift with the client.
3. Stand at the client's shoulder (for cervical implants) or at the foot of the bed (for head and neck implants) avoiding close contact with unshielded areas.
4. In case, if you must have prolonged contact with the client or if you will be exposed to an unshielded area, use a lead shield.
5. Do not care for more than one client with a radiation implant at one time.
6. All health care personnel should wear appropriate monitoring devices.
7. The room should be marked with appropriate signs stating the presence of radiation, do not allow children under 18 or pregnant women to visit; limit visitors' time to 30 minutes at a distance of at least 6 feet from the radioactive source; do not care for these patients if you (female nurse) are pregnant.
8. Carefully check all linens or other materials from the bed for the presence of implants.
9. Keep long handled forceps and lead-lined container available on the nursing unit or in the client's room while the implant is in place.

Nursing Management of Radiation Therapy

- Answer questions and allay fears of patient and family about the effects of radiation on others, on the tumor, and on normal tissues and organs

- Explain the procedure for delivering radiation. Describe the equipment, the duration of the procedure (often minutes), the possible need for immobilizing the patient during the procedure, and the absence of new sensations, including pain, during the procedure
- If a radioactive implant is used, inform patient about the restrictions placed on visitors and health care personnel and other radiation precautions as well as the patient's own role before, during, and after the procedure
- Maintain bed rest for patient with an intracavitary delivery device. Use the log-roll maneuver when positioning patient to prevent displacing the intracavitary device. Provide a low-residue diet and antidiarrheal agents to prevent bowel movements during therapy to prevent the radioisotopes from being displaced. Maintain an indwelling urinary catheter to ensure that the bladder empties
- Assess patient's skin, nutritional status, and general feeling of well-being
- Assess skin and oral mucosa frequently for changes (particularly if radiation therapy is directd to these areas). Protect the skin from irritation, and instruct patient to avoid using ointments, lotions, or powders on the area
- Assist the weak or fatigued patient with activities of daily living and personal hygiene, including gentle oral hygiene to remove debris, prevent irritation, and promote healing
- Reassure the patient by explaining that these symptoms are a result of the treatment and do not represent deterioration or progression of the disease
- Follow the instructions provided by the radiation safety officer from the radiology department, which identify the maximum time a health care provider can spend safely in the patient's room, the shielding equipment to be used, and special precautions and actions to be taken if the implant is dislodged. Explain the rationale for these precautions to patient.

For safety in brachytherapy, assign the patient to a private room, and post appropriate notices about radiation safety precautions. Have staff members wear dosimeter badges. Make sure that pregnant staff members are not assigned to this patient's care. Prohibit visits by children or pregnant women and limit visits from other to 30 minutes daily. Instruct and monitor visitors to ensure they maintain a 6-foot distance from the radiation source.

CHEMOTHERAPY

Chemotherapy is the systemic treatment of cancer with chemicals, i.e. drugs. Here the use of antineoplastic drugs to promote tumor cell destructions by interfering with cellular function and reproduction. It includes the use of various therapeutic agents and hormones.

The goal of chemotherapy is to destroy as many tumor cells as possible with minimal effect on healthy cells. It can be used for cure, control, and palliation. The objective of chemotherapy is to reduce the number of cancer cells present in the primary tumor site(s) and metastatic tumor site(s). Several factors will determine the response of cancer cells to chemotherapy as given below:

i. *Mitotic rate of the tissue* from which the tumor arises. The more rapid the mitotic rate, the greater response to chemotherapy. Chemotherapy is the treatment of choice for acute leukemia, choriocarcinoma of the placenta, Wilms' tumor (used in conjunction with surgery) and neuroblastoma. These cancer cells have a rapid rate of cellular proliferation.
ii. *Size of the tumor:* The smaller the number of cancer cells, the greater the response to chemotherapy.
iii. *Age of the tumor:* The younger tumor, the greater the response to chemotherapy. Younger tumors have a greater percentage of proliferating cells.
iv. *Location of the tumor:* Certain anatomic sites provide a protected environments from the effects of chemotherapy. For example, only few drugs cross the blood-brain barrier (nitrosoureas and bleomycin).
v. *Presence of resistant tumor cells:* Mutation of cancer cells within the tumor mass can result in varient cells that are resistant to chemotherapy. Resistance can also occur because of the biochemical inability of some cancer cells to convert the drug to its active form.
vi. *Physiologic and psychologic status of the host:* A state of optimum health and positive attitude will allow better withstand aggressive chemotherapy.

Classification of Chemotherapy

Chemotherapeutic agents generally are classified according to their pharmacologic action and effect on the cell generation cycles. However, the method by which cancer cells are inhibited or destroyed is not always unknown.

The two major categories of chemotherapeutic drugs are cell cycle-nonspecific and cell cycle-specifier. The cell cycle non-specifiers have their effect on the cells that are in the process of cellular replication and proliferation, as well as on the cells that are in the resting phase. The cell cycle-specific have their effect on cells that are in the process of cellular replication or proliferation. These drugs are effective at only one specific phase of cell cycle.

The common drugs used as chemotherapeutic agents are as follows:

1. Alkylating agent
   - Nitrogen mustard (Mechlorethamine)
   - Cyclophosphamide (Cytoxan)
   - Chlorambucil (Leukeran)
   - Busulfan (Myleran)
   - Melphalan (Alkeran)
   - Thiotepa (Thioplex)
   - Ifosfamide (Ifex).

2. Antimetabolites
   - Methotrexate
   - 6 Mercaptopurine (6 MP)
   - 6 Thioguanine (6 TG)
   - 5 Fluorouracil (5 Fu)
   - Cytosine arabinoside ((A-RA-C) Cytosar-4)
   - Fludarabine phosphate
   - Deoxycoformycin (Pentostatin).
3. Antitumor antibiotics
   - Daunorubicin (Cerubidine)
   - Doxorubicin (Adriamycin)
   - Dactinomycin (Cosmegen)
   - Bleomycin (Blenoxane)
   - Mitomycin (Mutamycin)
   - Plicamycin (Mithracin, mithramycin)
   - Idarubicin (Idamycin)
   - Mitoxantrone (Novantrone).
4. Hormonal agents
   i. Androgens
      - Testosterone propionate
      - Fluoxymesterone (Halotestin)
      - Dromostanolone (Drolban)
      - Testolactone (Teslac)
      - Methyltestosterone.

   ii. Corticosteroids
      - Cortisone acetate
      - Prednisone (Meticorten)
      - Dexamethasone (Decadron)
      - Methyl prednisolone sodium (Solu-Medrol)
      - Hydrocortisone sodium succinate (Solu-Cortef).

   iii. Estrogen
      - Diethylstilbestrol (DES)
      - Ethinyl estradiol (Estriny).

   iv. Progesterones
      - Hydroxyprogesterone caproate (Prodrox)
      - Megestrol (Megace)
      - Medroxyprogesterone (Provera)
      - Estramustine (Emcyt).

   v. Estrogen antagonists
      - Tamoxifen (Nolvadex)
      - Leuprolide (Lupron).

   vi. Antiadrenal
      - Aminoglutethimide.
5. Vinca alkaloids
   - Vincristine (Oncovin)
   - Vinblastine (Velban)
   - Vindesine sulfate.
6. Epipodophyllotoxins
   Etoposide (VP-16).

Nursing Management of Chemotherapy

- Assess patients nutritional and fluid and electrolyte status frequently. Use creative ways to encourage adequate fluid and dietary intake
- Due to increased risk of anemia, infection, and bleeding disorders, focus nursing assessment and care on identifying and modifying factors that further increase the risk
- Use aseptic technique and gentle handling to prevent infection and trauma
- Closely monitor laboratory test results (blood cell counts), and promptly report untoward changes and signs of infection or bleeding
- Carefully select peripheral veins and perform venipuncture, and carefully administer drugs. Monitor for indications of extravasation during drug administration (e.g. absence of blood return from the intravenous catheter, resistance to flow of intravenous fluid, or swelling, pain, or redness at the site)
- Assist patient with delayed nausea and vomiting (occurring later than 48 to 72 hours after chemotherapy) by teaching the patient to take antiemetic medications as necessary for the first week at home after chemotherapy and by teaching relaxation techniques and imagery, which can help to decrease stimuli contributing to symptoms
- Advise patient to eat small, frequent meals, bland foods and comfort foods, which may reduce the frequency or severity of these symptoms
- Monitor blood cell counts frequently, note and report neutropenia, and protect the patient from infection and injury, particularly while blood cell counts are depressed
- Monitor blood urea nitrogen (BUN), serum creatinine, creatinine clearance, and serum electrolyte levels, and report any finding that indicate decreasing renal function
- Provide adequate hydration and alkalinization of the urine to prevent formation of uric acid crystals, and administer allopurinol as ordered to prevent renal damage
- Monitor closely for signs of heart failure and for pulmonary fibrosis (e.g. pulmonary function test results)
- Inform patient and partner about potential changes in reproductive ability resulting from chemotherapy and options. (Banking of sperm is recommended for men before treatments.) Advise patient and partner to use reliable birth control while receiving chemotherapy because sterility is not certain
- Inform patient that the taxanes and plant alkaloids, especially vincristine, can cause peripheral neuropathies, loss of deep tendon reflexes, and paralytic ileus; these side effects are usually reversible and disappear after completion of chemotherapy
- Help patient and family plan strategies to combat fatigue
- Use precautions developed by the Occupational Safety and Health Administration (OSHA), Oncology Nursing Society

Box 8.7 Safety in administering chemotherapy

Safety recommendations from the Occupational Safety and Health Administration (OSHA), Oncology Nursing Society (ONS), hospitals, and other health care agencies for the preparation and handling of antineoplastic agents follow:
- Use a biologic safety cabinet for the preparation of all chemotherapy agents
- Wear surgical gloves when handling antineoplastic agents and the excretions of patients who received chemotherapy
- Wear disposable, long-sleeved gowns when preparing and administering chemotherapy agents
- Use Luer-Lock fittings on all intravenous tubing used to deliver chemotherapy
- Dispose of all equipment used in chemotherapy preparation and administration in appropriate, leak-proof, puncture-proof containers
- Dispose of all chemotherapy wastes as hazardous materials. When followed, these precautions greatly minimize the risk of exposure to chemotherapy agents

(ONS), hospitals, and other health care agencies to protect health care personnel who handle chemotherapeutic agents (Box 8.7).

If extravasation is suspected, stop the drug administration immediately and apply ice to the site (unless the extravagated vesicant is a vinca alkaloid).

Nursing Intervention in Chemotherapy

Alkalating agents are cell cycle non-specific and act against already formed nucleic acid by cross-linking DNA strands, thereby preventing DNA replication and transcription of RNA. The major toxin of alkalatings are dependent upon drugs given which include hematopoietic anemia, leukopenia, thrombocytopenia, GI-nausea and vomiting, diarrhea, reproductive-infertility, change in libido, GU-cystitis and renal toxicity.

The nursing intervention for these toxicities are:

i. Hematopoietic toxicity:
   - Monitor WBC, RBC, platelets count biweekly for pancytopenia
   - Observe for signs and symptoms of infections, bleeding, anemia
   - Provide rest periods and 8 hours sleep per night
   - Teach benefits of good personal hygiene
   - Provide comfort and suggestion measures.

ii. Gastrointestinal toxicity:
   - Document nausea and vomiting times and amount
   - Administer antiemetic drug PRN
   - Hydrate to 2000 mL/24 hour if not contradicted
   - Record intake and output
   - Avoid noxious odors
   - Use relaxation techniques or distractions
   - Provide small frequent meals.

iii. Reproductive toxicity:
   - Inform of possibility of temporary or permanent infertility and danger to growing fetus
   - Provide reproductive counseling as needed.

iv. Genitourinary toxicity:
   - Inform that hemorrhagic cystitis can occur with cytoxan and ifosfamide therapy
   - Administer mesna (urothelial protection agent) to help to prevent cystitis
   - Encourage hydration and complete and frequent emptying of bladder.

Antimetabolites act by interfering with synthesis of chromosomal nucleic acid, antimetabolites are analogs of normal metabolites and block the enzyme necessary for synthesis of essential factors or are incorporated into the DNA or RNA and thus prevent replication are cycle-specific.

The major toxicities of antimetabolities are dependent on drugs given, which are as follows:

- Hematopoietic
  - Bone marrow suppression
  - Anemia
  - Leukopenia
  - Thrombocytopenia
- Gastrointestinal
  - Mucositis/stomatitis
  - Diarrhea
  - Nausea and vomiting.

The nursing intervention of these toxicities are as stated in alkylating agents and in addition to the above, the following has to be performed.

For Mucositis and Stomatitis

- Inspect oral cavity daily for presence of sores, change in taste and sensation
- Teach oral care and encourage immediately after meals and at bed time, soft toothbrush and prescribed mouthwash (peroxide, oral saline, baking soda and water or provide anesthetic agent for mouth sores (e.g. stomatitic cocktail)
- Report signs and symptoms of oral infection
- Soft diet with non-irritating foods high in protein, calories, offer high caloric liquid supplements.

For Diarrhea

- Low residue diet, high protein and calories maintain hydration
- Monitor and document number and frequency stools
- Administer antidiarrheal medication as needed
- Provide meticulus skin care in perirectal area
- Promote good hygiene habits.

Antitumor antibiotics interfere with synthesis and function of nucleic acids and inhibit RNA and DNA synthesis. These are cycle-specific. The major toxicities of antitumor antibiotics include:

- Hematopoietic—bone marrow suppression
- GI—mucositis/stomatitis, anorexia, nausea and vomiting
- Integumentary—alopecia, tissue necrosis (if extravasate)
- Cardiac and pulmonary toxicity.

In addition to above stated nursing interventions, for other chemotherapeutics, the added nursing interventions for;

i. *Integumentary:* For alopecia, warn of potential for hair loss and ways of minimizing loss.
   For extravasation
   - Monitor IV infusion to prevent infiltration. When infiltrated stop immediately and institute agency protocol to prevent tissue necrosis-notify doctor immediately and keep extravasation kit available at all times.

ii. Cardiac toxicity may occur with bleomycin (pneumonitis and progressive pulmonary fibrosis), should not exceed a lifetime dose of 400 IU. Assess respiratory status and document changes.

Hormonal Agents

- Androgens alter pituitary function and directly affects the malignant cell. Toxicities of androgens include fluid retention and masculinization
- Corticosteroids use in lymphoid malignancies and have indirect effects on malignant cells. The major toxicities include fluid retention, hypertension, diabetes, and increased susceptibility to infection
- Estrogen and progesterone suppress testosterone production in males and alter the response of breast cancer to prolactin and promote differentiation of malignant cells. The major toxicities include fluid retention, feminization and uterine bleeding
- Estrogen antagonists compete with estrogens for binding with estrogen receptor sites on malignant cells. Toxicities are minimal with occasional headache and hot flash
- Antiadrenals produce the equivalent of a medical adrenalectomy, thereby inhibiting the formations of estrogen and androgenesis and function of nucleic acids and inhibit RNA and DNA synthesis. These agents are cycle non-specific toxicity in adrenal insufficiency.

The nursing interventions during chemotherapy with harmful agent are:

- For fluid retention
  - Warn of potential weight gain
  - Weight biweekly
  - Maintain intake and output if needed.
- For feminization in males
  - Inform about chance of gynecomastia—change in voice, distribution of body fat and hair and cardiovascular problem.
- Assess fears and concerns and provide psychological support as needed.
- For virilization in females
  - Discuss the risk for facial hair, lowered voice, clitorial enlargement—fluid retention
  - Assess fears and concerns and provide psychological support.
- For uterine bleeding
  - Prepare postmenopausal woman for occurrence
  - Provide support and reassurance.
- For diabetes
  - Inform patient of potential occurrence
  - Monitor blood sugar changes
  - Observe signs and symptoms of diabetes.
- For adrenal insufficiency
  - Instruct on need to comply with replacement therapy while on medication
  - Reassure that need for therapy will cease when drug is discontinued.

Vinca alkaloid bind to proteins within the cells causing metaphase arrest thus inhibiting RNA and protein synthesis. Major toxicities are bone marrow suppression and alopecia (see nursing intervention as stated above).

Epipodophyllotoxins cause breaks in DNA and RNA protein cross links. The major toxicities are neurological, i.e. neurotoxicity, muscle weakness, peripheral neurities, paralytic ileus, loss of deep tenden reflexes.

The nursing intervention for neurological toxicities will include:

- GI
  - Check for peristalsis frequently
  - Determine usual pattern of bowel elimination
  - Facilitate elimination with laxative regimens.
- Peripheral
  - Observe for numbness, tingling in extremities
  - Institute safety measure (e.g. wearing shoes, using cane or walker for ambulation)
  - Seek assistance for ambulation as needed
  - Teach signs and symptoms to report to concerned doctor
  - Provide supportive care and reassurance.

Guidelines for Care of Client with Chemotherapy

1. Teach the patient and significant others
   - Signs and symptoms of infection, thrombocytopenia
   - How to read thermometer and when to notify the doctor

- Good hygienic practices—cleansing the perinium from front to back, change underwear daily and handwashing
- Information about prescribed drugs—name, dose, side effects, importance of taking as prescribed
- Use of antiemetics
- Importance of medical follow-up and blood studies
- Available support group for chemotherapy patients.

2. Prevent infection
   - Good hygiene especially handwashing—patient, family, health personnel
   - Prevent exposure to people with known infection (other staff, family, etc.)
   - Meticulous aseptic technique during IV infusion and dressing changes
   - Avoid use of aspirin or acetaminophen to prevent masking fever
   - Maintain intact skin and mucous membrane
     - Avoid bumping and breaking the skin
     - No injections
     - Keep finger nails short, to prevent small skin breaks (nurses, patients other care givers)
     - Avoid anal intercourse
     - Avoid enemas, rectal medications, rectal thermometers
     - Avoid excessive friction and provide vaginal lubrication during sexual intercourse (use water soluble jelly...).
   - Maintain meticulous oral hygiene
     - Maintain teeth and gums in good condition
     - Use mouthwash or oral irrigations with normal saline... baking soda or sodium bicarbonate solution
     - Use mycostatin tablets or suspension as necessary
     - Relieve dryness, drink water and other fluids
     - Use artificial saliva as needed in form of spray
     - Stimulate saliva with gum, candies, buttermilk, yoghurt
     - Brush teeth with soft toothbrush (small soft bristle) or use foam stick or swab
     - Brush teeth in short horizontal strokes at least for 3 to 4 minutes, at least 3 times a day
     - Use fluoridated toothpaste or rinse to prevent caries
     - Use waterpik under low pressure or irrigation, if platelet count is low
   - Maintain optimal respiratory functions, encourage, turn, cough and deep breathe (if confined to bed).
3. Maintain optimal gastrointestinal function
   - Give antidiarrheal medication as needed
   - Plan daily bowel regimen for constipation, give stool softener as prescribed
   - Treat stomatitis coral nystatin, or other prescribes
   - Oral irrigations every 2 hours
   - Soft, bland foods, cold liquids, tolerated by some persons
   - Treat nausea and vomiting:
     - Give antiemetics 30 to 45 minutes before chemotherapy, use large doses
     - Use auditory or diversional stimulation (music slides, phonograph)
     - Give antiemetics around the clock for severe nausea and vomiting
     - Use texation techniques were hypnosis, therapeutic touch
     - Eat foods which can minimize nausea and vomiting.
4. Minimizing or preventing alopecia:
   - Encourage use of wigs, scarves, eyebrow pencils, false eyelashes
   - Avoid frequent shampooing, combing, or brushing
   - Use soft-bristle hair brush
   - Advise against permanent and hair coloring (increase rate of hair loss).
5. Minimizing or preventing urinary effects
   - Hemorrhage, cystitis, renal toxicity
   - Force fluids when take cyclophosphamide
   - Take cyclophosphamide early in the day
   - Check serum creatinine or 24 hours urine for creatinine clearance before giving cisplatin and streptozotocin.
6. Minimizing reproductive effects
   - Provide birth control information and reproductive counseling
   - Provide informatioan about sperm banking before initiation of therapy for male patients.

Administration of Chemotherapy

Chemotherapy can be administered by several routes.

• Oral	Ex. cyclophosphomide
• Intramuscular	Ex. bleomycin
• Intravenous	Ex. doxorubicin, vincristine
• Intracavitary (pleural, peritoneal)	Ex. radioisotopes, alkylating agents
• Intrathecal arbinoside	Ex. methotrexate, cytosine,
• Intraarterial	Ex. DTIC, 5-Fu, methotrexate, fluxuridine
• Perfusion	Ex. alkalinizing, alkylating agents
• Continuous infusion cytosine, arbinoside	Ex. 5-Fu, methostreate,
• Subcutaneous	Ex. cytosine arabinoside
• Topical	Ex. 5-Fu cream
• Intraperitoneal	Ex. methotrexate, 5-Fu

Mostly used common routes are IV and oral. One of the major concerns with the IV administration of antineoplastic drugs is possible irritation of vessel wall by the drugs, or even worse, extravasation (infiltration of drugs into tissues surrounding the infusion site), causing local tissue damage.

Many chemotherapeutic drugs are vesicants agents that when accidentally infiltrated into the skin cause severe local tissue breakdown and necrosis. Some guidelines to promote safe use of chemotherapeutic drugs by IV administration are as follows:

1. Know specifics about the safe administration of chemotherapy.
2. Start an IV infusion and normal saline solution or 5% dextrose in water or saline solution with a small-lumens short needle or catheter. Ensure that recent venipunctures have not been performed to the proximal to the IV. Avoid using on arm that has poor lymphatic drainage or that has previously received radiation therapy.
3. Select a vein that is larger enough to promote infusion without irritating the intima of the vein. When a vesicant is administered, avoid the veins in the hand, wrist and antecubital area.
4. Instruct the patient to immediately report any changes in sensation especially burning or stinging pain.
5. Check for blood return before infusing the chemotherapeutic drug. However, a blood return does not always indicate an intact vein.
6. If more than one drug is to be used, give the vesicant agents. First, when the vein is at its optimum integrity (note this method is controversial, so confirm with the concerned).
7. Slowly push those drugs that are to be given by the push or bolus method. Give in small increments (0.5 to 1.0 mL). Pause 30 to 60 seconds after each increment and allow the IV infusion to flush the vein, check blood returns, and again gently push 0.5 to 1.0 mL of the medication. Repeat until the medication has been given and allow the IV infusion to flush the vein for several minutes.
8. Avoid continuous peripheral IV infusion of vesicant agents. If given peripherally, the administration of vesicant agents must be motivated directly at all times.
9. Stop the IV infusion immediately if the patient complains of a burning or stinging pain or if an infiltration is suspected. If the drug is an irritant, check for blood return and if present continue to administer the drugs. If it is vesicant, stop the infusion and begin appropriate extravasation procedure.
10. If extravasation occurs:
    - Stop the IV infusion immediately; notify the doctor or use the standing written orders for the treatment related to the specific vesicant agent
    - Remove the IV infusion tubing and aspirate any remaining drug with a new syringe
    - Inject the prescribed antidote (if one is available) in the infusion needle or in a 'pincushion' fashion in the skin surrounding the needle site
    - Apply a topical corticosteroid cream, if prescribed
    - Elevate the site
    - Apply cold compresses for the first 24 to 48 hours unless a vinca alkaloid has been infiltrated; heat is applied following extravasation of vinca alkaloids
    - Document the extravasation
    - Observe site at designated intervals
    - A plastic surgeon may be consulted, depending on the extent of anticipated damage
    - If extravasation is suspected, the medication is stopped immediately and depend upon the drug, an attempt is made to aspirate any remaining drug from the extravasation site through the existing needle.

Principles of Chemotherapy Administration

1. Combination chemotherapy is far superior to single agent chemotherapy.
2. Complete remission is the minimum requisite for cure and even increased survival.
3. The first round chemotherapy offers the best chance for significant benefit, therefore, the initial therapy should be the type with maximum effectiveness.
4. Maximum doses of drugs are used to attain maximum tumor cell kill; Dose reduction to minimised toxicity has been called "killing patients with kindness".
5. Neoadjuvant or induction chemotherapy is always recommended for some specific cancer (e.g. breast cancer).
6. Chemoprevention shows promise in prevention of some second-primary cancers (head and neck).

Side effects of radiation therapy and chemotherapy: The common side effects of radiation therapy and chemotherapy classified according to systemwise are described further and also see Box 8.8 for predisposing cancer patients to infection.

Gastrointestinal System

i. *Dryness of the mucous membranes of the mouth:* When salivary glands are located in the radiation treatment field, they are frequently damaged. This may be a permanent side effect of the radiation therapy and it can be quite disturbing because it is difficult to eat, swallow, and talk when the mucous membranes are dry. Artificial saliva is available.
ii. *Stomatitis and mucositis:* This problem occurs when epithelial cells of the oral mucosa and intraoral soft tissue structures are destroyed by chemotherapy or radiation therapy. These cells are extremely sensitive because of their normal high cell turnover rate. Mucositis can precipitate complications of infection and hemorrhage.
iii. *Esophagitis:* Inflammation and ulceration of mucous membranes or esophagus as a result of rapid cell destructions occur as a side effect of chemotherapy and radioactive therapy to the area of the neck, chest and back.
iv. *Nausea and vomiting:* The vomiting center in the brain is stimulated by products of cellular breakdown that occurs in response to chemotherapy and radiation therapy.

Box 8.8 Factors predisposing cancer patients to infection

Factors	Underlying mechanisms
Impaired skin and mucous membrane integrity	• Loss of body's first line of defense against invading organisms
Chemotherapy	• Chemotherapy agents that cause mucositis impair skin and mucous membrane integrity • Organ damage associated with certain agents may also predispose patients to infection • Organ damage such as pulmonary fibrosis or cardiomyopathy that is associated with certain agents may also predispose patients to infection
Radiation therapy	• Radiation involving sites of bone marrow production may result in bone marrow suppression • May also lead to impaired tissue integrity
Biologic response modifiers	• Some biologic response modifiers may cause bone marrow suppression and organ dysfunction
Malignant	• Malignant cells may infiltrate the bone marrow and interfere with production of white blood cells and lymphocytes. Hematologic malignancies (leukemias and lymphomas) are associated with impaired function and production of blood cells
Malnutrition	• Malnutrition results in impaired production and function of cells of the immune response • It may contribute to impaired skin integrity
Medications	• Antibiotics disturb the balance of normal flora, allowing them to become pathogenic. This process occurs most commonly in the gastrointestinal tract
Urinary catheter	• Corticosteroids and nonsteroidal anti-inflammatory drugs (NSAIDs) mask inflammatory responses
Intravenous catheter	• The catheter creates a port and mechanism of entry for organisms
Other invasive procedure (e.g. surgery, paracentesis, thoracentesis, drainage tubes, endoscopy, mechanical ventilation)	• The catheter is a site of entry of organisms • These procedure create a port of entry and possible introduction of exogenous organisms into the system
Contaminated equipment	• Stagnant water in oxygen equipment is associated with growth of microorganisms
Age	• Increasing age is associated with declining organ function and decreased production and functioning of the cells of the immune system
Chronic illness	• Chronic illness is associated with impaired organ function and altered immune responses
Prior infection	• Recent infection may by associated with depleted immune responses and debilitation; prior infection may not have completely resolved; previous use of antibiotics may have altered normal flora allowing flora to become pathogenic
Recent travel	• Travel, especially to less developed areas, may have lead to exposure to microbial infection and disease
Pet excreta	• Exposure to pet excreta, especially in the immunocompromised patient, may be associated with infections such as *Toxoplasma gondii* (toxoplasmosis)
Prolonged hospitalization	• Hospitalization allows increased exposure to nosocomial infection and colonization by new organisms

The drugs used in chemotherapy also stimulate the vomiting center. Destruction of the epithelial lining of the GI tracts occurs in response to both these therapies to chest, abdomen and back. A strong psychologic impacts is associated with nausea and vomiting and the high stress level associated with concern cancer and cancer treatment.

v. *Anorexia:* It is site specific side effect of radiation therapy dry mouth, mucositis, esophagitis, nausea, vomiting, and diarrhea occur. Side effects of chemotherapy include nausea, vomiting, stomatitis, esophagitis, and diarrhea. Fatigue, pain and infection are present. Alteration in the sensation of taste occurs when tumors release waste products into the blood stream. Psychological and social impact of cancer and cancer therapy result in an increased level of stress and changes in the usual lifestyle pattern.

vi. *Altered taste sensations:* Due to destruction of the taste buds in the treatment field occurs in radiation therapy. The amount of taste alterations or loss depends on the radiation dosage and the extent field. Complete loss of taste often occurs. Taste changes may be a permanent outcome of therapy. Waste products occur in response to cellular destructions from radiation therapy and chemotherapy. These waste products are thought to be responsible for alteration in task sensations.

   Reduction in the amount of saliva occurs because of the locatioan of the salivary glands in the treatment field. Food must be in solution to be tasted.

vii. *Diarrhea:* Due to denuding of the epithelial lining of the small intestine occurs as a side effect of both the therapies to the abdomen or the lower back.

Box 8.9 Sources of fatigue in cancer patient

- Pain, pruritus
- Imbalanced nutrition related to anorexia, nausea, vomiting, cachexia
- Electrolyte imbalance related to vomiting, diarrhea
- Ineffective protection related to neutropenia, thrombocytopenia, anemia
- Impaired tissue integrity related to stomatitis, mucositis
- Impaired physical mobility related to neurologic impairments, surgery, bone metastasis, pain, and analgesic use
- Uncertainty and deficient knowledge related to disease process, treatment
- Anxiety related to fear, diagnosis, role changes, uncertainty of future
- Ineffective breathing patterns related to cough, shortness of breath and dyspnea
- Disturbed sleep pattern related to cancer therapies, anxiety, and pain

viii. *Constipation:* Due to dysfunction of the autonomic nervous system from neurotoxic effects of plant alkaloids (vincristine, vinblastine) occurs.

ix. *Hepatotoxicity:* Toxic effects of certain chemotherapy drugs such as methotrexate, mitomycin, 6-MP and cytosine arabinoside are product.

x. *Fatigue:* The sources of fatigue in cancer (Box 8.9).

Hematopoietic System

i. *Anemia:* These therapies result in depressant effect on bone marrow function. Malignant infiltration of bone marrow by cancer occurs. Ulceration, necrosis and bleeding of neoplastic growth occurs.

ii. *Leukopenia:* As stated earlier, these therapies result in depressant effect on bone marrow. The effect is especially significant because of the short span of white blood cells. Infection is the most frequent cause of morbidity and death in the patient with cancer. Usual sites of infection are the respiratory and genitourinary system.

iii. *Thrombocytopenia:* Depressant effect on bone marrow functions may lead to malignant infiltrations of the bone marrow. Abnormal destruction of circulating platelets is present. When platelet count decreases spontaneous bleeding can occur.

Integumentary System

i. *Alopecia:* Alopecia occurs as a side effect of some chemotherapy agents and radiation therapy to the skull. Hair loss that occurs in response to radiation therapy is usually permanent. The hair begins to fall out during the first week of therapy, and this may progress to complete hair loss.

ii. *Skin reaction:* Extravasation of vesicant chemotherapeutic drugs (e.g. doxorubicin) gives intravenously causes severe necrosis of tissues exposed to the drug.

Genitourinary Tract

i. *Cystitis:* This problem occurs when the epithelial cells of the lining of the bladder are destroyed as a side effect of chemotherapy (e.g. cyclophosphamide) and as a side effect of radiation therapy when the bladder located in the treatment field. Clinical manifestation of urgency, frequency, and hematuria are present.

ii. *Reproductive dysfunction:* This problem occurs as a result of the effect of chemotherapy on the cells of the testes or ova or as a result of the effect of radiation therapy when the cells of the testes or ova are located in the treatment field. Symptoms of cancer and cancer therapy include fatigue, diarrhea nausea, vomiting, anxiety, fear and pain.

iii. *Nephrotoxicity:* Necrosis of proximal renal tubules present as a result of an accumulation of drugs (e.g. cisplatin) in the kidney.

Nervous System

i. *Increased intracranial pressure:* This problem may result from radiation edema in the CNS. This phenomenon is not well understood but is easily controlled with steroids and pain medication.

ii. *Peripheral neuropathy:* Paresthesia, areflexia, skeletal muscle weakness and smooth muscle dysfunction (e.g. paralytic ileus, constipation) can occur as a side effect of plant alkaloids (e.g. vinblastine, vincristine) and cisplatin.

Respiratory System

i. *Pneumonitis:* When the lungs are located in the treatment field, radiation pneumonitis may develop 2–3 months after start of treatment. It is characterized by a dry, hacking cough, fever and exertional dyspnea.

After 6–12 months, fibrosis will occur and will be persistently evident on X-ray. The patient with fibrosis is more susceptible to respiratory infection. This problem can also occur as a result of chemotherapy (e.g. bleomycin, busulfan).

Cardiovascular System

i. *Pericarditis and myocarditis:* This problem is an infrequent complication when the chest wall is radiated. It may occur up to 1 year after treatment.

In additions, for problems caused by chemotherapy and radiation therapy follow Table 8.2 for management.

Procedure Guidelines: Administering IV Chemotherapy

a. Examine the site for erythema or selling. Over a period of days to weeks, the site can become mottled and lead to necrosis.
b. Stop the infusion of the chemotherapeutic agent.
c. Aspirate all residual chemotherapeutic agent in the IV needle/catheter.
d. Administer antidote (see accompanying Table 8.2) inject intradermally in circular motion around the extravasation site to prevent leakage of drug to surrounding tissues (if appropriate or inject via the IV catheter).
e. Antidote may prevent tissue necrosis. If unable to aspirate from IV catheter, catheter may be blocked and antidote will not reach extravasation.

Do not inject an antidote via the IV catheter if unable to aspirate the chemotherapeutic agent.

Remove the needle.

Apply ice or heat to the site, depending on the chemotherapeutic agent which has extravasated (Table 8.3).

TABLE 8.2: Nursing management of problems caused by chemotherapy and radiation therapy

Problem	Etiology	Nursing management
Gastrointestinal system		
Stomatitis, mucositis, esophagitis	• Epithelial cells are destroyed by chemotherapy or radiation treatment when located in field (e.g. head and neck, stomach, esophagus) • Inflammation and ulceration occur due to rapid cell destruction	• Assess oral mucosa daily and teach patient to do this • Be aware that eating, swallowing, and talking may be difficult (may require analgesics) • Encourage patient to use artificial saliva to manage dryness (radiation) • Discourage use of irritants such as tobacco and alcohol • Apply topical anesthetics (e.g. viscous lidocaine, oxethazine)
Nausea and vomiting	• Release of intracellular breakdown products stimulates vomiting center in brain • Drugs also stimulate vomiting center in brain • GI lining destroyed with radiation and chemotherapy	• Teach patient to eat and drink when not nauseated • Administer antiemetics prophylactically prior to chemotherapy and also on as needed • Use diversional activities (if appropriate)
Anorexia	• Release of TNF (Tumor necrosis factor) and Il-1 from macrophages has appetite-suppressant effect • Therapy-induced GI effects (mucositis, nausea, and vomiting, bowel disturbances) and anxiety that reduce appetite	• Monitor weight • Encourage patient to eat small, frequent meals of high-protein, high-calorie foods • Gently encourage patient to eat, but avoid nagging • Serve food in pleasant environment
Diarrhea	• Denuding of epithelial lining of intestines • Side effect of chemotherapy • Radiation to abdomen, pelvis, lumbosacral areas	• Give antidiarrheal agents as needed • Encourage low-fiber, low-residue diet • Encourage fluid intake of at least 3 L
Constipation	• Decreased intestinal motility related to autonomic nervous system dysfunction • Caused by neurotoxic effects of plant alkaloids (vincristine, vinblastine)	• Instruct patients to 1. Take stool softeners as needed 2. Eat high-fiber foods 3. Increase fluid intake
Hepatotoxicity	• Toxic effects from chemotherapy drugs (usually transient and resolves when drug is stopped)	Monitor liver function tests
Hematologic system		
Anemia	• Bone marrow depressed secondary to therapy • Malignant infiltration of bone marrow by cancer	• Monitor hemoglobin and hematocrit levels • Administer iron supplements and erythropoietin • Encourage intake of foods that promote RBC production
Leucopenia	• Depression of bone marrow secondary to chemotherapy of radiation therapy • Infection most frequent cause of morbidity and death in cancer patients • Respiratory and genitourinary system usual sites of infection	• Monitor WBC count, especially neutrophils • Teach patient to report temperature elevation and any other manifestations of infection • Teach patient to avoid large crowds and people with infections • Administer WBC growth factors • Do patient teaching

Contd...

Contd...

Problem	Etiology	Nursing management
Thrombocytopenia	• Bone marrow depressed secondary to chemotherapy • Malignant infiltration of bone marrow that crowds out normal marrow • Spontaneous bleeding can occur with platelet counts ≤ 20,000/μL	• Observe for signs of bleeding (e.g. petechiae, ecchymosis) • Monitor platelet counts • Do patient teaching
Integumentary system		
Alopecia	• Destruction of hair follicles by chemotherapy or radiation to scalp • Hair loss usually temporary with chemotherapy; usually permanent in response to radiation	• Suggest ways to cope with hair loss (e.g. hair pieces, scarves, wigs) • Cut long hair before therapy • Avoid excessive shampooing, brushing, and combing hair • Avoid use of electric hair dryers, curlers, and curling rods • Discuss impact of hair loss on self-image
Radiation skin changes (dry to moist desquamation)	• Radiation damage to skin	• Keep treatment field protected; do not apply any lotions, creams, cosmetics, or other products unless prescribed by physician • Additional patient management needed
Chemotherapy-induced skin changes	• Hyperpigmentation • Telangiectasias • Photosensitivity • Acneiform eruptions • Acral erythema	• Alert patient to potential skin changes • Encourage patient to avoid sun exposure • Implement symptomatic management as needed depending on specific skin effect (e.g. application of lotions, benzoyl peroxide for acne, corticosteroid creams)
Genitourinary tract		
Hemorrhagic cystitis	• Cells lining bladder destroyed chemotherapy (e.g. cyclophosphamide, ifosfamide) • Side effect of radiation when located in treatment field	• Monitor manifestations such as urgency, frequency, and hematuria • Administer cytoprotectant agent (mesna [Mesnex]) and hydration • Administer supportive care agents to manage symptoms (e.g. Urimax, flavozate)
Reproductive dysfunction	• Cells of testes or ova are damaged from therapy	• Discuss possibility with patients prior to treatment initiation • Offer opportunity for sperm and ova banking prior to treatment for patients of childbearing age
Nephrotoxicity	• Direct renal cell damage due to exposure to nephrotoxic agents (cisplatin and high-dose methotrexate) • Precipitation of metabolities of cellular breakdown (tumor lysis syndrome [TLS])	• Monitor BUN are serum creatinine levels • Avoid potentiating drugs • Alkalinize the urine with sodium bicarbonate and administer allopurinol or rasburicase for TLS prevention
Nervous system		
Increased intracranial pressure	• May result from radiation edema in central nervous system	• Monitor neurologic status • May be controlled with corticosteroids
Peripheral neuropathy	• Paresthesias, areflexia, skeletal muscle weakness, and smooth muscle dysfunction can occur as a side effect of plant alkaloids and cisplatin	• Monitor for these manifestations in patients on these drugs
Respiratory system		
Pneumonitis	• Radiation pneumonitis develops 2–3 months after start of treatment • After 6–12 months, fibrosis occurs and is evident on X-ray • Side effect of some chemotherapy drugs	• Monitor for clinical manifestations of these disorders

Contd...

Contd...

Problem	Etiology	Nursing management
Cardiotoxicity	• Some chemotherapy drugs (e.g. anthracyclines, taxanes) can cause ECG changes and rapidly progressive heart failure	• Monitor heart with ECG and cardiac ejection fractions • Drug therapy may need to be modified for symptoms or deteriorating cardiac function studies
Biochemical		
Hyperuricemia	• Increased uric acid levels due to chemotherapy induced cell destruction • Can cause secondary gout and obstructive uropathy	• Monitor uric acid levels • Allopurinol (Zyloprim) may be given as a prophylactic measure • Encourage high fluid intake
Psychoemotional		
Fatigue	• Anabolic processes resulting in accumulation of metabolites from cell breakdown	• Tell patient that fatigue is an expected side effect of therapy • Encourage patient to rest when fatigued, to maintain usual lifestyle patterns as closely as possible, and to pace activities in accordance with energy level

TABLE 8.3: Management of an extravasation

Chemotherapeutic agent	Local antidote	Method of administration
Decarbazine (DTIC) Dactinomycin (actinomycin D) Mitomycin C (mutamycin) Mechlorethamine (nitrogen mustard)	Isotonic sodium thiosulfate 10% Mixing 4.0 mL of sodium thiosulfate 10% with 6.0 mL sterile water for injection	1. Inject 5–6 mL mixture through the existing line and so in divided doses into the extravasated site with multiple injections. Repeat SQ dosing over several hours 2. Apply cold compresses 6–12 hours after the extravasation
Vinblastine (velban) Vincristine (oncovin) Temposide (Vm 26)	Hyaluronidase (Wydase) 150 units/mL Add 1 mL USP NaCl	1. Inject 1–6 mL (150–900 units) Sq into extravasated site with multiple injections 2. Apply warm compresses
Etoposide (vepesid) Streptozocin (zanosar) Mithramycin (mithracin)		
Daunorubicin (cerubidine) Doxorubicin (adriamycin) Mitoxantrone (novantrone) AMSA	Hydrocartisone 50-100 mg/mL	1. Inject 1/2 mL (50–100 mg) IV through the existing line and SQ into the extravasated site with multiple injections. Total dose not to exceed 100 mg 2. Apply cold compresses for 15 minute 4 times in a 24-hour period
BCNU (carmustine)	Sodium bicarbonate (0.5 mEq/mL) prefilled syringe	1. Inject 2–6 mL of mixture (1.0–3.0 mEq) IV through the existing IV line and into the extravasated site with multiple injections 2. Total dose not to exceed 10 mL of solution (5.0 mEq) 3. Apply cold compresses. Do not apply pressure
Pachtaxel (taxol)	None	1. Apply warm compresses to the extravasation site for 24 hours

Follow-up Phase

1. Document drug dosage, site and any occurrence of extravasation including estimated amount of drug extravasated, management. Photograph if possible.
2. Observe regularly after administration for pain, erythema, induration, and necrosis.
2. If only a small amount of drug extravasated and frank necrosis does not occur, phlebitis may still result, causing pain for several days or induration at the site that may last for weeks or months.
3. Monitor for other side effects of infusion.
   a. Patient may describe sensations of pain, stretching, or pressure within the vessel, originating near the venipuncture site or extending 7.5–12.5 cm (3–5 inches) along the vein.
   b. Discoloration-red streak following the line of the vein (called a flare reaction) or darkening of the vein.

c. Itching, urticaria, muscle cramps, or pressure in the arm.

3. a. Caused by irritation to the vein.
b. Flare reaction common with doxorubicin (andriamycin). Darkening of vein may occur with 5-fluorouracil (5-FU)
c. Caused by irritation of surrounding subcutaneous tissue.

NURSING RESPONSIBILITIES IN ONCOLOGICAL EMERGENCIES

Nurses have the responsibilities in managing oncological emergencies as listed in Table 8.4:

Nursing Management of Patient with Cancer

Assessment

Infection

- Assess patient for secondary problems, such as infection, reduced white blood cell (WBC) count, bleeding, skin problems, nutritional problems, pain, fatigue, and psychological stress
- Assess factors that can promote infection, such as impaired skin; chemotherapy radiation, and other therapy; malignancy; medications; age; chronic illness; intravenous line; urinary catheter; and other invasive procedures

TABLE 8.4: Manifestation and management of oncologic emergencies

Emergency oncologic	Clinical manifestations and findings	Management
Superior vena cava syndrome (SVCS)	**Clinical**	**Medical**
i. Compression or invasion of the superior vena cava by tumor, enlarged lymph nodes, intraluminal thrombus that obstructs venous circulation, or drainage of the head, neck, arms and thorax. Typically associated with lung cancer, SVCS can also occur with breast cancer, Kaposi's sarcoma, thymoma, lymphoma and mediastinal metastases. If untreated, SVCS may lead to cerebral oxygen reaches the brain, laryngeal edema, bronchial obstruction, and death	Gradually or suddenly impaired venous drainage giving rise to • Progressive shortness of breath (dyspnea), cough, hoarseness, chest pain, and facial swelling • Edema of the neck, arms, hands, and thorax and reported sensation of skin tightness and difficulty swallowing • Possibly engorged and distended jugular, temporal and arm veins • Dilated thoracic vessels causing prominent venous pattern on the chest wall • Increased intracranial pressure, associated visual disturbances, headache, and altered mental status Diagnosis is confirmed by • Clinical findings • Chest X-ray • Thoracic computed tomography (CT) scan • Thoracic magnetic resonance imaging (MRI) Intraluminal thrombosis is identified by venogram	• Radiation therapy to shrink tumor size and relieve symptoms • Chemotherapy for chemosensitive cancers, (e.g. lymphoma, small cell lung cancer) or when the mediastinum has been irradiated to maximum tolerance • Anticoagulant or thrombolytic therapy for intraluminal thrombosis • Surgery (less common), such as vena cava bypass graft (synthetic or autologous), to redirect blood flow around the obstruction • Supportive measures such as oxygen therapy, corticosteroids, and diuretics *Nursing interventions* • Identify patients at risk for SVCS • Monitor and report clinical manifestations of SVCS • Monitor cardiopulmonary and neurologic status • Avoid upper extremity venipuncture and blood pressure measurement • Facilitate breathing by positioning the patient properly. This helps to promote comfort and reduce anxiety produced by difficulty breathing resulting from progressive edema • Promote energy conservation to minimize shortness of breath • Monitor the patients fluid volume status and administer fluids cautiously to minimize edema • Assess for thoracic radiation-related problems such as dysphagia (difficulty swallowing) and esophagitis • Monitor for chemotherapy-related problems, such as myelosuppression • Provide postoperative care as appropriate

Contd...

Contd...

Emergency oncologic	Clinical manifestations and findings	Management
Superior vena cava syndrome (SVCS)	**Clinical**	**Medical**
ii. *Spinal cord compression:* Potentially leading to permanent neurologic impairment and associated morbidity and mortality, compression of the cord and its nerve roots may result from tumor, lymphomas, intevertebral collapse, or interruption of blood supply to the nerve tissues. The prognosis depends on the severity and rapidity of onset. About 60% of compressions occur at the thoracic level, 30% in the lumbosacral level, and 10% in the cervical region. Metastatic cancers (breast, lung, kidney, prostate, myeloma, lymphoma) and related bone erision are associated with spinal cord compression	• Local inflammation, edema, venous stasis, and impaired blood supply to nervous tissues • Local or radicular back or neck pain along the dematomal area innervated by the effected nerve root (Flounders, 2003a) (e.g. thoracic radicular pain extends in a band around the chest or abdomen) • Pain exacerbated by movement, supine recumbent position, coughing, sneezing, or the Valsalva maneuver • Neurologic dysfunction, and related motor and sensory deficits (numbness, tingling, feelings of coldness in the affected area, inability to detect vibration, loss of positional sense) • Motor loss ranging from subtle weakness to flaccid paralysis • Bladder and/or bowel dysfunction depending on level of compression (above S2, overflow incontinence; from S3 top S5, flaccid sphincter tone and bowel incontinence) *Diagnostic findings includes* • Percussion tenderness at the level of compression • Abnormal reflexes • Sensory and motor abnormalities • MRI, myelogram, spinal cord X-rays, bone scans, and CT scan	• Radiation therapy to reduce tumor size to halt progression and corticosteroid therapy to decrease inflammation and swelling at the compression site • Surgery if symptoms progress despite radiation therapy or if vertebral fracture leads to additional nerve damage; surgery is also an option when the tumor is not radio-sensitive or is located in an area that was previously irradiated Chemotherapy as adjuvant to radiation therapy for patients with lymphoma or small cell lung cancer • *Note:* Despite treatment, patients with poor neurologic function before treatment are less likely to regain complete motor and sensory function; patients who develop complete paralysis usually to not regain all neurologic function. *Nursing interventions* • Perform ongoing assessment of neurologic function to identify existing and progressing dysfunction • Control pain with pharmacologic and non-pharmacologic measures • Prevent complications of immobililty resulting from pain and decreased function (e.g. skin breakdown, urinary stasis, thrombophlebitis, decreased clearance of pulmonary secretions) • Maintain muscle tone by assisting with range-of-motion exercises in collaboration with physical and occupational therapies • Institute intermittent urinary catheterization and bowel training programs for patients with bladder or bowel dysfunction • Provide encouragement and support to patient and family coping with pain and altered functioning, lifestyle, roles and independence
iii. *Hypercalcemia:* In patients with cancer, hypercalcemia is a potentially life-threatening metabolic abnormality resulting when the calcium released from the bones is more than the kidneys can excrete or the bones can reabsorb. It may result from – Bone destruction by tumor cells and subsequent release of calcium – Production of prostaglandins and osteoclast-activating factor, which stimulate bone breakdown and calcium release – Tumors that produce parathyroid-like substanaces that promote calcium release	Fatigue, weakness, confusion, decreased level of responsiveness, hyporeflexia, nausea, vomiting, constipation, polyuria (excessive urination), polydipsia (excessive thirst), dehydration, and dysrhythmias *Diagnostic findings includes* Serum calcium level exceeding 11 mg/dL (2.74 mmol/L)	*Nursing interventions* • Identify patients at risk for hypercalcemia and assess for signs and symptoms of hypercalcemia • Educate patient and family prevention and early detection can prevent fatality • Teach at-risk patients to recognize and report signs and symptoms of hyper-calcemia • Encourage patients to consume 2–3 L of fluid daily unless contraindicated by existing renal or cardiac disease • Explain the use of dietary and pharma-cologic interventions such as stool softeners and laxatives for constipation

Contd...

Contd...

Emergency oncologic Superior vena cava syndrome (SVCS)	Clinical manifestations and findings Clinical	Management Medical
– Excessive use of vitamins and minerals and conditions unrelated to cancer, such as dehydration, renal impairment, primary hyperparathyroidism, thyrotoxicosis, thiazide diuretics, and hormone therapy		• Advise patients to maintain intake without restricting normal calcium intake • Discuss antiemetic therapy if nausea and vomiting occur • Promote mobility by emphasizing demineralization and breakdown of bones
iv. *Pericardial effusion and cardiac tamponade:* Cardiac tamponade is an accumulation of fluid in the pericardial space. The accumulation compresses the heart and thereby impedes expansion of the ventricles and cardiac filling during diastole. As ventricular volume and cardiac output fall, the heart pump fails, and circulatory collapse develops. With gradual onset, fluid accumulates gradually, and the outer layer of the pericardial space stretches to compensate for rising pressure. Large amounts of fluid accumulate before symptoms of heart failure occur. With rapid onset, pressures rise too quickly for the pericardial space to compensate Cancerous tumors, particularly from adjacent thoracic tumors (lung, esophagus, breast cancers), and cancer treatment are the most common causes of cardiac tamponade. Radiation therapy of 4000 cGy or more to the mediastinal area has also been implicated in pericardial fibrosis, pericarditis, and resultant cardiac tamponade Untreated pericardial effusion and cardiac tamponade lead to circulatory collapse and cardiac arrest	*Clinical management* • Neck vein distention during inspiration (Kussumaul's sign) • Pulsus paradoxus (systolic blood pressure decrease exceeding 10 mm Hg during inspiration; pulse gets stronger on expiration) • Distant heart sounds, rubs and gallops, cardiac dullness • Compensatory tachycardia (heart beats faster to compensate for decreased cardiac output) *Diagnostic findings includes* • Electorcardiography (ECG) helps diagnose pericardial effusion • In small effusion, chest X-rays show small amounts of fluid in the pericardium; in large effusions, X-ray films disclose "water-bottle" heart (obliteration of vessel contour and cardiac chambers) • CT scans help diagnose pleural effusions and evaluate effect of treatment • Narrow pulse pressure • Shortness of breath and tachypnea • Weakness, chest pain, orthopnea, anxiety, diaphoresis, lethargy, and altered consciousness from decreased cerebral perfusion	• Increased venous and vascular pressures • Pericardiocentesis (the aspiration or withdrawal of pericardial fluid by a large-bore needle inserted into the pericardial space). In malignant effusions, pericardiocentesis provides only temporary relief, fluid usually reaccumulates. Windows or openings in the pericardium can be created surgically as a palliative measures to drain fluid into the pleural space. Catheters may also be placed in the pericardial space and sclerosing agents (such as tetracycline, talc, bleomycin, 5-fluorouracil, or thiotepa) injected to prevent fluid from reaccumulating • Radiation therapy or antineoplastic agents, depending on how sensitive the primary tumor is to these treatments. In mild effusions, prednisone and diuretic medications may be prescribed and the patients status carefully monitored *Nursing interventions* • Monitor vital signs and oxygen saturation frequently • Assess for pulsus paradoxus • Assess heart and lung sounds, and skin color and temperature • Monitor and record intake and output • Review laboratory findings (e.g. arterial blood gas and electrolyte levels) • Elevate the head of the patients bed to ease breathing • Minimize patients physical activity to reduce oxygen requirements, administer supplemental oxygen as prescribed • Provide frequent oral hygiene • Reposition and encourage the patient to cough and take deep breaths every 2 hours • As needed, maintain patent IV access, measures and appropriate patient instruction
v. *Disseminated intravascular coagulation (DIC, also called consumption coagulopathy)*	*Chronic DIC:* Few or no observable symptoms or easy bruising, prolonged bleeding from venipuncture and injection sites, bleeding of the gums, and slow GI bleeding	• Chemotherapy, biologic response modifier therapy, or surgery is used to treat the underlying cancer • Antibiotic therapy is used for sepsis

Contd...

Contd...

Emergency oncologic Superior vena cava syndrome (SVCS)	Clinical manifestations and findings Clinical	Management Medical
Complex disorder of coagulation or fibrinolysis (destruction of clots), which results in thrombosis or bleeding. DIC is most commonly associated with hematologic cancers (leukemia); cancer of prostate, gastrointestinal (GI) tract, and lungs; chemotherapy (methotrexate, prednisone, l-asparaginase, vincristine, and 6-mercaptopurine); and disease processes such as sepsis, hepatic failure, and anaphylaxis Blood clots form when normal coagulation mechanisms are triggered. Once activated, the clotting cascade continues to consume clotting factors and platelets faster than the body can replace them. Clots are deposited in the microvasculature, placing the patient at great risk for impaired circulation, tissue hypoxia, and necrosis. In addition, fibrinolysis occurs, breaking down clots and increasing the circulating levels of anticoagulant substances, thereby placing the patient at risk for hemorrhage	*Acute DIC:* Life-threatening hemorrhage and infarction; clinical symptoms of this syndrome are varied and depend on the organ system involved in thrombus and infarction or bleeding episodes *Diagnostic findings includes* • Prolonged prothrombin time (PT or protime) • Prolonged partial thromboplastin time (PTT) • Prolonged thrombin time (TT) • Decreased fibrinogen level • Decreased platelet level • Decrease in clotting factors • Decreased hemoglobin • Decreased hematocrit • Elevated fibrin split products • Positive protamine sulfate precipitation test (thrombin activation tests)	• Anticoagulants, such as heparin or antithrombin III, decrease the stimulation of the coagulation pathways • Transfusion of fresh-frozen plasma or cryoprecipitates (which contain clotting factors and fibrinogen), packed red blood cells, and platelets may be used as replacement therapy to prevent or control bleeding • Although controversial, antifibrinolytic agents such as aminocaproic acid (Amicar), which is associated with increased thrombus formation, may be used *Nursing interventions* • Monitor vital signs • Measure and document intake and output • Assess skin color and temperature, lung, heart, and bowel sounds; level of consciousness, headache, visual disturbances, chest pain, decreased urine output, and abdominal tenderness • Inspect all body orifices, tube insertion sites, incisions, and bodily excretions for bleeding • Review laboratory test results • Minimize physical activity to decrease injury risks and oxygen requirements • Prevent bleeding; apply pressure to all venipuncture sites, and avoid nonessential invasive procedures; provide electric rather than straight-edged razors; avoid tape on the skin and advise gentle but adequate oral hygiene • Assist the patient to turn, cough, and take deep breaths every 2 hours • Reorient the patient, if needed; maintain a safe environment; and provide appropriate patient education and supportive measures
vi. *Syndrome of inappropriate secretion of antidiuretic hormone (SIADH)* The continuous, uncontrolled release of antidiuretic hormone (ADH), produced by tumor cells or by the abnormal stimulation of the hypothalamic-pituitary network, leads to increased extracellular fluid volume, water intoxication, hyponatremia, and increased excretion of urinary sodium. As fluid volume increases, stretch receptors in the right atrium respond by releasing a second hormone, atrial natriuretic factor (ANF). The release of ANF causes increased renal excretion of sodium, which worsens hyponatremia	*Serum sodium levels lower than* 120 mEq/L (120 mmol/L: symptoms of hyponatremia including personality changes, irritability, nausea, anorexia, vomiting, weight gain, fatigue, muscular pain (myalgia), headache, lethargy and confusion *Serum sodium levels lower than* 110 mEq/L (110 mmol/L): seizure, abnormal reflexes, papilledema, coma, and death, edema is rare	Fluid intake range limited to 500–1000 mL/day to increase the serum sodium level and decrease fluid overload. If water restriction alone is not effective in correcting or controlling serum sodium levels, demeclocycline is often prescribed to interfere with the antidiuretic action of ADH and ANF. If neurologic symptoms are severe, parenteral sodium replacement and diuretic therapy are indicated. Electrolyte levels are monitored carefully to detect secondary magnesium, potassium and calcium imbalances. After the symptoms of SIADH are controlled, the underlying cancer is treated. If water excess continues despite treatment, pharmacologic intervention (urea and furosemide) may be indicated

Contd...

Contd...

Emergency oncologic	Clinical manifestations and findings	Management
Superior vena cava syndrome (SVCS)	**Clinical**	**Medical**
The most common cause of SIADH is cancer, especially small cell cancers of the lung. Antineoplastics—vincristine, vinblastine, cisplatin, and cyclophosphamide and morphine also stimulate ADH secretions, which promotes conservation and reabsorption of water by the kidneys. As more fluid is absorbed, the circulatory volume increases, ANF is released, and sodium is actively excreted by the kidneys in compensation	*Diagnostic findings includes* • Decreased serum sodium level • Increased urine osmolality • Increased urinary sodium level • Decreased blood urea nitrogen (BUN), creatinine, and serum albumin levels secondary to dilution • Abnormal water load test results	*Nursing interventions* • Maintain intake and output measurements • Assess level of consciousness, lung and heart sounds, vital signs, daily weight, and urine specific gravity, also assess for nausea, vomiting, anorexia, edema, fatigue, and lethargy • Monitor laboratory test results, including serum electrolyte levels, osmolality, and BUN, creatinine, and urinary sodium levels • Minimize the patients activity; provide appropriate oral hygiene; maintain environmental safety; and restrict fluid intake, if necessary • Reorient the patient and provide instruction and encouragement as needed
vii. *Tumor lysis syndrome:* Potentially fatal complication associated with radiation or chemotherapy-induced cell destruction of large or rapidly growing cancers such as leukemia, lymphoma and small cell lung cancer. The release of intracellular contents from the tumor cells lead to electrolyte imbalances—hyperkalemia, hypocalcemia, hyperphosphatemia, and hyperuricemia—because the kidneys can no longer excrete large volume of the released intracellular metabolites	Clinical manifestations depend on the extent of metabolic abnormalities. • Neurologic: Fatigue, weakness, memory loss, altered mental status, muscle cramps, tetany, paresthesias (numbness and tingling), seizures • Cardiac: elevated blood pressure, shortened QT complexes, widened QRS waves, dysrhythmias, cardiac arrest • GI: Anorexia, nausea, vomiting, abdominal cramps, diarrhea • Renal: Flank pain, oliguria, anuria, renal failure, acidic urine pH *Diagnostic findings includes* Electrolyte imbalances identified by laboratory test results	• To prevent renal failure and restore electrolyte balance, aggressive fluid hydration is initiated 48 hours before and after the initiation of cytotoxic therapy to increase urine volume and eliminate uric acid and electrolyes. Urine is alkalinized by adding sodium bicarbonate to IV fluid to maintain a urine pH of 7 or higher; this prevents renal failure secondary to uric acid precipitation in the kidneys • Diuretic therapy, with a carbonic anhydrase inhibitor or acetazolamide, to alkalinize the urine • Allopurinol therapy to inhibit the conversion of nucleic acids to uric acid • Administration of a action-exchange resin, such as sodium polystyrene sulfonate (kayexalate) to treat hyperkalemia by binding and eliminating potassium through the bowel • Administration of hypertonic dextrose and regular insulin temporarily shifts potassium into cells and lowers serum potassium levels • Administration of phosphate-binding gels, such as aluminum hydroxide, to treat hyperphosphatemia by promoting phosphate exertion in the feces • Hemodialysis when patients are unresponsive to the standard approaches for managing uric acid and electrolyte abnormalities *Nursing interventions* • Identify at-risk patients, including those in whom tumor lysis syndrome may develop up to 1 week after therapy has been completed • Institute essential preventive measures (e.g. fluid hydration, allpurinol) • Assess patient for signs and symptoms of electrolyte imbalances • Assess urine pH to confirm alkalinization • Monitor serum electrolyte and uric acid levels for evidence of fluid volume overload secondary to aggressive hydration • Instruct patients to report symptoms indicating electrolyte disturbances

- Monitor laboratory studies (e.g. WBC count for leukopenia or neutropenia)
- Frequently assess common sites of infection (e.g. pharynx, skin, perianal area, urinary tract, respiratory tract) for signs of infection (fever, swelling, redness, drainage, pain)
- Monitor patient for sepsis, particularly if invasive catheters of infusion lines are in place.

Bleeding

- Assess patient for factors that may contribute to bleeding (e.g. bone marrow suppression from radiation, chemotherapy, and medications such as aspirin, dipyridamole [Persantinel], heparin, or warfarin [Coumadin])
- Monitor common bleeding sites (e.g. skin, mucous membranes; intestinal, urinary, and respiratory tracts; brain)
- Monitor and report gross hemorrhage as well as blood in the stools, urine, sputum, or vomitus (melena, hematuria, hemoptysis, hematemesis), oozing at injection sites, bruising (ecchymosis), petechiae, and changes in mental status.

Skin Breakdown

- Assess patient for risk factors for decreased skin integrity (e.g. therapy effects, invasive diagnostic procedures, nutritional deficits, bowel and bladder incontinence, immobility, immunosuppression, and changes related to aging).
- Note skin lesions or ulcerations secondary to the tumor or therapy, particularly alteration throughout the gastrointestinal tract (e.g. oral mucous membranes), as well as their effects on the patient's nutritional status and comfort level
- Note any alopecia (hair loss) and assess the psychological impact of this side effect on the patient and family.

Nutritional Status

- Assess patient's nutritional status (weight, caloric intake and diet history, anorexia, changes in appetite) and cachexia (wasting, emaciation). Impaired nutritional status may contribute to disease progression and a multitude of complications
- Assess situations and foods that aggravate or relieve anorexia
- Review patients medication history
- Determine difficulty in chewing or swallowing nausea, vomiting, or diarrhea
- Assess clinical and laboratory data related to nutritional status (e.g. anthropometric measurements [triceps skin fold and middle-upper arm circumference], serum protein levels [albumin and transferrin], lymphocyte count, skin response to intradermal injection of antigens, hemoglobin levels, hematocrit, urinary creatinine levels, and serum iron levels).

Pain, Fatigue, and Attitude

- Assess the level (pain assessment scale), source, and site of pain and factors that increase the patient's perception of pain (e.g. fear and apprehension, fatigue, anger, and social isolation)
- Assess for feelings of weariness, weakness, lack of energy inability to carry out necessary and valued daily functions, lack of motivation, and inability to concentrate
- Assess physiologic and psychological stressors that can contribute to fatigue, including pain, nausea, dyspnea, fear, and anxiety or constipation
- Assess patient's mood and emotional reaction to the results of diagnostic testing and prognosis
- Assess patient's progress through the stages of grief and ability to talk about the diagnosis and prognosis with family
- Identify potential threats to self-concept and body image, and assess patient's ability to cope with these changes.

Nursing Diagnoses

Based on the assessment data, nursing diagnoses of the patient with cancer may include the following:

- Impaired tissue integrity (oral mucous membranes, alopecia, malignant skin lesions) related to the effects of treatment and the disease
- Imbalanced nutrition: Less than body requirements related to anorexia, malabsorption, and cachexia
- Pain or chronic pain related to diseases and treatment effects
- Fatigue related to physical and psychological stressors
- Disturbed body image related to changes in appearance and role functions
- Anticipatory grieving related to expected loss and altered role function.

Based on the assessment data, potential complication that may develop include the following:

- Infection and sepsis
- Hemorrhage
- Superior vena cava syndrome
- Spinal cord compression
- Hypercalcemia
- Pericardial effusion
- Disseminated intravascular coagulation
- Syndrome of inappropriate secretion of antidiuretic hormone
- Tumor lysis syndrome.

Goals

The major goals of the patient may include maintenance of tissue integrity, management of stomatitis, maintenance of nutrition, relief of pain, relief of fatigue, improved body image, progression through the grieving process and absence of complication.

Objectives

- Maintains adequate tissue (skin and mucous membrane integrity)
- Maintains adequate nutritional status
- Achieves relief of pain and discomfort
- Demonstrates increased activity tolerance and decreased fatigue
- Progresses through grieving process
- Exhibits improved body image and self-esteem
- Experiences no complications, such as inflammation, infection, or sepsis, and no episodes of bleeding or hemorrhage.

(For Nursing care plan of cancer client see Table 8.5).

TABLE 8.5: Nursing care plan of cancer client

Problem	Reason	Objective	Nursing intervention	Evaluation
1. Pain related to effects of disease or its treatment	• As manifested by facial mask, complains of pain, guarding	• Reduction of pain to a tolerable and manageable level	• Assess the pain to provide a baseline treatment • Confront and correct fears of addiction to reduce the possibility of understanding the patient's pain • Use an analgesic ladder (1. non-opioid 2. weak opioid 3. strong opioid) • Teach patient complementary pain management techniques (imagery, relaxation, biofeedback, etc. to augment pain management strategies	
2. Altered nutrition, body requirement related to anorexia and other symptoms	• Anorexia nausea, vomiting as manifested by fatigue • Inadequate food intake requirement with or without weight loss	• Maintenance of body weight and adequate energy of ADL • Decreased episodes of nausea and vomiting	• Avoid punitive or judgemental statements about food intake or weight loss • Administer antiemetic medication as prescribed to minimize GI effects • Maintain pleasant, quiet, restful environment to avoid triggering nausea and vomiting and to allow maximum rest • Modify diet to include bland, lukewarm, high calorie, high protein foods to prevent triggering vomiting and provide additional calories • Try small frequent feedings every few hours rather than fewer larger meals to facilitate gastric emptying and prevent early satiety • Teach patient to eat and drink slowly to allow patient to enjoy taste and to prevent bloating • Ensure adequate fluid hydration with chemotherapy to dilute drug level and reduce stimulation of vomiting receptor • Provide a well-balanced diet that includes all food groups with increased protein-caloric intake to promote positive nitrogen balance • Gently encourage patient to eat but avoid nagging to prevent establishing a negative meal environment • Avoid foods that are gas forming, such as salads, cabbage, broccoli, fruits and bear, because they can promote nausea and a sense of fullness • Serve all foods attractively and in a pleasant environment to stimulate appetite • Teach the patient to sip the nutritional supplement slowly between meals to avoid bloating	

Contd...

Contd...

Problem	Reason	Objective	Nursing intervention	Evaluation
			• Teach the patient what to eat rather than stressing the fact that more food should be eaten (advise home prepared items)	
3. Ineffective management of therapeutic regimen related to lack of knowledge of long-term management of cancer	• As manifested by frequent questions by patients and care given regarding – Self care – treatment – Side effects – Observed inability, etc.	• Patient and nurses express confidence in management of cancer patient • Adequate knowledge base to provide care	• Determine the knowledge and technical skills needed by patient and nurses to plan needed instruction • Assess current level of knowledge and skill to determine the abilities and of patient and caregivers to perform tasks correctly • Teach required skills and provide information to patient and caregiver to increase their knowledge level • Provide opportunity for follow-up evaluation and teaching to increase patient/caregiver confidence and ensure correct performance task	
4. Altered oral mucous membrane related to chemotherapy or radiation therapy	• As manifested by verbalization or signs of pain or discomfort in mouth-coated tongue, xerostomia, halitosis, swollen membranes, oral lesions, hemorrhagic gingivitis, leukoplakia, stomatitis	• No oral pain • No infection in oral mucosa • No break in integrity of oral mucosa	• Assess oral mucosa daily • Teach patient to inspect oral cavity because stomatitis occurs 4 to 14 days after treatment begins • Remove dentures at night to avoid further irritation • Observe for dryness, redness and white or yellow membrane and the presence of any breaks in integrity of tissues • Distinguish stomatitis from candidiasis and other oral problems, such as xerostomia and herpes for appropriate treatment • Use mouthwashes of baking soda and lime, or normal saline solution every 2 hours to provide comfort • Use soft-bristle-toothbrushes, sponge-tipped applicators, or an irrigation syringe as cleansing agents to prevent trauma • Avoid the use of lemon and glycerin swabs for mouth care because they increase dryness and irritation • Apply topical anesthetics such as viscous xylocaine as ordered to provide pain relief • Modify diet to avoid hot, spicy acidic foods to avoid irritation • Discourage use of irritants such as tobacco and alcohol • Encourage drinking of water or other liquids at frequent intervals to keep moist the mucous membrane • Apply small amount of petroleum jelly lip gloss or moisturizes to lips to promote comfort and prevent dryness • Help patient select clothing and colors that minimize weightloss or effects of disfiguring surgery • Assure patient that value as a person is not associated with external appearance • Discuss expected physical changes with family members and advise them of ways to assist patient with acceptance to prepare the family and to foster family relationships	

Contd...

Contd...

Problem	Reason	Objective	Nursing intervention	Evaluation
5. Fatigue related to the effects of cancer or its treatment	As manifested by verbal report of lack of energy and inability to maintain usual routine	Satisfactory activity level relative to phase of disease or environment	• Inform the patient that fatigue is an expected side effects of therapy and that it usually begins during the first week of therapy, reaches its peak in 2 weeks, continues and then gradually disappears 2 to 4 weeks after treatment has been ended • Encourage patient to rest when fatigued, to maintain usual lifestyle pattern as closely as possible and to pace activities in accordance with energy level because rest periods are essential to conserve energy	
6. Ineffective individual coping related to depression secondary to diagnosis and treatment	• Uncertain outcome of treatment • Disruption in life-style, or • Financial burden as manifested by verbalized or observed inability to manage effective components of diagnosis and resulting symptoms, threats or attempts to commit suicide, concern over financial implications of disease	• Appropriate response to problems • Able to seek and/or accept support and assistance	• Have patient direct own care when possible to encourage patient independence. – Provide information to allow patient to make informed choices regarding treatment regimen and plan of care – Facilitate communication between patient and family to foster a supportive network – Assess and mobilize patient's support systems – Refer patient to social services for financial assistance if appropriate to provide additional resources – Assess need for further counseling	
7. Body-image disturbance related to hair loss, disfiguring surgery and weight loss	As manifested by expressions of concern with changes in body; refusal to interact with visitors, isolation, frequent crying, refusal to care of self or to look in mirror	Able to verbalize acceptance of changes in body appearance and function	• Provide psychologic support and prepare patient for expected hairloss to lessen shock of event when it occurs • Encourage patients to select a wig and begin to wear it before hair-loss begins and to wear a scarf or turban to conceal hair loss • Use a mild, motion-based shampoo, cream rinse, and hair conditioner every 4 to 7 days to avoid drying remaining hair • Avoid excessive shampooing, brushing and combing of hair to reduce hair loss • Avoid use of electric hair dryers, curlers, curling rods, and hair spray to minimize scalp irritations and decrease hair loss. • Help patient select clothing and colors that minimize weightloss or effects of disfiguring surgery • Assure patient that value as a person is not associated with external appearance • Discuss expected physical changes with family members and advise them of ways to assist patient with acceptance to prepare the family and to foster family relationships	

Contd...

Contd...

Problem	Reason	Objective	Nursing intervention	Evaluation
8. Altered family process related to cancer diagnosis of family member	As manifested by observed communication problem among family members, lack of family support related to physical, emotional and for spiritual needs of the patient	• Family members communicate about patient and cooperate in care of the patient • Family will seek outside help when needed	• Assess family structure and support system to determine amount and quality of support available to patient • Teach needed skills to family members • Provide opportunities for discussion of caregiving and emotional implications of role changes to promote verbalization of feelings and shared understanding of problems • Assist family members to set realistic expectations for patient and themselves • Provide guidance on course of disease and anticipated outcome so planning can be accomplished	
9. Risk for infection related to lukopenia, depressed immune system and multiple exposure to microscope	(Please see concerned chapters for NCP)			
10. Potential for bleeding related to thrombocytopenia				
11. Potential for hyperuricemia related to chemotherapy		• Monitor signs of hyperuricemia • Report deviations from acceptable parameters • Carry out medical and nursing interventions	• Monitor for high level uric acid excretion in urine, high serum uric acid excretion in urine, high serum uric acid, obstructed uropathy, decreased urine output, nausea vomiting, lethargy • Record intake and output to determine fluid balance • Encourage fluids to prevent uric acid crystals from causing obstruction • Evaluate blood urea nitrogen (BUN) and serum creatinin levels to identify early changes in renal functions • Administer allopurinol (Zyloprim) as ordered to reduce endogenous uric acid production	

Nursing Interventions

Maintaining Tissue Integrity

Some of the most frequently encountered disturbance include skin and tissue reactions to radiation therapy, mucositis, stomatitis, alopecia, and metastatic skin lesions.

- Provide careful skin care to prevent further skin irritation, drying, and damage. Handle skin over the affected area gently; avoid rubbing and use of hot or cold water, soaps, powders, lotions and cosmetics
- Instruct patient to wear loose-fitting clothes and avoid clothes that constrict, irritate, or rub the affected area
- Provide aseptic wound care (moisture, vapor-permeable dressing and topical antibiotics, as ordered) on area of moist desquamation (painful, red, moist skin).

Take care not to disrupt any blisters present to reduce the risk of introducing bacteria.

Managing Stomatitis

- Instruct patient on, and assist patient with good oral hygiene (brushing with soft-bristled toothbrush and nonabrasive toothpaste)
- Use oral swabs with spongelike applicators in place of a toothbrush for painful oral tissues, or tissues, or oral rinses with saline solution or tap water
- Assist patient with flossing, unless it causes pain or unless platelet levels are below 40,000/mm^3
- Avoid products or foods that irritate or traumatize oral tissues or impair healing, such as alcohol-based mouth rinses and food that is difficult to chew or too hot or spicy

- Lubricate patients lips to keep the tissues from becoming dry and cracked. Use a topical anti-inflammatory agent and anesthetic agents if prescribed. Products that coat or protect oral mucosa are used to facilitate comfort and to promote healing and minimize discomfort. Give systemic analgesics as required
- Encourage adequate fluid and food intake; administer parenteral hydration and nutrition as ordered
- Administer topical or systemic antifungal and antibiotic drugs or other medications, such as IV palifermin, to promote replacement of cells in the mouth and GI tract, as prescribed to treat local or systemic infections.

Addressing Alopecia

- Provide information about alopecia (include that hair usually begins to regrow after completing therapy, although the color and texture of the new hair may be different), and support the patient and family in coping with disturbing effects of therapy
- Encourage patient to acquire a wig or hairpiece before hair loss occurs so that the replacement matches patient's own hair. Suggest that the use of attractive scarves and hats may make the patient feel less conspicuous
- Refer patients to supportive programs.

Managing Malignant Skin Lesions

- Carefully assess and cleanse the skin, reducing superficial bacteria, controlling bleeding, reducing odor, and protecting skin from pain and further trauma
- Assist and guide the patient and family regarding care for these skin lesions at home; refer for home care as indicated.

Promoting Nutrition

- Assist in selecting foods that patient might eat despite altered sense of taste and smell and decreased appetite
- Explain how to prepare foods so they look and taste appealing; also discuss ways to avoid unpleasant smells
- Include family members in the plan of care to encourage adequate food intake
- Consider patient's preferences as well as physiologic and metabolic requirements in selecting foods
- Provide and encourage patient to eat small, frequent meals with supplements between meals
- Offer oral hygiene and pain relief measures before mealtime to make meals more pleasant
- Use additional strategies as indicated (e.g. changing the feeding schedule, using simple diets, and relieving diarrhea).
- Administer enzyme and vitamin replacement if ordered for malabsorption; administer parenteral nutrition (PN) if ordered for severe malabsorption
- Teach patient and family how to care for venous access devices and how to administer PN; refer for home care nurses to assist with or supervise PN in the home, as needed
- Before invasive nutritional strategies are instituted assess patient carefully and discuss the options with patient and family (creative dietary therapies, enteral [tube] feedings or PN)
- Direct nursing care toward preventing trauma, infection, and other complications that increase metabolic demands.

Relieving Pain

- Use a multidisciplinary team approach to determine optimal management of pain for optimal quality of life
- Help patient and family play an active role in managing pain
- Provide educations and support to correct fears and misconceptions about opioid use.

Decreasing Fatigue

- Help patient and family to understand that fatigue is usually an expected and temporary side effect of the cancer process and treatments
- Help patient to identify sources of fatigue and develop ways to conserve energy
- Help patient plan daily activities, alternating periods of rest and activity
- Encourage regular, light exercise, which may decrease fatigue and facilitate coping
- Encourage patient to maintain normal lifestyle as possible by continuing with activities he or she values and enjoys
- Encourage patient and family to plan to reallocate responsibilities, such as child care, cleaning, and preparing meals. A patient who is employed full-time may need to reduce to number of hours worked each week
- Assist patient and family in coping with these changing roles and responsibilities
- Address factors that contribute to fatigue and implement pharmacologic and nonpharmacologic strategies to manage pain
- Provide nutrition counseling to patient's who are not eating enough calories or protein; small, frequent meals require less energy for digestion
- Monitor serum hemoglobin and hematocrit levels for deficiencies, and administer blood products as prescribed
- Monitor patient for alterations in oxygenation and electrolyte balances
- Arrange for physical therapy and assistive devices if patient has impaired mobility.

Improving Body Image and Self-Esteem

A positive approach is essential when caring for the patient with a disturbed body image. To help the patient retain control and a sense of self-worth, encourage independence and continued participation in self-care and decision making.

- Assist patient to assume tasks and participate in activities that are valuable to him or her
- Encourage patient to express any negative feelings or threats to body image
- Serve as a listener and counselor to patient and family
- Refer patient and family to a support group for additional assistance in coping with the changes resulting from cancer or its treatment
- Consult with a cosmetologist, who might provide ideas about hair or wig styling, make-up and the use of scarves and turbans to help with body image concerns
- Encourage patients who are experiencing disturbances in sexuality and sexual function to share and discuss concerns openly with their partner. Explore alternative forms of sexual expression with patient and partner to promote self-worth and acceptance
- Assist patient and partner in seeking further counseling if serious physiological, psychological, or communication difficulties related to sexuality or sexual function are identified.

Assisting in Grieving

- Answer question and clarify information provided by the physician
- Assess response of patient and family to the diagnosis and planned treatment, and assist them in framing their questions and concerns
- Identify resources and support people (e.g. clergy, counselor, and other support available through hospitals and various community organizations)
- Assist patient and family with communicating and sharing their concerns with each other. Encourage patient and family to express their feelings in an atmosphere of trust and support
- If patient enters the terminal phase of disease, assist patient and family to come to grips with their reactions and feelings. (physical support, such as holding the patient's hand just being with the patient at home or at the bedside)
- Maintain contact with the surviving family members after death of the patient. This may help them to work through their feelings of loss and grief.

Monitoring and Managing Potential Complications

- Use strict asepsis when handling intravenous lines, catheters, and other invasive equipment
- Avoid exposing the patient to others with an active infection and to crowds
- Place patients with profound immunosuppression, such as recipients of bone marrow transplants, in a protective environment in which the room and its contents are sterilized and the air is filtered
- Provide immunosuppressed patients with low-bacteria diets. Avoid fresh fruits and vegetables
- Avoid invasive procedures, such as injections, vaginal or rectal examinations, rectal temperatures, and surgery
- Encourage patient to do coughing and deep-breathing exercises frequently to prevent respiratory problems
- Teach patients and family that cancer is not contagious
- Teach patient and family to recognize signs and symptoms of infection to report, to perform effective hand washing, to use antipyretic agents, to maintain skin integrity, and to self-administer hematopoietic growth factors when indicated.

Managing Septic Shock

- Assess frequently for infection and inflammation throughout the course of the disease
- Prevent septicemia and septic shock, or detect and report for prompt treatment
- Monitor for signs and symptoms of septic shock (altered mental status, either subnormal or elevated temperature, cool and clammy skin, decreased urine output, hypotension, dysrhythmias, electrolyte imbalances, and abnormal arterial blood gas values)
- Instruct patient and family about signs of septicemia, methods for preventing infection, and actions to take if infection or septicemia occurs.

Managing Bleeding and Hemorrhage

- Monitor laboratory values, and continue to asses patient for bleeding
- Prevent trauma and minimize the risk of bleeding by encouraging the patient to use a soft (not stiff) toothbrush and an electric (not straight-edged) razor
- Avoid unnecessary invasive procedures (e.g. rectal temperatures, intramuscular injections, and catheterization)
- Assist patient and family to identify and remove environmental hazards that may led to falls or other trauma
- Provide soft foods, increased fluid intake, and stool softeners, if prescribed, to reduce trauma to the gastrointestinal tract
- Handle and move the joints and extremities gently to minimize the risk for spontaneous bleeding
- Monitor serum hemoglobin and hematocrit carefully for changes indicating blood loss
- Test all urine, stool, and emesis for occult blood
- Perform neurologic assessments to detect changes in orientation and behavior
- Administer fluids and blood products as prescribed to replace any losses and vasopressor drugs and supplemental oxygen as prescribed to maintain blood pressure and ensure tissue oxygenation.

Promoting Home and Community-based Care

Teaching patients self-care

- Provide information needed by patient and family to address the most immediate care needs likely to be encountered at home
- Verbally review, and reinforce with written information, the side effects of treatments and changes in the patients status that should be reported
- Discuss strategies to deal with side effects to treatment with patient and family
- Identify learning needs based on the priorities identified by patient and family as well as on the complexity of home care
- Instruct patient and family and provide ongoing support that allows them to feel comfortable and proficient in managing treatments at home
- Refer for home care nursing to provide care and support for patients receiving advanced technical care
- Provide follow-up visits and phone calls to patient and family, and evaluate patient progress and ongoing needs.

Continuing Care

- Refer patient for home care (assessment of the home environment, suggestions for modifications to assist patient and family in addressing patients physical needs, care, and ongoing assessment of the psychological and emotional effects of the illness on patient and the family)
- Assess adequacy of pain management and the effectiveness of other strategies to prevent or manage side effects of treatment
- Help coordinate patient care by maintaining close communication with all health care providers involved in the patients care
- Make referrals and coordinate available community resources (e.g. local office of the American Cancer Society, home aides, church groups, and support groups) to assist patients and caregivers.

CHAPTER

9

Respiratory Nursing

INTRODUCTION

The act of breathing involves two inter-related processes, ventilation and respiration—ventilation is the movement of air into and out of lungs. Respiration refers to the exchange of oxygen and carbon dioxide across cell membrane. The primary purpose of the respiratory system is gas exchange, which involves the transfer of oxygen and carbon dioxide between the atmosphere and blood. The respiratory system is divided into two parts, i.e. the upper respiratory tract and lower respiratory tract. The upper respiratory tract includes the nose, pharynx, adenoids, tonsils, epiglottis, larynx and trachea. The lower respiratory tract consists of bronchi, bronchioles, alveolar ducts and alveoli. With the exception of the right and left main stem bronchi, all lower airway structures are contained in the lungs. The right lung is divided into three lobes—upper, middle and lower and the left lung into two lobes—upper and lower. The structure of the chest walls (ribs, pleura, muscle of respiration) are also essential to respiration (Fig. 9.1).

ASSESSMENT OF RESPIRATORY SYSTEM

Respiratory assessment should be tailored to the individual's health status. The most common symptoms or reasons, a person seeks health care include dyspnea, cough, sputum production, hemoptysis, wheezing or chest pain. Upper airways symptoms may include obstruction of noses, nasal discharge, sinus pain, sore throat or hoarseness.

Dyspnea

Dyspnea means breathlessness, but the terms used to describe difficult or labored breathing observable by others. It may cause other problems such as constipation or poor nutrition, as well as psychosocial problem related to poor self-esteem or changes in lifestyle. Individuals experiencing pulmonary dysfunctions, such as breathlessness, tend to perceive their illness in terms of its impact on their ability to carry out activities of daily living. Which includes:

- Bathe, dress and groom
- Walk or exercise
- Prepare meals and rest
- Getting into home or
- Sleep
- Perform chores or hobbies
- Get to the bathroom
- Maintain family and social relationships
- Maintain employment climbing stairs
- Perform scanality
- Attend activities away from home.

Analysis of dyspnea according to its time and characteristics:

i. *Timing:* Chronic or acute, episodic or paroxysmal, onset, duration and frequency.
ii. *Characteristics:*
   - Perceived severity
   - Phases of respiratory cycle—inspiratory, expiratory, throughout cycle.

Other symptoms related to dyspnea:

- *Associated factors:*
  - Time of day
  - Seasonal or weather changes
  - Environmental irritants
  - Anxiety
  - Body position
    - Paroxysmal nocturnal dyspnea (PND). Sudden onset while sleeping in recumbent position.
    - Orthopnea: Breathlessness on assuming recumbent position.
  - Activity.

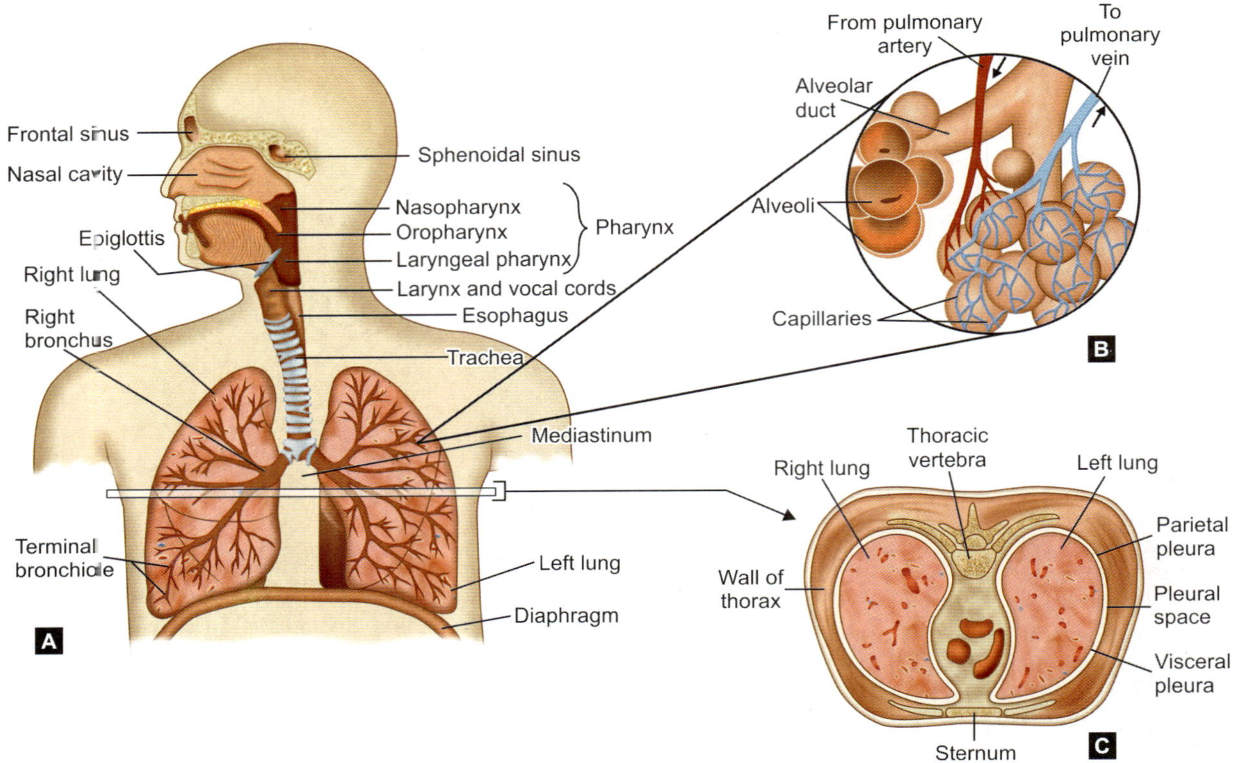

FIGS 9.1A TO C: The respiratory system. (A) Upper respiratory structures and the structures of the thorax; (B) Alveoli; (C) A horizontal cross section of the lungs

Cough

Coughing has two main functions. It protects the lungs from aspiration and it helps propel foreign matter and excess mucus up through the airways. The individual can describe the cough in terms of timing and characteristics as follows:

i. *Timing:* Chronic, acute, paroxysmal (periodic forceful episode difficult to control) onset (gradual or sudden).
ii. *Characteristics:*
   - Perceived severity
   - Pattern, occasional, upon rising, with activity (talking, exercising, eating)
iii. *Quality:*
   - Productive, non-productive
   - Dry progression to productive
   - Barking
   - Hoarse
   - Hacking
iv. *Other symptoms:*
   - Chest tightness
   - Fever, coryza
   - Choking.

Sputum Production

The mucus blanket lines the epithelial layer of the tracheobronchial tree and cleanses it of inhaled particles and debris. Mucus is produced by the goblet cells and submucosal glands. The cilia propel the mucous (which contains foreign particles, pus, blood and debris) upward toward the pharynx where it is coughed up, suctioned or swallowed. Normal sputum is clear and thin and average 100 mL/day. However, individuals with pulmonary disease often have sputum associated with these conditions making it important to assess the baseline super characteristics, describes as thick, viscous (gelatinous) tenacious (sticky), frothy, mucoid (colorless, clear, non-infectious watery, mucopurulent, and casts (from bronchioles, rubbery).

The mucopurulent sputum may be:

- *Creamy yellow: Staphylococcus pneumoniae*
- *Green: Pseudomonas pneumoniae*
- *Currentjelly: Klebsiella pneumoniae*
- *Rusty:* Pneumococcal pneumonia
- *Pink frothy:* Pulmonary edema.

The quantity of amount of sputum may be teaspoon, tablespoon or cups used as a measurement.

Hemoptysis

Hemoptysis is the coughing up of blood or blood-tinged sputum. It may contain air bubbles. The source of bleeding may be from anywhere in the upper or lower airways or from the lung parenchyma. Blood that originates in the GI tract and is coughed up as dark brown or resembling coffee grains in appearance termed as 'hematemesis'. It is usually never frothy, may be mixed with food particles, pH acidic dark-red or coffee colored. Bleeding from the nares (epistaxis) should be assessed as a cause for coughing up blood or vomiting of blood.

In hemoptysis, blood is usually frothy, pH alkaline, bright red. The coughing up of 400–1600 mL of blood in 24 hours period is considered massive and severe, needs immediate medical attention.

Wheezing

Wheezing is a continuous high-pitched, whistling sound produced when air passes through narrowed or obstructed airways. It is generally occurring during expiration, however, wheezing can be heard throughout respiratory cycle. Wheezing is usually heard with a stethoscope; however, wheezing may be audible to the person or heard by others in close proximity to the person. An analysis of this symptom should include factors that can cause bronchospasm and produce wheezing such as asthma, exposure to physiological irritants, stress, anxiety. Snoring or stridor cloud snoring may be experienced.

Chest Pain

Chest pain can result from several conditions. Chest pain may be cardiac origin. The chest pain of pulmonary origin can originate from the chest wall. Parietal pleura or lung parenchyma. The characteristics of pulmonary chest pain are:

- Pain from the chest wall is well-localized, constant ache increasing with movement. It may be due to trauma, cough and herpes zoster
- Pain in parietal pleura is a sharp, abrupt onset, increasing with inspiration or with sudden ventilatory effort (cough, sneeze) unilateral
- Pain from lung parenchyma is dull, constant poorly localized in benign pulmonary tumors and carcinoma; well-localized sharp, sudden onset in pneumothorax; sudden onset, increasing stabbing pain on inspiration, may radiate in cases of pulmonary embolus and infarction.

In addition to review of symptom or reason the person is seeking health care, the person should be interviewed about risk factors associated with respiratory dysfunction, including smoking, past pulmonary illnesses or exposure to respiratory infections, predisposition to genetic disorders, exposure to environmental irritants (dust, fume, gases, etc.) and the psychosocial effects of respiration disorders.

The emotional responses include anxiety, depression, hostility, fear or panic, etc. and ask the person's problems with swallowing and ambulating as well as neuromuscular diseases.

The common abnormalities of the thorax and lungs found by physical examinations are as follows:

Inspection

- *Pursed-lip breathing:* It is an exhalation through mouth with lips pursed together to slow exhalation. As seen in chronic obstructive pulmonary disease (COPD), asthma suggests increasing breathlessness. Strategy taught is slow expiration, decrease dyspnea
- *Tripod position:* Inability to be flat, i.e. leaning forward, with arms and elbows supported on overbed table. Seen in COPD, asthma in exacerbations, pulmonary edema, indicates moderate to severe respiratory distress
- *Accessory muscle use:* In intercostal retractions neck and shoulder muscles are used to assist breathing. Muscles between ribs pull in during respiration. Due to COPD, asthma in exacerbation—secretion retention, indicate severe respiratory distress, hypoxemia
- *Splinting:* A voluntary decrease in tidal volume to decreased pain on chest expansion. It is due to thoracic or abdominal incisions, chest trauma, pleurisy
- *Increased AP diameter:* AP chest diameter equal to the lateral, slope of ribs more horizontal (90°) or spine. One to COPD, asthma, cystic fibrosis, lung hyperinflation, advanced age
- *Tachypnea:* Increased rate of 20 breaths/minute >25 breath/minute in elderly. Due to fever, anxiety, hypoxemia, restrictive lung disease. Magnitude of increasing above normal rate reflects increased work of breathing
- *Kussmaul's respiration:* Regular rapid and deep respirations are due to metabolic acidosis. Increase in rate aids body in CO_2 excretion
- *Cyanoses:* Refer to a bluish color of skin best seen in earlobes, under eyelids or nailbeds. It is due to decreased oxygen transfer of lungs, decreased cardiac output, nonspecific unreliable indicator
- *Clubbing of fingers:* Refer to increased depth, bulk, sponginess, of distal digit finger. It is due to chronic hypoxemia, cystic fibrosis, lung cancer, bronchiectasis
- *Abdominal paradox:* An inward (rather than normal outward) movement of abdomen during inspiration. It is due to insufficient and ineffective breathing pattern—nonspecific indicator of severe respiratory distress.

Palpation (Fig. 9.2)

- Tracheal deviation is a leftward or rightward movement of trachea from normal midline position. It is non-specific indicator of change in position of mediasternoid structure, medical emergency if caused by tension pneumothorax.

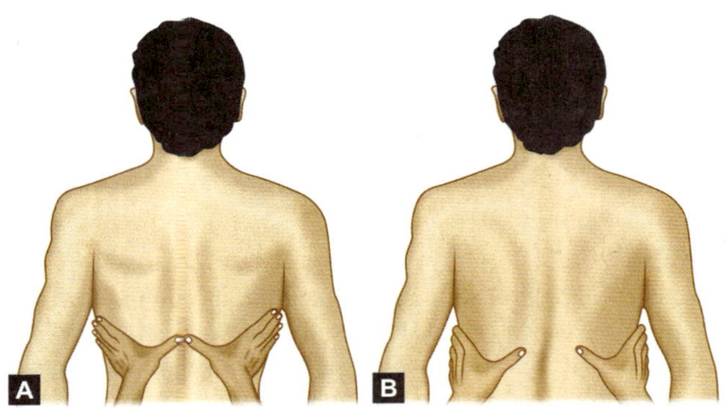

FIGS 9.2A AND B: Palpation of respiratory excursion. (A) During exhalation; (B) After inhalation

- Altered tactile fremitus is increased or decreased in vibrations. It is due to increased in pneumonia, pulmonary edema; decreased in pleural effusion, atelectic area, lung hyperinflation, absent in pneumothorax, large atelectasis
- Altered chest movements, i.e. unequal or equal but diminished movement of two sides of chest with inspiration.

  Usually unequal movement caused by atelectasis, pneumothorax, pleural effusion, splinting, equal but diminished movement caused by barrel chest, restrictive disease and neuromuscular disease.

Percussion

- Hyper-resonance is loud, lower-pitched sound over areas that normally produces a resonance sound. It is due to lung hyper inflation (COPD), lung collapse (pneumothorax) air trapping (asthma)
- Dullness is medium-pitched sound over areas that normally produce a resonant sound. It is due to increased density (pneumonia, large atelectasis). Increased fluid pleural space (pleural effusion).

Auscultation (Fig. 9.3)

- Fine crackles are series of short explosive, high-pitched sounds heard just before the end of inspiration: result of rapid equalisation of gas pressure when collapsed alveoli or terminal bronchioles suddenly snap open similar sound to that made by rolling hair between fingers just behind ear. Can be heard in fibrosis (asbestos interstitial edema, early pulmonary edema), alveolar filling (pneumonia) loss of lung volume (atelectasis), early phase of congestive heart failure
- Coarse crackles are series of short, low-pitched sounds caused by air passing through airway intermittently occluded by mucus unstable bronchial wall, of fold of mucosa, evident on inspiration and at times, expiration; similar sound to bowling quality with more fluid. These can be heard in congestive heart failure, pulmonary edema, pneumonia with severe congestion, COPD
- Ronchi are continuous rumbling, snoring, or rattling sounds from obstructions of a large airways with secretions most prominent on expiration; change often evident after coughing or suctioning. These are heard in COPD, cystic fibrosis, pneumonia, bronchietasis
- Wheezing are continuous musical sound of constant pitch: result of partial obstruction of larynx or trachea. It is due to epiglottis, vocal cord edema after extubation, foreign body
- Absent breath sounds, no sound evident over entire lung or area of lung. It is due to pleural effusion, main stem bronchi, obstruction, large atelectasis, pneumonectomy, lobectomy
- Pleural friction rub is cracking or grating sound from roughened inflamed surfaces of the pleura rubbing together, evident during inspiration. It is due to pleurasy, pneumonia, pulmonary infarction
- Bronchophony, whispered pectoriloguy a spoken or whispered syllable more distinct than normal on auscultation as in pneumonia
- Egophony is a spoken "e" similar to "a" on auscultation because of altered transmission of voice sounds seen in pneumonia, pleural effusion.

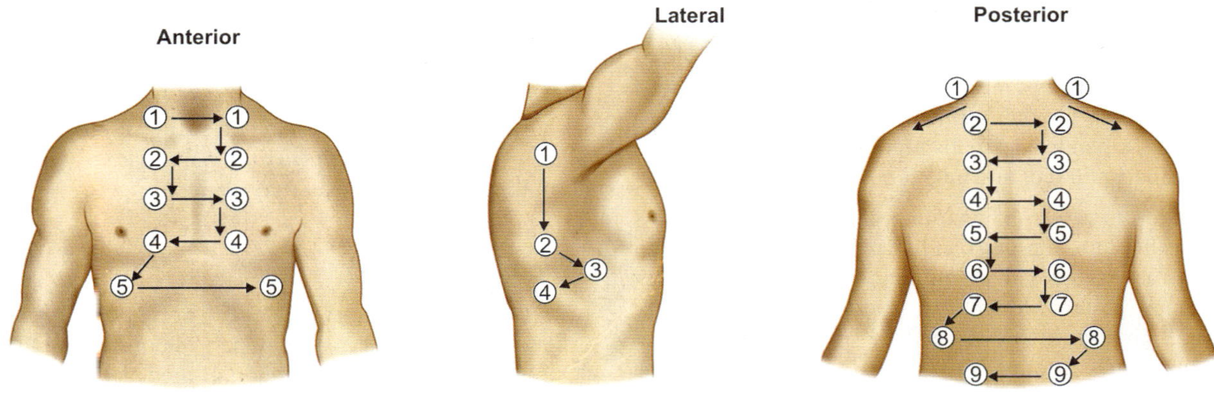

FIG. 9.3: Auscultation of the chest. Use a systematic approach to auscultate the chest, comparing sounds from side to side

DIAGNOSTIC STUDIES OF RESPIRATORY SYSTEM

Blood Studies

i. Hemoglobin test reflects amount of hemoglobin available for combination with oxygen. Venous blood is used. The normal level of adult man is 135–180 g/dL (13.5–18 g/L) = Normal level of adult woman is 12–16 g/dL (120–160 g/L). The nursing responsibilities during the procedure is to explain the procedure and its purpose. No special care is required.

ii. Hematocrit test reflects ratio of red blood cells to plasma increased hematocrit (polycythemia) found in chronic hypoxemia. Venous blood is used. Normal for adult man is 40–54 percent and woman is 38–47 percent. The nursing responsibility is as in Hb%.

iii. Antitrypsin assay is valuable in the identification of individuals with the genetic abnormality that leads to emphysema. This is a globulin that inhibits certain enzymes. The normal values of α_1-antitrypsin assay.

MM genotype: 2.1–3.8 U/mL

M2 phenotype: 1.05–2.1 U/mL

22 phenotype:0.5–0.7 U/mL

The nursing care includes as in hemoglobin. No food or fluid restrictions are necessary.

iv. Complete blood count: The normal counts of RBCs in male 4.6–6.2 million/D. 4.2–5.4 million/L in females. The normal level of WBC 4.0–11.0 × 10^3/L.

v. Arterial blood gases (ABG): Arterial blood is obtained through puncture of radial or femoral artery or through arterial catheter. ABGs are performed to assess acid-base-balance, ventilation status, need for oxygen therapy, change in oxygen therapy, or change in ventilation settings. Continuous ABG monitoring is also possible via a sensor or electrode inserted into the arterial catheter.

Nursing responsibility in this test, thus includes.

Explain the purposes of the test and its procedure to the patient in using oxygen (percentage, L/min). Avoid changing it for 20 minutes before obtaining sample. Assist with positioning (e.g. palm up, wrist slightly hyperextended if radial artery is used). Collect blood into heparinized syringe. To ensure accurate results, expel all air bubbles, and place sample in ice, unless it will be analyzed in less than 1 minute. Apply pressure to artery for 5 minutes after specimen is obtained to prevent hematoma at the arterial puncture site.

The normal values, parameters of ABGs are (Box 9.1):

- *Acid-base-balance* measured as pH (hydrogen ion concentration). Normal 7.35–7.45. Alkalemia increased 7.45. Acedemia decreased 7.35.

Box 9.1 Arterial blood gas analysis

	Normal values	Interpretation
PaO_2	75–100 mm Hg	↑ in hyperventilation ↓ in impaired respiratory function
$PaCO_2$	35–45 mm Hg	↑ in impaired gas exchange ↓ in hyperventilation
pH	7.35–7.45	↑ in respiratory alkalosis with low $PaCO_2$ ↓ in respiratory acidosis with high $PaCO_2$
HCO_3^-	22–26	↑ to buffer $PaCO_2$ in acidosis ↓ to buffer $PaCO_2$ in alkalosis
Oxygen saturation	95%–100%	↑ in hyperventilation ↓ in impaired respiratory function

- *Oxygenation* PaO_2 (partial pressure of dissolved O_2 in blood. Normal 80–100 mm Hg. Hyperoxemia ↑ 100 mm Hg, hypoxemia ↓ 80 mm Hg.
- *Ventilation* SaO_2 percentage of O_2 bound hemoglobin. $PaCO_2$ partial pressure of CO_2 dissolved in blood. The normal SaO_2 is 95–98 percent. The normal $PaCO_2$: 35–45 mm Hg, hypercapnia ↑ 45 mm Hg. Hypocapnia ↓ 35 mm Hg.

vi. *Oximetry:* Test monitors arterial or venous oxygen saturation device attached to the ear lobe, finger or nose for SPO_2 monitoring or is contained in a pulmonary artery catheter for SVO_2 monitoring. Oximetry is used for continuous monitoring in ICUs, inpatient and outpatient sortings and exercise testing.

The nursing responsibilities include, applying probe to finger, forehead, earlobe or bridge of nose. When interpreting SPO_2 and SVO_2 values, first assess patient status and presence of factors that can alter accuracy of pulse oximeter reading. For SPO_2, these include motion, low perfusion, bright lights, use of intravascular dyes, acryling nails, dark skin color. For SVO_2 these include change in O_2 delivery or O_2 consumptions. For SPO_2 notify physician of ± 4 percent change from baseline or decrease to less than 90 percent. For SVO_2 notify physician of ± 10 percent change from baseline or decrease to less than 60 percent.

Sputum Analysis

The nursing responsibilities include explain purposes. Some tests require specimens, collected in consecutive days usually 4 mL of sputum is sufficient. Coughing upon awakening is more likely to result in collecting sputum and not saliva. Instruct individual to rinse the mouth with water, demonstrate effective deep breathing and coughing, have individual practice deep breathing and coughing, instruct individual to notify staff as the specimen is collected. Following are different tests and nursing care:

i. Culture and Sensitivity

Single sputum specimen is collected in a sterile container. For diagnosing bacterial infection, select antibiotic and evaluate treatment. Here instruct patients on how to produce of good specimen for Gram stain test as given below if patients cannot produce specimen bronchoscopy may be used.

ii. Gram Stain

Staining of sputum permits classification of bacteria into gram- negative and gram-positive types. Results guide therapy until culture and sensitivity results are obtained. Here nurse instructs patient to expectorate sputum into the container after coughing deeply. Obtain sputum in early morning because secretions collect during night. If unsuccessful try increasing oral fluids, intake unless fluids are restricted. Collect sputum in sterile container (sputum trap) during suctioning or by aspirating secretions from the trachea. Send specimen to laboratory promptly.

iii. Acid-fast Smear Culture

Test is performed to collect sputum for acid-fast bacili (AFB). A series of three early morning specimen is used. Nursing responsibility as in Gram stain and cover specimen and send to laboratory for analysis.

iv. Cytology

In this, single sputum specimen is collected in special container with fixative solution. Purpose is to determine presence of abnormal cells that may indicate malignant condition. The nurse should send specimens to laboratory promptly and take measure in other tests.

Radiological Studies

Chest X-ray

Test is used to screen, diagnose, and evaluate change. Most common views are posteroanterior and lateral. In this, nurse instructs patient to undress to waist, put on gown, and remove any metal between neck and waist.

Computed Tomography (CT)

Test is performed for diagnostic of lesions difficult to assess by conventional X-ray studies, such as those in the hilum, mediastinum, and pleura. Images show structures in cross-section. Nursing care is same as for chest X-ray.

Magnetic Resonance Imaging (MRI)

Test is used for diagnosis of lesions difficult to assess by CT scan (e.g. lung apex near the spine). Here, nurse explains purpose, takes measures as in chest X-ray and instructs the patient to remove all metal (e.g. jewelery, watch) before test. It takes about an hour.

Ventilation/Perfusion (V/P) Lung Scan

Test is used to identify areas of the lung not receiving air flow (ventilator) or blood flow (perfusion). It involves injection of radioisotope and inhalation of small amount of radioactive gas (Xenon). A gamma detecting device is used to record radioactivity. Ventilation without perfusion suggests pulmonary embolus. The nursing measures are as for chest X-ray. Also check for dye allergy. Obtain an accurate weight so that the dosage of radioactive agent can be calculated. No special care or precaution is needed afterwards (post test) because the gas and isotope transmit radioactivity for only brief interval.

Pulmonary Angiogram

Study is used to visualize pulmonary vasculature and locate obstructions or pathologic conditions such as pulmonary embolus. A radio-opaque dye is injected, usually through a catheter into the pulmonary artery or right side of the heart. Nursing measures same as chest X-ray. Know that dye injection may cause flushing, warm sensation and coughing. Check pressure dressing site after procedure. Monitor blood pressure, pulse rate and circulation distal to injection site. Report and record significant changes.

Positron Emission Tomography (PET)

Test is used to distinguish benign and malignant lung nodules. It involves IV injection of a radioisotope with short half-life. Nursing measures same as V/P.

Endoscopic Examination

Bronchoscopy

This study is typically performed in outpatient procedure room. Flexible fiberoptic scope is used for diagnosis, biopsy, specimen collection, or assessment of changes. It may also be done to suction mucous plugs or to remove foreign objects. In this examination, the nurse instructs patient to be on NPO status for 6–12 hours. Obtain signed permit (consent). Give diazepam if ordered by physician before procedure to aid relaxation. After procedure, keep patient NPO until gag-reflex returns and monitor for laryngeal edema. If biopsy was done, monitor for hemorrhage and pneumothorax. Please note that sedation given to patient with respiratory insufficiency may precipitate respiratory failure.

Mediastinoscopy

Test is used for inspection and biopsy of lymph nodes in mediastinal area. Nurse prepares patient for surgical intervention, obtains signed permit. Afterwards monitor as for bronchoscopy.

Biopsy

In lung biopsy specimen may be obtained by transbronchial or open-lung biopsy. This test is used to obtain specimens for laboratory analysis. Nursing measures same as bronchoscopy (Fig. 9.4).

Others

Thoracentesis

Test is used to obtain specimen of pleural fluid for diagnosis, to remove pleural fluid or to instill medication. The physician inserts a large bore needle through chest wall into pleural space (Fig. 9.5). Chest X-ray is always obtained after procedures to check pneumothorax. Nursing responsibility includes explaining procedures to patient and obtain signed permit prior to procedure. Position patient upright, instruct not to talk or cough, and assist during procedure. If large volume of fluid is removed, monitor for decrease in shortness of breath, send labeled specimen to laboratory.

Pulmonary Function Test

It is used to evaluate lung function. It involves use of a spirometer to diagram air movement as patient performs prescribed respiratory maneuvers. Nurse has to avoid scheduling immediately after meals times. Avoid administration of inhaled bronchiodilator for 6 hours before procedure.

Explain procedure to patient. Provide rest after procedure.

DISORDERS OF NOSE AND SINUSES

Deviated Septum

Deviated septum is deflection of the normally nasal septum. It is most commonly caused by trauma to the nose or congenital disproportion, a condition in which the size of the septum is not proportioned to the size of the nose.

On inspection, septum is to one side, altering the air passage symptoms are variable. The patient may experience obstruction to nasal breathing, nasal edema, or dryness of the nasal mucosa with crusting and bleeding (epistaxis). A severely deviated septum may block drainage of mucus from the sinus cavities, resulting in infection (sinusitis). Nasal breathing is subjective and only the patient can gauge the degree of obstruction and amount of discomfort it causes.

Health promotion is aimed at prevention of precipitating factors such as accidental falls in childhood. Medical management of deviated septum includes the use of decongestants or a nasal corticosteroid only to reduce nasal edema. Before using the inhaler, ask the person to gently blow their nose, making sure that their nostrils are clear. Then follow these steps:

- Remove the cap from the nasal inhaler
- Shake the container well
- Hold the inhaler between the thumb and forefinger

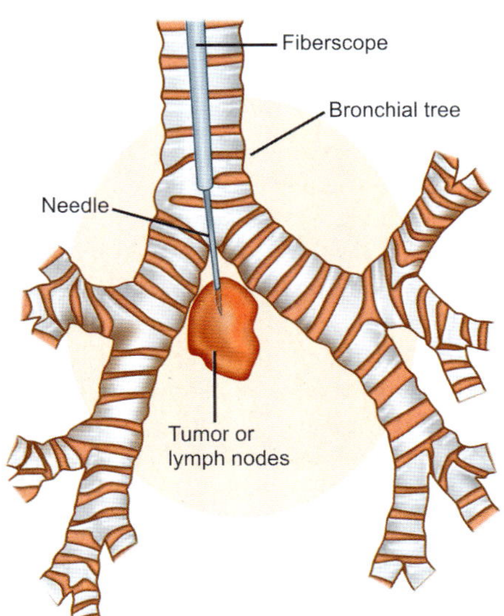

FIG. 9.4: Transbronchial needle biopsy. The diagram shows a transbronchial biopsy needle penetrating the bronchial wall and entering a mass of subcranial nodes or tumor

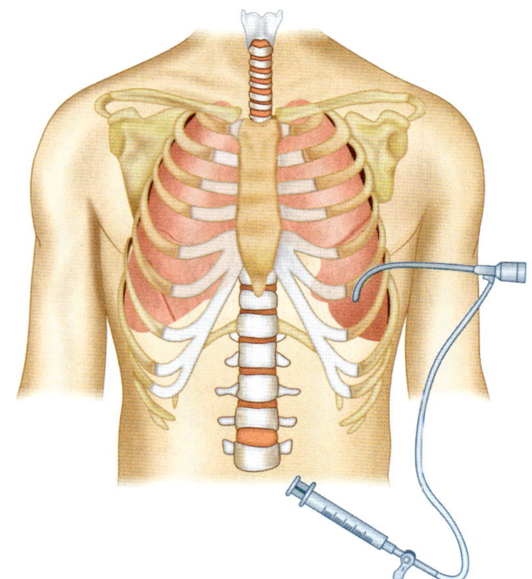

FIG. 9.5: Thoracentesis. A catheter is positioned in the pleural space remove accumulated fluid

- Tilt the head back, slightly and insert the end of the inhaler into the nostril, painting it slightly towards the outside nostril wall. Hold the nostril closed with one finger
- Press down the container to release one dose and at the same time inhale gently
- Ask patient to hold the breath for a few seconds then breathe out slowly through the mouth
- Withdraw the inhaler from the nostril and repeat the process for the other nostril if more than one puff is prescribed for nostril repetition
- Replace the protective cap on the inhaler.

Surgery is an option for patient with severe symptoms. A nasal septoplasty is performed to reconstruct and properly align the deviated septum. Nasal septoplasty can be performed alone or with a rhinoplasty.

Nasal Fracture

Nasal fracture is most often caused by trauma of substantial force to the middle of the face. Complications of the fracture include airway obstruction, epistaxis and cosmetic deformity. Nasal fractures are classified unilateral, bilateral or complex. A unilateral fracture typically produces little or no displacement. Bilateral fractures, the most common fractures, give the nose a flattened look. Powerful frontal blows cause complex fractures, which may also shatter frontal bones. Diagnosis is based on the health history, direct observation and X-ray finding.

On inspection, nurse should assess the patient's ability to breathe through each side of the nose and note the presence of edema, bleeding, or hematoma. There may be ecchymosis under one or both eyes. The nose is inspected internally for evidence of septal deviation, hemorrhage or clear drainage, which suggest leakage of CSF. If clear drainage is observed, a specimen may be sent for determining CSF. Injury of sufficient force to fracture nasal bones results in considerable swelling of soft tissues. With extensive swelling, it may be difficult to verify the extent of deformity or the repair the fracture until several days later when edema is subsiding.

The goals of nursing management are to reduce edema, prevent complications, educate the patient and provide emotional support. Ice may be applied to the face and nose to reduce edema and bleeding. When a fracture is confirmed, the goal of management is realignment of the fracture using closed or open reduction (septoplasty, or rhinoplasty). These procedures re-establish cosmetic appearance and proper function of the nose and provide an adequate airway.

Nursing management of nasal surgery (rhinoplasty, septoplasty, or nasal fracture reductions) includes the following:

- Before surgery, the patient should be instructed to avoid taking aspirin-containing drugs for 2 weeks to reduce bleeding
- In postoperative period, include assessment of respiratory status, pain management, and observation of the surgical site for hemorrhage and edema
- Health teaching is important, because, these procedures involve a short hospital stay and the patient must be able to detect early and late complications.

The problem of patient undergoing surgery may have certain problems needing nursing care.

- *Altered health maintenance* related to lack of knowledge of the procedure, for which nurse has to explain the procedure, expected postoperative course, and required self-care to decrease anxiety and increase patient cooperation. Answer questions as needed and assess the patient perception about body image and expectation of surgery to obtain information to use in patient care.
- *Ineffective breathing pattern related to presence of packaging,* nasal edema, intranasal splints, as manifested by complaints of shortness of breath, alterations in respiration rate, rhythm or depth. Here, the nurse has to assess for respiratory distress, elevate head of bed, provide supplemental oxygen (if prescribed).

  Instruct the patient to blow nose, open mouth when sneezing, and coughing to maintain correct position of packing. Apply cold compress to incisional area to promote vasoconstriction and reduce edema. Instruct the patient to call nurse for any untoward effects.
- *Pain related to edema* from surgical procedure, for which nurse should teach patient correct analgesic schedule, describe to patient the amount of pain expected, and teach patients non-pharmacological measures (elevation of head, cold compress) and avoid using aspirin on NSAIDs. Teach patient gentle cleaning techniques such as use of cotton swabs, with hydrogen peroxide to clean crusting and application of water-soluble jelly to lubricate when packing has been removed to promote cleanliness and prevent infection and promote use of bedside humidifier to decrease drying of mucosa and promote comfort and management of nasal hemorrhage or epistaxis.

Simple first aid measures should be used first to control epistaxis. The nurse should keep the patient quiet, position the patient in a sitting stature, leaning forward, or if not possible, in a reclining position with head and shoulders elevated; apply direct pressure by pinching the entire soft laven portion of the nose for 10 to 15 minutes; apply ice compresses to the nose, and have the patient suck on ice; partially insert a small gauze pad into the bleeding nostril and apply digital pressure if bleeding continues and obtain medical assistance, if bleeding does not stop. When first aid measure is not effective, management involves localization of the bleeding site and application of a vasoconstrictive agent cauterization or anterior packing indicated. Anterior packing may consist of ribbon guaze impregnated with antiseptic ointments that is wedged firmly in the desired location and remain in place for 48 to 72 hours. If posterior packing is required, the patient should be hospitalized. Inflatable balloons may be used as the nasal pack on gauze rolls may be inserted. Stringes attached to the packaging are brought to the outside and taped to check for ease of removal. A nasal sling (folded 2 × 2 in gauze pad) should be taped over the nares to absorb drainage. Since packing is painful, mild narcotic analgesic is administered.

Failure of posterior packing indicates surgical correction.

Rhinitis

Rhinitis refers to inflammation of the mucous membrane of the nose. It may be acute or chronic or allergic rhinitis. All forms of rhinitis cause sneezing, nasal discharge with nasal obstruction and headache. Etiology, pathophysiology and diverse manifestations are according to this type as follows:

Acute Rhinitis

Etiology

Acute rhinitis (coryza, common cold) is caused by viruses that invade the upper respiratory tract. It is an inflammatory, condition of the mucous membrane of the nose and accessory sinuses caused by a filterable virus. It affects almost everyone at some time and occurs most often in winter with additional high incidences in early rain fall and spring. Some of the known causes of the common cold are 100 serotypes of rhinoviruses, coronoviruses, adenoviruses, echoviruses, influenza and parainfluenza viruses and coxsackieviruses.

It is the most prevalent infectious disease and is spread by airborne droplet sprays emitted by the infected person while breathing talking, sneezing or coughing or by direct hand contact. Frequency increases in winter months, when people stay indoors and overcrowding is more common. Other factors such as chilling, fatigue, physical and emotional stress and the patient compromised immune status, may increase susceptibility. Pathophysiologic process of rhinitis in shown in Figure 9.6.

Clinical Manifestations

The patient with acute viral rhinitis typically first experiences tickling, irritation, sneezing or dryness of the nose or nasopharynx followed by copious nasal secretions, some nasal obstruction, watery eyes, elevated temperature, general malaise, and headache. After the early profuse secretions, the nose becomes more obstructed and the discharge is thicker, within few days, the general symptoms improve, nasal passages reopen, and normal breathing is established. Secondary invasion by bacteria may cause pneumonia, acute bronchitis sinusitis and otitis media.

Management

No specific treatment exists for the common cold. The goals of treatment are to:

- Relieve symptoms
- Inhibit spread of infections, and
- Reduce the risk of bacterial complications.

Rest, fluids, proper diet, antipyretics and analgesics are helpful. Complications of acute rhinitis include pharyngitis, sinusitis, otitis media, tonsilitis, and chest infection. Treat with proper antibiotic therapy. Antibiotics have no effect on virus if taken unjudiciously, may produce resistance organisms.

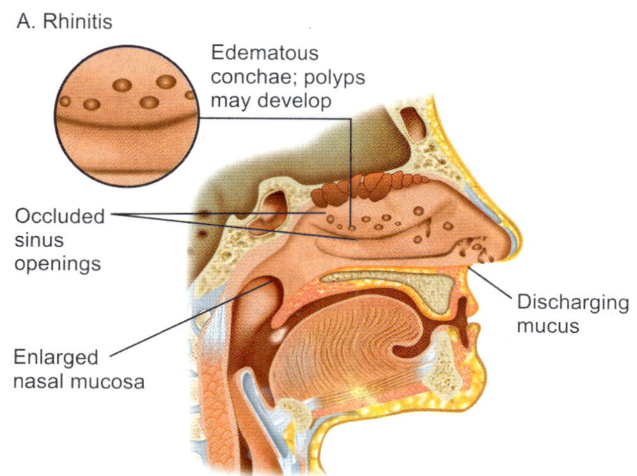

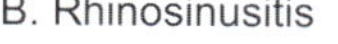

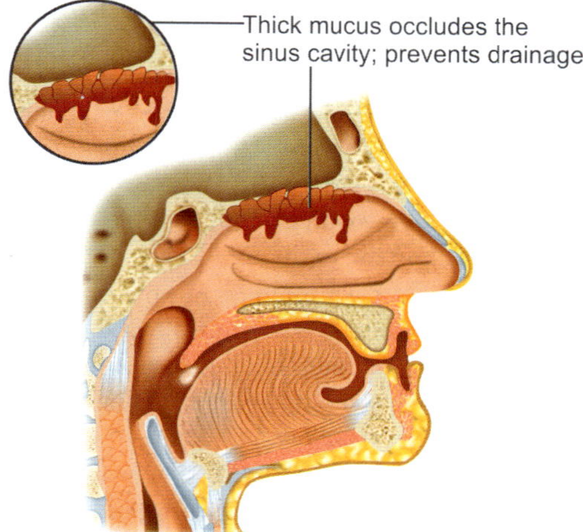

FIGS 9.6A AND B: Pathophysiologic processes in rhinitis and rhinosinusitis. Although pathophysiologic processes are similar in rhinitis and rhinosinusitis, they affect different structures. (A) In rhinitis, the mucous membranes lining the nasal passages become inflamed, congested, and edematous. The swollen nasal conchae block the sinus openings, and mucus is discharged from the nostrils; (B) Rhinosinusitis is also marked by inflammation and congestion, with thickened mucous secretions filling the sinus cavities and occluding the openings

Allergic Rhinitis

Etiology

Allergic rhinitis (hayfever) is a type I-hypersensitive reaction. It is the reaction of the nasal mucosa to a specific antigen (allergen). Attacks of seasonal rhinitis usually occur in spring and fall and are caused by allergy to pollens from trees, flowers or grasses or weeds. Inhaled allergens are classified as outdoor (seasonal) also called acute or indoor (perennial), also called chronic. The outdoor allergens are pollen of trees, grasses or weeds. Inhaled allergens are classified as outdoor (seasonal) also called acute or indoor (perennial lasting for long time), also called chronic. The outdoor allergens are pollen of trees, grasses or weeds. The indoor allergens are spores of molds, dustmites, and animal danders.

Clinical Manifestation

Manifestations of allergic rhinitis are nasal congestion, sneezing, watery, itchy eyes and nose, altered sense of smell and thin watery nasal discharge. The nasal turbinates appear pale, boggy and swollen. The turbinates may fill the air space and press against the nasal septum. The posterior ends of the turbinates can become so enlarged that they obstruct sinus aeration or drainage and result in sinusitis. With chronic exposure to allergens the patient responses include, headache, congestion, pressure and postnasal drip. The patient may complain of cough, hoarseness, or the recurrent need to clear throat. Congestion may be sufficient to cause snoring. Nasal polyps may be present if the allergy has persisted for a long time.

Management

There are several measures used in management of allergic rhinitis. The measures to reduce symptoms of allergic rhinitis are:

- Avoidance is the best treatment
- *Avoid house dust:* Use the approach "less is best". Focus on the bedroom. Remove carpeting. Limit furniture. Enclose the pillows, mattresses and springs in airtight, zipper-sealed, vinyl cloth bags, install an airfilter if possible. Close the airconditioning vent into the room
- *Avoid house dust-mites:* Wash building in hot water (130°F) weekly. Wear a mask when vacuuming. Double bag the vacuum-cleaner. Install a filter on the outlet post of the vacuum cleaner. Avoid sleeping or lying on upholstered furniture. Remove carpets that are laid down on concrete. If possible, have someone else for cleaning the house
- *Avoid mold spores:* The three 'D's that promote growth of mold spores are darkness, dampness, and drafts. Avoid places where humidity is high (e.g. basements, camps on the lake, clothe hampers, greenhouses, stables, barns)

  Dehumidifiers are rarely helpful. Ventilate closed rooms, open doors and install fans. Consider adding windows to dark room. Consider keeping lights on in closets. A basement light with a timer that provides light several hours a day decreases mold growth
- *Avoid pollens:* Stay inside with closed doors and windows during high-pollen season. Avoid the use of fans. Install an airconditioner with a good airfilter. Wash filter weekly during high pollen season. Put the car air-conditioner on "recirculate" when driving
- *Avoid pet allergens:* Remove pets from the interior of the home. Clean the living area thoroughly. Do not expect instant relief. Symptoms usually do not improve signi-ficantly for 2 months following pet removal
- *Avoid smoke:* The presence of a smoker will sabotage the best of all possible symptoms reduction program. The drug therapy involves the use of antihistamines, decongestants and nasal sprays. An oral antihistamine or oral decongestant is typically used first. If therapy is not effective, a nasal corticosteroid spray may be used to decrease inflammation. Corticosteroid administered by a nasal spray are purely absorbed in the system in circulation
  - *Antihistamines* bind with H_1 receptors on target cells, block of histamine binding. Relieve acute symptoms of allergic response (itching, sneezing, excessive secretions, mild congestions) may cause sedation (diminished alertness, slow reaction time, somnolence) and stimulation (restlessness, nervous insomnia) and may cause palpitation tachycardia, urinary retention or frequency. So, the nurse warns the patient regarding side effects and teaches the patient to report palpitations, change in heart rate, change in bowel, bladder habits and instruct the patient not to use alcohol with antihistamines because of additive depressive effects

    An example of antihistamine includes first generation agents such as ethanolamines (e.g. benzedrine) ethylenediamines, alkylamines (chloropheniramine) piperazines, piperidine, phenothazine (phenergan), etc. The second generation agents such as astemizole, loratadine, cetrizone, etc.
  - *Decongestants* stimulate adrenergic receptors on blood vessels promote vasoconstriction and reduce nasal edema and rhinorrhea. Example, oral pseudoephedrin (sudafed), topical-nasal-spray: e.g. oxymetazoline, phenylephrine. The side effects include CNS stimulation causing insomnia, excitation, headache, irritability, increased blood and ocular pressure, dysuria, palpitations, tachycardia. Here the nurse advises patient of adverse reactions. Advise some preparations are contraindicated for patients with cardiovascular diseases, hypertension, diabetes, glaucoma, prostate hyperplasia, hepatic and renal disease. Teach patient that these drugs should not be used for more than 3 days or more than 3–4 times a day. Longer use increases risk of rhinitis medicamentosa
  - *Corticosteroids* nasal spray inhibits inflammatory response. At recommended dose, systemic side effects are unlikely because of low systemic absorption. If used

greater than prescribed dose, mild transient nasal burning and stringing occurs. Here nurse should teach patient correct use instruct patient to use on regular basis and not prn reinforce that spray acts to decrease inflammation, and discontinue the use of nasal infection to develop

- *Mast cell stabilizer,* i.e. nasal spray (cromolyn spray, nidocromia spray) inhibits degranulation of sensitized mast cells which occurs after exposure to specific antigen. Has minimal side effects. Teach patient correct use, explain occurrence of nasal irritation or burning
- *Anticholinergic* nasal spray (ipratropium bromide), blocks hypersecretory effects by competing in binding sites on the cell. Reduces rhinorrhea and common cold, allergic and non-allergic rhinitis. The side effects include dryness of mouth and nose. Does not cause systemic side effects.

Chronic rhinitis is a chronic inflammation of the mucous membrane with increased nasal mucosa caused by repeated acute infections, by an allergy or by vasomotor rhinitis. The cause of vasomotor rhinitis is unclear but this condition may result from an instability of the autonomic nervous system caused by stress, tension or some endocrine disorders. Rhinitis may also be caused by the overuse of nose drops.

In addition to measures of management of rhinitis, suggestion is made in acute allergic rhinitis, that the patient should be taught to self-administration of nose drops as given below:

- Wash hands
- Assume a position that will facilitate flow of medication:
  - Sit on chair and tip head well backward, or
  - Lie down with head extended over the edge of bed, or
  - Lie down with pillow under shoulders and head tipped backwards
- Turn head to side that will receive the drops
- Place no more than three drops of solution into each nostril at one time (unless otherwise prescribed)
- Remaining position with head tilted backward for 3 to 5 minutes to permit solution to reach posterior nares
- If marked congestion is still present 10 minutes after nose drop insertion, another drop or two of solutions may be administered (nasal constriction from first insertion may facilitate additional drops reaching posterior nares).

And advise the person with rhinitis regarding—

- Obtain additional rest
- Drink at least 2 to 3 liters of fluid daily
- Medications: Use nasal spray or nose drops two or three times per day as ordered
- Prevention of further infection
  - Blow nose with both nostrils open to prevent infected matter from being forced into Eustachian tube
  - Cover mouth with disposable tissues when coughing and sneezing to prevent droplet nuclei from contaminating the air
  - Dispose of used tissues carefully
  - Avoid exposure when possible (i.e. avoid crowds, people with cold specific allergens). Elderly persons and those with chronic lung diseases are particularly vulnerable and should have a flu shot yearly
  - Wash hands frequently and especially after coughing, blowing the nose, sneezing, and so on. Evidences suggest that several types of colds are transmitted from person to person by hand contact and from touching objects handled by persons with a cold
  - Seek medical attention if the following are present:
    - High fever, severe chest pain, earache
    - Symptoms lasting longer than 2 weeks
    - Recurrent cold.

Sinusitis

The sinuses are airfilled cavities lined with nucleus membranes. Any inflammation of the mucous membrane of the sinuses is termed as "Sinusitis". Figure 9.7 shows paranasal sinuses. For causes see Box 9.2.

Etiology

Sinusitis develops when the ostia (exit) from the sinuses is narrowed or blocked by inflammation or hypertrophy (swelling) of the mucosa. The secretions that accumulate behind the obstruction provide a rich medium for growth of bacteria, viruses and fungi all of which cause infections.

Box 9.2 Causes of rhinosinusitis

Category	Causes
Vasomotor	Idiopathic Abuse of nasal decongestants (rhinitis medicamentosa) Psychological stimulation (anger, sexual arousal) Irritants (smoke, air pollution, exhaust fumes, cocaine)
Mechanical	Tumor Deviated septum Crusting Hypertrophied turbinates Foreign body Cerebrospinal fluid leak
Chronic inflammatory	Polyps (in cystic fibrosis) Sarcoidosis Wegener's granulomatosis Midline granuloma
Infections	Acute viral infection Acute or chronic rhinosinusitis Rare nasal infection (syphilis, tuberculosis)
Hormonal	Pregnancy Use of oral contraceptives Hypothyroidism

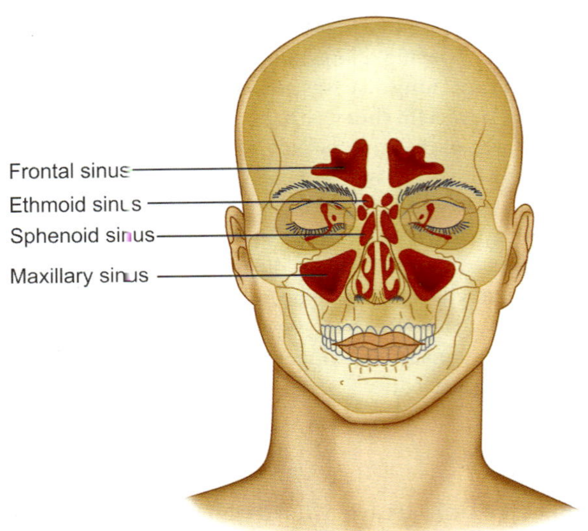

FIG. 9.7: Paranasal sinues

- Bacterial sinusitis is most commonly caused by *Streptococcus pneumoniae, Haemophilus influenzae,* or *Moraxella catarrhalis,* beta-hemolytic *Streptococcus, Klebsiella pneumoniae,* anareobic organism.
- Viral sinusitis follows an upper respiratory infection in which the virus penetrates the mucous membrane and decreases ciliary transports, e.g. rhinovirus, parainfluenza, adenovirus
- Fungal sinusitis is uncommon and is usually found in patients who are debilitated or immunocompromised.

Acute sinusitis usually results from an URI, allergic rhinitis, swimming or dental manipulations all of which cause inflammatory changes and retention of secretions. Chronic sinusitis generally results from repeated episodes of a acute sinusitis that result in irreversible loss of the normal ciliated epithelium lining the sinus cavity.

Pathophysiology

The first symptom of acute bacterial sinusitis is usually a stuffy nose followed by slowly developing pressure over the involved sinus. Other signs and symptoms include general malaise and toxicity, persistent cough, postnasal drip, headache slightly elevated or normal temperature and mild leukopenia. Symptoms worsen over 48 to 72 hours culminating in severe localized pain and tenderness over the involved sinus. The patient often believes that the pain is due to an infected tooth.

In acute frontal and maxillary sinusitis pain usually does not appear until 1 to 2 hours after awakening. It increases for 3 to 4 hours after awakening and then becomes less severe in the afternoon and evening. There may be bloody or blood-tinged discharge from the nose in the first 24 to 48 hours. The discharge rapidly becomes thick, green and copious, blocking the nose. The throat may become inflamed and sore on one side, because of the purulent discharge.

Clinical Manifestation

Acute sinusitis causes significant pain over the affected sinus purulent nasal drainage, nasal obstruction, congestion, fever and malaise. The patient looks and feels sick. Assessment involves inspection of the nasal mucosa and palpation of the sinus points for pain. Findings that indicate acute sinusitis include a hyperemic and edematous mucosa, enlarged turbinates and tenderness over the involved sinuses. Pain is caused by the accumulation of pus and absorption of air behind a blocked ostium. The patient also experiences recurrent headaches that change in intensity with position or when secretions drain.

Management

For most patients, diagnosis is made without any studies. Certain cases of radiographic studies are indicated particularly chronic sinuses, conventional sinus X-rays, computed tomography (CT) and MRI. Fibrocystic examination of the nose (Rhinoscopy) may also be used. Management of acute bacterial sinusitis centers on relief of pain and shrinkage of the nasal mucosa. Ibuprofen and oral decongestant such as pseudoephedrine are commonly prescribed. In some patients, codeine may be required for pain relief. The antibiotic of choice is limited for 10 days. If patient does not improve after 5 days of amoxicilline a changes of antibiotics may be necessary, which includes Loracarbef amoxicillin clavulanate potassium (Augmentin), cefacler, doxycycline, trimethoprim, and sulfamethoxazole, clarithromycin, azithromycin (5 days).

Patient may obtain relief from saline nasal sprays steam, from a shower, or a humidifier. Hot wet packs applied to the face over the infected sinus (es) either continuously or for 1 to 2 hours at a time for four times a day may provide symptomatic relief. A washcloth wrung out in hot water is convenient way to provide wet pack.

Acute frontal sinusitis with pain, tenderness and edema of the frontal or sphenoid sinus may require hospitalization because of the risk of intracranial complications and osteomyelitis. High dose of intravenous antibiotic and nasal congestants orally or spray may be ordered.

Fungal sinusitis can range from mild infections resembling chronic sinusitis to severe life-threatening invasive infections, needs prolonged and necessary antibiotics or surgical drainage of sinuses.

Invasive fungal sinusitis is most likely to occur in transplant patients, patients on chemotherapy, patients with AIDS, or persons with controlled diabetes. Aspergillus and Mucor are two types of fungi most prone to cause invasive disease. Symptoms include facial fullness, cranial neuropathies, and pain.

Proptosis of the eye, facial swelling and blood-stinged discharge may be present. These patients need hospitalization.

Treatment includes IV amphotericin B, aggressive surgical management are required.

The types of sinus surgery are:

- *Functional endoscopic sinus surgery (FESS):* Here sinus endoscope enters sinus and removes diseased mucosa and opens ostia. It is used for chronic sinusitis and removal of polyps
- *Caldwell-Luc (radical antrum perforation):* Here clearing out of maxillary sinus through incision under upper lip. It is used as chronic maxillary sinusitis
- *Transnasal external or transantral ethimoidectomy:* Various approaches used to excise inject ethmoid and sphenoid cells. It is used in chronic ethimoid and sphenoid sinusitis
- *Frontal sinusectomy:* A complete removal of diseased mucosa of both frontal sinus, space packed with subcutaneous fat from abdomen. Performed in chronic frontal sinusitis
- *Ethmoid sinus surgery:* Ethmoid sinus removed and anterior wall of sphenoid sinus opened. Performed in chronic sphenoid sinusitis

The nurse has to perform preoperative teaching for the person undergoing sinus surgery, which includes:

- Determine patients' understanding about the surgical procedure. Clarify misconceptions and answer patients' and family questions. Explain that the patient will:
  - Have nothing to eat or drink for 6 to 8 hours preoperatively
  - Receive a sedative before surgery
  - Feel pressure, not pain during surgery
  - Have a nasal pack for 24 to 48 hours postoperatively and may feel like he or she has a "head cold"
  - Have "black eyes" and swelling around the nose and eyes for 1 to 2 weeks postoperatively
  - Have prescription for pain medication as needed.

Postoperative care of the person undergoing sinus surgery will include:

- After general anesthesia, position patient well into the side to prevent swelling of aspiration of blood drainage
- Administer cool mist via face tent or collar, or provide humidifier
- When the patient is awake, remind him or her to expectorate secretions and not swallow them
- Encourage mid-Fowler's position when fully awake to promoted drainage and decrease edema
- Apply ice compresses over nose (or ice bag over nose, (or ice bag over maxillary and frontal sinuses) in the early postoperative period
- Monitor patient for:
  - Excessive bleeding from nose (may be evidence of repeated swallowing)
  - Decreased visual acuity, especially diplopia, indicating damage to optic nerve or muscles of globe of eye
  - Complaint of pain over the individual sinus, which may indicate infection or inadequate drainage
  - Fever-take temperature rectally
- Give frequent mouth care using a soft toothbrush. If there is an oral incision, mouthcare is given before meals to improve appetite and after meals to decrease danger of infection
- Change nasal pad when it is soiled
- Apply ice compresses to ecchymosis areas to constrict blood vessels, decrease oozing and edema, and help relieve pain
- Encourage liberal fluid intake. Patient may be very thirsty because of dry mouth from mouth breathing
- Teach patient to:
  - Avoid blowing nose for at least 48 hours after packing is removed to prevent bleeding
  - Avoid sneezing: If the patient must sneeze he or she should keep mouth open
  - Avoid lifting heavy objects
  - Report signs of infection—fever, purulent discharge to surgeon
  - Expect tarry stools from swallowed blood for a few days
  - Avoid constipation (Valsalvas maneuver, i.e. straining can cause bleeding)
  - Expect that ecchymosis of nose and eyes will begin to change color over next 1 to 2 weeks
  - Take prophylactic antibiotics as prescribed. Do not stop until all medication is taken.

In addition, patients are advised to take more rest to heal; precaution to be given blowing and sneezing. Keep head elevated for proper breathing, small dressing pad around dressing to absorb drainage, and instruct the patient not to take aspirin or any product containing aspirin, which can cause bleeding and caution with oral hygiene to avoid injury to the incisions.

EPISTAXIS (NOSEBLEED)

Epistaxis is a hemorrhage from the nose caused by the rupture of tiny, distended vessels in the mucous membrane of any area of the nasal passage. The anterior septum is the most common site. Causes include trauma, infection, drugs, cardiovascular diseases, blood dyscrasias, nasal tumors, low humidity, foreign body, and deviated nasal septum. Vigorous nose blowing and nose picking are additional causes. Risk factors for epistaxis are listed in Box 9.3.

Medical Management

The bleeding site is determined by using a nasal speculum or headlight. The patient sits upright with the head tilted forward to prevent swallowing and aspiration of blood. Then direct pressure is applied to the site by compressing the soft outer portion of the nose against the midline septum for 5 or 10 minutes continuously.

Vessels involved in anterior nosebleeds are cauterized by chemical agents (e.g. silver nitrate and Gelfoam) or electrocautery; topical vasoconstrictors, such as adrenaline (1:1,000), cocaine (0.5%), and phenylephrine, are also used.

Box 9.3 Risk factors for epistaxis

- Local infections (vestibulitis, rhinitis, sinusitis)
- Systemic infections (scarlet fever, malaria)
- Drying of nasal mucous membranes
- Nasal inhalation of illicit drugs (e.g. cocaine)
- Trauma (digital trauma as in picking the nose; blunt trauma; fracture; forceful nose blowing)
- Arteriosclerosis
- Hypertension
- Tumor (sinus or nasopharynx)
- Thrombocytopenia
- Use of aspirin
- Liver disease
- Redu-Osler-Weber syndrome (hemorrhagic telangiectasia)

For posterior nosebleeds cotton pledgets moistened with vasoconstricting solution are inserted into the nostril to control bleeding. Antibiotics may by given to manage or prevent infection.

Nursing Management

- Monitor vital signs and assist in control of bleeding
- Provide tissues and an emesis basin for expectoration of blood
- Reassure patient that bleeding can be controlled
- Packing to control bleeding from posterior nose (Fig. 9.8)
- Maintain a calm, efficient manner
- Teach patient to provide self-care by reviewing ways to prevent epistaxis: avoid forceful nose blowing, straining, high altitudes, and nasal trauma (including nose picking)
- Provide adequate humidification to prevent drying of nasal passages
- Instruct patient how to apply direct pressure to nose with thumb and index finger for 15 minutes if nosebleed recurs. Instruct patient to seek medical attention if recurrent bleeding cannot be stopped.

ACUTE PHARYNGITIS

Acute pharyngitis is an acute inflammation of the pharyngeal walls. It may include the tonsils, palate, and uvula.

Etiology

It may be caused by hemolytic streptococci, staphylococci, other bacteria, filterable virus or fungi. Acute follicular pharyngitis (strep throat) results from beta hemolytic streptococcal invasion. Neisseria gonorrhea and corynebacterium diphtheria and other bacteria causing pharyngitis. Fungal pharyngitis caused by candidiasis can develop prolonged use of antibiotics or inhaled corticosteroids as in immunosuppressed patient (e.g. AIDS). Acute pharyngitis is an infection or inflammation in the throat, usually (70%) caused by a viral organism. The inflammatory response results in sore throat with pain, fever, vasodilation, edema and tissue damage (redness and swelling in the tonsillar pillars, uvula, and soft, palate). Uncomplicated viral infections usually subside within 3 to 10 days after onset. When caused by bacteria, the most common organism is group A streptococcus (strep throat). Pharyngitis caused by streptococcus is a more severe illness because of dangerous complications, including sinusitis, otitis media, mastoiditis, cervical adenitis and peritonsillar abscess. Rarely, infection may lead to bacteremia, rheumatic fever, meningitis, pneumonia and nephritis.

Pathophysiology

Dryness of the throat is common complaint. The throat appears red, and soreness may range from slight scratchiness to severe pain with difficulty in swallowing. A hacking cough may be present. Children often develop a very high fever, whereas adults may have only a mild elevation of temperature, symptoms usually precede or occur simultaneously with the onset of acute rhinitis or acute sinusitis.

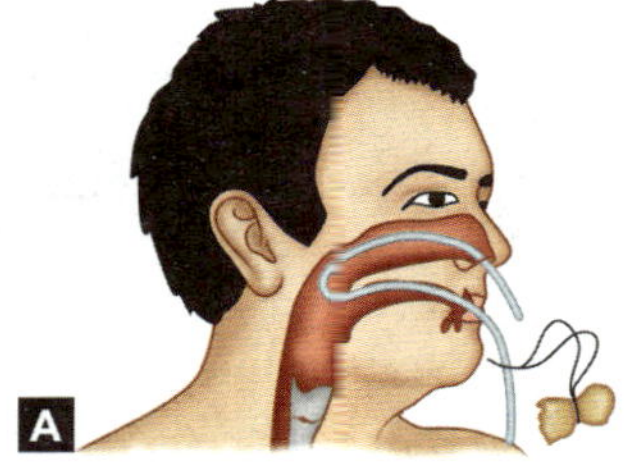

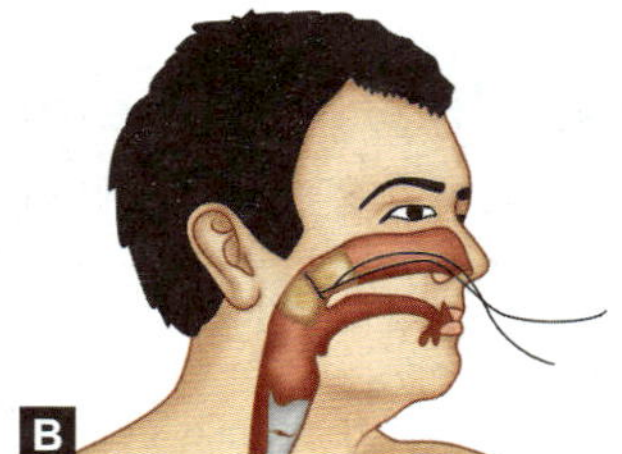

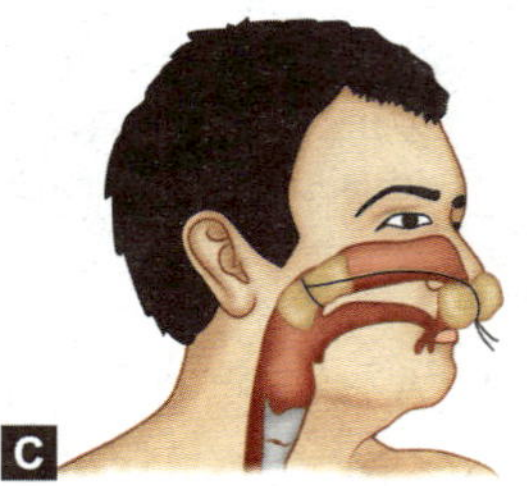

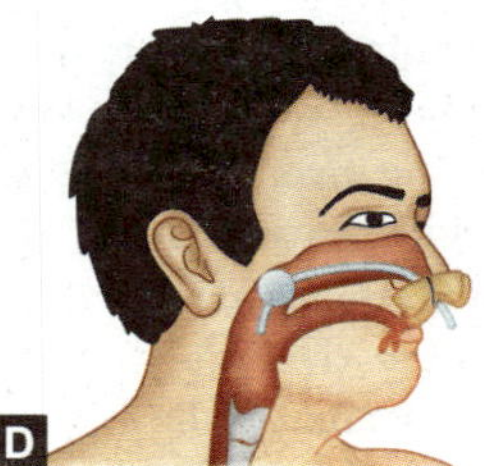

FIGS 9.8A TO D: Packing to control bleeding from the posterior nose. (A) Catheter is inserted and packing is attached; (B) Packing is drawn into position as the catheter is removed; (C) Strip is tied over a bolster to hold the packing in place with an anterior pack installed "accordion pleat" style; (D) Alternative method, using a balloon catheter instead of gauze packing

Clinical Manifestation

- Fiery red pharyngeal membrane and tonsils
- Lymphoid follicles swollen and freckled with white purple exudate
- Cervical lymph nodes enlarged and tender
- Fever, malaise and sore throat
- Hoarseness.

In follicular pharyngitis uniform infection of pharyngeal walls, purulent exudate, edema of lymphoid tissue of palate, tonsils uvula, occur and show sore throat, slightly elevated temperature, and malaise.

In gonococcal or viral pharyngitis, vesicles may be present on pharyngeal walls and tonsils occur. There will be minimal discomfort, fever, diffuse sore throat.

In infectious mononucleosis (Epstein-Barr virus), exudate on pharyngeal walls and tonsils, spleen may be enlarged. There will be a sore throat, cervical lymphadenopathy, and fever.

Fungal pharyngitis (e.g. especially candidiasis-thrush) develop in patient who is immune suppressed and in prolong antibiotics. There will be pus, dysphagia, white plaque, in mouth or on pharyngeal walls.

Management

- Rapid screening test for streptococcal antigens, optical immunoassay (OIA), streptolysin titers, and throat cultures
- Nasal swabbings and blood cultures.

Medical Management

Viral pharyngitis is treated with supportive measures, whereas antibiotic agents are used to treat pharyngitis caused by bacteria: penicillin for group A streptococci and cephalosporins for patients with penicillin allergies or erythromycin resistance. Antibiotics are administered for at least 10 days. In addition, liquid or soft diet is recommended during the acute stage. In some instances, intravenous fluids are administered if the patient cannot swallow. If the patient can swallow, he or she is encouraged to drink 2,000 to 3,000 mL of fluid daily.

Analgesic medications are given at 3- to 6-hour intervals, and antitussive medications (codeine, dextromethorphan [Robitussin DM] or hydrocodone [Hycodan]) are given to control persistent and painful cough.

Acute pharyngitis is usually relieved by hot saline throat gargles. An ice collar may make the person feel more comfortable. For adults acetylsalicylic acid administered orally. Aspergum may be prescribed. Lozenges containing a mild anesthetic may help relieve local soreness. Moist inhalations may help relieve local soreness. A liquid diet usually is better tolerated than solid food and fluids to at least 2.5 liter per day is encouraged.

Oral hygiene may prevent drying and cracking of the lips and usually refreshes the mouth. If the temperature is elevated, the person should remain in bed and even if ambulatory and a febrile, should have extra rest.

A throat culture is necessary to identify the offending organism. For follicular pharyngitis, the choice of antibiotic is penicillin. If person is allergic to penicillin, erythromycin or other antibiotic is prescribed. Candida infections are treated with nystatin and antifungal, antibiotic.

Nursing Management

- Encourage bed rest during febrile stage of illness
- Implement secretion precautions to prevent spread of infection
- Examine skin once or twice daily for possible rash because acute pharyngitis may precede some other communicable disease.

Secure nasal swabbings and throat and blood specimens for culture as needed.

Administer warm saline gargles or irrigations (150°F - 110°F [40.5°-43.3°C]) to ease pain. Also instruct patient regarding purpose and technique for warm gargles (as warm as patient can tolerate) to promote maximum effectiveness.

- Apply an ice collar for symptomatic relief
- Administer analgesic drugs or antitussive medications
- Perform mouth care to prevent fissures of lips and inflammation in the mouth
- Permit gradual resumption of activity
- Advise patient of importance of taking the full course of antibiotic therapy
- Inform patient and family of symptoms to watch for that may indicate development of complications, including nephritis and rheumatic fever.

The goals of nursing management are infection control, symptomatic relief and prevention of secondary complications. The patient should be encouraged to increase fluid intake, cool, bland liquids and gelatin will not irritate pharynx. Citrus fruits juice should be avoided because they irritate the mucous membrane. And make the patient understand the need to take prescribed antibiotic until the course is completed.

CHRONIC PHARYNGITIS

Chronic pharyngitis is common in adults who work or live in dusty surroundings, use their voice to excess, suffer from chronic cough, and habitually use alcohol and tobacco. Three types are recognized; hypertrophic, a general thickening and congestion of the pharyngeal mucous membranes; atrophic, a late stage of type 1; and chronic granular, marked by numerous swollen lymph follicles of the pharyngeal wall.

Clinical Manifestations

- Constant sense of irritation of fullness in the throat
- Mucus that collects in the throat and is expelled by coughing
- Difficulty in swallowing.

Medical Management

Treatment is based on symptom relief, avoidance of exposure to irritants, and correction of any upper respiratory, pulmonary or cardiac condition that might be responsible for chronic cough. Nasal sprays (ephedrine sulfate or phenylephrine hydrochloride) are used to relieve nasal congestion . Aspirin (adults only) or acetaminophen may be recommended to control inflammation and relieve discomfort.

Nursing Management

- Advise patient to avoid contact with others until fever has subsided completely to prevent infection from spreading
- Instruct patient to avoid alcohol, tobacco, secondhand smoke, exposure to cold, and environmental and occupational pollutants. Suggest wearing a disposable mask for protection
- Encourage patient to drink plenty of fluids, and encourage gargling with warm salt water to relieve throat discomfort. Using lozenges may help to keep the throat moist.

ACUTE FOLLICULAR TONSILLITIS

Acute follicular tonsillitis is an acute inflammation of the tonsils and their crypts. It is usually caused by the streptococcus organism. It is more likely to occur when the persons's resistance is low, and it is common in children.

Pathophysiology and Clinical Manifestation

The onset is almost always sudden, and symptoms include sore throat, pain on swallowing, fever, chills, general muscle aching and malaise. These systems often last for 2 to 3 days. The pharynx and tonsils appear red, and the peritonsillar tissues are swollen. Sometimes a yellowish exudate drains from crypts in the tonsils. A throat culture usually is taken to identify the offending organism.

Complications of untreated tonsillitis include heart and kidney damage, chorea and pneumonia. Incidence of these complications is decreasing with early diagnosis and wide-spread use of penicillin. Recurrent attacks of tonsillitis need to undergo tonsillectomy. This procedure is usually performed from 4 to 6 weeks after an acute attack is subsided.

Peritonsillar abscess typically occurs as a complication of acute pharyngitis and acute tonsillitis if bacterial invasion of one or both tonsils. The tonsils may enlarge sufficiently to threaten airway patency. Infections extend from the tonsils to form an access in the surrounding tissues. The presence of pus behind the tonsils causes difficulty in swallowing, talking and opening the mouth, the difficulty in swallowing may be so great that the person is unable to swallow. Pain is severe and may extend to the ear on the affected side. The patient will experience high fever, leukocytosis and chills.

Management

The patient with acute tonsillitis is encouraged to rest and take generous amounts of fluid orally. Warm saline throat gargle (irrigation) may be ordered, and antibiotics are given for streptococcal pharyngitis, acetaminophen (tyclerol) and codeine sulfate may be ordered for pain and discomfort. An ice collar applied to the neck may relieve discomfort.

Early detection and treatment with IV antibiotic therapy may clear the infection and prevent abscess development. If antibiotics to which the offending organism is sensitive are administered early, infection subsides. If the peritonsillar abscess caused by anerobic organisms hydrogen peroxide (an oxidizing agent) in the form of mouthwash may help to relieve symptoms. If an abscess develops incision and drainage are required. An emergency tonsillectomy may be performed, or an elective tonsillectomy may be scheduled after the infection subsided.

CHRONIC ENLARGEMENT OF ADENOIDS AND TONSILS

Tonsils and adenoids are lymphoid structures located in the oropharynx and nasopharynx. They reach full size in childhood and then begin to atrophy during puberty. When adenoids enlarge, usually results of chronic infections but sometimes for no known reason they cause nasal obstructions. The person breathes through mouth, snores loudly, may have a dull facial expression and may have reduced appetite, because the blocked nasopharynx can interfere with swallowing. Hypertrophy of the tonsils does not usually block the oropharynx but may affect speech and swallowing and cause mouth breathing.

Pathophysiology

The tonsils are red and swollen with yellow or white exudate found mainly in the crypts of the tonsils. Signs and symptoms include fever, dry throat, malaise, dysphagia, otalgia, and a feeling of fullness in the throat. Lymph nodes in upper part of the neck is swollen and palpable.

Management

The tonsils and adenoids are removed when they become enlarged and cause symptoms of obstruction, when they are chronically infected. When the person has repeated attacks of tonsillitis or after repeated peritonsillar abscess. Chronic infections of these structures usually do not respond to antibiotics and may become foci of infections by spreading organisms to other parts of the body such as heart and kidney.

Tonsillectomy is performed with either general or local anesthesia. After tonsils are removed, pressure is applied to stop superficial bleeding. Bleeding vessels are tied off with sutures or by electrocoagulation. The person is monitored carefully for hemorrhage, especially when sleeping, because a large amount of blood may be lost without any external evidence of bleeding. The person who is bleeding excessively often is returned to the operating room for surgical treatment to stop the hemorrhage. If sutures are used, the person will have more pain and discomfort than that occurring after simple tonsillectomy and may be unable to take solid food for several days.

The tough, yellow, fibrous membrane that forms over the operative site begins to break away between the fourth and eight postoperative days and hemorrhage may occur. The separation of the membranes accounts for throat being more painful at this time.

Pink granulation tissue soon becomes apparent and by the end of the third postoperative week, the area is covered with normal mucous membrane.

The following points to be kept in mind while taking care of a person after tonsillectomy:

- Position patient on side until fully awake after general anesthesia of in mid-Fowler's position when awake
- Monitor for hemorrhage
  - Frequent swallowing (inspect throat)
  - Bright red vomitus
  - Rapid pulse
  - Restlessness
- Comfort
  - Give 30 percent cool mist via collar
  - Apply ice collar to neck (will also reduce bleeding by vasoconstriction)
  - Use acetaminophen in place of aspirin (in tendency on bleeding)
- Food and fluids
  - Give ice-cold fluids and bland foods during initial period (e.g. ice chips, popsicles, jella)
  - Milk is usually not given, because it may increase mucus and cause the patient to clear the throat
  - Advance to normal diet as soon as possible
- Patient and family teaching
  - Avoid attempting to clear throat immediately after surgery (may initiate bleeding)
  - Avoid coughing, sneezing, vigorous nose blowing and vigorous exercise for 1 to 2 weeks
  - Drink fluids (2 to 3 L/day) until mouth odor disappears
  - Avoid hard, scratchy foods such as pretzels, popcorn or toast, until throat is healed
  - Report signs of bleeding to physician immediately
  - Expect more throat discomfort between 4th and 8th postoperative days because of membrane separation
  - Expect stool to be black or dark for a few days because of swallowed blood
  - Resume normal activity immediately as long as it is not stressful and does not require straining.

ACUTE LARYNGITIS

Acute laryngitis is an inflammation of the mucous membrane lining of the larynx accompanied by edema of the vocal cords. It may be caused by cold, by sudden changes in temperature or by irritating fumes.

Pathophysiology/Clinical Manifestation

Symptoms vary from a slight huskiness to complete loss of voice. The throat may be painful and feel scratching, and a cough may be present.

Management

Laryngitis management requires only symptomatic treatment. The person is advised to remain indoors in an even temperature and to avoid talking for several days or weeks, depending on the severity of the inflammation. Steam inhalation may be soothing and cough syrups or home remedies for cough to provide relief to some patients. Smoking should be avoided. Additional fluids by mouth help prevent dehydration and drying of throat.

The nursing role is mainly patient teaching, which could include the following:

- Need to take antibiotics as prescribed (full course as prescribed)
- Need to increase fluid intake
- Need to stop smoking for smokers
- Need to avoid smoky environment
- Referral to a support group of persons wanting to stop smoking
- Precautions to be observed in using steam inhalations.

Chronic laryngitis may occur in persons who use their voices excessively, who smoke a great deal or who work continuously where there are irritating fumes. Hoarseness usually is worse in early morning and evening. There may be dry, harsh cough. Treatment of chronic laryngitis includes removal of irritants, voice test, correction of faulty voice habits, steam inhalation. Additional fluid by mouth care are encouraged.

Laryngeal Paralysis

Laryngeal paralysis may result from disease or injury of either the laryngeal nerves or the vagus nerve.

Etiology

Laryngeal paralysis may be caused by
- Aortic aneurysm
- Mitral stenosis
- Laryngeal cancer (Box 9.4)
- Subglottic or cervical esophageal tumors
- Bronchial carcinoma
- Neck injury
- Severing or stretching of the recurrent laryngeal nerve during thyroidectomy
- Prolonged intubation of patients in intensive care units.

Pathophysiology

Either one or both vocal cords may be paralyzed. If only one cord is affected, the airway is adequate and now the voice may be affected. Efforts to improve the voice in persons with unilateral cord paralysis have been accomplished by injecting a small quantity of Gelfoam or Teflan into paralyzed cord. This swells the cord and pushes it towards the midline where the other cord can approximate it better during phonation.

Bilateral paralysis causes a poor airway that results in incapacitating dyspnea, stridor on exertion and a weak voice. A sudden bilateral vocal cord paralysis is not common and usually a result of massive cerebrovascular accident or blunt trauma both of which are incompatible with life.

Management

Diagnostic tests performed include:
- Indirect laryngoscopy to diagnose vocal cord abnormality
- Videostroboscopy (observe vocal cords vibration during phonation). Here fiberoptic laryngoscope is attached to videotape to record actual cord motion. This is to diagnose abnormal vibrations of cord
- Electromyography to determine innervation and thus movement of vocal cords
- CT scan to determine cause of vocal cord paresis or paralysis such as tumor or aneurysm along course of recurrent laryngeal nerve.

Box 9.4 An overview of laryngeal cancer

Signs and symptoms	Hoarse voice Pain Cough Shortness of breath Difficulty swallowing Weight loss Foul breath
Diagnostic tests	Examination with laryngeal mirror Laryngoscopy with biopsy Additional blood and radiographic studies to detect metastasis
Therapeutic measures	Radiation therapy Chemotherapy (adjunct to radiation or surgery) Endoscopic laser surgery to destroy tumor Partial laryngectomy (preserves some voice) Radical neck dissection with total laryngectomy (loss of voice)

Treatment of laryngeal paralysis is symptomatic:
- Antacids are used if patient experiencing gastroesophageal reflux which neutralize gastric acid
- H_2 inhibitor, used to reduce the amount of gastric acid produced
- Antibiotics are used for infection
- Tracheostomy may be necessary to maintain airway
- Other procedures are followed according to causes.

Complete removal of the larynx (total laryngectomy) can provide the desired cure in most advanced laryngeal cancers, when the tumor extends beyond the vocal cords, or for cancer that recurs or persists after radiation therapy. In a total laryngectomy, the laryngeal structures are removed, including the hyoid bone, epiglottis, cricoid cartilage, and two or three rings of the trachea. The tongue, pharyngeal walls and trachea are preserved. A total laryngectomy results in permanent loss of the voice and a change in the airway, requiring a permanent tracheostomy (Fig. 9.9). Occasionally, patients continue to have a laryngectomy tube in the stoma. Laryngectomy tubes are similar in appearance to tracheostomy tubes; however, a laryngectomy tube can be distinguished from a tracheostomy tube because the patient is unable to speak or breathe when the laryngectomy require alternatives to normal speech; these may include a prosthetic device, such as the Blom-Singer valve, to speak without aspirating.

Surgery is more difficult when the lesion involves the midline structures of both vocal cords. With or without neck dissection, a total laryngectomy requires a permanent tracheal stoma because the larynx that provides the protective sphincter is no longer present. The tracheal stoma prevents the aspiration of food and fluid into the lower respiratory tract. The patient has no vice but has normal swallowing. A total laryngectomy changes the manner in which airflow is used for breathing and speaking, as depicted in Figure 9.10. The patient has significant loss of the natural voice and the need to breathe through an opening (stoma) created in the lower neck. Complications that may occur include a salivary leak, wound infection from the development of a pharyngocutaneous fistula, stomal stenosis, and dysphagia secondary to esophageal stricture. Despite these changes and potential complications, many patients who have undergone a total laryngectomy maintain a good quality of life overall.

In some cases, the patient may be a candidate for a near-total laryngectomy. In this situation, the patient would be a candidate for chemotherapy and radiotherapy regimens postoperatively. Voice preservation can be achieved in most cases.

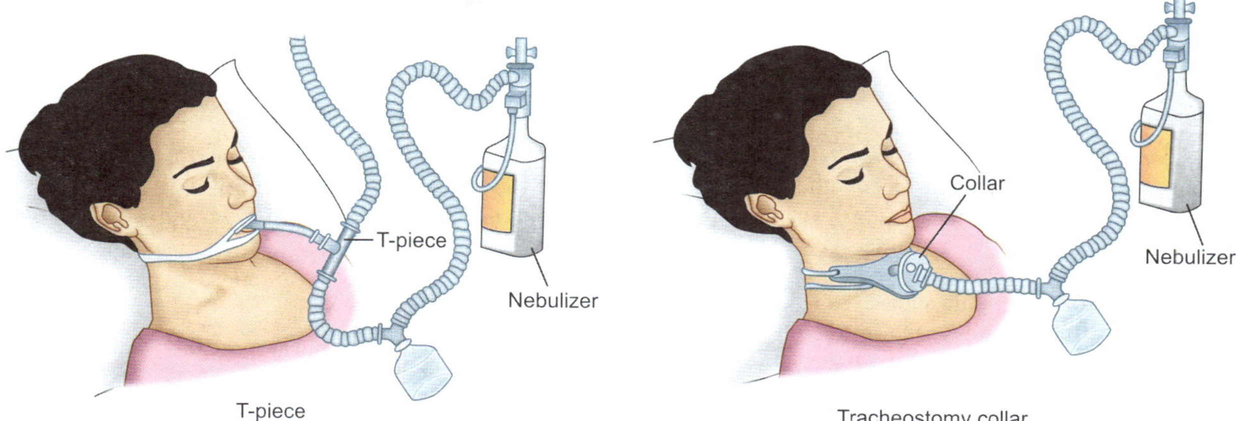

FIG. 9.9: Pieces and tracheostomy collars are devices used when weaning patients from mechanical ventilation

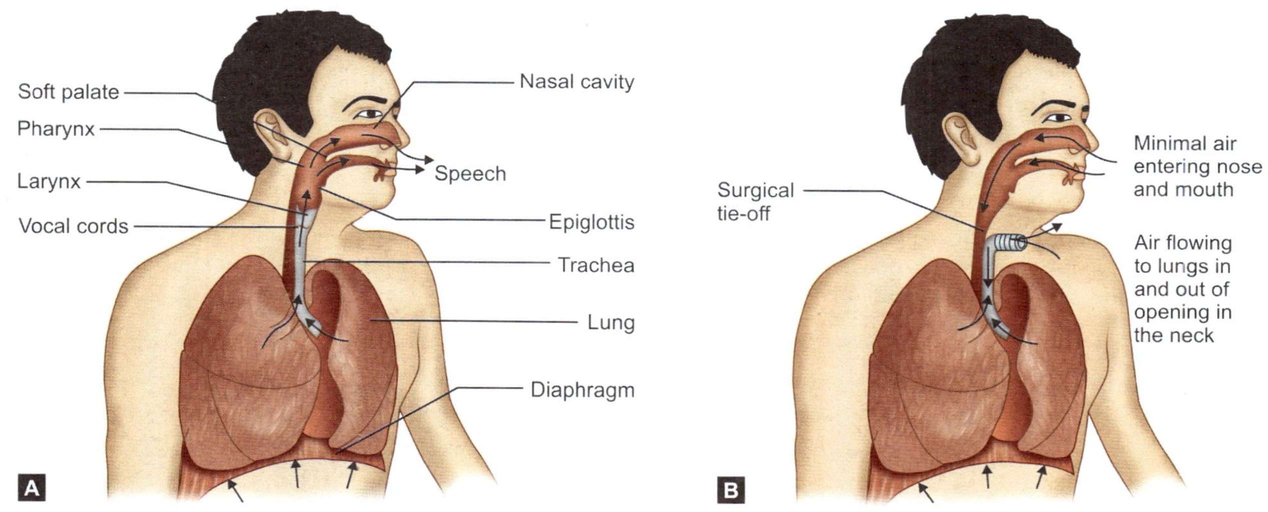

FIGS 9.10A AND B: Total laryngectomy produces a change in airflow for breathing and speaking. (A) Normal airflow; (B) Airflow after total laryngectomy

Advances in surgical techniques for treating laryngeal cancer may minimize the cosmetic and functional deficits previously seen with total laryngectomy. Some microlaryngeal can be performed endoscopically.

Laryngeal Edema

Acute laryngeal edema may be caused by anaphylaxis, urticaria, acute laryngitis, scream inflammatory diseases to the throat or edema after intubation. It causes the airway to narrow or close and required immediate restoration of the airway.

Treatment of acute laryngeal edema consists of administration of an adrenocorticosteroid or epinephrine. Intubation or tracheostomy may be necessary.

Airway Obstruction

Airway may be complete or partial. Complete airway obstruction is medical emergency. Partial airway obstructions may occur as a result of aspiration of food as foreign body. In addition, partial airway obstruction may result from laryngeal edema following extubation laryngeal or tracheal stenosis, and neurologic depression.

Symptoms include stridor, use of accessory muscles, suprasternal and intercoastal retractions, wheezing, restlessness, tachycardia and cyanosis.

Management

Prompt assessment and treatment are essential because partial obstructions may quickly progress to complete destruction. Interventions to maintain a patient airway include use of obstructed airway (Heimlich) maneuver, endotracheal intubation and tracheostomy.

An endotracheal tube is usually chosen initially as a means of providing airway, tracheostomy is performed only if airway maintenance is necessary for longer than 10 to 14 days or if trauma to the airway prevents the use of an endotracheal tube.

In endotracheal intubation, a tube is passed through either the nose or mouth into the trachea, whereas in a tracheostomy, an artificial opening is made in the trachea into which a tracheostomy tube is inserted. The procedures are used to:

- Establish and maintain patent airway
- Prevent aspiration by sealing off the trachea from digestive tract in the unconscious or paralyzed person
- Permit removal of tracheobronchial secretions in the person who cannot cough adequately, and
- Treat the patient who requires positive pressure mechanical ventilation that cannot be given effectively by masks.

The endotracheal tubes is made of plastic with an inflatable cuff so that a closed system with the ventilator may be maintained. The tube is inserted via the mouth or nose through the larynx into the trachea. If an oral endotracheal tube is used, a rubber airway or bite block is often necessary to prevent the patient from biting down on the tube and obstructing the airway.

Tracheostomy

A tracheostomy is a surgical incision into the trachea for the purpose of establishing an airway. It is the stoma (an opening) that results from the tracheostomy. Indications for a tracheostomy are to:

- Bypass an upper airway obstruction
- Facilitate removal of secretions
- Permit long-term mechanical ventilation, and
- Permit oral intake and speech in the patient who requires long-term mechanical ventilation (Fig. 9.9).

Nursing Care

Before the procedure the nurse should explain to the patient and the family the purpose of the procedure and inform them that the patient will not be able to speak if an inflated cuff is used.

The patient and family should be informed the normal speech will be possible as soon as the cuff can be deflated.

A variety of tubes are available to meet individual patient needs, which include (Fig. 9.11):

i. Tracheostomy tube with cuff and inflated balloons: When properly inflated, lower pressure, high-volume cuff distributes cuff pressure over large areas, minimizing pressure on tracheal wall.

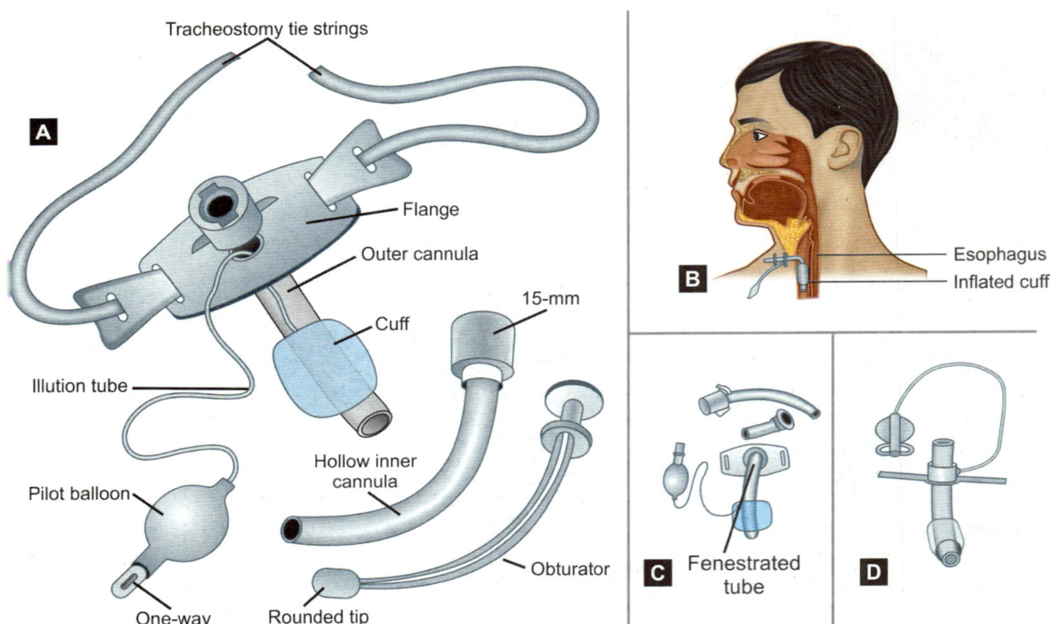

FIGS 9.11A TO D: Types of tracheostomy tubes. (A) Parts of a tracheostomy tube; (B) Tracheostomy tube inserted in airway with inflated cuff; (C) Fenestrated tracheostomy tube with cuff, inner cannula, decannulation plug, and pilot ballon; (D) Trachestomy tube with foam cuff and obturator (one cuff is deflated on tracheostomy tube)

ii. Fenestrated tracheostomy tube with cuff and inner cannula and decannulation plug: When inner cannula is removed, cuff deflated, and decannulation plug inserted, air flows around the tube through fenestration in outer cannula and up over vocal cords. Patient can then speak.
iii. Speaking tracheostomy tube (Portex, National) with cuff, two external tubings; It has two tubings, one leading to cuff and second to opening above the cuff. When port is connected to air source, air flows out of opening and up over the vocal cords, allowing speech in the cuff inflated.
iv. Tracheostomy tube (Bivona Fome-cuff) foam filled cuff: This cuff is filled with plastic foam. Before insertion, cuff is deflated. After insertion, cuff is allowed to fill passively with air. Pilot tubing is not capped and no cuff pressure monitoring is required.

All tracheostomy tubes contain a face plate or flange, which rests on the neck between the clavicles and outer cannula. In addition, all tubes have an obturator, which is used when inserting the tube. During insertion of the tube, the obturator is placed inside the outer cannula with its rounded tip protruding from air end of the tube to ease insertion. After insertion, the obturator must be immediately removed so that air can flow through the tube. The obturator should be kept in an easily accessible place at the bedside (e.g. taped to the wall) so that it can be used quickly in case of accidental decannulation.

Nursing Management of Endotracheal or Tracheostomy Tube

An endotracheal or tracheostomy tube provides a direct route for introduction of pathogen, into the lower airway, increasing the risk of infection. It is essential that the following preventive nursing intervention be consistently implemented.

1. Minimize infection risk
   - Endotracheal airways irritate the trachea resulting in increased mucus production. Assess the patient regularly for excess secretions and suction as often as necessary to maintain a patent airway.
   - Provide constant airway humidifications. Endotracheal airways bypass the upper airway which normally humidifies and warms inspired air. An external source of cool, humidified air must be provided to avoid thickening and crusting of bronchial secretions.
   - All respiratory therapy equipment should be changed every 6 hours. In addition:
     - Replace any equipment that touches the floor
     - Remove water that condenses in equipment tubing. Do not pour condensed water back into humidifier reservoir, because it may contain pathogens.
   - Provide frequent mouth care. Secretions tend to pool in the mouth and in the pharynx, particularly if the cuff of the tube is inflated. An endotracheal tube or oral airway increases the risk of ulceration or abrasion of the lips and oropharynx.
     - Gently suction oropharynx as needed
     - Inspect the lips, tongue and oral cavity regularly
     - Clean the oral cavity with swab soaked in saline
     - Apply moisturising agent to cracked lips.
   - Maintain adequate nutrition levels.
     a. The person with endotracheal tube is allowed nothing by mouth. Nourishment will be given parenterally or gastrointestinal feedings. Gastrointestinal supplemental feedings are preferred because they maintain the function of the gut, propose less infection risk, and more economical than IV fluids. While administering GI feeding to the intubated patient, nurse will:
        - Assess for bowel sounds and tube placement,
        - Elevate head of the bed at least 45 degrees, and
        - Inflate the tracheostomy tube cuff
          - If using a Salem sump nasogastric tube, check the amount of residual feeding. If the half volume of the feeding to be given remains, the tube feeding is withheld
          - Administer the tube feeding over 20–30 minutes
          - Keep head of bed elevated for 45–60 minutes after feeding
          - Assess at regular intervals for aspiration
          - Regularly assess for tube placement and residual stomach contents.

     b. The patient with a tracheostomy tube is usually able to swallow and have a normal oral intake. Some experts prefer that the cuff on the tracheostomy tube be inflated while the patient is eating to prevent aspiration. Others believe that cuff bulges into esophagus and make swallowing more difficult, and they therefore prefer that cuff be deflated. Nursing assessment will determine which technique to be used. Methylene blue dye can be swallowed before each feeding or mixed with tube feeding. If the dye does not appear in tracheal secretions, it is safe to proceed with the meal.
2. Ensure adequate ventilation and oxygenation
   - Assess lung sounds regularly. Unless the individual's underlying pathology alters lung ventilations, sounds should be heard bilaterally, and chest expansion should be symmetrical. If an endotracheal tube is inserted too far it will slip into one of the mainstems of bronchi (usually the night) and occlude the opposite bronchus and lung resulting in atelectasis on the obstructed side. Even if the endotracheal tube is still in the trachea, airway obstruction will result if the end of the tube is located on the carina. This will result in dry secretions that obstruct both bronchi. So the tube is pulled back until it is positioned below the larynx and above the carina. The tube is then fastened securely in place
   - Turn and reposition the patient every 2 hours for maximum ventilation and lung perfusion

- Assess respiratory frequency, tidal volume and viral capacity
- Perform postural drainage, percussion and vibration as appropriate.

3. Provide safety and comfort
   - Most endotracheal and tracheostomy tubes have cuffs for the following reasons:
     - To provide a sealed airway for positive pressure mechanical ventilation, and
     - To prevent aspirations in the unconscious person during tube feedings
   - Assess tube placement in regular intervals
     - The tube is secured around neck with tape or especially designed ties, and
     - The endotracheal tube is marked to establish a landmark for position comparison and to measure and document the length of the tube that extends beyond the patient lips.
   - Change tapes or ties whenever soiled to decreased skin irritation.
   - Always keep a spare tube at the bedside.
   - Minimize sensory deprivations. Because patients with these tubes with cuff-inflated cannot talk. Therefore, an acceptable communication mode must be established as follows:
     - Organise questions so that patient can use a simple 'Yes' or 'No' response (nodding head, using hand signals, or squeezing the nurse's hand)
     - The patient may be able to use an erasable board or note pad to communicate
     - Always talk to the patient and explain all procedures
     - Reorient the patient frequently
     - Encourage family and friends to talk to patient and offer encouragement
     - Keep call light (or tap bell) within the patient's reach
     - Reinforce that the ability to speak will return when the tube is removed.
4. Observe special precautions during the immediate extubation period
   - Monitor for signs such as increased respiratory distress, increased restlessness, hoarseness and laryngeal stridor indicating upper airway obstruction secondary to laryngeal edema
   - Assess for adequacy of cough and gag reflex
   - After removal of a tracheostomy tube there is a temporary air leak at the incision site. To speak, the patient will have to occlude the opening with a finger
   - The tracheal stoma can be suctioned. However, frequent use of the stoma for suctioning can delay closure and healing of tracheostomy incisions.

Procedure for Suctioning a Tracheostomy Tube (Fig. 9.12)

1. Assess the need for suctioning 4th hourly. Indications include coarse crackles or rhonchi over large airways, moist cough, increase in peak inspiratory pressure and mechanical ventilator and restlessness or agitation if accompanied by decrease in SPO_2 or PaO_2. Do not suction routinely or if patient is able to clear secretion with cough.
2. If suctioning indicated, explain the procedure to the patient.
3. Collect necessary equipment; suction catheters no larger than half the lumen of the tracheostomy tube), gloves, water, cup, and drape. If a closed tracheal suction is used, the catheter is enclosed in a plastic sleeves and reused for 24 hours. No, additional equipment is needed.
4. Check suction source and regulator. Adjust suction pressure until the dial reads-120 to 150 mm Hg pressure with tubing occluded.
5. Wash hands, put on goggles and gloves.
6. Use sterile technique to open package, fill cup with water, put on gloves, and connect catheter to suction. Designate on hand as contaminated for disconnecting, bagging and operating the suction control. Suction water through the catheter to test the system.
7. Assess SPO_2 heart rate and rhythm to provide baseline for etecting change during suctioning.
8. Provide preoxygenation by (i) adjusting ventilator to deliver 100 percent O_2, (ii) using reservoir-equipped manual resuscitate bag (MRB) connected to 100 percent O_2; or (iii) asking patient to take 3–4-deep breaths. While administering oxygen, the method chosen will depend on the patient's underlying disease and ability or illness. The patient who has tracheostomy for an extended period of time and is not acutely ill, may be able to tolerate suctioning without use of an MRB or the ventilator.
9. Gently insert the catheter without suction to minimize the amount of oxygen removed from the lungs. Insert the catheter approximately 5-6 inches. Stop if any obstruction is met.
10. Withdraw the catheter 1–2 cm and apply suction intermittently, while withdrawing catheter in a rotating manner. If secretion volume is large, apply suction continuously.
11. If the patient develops mucus plugs or thick secretions a 3–5 mL bolus of normal saline may be instilled into the airway to loosen secretions sufficiently to clear the airway either through coughing or suctioning.
12. Limit suction time to 10 seconds. Discontinue suctioning if heart rate decreases from baseline by 20 beats, increases from baseline by 40 beats per minute, an arrhythmias or SPO_2 decreases to less than 90 percent.

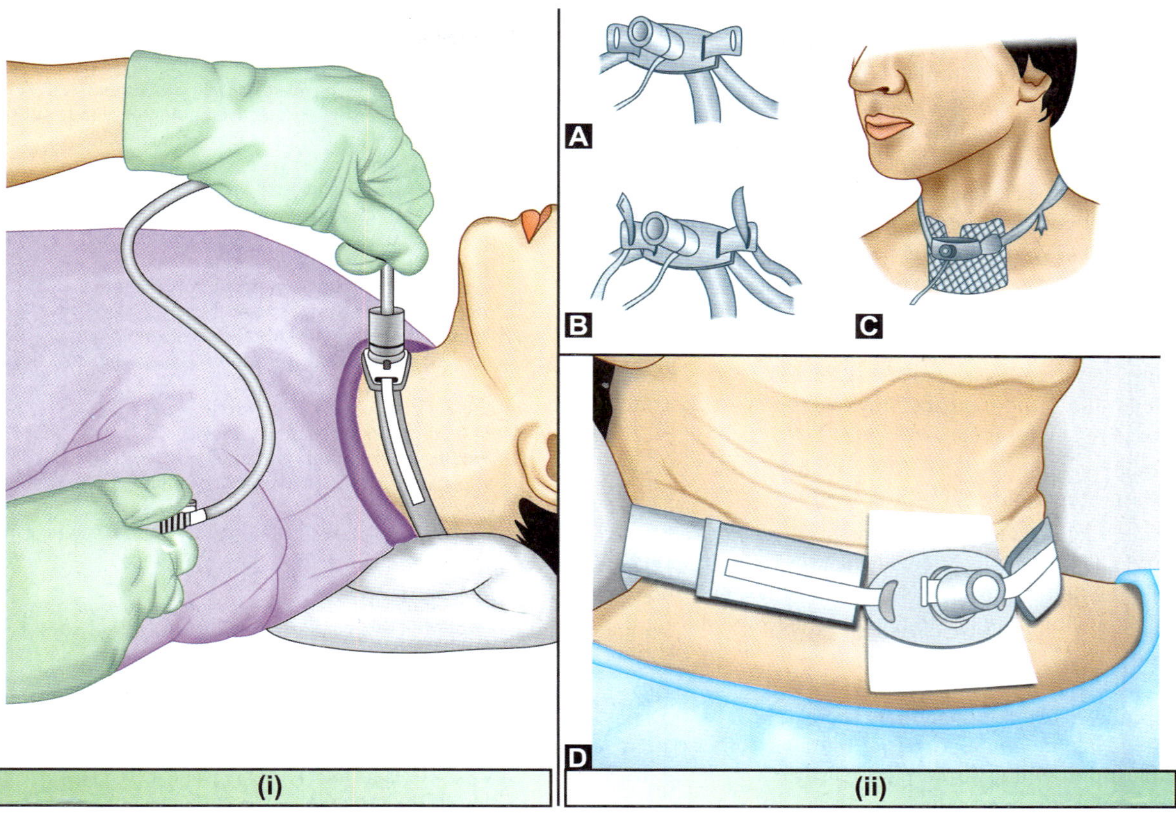

FIGS 9.12: (i) Suctioning a trachesostomy. Using sterile technique, the suction catheter is being withdrawn from the airway while suction is applied. The pilot ballon tubing may be seen lying on the patient's chest; (ii) Changing tracheostomy ties. (A) A slit is cut about 1 inch (2.5 cm) from the end. The slit end is put into the opening of the cannula. (B) A loop is made with the other end of the tape. (C) The tapes are tied together with a double knot on the side the neck. (D) A tracheostomy tube holder can be used in place of twill ties to make tracheostomy tube stabilization more secure

13. After each suction—pass, oxygenate with 3–4 breaths by ventilator, MRB or deep breaths with oxygen.
14. Rinse catheter with sterile water.
15. Repeat procedure until airway is clear. Limit insertions of suction catheter to three passes.
16. Return oxygen concentration to prior setting.
17. Rinse catheter and suction the oropharynx or use mouth suction.
18. Dispose of catheter by wrapping it around fingers of gloved hand and pulling glove over catheter. Discard equipment in proper waste container.
19. Auscultate to assess changes in lung sounds. Record time, amount, and character of secretions and response to suctioning.

Tracheostomy Care

Although nursing care of persons with either endotracheal or tracheostomy tube is similar, patients with tracheostomies have additional nursing care needs. Nursing care includes maintaining air humidification, providing nourishment, and weaning for the tracheostomy tube. The care of the tracheostomy tube. The care of the tracheostomy is as follows:

1. Explain procedure to the patient.
2. Collect necessary sterile equipment (e.g. suction catheter, gloves, water, basin, drape, tracheostomy-ties, tube brush or pipe cleaners, 4x4s, hydrogen peroxide 3 percent, sterile water and tracheostomy dressing (optional).

   Note: Clean rather than sterile technique is used at home.
3. Position patient in semi-Fowler's position.
4. Assemble needed materials on bedside table next to patient.
5. Wash hands, put on goggles and gloves.
6. Auscultate chest sounds. If rhonchi or coarse crackles are present suction the patient if unable to cough up secretions.
7. Unlock and remove inner cannula, if present. Many tracheostomy tubes do not have inner cannula. Care for

these tubes includes all steps except for inner cannula care.

8. If disposable inner cannula is used, replace with new cannula. If non-disposable cannula is used:
   - Immerse inner cannula in 3 percent hydrogen peroxide and clean inside and outside of cannula using tube brush or pipe cleaner
   - Drain hydrogen peroxide from cannula. Immerse cannula in sterile water and shake to dry
   - Insert inner cannula into outer cannula with the curved part downward and lock in place.
9. Remove dried secretions from stoma using 4 × 4 soaked in sterile water. Gently pat area around the stoma dry. Be sure to clear under the tracheostomy face plate, using cotton swabs to reach this area.
10. Maintain position of tracheal retention sutures if present, by taping above and below the stoma.
11. Change tracheostomy ties. Tie tracheostomy ties securely with room for one finger between ties and skin. To prevent accidental tube removal, secure the tracheostomy tube by gently applying pressure to flange of the tube during the tie changes. Do not change tracheostomy ties for 24 hours after the tracheostomy procedure.
12. As an alternative some patients prefer tracheostomy ties made of velero, which are easier to adjust, other patients use plastic IV tubing because it is easily cleaned and dries without need to replace the ties.
13. Unless excessive amounts of exudate are present avoid using a tracheostomy dressing since this keeps the site moist and may predispose to infection.
14. If drainage is excessive, place dressing around tube. A tracheostomy dressing or unlined gauze should be used. Do not cut the guaze because threads may be inhaled or wrope around the tracheostomy tube. Change the dressing frequently. Wet dressings promote infection and stoma irritation
15. Repeat care three times a day and as needed and also follow manufacturers' instructions (Box 9.5).

Box 9.5 Tracheostomy cleaning procedure

1. Assemble equipment: Tracheostomy care kit, new inner cannula (if disposable), sterile water or saline, hydrogen peroxide, suction equipment, personal protective equipment (gown, goggles, face shield) as indicated by patient's condition
2. Put on personal protective equipment as necessary
3. Explain the procedure to the patient
4. If patient is receiving oxygen, keep mask intact as much as possible. If mask must be removed for care, replace immediately between each step of procedure
5. Suction inner cannula if necessary. See Figure 9.12 of suctioning procedure for the patient with a tracheostomy
6. Open and prepare the kit, keeping all equipment sterile. Fill one side of basin with half peroxide and half saline and the other with saline
7. Don clean gloves
8. Remove old tracheostomy dressing
9. Remove inner cannula from tracheostomy tube and discard (if disposable) or place it in peroxide solution (if nondisposable)
10. Don sterile gloves
11. Use brush and pipe cleaners to clean reusable inner cannula. Place in water or saline to rinse. Dry inside of cannula with pipe cleaner
12. Reinsert new or cleaned inner cannula into tracheostomy tube
13. Use cotton swab and sterile gauze with sterile peroxide and saline to clean around tracheostomy site. Rinse with saline to prevent skin irritation
14. Replace ties or Velcro stabilizer. Remove old ties after new ties are securely in place
15. Apply sterile tracheostomy dressing (drain sponge or 'trach pants'). Use precut or folded dressing (cutting gauze creates fibers that can enter the tracheostomy.)

ACUTE BRONCHITIS

Bronchitis is an inflammation of the lower respiratory tract that is usually due to infection and occurs most frequently in patients with chronic respiratory disease. Bronchitis can be acute or chronic bronchitis.

Acute bronchitis is an inflammation of the bronchi and usually the trachea (tracheobronchitis).

Etiology

Acute bronchitis occurs most often in persons with chronic lung disease. It also occurs as an extension of the URI in persons without underlying any lung disease, and is therefore communicable. It may be caused by physical and chemical agents such as dust, smoke, or volatile fumes. As air pollution increases, the incidence of acute bronchitis increases.

Acute bronchitis is typically viral, but bacterial pathogens such as *Streptococcus pneumoniae* and *Haemophilus influenzae* may also cause bronchitis, either primary or secondary infections which includes:

- *Viruses:* Rhinovirus, adenovirus, influenza A and B, parainfluenza virus and respiratory syncytial virus (RSV).
- *Bacteria: Streptococcus pneumoniae, Haemophilus influenzae, Moraxella catarrhalis, Bordetella pertussis, Mycoplasma pneumoniae, Chlamydophila pneumoniae.*

Pathophysiology

As a part of the inflammatory process, there is increased blood flow to the affected area, causing an increased pulmonary secretions. A painful cough with sputum productions, low-grade fever, and malaise are common symptoms. The patient may have pain beneath the sternum caused by inflammation of the tracheal wall. Bronchitis without tracheitis never seen, and tracheobronchitis is more appropriate term for this condition. Symptoms usually last 1 for 1 to 2 weeks but may continue for 3 to 4 weeks. Rhonchi and wheezes heard on chest examination. If symptoms worsen and there is a high fever, shortness of breath, pleuritic chest pain (pain on inspiration) rapid respirations and rales or sign if consolidation on physical examination of the chest, pneumonia suspected (Fig. 9.13).

Management

Treatment of acute bronchitis is mainly supportive and includes the following:

- Codeine or dextromethorphan is prescribed for nocturnal cough
- Bronchodilator therapy is prescribed for patients who are wheezing and for those whose peak expiratory rate prolonged, e.g. albuterol or ipratropium
- Decongestants and antihistamines are used sparingly, if at all, because they tend to dry secretions and make them more difficult to remove
- Oral fluids intake of 2 to 3 liter per day is encouraged if there is no contraindications to it
- Aspirin helps to reduce fever and alleviate some of the symptoms and inflammation
- Patients who are smokers are urged to quit
- Antibiotics are usually not prescribed unless there is evidence of bacterial infections
- Rest is encouraged to give the body a chance to heal.

Nursing care is supportive and is directed towards helping the patient with prescribed therapy and avoiding future infections. Emphasis on assisting the patient to cough effectively, assisting with comfort, assisting with activities of daily living and teaching the patient and family.

To produce an effective cough, a deep inspiration must be followed by maximal expiratory effort against a closed glottis. This results in a tremendous increase in intrathoracic pressure. As glottis opens, mucus and inhaled particles are forced out of the airways at a high velocity. Persistent coughing can be annoying and tiring to the patient and those around him or her. Complications of persistent coughing includes, insomnia, exhaustion vomiting, urinary incontinence, rib or muscle trauma, pneumothorax, and fainting. If cough persists, give cough medication as prescribed. A semi-Fowler's position or high-Fowler's position usually facilitates breathing. Provide for good drainage of tracheobronchial secretions and give antibiotics as ordered and assist in ADL.

PNEUMONIA

Pneumonia or pneumonitis is an acute inflammation of the lung tissue (lung parenchyma). Pneumonia is an inflammation of the lung parenchyma commonly caused by microbial agents. Classically, pneumonia has been categorized as being bacterial or typical, atypical, anaerobic/cavitary, or opportunistic. Another classification scheme categorizes pneumonias as

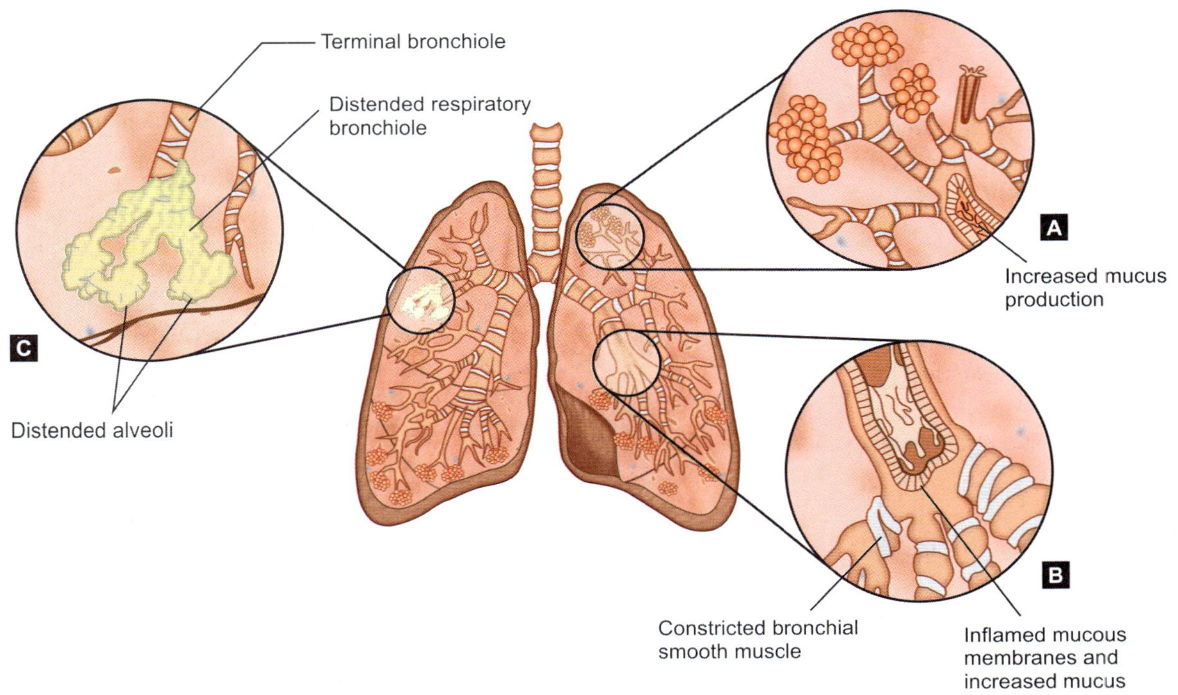

FIGS 9.13A TO C: (A) Chronic bronchitis: Note inflamed airways and excessive mucus; (B) Asthma: Note narrowed bronchial tubes and swollen mucous membranes; (C) Emphysema: Note distended respiratory bronchioles and alveoli

community-accquired (CAP), hospital acquired (HAP or nosocomial), pneumonia in the immunocompromised host, and aspiration pneumonia. Those at risk for pneumonia often have chronic underlying disorders, severe acute illness, a suppressed immune system from disease or medications, immobility, and other factors that interfere with normal lung protective mechanisms.

Etiology

Pneumonia is resulting from inhalation or transport via the bloodstream of infectious agents or noxious fumes or from radiation treatment. Pneumonia is classified according to whether infection was acquired in the community or in the hospital. Thus pneumonia is classified as "community-acquired pneumonia (CAP) or hospital acquired pneumonia (HAP)". HAP is also called nosocomial pneumonia. The causes of pneumonia are as follows:

i. Community-acquired pneumonia caused by:
   - *Streptococcus pneumoniae*
   - *Haemophilus influenzae*
   - *Mycoplasma pneumoniae*
   - Respiratory viruses
   - *Chlamydia pneumoniae*
   - *Legionella pneumophila*
   - Oral anaerobes
   - *Moraxella catarrhalis*
   - *Staphylococcus aureus*
   - *Nocardia*
   - Enteric aerobic Gram-negative bacteria (e.g. *Klebsiella*)
   - Fungi
   - *Mycobacterium tuberculosis.*

ii. Hospital-acquired pneumonia caused by:
   a. *Pseudomonas aeruginosa*
   b. Enterobacter
   c. *Escherichia coli*
   d. *Proteus*
   e. *Klebsiella*
   f. *Staphylococcus aureus*
   g. *Streptococcus pneumoniae*
   h. Oral anaerobes.

The risk factors which predispose to pneumonia are:

- Smoking
- Air pollution
- Altered consciousness: Alcoholism, head injury, seizures, anesthesia, drug overdose
- Tracheal intubation (endotracheal intubations, tracheostomy)
- Upper respiratory tract infection
- Chronic diseases: Chronic lung diseases, diabetes mellitus, heart disease, uremia, cancer
- Immunosuppression
  - Drugs (carciosteroids, cancer chemotherapy, immunosuppressive therapy after organ transplant)
  - HIV
- Malnutrition
- Inhalation of aspiration of noxious substances
- Debilitating illness
- Bedrest and prolonged immobility
- Altered oropharyngeal flora.

The risk factors for hospital acquired pneumonia are:

- Residence in an ICU
- Mechanical ventilation (those who required 48 hours or more ventilation)
- Endotracheal intubation or tracheostomy
- Recent surgery
- Debilitation, i.e. malnutrition
- Invasive devices
- Neuromuscular disease
- Depressed level of alertness
- Aspiration
- Antacid use
- Age 60 or older
- Prolonged hospital stay
- Any serious underlying disease.

Pathophysiology

An inflammatory reaction may occur in the alveoli, producing an exudate that partially occludes the bronchi or alveoli; bronchospasm may also occur if the patient has reactive airway disease that interferes with gas exchange (bronchopneumonia, the most common form, is distributed in a patchy fashion extending from the bronchi to surrounding lung parenchyma. Lobar pneumonia is the term used if a substantial part of one or more lobes is involved). The elderly are also at high risk. Pneumonias are caused by a variety of microbial agents in the various settings. Common organisms include *Pseudomonas aeruginosa* and *Klebsiella* species, *Staphylococcus aureus, Haemophilus influenzae, Staphylococcus pneumonia,* and enteric gram-negative bacilli, fungi and viruses (most common in children).

Normally, the airway distal to the larynx is sterile because of protective defence mechanisms. These mechanisms include:

- Filtration of air
- Warming and humidification of inspired air
- Epiglottis closure over the trachea
- Cough reflex
- Mucociliary escalator mechanism
- Secretion of immunoglobulin A
- Alveolar macrophages.

Pneumonia results in inflammation of lung tissue. Depending on the particular pathogen and the hosts' physical status, the inflammatory process may involve different anatomical areas of the lung parenchyma and the pleurae. The normal function of respiratory system and primary pathophysiology and clinical manifestation are as follows:

i. Normally 'mucociliary system' cleanses inhaled air by trapping particles. In pneumonia, hypertrophy of mucous membrane lining lung, resulting in hypersecretions leads to increased sputum production and cough:
   - Anerobic—foul-smelling, sputum
   - *Klebsiella*—current jelly color
   - *Staphylococcus*—creamy yellow
   - *Pseudomonas*—green
   - Viral/mucopurulent

   And bronchospasms from increased secretions, leads to localized or diffuse wheezing dyspnea.
ii. Generally 'alveolocapillary membrane' exchanges oxygen-carbon dioxide. In pneumonia, there is increased permeability resulting in excess fluid in interstitial space, shows consolidation (in chest X-ray films) localized/bacterial; diffuse/viral, and also there is decreased surface area for gas exchange leads to hypoxemia.
iii. Normally pleura maintains close approximation of lungs and chest wall; minimizes friction during lung expansion and contraction. In pneumonia, there is inflammation of the pleura which shows, chest pain, especially on inspiration, pleural effusion, dullness on percussion, decreased breath sounds and decreased vocal fremitus.
iv. Normally, respiratory muscle expands and contracts chest wall and thus pleura and lungs. In pneumonia, there is hypoventilation and respiratory acidosis (in presence of underlying disease) leads to decreased chest expansion and hypercapnea and low arterial blood pH.
v. The lung defense system protects normally sterile lung from invasion. In pneumonia, there is bacteremia, shows elevated blood cell counting; leukocytes (15,000 to 25,000/mm), neutrophilia and tachypnea and fever.

In pneumococcal pneumonia, there is congestion, red hepatization and gray hepatization.

Clinical Manifestation

Community acquired pneumonia (CAP) has been traditionally thought to present any two syndromes; typical and atypical, although the distinctions are not clear.

Typical pneumonic syndrome is characterized by sudden onset of fever, chills, cough productive of purulent sputum, and pleuritic chest pain (in some cases). On physical examination signs of pulmonary consolidations such as dullness, percussion, increased fermitus, bronchial breath sounds, and crackles may be found. In elderly or debilitated patient, confusion or stupor may be predominant. Usually two types of pneumonia caused by *S. pneumoniae* and *H. influenzae*.

Clinical features vary depending on the causative organism and the patients disease.

- Sudden chills, rapidly rising fever (38.5°C to 40.5°C) and profuse perspiration
- Pleuritic chest pain aggravated by respiration and coughing
- Severely ill patient has marked tachypnea (25 to 45 breath/min) and dyspnea; orthopnea when not propped up
- Pulse rapid and bounding; may increase 10 beats/min per degree of temperature elevation (Celsius)
- A relative bradycardia for the amount of fever suggests viral infection or *Mycoplasma* or *Legionella* species infection
- Sputum purulent, rusty, blood tinged, viscous or green depending on etiologic agent
- Other signs: Fever, headache and myalgia, crackles, and signs of lobar consolidation; initial upper respiratory tract symptoms (nasal congestion, sore throat)
- Severe pneumonia: Flushed cheeks; lips and nail beds demonstrating central cyanosis.

The atypical syndrome is characterized by a more gradual onset dry cough, and extrapulmonary manifestation such as headache, myalgia, fatigue, sore throat, nausea, vomiting and diarrhea. On physical examination, crackles are often heard. This type is classically produced by *Mycoplasma pneumoniae*, *Legionella* and *Chlamydia pneumoniae*. Viral pneumoniae are characterized by an atypical presentation with chills, fever, dry non-productive cough and extrapulmonary symptoms. Most of the pneumoniae run uncomplicated. If occurs, the complications are pneumonia including pleurisy, pleural effusion, atelectasis, delayed resolution, lung abscess, empyema, pericarditis, arthritis, meningitis and endocarditis.

Management

History, physical examination and chest X-ray often provide enough information to take management decisions without costly laboratory tests. Diagnostic tests include:

- Chest X-ray film to conform consolidation and distribution and pleural effusions
- Sputum studies for culture and sensitivity if unable to obtain specimen by usual means, may use
  - Transtracheal aspiration
  - Bronchoscopy with aspiration, biopsy or bronchial brushings
- Arterial blood gas studies or pulse oximetry
- Hematology: WBC count, cole agglutinin and compliment fixation for viral studies
- Thoracentesis to obtain pleural fluid specimen if pleural effusion is present.

Medical Management

Antibiotics are prescribed based on Gram stain results and antibiotic guidelines (resistance patterns, risk factors, etiology must be considered). Combination therapy may also be used.

- Supportive treatment includes hydration, antipyretics, antihistamines, or nasal decongestants
- Bed rest is recommended until infection shows signs for clearing
- Oxygen therapy is given for hypoxemia
- Respiratory support includes endotracheal intubation, high inspiratory oxygen concentrations and mechanical ventilation
- Treatment of atelectasis, pleural effusion, shock, respiratory failure, or superinfection is instituted, if needed
- For groups at high risk for community-acquired pneumonia, pneumococcal vaccination is advised.

The possible nursing diagnosis on the basis and assessment will be:

- Airway clearance, ineffective related to decreased energy, fatigue, tracheobronchial inflammation
- Impaired gas exchange related to alveolar capillary membrane changes altered oxygen delivery
- Pain related to pleural inflammation, coughing paroxysms
- Rest for infection related to compromised lung defense system
- Knowledge deficient related to condition, treatment
- Anorexia related to infection process-sputum production
- Altered nutrition/body requirement related to increased metabolic needs.

Prompt treatment with the appropriate antibiotic almost always cures bacterial and mycoplasmal pneumonia. In uncomplicated cases, the patient responds to drug therapy within 48 to 72 hours. Indications for improvement including decreased temperature, improved breathing, and reduced chest pain.

Abnormal physical finding lasts for more than 7 days. The nursing intervention includes:

i. Maintaining effective airway clearance
   - Monitor for increased respiratory distress
   - Assist patient to cough effectively
   - If unable to clear down airway, suction airway using sterile technique
   - Assist with nebulizer therapy
   - Administer bronchiodilator as ordered. Monitor for side effects and response to therapy
   - Change position frequently to assist in mobilizing secretions
   - Ensure fluid intake adequate to thin secretions.

ii. Facilitate breathing
   - Help the patient breathe deeply and expand the chest to increase ventilation
   - Place the patient in position to facilitate breathing, usually upright or semiupright position
   - A pillow may be placed lengthwise at the patient's back to provide support and thrust thorax slightly towards allowing free use of the diaphragm
   - The patient who must be upright to breathe may find it restful to place head and arms on a pillow placed on an overbed table
   - For the patient with severe hypoxemia, side rails should be in place. The patient can use them to assisting about in bed
   - Some patients who breathe best when sitting up in a large armchair while leaning on a smaller chair. Placed in front of that. This chair is blocked to prevent it from slipping
   - Assist with ADL pacing activities to prevent fatigue and respiratory distress.

iii. Administration of medication and treatment
   - Before starting prescribed antibiotic, collect sputum for culture and blood for culture if ordered
   - Maintain antibiotic blood levels by giving antibiotic at scheduled time
   - Give medication prescribed to relieve pain. Codeine may be ordered because it is less likely to inhibit cough reflex than more potent narcotics
   - Begin oxygen therapy.

iv. Administering oxygen therapy

v. Promoting comfort
   - Place in position of comfort. Preferably head of bed elevated 45 to 90 degrees
   - Assess character and location of chest pain
   - Administer analgesic for chest pain, e.g. acetylsalicylic acid, acetominophen and codeine
   - Splint chest with hands when patient coughs.
   - Administer frequent mouth care. Protect lips and nares with lubricants
   - Keep patient warm and dry and avoid chilling.

vi. Preventing spread of infection
   - Standard precautions are used.

vii. Facilitating learning
   - The major teaching emphasis is on prevention
   - Assess patient's understanding of pneumonia with questions concerning such information on how pneumonia is transmitted and risk factor
   - Teach proper handling of secretions. Cover nose and mouth with tissue when coughing or sneezing. Discard tissues in paper or plastic bag for disposal. Expectorate into specimen container provided
   - Stress importance of handwashing after coughing, sneezing and expectorating
   - Reinforce importance and follow-up care
   - Reinforce the need for immunization, i.e. inlfuenza vaccine and pneumococcal vaccine. Pneumonia Polysaccaride vaccine is given only every 3 to 5 years.

viii. Promoting adequate hydration and nutrition
   - Encourage oral fluids. If patient is receiving IV fluids, monitor rate. Observe for signs of fluid volume deficit or excess
   - Ask patient what foods he or she would like to eat
   - Offer small, frequent feedings
   - Encourage high-carbohydrate and high-protein foods.

TUBERCULOSIS

Tuberculosis is an infectious disease caused by *Mycobacterium tuberculosis*. It usually involves the lungs, but it also occurs in the kidneys, bones, adrenal glands, lymph nodes and meninges and can be disseminated throughout the body.

Etiology

Mycobacterium tuberculosis, a gram-positive, acid-fast bacillary, is usually spread via air-borne droplets, which are produced when the infected individual coughs, sneezes or speaks. Once released into a room, the organisms are dispersed and can be inhaled. Brief exposure to a tubercle bacilli rarely causes an infection. Rather it is more commonly spread to the individual who has had repeated close contact with an infected person. It is not highly infective and transmitted. It usually requires close, frequent or prolonged exposure. The disease cannot be spread by hands, books, glasses, dishes or other fomites.

Risk Factors

- Close contact with someone who has active TB. Injection drug use and alcoholism
- Residence in overcrowded, substandard housing or institutions (e.g. long-term care patients, psychiatric patients, prison inmates)
- Immunocompromise (e.g. elderly, cancer, corticosteroid therapy and HIV)
- Patients with pre-existing medical conditions, including diabetes, chronic renal failure, silicosis, and malnorishment
- Immigrants from countries with a high incidence of TB (e.g. Haiti, Southeast Asia)
- People lacking adequate health care (e.g. homeless or impoverished, minorities, children and young adults)
- Occupation (e.g. health care workers, particularly those performing high-risk activities).

Pathophysiology

Tuberculosis (TB), an infectious disease primarily affecting the lung parenchyma, is most often caused by *Mycobacterium tuberculosis*. It may spread to almost any part of the body, including the meninges, kidney, bones and lymph nodes. The initial infection usually occurs 2 to 10 weeks after exposure. The patient may then develop active disease because of a compromised or inadequate immune system response. The active process may be prolonged and characterized by long remissions when the disease is arrested, only to be followed by periods of renewed activity. TB is a worldwide public health problem and the leading cause of death among HIV-positive patients. Mortality and morbidity rates continue to rise.

TB is transmitted when a person with active pulmonary disease expels the organisms. A susceptible person inhales the droplets and becomes infected. Bacteria are transmitted to the alveoli and multiply. An inflammatory reaction results in exudate in the alveoli and bronchopneumonia, granulomas, and fibrous tissue. Onset is usually insidious.

When an individual with no previous exposure to TB (negative tuberculin reactor) inhales a sufficient number of tubercle bacilli into the alveoli, tuberculosis infection occurs. The body's reaction to the TB bacilli depends on the susceptibility of the individual, the size of the dose and the virulence of the organisms. Inflammation occurs within the alveoli (parenchyma) of the lungs, and natural body defenses attempt to counteract the infection.

When the bacilli is inhaled, they pass down the bronchial system and implant themselves on the respiratory bronchioles or alveoli. The lower part of the lungs are usually the site of initial bacterial implantation. After implantation, the bacilli multiply with no initial resistance from the host. The organisms are engulfed by phagocytosis (initially neutrophils and later macrophages) and may continue to multiply within the phagocytes.

Macrophages ingest the organism and present the micro-bacterial antigens to the T cells. CD4 cells secrete lymphothine than enhance the capacity of the macrophages to ingest and kill bacteria. Lymph nodes in the hilar region of the lung become enlarged on their filter drainage from the infected site. The inflammatory process and the cellular reaction produce a small, firm, white nodules called the 'primary tubercle'. The center of the nodules contain tubercle bacilli cells gather around the centre and usually the outer portion becomes fibrosed. Thus, blood vessels are compressed, nutrition of tubercle is impaired, and necrosis occurs at the center. The area becomes walled off by fibrotic tissue, and the center gradually becomes soft and cheesy in consistency. This later process is known as "Caseation necrosis". This material may become calcified (calcium deposits) or it may liquify (liquification necrosis). The liquified material may be coughed up, leaving a cavity or hole in the parenchyma of the lung. This cavity or cavities are visible on chest X-ray films and results in the diagnosis of cavitary disease. The only X-ray evidence of TB infection is a calcified nodule known as "Ghon's tubercle". Ghon's tubercle is referred to as the "primary complex". When a tuberculosis lesion regresses and heals, the infection enters a latent period in which it may persist without producing a clinical illness. The infection may develop into clinical disease if the persisting organism begins to multiply rapidly, or it may remain dormant. If the initial immune response is not adequate, control of the organisms is not maintained and clinical disease results. Certain individuals are at a higher-risk for clinical disease including those who are immunosuppressed, e.g. HIV, cancer, person who received chemotherapy or corticosteroid therapy) or have diabetes mellitus. Dormant but viable organism persists for years. Reactivation of TB can occur if the host defense mechanisms become impaired.

Clinical Manifestation

In the early stages of TB, the person is usually free of symptoms. Many cases, if it is found that incidentally when routine chest X-rays are taken, especially in older adults. Systemic manifestation may initially consist of fatigue, malaise, anorexia, weight loss, low grade fever (especially in late afternoons) and night sweats. The weight loss may not be excessive until late in the disease and is often attributed to overwork or other factors. Irregular menses may also be present in premenopausal women.

A characteristic pulmonary manifestation is cough that becomes frequent and produce mucoid or macopurulent's sputum. Chest pain characterised as dull or tight may also be present. Hemoptysis is not a common finding and is usually associated with more advanced cases. Sometimes TB has more acute, sudden manifestation, the patient has high fever, chills, generalized of the like symptoms, pleuritic pain and a production of cough.

The complication of TB are miliary tuberculosis, pleural effusion, TB pneumonia, involvement of other organs, e.g. bone, kidney, brain, etc.

Management

This will be diagnosed by taking prompt health history and physical examination. The diagnostic studies of TB include:

- Tubercular skin testing, montoux test
- Chest X-rays
- Bacteriological studies—sputum smear, sputum
- WBC Serologic test by ELISA (enzyme-linked immunosorbent assay)
- CSF.

The common drugs used for management of tuberculosis are (Box 9.6):

i. Isoniazid (INH): It interferes with DNA metabolism and tubercle bacilli. It is bactericidal, penetrates all body tissues and fluids, including CSF. The side effects include peripheral nueritis, hepatotoxicity, hypersensitivity (skin rash, arthralgin, fever). Optic neuritis, vitamin B_6 neuritis. INH metabolizes primarily by liver and excretion by kidneys, pyridoxine (vitamin B_6) administration during high-dose therapy as prophylactive measure, use as single prophylactic agent. For active TB in individuals whose PPD converts to positive, ability to cross blood-brain barrier. Avoid alcohol and antacids during therapy. Daily alcohol intake interferes with metabolism of isoniazid and increases risk of hepatitis, antacids containing aluminium hydroxide also interferes with absorption of INH.

Box 9.6 Antibiotics used to treat tuberculosis

First-line drugs
Isoniazid
Rifampin
Ethambutol
Pyrazinamide

Second-line drugs
Rifabutin
Rifapentine
Para-aminosalicylic acid
Streptomycin
Levofloxacin
Ethionamide
Amikacin
Others

ii. Rifampin has broad spectrum effects, inhibits RNA polymerase of tubercle bacillus. It is bactericidal, penetrates all body tissues, including CSF. It is most commonly used with INH, low incidence of side effects, suppression of effects of birth control pills, possible orange urine. The other side effects may develop are hepatitis, febrile reactions, thrombocytopenia (Rare) GI disturbance, peripheral neuropathy, hypersensitivity, hepatotoxicity increases when given with INH. During its therapy, urine, sweat, tears may turn orange temporarily decrease effectiveness of oral contraceptives, anticoagulants, corticosteroids, barbiturates, hypoglycemics and digitalis.

iii. Ethambutol inhibits RNA synthesis and a bacteriostatic for the TB bacilli and does not penetrate all body fluids except CSF. The common side effects are skin rash, GI disturbance, malaise, peripheral neuritis, and optic neuritis. It has no significant reaction with other drugs. Should be given with food. Periodic checking of vision needed. It is most commonly used as substitute drug when toxicity occurs with rifampin and INH.

iv. Streptomycin inhibits protein synthesis and is bactericidal. Poor penetration into body tissues and CSF. The side effects of streptomycin and INH include (eighth cranial nerve damage streptomycin vestibular or occular) damage often irreversible, nephrotoxicity and hypersensitivity. It should be used cautiously in older adults those with renal disease and pregnant women; must be given parenterally. During its use patient should be monitored monthly for kidney function, vestibular function with caloric stimulation test, and hearing with audiogram.

v. Pyrazinamide is bacteriostatic or bacteriocidal depending on susceptibility of *Mycobacterium* (exact mechanism not known). Usual side effects of fever, skin rash, hyperuricemia, jaundice (rare) hepatitis, arthralgia, GI irritation. High rate of effectiveness when used with streptomycin or capreomycin.

In addition, ethionamide, capromycine, kanamycin and para-aminosalicylic acid (PAS) cycloserine (seromycin) and used as second line of drugs for TB treatment.

A problem with antituberculosis therapy is the length of time medication must be taken. In the past, 18 to 26 months was the usual period of time required for individuals to adhere to the medical regiment. Shorter courses of therapy (6 to 9 months) have been shown to be effective. Now three options for treatment are available. Regimen option for the initial treatment of tuberculosis include:

Option 1: Four drug regimen consisting of isoniazid, rifampin, pyrazinamide and either ethambutol or streptomycine. Therapy may be given daily or 2–3 times weekly if DOT (directly observed therapy). Ethambutol or streptomycin may be discontinued if susceptibility to isoniazid or rifampin is documented. Pyrazinamide should be discontinued after 8 weeks. The total duration of the therapy should be at least 6 months and at least 3 months after sputum culture converts to negative. Fixed dose combination of all these drugs are available to simplify therapy.

Option 2: Daily isoniazid, rifampin, pyrazinamide and streptomycin or ethambutol for 2 weeks followed by DOT twice weekly administration of the same drugs for 6 weeks followed by rifampin for 16 weeks.

Option 3: DOT 3 times/weekly administration of isoniazid, rifampin, pyrazinamide, and ethambutol or streptomycin for 6 months.

For TB with HIV infection cases, option 1, 2, 3 can be used, but treatment regimens should continue for a total of 9 months and at least 6 months beyond culture conversion.

Medical therapy is the primary treatment of tuberculosis, but surgery may be used to remove residual pulmonary lesions and patients. The surgical procedures then are used to include wedge resection, segmental resection, lobestomy, etc.

A well-balanced diet containing the essential food groups with a vitamin supplement is recommended. Those who are poorly nourished or underweight may benefit from six small feedings of high-calorie, high protein foods daily rather than three meals.

Nursing Interventions

Promoting Airway Clearance

- Instruct about best position to facilitate drainage
- Encourage increased fluid intake.

Promoting Activity and Adequate Nutrition

- Plan a progressive activity schedule with the patient to increase activity tolerance and muscle strength
- Devise a complementary plan to encourage adequate nutrition. A nutritional regimen of small, frequent meals and nutritional supplements may be helpful in meeting daily caloric requirements.

Advocating Compliance and Prevention

- Explain that TB is a communicable disease and that taking medications is the most effective way of preventing transmission
- Instruct about hygiene measures, including mouth care covering mouth and nose when coughing and sneezing proper disposal of tissues, and hand washing
- Instruct about medications, schedule, and side effects.

Monitoring and Managing Potential Complications

- Strategize with health care team to ensure adequate nutritional intake and availability of nutritious foods and high-calorie nutritional supplements
- Assess for side effects of medication therapy and signs of multidrug resistance
- Encourage patient to obtain liver and kidney function follow-up studies
- Monitor sputum culture results to evaluate effectiveness of therapy
- Teach patient to take medications on empty stomach or 1 hour before meals, because food interferes with drug absorption
- Teach patients taking INH to avoid foods containing tyramine and and histamine (tuna fish, aged cheese, yeast extract)
- Inform patient that rifampin may discolor tears and contact lenses. Eyeglasses may be substituted for contact lenses
- Instruct patient about risk of drug resistance if regimen is not followed continuously; failure to comply results in multidrug resistance
- Caution about the spread of TB infection from lungs to other body sites, a consequence of late reactivation of dormant infections.

Promoting Home and Community-based Care

Teaching patient's self-care

- Assess patient's ability to continue therapy at home
- Instruct patient and family about infection control procedures; cover mouth when coughing; use disposable tissues, place in paper bag and discard
- Teach and use universal precautions for body fluids, including sputum
- Demonstrate and stress good hand hygiene.

Continuing Care

- Evaluate patient's environment to identify other potentially infected people, and arrange follow-up screening for them.
- Emphasize importance of keeping scheduled appointments with health care providers.

The major nursing responsibility is to teach the patient about TB and how it is transmitted. Preventing contamination of air with tubercle bacilli is accomplished by treating the patient antituberculosis drugs and teaching the patient to cover the nose and mouth with tissues when sneezing and coughing. Advise the patient, he must take antituberculosis drugs as prescribed and drugs are always taken as combination of at least four drugs initially and drugs must be taken uninterruptedly.

To improve airway clearance, the patient is taught to sit upright in a chair or bed. If the patient is confined to bed at home, he or she may find it helpful to sit on the side of the bed with the feet on a chair. The patient may be taught to take two or three deep breaths, cover the mouth with tissues and then cough. Using this method when coughing decreases fatigue because it requires less expenditure of energy than does repeated ineffective coughs. Many patients can cough most effectively when the mouth is moist and sips of water or a warm beverage such as tea or coffee can be encouraged before coughing.

For patients with thick tenacious sputum, fluid intake is encouraged to thin the secretions and make them easier to expectorate. Water is considered by many experts to be the most effective sputum liquifying agent.

To reduce fear about the disease and what lifestyle changes it will require, patients are encouraged to ask questions about anything they do not understand or anything that concerns them. The nurse who sits while talking with the patients signals them he or she will take the time to listen to the patient. All questions should be answered as completely as possible, supplying information appropriate to the patients' educational level and ability to comprehend what is being taught. Written materials with diagram and drawings that reinforce what is being taught are helpful. The materials are given to the patient for use later on.

Nurses and other health care workers need to know the protective measures they can use when caring for patients who have a positive TB smear or culture.

BRONCHIECTASIS

Bronchiectasis is a disorder characterized by permanent, abnormal or irreversible dilation of the bronchial tree or one or more large bronchi. Bronchiectasis is a chronic, irreversible dilation and impaired mucociliary clearance of the bronchi and bronchioles. The result is retention of secretions, obstruction, and eventual alveolar collapse. Bronchiectasis may be caused by a variety of conditions, including pulmonary infections and obstruction of the bronchus; diffuse airway injury; genetic disorder (e.g. cystic fibrosis); and abnormal host defense (e.g. humoral immunodeficiency). Bronchiectasis is usually localized in a lobe or segment of a lung (frequently the lower lobes). A person may be predisposed to bronchiectasis (history of recurrent respiratory infections, measles, influenza, tuberculosis and immunodeficiency disorders). Patients with bronchiectasis almost always have bronchitis.

Pathophysiology

When infection attacks the bronchial lining, inflammation occurs, and an exudate forms. The progressive accumulation of secretions obstructs the bronchioles. The obstructed bronchioles then breakdown, and ciliated columnar epithelium is replaced by non-ciliated cuboidal epithelium and sometimes fibroitic tissue, resulting in localized areas of dilations or saccules. The pathologic changes result in dilation and destruction of the elastic and muscular structures of the bronchial wall.

There are two pathological types of bronchiectasis, i.e. saccular and cylindrical. Saccular bronchiectasis occurs mainly in large bronchi and is characterized by cavity-like dilations. The affected bronchi end in large sacs. Cylindrical bronchiectasis involve medium-sized bronchi that are mildly to moderately dilated. Fusiform bronchiectasis occurs mainly in large bronchi and is characterized by cavity-like dilations. The affected bronchi end in large sacs cylindrical bronchiectasis involves medium sized bronchi that are mildly to moderately dilated. Fusiform bronchiectasis a subtype of cylindrical tends to involve more 'pouching' of the bronchi. The explosive force of the bronchioles is diminished and they may remain filled with exudate. Only forceful coughing and postural drainage will empty them. Almost all forms of bronchiectasis are associated with bacterial infections and viral infections (adenovir, influenza).

Clinical Manifestations

The condition may develop so gradually that the person is unable to tell when the symptoms first began. Signs and symptoms of bronchiectasis vary with the severity of the conditions and may include the following:

- Chronic cough and production of copious purulent sputum, which has a quality of "layering out" into three layers on standing: a frothy top layer, a middle clear layer, and a dense particulate bottom layer
- Hemoptysis, clubbing of the fingers, and repeated episodes of pulmonary infection.

Signs

- Cyanosis
- Clubbing of fingers
- Find crackles and coarse rhonchi
- Dull or flat sound over the areas of mucus plugs

- Increased vocal and tactile fermitus over the middle and lower lobes
- Decreased diaphragmatic excursion
- Paroxysms of coughing on rising in morning and when lying down.

Symptoms

- Severe coughing productive of copious amounts of purulent sputum
- Hemoptysis
- Dyspnea
- Fatigue and weakness
- Loss of appetite and weight loss.

The diagnostic studies used to diagnose bronchiectasis are chest X-ray, bronchography, sputum examination and CT scanning.

Management

Medical Management

- Objectives of treatment are to prevent and control infection and to promote bronchial drainage
- Chest physiotherapy with percussion; postural drainage, expectorants, or bronchoscopy to remove bronchial secretions
- Antimicrobial therapy guided by sputum sensitivity studies
- Year-round regimen of antibiotics, alternating types of drugs at intervals
- Vaccination against influenza and pneumococcal pneumonia
- Bronchodilators; sympathomimetics (beta-adrenergic agonists)
- Increased oral fluid intake
- Smoking cessation
- Surgical intervention (segmental resection of lobe or lung removal), used infrequently
- In preparation for surgery; vigorous postural drainage, suction through bronchoscope and antibacterial therapy.

Treatment of bronchiectasis includes:

- Administration of antibiotics on the basis of sputum culture results
- Administering of bronchodilator, mucolytic agents and expectorants
- Postural drainage (Fig. 9.14) to assist in mobilizing secretions to larger airways where they can be coughed up
- Bronchoscopy to remove thicker secretions
- Maintaining good hydration to liquify secretion
- Maintaining good general hygiene including oral hygiene may contribute to relief symptoms
- Adequate rest, diet, exercise and diversional activities
- Avoiding superimposed infections such as colds

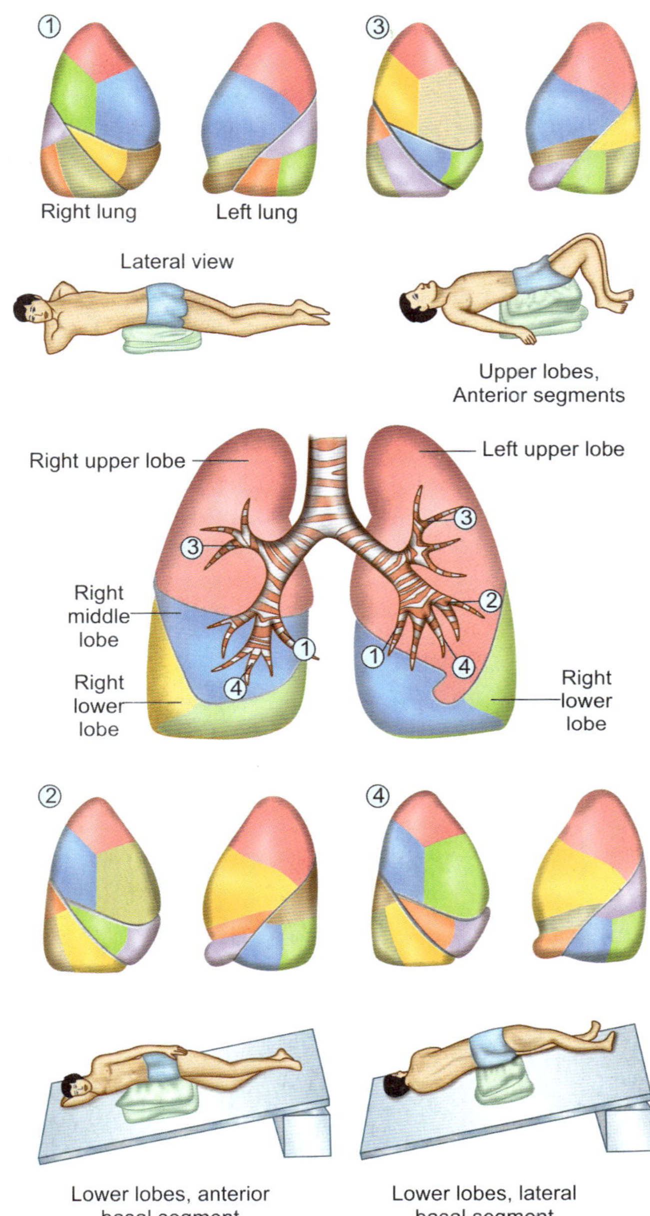

FIG. 9.14: Postural drainage positions. Anatomic segments of the lung with four postural drainage positions. The numbers relate the position to the corresponding anatomic segment of the lung

- Individual should reduce exposure to excessive air pollutants and irritants, avoid cigarette smoking and obtain pneumococcal and influenza vaccinations.

Surgical resection of the parts of the lungs, necessary when signs and symptoms of bronchiectasis persists despite medical therapy. The goal of surgery is to preserve as much functional lung as possible. Therefore, segmentectomy or lobectomy is given priority.

Nursing Management

See Nursing Management and Patient Education under Chronic Obstructive Pulmonary Disease and Preoperative and Postoperative Nursing Management for additional information.

EMPYEMA

Empyema is pus within a body cavity most often the pleural cavity. It usually occurs after pleural effusion secondary to other respiratory diseases such as pneumonia, lung abscess, TB and fungal infections of the lung and also after thoracic surgery or chest trauma.

Empyema is a collection of purulent (infected) liquid or pus in the pleural cavity. At first the pleural fluid thin, but it progresses to a fibropurulent stage and then to a stage at which it encloses the lung with a thick exudative membrane (loculated empyema)

Clinical Manifestation

The patient with a lung infection or chest injury may develop empyema and should be observed closely for the following signs and symptoms of empyema:

- Cough (usually nonproductive)
- Dyspnea
- Tachypnea
- Tachycardia
- Elevation of temperature
- Unilateral chest expansion
- Malaise
- Decreased appetite
- Fever, night sweats, pleural pain, cough dyspnea, anorexia and weight loss
- Decreased or absence of breath sounds; dullness on chest percussion; decreased fremitus
- Symptoms vague (immunocompromised patient) or less obvious if patient has received antimicrobial therapy.

The diagnosis can usually be made from the signs and symptoms and the medical history, but it is confirmed by a chest X-ray film that demonstrates the presence of a pleural exudate. A thoracentesis is performed to obtain sample of the pus for culture and sensitivity studies and to relieve the patients' respiratory symptoms.

- Chest auscultation, which demonstrates decreased or absent breath sounds over the affected area; dullness on chest percussion; decreased fremitus
- Chest radiographs, chest CT and thoracentesis

Management

Medical Management

Objectives of management are to drain the pleural cavity and to achieve full expansion of the lung. This is accomplished by adequate drainage, antibiotics (large doses), streptokinase, or a combination of these. Drainage of the pleural fluid depends on the stage of the disease and is accomplished as follows:

- Needle aspiration (thoracentesis) if fluid is not too thick
- Tube thoracostomy water-seal chest drainage, with fibrinolytic agents instilled through chest tube when indicated
- Open chest drainage to remove thickened pleura, pus and debris and to remove the underlying diseased pulmonary tissue
- Decortication, surgical removal, if inflammation has been long-standing.

The aim of treatment of empyema is to obliterate the pleural space by draining the empyema cavity completely. The cavity can be drained in the following ways:

- Initial treatment is often daily thoracentesis with aspiration of the cavity and instillation of antibiotics into the pleural space. Oral or IV antibiotics may also be given
- If the cavity cannot be evacuated within a few days and if the lung fails to re-expand to obliterate then space surgery is necessary. The types of surgery depends on the situation and may include:
  - Closed chest drainage
  - Rib resection
  - Decortication and
  - Thoracoplasty.

Nursing Management

- Provide care specific to method of drainage of pleural fluid
- Help patient cope with condition; instruct in lung expansion breathing exercises (pursed-lip and diaphragmatic breathing). See Perioperative Nursing Management for additional information.
- Instruct patient and family about care of drainage system and drain site and measurement and observation of drainage.
- Teach patient and family signs and symptoms of infection and how and when to contact the health care provider.

Nursing depends on the type and effectiveness of the procedure and the patient's symptoms. Some patients require oxygen therapy. Bedrest and coughing and deep breathing exercises may be indicated to improve ventilations. In some cases, the patient will go through several treatments before the empyema in space is closed. This can be frustrating, and the patient can become very discouraged. A major nursing role is to support the patient and family during the various procedure.

LUNG ABSCESS

Lung abscess is a pus-containing lesion of the lung parenchyma that gives rise to a cavity. The cavity is formed by necrosis of the lung tissue. A lung abscess is a localized necrotic lesion of the lung parenchyma containing purulent materials; the lesion collapses and forms a cavity. Most lung abscesses occur because of aspiration of nasopharyngeal or oral anaerobes into the lung. Abscesses may also occur secondary to mechanical or functional obstruction of the bronchi. At-risk patients include those with impaired cough reflexes, loss of glottal closures, or swallowing difficulties, which may cause aspiration of foreign material. Other at-risk patients include those which central nervous system disorders (seizure, stroke, altered mental status, drug or alcohol addiction) or esophageal disease, those with compromised immune function and those fed by nasogastric tube. The site of lung abscess is related to gravity and is determined by the patient's position. For patient in a recumbent position, the posterior segment of the upper right lobe is the most common site. The organisms most frequently associated with lung abscess are *Klebsiella* species and *Staphylococcus aureus*.

Etiology

In many cases, the causes and pathogenesis of lung abscess are similar to those of pneumonia. The more common contributing factor to a lung abscess is aspiration of material into the lungs. Risk factors for aspiration include alcoholism, seizure disorder, drug overdose, general anaesthesia, and cerebrovascular accidents. Most of the lung abscesses are caused by infectious agents, i.e. *Klebsiella, S. aureus*, anerobic bacilli. Lung abscess also can result from hematogenously spread lung infarct secondary to pulmonary embolus, malignant growth, TB and various fungus and parasitic diseases of the lung.

Pathophysiology

The areas of the lung most commonly affected are the atypical segments of the lower lobes and the posterior segments of the upper lobes. Fibrous tissues usually form around the abscess in an attempt to wall it off. The abscess may erode into the bronchial system, causing the production of foul-smelling sputum. It may grow towards the pleura and cause pleuritic pain. Multiple small abscesses can occur within the lung.

Clinical Manifestation

- The clinical features vary from a mild productive cough to acute illness
- Fever is accompanied by a productive cough of moderate to copious amounts of foul-smelling sputum, often bloody
- Pleurisy, or dull chest pain, dyspnea, weakness, anorexia and weight loss are common
- Chest dullness on percussion and decreased or absent breath sounds are found, with an intermittent pleural friction rub and possibly crackles on auscultation.

The onset of a lung abscess is usually insidious, especially if anaerobic organisms are the primary cause. A more acute onset occurs with aerobic organisms. The most common manifestation is cough-producing, purulent (often dark brown) that is foul-smelling and foul tasting. Hemoptysis is common especially at the time that an abscess ruptures into a bronchus. Other common manifestations are fever, chills, prostration, pleuritic pain, dyspnea, cough and weight loss. History may reveal a predisposing condition such as alcoholism, pneumonia or oral infections.

Physical examination of the lungs indicate the dullness to percussion and decreases breath sounds on auscultation over the segment of lung involved. There may be transmission of breath sounds to the periphery if the communicating bronchus becomes patent and drainage of the segment begins. Crackle may also be present. Oral examination often reveals dental caries, gingivitis and periodontal infection.

Complication can occur, which include chronic pulmonary abscess, hemorrhage from abscess erosion into blood vessels, brain abscess, bronchopleural fistula and empyema.

Management

Chest radiograph, sputum culture, and fiberoptic bronchoscope are performed. A computed tomography (CT) scan of the chest may be required.

Medical Management

Prevention

To reduce the risk for lung abscess, given appropriate antibiotic therapy before dental procedures and maintain adequate dental and oral hygiene. Give appropriate antimicrobial therapy pneumonia.

Treatment

Findings of the history, physical examination, chest radiograph and sputum culture indicate type of organism and treatment.

- Coughing, postural drainage (chest physiotherapy), and possible percutaneous catheter placement or, infrequently bronchoscopy for abscess drainage are used
- The patient is advised to eat a high-protein, high-calorie diet
- Surgical intervention is rare. Pulmonary resection (lobectomy) is performed when there is massive hemoptysis or no response to medical management.

Pharmacologic Theraphy

- Intravenous antimicrobial therapy; clindamycin (Cleocin) the medication of choice. Meropenem (Merrem) or piperacillin/tazobactam (Zosyn) is also prescribed. Large intravenous doses are required because the antibiotic must penetrate necrotic tissue and abscess fluid
- Antibiotics are administered orally instead of intravenously after signs of improvement (normal temperature, lowered white blood cell count and improvement on chest X-ray [reduction in size of cavity]). Antibiotic therapy may last 4 to 8 weeks.

Diagnosis is made on the basis of physical examination, chest X-ray, sputum culture and sensitivity. Prolonged administration of antibiotics (6 to 8 weeks). Penicillin is the choice antibiotics. Recently, clindamycin or metronidazole in combination with penicillin are used.

The patient should be taught how to cough effectively. Chest physiotherapy and postural drainages are helpful. Frequent mouth care (every 2 to 3 hours) is needed to relieve the foul-smelling odor and taste from the sputum. Diluted hydrogen peroxide and mouthwash are often effective. Rest, good nutrition, adequate fluid intake are all supportive measures to facilitate recovery. If dentition is poor and dental hygiene is not adequate and the patient should be encouraged to obtain dental care.

Surgery is indicated but occasionally may be necessary if reinfection of a large cavity lesion occurs.

Nursing Management

- Administer antibiotic and intravenous therapy as prescribed and monitor for any adverse effects
- Initiate chest physiotherapy as prescribed to drain abscess
- Teach patient deep-breathing and coughing exercises
- Encourage diet high in protein and calories
- Provide emotional support; abscess may take a long time to resolve
- Teach patient or caregiver how to change dressing to prevent skin excoriation and offensive odor
- Perform deep-breathing and coughing exercises every 2 hours during the day
- Teach postural drainage and percussion techniques to caregiver
- Provide counselling for attaining and maintaining an optimal state of nutrition
- Emphasize importance of completing antibiotic regimen, rest and appropriate activity levels to prevent relapse
- Arrange home health nursing and visits by an intravenous therapy nurse to administer intravenous antibiotic therapy.

OCCUPATIONAL LUNG DISEASES

Occupational or environmental lung diseases result from inhaled dust or chemicals. The duration of exposure and the amount of inhalant have a major influence on whether the exposed individual will have lung damage. Another factor is the susceptibility of the host.

Etiology

Many pulmonary diseases are believed to be caused by substances inhaled in the work place. Occupational lung disease are more common in:

- Blue-collar workers than white collar workers
- Industrial areas than in rural areas
- Small and medium-sized business than in larger industrial plants.

In some instances, it is debatable whether a person's lung disease is clearly occupation specific. This is true in cases of bronchitis, asthma, emphysema, or cancer, because all of these conditions can be caused or aggravated by several factors found in many different occupations and by non-occupational factors such as smoking and air pollution.

Types

Occupational lung disease can be divided into several categories. The major ones are:

- The pneumoconiosis (black lung disease)
- Asbestos-related lung diseases
- Hypersensitivity diseases including occupational asthma allergic alveolitis
- Byssinosis (brown lung disease).

Pathophysiology

The pathophysiology, clinical manifestation and prevention of some common occupational diseases are as follows:

i. Pneumoconiosis also known as 'dust in the lungs' is called by inhalation and retention of dust particles. Examples of this condition are: Silicosis, asbestosis and Byssinosis.
   - Silicosis caused if inhaled silica dust, most common form seen in miners, foundry workers, and others who inhaled relatively low concentration of dust for 10–20 years.

     In this, dust accumulation is tissue or tissue reaction with whorl-shaped nodules throughout lungs. In complicated silicosis, there is progressive massive fibrosis throughout lungs decreased lung function and cor pulmonale. In acute silicosis, there is inflammatory reaction within alveoli, diffuse fibrosis. Rapid progression to respiratory failure. The clinical manifestation will include, breathlessness, weakness, chest pain, productive cough with sputum, dies of cor pulmonale and respiratory failure. The preventive measures include dust control and improved ventilation can reduce dust levels. Sand blasters in enclosed spaces can use special suits and breathing apparatus. The complicated progressive massive fibrosis shortens life-span.

ii. Asbestos-related lung disease: Asbestos caused lung cancer, malignant mesothelioma of pleura and periosteum, cancer of the larynx, and certain gastrointestinal cancer, also cause asbestosis of fibrotic lung disease.

Fibrosis caused by asbestos called asbestosis, asbestos fibers, accumulated around terminal bronchioles, surrounds fibers with iron rich tissue, forming asbestos body with characteristic picture on X-ray, more asbestos bodies as more fibers are inhaled, after 20–30 years of exposure fibrosis begins in lungs, interstitial fibrosis develops. Pleural plaques, which are calcified lesions develop on pleura. Dyspnea, basal crackles and decreased vital capacity are early manifestation. The complications include diffused interstitial pulmonary fibrosis. Lung cancer especially in cigarette smokers, mesothelioma (cancer affecting pleura and peritonial membrane).

Treatment with radical pleurectomy and pneumonectomy survival only for 1–2 years. Preventive measures include enforcement for regulations governing mining milling and use of asbestos. Protective masks must be used when working with asbestos.

iii. Hypersensitivity diseases fall into occupational category when can occur in bronchi, bronchioles or alveoli, coarse dust causes bronchial reactions, fine dust previous small airway and alveolar reactions.

- In occupational asthma, hypersensitivity reaction mediated by histamine bronchoconstriction and increased mucus production repeated attacks if cause unrecognized and asthma is untreated, may lead to permanent obstructive lung disease; asthmatic response that is well established can be provoked by other factors (i.e. house dust, cigarette smoke) and by fatigue, breathing cold air and coughing where wheezing is major symptom. It can be prevented by total elimination of antigen, desensitization not successful
- In farmer's lung (hypersensitivity pneumonitis or allergic alveolitis), alveoli are inflamed, inundated by WBCs, sometimes filled with fluid, if exposure infrequent or level of dust low, symptoms are mild, and treatment not sought, chronic form develops over a period of time eventually fibrosis occurs, and fibrosis may be so well established that it cannot be arrested.

Symptoms begin some hours after exposure to offending dust and include fatigue, shortness of breath, dry cough, fever and chills. Symptoms may be severe enough to require emergency treatment and hospitalization; acute attacks treated with steroids, recovery may take 6 weeks and patient may have residual lung damage, real cure is permanent separation of patient and antigen.

Preventive measures include properly dried and stored farm products (hay, straw, sugar cane) do not cause allergic alveolitis presumably fungi only grow in moist condition.

iv. Byssinosis (Brown lung disease) is occupational disease. Occurs in textile workers; mainly in cotton workers but also afflict workers in flax and hemp industries; cause is found in bales of raw cotton.

In this, chronic bronchitis and emphysema develop in time. Constriction of bronchioles in response to something in crude cotton. Symptoms of asthma and allergy persists long there is exposure to cotton antigen.

Clinical manifestations that develop are tightness in chest on returning to work after a weekend away (Monday fever), strong relationship between amount of dust inhaled and symptoms. Persistent of symptom increases tightness of chest with chronic bronchitis and emphysema, person leaves industry as respiratory cripple.

The preventive measures include–dust control measures, pretreating bales of cotton by washing with steam and other agents may inactivate causative agent, try to detect persons who are likely to become sensitized to cotton dust and keep them out of high risk areas.

Management

Medical therapy of these patients depend on the patient's signs, symptoms and complications. The major role of nurses is to be knowledgeable about the cause and prevention of occupational lung diseases, so that appropriate information and teaching can be presented to community. The best approach to management is to try to prevent or decrease environmental and occupational risks. Well-designed effective ventilation system can reduce exposure to irritants, wearing mask is appropriate in some occupations. Cigarette smoking must be avoided.

Early diagnosis is essential if the disease process is to be halted. The best treatment is to decrease or stop exposure to the harmful agents. Some places of employment at which there is a known risk of lung disease may require periodic chest

X-rays and pulmonary function studies for exposed employees. There is no specific treatment for most environmental lung diseases. Treatment is directed towards symptomatic relief. If there is coexisted problem such as pneumonia, chronic bronchitis, emphysema, or asthma, they are treated on providing nursing care accordingly.

LUNG CANCER

Cancer of the lung may be either metastatic or primary. Metastatic tumours may follow malignancy anywhere in the body. Metastasis forms the colon and kidney are common. Metastasis to the lung may be discovered before the primary lesion is known, and sometimes locations of the primary lesion may be found only at autopsy. Predominant sites of lung cancer are shown in Figure 9.15.

Etiology

Cigarette smoking as a chronic respiratory irritant is by far the major risk factor in the development of lung cancer. Heredity may play a role in both the tendency to smoke and the predisposition to develop lung cancer. Another possible risk factor is pre-existing pulmonary disease such as TB, pulmonary fibrosis, bronchiectasis and COPD.

Pathophysiology

The pathogenesis of primary lung cancer is not well understood. Usually cancers originate from the epithelium of the bronchus (bronchogenic). They grow slowly and it takes 8 to 10 years for a tumor to reach 1 cm in size, which is smallest detectable lesion on an X-ray. Lung cancer occurs primarily in the segmental bronchi or beyond and have a preference for the upperlobes of the lungs. Pathologic changes in the bronchial system show non-specific inflammatory changes with hypersecretions of mucus, desquamation of cells, reactive hyperplasia of the basal cells, and metaplasia of normal respiratory epithelium to stratified squamous cells. Lung cancers metastasize primarily by direct extension and via the blood circulation and the lymph system. The common sites for metastatic growth are the liver, brain, bones, scalene lymph nodes and adrenal glands. Stages of lunge cancer are listed in Box 9.7.

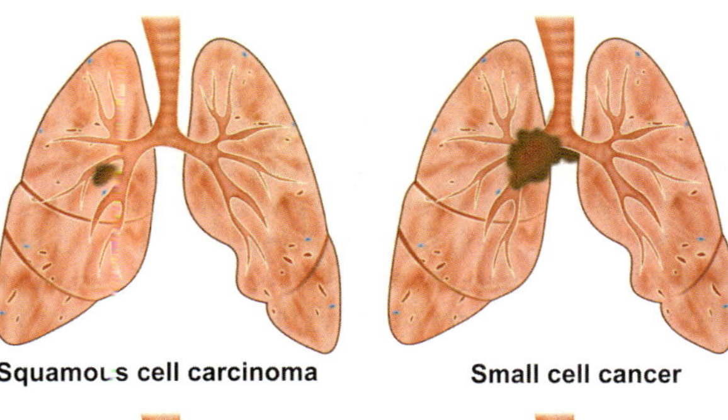

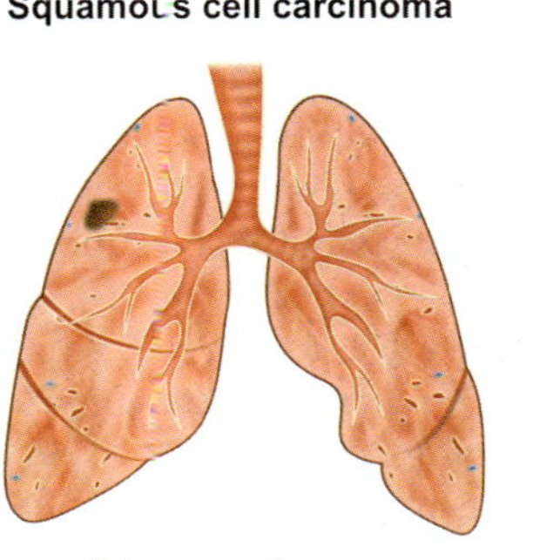

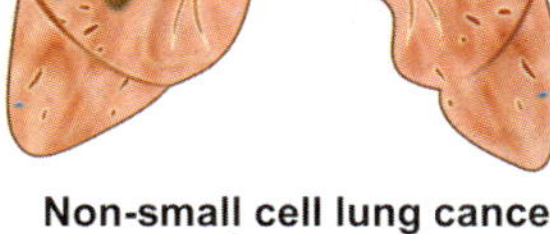

FIG. 9.15: Predominant sites of types of lung cancer

Box 9.7 Stages of lungs cancer

Cancer type	Stage	Characteristics
Non-small cell lung cancer	I	No metastasis to lymph nodes Atelectasis or pneumonia may be present
	II	Cancer has spread to local lymph nodes or chest wall
	III	Cancer has invaded chest wall and mediastinum and usually has spread to lymph nodes
	IV	Tumor has metastasized to distant organs and lymph nodes
Small cell lung cancer	Limited	Cancer is limited to one side of the chest
	Extensive	Cancer cells are found outside one side of the chest or in distant sites

Certain lung cancers cause the paraneoplastic syndrome, which is characterized by various manifestations caused by certain substances (e.g. hormones, enzymes and antigens) produced by the tumor cells. Small cell lung cancer most commonly is associated with it.

Clinical Manifestation

Lung cancer is clinically silent for most individuals for the majority of its course. The clinical manifestations of lung cancer are usually non-specific and appear late in the disease process. A patient's signs and symptoms depend on several factors including location of the lesion. Signs and symptoms of lesion in the bronchus and lung include:

- Approximately 10 percent of patients are asymptomatic and cancer is identified on routine chest X-ray film
- Approximately 75 percent have a cough
- Approximately 50 percent have a hemoptysis
- Shortness of breath and a unilateral wheeze are common.

Peripheral lesions that perforate into pleural space shows extrapulmonary intrathoracic signs and symptoms. These include (Box 9.8):

- Pain on inspiration
- Friction rub
- Pleural effusion

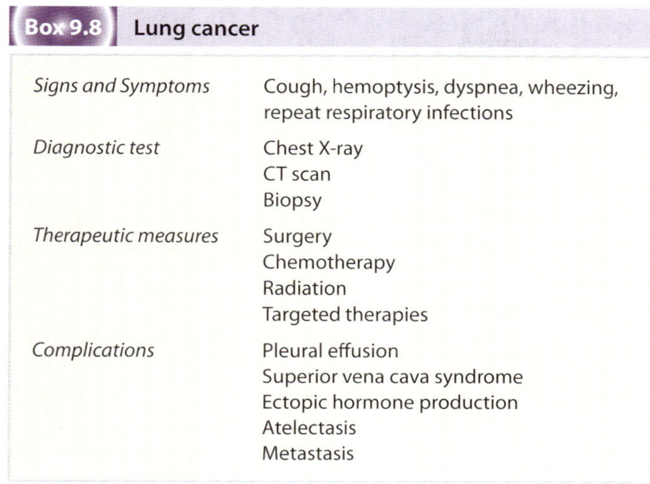

Box 9.8 Lung cancer

Signs and Symptoms	Cough, hemoptysis, dyspnea, wheezing, repeat respiratory infections
Diagnostic test	Chest X-ray CT scan Biopsy
Therapeutic measures	Surgery Chemotherapy Radiation Targeted therapies
Complications	Pleural effusion Superior vena cava syndrome Ectopic hormone production Atelectasis Metastasis

- Edema of face and neck when superior vena cava is involved
- Fatigue
- Clubbing fingers.

Later manifestations include non-specific system and symptoms such as anorexia, fatigue, weight loss, nausea and vomiting. Hoarseness may be present as a result of involvement of the recurrent laryngeal nerve. Unilateral paralysis of the diaphragm, dysphagia and superior vena cava obstruction may occur because of the intrathoracic spread of the malignancy (Box 9.8).

Management

Diagnosis may be confirmed by taking accurately the:

- Health history and physical examination
- Chest X-ray to depict tumor
- Sputum in cytologic study—for examining bacteria and cancer cells
- Bronchioscopy
- CT scan
- MRI
- Positron emission tomography (PET)
- Spirometry (preoperative)
- Mediastinoscopy
- Pulmonary angiography
- Lung scan.

Fine-Needle Aspiration

Surgical resection is usually the only hope for cure in lung cancer. The types of thoracic surgery and indications for their use are as follows:

- Exploratory thoracotomy is performed to confirm suspected diagnosis of lung or chest disease, especially carcinoma; to obtain a biopsy; being replaced by non-invasive procedure (thoracoscopy)
- Pneumonectomy is removal of a lung, bronchogenic carcinoma when lobectomy will not remove all of lesion, tuberculosis when other surgery will not remove all of diseased lung
- Pneumonectomy is lung reduction surgery to reduce lung volume and decrease tension on respiratory muscle in persons with emphysema
- Lobectomy is removal of one lobe of lung, bronchogenic carcinoma confined to a lobe, bronchiectasis, emphysematous blebs or bullae, lung abscess; fungal infections, benign tumors, and tuberculosis (Fig. 9.16)
- Bilobectomy in removal of two lobes from right lungs, bronchogenic carcinoma when lobectomy will not remove all of disease
- Sleeve lobectomy in the resection of main bronchus or distal trachea with reanastomosis to a distal uninvolved bronchus, bronchogenic carcinoma to preserve functional parenchyma
- Segmental resection is known as segmentectomy, that is removal of one or more lung segments; bronchiectasis, lung abscess or cyst; metastatic carcinoma and tuberculosis

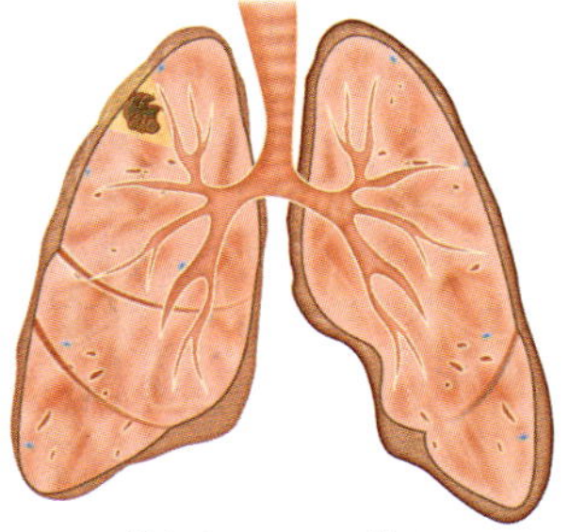

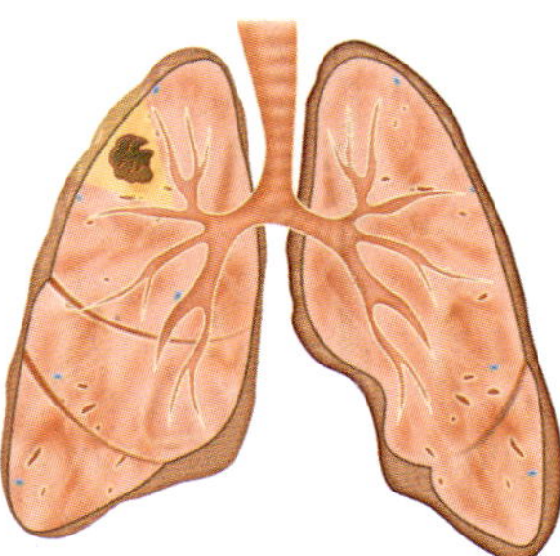

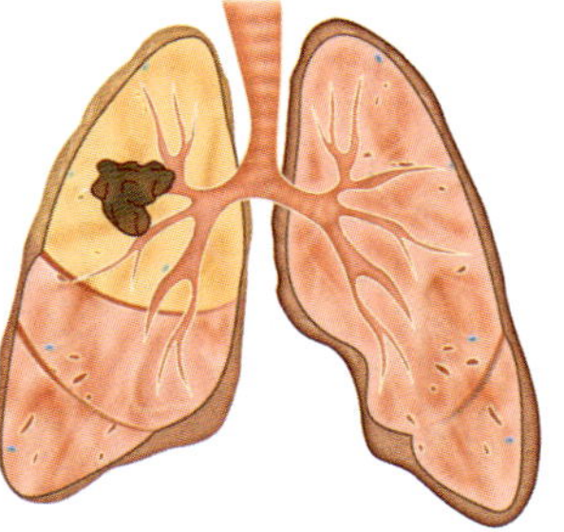

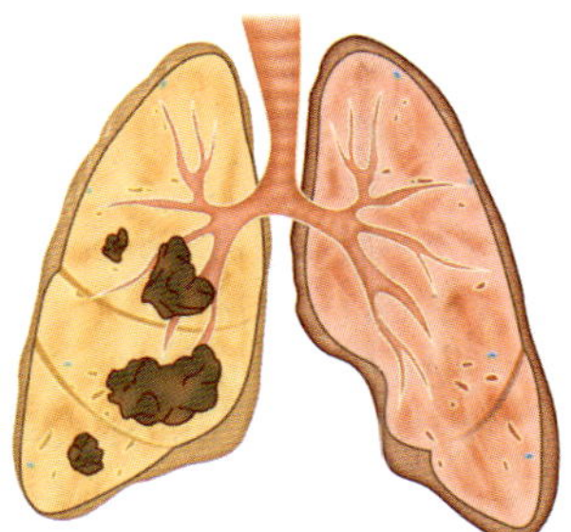

FIG. 9.16: Types of surgery of lung

- Wedge resection is a removal of pie-shaped section from surface of lung, well-circumscribed benign tumors, metastatic tumors or localized inflammatory disease, including TB
- Decortication is removal of fibrinous peel from visceral pleura; chronic empyema
- Thoracoplasty is removal of ribs, residual airspace after resectional surgery; chronic empyema space.

Radiation therapy is used as curative approach in the individual who has resectable tumor but who is considered a poor surgical risk. It is also used as palliative procedure to reduce distressing symptoms such as cough, hemoptysis, bronchial obstruction and superior vena cava syndrome.

Chemotherapy may be used in the treatment of non-resectable tumors or as adjuvant therapy to surgery in non-small cell lung carcinoma.

Biologic therapy used as adjuvant therapy.

Phototherapy, i.e. laser surgery with use of the Nd:YAG also useful in some cases.

The best way to prevent lung cancer is to abstain from smoking. When it is confirmed, nurse has to assist in supporting the patient in all above stated procedures and take suitable nursing measures accordingly.

NURSING MANAGEMENT IN THORACIC SURGERY

Preoperative Care

Preoperative teaching is essential for patients who are undergoing thoracic surgery. The goal of teaching is to prepare the patient for what he or she is expected to do postoperatively. The nurse who is caring for the patient is responsible for determining what the patient understands about the impending surgery and to be sure that preoperative teaching is completed. The points to be discussed in teaching include:

- Patient's knowledge of procedure
- Explanation of procedure is necessary, including intubation for anesthesia, site of incision and chest tube(s) and drainage system
- Oxygen
- Blood administration and IV
- Pain medication, including PCA if used
- What the patient will be asked to do:
  - Coughing and deep breathing
  - Arm exercise
  - Ambulation
- Where patient will be taken after surgery:
  - To recovery–how long
  - To ICU–for how long
- Where family can wait during surgery?

The other routines of preoperative care of any surgery has to be followed.

Postoperative Care

The care of the patient after thoracic surgery centers on promoting ventilation, and re-expansion of the lung by maintaining a clear airway, maintaining the closed drainage system, promoting nutrition, monitoring the incision for bleeding and subcutaneous emphysema.

In most of the hospitals, the patient is taken from the recovery room to the ICU. The immediate postoperative nursing cares are as follows:

Oxygen Therapy

Oxygen is attached to the endotracheal tube in the immediate postoperative period. After extubation, humidified oxygen is given by cannula, usually at 6 L/minute. Oxygen mask should not be used to avoid cough and to rouse secretion.

Hemodynamic Monitoring

The patient is usually attached to a cardiac monitor. A Swan-Ganz catheter and central venous pressure line are used for hemodynamic monitoring.

Position of the Patient in Bed

The patient is kept flat in bed or with head elevated slightly (20 degrees) until blood pressure is stabilized to preoperative levels. Once blood pressure is stabilized, the patient can usually breathe best in semi-Fowler's position with a pillow under the head and neck but not under the shoulders and back, because of the subscapular incision.

Monitoring Vital Signs

Vital signs are taken every 15 minutes until the patient is well recovered from anesthesia, every hour until condition has stabilized, and then every 2 to 4 hours. Any deviation should be reported immediately to take suitable measures.

Initiating Coughing and Deep Breathing Exercises

The patient should be assisted to cough as soon as conscious and extubated. If blood pressure is stable, the patient is assisted to sitting position, and the incision is supported anteriorly and posteriorly by the nurse's hands. Firm, even pressure over the incisions with the open palm of the hands is most effective method. The nurse's head should be behind the patient when the patient is coughing. The patient is encouraged to breathe deeply, exhale and then cough. Sips of fluid especially warm ones such as tea or coffee often facilitate coughing. Deep breathing or coughing keep the airway patent, prevent atelectasis and facilitate reexpansion of the lung. Patient is assisted every 2 to 4 hours around the clock. When a patient is unable to cough effectively, tracheobronchial suctioning is performed (Box 9.9).

Box 9.9 Breathing exercises

General instructions
- Breathe slowly and rhythmically to exhale completely and empty the lungs completely
- Inhale through the nose to filter, humidify, and warm the air before it enters the lungs
- If you feel out of breath, breathe more slowly by prolonging the exhalation time
- Keep the air moist with a humidifier

Diaphragmatic breathing
Goal: To use and strengthen the diaphragm during breathing
- Place one hand on the abdomen (just below the ribs) and the other hand on the middle of the chest to increase the awareness of the position of the diaphragm and its function in breathing
- Breathe in slowly and deeply through the nose, letting the abdomen protrude as far as possible
- Breathe out through pursed lips while tightening (contracting) the abdominal muscles
- Press firmly inward and upward on the abdomen while breathing out
- Repeat for 1 minute; follow with a rest period of 2 minutes
- Gradually increase duration up to 5 minutes, several times a day (before meals and at bedtime)

Pursed-lip breathing
Goal: To prolong exhalation and increased airway pressure during expiration, thus reducing the amount of trapped air and the amount of airway resistance.
- Inhale through the nose while slowly counting to 3—the amount of time needed to say "smell a rose"
- Exhale slowly and evenly against pursed lips while tightening the abdominal muscles (pursing the lips increases intratracheal pressure; exhaling through the mouth offers less resistance to expired air)
- Count to 7 slowly while prolonging expiration through pursed lips—the length of time to say "blow out candle"
- While sitting in a chair
  - Fold arms over the abdomen
  - Inhale through the nose while counting to 3 slowly
  - Bend forward and exhale slowly through pursed lips while counting to 7 slowly
- While walking
  - Inhale while walking two steps
  - Exhale through pursed lips while walking four or five steps

Promoting Abdominal Breathing

Abdominal breathing exercises are a valuable adjunct to the care of the patient with chest surgery, because it improves ventilation without increasing pain assist in coughing more effectively.

Promoting Comfort by Pain Relief

Medication for pain should be given as needed and may be required as often as every 3 to 4 hours during the first 48 to 72 hours. PCA and epidural catheters are widely used for pain medication management. Usually morphine is ordered for pain. If medication for pain fails intercostal nerve block may be performed.

Promoting Arm Exercises

Passive arm exercises are usually started in the evening of surgery. The purpose of pulling the patient's arm through range of motion is to prevent restriction of function.

Promoting Nutrition

The patient is encouraged to take fluids postoperatively and to progress to general diet as soon as it is tolerated. Fluid helps liquefy secretions and make them easier to expectorate. A diet adequate in protein and vitamins (especially vit C) facilitates wound healing.

Monitoring the Incision for Bleeding or Subcutaneous Emphysema

The dressing is checked periodically for bleeding. Blood on the dressing is unusual and should be reported to the surgeon at once. The time and amount of blood are recorded in the patient's record. Air leak from the pleural space through the thoracotomy incision or around the chest tubes into the soft tissues indicates subcutaneous emphysema. The presence of air under the skin is readily detected and has been described as feeling like 'tissue paper' "rice krispies" under the skin.

Maintaining Chest Tube(s) and Drainage (Table 9.1 and Fig. 9.17)

All patients who have resectional surgery of the lung, except those having a pneumonectomy will require drainage of the pleural space by one or two chest tubes connected to closed drainage. Precautions to be observed with any type of closed drainage system are as follows (Box 9.10):

- Monitor drainage system for tidaling (fluctuating) in one waterseal chamber:
  - Be sure the patient is not lying on the tubes
  - Check connections to be sure the chest tube system is intact
  - Ask patient to cough or change position to see if tidaling is resorted
  - Tidaling will stop when the lung is re-expanded
- Never lift the closed drainage system above the level of the patient's chest, because this allows fluid to be pulled into the pleural space
- Never clamp chest tubes without a written order from the surgeon because air (positive pressure) will be trapped in the pleural space, further collapsing the lung

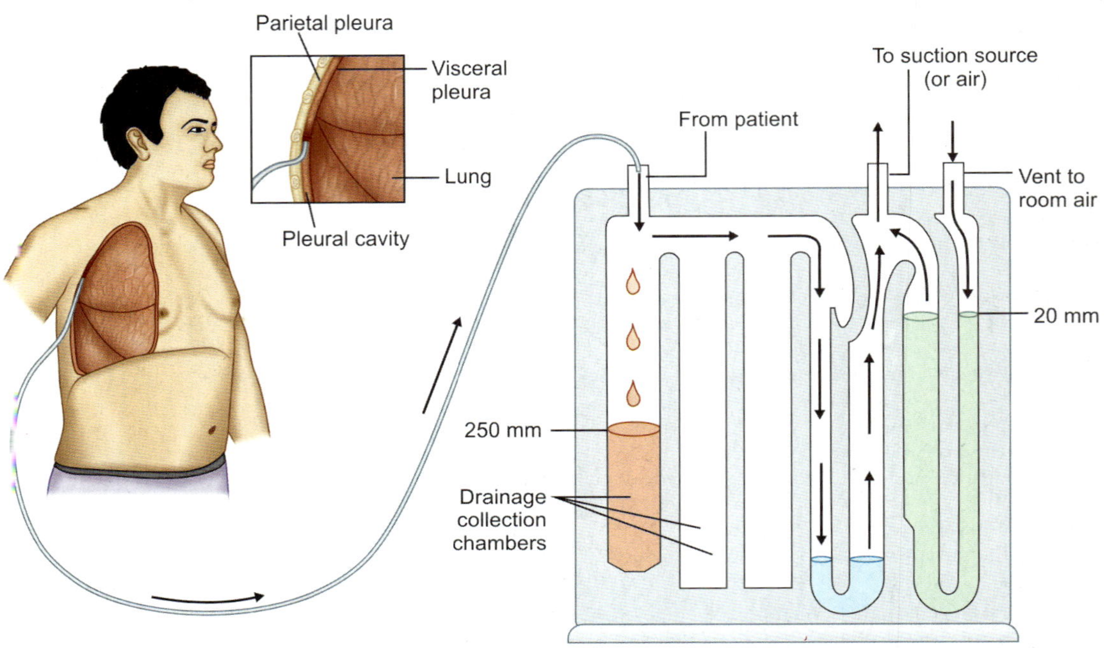

FIG. 9.17: Example of a disposable chest drainage system

Box 9.10 Care of the patient with a chest drainage system

Assess the patient according to institution policy. Start with the patient and move toward the drainage system.

1. Observe respiratory rate, effort and symmetry
2. Assess shortness of breath, pain, anxiety or other discomfort
3. Auscultate lung sounds (lung sound may initially be muffled or absent on the side of a collapsed lung but should gradually return to normal as the lung reinflates.
4. Confirm that dressing is intact; observe for drainage. If necessary, reinforce the dressing and notify the physician. Do not change the dressing unless specifically ordered to and trained to do so
5. Palpate around insertion sites for crepitus
6. Check all tubing for kinks, breaks, or broken connections. Verify that all connections are securely taped
7. Ensure that there are no dependent loops of tubing. Excess tubing should be coiled on the bed
8. Verify that drainage system is below level of patient's chest at all times
9. Check drainage system or bottles for cracks or leaks
10. Check water seal chamber for correction of water level and for tidaling (unless lung reinflated). Add water if evaporation has decreased level. If continuous bubbling is present, check entire system for leaks and notify physician
11. Check suction control chamber for gentle bubbling (or open to air). Confirm correct amount of water as ordered. Add water if needed
12. Check and mark amount of drainage in collection chamber every 8 hours and prn or as ordered. Report any marked increase in bloody drainage. Record drainage as output
13. Document finding
    Notify RN or physician if any of the following occur
    - The patient suddenly reports increasing dyspnea
    - There is a change in the patient's assessment findings
    - The drainage chamber is full and needs to be changed.

TABLE 9.1: Guidelines for managing chest drainage systems (Fig. 9.17)

Equipment
- Chest tube insertion tray (contains chest tube, scalpel, gloves)
- Antiseptic solution
- Local anesthetic agent
- Chest drainage system
- Adhesive tape

Implementation

Actions	*Rationale*
1. If using a chest drainage system with a water seal, fill the water seal chamber with sterile water to the level specified by the manufacturer	Water seal drainage allows air and fluid to escape into a drainage chamber. The water acts as a seal and keeps the air from being drawn back into the pleural space
2. When using suction in chest drainage systems with a water seal, fill the suction control chamber with sterile water to the 20 cm level or as prescribed. In systems without a water seal, set the regulator dial at the appropriate suction level	The water level regulator dial setting determines the degree of suction applied
3. Attach the drainage catheter exiting the thoracic cavity to the tubing coming from the collection chamber. Tape securely with adhesive tape	In chest drainage units, the system is closed. The only connection is the one to the patient's catheter
4. If suction is used, connect the suction control chamber tubing to the suction unit. If using a wet suction system, turn on the suction unit and increase pressure until slow but steady bubbling appears in the suction control chamber. If using a chest drainage system with a dry suction control chamber, turn the regulator dial to 20 cm H_2O	With a wet suction system, the degree of suction is determined by the amount of water in the suction control chamber and is not dependent on the rate of bubbling or the pressure gauge setting on the suction unit. With a dry suction control chamber, the regulator dial replaces the water
5. Mark the drainage from the collection chamber with tape on the outside of the drainage unit. Mark hourly/daily increments (date and time) at the drainage level	This marking shows the amount of fluid loss and how fast fluid is collecting in the drainage chamber. It serves as a basis for determining the need for blood replacement, if the fluid is blood. Visibly bloody drainage will appear in the chamber in the immediate postoperative period but should gradually becomes serous. If the patient is bleeding as heavily as 100 mL every 15 minutes, check the drainage every few minutes. A reoperation or autotransfusion may be needed. The transfusion of blood collected in the drainage chamber must be reinfused within 4 to 6 hours. Usually, however, drainage decreases progressively in the first 24 hours
6. Ensure that the drainage tubing does not kink, loop, or interfere with the patient's movements	Kinking, looping, or pressure on the drainage tubing can produce back-pressure, which may force fluid back into the pleural space or impede its drainage
7. Encourage the patients to assume a comfortable position with good body alignment. With the lateral position, make sure that patient body does not compress the tubing. The patient should be turned and repositioned every 1.5 to 2 hours. Provide adequate analgesia	Frequent position changes promote drainage, and good body alignment helps prevent postural deformities and contractures. Proper positioning also helps breathing and promotes better air exchange. Analgesics may be needed to promote comfort
8. Assist the patient with range-of-motion exercises for the affected arm and shoulder several times daily. Provide adequate analgesia	Exercise helps to prevent ankylosis of the shoulder and to reduce post-operative pain and discomfort. Analgesics may be needed to relieve pain
9. Gently "milk" the tubing in the direction of the drainage chamber as needed	Milking prevents the tubing from becoming obstructed clots and fibrin. Constant attention to maintaining the patency of the tube facilitates prompt expansion of the lung and minimizes complications
10. Make sure there is fluctuation (tidaling) of the fluid level in the water seal chamber (in wet systems), or check the air leak indicator for leaks (in dry systems with a one-way valve). Note: Fluid fluctuations in the water seal chamber or air leak indicator area will stop when: a. The lung has re-expanded b. The tubing is obstructed by blood clots, fibrin, or kinks c. A loop of tubing hangs below the rest of the tubing d. Suction motor or wall suction is not working properly	Fluctuation of the water level in the water seal shows effective connection between the pleural cavity and the drainage chamber and indicates that the drainage system remains patient. Fluctuation is also a gauge of intrapleural pressure in systems with a water seal (wet and dry, but not with the one-way valve)

Contd...

Contd...

11. With a dry system, assess for the presence of the indicator (bellows or float device) when setting the regulator dial to the desired level of suction	An air leak indicator shows changes in intrathoracic pressure in dry systems with a one-way valve. Bubbles will appear if a leak is present. The air leak indicator takes the place of fluid fluctuations in the water seal chamber
12. Observe for air leaks in the drainage system; they are indicated by constant bubbling in the water seal chamber, or by the air leak indicator in dry systems with a one-way valve. Also assess the chest tube system for correctable external leaks. Notify the physician immediately of excessive bubbling in the water seal chamber not due to external leaks	The indicator shows that the vacuum is adequate to maintain the desired level of suction Leaking and trapping of air in the pleural space can result in tension pneumothorax
13. When turning down the dry suction, depress the manual high-negativity vent, and assess for a rise in the water level of the water seal chamber	A rise in the water level of the water seal chamber indicates high negative pressure in the system that could lead to increased intrathoracic pressure
14. Observe and immediately report and shallow breathing, cyanosis, pressure in the chest, subcutaneous emphysema, symptoms of hemorrhage, or significant changes in vital signs	Many clinical conditions can cause these signs and symptoms, including tension pneumothorax, mediastinal shift, hemorrhage, severe incisional pain, pulmonary embolus, and cardiac tamponade. Surgical intervention may be necessary
15. Encourage the patient to breathe deeply and cough at frequent intervals. Provide adequate analgesia. If needed, request an order for patient-controlled analgesia. Also teach the patient how to perform incentive spirometry	Deep breathing and coughing help to raise the intrapleural pressure, which promotes drainage of accumulated fluid in the pleural space. Deep breathing and coughing also promote removal of secretions from the tracheobronchial tree, which in turn promotes lung expansion and prevents atelectasis (alveolar collapse)
16. If the patient is lying on a stretcher and must be transported to another area, place the drainage system below the chest level. If the tubing disconnects, cut off the contaminated tips of the chest tube and tubing, insert a sterile connector in the cut ends, and reattach to the drainage system. Do not clamp the chest tube during transport	The drainage apparatus must be kept at a level lower than the patient's chest to prevent fluid from flowing backward into the pleural space. Clamping can result in a tension pneumothorax
17. When assisting in the chest tube's removal, instruct the patient to perform a gentle Valsalva maneuver or to breathe quietly. The chest tube is then clamped and quickly removed. Simultaneously, a small bandage is applied and made airtight with petrolatum gauze covered by a 4 × 4 inch gauze pad and thoroughly covered and sealed with nonporous tape	The chest tube is removed as directed when the lung is re-expanded (usually 24 hours to several days), depending on the cause of the pneumothorax. During tube removal, the chief priorities are preventing air from entering the pleural cavity as the tube is withdrawn and preventing infection

- One liter bottle of sterile water is kept at the bedside at all times. If the patient's chest drainage system cracks or breaks.
  - Insert patiently chest tube into the bottle of sterile water
  - Remove the cracked or broken system
  - Obtain new system and connect it to patient's chest tube as soon as possible
- If the patient's tube is accidentally pulled out of the chest (rarely occurs)
  - Apply gloves in accordance with body substance isolation policy
  - Pinch skin opening together with fingers
  - Apply occlusive dressing
  - Cover dressing with overlapping pieces of 2-inch tape
  - Call surgeon immediately.

Chest tubes are removed when there is no tidaling of fluid in the water-sealed chamber and when X-ray films confirm the full re-expansion of the lung.

CHEST TRAUMA AND THORACIC INJURIES

Chest trauma is a major problem often seen in the casualty. Injury to the chest may affect the bony chest cage, pleura and lungs, diaphragm, or mediastinal contents.

Etiology

Injury to the chest are broadly classified into two groups— blunt and penetrating.

i. Blunt trauma or non-penetrating injuries damage the structures within the chest cavity without disrupting chest wall integrity. Blunt injury occurs when the body is struck by a blunt object, such as steering wheel. The external injury may appear minor but the impact may cause severe, life-threatening internal injuries such as ruptured spleen.

- Blunt steering wheel injury to chest may lead to rib fracture, flail chest, pneumothorax, hemopneumo thorax, cardiac contusion, pulmonary contusion, cardiac tamponade, great vessel tears
- Shoulder harness seat belt injury may lead to fractured clavicle, dislocated shoulder, rib fractures, pulmonary contusion, pericardial contusion, cardiac tamponade
- Crush injury (e.g. heavy equipment, crushing thorax) leads to pneumothorax and hemopneumothorax, flail chest, great vessel tears and rupture, decreased blood returned with decreased cardiac output
- Countrecoup trauma—a type of blunt trauma, is caused by the impact of parts of the body against other objects. Examples are many head injuries caused by countrecoup trauma
- The causes of blunt injuries are, motor vehicle accident, pedestrian accident, fall, assault with blunt object, crush injury and explosion.

ii. Penetrating trauma or injuries disrupt chest wall integrity and result in alteration in intrathoracic pressures. It occurs when a foreign body impales or passes through the body tissue, e.g. gunshot wound, stabbing with knife, gunshot, stick, arrow and other missiles. Gunshot or stab wound to chest may lead to open pneumothorax, tension pneumothorax, hemopneumothorax, cardiac tamponade, esophageal damage, tracheal tear, great vessel tears.

Emergency care of the patient with chest trauma requires an accurate assessment of respiratory, cardiovascular and surface finding which include:

- Respiratory
  - Dyspnea, respiratory distress
  - Cough with or without hemoptysis
  - Cyanosis of the mouth, face, nail beds, mucous membrane
  - Tracheal deviation
  - Audible air escaping from the chest wound
  - Decreased breath sounds on side of injury
  - Decreased oxygen saturation
  - Frothy secretions
- Cardiovascular
  - Rapid, thready pulse
  - Decreased blood pressure
  - Narrowed pulse pressure
  - Asymmetric blood pressure value in arms
  - Distended neck veins
  - Muffled heart sounds
  - Chest pain
  - Crunching sounds synchronous with heart sounds
  - Arrhythmias.
- Surface findings
  - Bruising
  - Abrasions
  - Open chest wounds
  - Asymmetric chest movement
  - Subcutaneous emphysema.

Nursing Intervention

The emergency care are:

- Ensure patient airway
- Administer high-flow O_2 with non-rebreather mask
- Establish IV access with two large-bore catheters. Begin fluid resuscitation as appropriate
- Remove clothing to assess injury
- Cover sucking chest wound with non-porous dressing taped on three sides
- Stabilize impaled objects with bulky dressings. Do not remove
- Assess for other significant injuries and treat appropriately
- Stabilize flail rib segment with hand followed by application of large pieces of tape horizontal across the flail segment
- Place patient in a semi-Fowler's position or position the patient on injured side if breathing is easier after carvical spine injury has been ruled out.

An ongoing monitoring will include:

- Monitor vital signs, level of consciousness, oxygen saturation, cardiac rhythm, respiratory status and urinary output
- Anticipate intubation for respiratory distress
- Release dressing if tension pneumothorax develops after sucking chest wound is covered.

Thorax injuries range from single rib fracture to the life-threatening tears of aorta, vena cava, and other major vessels. The most coronary thoracic emergencies are discussed further:

RIB FRACTURES

Rib fractures are the most common type of chest injury (blunt injury), resulting from trauma ribs (4–9) 3rd to 10th are most commonly fractured because they are least protected by chest muscles. If the fractured rib is splintered or displaced, it may damage the pleura and lungs.

Ribs usually function at the point of maximum impact, but they may fracture at a site distant from impact. Rib fractures are caused by blows, crushing injuries, or strain caused by severe coughing or sneezing spells. When the rib is splintered or the fracture displaced, sharp fragments may penetrate the pleura and lungs, resulting in a hemothorax (blood in the pleural space) or pneumothorax (air in the pleural space) which are penetrating injuries.

Clinical manifestation of fractured ribs include:

- Pain at the site of injury, especially increasing on inspiration
- Localized tenderness and crepitus on palpation
- Splinting of chest and shallow breathing.

Fractures are confirmed by chest X-ray.

The main goal in treatment is to decrease pain so that patient can breathe adequately to promote good chest expansion. Intercostal nerve blocks with local anesthesia (1% procaine) may be used to provide pain relief and analgesics is given to relieve pain so that the patient can be encouraged to breathe more rapidly.

The patient is observed for splinting of the chest and shallow breathing to which could lead to atelectasis. To improve breathing, the patient is placed in a position of comfort. Most of the patients are able to breathe best in Fowler's or semi-Fowler's positions.

The patient and family should be educated regarding:

- The patient should rest and do nothing strenuous for several days
- The patient should take deep breath every hour
- Narcotic drug therapy must be individualized and used with caution because these drugs can depress respiration
- The pain is not relieved if analgesic call physician
- If shortness of breath, sudden sharp chest pain, coughing up blood occurs, rush to casualty part of hospital.

FLAIL CHEST

Flail chest results from multiple rib fractures and thereby causing instability of the chest wall.

When multiple ribs or the sternum is fractured in more than one places, a portion of the chest wall becomes separated from the chest cage, resulting in a flail chest. The chest wall cannot provide the bony structures necessary to maintain bellows action and ventilation. The affected (flail) area will move paradoxically the intact portions of the chest during respiration. During inspiration the affected portion is sucked in, and during expiration it bulges out. This paradoxical chest movement prevents adequate ventilation of the lung in the injured area. The underlying lung may or may not have a serious injury. Associated pain and any lung injury give rise to loss of compliance, will contribute to an alteration in breathing pattern and lead to hypoxemia. And may also develop hypercapnia and respiratory acidosis due to increased work of breathing (Fig. 9.18).

Clinical Manifestations

- Severe chest pain
- Paradoxical breathing (asymmetrical chest movement)
- Oscillation of mediastinum
- Increasing dyspnea
- Rapid shallow respiration
- Accessory muscle breathing
- Restlessness
- Decreased breath sounds on auscultation
- Cyanosis
- Anxiety related to difficult breathing.

Management

- Stabilizing the flail segment position end-expiratory pressure (PEEP) used with mechanical ventilation to improve oxygenation will maintain pressure in the lungs throughout the respiratory cycle
- Provide supplemental oxygen: Monitor with pulse oximetry
- Correct acid-base balance by mechanical ventilation
- Provide analgesic for pain control
- For severe pain, epidural anesthesia may be used
- Avoid fluid overload
- Patient should be confined to bed as he or she is on a ventilator.

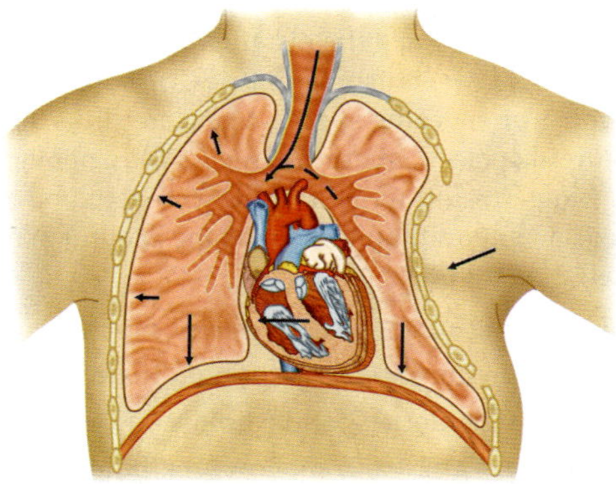

Inspiration

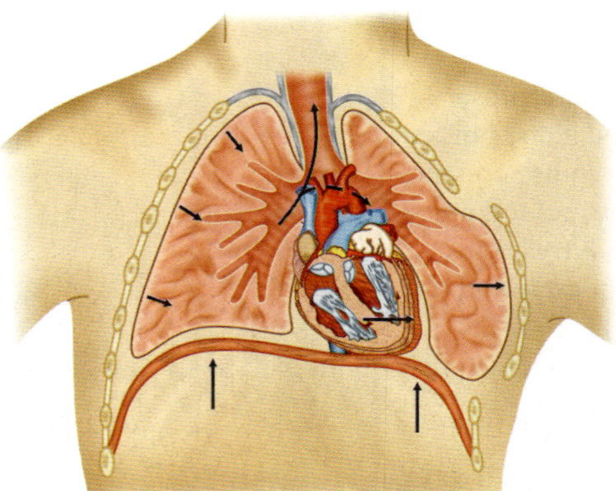

Expiration

FIG. 9.18: Flail chest produces paradoxic respiration, the flail section sinks in with mediastinal shift to the uninjured side. On expiration, the flail section bulges outward with mediastinal shift to the injured side

PNEUMOTHORAX

A pneumothorax is a complete or partial collapse of a lung as a result of an accumulation of air in the pleural space. Pneumothorax may be closed or open (Box 9.11).

Pneumothorax occurs when the parietal or visceral pleura is breached and the pleural space is exposed to positive atmospheric pressure. Air enters the pleural space, and lung or a portion of it collapses. Types of pneumothorax include simple, traumatic and tension pneumothorax. A simple pneumothorax may occur in an apparently healthy person or may be associated with interstitial lung disease or emphysema. A traumatic pneumothorax can occur with blunt chest trauma, penetrating trauma to the chest, abdominal or diaphragmatic tears, or invasive thoracic procedures. An open traumatic pneumothorax includes a mediastinal swing that process serious circulatory problems. Hemothorax is the collection of blood in the chest cavity because of torn intercostal vessels or laceration of the lungs injured through trauma. Often both blood and air are found in the chest cavity (hemopneumothorax).

Closed Pneumothorax

The common form is:

- Spontaneous pneumothorax, which is caused by rupture of small blebs on the visceral pleural space. The cause of the bleb is unknown. This condition occurs most commonly in male cigarette smokers between 20–40 years of age. The other causes include:
  - Injury to the lungs from mechanical ventilation
  - Injury to the lungs from insertion of a subclavian catheter
  - Perforation of esophagus
  - Injury to the lungs from broken ribs
  - Receptive blebs or bullae in a patient with COPD (e.g. asthma).

Box 9.11 Overview of pneumothorax

Signs and symptoms	Sudden-onset dyspnea, chest pain, tachypnea Asymmetrical chest expansion Diminished or absent breath sounds on affected side
Diagnostic tests	Ultrasound Chest X-ray, CT scan ABGs
Therapeutic measures	Chest tube and water seal drainage Pleurodesis for recurrent pneumothorax
Complications	Tension pneumothorax Shock

Clinical Manifestation

Signs and symptoms associated with pneumothorax depend on its size and cause:

- Pleuritic pain of sudden onset
- Minimal respiratory distress with small pneumothorax; acute respiratory distress if large
- Anxiety, dyspnea, air hunger, use of accessory muscles, and central cyanosis (with severe hypoxemia), accompanied by tachypnea, tympanic sound on percussion of the chest wall, decreased or absent breath sound, and tactile fremitus of affected side.

Small or slowly developing pneumothorax may produce no symptoms, but in large or rapidly developing pneumothorax results in:

- Sharp pain on respiration
- Increasing dyspnea
- Increasing restlessness
- Diaphoresis
- Hypotension
- Tachycardia
- Absence of chest movement in affected side
- Hyperresonance on affected side (to percussion).

The goal is evacuation of air or blood from the pleural space while maintaining fluid balance.

- A large-diameter chest tube is inserted, usually in the fourth or fifth intercostal space, for hemothorax
- A small chest tube is inserted near the second intercostal space for a pneumothorax
- Autotransfusion is begun if excessive bleeding from chest tube occurs
- Traumatic open pneumothorax is plugged (petroleum gauze); patient is asked to inhale and strain against a closed glottis to eject air from the thorax until the chest tube is inserted, with water-seal drainage.

Management of closed pneumothorax will include:

- Observation on outpatient basis
- Giving supplemental oxygen
- Needle aspiration of air from pleural space, if present, insertion of chest catheter connected to a flutter valve or closed drainage system (suction or vented drainage).

Open Pneumothorax (Fig. 9.19)

Open pneumothorax is an opening in the chest wall large enough to allow air to pass freely in and out of the thoracic cavity with respiration (sucking wounds). The lung is collapsed; the heart and great vessels are shifted toward the uninjured side with each inspiration and in the opposite direction with expiration (mediastinal flutter).

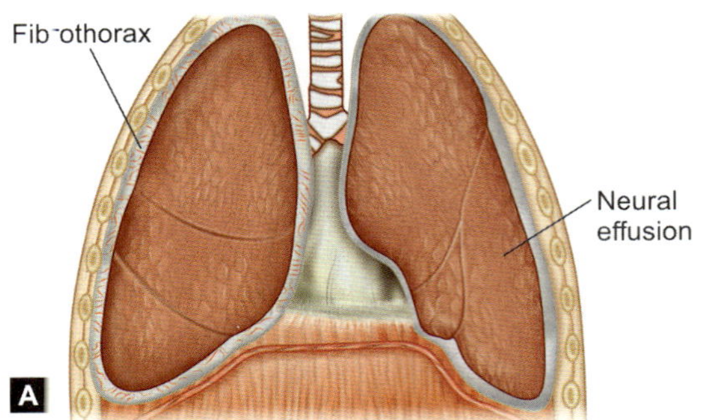

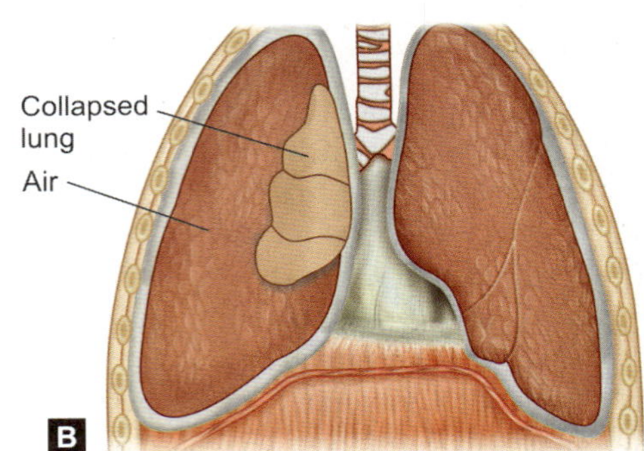

FIGS 9.19A AND B: Disorder of the pleura. (A) Fibrothorax resulting from an organization of inflammatory exudate, and pleural effusion; (B) Open pneumothorax resulting from collapse of lung due to disruption of chest wall and outside air entering

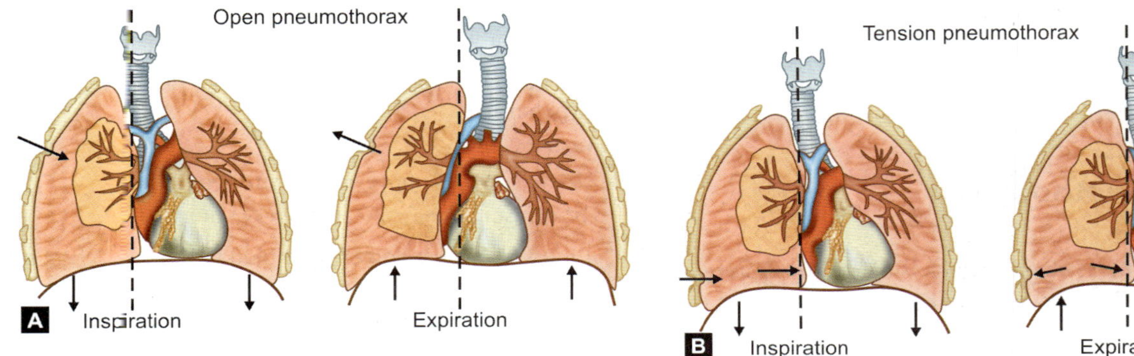

FIGS 9.20A AND B: Open pneumothorax (A) and tension pneumothorax. In open pneumothorax, air enters the chest during inspiration and exits during expiration. A slight shift of the affected lung may occur because of a decrease in pressure as air moves out of the chest. In tension pneumothorax, air enters but cannot leave the chest. As the pressure increases, the heart and great vessels are compressed and the mediastinal structures are shifted toward the opposite side of the chest. The trachea is pushed from its normal midline position toward the opposite side of the chest, and the unaffected lung is compressed

Open pneumothorax occurs when air enters the pleural space through an opening in the chest wall. For example, gunshot or stab wound to chest in surgical thoracotomies. A penetrating chest wound is often referred to as a "sucking chest wound, because each time the person inspires, air is sucked into pleural space. In which, sucking sounds at wound site with respiration and tracheal deviation (trachea moves towards unaffected area during inspiration and returns towards midline inspiration are the clinical manifestations (Fig. 9.20).

This will be managed by occlusion of open wound and use other measures as in closed pneumothorax. To stop the flow of air through the opening in the chest wall, use anything large enough to fill the hole (towel, handkerchief, heel of hand). Have patient inhale and strain against a closed glottis (if conscious). When possible, plug the opening by sealing with petrolatum-impregnated gauze. Apply pressure dressing.

Medical Management

Traumatic open pneumothorax call for emergency interventions. Stopping the flow of air through the opening in the chest wall is a life saving measure.

A thoracotomy is performed or a chest tube is connected to water-seal drainage for exit of air and fluid, and antibiotics are administered to combat infection from contamination. Autotransfusion is performed if bleeding is excessive.

Nursing Management

- Promote early detection through assessment and identification of high-risk population; report symptoms
- Assist in chest tube insertion; maintain chest drainage or water-seal

- Monitor respiratory status and reexpansion of lung, with interventions (pulmonary support) performed in collaboration with other health care professionals (e.g. physician, respiratory therapist, physical therapist).
- Provide information and emotional support to patient and family.

TENSION PNEUMOTHORAX (FIG. 9.21)

A tension pneumothorax occurs when air is drawn into the pleural space and is trapped with each breath. Tension builds up in the pleural space, causing lung collapse. Mediastinal shift (shift of the heart and great vessels and trachea toward the unaffected side of the chest) is a life-threatening medical emergency. Both respiratory and circulatory functions are compromised.

Tension pneumothorax may result from either in open or a closed pneumothorax. It occurs when air enters the pleural space on inspiration but cannot leave it on expiration. Although usually a result of a closed pneumothorax, a tension pneumothorax can be caused by a penetrating chest injury. The accumulated air builds up positive pressure in the chest cavity resulting in the following:

- Lung collapse on the affected side
- Mediastinal shift towards the unaffected side
- Compression of mediastinal contents (heart, great vessels) resulting in decreased cardiac output and decreased venous return.

The clinical manifestation, tension pneumothorax will include:

- Air hunger, anxiety and agitation
- Increasing hypoxemia, cyanosis

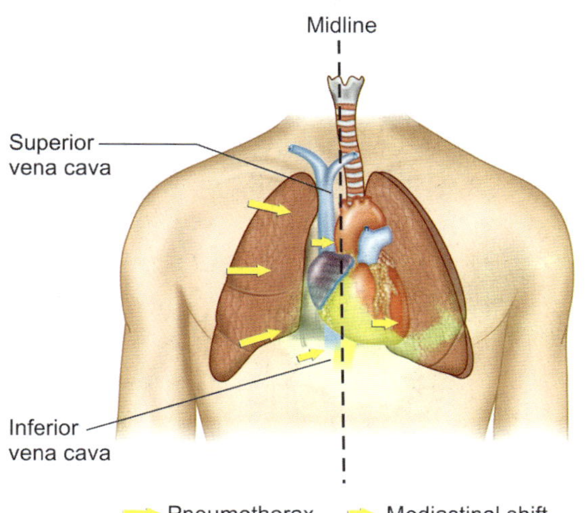

FIG. 9.21: Tension pneumothorax. As pleural pressure on the affected side increases, mediastinal displacement ensuses with resultant respiratory and cardiovascular compromise

- Hypotension, tachycardia and profuse diuresis
- Tracheal shift away from the affected side
- Severe dyspnea
- Agitation
- Trachea deviated from midline toward unaffected lung mediastinal shift
- Jugular venous distention
- Absence of chest movement on affected side
- Hypotension, tachycardia
- Breath sounds absent on affected side
- Hyperresonance on affected side
- Diminished heart sounds
- Shock
- Subcutaneous emphysema
- Ineffective ventilation.

Tension pneumothorax is a medical emergency because both the respiratory and circulatory systems are affected. If the tension of the pleural space is not relieved, the patient is likely to die from inadequate cardiac output or marked hypoxemia. Nurses are now being trained to insert large bore needle and chest tube into the chest walls to release the trapped air. Tension of pneumothorax usually occurs during mechanical ventilation or resuscitative efforts. Since it is the emergency defect in chest wall, covered with a sterile dressing, and insertion of chest tube connected to a flutter valve or closed drainage system.

- Pulse oximetry is used to monitor blood oxygen levels in cases of hypoxia
- Conversion to simple pneumothorax is accomplished by insertion of a large-bore needle into the pleural space to relieve pressure
- Chest tube is inserted with suction to remove remaining and fluid
- Surgery may be necessary to close the leak.

HEMOTHORAX

Hemothorax is an accumulation of blood in the intrapleural space. It is frequently found in association with open pneumothorax. It may be due to chest trauma, lung malignancy, complication of anticoagulative therapy, pulmonary embolus, and tearing of pleural adhesions.

The clinical manifestations are:

If it is small mild tachycardia, and dyspnea, air present. If it is large, respiratory distress may be present, which include shallow, rapid, respiration, dyspnea and air hunger. Chest pain or cough with or without hemoptysis. No breath sounds heard on auscultation.

If tension pneumothorax develops, feature of these also develop as a clinical manifestation.

Treatment of hemopneumothorax depends on air severity of the pneumothorax and the nature of the underlying disease.

An emergency management will include chest insertion, autotransfusion of collected blood, treatment of hypovolemia as necessary. Repeated spontaneous pneumothorax may need to be treated surgically by a partial pleurectomy, stapling or laser pleurodesis to promote adherence of the pleurae to one another. The injection of doxycycline (dry) an irritating agent can be used for pleurodesis.

Nursing intervention for closed, tension and open pneumothorax are as follows:

- Closed pneumothorax patient if he or she admitted performing the following:
  - Place the patient in semi-Fowler's position
  - Administer oxygen
  - Obtain thoracentesis tray and closed drainage equipment.

  For outpatients or for patients after chest tube removal, instruct the patient to:
  - Report any increased dyspnea to physician
  - Avoid strenous exercises or activity that increases rate and depth of breathing
  - Avoid holding breath
  - Follow physician's instructions about resuming normal activity.
- Tension pneumothorax is life-threatening event; imperative that intervention be carried immediately to relieve increased intrapleural pressure; intervention same as those listed CP and performed the following:
  - Monitor vital signs frequently
  - Observe for cardiac dysrhythmias
  - Palpate for subcutaneous emphysema in upper chest and neck
  - Use same discharge instruction as in CP (above).
- Open pneumothorax-performed the following:
  - Occlude wound on the non-porous covering
  - Same intervention as CP (closed pneumothorax), and
  - Same discharge instruction as CP.

PLEURAL EFFUSION

The pleural space lies between the lung and chest wall and normally contains a very thin layer fluid. Pleural effusion is a collection of fluid in the pleural space. It is not a disease but rather a sign of a serious disease. Pleural effusion is frequently classified as transudative or exudative according to whether the protein content of the effusion is low or high, respectively. A transudate occurs primarily in noninflammatory conditions and is an accumulation of protein-poor, cell-poor fluid. Transudative pleural effusions (also called hydrothoraces) are caused by (1) increased hydrostatic pressure found in heart failure (HF), which is the most common cause of pleural effusion, or (2) decreased oncotic pressure (from hypoalbuminemia) found in chronic liver or renal disease. In these situations, fluid movement is facilitated out of the capillaries an into the pleural space.

Pathophysiology

In certain disorders, fluid may accumulate in the pleural space to a point at which it becomes clinically evident. This almost always has pathologic significance. The effusion can be a relatively clear fluid, or it can be bloody or purulent. An effusion of clear fluid may be a transudate or an exudate. A transudate (filtrate of plasma that moves across intact capillary walls) occurs when factors influencing the formation and reabsorption of pleural fluid are altered, usually by imbalances in hydrostatic or oncotic pressures. The finding of a transudative effusion generally implies that the pleural membranes are not diseased. A transudative effusion most commonly results from heart failure. An exudate (extravasation of fluid into tissues or a cavity) usually results from inflammation by bacterial products or tumors involving the pleural surfaces (Fig. 9.22).

Pleural effusion, a collection of fluid in the pleural space, is usually secondary to other diseases (e.g. pneumonia, pulmonary infections, nephrothic syndrome, connective tissue disease, neoplastic tumors, congestive heart failure). The effusion can be relatively clear fluid or it can be blood or pus, which may be a transudate due to altered or reabsorption of pleural fluid or an exudate resulting from inflammation by bacterial products or tumors, or it can be blood or pus. Pleural fluid accumulates due to an imbalance in hydrostatic or oncotic pressures (transudate) or as a result inflammation by bacterial products or tumors (exudate).

An exudative effusion is an accumulation of fluid and cells in an area of inflammation. An exudative pleural effusion results

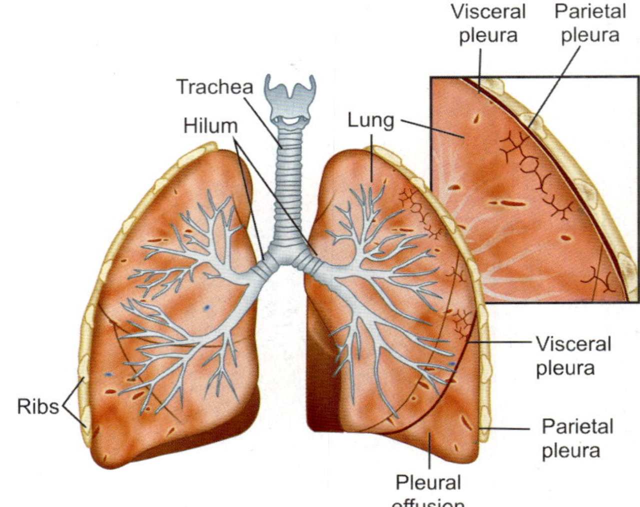

FIG. 9.22: In pleural effusion, an abnormal volume of fluid collects in the pleural space, causing pain and shortness of breath. Pleural effusion is usually secondary to other disease processes

from increased capillary permeability characteristic of the inflammatory reaction. This type of effusion occurs secondary to conditions such as pulmonary malignancies, pulmonary infections, pulmonary embolization, and GI disease (e.g. pancreatic disease, esophageal perforation).

The type of pleural effusion can be determined by a sample of pleural fluid obtained via thoracentesis (a procedure done to remove fluid from the pleural space). Exudates have a high protein content, and the fluid is generally dark yellow or amber. Transudates have a low protein content or contain no protein, and the fluid is clear or pale yellow. The fluid can also be analyzed for RBCs and WBCs, malignant cells, bacteria and glucose.

An empyema is a pleural effusion that contains pus. It is caused by conditions such as pneumonia, TB, lung abscess, and infection of surgical wounds of the chest. A complication of empyema is fibrothorax, in which there is fibrous fusion of the visceral and parietal pleurae.

Clinical Manifestations

Some symptoms are caused by the underlying disease. Pneumonia causes fever, chills and pleuritic chest pain. Malignant effusion may result in dyspnea and coughing. The size of effusion and the time course of development determine the severity of symptoms.

- Large effusion: Shortness of breath to acute respiratory distress
- Small to moderate effusion: Dyspnea may not be present
- Dullness of flatness to percussion over areas of fluid, minimal or absence of breath sounds, and tracheal deviation away from the affected side.

Common clinical manifestations of pleural effusion are progressive dyspnea and decreased movement of the chest wall on the affected side. There may be pleuritic pain from the underlying disease. Physical examination of the chest will indicate dullness to percussion and absent or decreased breath sounds over the affected area. The chest X-ray will indicate an abnormality if the effusion is greater than 250 mL. Manifestations of empyema include the manifestations of pleural effusion, as well as fever, night sweats, cough and weight loss. A thoracentesis reveals an exudates containing thick, purulent material.

If the cause of the pleural effusion is not known, a diagnostic thoracentesis is needed to obtain pleural fluid for analysis. If the degree of pleural effusion is severe enough to impair breathing, a therapeutic thoracentesis is done to improve breathing and to remove fluid for analysis.

Diagnostic studies will be:

- Chest X-ray (lateral decubitus)
- Chest CT scan
- Ultrasound
- Thoracentesis
- Pleural biopsy
- Pleural fluid analysis (culture, chemistry, cytology).

A thoracentesis is performed by having the patient sit on the edge of a bed and lean forward over a bedside table. The puncture site is determined by chest X-ray, and percussion of the chest is used to assess the maximum degree of dullness. The skin is cleaned with an antiseptic solution and anesthetized locally. The thoracentesis needle is inserted into the intercostal space. Fluid can be aspirated with a syringe, or tubing can be connected to allow fluid to drain into a sterile collecting bottle. After the fluid is removed, the needle is withdrawn, and a bandage is applied over the insertion site. Usually only 1,000 to 1,200 mL of pleural fluid are removed at one time. Because high volumes are removed, rapid removal can result in hypotension, hypoxemia, or pulmonary edema. A follow-up chest X-ray should be done to detect a possible pneumothorax that could have been induced by perforation of the visceral pleura. During and after the procedure, vital signs and pulse oximetry are monitored, and the patient should be observed for any manifestations of respiratory distress.

Management of Pleural Effusion

Objectives of treatment are to discover the underlying cause, prevent reaccumulation of fluid, and to relieve discomfort, dyspnea and respiratory compromise. Specific treatment is direct at the underlying cause.

- Thoracentesis is performed to remove fluid, collect specimen for analysis and relive dyspnea
- Chest tube and water-seal drainage may be necessary for drainage and lung re-expansion
- Chemical pleurodesis: Adhesion formation is promoted when drugs are instilled into the pleural space to obliterate the space and prevent further accumulation of fluid
- Other treatment modalities include surgical pleurectomy (insertion of a small catheter attached to a drainage bottle). Educate patient and family about management of catheter and drainage system with outpatient therapy.

The main goal of management of pleural effusions is to treat the underlying cause. For example, adequate treatment of HF with diuretics an sodium restriction will result in decreased pleural effusions. The treatment of pleural effusions secondary to malignant disease represents a more difficult problem. These types of pleural effusions are frequently recurrent and accumulate quickly after thoracentesis. Chemical pleurodesis may be used to sclerose the pleural space and prevent reaccumulation of effusion fluid. Although doxycycline (Vibramycin) and bleomycin (Blenoxane) have been used for sclerosing with good results, talc appears to be the most effective agent for pleurodesis.

Nursing Management

- Implement medical regimen: Prepare and position patient for thoracentesis and offer support throughout the procedure
- Assist patient in pain relief: Assist patient to assume positions that are least painful. Administer pain medication as prescribed and needed to continue frequent turning and ambulation
- Monitor chest tube drainage and water-seal system; record amount of drainage at prescribed intervals
- Administer nursing care related to the underlying cause of the pleural effusion.

Thoracoscopy can be used to perform talc pleurodesis after inspection of the pleural space. After instillation of the sclerosing agent, patients may be instructed to rotate their positions to spread the agent uniformly throughout the pleural space. The decision to rotate the patient from side to side to back depends on physician preference and the patients ability to tolerate turning. Chest tubes are left in place after pleurodesis until fluid drainage is less than 150 mL/day and no air leaks are noted. A more rapid completion of the pleurodesis procedure, in less than 24 hours, is reported in the literature with good results, and this limited admission for symptomatic malignant effusions may become more frequent.

Treatment of empyema is generally with chest tube drainage. Appropriate antibiotic therapy is also needed to eradicate the causative organism. A condition called trapped lung can occur with effusions and empyemas. This is a fibrous peel around the pleura that can cause serve pulmonary restriction. A decortication surgical procedure to remove the pleural peel may need to be performed.

The other conditions of lungs briefed here as pleurisy and atelectasis.

PLEURISY

Pleurisy refers to inflammation of both the visceral and parietal pleurae. When inflamed, pleural membranes rub together. The result is severe, sharp, knifelike pain with breathing that is intensified on inspiration. Pleurisy may develop with pneumonia or upper respiratory tract infection, tuberculosis, or a collagen disease; after chest trauma, pulmonary infarction, or embolism in primary and metastatic cancer; and after thoracotomy.

Clinical Manifestations

- Pain usually occurs on one side and worsens with deep breaths, coughing, or sneezing
- Pain is decreased when the breath is held. Pain is localized or radiates to the shoulder or abdomen
- As pleural fluid develops, pain lessen. A friction rub can be auscultated but disappears as fluid accumulates.

Assessment and Diagnostic Methods

- Auscultation for pleural friction rub
- Chest X-rays
- Sputum culture
- Thoracentesis, pleural fluid examination, pleural biopsy (less common).

Medical Management

Objectives of management are to discover the underlying condition causing the pleurisy and to relieve the pain.

- Patient is monitored for signs and symptoms of pleural effusion: shortness of breath, pain and decreased excursion of the chest
- Prescribed analgesics, such as nonsteroidal anti-inflammatory drugs (NSAIDs), are given to relive pain and allow effective coughing
- Applications of heat or cold are provided for symptomatic relief
- A procaine intercostal nerve block is done for severe pain.

Nursing Management

- Enhance comfort by turning patient frequently on affected side to splint chest wall
- Teach patient to use hands to splint rib cage while coughing
- Position patient to decrease pain.

Pleurisy (pleuritis) is an inflammation of the pleura. The most common causes are pneumonia, TB, chest trauma, pulmonary infarctions and neoplasms. The inflammation usually subsides with adequate treatment of the primary disease. The pain of pleurisy is typically abrupt and sharp in onset and is aggravated by inspiration. The patients breathing is shallow and rapid to avoid unnecessary movement of the pleura and chest wall. A pleural friction rub may occur, which is the sound over areas where inflamed visceral pleura and parietal pleura rub over one another during inspiration. This sound is usually loudest at peak inspiration but can be heard during exhalation as well.

Treatment of pleurisy is aimed at treating the underlying disease and providing pain relief. Taking analgesics and lying on or splinting the affected side may provide some relief. The patient should be taught to splint the rib cage when coughing. Intercostal nerve blocks may be done if the pain is severe.

Atelectasis is a condition of the lungs characterized by collapsed, airless alveoli. The most common cause of atelectasis is airway obstruction that results from retained exudates and secretions. This is frequently observed in the postoperative patient. Normally the pores of Kohn provide for collateral passage of air from one alveolus to another. Deep inspiration is necessary to open the pores effectively. For this reason, deep-breathing exercises are important in preventing atelectasis in the high-risk patient (e.g. postoperative, immobilized patient).

INTERSTITIAL LUNG DISEASES

Many acute and chronic lung disorders with variables degrees of pulmonary inflammation and fibrosis are collectively referred to as interstitial lung diseases (ILD) or diffuse parenchymal lung diseases. ILDs have been difficult to classify because more than 200 known diseases have diffuse lung involvement. The lung involvement may occur either from the primary condition or as a significant part of a multiorgan process, as may occur in connective tissue disorders (e.g. systemic lupus erythematosus, rheumatoid arthritis).

Among the ILDs of known cause, the largest group comprises occupational and environmental exposures, especially the inhalation of dusts and various fumes or gases. The most common ILDs of unknown etiology are idiopathic pulmonary fibrosis and sarcoidosis.

i. *Idiopathic pulmonary fibrosis (IPF)* is characterized by scare tissue in the connective tissue of the lungs as a sequela to inflammation or irritation. A common risk factor for IPF is environmental or occupational inhalation of organic and inorganic substances. Other risk factors include cigarette smoking and history of chronic aspiration. There also may be genetic risk factors.

   Clinical manifestations of IPF include exertional dyspnea, non-productive cough, and inspirational crackles with or without clubbing. Chest X-ray shows changes characteristic of IPF. High-resolution CT scan is the most definitive diagnostic study. Pulmonary function tests show a typical pattern characteristic of restrictive lung disease. Open lung biopsy using VATs may help to differentiate the specific pathology.

   The clinical course is variable and the prognosis poor, with a 5-year survival rate of 30 to 50 percent after diagnosis. Treatment includes corticosteroids, cytotoxic agents (azathioprine [imuran], cyclophosphamide [cytoxan]), and antifibrotic agents (colchicines). However, there is no good evidence that any of these treatments improves survival or quality of life. Lung transplantation is an option that should be considered for those who meet the criteria. (Lung transplantation is discussed later in this chapter).

ii. *Sarcoidosis* is a chronic, multisystem granulomatous disease of unknown cause that primarily affects the lungs. The disease may also involve the skin, eyes, liver, kidney, heart and lymph nodes. It is seen worldwide, can be familial, and is 3 to 4 times more common among African Americans. The lifetime risk of sarcoidosis in African Americans in the United States is 2.4%, compared to a risk of 0.85% for whites. Spontaneous resolution of the disease is common, but progressive and disabling organ failure can occur in up to 10% of patients The disease is often acute or subacute and self-limiting, but in other patients it is chronic, with remissions and exacerbations.

   Marked pulmonary fibrosis can be present with severe restrictive lung disease. Cor pulmonale (right-sided heart failure) and bronchiectasis can develop in the advanced stages. Corticosteroids are the most commonly used agents for the treatment of pulmonary sarcoidosis. A trial of methotrexate may be considered if the patient does not respond to or cannot tolerate corticosteroid therapy. If this is ineffective or not tolerated, cyclophosphamide (cytoxam) or azathioprine (imuran) may be initiated. Nonsteroidal anti-inflammatory agents, such as ibuprofen (Motrin), may help decrease acute inflammation or relieve symptoms but are not a treatment of sarcoidosis. Disease progression is monitored by pulmonary function tests, chest X-ray, and CT scan.

VASCULAR LUNG DISORDERS

Pulmonary edema is an abnormal accumulation of fluid in the alveoli and interstitial spaces of the lungs. It is a complication of various heart and lung, diseases. It is considered a medical emergency and may be life threatening.

Causes of Pulmonary Edema

- Heart failure
- Over hydration with intravenous fluids
- Hypoalbuminemia: Nephritic syndrome, hepatic disease, nutritional disorders
- Altered capillary permeability of lungs: Inhaled toxins, inflammation (e.g. pneumonia), severe hypoxia, near-drowning
- Malignancies of the lymph system
- Respiratory distress syndrome (e.g. O_2 toxicity)
- Unknown causes: Neurogenic condition, opioid overdose, re-expansion pulmonary edema, high altitude.

Normally, there is a balance between the hydrostatic and colloidal oncotic pressure in the pulmonary capillaries. If the hydrostatic pressure increases or the colloidal oncotic pressure decreases, the net effect will be fluid leaving the pulmonary capillaries and entering the interstitial space. This stage is referred to as interstitial edema. At this stage, the lymphatics can usually drain away the excess fluid. If fluid continues to leak from the pulmonary capillaries, it will enter the alveoli. This stage is referred to as alveolar edema. Pulmonary edema interferes with gas exchange by causing an alteration in the diffusing pathway between the alveoli and the pulmonary capillaries. The most common cause of pulmonary edema is left-sided HF.

PULMONARY EMBOLISM

Pulmonary hypertension is a condition that is not clinically evident until late in the disease. The systolic pulmonary artery pressure exceeds 30 mm Hg, and the mean pulmonary artery pressure is higher than 25 mm Hg at rest or 30 mm Hg with activity. There are two forms—primary (idiopathic) and secondary. Primary pulmonary hypertension is uncommon; diagnosis made by exclusion. The exact cause is unknown. The clinic presentation exists with no evidence of pulmonary and cardiac disease or pulmonary embolism. It occurs most often in women between ages 20 and 40 and is usually fatal within 5 years of diagnosis. Secondary pulmonary hypertension is more common and results from existing cardiac or pulmonary disease. The prognosis depends on the severity of the underlying disorder and the changes in the pulmonary vascular bed.

Pulmonary embolism (PE) is the blockage of pulmonary arteries by a thrombus, fat or air embolus or tumor tissue. The word embolus derives from a Greek word meaning "plug" or "stopper". A pulmonary embolus consists of material that gains access to the venous system and then to the pulmonary circulation. The material eventually reaches a section of the pulmonary arterial vessels, where it lodges, thus obstructing perfusion (Fig. 9.23).

Most pulmonary emboli arise from thrombi in the deep veins of the legs. Other sites of origin include the right side of the heart (especially with a trial fibrillation), the upper extremities (rare), and the pelvic veins (especially after surgery or childbirth). Lethal pulmonary emboli most commonly originate in the femoral or iliac veins. Embolic are mobile clots that generally do not stop moving until they lodge at a narrowed part of the circulatory system. The lungs are an ideal location for emboli to lodge because of their extensive arterial and capillary network.

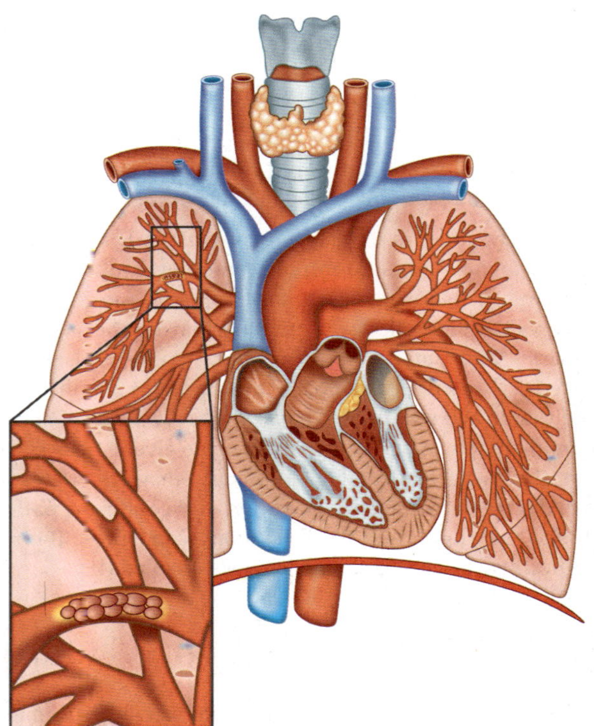

FIG. 9.23: Pulmonary embolism

The lower lobes are most frequently affected because they have a higher blood flow than the other lobes.

Thrombi in the deep veins can dislodge spontaneously. However, a more common mechanism is jarring of the thrombus by mechanical forces, such as sudden standing, and by changes in the rate of blood flow, such as those that occur with the valsalva maneuver. The majority of patients with PE due to deep vein thrombosis (DVT) have no leg symptoms at the time of diagnosis.

In addition to dislodged thrombi, less common causes of PE include fat emboli (from fractured long bones), air emboli (from improperly administered IV therapy), bacterial vegetations, amniotic fluid and tumors. Tumor emboli may originate from primary or metastatic malignancies.

The most common risk factors for PE are immobilization, surgery within the last 3 months, stroke, history of DVT and malignancy. The Nurse's Health Study reported an increased risk of PE in women associated with obesity, heavy cigarette smoking and hypertension. More than 95% of pulmonary emboli arise from thrombi in the deep veins of the lower extremity. Generally, the DVTs that are below the knee have not been considered a risk factor for PE since they rarely migrate to the pulmonary circulation without first extending above the knee. Upper extremity DVT occasionally occurs in the presence of central venous catheters or cardiac pacing wires. These cases may resolve with removal of the catheter. The highest rate of DVT is seen in spinal cord injury patients.

Clinical Manifestations

The signs and symptoms of PE are generally subtle and nonspecific, making diagnosis difficult. The classic triad of dyspnea, chest pain, and hemoptysis occurs in only about 20% of patients. The most common manifestations of PE are anxiety and the sudden onset of unexplained dyspnea, tachypnea, or tachycardia. A mild to moderate hypoxemia with a low $PaCO_2$ is a common finding. Other manifestations are cough, pleuritic chest pain, hemoptysis, crackles, fever, accentuation of the pulmonic heart sound, and sudden change in mental status as a result of hypoxemia.

Massive emboli may produce sudden collapse of the patient with shock, pallor, severe dyspnea, hypoxemia, and crushing chest pain. However, some patients with massive PE do not have pain. The pulse is rapid and weak, the BP is low, and ECG indicates right ventricular strain. When rapid obstruction of 50% or more of the pulmonary vascular bed occurs, acute cor pulmonale may result because the right ventricle can no longer pump blood into the lungs. The mortality rate of persons with massive PE and shock is approximately 33%.

Medium-sized emboli often cause pleuritic chest pain, dyspnea, slight fever and a productive cough with blood-streaked sputum. A physical examination may reveal tachycardia and a pleural friction rub. Small emboli frequently are undetected or produce vague, transient symptoms. The exception to this is the patient with underlying cardiopulmonary disease, in whom even small- or medium-sized emboli may result in severe cardiopulmonary compromise. However, repeated small emboli gradually cause a reduction in the capillary bed and eventual pulmonary hypertension. An ECG and chest X-ray may indicate right ventricular hypertrophy secondary to pulmonary hypertension.

Complications

Pulmonary infarction (death of lung tissue) is most likely when the following factors are present: (1) occlusion of a large or medium-sized pulmonary vessel (>2 mm in diameter), (2) insufficient collateral blood flow from the bronchial circulation, or (3) pre-existing lung disease. Infarction results in alveolar necrosis and hemorrhage. Occasionally the infracted tissue becomes infected, and an abscess may develop. Concomitant pleural effusion is frequently found.

Pulmonary hypertension occurs when more than 50% of the area of the normal pulmonary bed is compromised. Pulmonary hypertension also results from hypoxemia. As a single event, an embolus does not cause pulmonary hypertension unless it is massive. However, recurrent small- to medium-sized emboli may result in chronic pulmonary hypertension. Pulmonary hypertension eventually results in dilation and hypertrophy of the right ventricle. Depending on the degree of pulmonary hypertension and its rate of development, outcomes can vary, with some patients dying within months of the diagnosis and others living for decades.

Diagnostic Test

A ventilation-perfusion lung scan is the most frequently used test to aid in the diagnosis of PE. The lung scan has two components and is most accurate when both are performed:

1. Perfusion scanning involves IV injection of a radioisotope. A scanning device detects the adequacy of the pulmonary circulation.
2. Ventilation scanning involves inhalation of a radioactive gas such as xenon. Scanning reflects the distribution of gas through the lung. The ventilation component requires the cooperation of the patient and may be impossible to perform in the critically ill patient, particularly if the patient is intubated.

D-dimer testing may be recommended when a PE is initially suspected. D-dimer is a degradation product rarely found in healthy individuals. However, levels of D-dimer are elevated in any condition involving degradation of fibrin (infection, cancer, surgery, heart failure). They are elevated 8 times higher in venous thromboembolism. When D-dimer levels are normal (< 250 mcg/L), it is highly unlikely that the patient has a PE. Thus a normal or near-normal D-dimer level can rule out a PE. In the event that the D-dimer levels are elevated, a noninvasive venous study is indicated to look for a DVT as the likely source of a PE. If a DVT is located by venous ultrasound, the index of suspicion for PE is very high and anticoagulant treatment should be initiated immediately. Patients with an elevated D-dimer level but normal venous ultrasound need a lung scan or spiral CT scan.

If the lung scan is inconclusive, pulmonary angiography is recommended. Pulmonary angiography is an invasive procedure that involves the insertion of a catheter through the antecubital or femoral vein, advancement to the pulmonary artery, and injection of contrast medium. This allows visualization of the pulmonary vascular system and location of the embolus.

The use of computed tomography (CT) has revolutionized the diagnosis of PE. A spiral (or helical) CT scan, a noninvasive diagnostic test, may also be used to diagnose PE. Conventional CT scans rotate a frame 360 degrees in one direction, stop, make an image (called a slice), and then spin back in the opposite direction to make another slice after again stopping. The spiral CT scan is able to continuously rotate while obtaining slices and does not have to start and stop between each slice. This allows visualization of entire anatomic regions such as the lungs. The data can be computer reconstructed to allow for a three-dimensional picture of the area being imaged and assist in emboli visualization.

ABG analysis is important, but not diagnostic. The PaO_2 is low because of inadequate oxygenations secondary to an occluded pulmonary vasculature. The $PaCO_2$ is usually low because of hyperventilation. The pH remains normal unless respiratory alkalosis develops as a result of prolonged hyperventilation or to compensate for lactic acidosis caused by shock. Abnormal findings are usually reported on the chest X-ray (atelectasis, pleural effusion) and the ECG (ST segment and T wave changes), but they are not diagnostic for PE. Serum troponin levels are elevated in 30 to 50% of patients with PE, and, although not diagnostic, they are predictive of an adverse prognosis. Serum b-type natriuretic peptide (BNP) levels, while not diagnostic, may be helpful in identifying the severity of the clinical course (Box 9.12).

Box 9.12 Pulmonary embolism

Signs and symptoms	Sudden-onset dyspnea, tachypnea Tachycardia Hemoptysis Crackles History of blood clot
Diagnostic tests	D-dimer CT scan Ventilation-perfusion lung scan Angiogram
Therapeutic measures	Thrombolytic therapy Anticoagulants Oxygen
Complication	Pulmonary hypertension

Management of Pulmonary Emboli

When the diagnosis of PE has been made, treatment should be instituted immediately. The objectives of treatment are to (1) prevent further growth or multiplication of thrombi in the lower extremities, (2) prevent embolization from the upper or lower extremities to the pulmonary vascular system, and (3) provide cardiopulmonary support if indicated.

Conservative Therapy

Supportive therapy for the patients cardiopulmonary status varies according to the severity of the PE. The administration of supplemental O_2 by mask or cannula may be adequate for some patients. Oxygen is given in a concentration determined by ABG analysis. In some situations, endotracheal intubation and mechanical ventilation may be needed to maintain adequate oxygenation. Respiratory measures such as turning, coughing and deep breathing are necessary to prevent or treat atelectasis. If symptoms of shock are present, vasopressor agents may be necessary to support the systemic circulation. If heart failure is present, diuretics are used. Pain resulting from pleural irritation or reduced coronary blood flow is treated with opioids, usually morphine.

Drug Therapy

Properly managed anticoagulant therapy is effective in the treatment of many patients with PE. Although unfractionated heparin has been traditionally used for PE, low-molecular-weight heparin (e.g. enoxaparin [Levenox]) is becoming more commonly used in the treatment of PE. Warfarin (Coumadin) should be initiated within the first 24 hours and is typically administered for 3 to 6 months. Factor Xa inhibitors and direct thrombin inhibitors are also being used in the treatment of PE.

The dosage of heparin is adjusted according to the activated partial thromboplastin time (apt), while warfarin dose is determined by the international normalized ration (INR). Frequent changes and titrations of heparin doses are needed initially in order to obtain a therapeutic apt level. The heparin works to prevent future clots, but does not dissolve existing clots. Anticoagulant therapy may be contraindicated if the patient has blood dyscrasias, hepatic dysfunction causing alteration in the clotting mechanism, injury to the intestine, overt bleeding, a history of hemorrhage stroke, or neurologic conditions.

Fibrinolytic agents, such as tissue plasminogen activator (tPA) or alteplase (activase), dissolve the pulmonary embolus and the source of the thrombus in the pelvis or deep leg veins, thereby decreasing the likelihood of recurrent emboli. Indications for thrombolytic therapy in PE include hemodynamic instability and right ventricular dysfunction.

Surgical Therapy

If the degree of pulmonary arterial obstruction is severe and the patient does not respond to conservative therapy, an immediate embolectomy may be indicated. Pulmonary embolectomy, a rare procedure, has a 50% mortality rate. Preoperative pulmonary angiography is necessary to identify and locate the site of the embolus. When a pulmonary embolectomy is performed, the patient also has placement of a vena cava filter.

To prevent further pulmonary embolization, an inferior vena cava (IVC) filter may be warranted. This device prevents migration of large clots into the pulmonary system, is easily and safely placed percutaneously, is biocompatible, and does not require the patient be anticoagulated. It can be used for patients who have an absolute contraindication to anticoagulant therapy. In addition, it may be used as a prophylactic measure for patients at high risk of PE (e.g. those with spinal cord injury or cor pulmonale). The complications associated with this device are rare and include misplacement, migration and perforation. The spinal cord injury patient with an IVC filter cannot have assisted cough (quad cough) to mobilize secretions since the quad cough procedure can displace the filter.

Nursing Interventions (Also see Table 9.5)

Nursing measures aimed at prevention of PE parallel those for prophylaxis of deep vein thrombosis.

Acute intervention: The prognosis of a patient with PE is good if therapy is promptly instituted. The patient should be kept on bed rest in a semi-Fowler's position to facilitate breathing. An IV line should be maintained for medications and fluid therapy. The nurse should know the side effects of medications and observe for them. Oxygen therapy should be administered as ordered. Careful monitoring of vital signs, cardiac dysrhythmia monitoring, pulse oximetry, ABGs, and lung sounds is critical to assess the patients status. Laboratory results are monitored to assure normal ranges of aPPT and INR. Nursing care includes assessing for the complications of anticoagulant therapy (e.g. bleeding, hematomas, bruising) and PE (e.g. atelectasis, pneumonia). The nursing care plan includes interventions related to immobility and fall precautions.

The patient is usually anxious because of pain, sense of doom, inability to breathe and fear of death. The nurse carefully explains the situation and provide emotional support and reassurance to help relieve the patients anxiety.

The patient affected by thromboembolic processes may require psychologic and emotional support. In addition to the thromboembolic problems, the patient may have an underlying chronic illness requiring long-term treatment. To provide supportive therapy, the nurse must understand and differentiate between the various problems caused by the underlying disease and those related to thromboembolic disease. Patient teaching regarding long-term anticoagulant therapy is critical. The anticoagulant therapy continues for at least 3 to 6 months; patients with recurrent emboli are treated indefinitely. Warfairn blood levels are initially drawn monthly, and patients may have follow-up appointments at a nurse-managed anticoagulation clinic to monitor their medication and adjust dosages.

Long-term management is similar to that for the patient with DVT. Discharge planning is aimed at limiting progression of the condition and preventing complications and recurrence. The nurse must reinforce the need for the patient to return to the health care provider for regular follow-up examination.

PULMONARY HYPERTENSION

Pulmonary hypertension is a condition that is not clinically evident until late in the disease. The systolic pulmonary arteria pressure exceeds 30 mm Hg, and the mean pulmonary artery pressure is higher than 25 mm Hg at rest or 30 mm Hg with activity. There are two forms: primary (idiopathic) and secondary. Primary pulmonary hypertension is uncommon; diagnosis made by exclusion. the exact cause is unknown. The clinical presentation exists with no evidence of pulmonary and cardiac disease or pulmonary embolism. It occurs most often in women between ages 20 and 40 and is usually fatal wit in 5 years of diagnosis. Secondary pulmonary hypertension is more common and results from existing cardiac or pulmonary disease. The prognosis depends on the severity of the underlying disorder and the changes in the pulmonary vascular bed.

Pulmonary hypertension is elevated pressures resulting from an increase in pulmonary vascular resistance to blood flow. The disease commonly presents with shortness of breath and fatigue. Pulmonary hypertension can occur as a primary disease (primary pulmonary hypertension) or as a secondary complication of a respiratory, cardiac, autoimmune, hepatic, or connective tissue disorder (secondary pulmonary hypertension).

Primary Pulmonary Hypertension

Primary pulmonary hypertension (PPH) is a severe and progressive disease. PPH is characterized by mean pulmonary arterial pressure greater than 30 mm Hg with exercise in the absence of a demonstrable cause. Until the last decade, this disorder was rapidly progressive with right-sided heart failure and death. The median survival if untreated was 2.8 years. Epoprostenol (Flolan) therapy, introduced in the 1990s, greatly survival rates. Unfortunately, the disease remains incurable despite these advances.

Etiology

The exact etiology of PPH is unknown. It is rare and potentially fatal disease. PPH has been linked to the use of fenfluramine in the drug Fen-Phen, which was used as an appetite suppressant to treat obesity. The drug was withdrawn from the market in 1996. PPH affects more women than men; the mean age at diagnosis is 36 years old. It may have a genetic component as the incidence is higher in families.

Pathophysiology

A common cause is pulmonary artery constriction due to hypoxia from chronic obstructive pulmonary disease (COPD). When the pulmonary vascular bed is destroyed or obstructed its ability to handle the blood volume received is impaired. The increased blood flow increases the pulmonary artery pressure and pulmonary vascular resistance and pressure (hypertension).

Normally the pulmonary circulation is characterized by low resistance and low pressure. In pulmonary hypertension, the pulmonary pressures are elevated. Until recently the pathophysiology of PPH was poorly understood. Recently it was discovered that a key mechanism involved in PPH is a deficient release of vasodilator mediators from the pulmonary epithelium, with a resultant cascade of injury. Vasoconstriction, remodeling of the walls of the pulmonary vessels, and thrombosis in situ are the three elements that combine to cause the increased vascular resistance. The remodeling process is a complex set of events involving endothelial cell injury that results in intimal/medial wall thickening.

Clinical Manifestations

- Dyspnea, the main symptom, is noticed first with exertion and then at rest
- Substernal chest pain is common (25–50% of patients)
- Weakness, fatigability, syncope and occasional hemoptysis may occur
- Signs of right-sided heart failure (peripheral edema, ascites, distended neck veins, liver engorgement, crackles, heart murmur) are noted
- Electrocardiogram (ECG) changes (right ventricular hypertrophy) are seen, with right axis deviation and tall, peaked P waves in inferior leads and tall anterior R waves and ST-segment depression or T-wave inversion anteriorly. PaO_2 is decreased (hypoxemia).

Classic symptoms of pulmonary hypertension are dyspnea on exertion and fatigue. Exertional chest pain, dizziness and exertional syncope are other symptoms. These symptoms are related to the inability of cardiac output to increase in response to increased oxygen demand. Eventually, as the disease progresses, dyspnea occurs at rest. Pulmonary hypertension increases the workload of the right ventricle and causes right ventricular hypertrophy (a condition called cor pulmonale) and eventually heart failure. A chest X-ray generally shows enlarged central pulmonary arteries and clear lung fields. An enlarged right heart may be seen. Echocardiogram usually reveals right ventricular hypertrophy. The mean time between onset of symptoms and the diagnosis is 2 years. By the time patients become symptomatic, the disease is already in the advanced stages and the pulmonary artery pressure is 2 to 3 times normal.

Management of Primary Pulmonary Hypertension

The PPH is a diagnosis of exclusion. All other conditions must be ruled out. Diagnostic evaluation includes ECG, chest X-ray, pulmonary function tests, echocardiogram, and spiral CT. Cardiac catheterization is done to measure pulmonary artery pressure, cardiac output and left ventricular filling pressure. Early recognition of pulmonary hypertension is essential to interrupt the vicious cycle responsible for the progression of the disease.

Medical Management

Objective of treatment is to manage the underlying cardiac pulmonary condition. In all cases, management includes continuous oxygen therapy for progressive disease to decrease vasoconstriction and reduce pulmonary hypertension.

Treatment when hypertension results from cor pulmonale including:

- Fluid restriction
- Cardiac glycosides (digitalis)
- Calcium channel blockers for vasodilation
- Rest
- Diuretics to decrease fluid accumulation.

Treatment when hypertension results from primary pulmonary hypertension includes:

- Vasodilators (calcium channel blockers, intravenous prostacyclin); also bosentan, an endothelin receptor antagonist
- Anticoagulants (warfarin [Coumadin])
- Heart-lung transplantation when not responsive to other therapies.

Nursing Management

- Identify patients at high risk for developing pulmonary hypertension (i.e. those with COPD, pulmonary emboli congenital heart disease, and mitral value disease)
- Be alert for signs and symptoms
- Administer prescribed oxygen therapy appropriately
- Inform and instruct patient and family about home oxygen supplementation.

Although there is no cure of PPH treatment can relieve symptoms, increase quality of life and prolong life. Diuretic therapy relieves dyspnea and peripheral edema and may be useful in reducing right ventricular volume overload. Anticoagulation therapy is recommended for patients with severe pulmonary hypertension to prevent in situ thrombus formation and venous thrombosis. Warfarin is given to keep the INR in the 2 to 3 range. Hypoxia is a potent pulmonary vasoconstrictor and use of low-flow oxygen provides symptomatic relief. The goal is to keep oxygen saturation at ≥ 90%.

Vasodilator therapy is used to reduce right ventricular overload by dilating pulmonary vessels and reversing remodeling. Some patients with pulmonary hypertension can be effectively managed with calcium channel blocker therapy, such as sustained-release nifedipine (Procardia) or diltiazem (Cardizem).

Epoprostenol (Flolan) has revolutionized the management of PPH. It is a prostacyclin that promotes pulmonary vasodilation and reduces pulmonary vascular resistance. Continuous epoprostenol has been shown to result in significant improvement in clinical symptoms and long-term survival. It is now the treatment of choice for selected patients who are unresponsive to calcium channel blockers. Its administration requires the placement of an indwelling central line catheter and continuous infusion pump. The patient and the family must be trained to use the portable intravenous infusion pump, mix medications, manage the central line and monitor for complication. The half-life of the drug is less than 6 minutes. If the central line is disrupted, stopped or dislodged for any reason, clinical deterioration from abrupt withdrawal of epoprostenol can occur. This is a serious event with potential rebound pulmonary hypertension and clinical deterioration developing within minutes. The patient will have signs and symptoms of right-sided heart failure, including dyspnea, cyanosis, cough, syncope and weakness. If the patient loses significant weight, the dosage, which is weight based, may become excessive. Symptoms of over-dose include flushing, hypotension and tachycardia. The major problems have been infectious related to vascular access and broken central lines.

Epoprostenol has been successful in improving the quality of life of patients with PPH. The drug was developed as a bridge to lung transplantation but is now a standard of care. Although the patient and family teaching is extensive, the patient on continuous epoprostenol therapy can be successfully managed with an interdisciplinary health care team.

Treprostinil (Remodulin), a prostacyclin, is used a continuous subcutaneous injection. It causes vasodilation of the pulmonary arterial system and inhibits platelet aggregation. The subcutaneous route had drawbacks, including needles that could dislodge and infusion site pain and reactions. The drug has recently been approved for continuous intravenous use. This drug is stable at room temperature and has a longer half-life than epoprostenol. It may be a reasonable alternative to epoprostenol for some patients.

Bosentan (Tracleer), a form of prostacyclin, is the only oral vasodilator currently approved for the treatment of pulmonary hypertension. It is an active endothelin receptor antagonist and works by blocking the hormone endothelin, which antagonist and works by blocking the hormone endothelin, which causes blood vessels to constrict. Monthly liver function tests are needed since there is a risk of hepatotoxicity. Sildenafil (Revatio) is an oral phosphodiesterase inhibitor that prolongs the vasodilatory effect of nitric oxide and appears to be as effective in decreasing pulmonary vascular resistance. It should not be taken by patients using nitrates because severe hypotension may develop. Iloprost (Ventavis) is in inhaled form of prostacyclin in an aerosolized preparation. It is taken 6 to 9 times a day using a disk inserted into a nebulizer. Because of the risk of orthostatic hypotension, iloprost should not be taken by patients with low systolic blood pressure (<85 mm Hg). Beraprost (an oral formulation of prostacyclin) is undergoing clinical trials for the treatment of early-stage pulmonary hypertension.

Surgical interventions for pulmonary hypertension include atrial septostomy (AS), pulmonary thromboendarterectomy (PTE), and lung transplantation. AS involves the creation of an intra-atrial right-to-left shunt to decompress the right ventricle. It is indicated for a select group of patients awaiting lung transplantation. PTE may provide a potential cure for those patients suffering from chronic thromboembolic pulmonary hypertension. It is only recommended for patients with operable sites where the emboli can be surgically removed by embolectomy.

Lung transplantation has been the mainstay of treatment for pulmonary hypertension for those patients who do not respond to drug therapy and progress to severe right-sided heart failure. Recurrence of the disease has not been reported in individuals who have undergone transplantation. A patient education and support website for pulmonary hypertension is located.

Secondary Pulmonary Hypertension

Secondary pulmonary hypertension (SPH) occurs when a primary disease causes a chronic increase in pulmonary artery pressures. Secondary pulmonary hypertension can develop as a result of parenchymal lung disease, left ventricular dysfunction, intracardiac shunts, chronic pulmonary thromboembolism, or systemic connective tissue disease. The specific primary disease pathology can result in anatomic or vascular changes causing the pulmonary hypertension. Anatomic changes causing the increased pulmonary vascular resistance include (1) loss of capillaries as a result of alveolar wall damage (e.g. COPD), (2) stiffening of the pulmonary vasculature (e.g. pulmonary fibrosis connective tissue disorders), and (3) obstruction of blood flow (chronic emboli).

Vasomotor increases in pulmonary vascular resistance are found in conditions characterized by alveolar hypoxia. Hypoxia causes localized vasoconstriction and shunting of blood away from poorly ventilated alveoli. Alveolar hypoxia can be caused by a wide variety of conditions. It is possible to have a combination of both anatomic changes and vasomotor constriction. This is found in the patient with long-standing chronic bronchitis who has chronic hypoxia in addition to loss of lung tissue.

The symptoms can reflect the underlying disease, but some are directly attributable to SPH, including dyspnea, fatigue, lethargy and chest pain. The initial physical findings can include right ventricular hypertrophy and signs of right ventricular failure (increased pulmonic heart sound, right-sided fourth heart sound, peripheral edema, hepatomegaly). Diagnosis of SPH is similar to that of PPH. Treatment of SPH consists mainly of treating the underlying primary disorder. When irreversible pulmonary vascular damage has occurred, therapies used for PPH are initiated. The efficacy of treatment for pulmonary hypertension has been primarily evaluated for PPH, and there are limited data on the effectiveness of these therapies for SPH. Epoprostenol is used in the management of SPH. More studies are ongoing into effective therapies for SPH.

COR PULMONALE (RIGHT HEART FAILURE)

Cor pulmonale is a condition in which the right ventricle enlarged (with or without right heart failure), as a result, affects the structure or function of the lung or its vasculature. A mean pulmonary artery pressure of 45 mm Hg or more may occur. The most frequent cause is chronic obstructive pulmonary disease (COPD). Other causes are conditions that restrict or compromise ventilatory function (massive obesity, deformities of the thoracic cage) or that reduce the pulmonary vascular bed (pulmonary embolus), causing primary pulmonary hypertension. Certain disorders of the nervous system, respiratory muscles, chest wall, and pulmonary arterial tree may also be responsible for cor pulmonale. Prognosis depends on reversing the hypertensive process.

Cor pulmonale is enlargement of the right ventricle secondary to diseases of the lung, thorax or pulmonary circulation. Pulmonary hypertension is usually a pre-existing condition in the individual with cor pulmonale. Cor pulmonale may be present with or without overt cardiac failure. The most common cause of cor pulmonale is COPD. Almost any disorder that effects the respiratory system can cause cor pulmonale.

Clinical Manifestations

Symptoms are usually those of the underlying lung disease:

- Clinical features include COPD, shortness of breath and cough
- Right ventricular failure develops (edema of the feet and legs, distended neck veins, enlarged palpable liver, pleural effusion, ascites and a heart murmur)
- Headache, confusion and somnolence from carbon dioxide narcosis may occur.

Clinical manifestations of cor pulmonale include dyspnea, chronic productive cough, wheezing respirations, retrosternal or sub-sternal pain, and fatigue. Chronic hypoxemia leads to polycythemia and increased total blood volume and viscosity of the blood (polycythemia is often present in cor pulmonale secondary to COPD). Compensatory mechanisms that are secondary to hypoxemia can aggravate the pulmonary hypertension. Episodes of cor pulmonale in a person with underlying chronic respiratory problems are frequently triggered by an acute respiratory tract infection.

Management

Objectives of treatment are to improve ventilation and to treat both the underlying lung disease and the manifestations of heart disease.

- Oxygen is given to reduce pulmonary arterial pressure and pulmonary vascular resistance. Continuous (24-h/day) oxygen therapy is provided for severe hypoxia
- Blood oxygen levels are assessed with pulse oximetry and arterial blood gas (ABG) analysis
- Bronchial hygiene, bronchodilators and chest physical therapy may be instituted
- If respiratory failure occurs, intubation and mechanical ventilation may be necessary
- If heart failure occurs, hypoxemia and hypercapnia must be relieved to improve cardiac output
- Peripheral edema and circulatory load on the right side of the heart are reduced with bed rest, sodium restriction, and diuretics
- If indicated (e.g. in left ventricular failure), digitalis may be given
- The electrocardiogram (ECG) is monitored
- Pulmonary infections must be treated promptly (it will exacerbate hypoxemia and cor pulmonale).

The primary management of cor pulmonale is directed at treating the underlying pulmonary problem that precipitated the heart problem. Long-term low-flow O_2 therapy is used to correct the hypoxemia and reduce vasoconstriction in chronic states of respiratory disorders. If fluid, electrolyte and acid-base imbalances present, they must be corrected. Diuretics and a low-sodium diet will help decrease the plasma volume and the load on the heart. Bronchodilator therapy is indicated if the underlying respiratory problem is due to an obstructive disorder. Digoxin use is controversial. However, studies have confirmed a modest effect of digoxin on the failing right ventricle in chronic cor pulmonale. Other treatments include those for pulmonary hypertension, such as vasodilator therapy, calcium channel blockers and anticoagulants. Theophylline may help due to its weak inotropic effect on the heart. When medical treatment fails, lung transplantation is an option for some patients.

Chronic management of cor pulmonale resulting from COPD is similar to that described for COPD. Continuous low-flow O_2 during sleep, exercise, and small, frequent meals may allow the patient to feel better and be more active.

Nursing Management

See Nursing Management of Heart Failure for additional information

- If required, assist with intubation and mechanical ventilation. Support patient physically and emotionally
- Assess respiratory and cardiac status
- Instruct patient about the importance of close monitoring and adherence to the therapeutic regimen, especially oxygen
- Explore and address factors that affect the patient's adherence to the treatment regimen
- Advise patient and family that management is long-term and that most care and monitoring will be performed at home for this chronic disorder
- Advise patient to avoid activities that irritate airway if COPD exists
- Administer continuous oxygen and instruct how to use
- Urge patient to stop smoking, if appropriate; refer patient to smoking cessation or community support group
- Counsel patient about nutrition if a sodium-restricted diet or a diuretic medication is part of treatment
- If patient's physical condition warrants close assessment or if patient cannot manage self-care, refer the patient for home care.

If the patient has coincident left ventricular failure, supraventricular dysrhythmia, or right ventricular failure and is not responsive to other therapy administer digitalis, if prescribed, with extreme caution because pulmonary heart disease appears to enhance susceptibility to digitalis toxicity.

LUNG TRANSPLANTATION

Lung transplantation has become an important mode of therapy for patients with a variety of end-stage lung diseases. A variety of pulmonary disorders are potentially treatable with some type of lung transplantation. Improved patient selection criteria, technical advances, and better methods of immunosuppression have resulted in improved survival rates. Four types of transplant procedures are available: single-lung transplantation, bilateral lung transplantation, heart-lung transplantation, and transplantation of lobes from a living related donor.

Indications for Lung Transplantation

- α1-antitrypsin deficiency
- Bronchiectasis
- Cystic fibrosis
- Emphysema
- Idiopathic pulmonary fibrosis
- Interstitial lung disease
- Pulmonary fibrosis secondary to other diseases (e.g. sarcoidosis)
- Pulmonary hypertension.

Single-lung transplantation involves an incision on the side of the chest. The opposite lung is ventilated while the diseased lung is excised. The lung is removed and the donor lung implanted. Three anastomoses are done: the bronchus, pulmonary artery, and pulmonary veins. In a bilateral lung transplantation, the incision is made across the sternum and the donor lungs are implanted separately. A median sternotomy incision is used for a heart-lung transplant procedure. Chest tubes are placed around the donor lungs to help them re-expand with air. Lobar transplantation from living donors is reserved for candidates who urgently need transplantation and are unlikely to survive until a donor becomes available. The majority of these transplant recipients are patients with cystic fibrosis, and their parents or relatives are donors.

Patients being considered for lung transplantation need to undergo extensive evaluation. The candidate for lung transplantation should not have a malignancy or recent history of malignancy (within the last 2 years), renal or liver insufficiency, or HIV. Typically patients wait an average of 12 to 18 months for a donor lung.

The candidate and the family undergo psychologic screening to determine the ability to cope with a postoperative regimen that requires strict adherence to immunosuppressive therapy, continuous monitoring for early signs of infection, and prompt reporting of manifestations of infection for medical evaluation. Many transplant centers require preoperative outpatient pulmonary rehabilitation to maximize physical conditioning.

Early postoperative care includes ventilatory support, fluid and hemodynamic management, immunosuppression, detection of early rejection and prevention or treatment of infection. Pulmonary clearance measures, including aerosolized bronchodilators, chest physiotherapy, and deep-breathing and coughing techniques, minimize potential complications. Maintenance of fluid balance is vital in the postoperative phase.

Lung transplant recipients are at high risk for bacterial, viral, fungal, and protozoal infections. Infections are the leading cause of death in the early period after the transplant. Gram-negative bacterial pneumonia is common. Among potential causes of viral infections, cytomegalovirus (CMV) is the most important in lung transplantation patients, usually seen 4 to 8 weeks postoperatively. Clinical manifestations of CMV infection include fever, bone marrow suppression, hepatitis, enteritis and pneumonitis. *Aspergillus* is the most common fungal infection.

Immunosuppressive therapy usually includes a three-drug regimen of cyclosporine or tacrolimus, azathioprine (Imuran) or mycophenolate mofetil (CellCept), and prednisone. However, because of an array of potential adverse effects and drug interactions, there are limitations to immunosuppressive therapy. Drug levels are monitored on a regular basis. Lung transplant recipients are usually maintained on higher levels of immunosuppressive therapy than other organ recipients.

Acute rejection is fairly common in lung transplantation and can be seen as soon as 5 to 7 days after surgery. It is characterized by low-grade fever, fatigue, and oxygen desaturation with exercise. Accurate diagnosis is by transtracheal biopsy. Treatment is high doses of corticosteroids administered IV for 3 days. In patients with persistent or recurrent acute rejection, other strategies may include antilymphocyte antibodies or changing maintenance immunosuppressive drugs.

Bronchiolitis obliterans (an obstructive airway disease causing progressive occlusion) is thought to be a manifestation of chronic rejection in lung transplant patients. The onset is often subacute, with gradual onset of progressive obstructive airflow defect, including cough, dyspnea and recurrent lower respiratory tract infection. Treatment involves optimum maintenance immunosuppression.

Discharge planning begins in the preoperative phase. Prior to discharge, the patient needs to be able to perform self-care activities, including medication management and activities of daily living, and to accurately identify when to call the transplant team physician. Patients are placed in an outpatient rehabilitation program to improve physical endurance. Home spirometry has been useful in monitoring trends in lung function. Patients are taught to keep medication logs, laboratory results and spirometry records. The average lung transplant patient takes 13 medications (range, 5 to 24) a day. After discharge, the patients are followed by the transplant team for transplant-related issues. The patients return to their primary care team for their health maintenance and routine illnesses. As transplant procedures become more frequent, transplant patients will return to hospitals for other routine procedures. Coordination of care between the transplant team, primary care team, and inpatient teams is essential for ongoing successful management of these patients.

PULMONARY CONTUSION

A penetrating injury may cause contusion of the lung or pleura. Pulmonary contusion usually results from sudden compression followed by rapid compression of the thoracic cavity, causing blood to extravasate into pulmonary tissue.

The contusion is usually self-limiting because the pulmonary vasculature is a low-pressure system. However, extensive contusion can precipitate pulmonary edema with resultant hypoxemia, hypercapnea, and respiratory acidosis.

Clinical Manifestation

Pulmonary contusion may vary from total absence of symptoms to the full spectrum of symptoms associated with non-cardiogenic pulmonary edema. Signs and symptoms (some of which may be delayed) include the following:

- Increasing dyspnea
- Tachypnea
- Increasing restlessness
- Crackles notes on auscultations
- Hemoptysis.

Management

Medical treatment of pulmonary contusion depends on the severity of the injury. Treatment may vary from outpatient monitoring to intubation and mechanical ventilating support when pulmonary edema present. The nursing care includes the following:

- Administer analgesic as ordered every 3 hours
- Monitor for fluid overload
  - Keep accurate records of all intake and output
  - Monitor vital signs every 30 minutes. Report increased pulse and respiration
  - Monitor breath sound every 30 minutes
- Monitor ventilating status
  - Check for signs of respiratory distress—dyspnea, increased inspiration, changes in breath sound
  - Check ABG results
- Monitor for sign of symptom of flail chest
- Support patient to stay in bed until physical status is stabilized
  - Stay with patient, listen to patient's concern, explain what is planned
  - Assist with ADL
- Teach patient/family how to support pulmonary contusion.

OBSTRUCTIVE LUNG DISEASES

Chronic obstructive pulmonary disease (COPD) is defined as a disease state characterized by airflow obstruction resulting from chronic bronchitis or emphysema. The airflow obstruction is generally progressive, may be accompanied by airway hyperactivity and may be partially reversible.

CHRONIC BRONCHITIS

Chronic bronchitis is defined by the presence of chronic productive cough for minimum of 3 months per year for at least 2 consecutive years in patients in whom other causes have been excluded, it is characterized by physiologically by hypertrophy and hypersecretion of the bronchial mucous glands and structural alterations of the bronchi and bronchioles.

Etiology

Chronic bronchitis is caused by the inhalation of physical or chemical irritants or by viral or bacterial infections. The most common inhaled irritant is cigarette smoke—heavy cigarette smoking.

Pathophysiology

In chronic bronchitis, there is pathologic changes in the lung consisting of:

- Hyperplasia of mucus secreting glands in the trachea and bronchi
- Increase in goblet cells
- Disappearance of cilia
- Chronic inflammatory charges and narrowing of small airways
- Altered functions of alveolar macrophages, leading to increased bronchial infections.

Frequently airways are colonized with microorganisms. Infection occurs when the organisms increase. Most common infecting agents are *S. pneumoniae* and *H. influenzae*. Excess amounts of mucus are found in the airways and sometimes may occlude small bronchioles and scarring the bronchiole wall may occur chronic inflammation in the primary pathologic mechanism involved in causing the changes characteristics of chronic bronchitis.

Clinical Manifestation

The earliest symptom in chronic bronchitis is usually a frequent, productive cough during most winter months. It is often exacerbated by respiratory irritants and cold, damp air. Bronchospasm can occur at the end of paroxysms of coughing. Frequent respiratory infections are other common manifestation. Somewhat later, dyspnea on exertion may develop. Unfortunately a patient often attributes chronic cough to smoking rather than lung disease, thus delaying initiation of treatment. In addition, the patient may not be aware of the cough because he/she becomes accustomed to it.

Hypoxemia and hypercapnea result from hypoventilation caused by increased airway resistance. The bluish red color of the skin results from polycythemia and cyanosis. Polycythemia develops as a result of increased production of red blood cells secondary to the body's attempt to compensate for chronic hypoxemia. Hemoglobin concentration may reach 200 g/L. Cyanosis develops when there is at least 5 g/dL or more of circulating unoxygenated hemoglobin.

The complication of chronic bronchitis are cor pulmonale, acute exacerbation of chronic bronchitis, and acute respiratory failure, peptic ulcer, and GERD, and pneumonia.

Management

Diagnostic studies of COPD include:

- Chest X-ray film, typical finding in chronic bronchitis and increased bronchovascular markings
- Sputum studies for culture and sensitivity. Neutrophils and bronchial epithelial cells usually occurs in chronic bronchitis
- ABG
- ECG
- Exercise testing with oximetry (if indicated)
- EEG or cardia nuclear scan (if indicated).

The primary goal of care for COPD patients are to:

- Improve ventilation
- Promote secretion removal

- Prevent complication and progression of symptoms
- Promote patient comfort and participation in care
- Improve quality of life as much as possible.

Main objectives of treatment are to keep the bronchial tubes open and functioning, facilitate removal of secretions, and prevent disability.

- Note changes in sputum (nature, color, amount, thickness) and in the cough pattern
- Treat recurrent bacterial infections with antibiotic therapy
- Facilitate removal of secretions (bronchodilators)
- Provide for postural drainage and chest percussion
- Give fluids orally or parenterally to liquefy secretions
- Use steroid therapy when conservative measures fail. Patient must stop smoking (causes bronchoconstriction)
- Counsel patient to avoid respiratory irritants (e.g. tobacco smoke).

Medical therapy of chronic bronchitis depends on symptoms. Pulmonary function tests results in ABG findings. Therapy may include all or some of the modalities outlined here:

i. Supportive measures:
   Education of patient and family about the following:
   - Avoidance of cigarette smoke
   - Avoidance of other inhaled irritants
   - Avoidance of persons with upper respiratory infections
   - Control of environmental temperature and humidity
   - Proper nutrition
   - Adequate hydration.
ii. Specific therapy: Medication such as
   - Bronchiodilator-α antitrypsin replacement for those with ↓ levels
   - Antimicrobials—ampicillin or another broad-spectrum antibiotic
   - Corticosteroids—to alleviate acute symptoms e.g. prednisone
   - Digitalis—to treat LVF if present.
iii. Respiratory therapy in aerosol therapy used to deliver bronchiodilator, through metered cartridge device with spacer at rest.
   - Oxygen therapy for patients who are unable to maintain PaO_2.
iv. Relaxation exercises
   - Meditation for relax.
v. Breathing retraining.
vi. Rehabilitation.

EMPHYSEMA

Emphysema is defined pathologically by destructive changes in alveolar walls and enlargement of air spaces distal to the terminal non-respiratory bronchioles. It is characterized physiologically by increased lung compliance, decreased diffusing, capacity and increased airway resistance.

Pulmonary emphysema is defined as a nonuniform pattern of abnormal, permanent distension of the air spaces with destruction of the alveolar walls and eventually a reduced pulmonary capillary bed. It appears to be the end stage of a process that has progressed slowly for many years. Smoking is the major cause. In a few patients, there is a familial predisposition associated with a plasma protein abnormality (deficiency of alphal-1-antitrypsin), making the person sensitive to environmental factors (air pollution, infectious agents, allergens). Emphysema manifests commonly in the fifth decade of life and is classified as follows (Fig. 9.24):

- *Panlobular (panacinar):* Characterized by destruction of the respiratory bronchiole, alveolar duct, and alveoli; air spaces within the lobule are enlarged, with little inflammatory disease
- *Centrilobular (centriacinar):* Causes pathlogic changes in the center of the secondary lobule, producing chronic hypoxemia, hypercapina polycythemia, and episodes of right-sided heart failure.
- Both types of emphysema can occur together.

Etiology

The cause of emphysema is not known. However, evidence suggests that proteases released by polymorph nuclear leukocytes or alveolar macrophages are involved in the destruction of the connective tissue of the lungs. Cigarette smoking, infections, ambient air pollution and heredity (AAT-α, antitrypsin) are the other causes of emphysema.

Pathophysiology

Emphysema is a condition of the lungs characterized by abnormal permanent enlargement of the airspaces distal to the terminal bronchioles, accompanied by destruction of these walls and without obvious fibrosis. Structural changes include

- Hyperinflation of alveoli
- Destruction of alveolar walls
- Destruction of alveolar capillary walls
- Narrowed tortuous, small airways, and
- Loss of lung elasticity.

There are two types of emphysema centrilobular and panlobular. In centrilobular emphysema, the primary area involvement is the central part of the lobula. Respiratory bronchioles enlarge, the walls are destroyed, and the bronchioles become confluent, chronic bronchioles associate with centrilobular types.

Panlobular emphysema, involves distentions and destruction of the whole lobule. Respiratory bronchioles, alveolar ducts and sacs and alveoli are all affected. There is a progressive loss

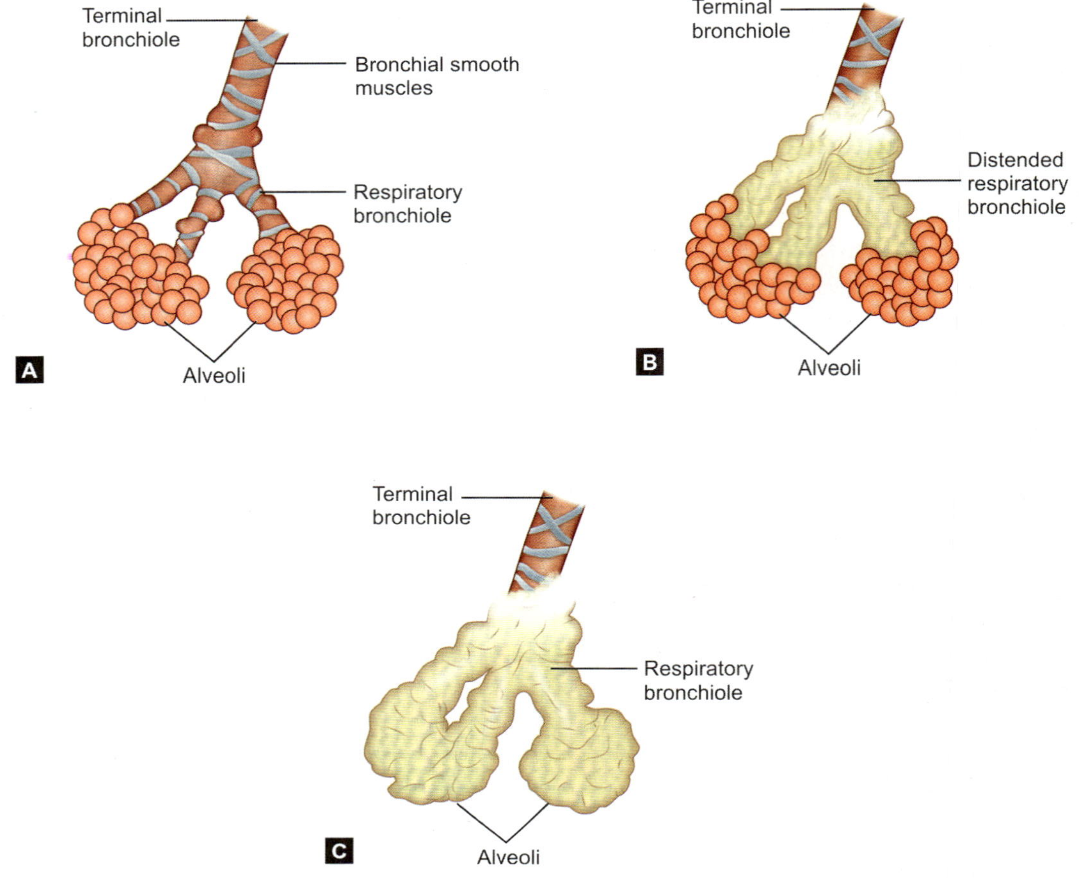

FIGS 9.24A TO C: Types of emphysema. (A) Normal lungs; (B) Centrilobular emphysema; (C) Panlobular emphysema

of lung tissue and decreased alveolar-capillary surface area. Severe panlobular emphysema/usually found in persons with AAT (alpha-antitrypsin) deficiency.

Clinical Manifestation

An early symptom of emphysema is dyspnea, which becomes progressively more severe. The patient will first complain of dyspnea on exertion that progresses to interfering with ADL to dyspnea at rest. Minimal coughing is present, with no sputum or smell amounts of mucoid sputum. As more alveoli becomes over distended increasing amount of air are trapped. This causes flattened diaphragm and an increased anteroposterior diameter of the chest, forming the typical barrel chest.

- Dyspnea with insidious onset progressing to severe dyspnea with slight exertion (major symptom)
- Chronic cough, sputum production, wheezing, dyspnea, fatigue, and tachypnea
- On inspection, hyperinflated "barrel chest" due to air trapping, muscle wasting and pursed-lip breathing
- On auscultation, diminished breath sounds with crackles, wheezes, rhonchi, and prolonged expiration
- Hyperresonance with percussion and a decrease in fremitus
- Anorexia, weight loss, weakness and inactivity
- Hypoxemia and hypercapnia, morning headaches in advanced stages
- Inflammatory reactions and infections from pooled secretions.

Effective abdominal breathing decreased. The person becomes more of chest breather, relying on the intercostal and accessory muscles. Hypoxemia may be present. The person is characteristically thin and underweight. The person may suffer from protein-caloric malnutrition. Later clubbing finger may develop. The complications as in chronic bronchitis.

Medical Management

The major goals of medical management are to improve quality of life, slow progression of the disease, and treat obstructed airways to relieve hypoxia. Treatment is directed at improving ventilation, decreasing work of breathing and preventing infection.

- Smoking cessation
- Physical therapy to conserve and increase pulmonary ventilation
- Maintenance of proper environmental conditions to facilitate breathing
- Psychological support
- Ongoing program of patient education of rehabilitation
- Bronchodilators and metered-dose inhalers (aerosol therapy dispensing particles in fine mist)
- Treatment of infection (antimicrobial therapy at the first sign of respiratory infection)
- Oxygenation in low concentrations for severe hypoxemia.

Management of emphysema is same as in chronic bronchitis. Nursing intervention for persons with chronic bronchitis and pulmonary emphysema are also the same, which include administration of medication such as digitalis and diuretics as prescribed, improving gas exchange, oxygen therapy, improving efficiency for breathing pattern (pursed lip-breathing, forward-leaving position, abdominal breathing and exercise, pulmonary physiotherapy, segmental postural drainage), improving airway clearance, improving nutrition, preventing infection, preventing fluid volume excess, assisting with breathing in rest, assisting with central of environment, and mounting temperature and humidity, etc.

And teach the following:

i. Progressive relaxation exercise.
   - Contract each muscle to a count of 10 and then relax it
   - Do exercises in quiet room while sitting or lying in a comfortable position
   - Do exercises for relaxing muscle, if desired
   - Have another person serve as a "coach" by giving command to contract specific muscles, count to 10 and relax muscle
   - The following are the examples of exercises helpful to some person with (COPD)
     - Raise shoulders, shrug them, and relax for 5 seconds, then relax them completely
     - Make a first of both hands. Squeeze them lightly for 5 seconds and relax them completely.

ii. Meditation exercises:
   - Sit or lie quietly with eyes closed and attempt to relax all muscles beginning with feet and moving upward
   - Breathe in through the nose slowly (may help to count slowly to 4 on inhalation) and exhale slowly through pursed lips (mentally count to 6) with a natural rhythm, relaxed and peaceful (this can be coached or performed without assistance)
   - Survey the body points of tension, consciously relax the tense areas. The body is peaceful and relaxed
   - Continue breathing as above. Aware of the feeling of well-being throughout your body. This can be used for 10 to 20 minutes or after 5 minutes go to step 5
   - Listen for (or visualize) a special relaxation sound (or image). Listen to it closely (or visualise) all the while breathing as above
   - At this point, positive suggestion can be used, for example, I am in control of my body. When I find myself getting tense, I can take moment to stop and breathe in all the air that I need and let the tension flow away
   - After mental suggestion, continue breathing easily and slowly come back to normal alert to mental state
   - Meditation can be used at any time to induce relaxed state of mind (e.g. to promote sleep)

   While taking care of the person with COPD, nurse has to take the following areas and should address in a typical teaching program for persons with chronic bronchitis or emphysema
     - Patients should be able to explain in lay terms, the basic functions and pathology of their lungs
     - Avoidance of respirative irritants and maintenance of a proper environment should be emphasised to people with COPD. Inhaled irritants (especially cigarette smoke) pose a serious threat to these persons. Steps the patient can take to reduce or avoid exposure to these irritants
       - Stop smoking. The nurse should be familiar with community programs and give a list of them to the patient, to involve in it
       - Ask other persons not to smoke in the patient's room. Inhalation of secondary smoke can exacerbate symptoms
       - Pay heed to announcement on radio and TV warning of pollution alert. Do not go outside during an alert
       - Use an air-conditioner or HEPA filter or electrostatic filter to remove particular matter from air
         - Keep filters clean and follow manufacturers' directions for use
         - Use an activated charcoal filter if offending odors or gas pollutants are a problem
       - Avoid abrupt environmental temperature or humidity changes, because they can increase sputum production and cause bronchospasms
         - Use an airconditioner in hot weather
         - Use a face mask when going out in cold weather
         - Use a dehumidifier or humidifier as appropriate to maintain a humidity of 30 to 50 percent

  - If air travel is required, check with physician about need for suplemental oxygen
  - Avoid large growds, especially during known influenza
    - Avoid contact with people who have an upper respiratory infection
    - Receive influenza and pneumonia immunization

iii. The patient should be able to explain the following aspects of the home medication or treatment regimen
   - State name, dose, action and side effects of each infection
   - Explain how and where to use medication ordered on an as needed basis (e.g. bronchodilators, antibiotics, steroids, antacids)
   - Describe how to obtain and maintain any needed equipment or supplies (e.g. oxygen, nebulizers, humid fiers, aerosols IPPB machines and syringes medications)

iv. The patient should demonstrate how to carry out the specific home exercise program:
   - Specific exercises to be completed
   - Frequency of exercise
   - Monitor physical response to exercises, such as heart rate increase, increase respiratory rate, or perceived fatigue

v. The patient should be able to list the names and telephone numbers of the appropriate support services.

See Nursing Management under Chronic Obstructive Pulmonary Disease for additional information.

ASTHMA

Asthma is an inflammatory disease characterized by hyper-responsiveness of the airways and periods of bronchospasm, resulting in intermittent airway obstruction. The onset of asthma is sudden, contrary to the slow, insidious progression of symptoms seen in chronic bronchitis and emphysema.

Asthma is a chronic inflammatory disease of the airways characterized by hyperresponsiveness, mucosal edema and mucus production. Inflammation leads to obstruction from mucosal edema, reducing airway diameter, and contraction of bronchial smooth muscle. Acute exacerbations last from minutes to hours to days, and are interspersed with symptom-free periods.

Asthma can begin at any age. It is the most common chronic disease of childhood. Risk factors for asthma include family history, allergy (strongest factor), and chronic exposure to airway irritants or allergens (e.g. grass, weed pollens, mold dust or animals). Common triggers for asthma symptoms and exacerbations include airway irritants (e.g. pollutants, cold, heat, strong odors, smoke, perfumes), exertion, stress, sinusitis, and esophageal reflux.

Etiology

Asthma is caused by increased responsiveness of the trachea and bronchi to various stimuli that cause narrowing of the airways and difficulty in breathing. The common factors triggering an asthma attack include:

- Environmental factors
  - Change in temperature especially cold air and
  - Change in humidity; dry air
- Atmospheric pollutants
  - Cigarette and industrial smoke, ozone, sulfur dioxide, formaldehyde
  - Exhaust fumes, oxidants, aerosol sprays
- Strong odors, perfumes
- Allergen inhalation.
  - Feathers, animal danders, dust mites molds allergens
  - Foods treated with sulfites, beer, wine fruit juices, snack foods salads, potatoes, shellfish, fresh and dried fruits) and metabisulfites, bisulfites, tartrazine
- Exercise and cold, dry air
- Stress or emotional upset
- Infection: Vital upper respiratory infection, sinusitis
- Medications: Aspirin and NSAIDs, β-blockers (including eyedrops of glaucoma)
- Enzymes: Including those in laundry detergents
- Occupational exposure: Metal salts, wood and vegetable dust, industrial chemicals and plastics
- Chemicals, toluene and others used in solvents, paints, rubber and plastics
- Hormones, menses
- Gastroesophageal reflex (GER).

Pathophysiology

The mechanism that induces asthma remains unknown. There are two types of asthma. Extrinsic (atopic) and intrinsic (non-atopic).

Extrinsic asthma results from an inflammatory response of the airway caused by mast cell activation, eosinophil infiltration, and epithelial slughing. An attack is triggered by environmental allergen (dust, pollen, molos, animal dander and foods). An initial encounter with an allergen stimulates plasma cells to produce antigen-specific IgE, antibodies that bind mast cells in airways. When exposed to the allergen IgE antigen binding causes mast cell deregulation and release of inflammatory mediators. The result is an intense inflammatory response in the airways.

Intrinsic asthma occurs in adults 35 years of age in older, the asthma attack is often severe. Factors that precipitate attacks include respiratoy tract infections, drugs (aspirin, β-adrenergic antogonism), environmental irritants, (occupational chemicals) air pollutions, cold, dry, air, exercise and emotional stress.

Chemical mediator, interacts with the autonomic nervous systems causing inflammation and bronchoconstriction.

An asthmatic attack results from several physiological alterations, include altered immunological response increased airway resistance, increased lung compliance, impaired mucociliary function and altered carbon dioxide exchange.

The primary pathophysiologic process in asthma is chronic inflammation, which leads to airway hyperresponsiveness (hyperreactivity) and acute airflow limitation. Exposure to allergens or irritants initiates the inflammatory cascade. A variety of inflammatory cells are involved in asthma. Examples of inflammatory cells in asthma are mast cells, macrophages, eosinophils, neutrophils, T and B lymphocytes, and epithelial cells of the airways.

As the inflammatory process begins, mast cells (found beneath the basement membrane of the bronchial wall) degranulate and release multiple inflammatory mediators (Fig. 9.25). Common inflammatory mediators are leukotrienes, histamine, cytokines (e.g. interleukins 4 and 5), prostaglandin's, and nitric oxide. Some inflammatory mediators have effects on the blood vessels, causing vasodilation and increasing capillary permeability. Some mediators result in the airways being infiltrated by eosinophils, lymphocytes, and neutrophils. The resulting inflammatory process results in vascular congestion; edema formation; production of thick, tenacious mucus; bronchial muscle spasm; thickening of airway walls; and increased bronchial hyperresponsiveness (Fig. 9.26). This whole process is sometimes referred to as the *early-phase response* in asthma. Clinically it can occur within 30 to 60 minutes after exposure to the allergen or irritant.

Symptoms can recur 4 to 10 hours after the initial attack because of eosinophil and lymphocyte activation and further release of more inflammatory mediators. The epithelial cells also produce cytokines and other inflammatory mediators. This delayed response is called the *late-phase response* in asthma. Only about 30 to 50 percent of patients experience this delayed response. It can be more severe than the early-phase response and persist for 24 hours or more. It is characterized by a self-sustaining cycle of inflammation. Airflow may be limited from the swelling of the airways with or without bronchoconstriction. Corticosteroids are effective in treating this inflammation.

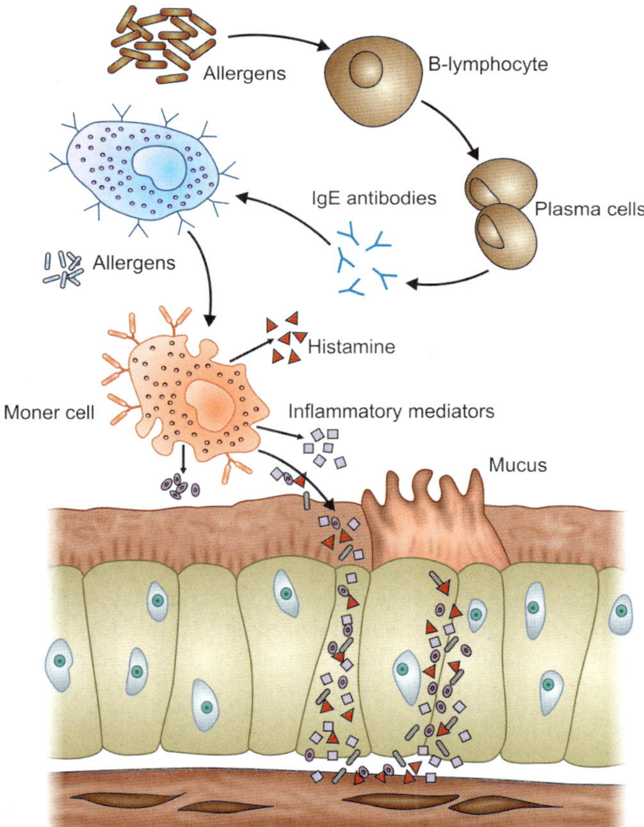

FIG. 9.25: Allergic asthma is triggered when an allergen cross-links IgE receptors on mast cells, which are then activated to release histamine and other inflammatory mediators (early-phase response). A late-phase response may occur due to further inflammation

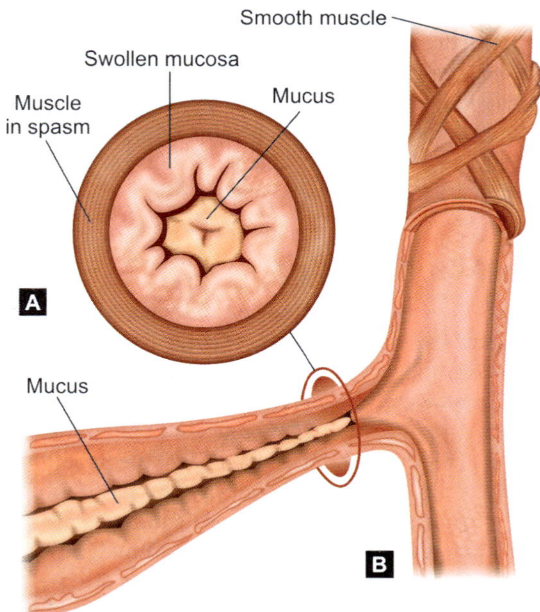

FIGS 9.26A AND B: Factors causing obstruction (especially expiratory obstruction) in asthma. (A) Cross-section of a bronchiole occluded by muscle spasm, swollen mucosa, and mucus in the lumen; (B) Longitudinal section of a bronchiole

Untreated inflammation can lead to long-term damage that is irreversible. Chronic inflammation resulting in structural changes in the bronchial wall is known as remodeling. The bronchial smooth muscle hypertrophies and collagen is deposited in the airway walls. The mechanisms responsible for remodeling are thought to be related to chronic or recurrent inflammation of the airways. The combination of damage to the epithelium of the airways, prolonged repair of the epithelium, fibrosis and increased types of fibroblasts are central to remodeling. The airway smooth muscles hypertrophy and mucus-secreting cells undergo hyperplasia in remodeling. There is some evidence that remodeling can occur even in mild asthma of recent onset, but it can be prevented by early introduction of inhaled corticosteroids.

Hyperventilation occurs during an asthma attack as lung receptors respond to increased lung volume from trapped air and airflow limitation. Decreased perfusion and ventilation of the alveoli and increased alveolar gas pressure lead to ventilation-perfusion abnormalities in the lungs. The patient will be hypoxemia early on with decreased $PaCO_2$ and increased pH (respiratory alkalosis) as he or she is hyperventilating. As the airflow limitation worsens with air trapping, the patient works much harder to breathe. The $PaCO_2$ will normalize as the patient tires, and then it will rise to produce respiratory acidosis, which is an ominous sign signifying respiratory failure.

Alterations in the neural control of the airways also occur in asthma. The automatic nervous system, consisting of the parasympathetic and sympathetic systems, innervates the bronchi. Airway smooth muscle tone is regulated by the parasympathetic nervous system via the vagus nerve. Afferent and efferent impulses are conducted through the vagus nerve to the medulla and back to the lungs. When airway nerve endings are stimulated by mechanical or chemical stimuli (e.g. air pollution, cold air, dust, allergens), increased release of acetylcholine causes bronchoconstriction.

Clinical Manifestation

Asthma is characterized by an unpredictable and variable course. It causes recurrent episodes of wheezing, breathlessness, chest tightness, and cough, particularly at night and in the early morning. An attack of asthma may have an abrupt onset or it may be more gradual. Attacks often occur at night may last for a few minutes to several hours. In between, the patient may be asymptomatic with normal and abnormal pulmonary function. However, in some persons, compromised pulmonary functions may result in a state of continuous asthma and chronic debilitation characterized by irreversible airway disease.

The characteristic clinical manifestation of asthma are wheezing cough, dyspnea, and chest tightness after exposed to a precipitating factor or trigger. Expiration may be prolonged.

- Most common symptoms of asthma are cough (with or without mucus production), dyspnea, and wheezing (first on expiration, then possibly during inspiration as well)
- Asthma attacks frequently occur at night or in the early morning
- An asthma exacerbation is frequently preceded by increasing symptoms over days, but it may begin abruptly
- Chest tightness and dyspnea occur
- Expiration requires effort and becomes prolonged
- As exacerbation progresses, central cyanosis secondary to sever hypoxia may occur
- Additional symptoms, such as diaphoresis, tachycardia, and a widened pulse pressure, may occur
- A severe, continuous reaction, status asthmaticus, may occur. It is life-threatening
- Eczema, urticarial and temporary edema are allergic reactions that may be noted with asthma.

Instead of normal inspiratory-expiratory ratio of 1:2 it will be prolonged to 1:3 or 1:4. Normally, the bronchioles constrict during expiration. However, as a result of bronchospasm, edema and mucus in the bronchioles, the airways become narrower than usual. This takes longer for the air to move out of the bronchioles. This produce the characteristic wheezing, air trapping and hyperinflation.

The normal $PaCO_2$ during an asthma attack may be a signal of impending respiratory failure.

The signs and symptoms associated with asthma are correlated with normal lung functions and underlying pathophysiological origins (see etiology). The character of asthmatic attacks can vary on a continuum from chronic or acute mild intermittent attacks to life-threatening status asthmaticus. Severe acute asthma can result in complication such as rib fractures, pneumothorax, pneumomediastinum, atelectasis, pneumonia and *status asthmaticus.*

Status asthmaticus is a severe, life-threatening asthma attack that is refractory to usual treatment and places the patient at risk for developing respiratory failure. The causes of which include viral illnesses, ingestion of aspirin or other NSAIDs, emotional stress, increase in environmental pollutants or other allergen exposure, abrupt discontinuation of aerosal medication and ingestion of beta adrenergic blocking agent. In this exhaustion, diminished breath sounds, intubation and mechanical ventilation, complications of status asthmaticus include pneumothorax, pneumomediastenum, acute cor pulmonale with RVF and severe respiratory muscle fatigue leading to respiratory arrest. Death from status asthmaticus is usually the result of respiratory arrest or cardiac failure (Box 9.13).

Management

For diagnosis of asthma

- Family, environment and occupational history is essential
- During acute episodes, sputum and blood test, pulse oximetry, arterial blood gases (ABGs), and hypocapnia and respiratory alkalosis and pulmonary function (FEV and FVC decreased) tests are performed.

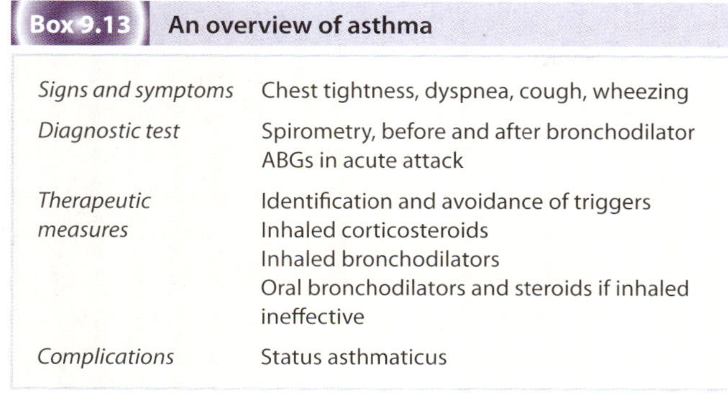

Box 9.13 An overview of asthma

Signs and symptoms	Chest tightness, dyspnea, cough, wheezing
Diagnostic test	Spirometry, before and after bronchodilator ABGs in acute attack
Therapeutic measures	Identification and avoidance of triggers Inhaled corticosteroids Inhaled bronchodilators Oral bronchodilators and steroids if inhaled ineffective
Complications	Status asthmaticus

The objective of medical management of asthma is to promote normal functioning of the individual, prevent recurrent symptoms, prevent severe attacks and prevent side effects of medication. The chief aim of various medication is to afford the patient immediate, progressive ongoing bronchial relaxation.

Medical Management

Pharmacologic Therapy

There are two classes of medications—long-acting control and quick-relief medications—as well as combination products.

- Leukotriene modifiers inhibitors/antileukotrienes block receptors to prevent bronchoconstriction
- Beta-adrenergic agonists
- Methylxanthines
- Anticholinergics
- Corticosteroids: Metered-dose inhaler (MDI)
- Mast cell inhibitors.

One approach to treat an acute asthmatic attack is as follows: Inhalation of beta-agonist such as albuterol sulfate (proventil, ventolin), salmeterol (Serevent), or metaproterenol sulfate in normal saline. Which stimulates beta 2-receptors in bronchial smooth muscle resulting in smooth muscle relaxation. It starts to act in 10 minutes, effects last 4–6 hours. Here, the nurse has to monitor vital signs, lung sounds, and peak expiratory flow rate (PEFR) before and after treatment. If this is not successful: Go for the following:

a. Methylprednisolone IV loading dose 2 mg/kg or about 125 mg 6th hours/then 60–125 mg 6th hourly for 48 hours total or until patient is stable, which reduces inflammation and edema of airway and decreases hyperactivity of airway. The benefits seen within 6 hours full effect in 6–8 hours.

   When patient is stabilized, change IV to 60 mg oral prednisolone by mouth daily or every other day. The oral prednisolone should be tapered off by 7–10 days, Taper 60 mg over 2 days, 40 mg over 2 days, 30 mg over 2 days and 10 mg over 2 days.

b. Nebulized atrophine sulfate may be tried, or aminophylline may be given IV a pump is used for better control of infusion... which relax bronchial smooth muscle.

Loading dose of aminophylline 4 to 6 mg/kg over 15 to 30 minutes and then continuous infusion of 0.45 to 0.70 mg/kg/h. Patients who have been taking aminophylline at home will be placed on continuous IV therapy. Rate of infusion is 10–20 mg/mL. Too rapid an infusion may cause severe hypotension, premature ventricular contractions, and cardiac arrest.

Here, the nurse has to monitor heart rate and rhythm closely, and report any change immediately to the concerned. Theophylline metabolized by the liver. For persons with liver disease, small doses are used. Patient taking cemitidene, erythromycin or ciprofloxacin require smaller doses. Smokers and those taking phenytoin require larger doses to maintain blood level.

Other common medications for asthma are as follows:

- NSAIDs such as cromolym, nedocromil, administered through metered dose inhaler (MDI) or nebulizer, decreases airway inflammation and irritation, headache, bad taste in mouth
- Corticosteroids (dexamethasone, triamcinolone acetonide, Flunisolide, fluticasone) administered through MDI has an anti-inflammatory action. Side effects are sore throat, hoarseness, cough, oral thrush
- Leukotriene inhibitors/receptor antagonists such as zafirlukast, zilenton, are anti-inflammatory used orally. Adverse efforts include headache, nausea, diarrhea, dizziness, myalgia, fever, dyspepsia, elevated glanine aminotransferase level
- Theophylline can be administered orally or parenterally. It is long acting, bronchiodilator. Side effects are nausea, vomiting, stomach cramps, diarrhea, headache, muscle cramps, tachycardia, irritability, restlessness, serum blood levels should be checked for therapeutic range
- Anticholinergics (spray) administered through MDI or nebulizer or nasal spray. It is short-acting bronchiodilator. Side effects are nervousness, dizziness, headache, palpations, blurred vision, nausea, GI distress and dry mouth
- Beta 2-agonist such as salmeterol administered through MDI. It is long-acting bronchiodilator; may lead to adverse effects—headache, tremor, tachycardia, palpations, nasopharyngitis, stomachache, cough, rash.

When administering the above drugs, nurse has to monitor the responses and side effects of the medication and act accordingly. And when using a metered-dose inhaler (MDI) the nurse has to teach the patient as follows (Figs 9.27 and 9.28):

- Inhale through nose, then slowly exhale
- Place inhaler 1 to 2 inches off the mouth
- Press down inhaler while simultaneously inhaling one puff deeply. Breath in air from around the mouth piece while inhaling
- Hold breath for 5 to 10 seconds to allow medication to reach lung
- Repeat second puff if one is ordered
- If any untoward effects, stop administering of MDI.

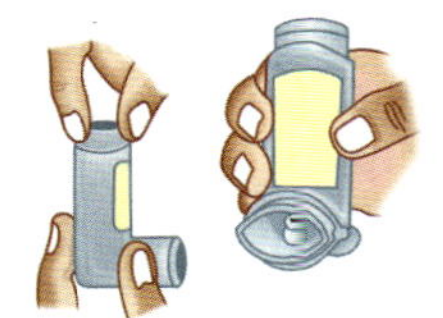

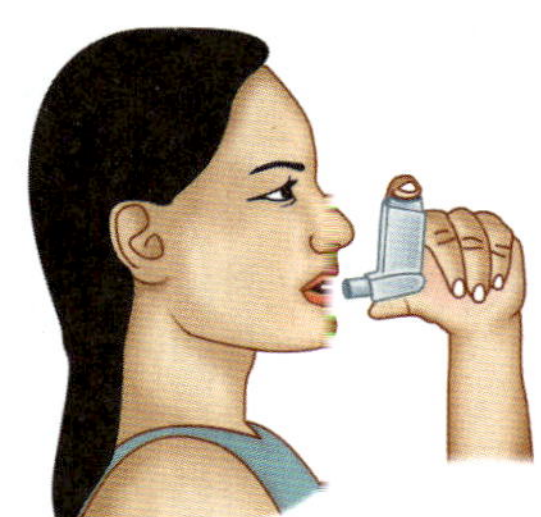

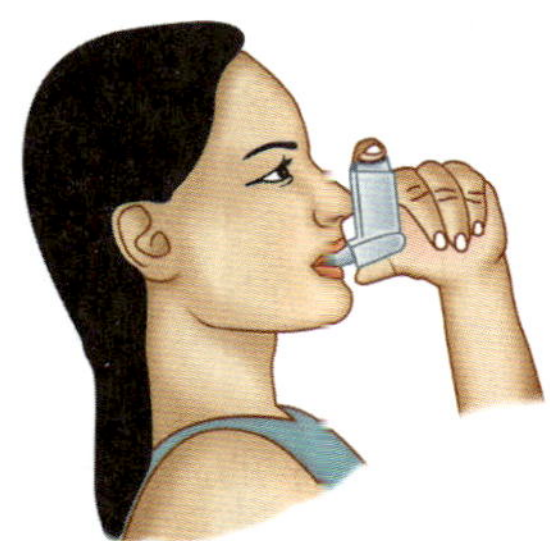

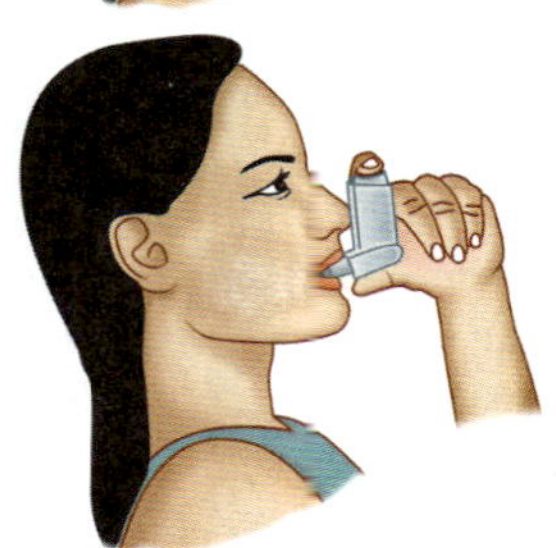

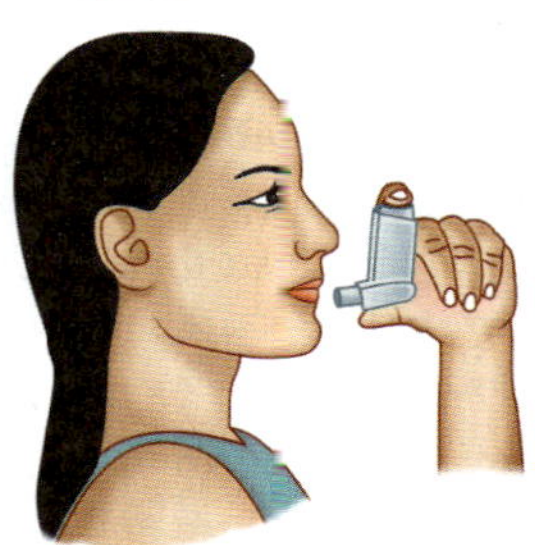

FIG. 9.27: Instructions for use of a metered-dose inhaler

Nursing Management

Assessment

- Evaluate and identify substances that precipitate attacks (obtain history of exacerbations, family, environment, health history)

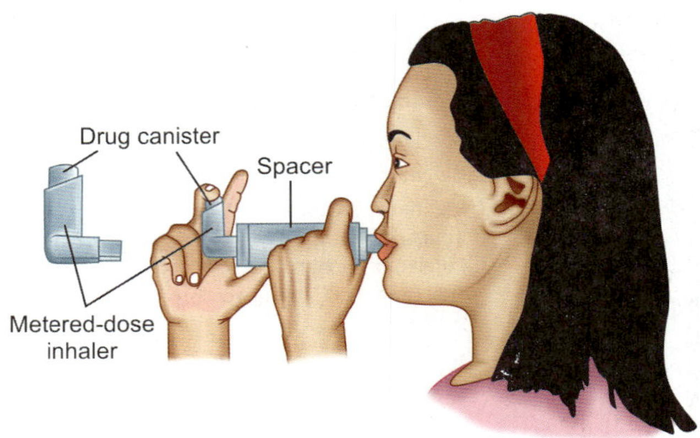

FIG. 9.28: Use of a spacer increase the amount of medication that gets to the lungs

- Monitor respiratory status for progression or resolution of asthma attack (e.g. breath sounds, pulse oximetry, vital signs, peak flow)—daily monitoring
- Obtain medical history and history of medication allergy.

Nursing Diagnoses

- Ineffective airway clearance related to airway constriction and execs mucus production
- Anxiety related to fear of death
- Risk for ineffective management of treatment regimen.

Nursing Interventions

Promoting Airway Clearance

- Administer prescribed therapy, and monitor patient responses
- Administer fluids and antibiotics (if infection present)
- Assist with intubation and respiratory support as needed.

Minimizing Anxiety

- Provide nursing care, using a calm approach
- Keep patient and family informed about procedures.

Teaching Patients Self-care

- Teach patient and family about asthma (chronic inflammatory), purpose and action of medications, triggers to avoid (e.g. exposure to offending pollens—stay in air-conditioned rooms during pollen season or, if feasible, change climate zone)
- Instruct patient and family about peak-flow monitoring

- Teach patient how to implement an action plan and how and when to seek assistance
- Emphasize adherence to prescribed therapy, preventive measure and need for follow-up appointments.

Continuing Care

- Refer for home health nurse as indicated
- Home visit to assess for allergens may be indicated (with recurrent exacerbations)
- Encourage patient to maintain good physical and mental health because attacks may be induced by suggestion alone
- Refer patient to community support groups.

Status asthmaticus is severe persistent asthma that is unresponsive to conventional therapy; it can last longer than 24 hours. Infection, anxiety, nebulizer abuse, dehydration, increased adrenergic block, and nonspecific irritants may contribute to these episodes. An acute episode may be precipitated by hypersensitivity to aspirin. Two predominant pathologic problems occur a decrease in bronchial diameter and a ventilation-perfusion abnormality. Symptoms are same as those in severe asthma.

- No correlation between severity of attack and number of wheezes; with greater obstruction, wheezing may disappear possibly signalling impending respiratory failure
- Initial treatment: Beta-adrenergic agonists, corticosteroids, supplemental oxygen and IV fluids to hydrate patient. Sedatives are contraindicated
- Start with low-flow humidified oxygen by mask or nasal catheter; flow rate determined by ABG values (PaO_2 65 to 85 mm Hg)
- Hospitalization if blood gas levels deteriorate or pulmonary function scores are low
- Mechanical ventilation if patient is tiring or in respiratory failure or if condition does not respond to treatment.

CYSTIC FIBROSIS

Cystic fibrosis is an autosomal recessive, multisystem disease characterized by altered function of the exocrine glands involving primarily the lungs, pancreas, and sweat glands. Abnormally thick, abundant secretions from mucus glands can lead to a chronic, diffuse, obstructive pulmonary disorder in almost all patients.

Etiology

Cystic fibrosis is an autosomal recessive disease resulting from mutations in a gene located on chromosome 7. The most common mutations in the CF gene is known as the CF transmembrane regulator (CFTR). The primary defect in the CF is abnormally regulated chloride channel activity. This defect alters ionic transport of sodium and chloride across epithelial surfaces. The high concentration of NaCl in the sweat of the patients with CF results from decreased chloride reabsorption in the sweat duct. The basic pathophysiologic mechanism is obstruction of exocrine gland duct with thick viscous secretions that adhere to the lumen of the ducts. The glands distal to the duct eventually undergo fibrosis.

Pathophysiology

Cystic fibrosis is an exocrine gland disease involving various systems, i.e. pulmonary, pancreatic/hepatic, GI, reproductive obstruction of the exocrine glands duct or passage ways occurs in nearly all adult patients with CF. Exocrine gland secretions are known to have a decreased water content, altered electrolyte concentration and abnormal organic constituents (especially no mucus glycoproteins), however, the specific biochemical or physiological defect that leads to obstruction is not known.

The following physiological alterations are found in adults with CF include:

- Pulmonary damage
- Gastrointestinal and pancreatic involvement
- Glucose intolerance.

Clinical Manifestations

The specific clinical manifestation by symptoms are:

- Pulmonary signs and symptoms of CF includes
  - Chronic productive cough and/or recurrent bronchitis or pneumonia
  - Crackles and rhonchi decreased pulmonary compliance, digital clubbing
  - Shortness of breath and dyspnea on exertion, wheezing, and weight loss occurs with respiratory complication and usually indicate need for vigorous therapy
- Gastrointestinal signs and symptoms include the following:
  - Frequent, bulky, greasy stools
  - Weight loss
  - Cramps and abdominal pain should arouse suspicion of obstruction
- Glucose intolerance signs and symptoms include:
  - Polyuria, polydipsia, polyphagia
  - Absence of ketoacidosis even with above signs.

Normally, mucus production by goblet cells lubricate airways and entraps foreign particles. In CF, excessive amounts of mucus production leads to increased cough and mucus production, inflammation of small airways causing hyperinflation of alveoli give rise to fatigue, shortness of breath, chronic bacterial infections leading to fever, fatigue, shortness of breath, and eroding of a major blood vessel and secondary infection may lead to hemoptysis.

Management

The goals of medical management of CF are to minimize bronchial plugging and to inhibit bacterial colonization. Measures to minimize bronchial plugging include:

- Chest physiotherapy with chest percussion and postural drainage are performed for 20 minutes two or three times daily and some time much more frequently
- Administer dornase-alfa 2.5 mg ampule in compressed air-driven nebulizer for reducing visco-elasticity of CF secretion
- Mucolytic agents may be ordered to thin secretions
- Humidification of air, according to some physicians
- Antibiotics for infection

  Nursing measures include preventing pulmonary infections, care of hemoptysis, care of pneumothorax and care of cor pulmonale diet, activity and regimen
- Prevention of pulmonary infection can be made best by:
  - Vigorous postural drainage and percussing
  - Room humidification if ordered
  - Aerosols with a bronchodilator, and
  - Monitoring for infection-and take suitable measure accordingly
- Nursing care and medical care during hemoptysis include:
  - Elevate head of bed 45 to 90 degrees
  - Turn patient's head to left side to facilitate expectoration of blood
  - Provide clean basin frequently so that patient is not made more anxious by amount of blood
  - Measure amount of hemoptysis and record time and amounts
  - Postural drainage and percussion are contraindicated if hemoptysis present
  - Vitamin K as ordered by mouth or subcutaneously to check bleeding
  - Stay with the patient until bleeding has subsided and made comfortable to less fearful
  - Bronchioscopy with endobronchial tamponade may be successful
- Care of pneumothorax includes proper care for chest tube connected to closed drainage system and other measure used in pneumothorax
- Care of cor pulmonale includes supplement oxygen, long-term diuretic therapy. Digoxin if or as ordered by the physician
- Promoting adequate nutrition-supplemental fat soluble vitamins and multivitamins and vitamin E. Pancreatin enzyme supplemented
- Patient should be encouraged to be upright position as a tolerated
- Patient and family educated about taking care of CF cases.

RESPIRATORY FAILURE

Acute respiratory failure (ARF) is used to describe any rapid change in respiration resulting in hypoxemia, hypercapnia, or both. ARF can be classified as hypoxemia or hypercapnia.

Hypoxemic respiratory failure is also related to an oxygenation failure, because the primary problem is inadequate O_2 transfer. This can be defined as a PaO_2 of 60 mm Hg or less when the patient is receiving an inspired O_2 concentration of 60 per cent or greater.

Hypercapnic respiratory failure is also referred to as ventilatory failure because the primary problem is insufficient CO_2 removal. It is defined as a $PaCO_2$ above normal (> 45 mm Hg) in combination with acedemia (pH < 7.35).

Etiology

Many disorders can lead to or associated with respiratory failure which can be divided into pulmonary and nonpulmonary diseases.

i. Pulmonary disorders
   - Severe infection
   - Pulmonary edema
   - Pulmonary embolus
   - COPD - Chronic obstructive pulmonary disease
   - CF - Cystic fibrosis
   - ARDS - Acute respiratory distress syndrome
   - Cancer
   - Chest trauma (flail chest)
   - Severe atelectasis
   - Airway compromise, secondary to trauma, infection or surgery.

ii. Non-pulmonary disorders
   - CNS disturbance secondary to drug overdose, anesthesia, head injury
   - Neuromuscular disorders, i.e. Guillain-Barré syndrome. Myasthenia gravis, multiple sclerosis, poliomyelitis, muscular disatrophy, spinal cord injury
   - Postoperative reduction in ventilation following thoracic and abdominal surgery
   - Prolonged mechanical ventilation.

Pathophysiology

The respiratory system is made up of two basic parts, the gas exchange organ (lung) and the pump (the respiratory muscles and the respiratory control mechanism). Any alteration in the function of gas exchange unit or pump can result in respiratory insufficiency or respiratory failure. Regardless of the underlying condition, the resultant events or processes that occur in respiratory failure are the same. With inadequate ventilation, the arterial oxygen falls and tissue cells become hypoxic. Carbon dioxide accumulates, leading to a fall in pH and respiratory acidosis.

Lung or gas exchange unit respiratory failure is usually seen in person with underlying primary pulmonary disease such as COPD. In this situation respiratory failure as a result of pathology directly affects the respiratory unit.

Pump failure is associated with extrapulmonary disorders that may precipitate respiratory failure. In this situation the underlying disorder decreases the ability of lungs to move oxygen and carbon dioxide into and out of the lungs by altering either the central ventilatory control mechanism (e.g. drug overdose) neuromuscular function (e.g. Gullain-Barré syndrome) or chest wall movement (flail chest).

Acute respiratory failure is defined by predetermined physiological criteria, i.e. sudden onset of the following.

- PaO_2 50 mm Hg or less (measured in room air)
- $PaCO_2$ 50 mm Hg or more
- pH 7.35 or less.

Clinical Manifestations

The sign and symptoms associated with hypercapnia, hypoxemia and respiratory acidosis are:

- Headache
- Irritability
- Increasing somnolence coma
- Asterixis (flapping tremor)
- Cardiac dysrhythmias
- Tachycardia
- Hypotension
- Cyanosis.

Management

The management of respiratory failure includes the following.

1. Medical therapy is based on degree of severity.
   - Severe acute respiratory failure, focus on immediate oxygenation and ventilation
   - Less severe acute respiratory failure: Underlying cause determined and treated concurrently while treating hypoxemia and hypercapnia.
2. Clinical evaluation
   a. Diagnosis studies include—ABGs, chest X-ray film, bedside pulmonary spirometry, sputum for culture and sensitivity
   b. Treatment includes
      - Oxygen therapy
      - Ventilation: May require intubation and mechanical ventilatory supports
      - Treatment of underlying causes.

Nursing care includes improving gas exchange, ventilatory support, mechanical ventilation, improving airway clearance, improving breathing pattern, improving cardiac output, maintaining adequate nutrition, health promotion and prevention.

ACUTE RESPIRATORY DISTRESS SYNDROME

Acute respiratory distress syndrome (ARDS; noncardiogenic pulmonary edema) is a clinical syndrome characterized by sudden and progressive edema, increasing bilateral infiltrates, reduced lung compliance, and hypoxemia refractory to oxygen supplementation. ARDS results from an inflammatory trigger that causes injury to the alveolar capillary membrane. People at risk for ARDS are those experiencing direct injury to the lungs (e.g. aspiration, smoke inhalation) or indirect insult to the lungs (e.g. shock). Death results mainly from multi-system organ failure with sepsis. The mortality rate of ARDS may be as high as 50 to 60 percent.

Clinical Manifestations

- Rapid onset of severe dyspnea, usually 12 to 48 hours after an initiating event
- Intercostal retractions and crackles
- Arterial hypoxemia not responsive to oxygen supplementation
- Labored breathing and tachypnea
- Based on clinical criteria; history of risk factors, acute onset of respiratory distress, bilateral pulmonary infiltrates, absence of left heart failure, and severe refractory hypoxemia ($PaO_2/FiO_2 < 200$ mm Hg)
- Chest X-ray shows bilateral infiltrates and pulmonary edema.

Medical Management

- Identify and treat the underlying condition; ensure early detection; use aggressive supportive treatment; prevent infection (intubation and mechanical ventilation)
- As disease progresses, use positive end-expiratory pressure (PEEP)
- Neuromuscular blocking agents such as pancuronium (Pavulon) and vecuronium (Norcuron) may be used to paralyze patient for easier ventilation
- Monitor arterial blood gas values, pulse oximetry, and pulmonary function testing
- Provide circulatory support; treat hypovolemia carefully; avoid overload
- Provide adequate fluid management; administer intravenous solutions
- Provide nutritional support (35 to 45 kcal/kg daily)

- Pharmacologic therapy may include human recombinant interleukin-1 receptor antagonist, neutrophil inhibitors, pulmonary-specific vasodilators, surfactant replacement therapy, antisepsis agents, antioxidant therapy, and corticosteroids (late in the course of ARDS).

Nursing of Management (see also Table 9.4)

Assessment

- Monitor patient closely because ARDS can quickly progress to a life-threatening situation
- Note agitation and anxiety and minimize.

Nursing Diagnoses

- Impaired gas exchange related to congestion
- Anxiety related to fear of death.

Planning

The goals of patient care may include achieving adequate spontaneous, nonlabored ventilation; maintaining arterial blood gas values within normal limits for patient without ventilator assistance; and ensuring that patient experience minimal anxiety.

Objectives

- Nonlabored spontaneous respirations
- Arterial blood gases, pulse oximetry and pulmonary function tests within normal limits.

Nursing Interventions

Promoting Adequate Ventilation

- Facilitate respiratory management; position patient to maximize respiration, oxygen, endotracheal intubation, tracheostomy, suctioning, and mechanical ventilation with sedation and paralytics as needed
- Chest physiotherapy (monitor closely for deterioration in oxygenation with changes in position)
- Provide safety interventions related to ventilator care
- Encourage rest to limit oxygen consumption
- Encourage oral fluid intake if patient is not ventilated.

Minimizing Anxiety

- Provide emotional support and reduce patient anxiety
- Explain all procedures and deliver care in calm, reassuring manner.

CHRONIC OBSTRUCTIVE PULMONARY DISEASE

Chronic obstructive pulmonary disease (COPD) is a preventable and treatable disease state characterized by airflow limitation that is not fully reversible. The airflow limitation is usually progressive and associated with an abnormal inflammatory response of the lungs to noxious particles or gases, primarily caused by cigarette smoking. Although COPD affects the lungs, systemic consequences also develop.

The term chronic obstructive pulmonary disease encompasses two types of obstructive airway diseases, chronic bronchitis and emphysema. Chronic bronchitis is the presence of chronic productive cough for 3 months in each of 2 consecutive years in a patient in whom other causes of chronic cough have been excluded. Emphysema is an abnormal permanent enlargement of the air spaces distal to the terminal bronchioles, accompanied by destruction of their walls and without obvious fibrosis. Only about 10% of patients with COPD have pure emphysema. Patients with COPD may have a predominance of one of these conditions, but in reality it is often difficult to determine because the conditions unusually coexist. COPD is discussed in this session as one disease state from the standpoint of pathophysiology and management.

Patients with COPD may have asthma, and some patients with asthma may go on to develop fixed or irreversible airflow obstruction. It may be nearly impossible to differentiate asthma from COPD, especially if the individual has a history of cigarette smoking.

Etiology

Chronic obstructive pulmonary disease (COPD) is a disease characterized by airflow limitation that is not fully reversible. The airflow obstruction is usually progressive and associated with airway hyperreactivity, resulting in narrowing of peripheral airways, airflow limitation, and changes in the pulmonary vasculature. Asthma is now considered a separate disorder, although symptoms overlap with symptoms of COPD. Cigarette smoking, air pollution, and occupational exposure (coal, cotton, grain) are important risk factors that contribute to COPD development, which may occur over a 20- to 30-year span. Complications of COPD vary but include respiratory insufficiency and failure (major complications) as well as pneumonia, atelectasis, and pneumothorax.

Cigarette Smoking

The major risk factor for developing COPD is cigarette smoking. It is still a major public health concern, especially among young people. Nearly all first-time use of tobacco occurs before high school graduation, and each day 2000 teens will become regular, daily smokers, with one third of them eventually dying because of a smoking-related disease. Clinically significant airway obstruction develops in approximately 15 to 20 percent of smokers, hospitalizations and loss of many years of productivity. Cigarette smoking remains the most preventable cause of premature death in the United States. In addition to being linked with COPD and lung cancer, cigarette smoking has also been implicated as a factor in cancers of the mouth, pharynx, larynx, esophagus, pancreas, kidney, stomach, colon, cervix, uterus, and bladder. When cigarettes are smoked, tar is inhaled, which contains approximately 4000 chemicals. Over 60 carcinogens have been isolated from cigarette smoke, including cyanide, formaldehyde and ammonia. Nicotine is probably not a carcinogen, but it has other deleterious effects. It acts by stimulating the sympathetic nervous system, resulting in increased heart rate, increased peripheral vasoconstriction, increased BP, and increased cardiac workload. Nicotine also decreases the amount of functional hemoglobin and increases platelet aggregation. These effects of nicotine compound the problems in a person with coronary artery disease.

Cigarette smoke has several direct effects on the respiratory tract. The irritating effect of the smoke causes hyperplasia of cells, including goblet cells, which subsequently result in increased production of mucus. Hyperplasia reduces airway diameter and increases the difficulty in clearing secretions. Smoking reduces the ciliary activity and may cause actual loss of ciliated cells. Smoking also produces abnormal dilation of the distal air space with destruction of alveolar walls. Many cells develop large, atypical nuclei, which are considered a precancerous condition. After a short time of smoking, changes in small airway function can develop. In the early stages these changes are mostly inflammatory with mucosal edema and an influx of inflammatory cells. In later stages, however, thickening of the airway wall occurs by a remodeling process related to tissue repair and the inability of cilia to clear mucus, thus resulting in accumulation of inflammatory exudates in the airway lumen. Quitting smoking can prevent or delay the development of airflow limitation or reduce its progression.

Carbon monoxide (CO) is a component of tobacco smoke. CO has a high affinity for hemoglobin and combined with it more reality than does O_2, thereby reducing the smokers O_2-carrying capacity. The smoker inhales a lower percentage of O_2 than normal, resulting in less O_2 available at the alveolar level. The hearts need for O_2 is increased because of the stimulatory effect of nicotine on the sympathetic nervous system. Because the bloods O_2-carrying capacity is reduced, the heart must pump more rapidly to adequately supply tissues with O_2. CO also seems to impair psychomotor performance and judgment.

Passive smoking is the exposure of nonsmokers to cigarette smoke, also known as environmental tobacco smoke (ETS) or secondhand smoke. In adults, involuntary smoke exposure is associated with decreased pulmonary function, increased respiratory symptoms, and severe lower respiratory tract infections such as pneumonia. ETS also is associated with increased respiratory symptoms, and severe lower respiratory tract infections risk for lung cancer and nasal sinus cancer. The cardiovascular system is affected by ETS with increased heart rate and blood pressure and decreased levels of high-density lipoproteins (HDLs).

Occupational Chemicals and Dusts

If a person has intense or prolonged exposure to various dusts, vapors, irritants, or fumes in the workplace, COPD can develop independently of cigarette smoking. If the person smokes, the risk of COPD increases. Exposure to these irritants causes the airways to be hyperresponsive.

Air Pollution

High levels of urban air pollution are harmful to persons with existing lung disease. However, the effect of outdoor air pollution as a risk factor for COPD appears to be small compared to the effect of cigarette smoking. Another risk factor for COPD development is fossil fuels that are used for indoor heating and cooking. Many women, particularly because of cooking with these fuels in poorly ventilated areas.

Infection

Infections are a risk factor for developing COPD. Severe recurring respiratory tract infections in childhood have been associated with reduced lung function and increased respiratory symptoms in adulthood. Recurring infections impair normal defense mechanisms, making the bronchioles and alveoli more susceptible to injury. The person with COPD is prone to acute exacerbations of the disease, with 50 to 75 percent of cases thought to be caused by bacteria. These respiratory infections subsequently intensify the pathologic destruction of lung tissue and the progression of COPD. The most common causative organisms are *Haemophilus influenzae, Streptococcus pneumoniae,* and *Moraxella catarrhalis.*

Heredity

α_1-Antitrypsin (AAT) deficiency is the genetic risk factor that leads to COPD. AAT deficiency, an autosomal recessive disorder, accounts for 1 to 2 percent of COPD cases. Also known as α_1-protease inhibitor, AAT is a serum protein produced by the liver and normally found in the lungs. Severe AAT deficiency leads to premature bullous emphysema in the lungs found via radiologic testing. Normally, AAT inhibits the lysis of lung tissues by proteolytic enzymes from neutrophils and macrophages. Emphysema occurs because of the AAT deficiency. Lower levels of AAT result in insufficient inactivation and subsequent destruction of lung tissue. Smoking greatly exacerbates the disease process in these patients.

The level of AAT is controlled by a pair of autosomal co-dominant genes. Low levels of AAT are related to homozygosity for the deficiency gene (ZZ), intermediate levels to heterozygosity (MZ), and normal values to homozygosity for the normal gene (MM). In the recessive gene homozygous group (ZZ), many individuals may have relatively normal lung function, especially those who never smoked. However, those with ZZ have the most severe disease. Clues to AAT deficiencies are the onset of symptoms often occurring by age 40, minimal to no tobacco use, and family history of emphysema. Chronic lever disease as an infant or adult with increased liver enzyme tests may also be seen. The people with this type of emphysema are primarily of northern European origin. A simple blood test can determine low levels of AAT. Those with borderline or low levels can then be genetically tested. IV-administered AAT (Prolastin) augmentation therapy is approved for persons with AAT deficiency. The infusions are administered weekly. Its effectiveness in slowing the progression of the disease continues to be evaluated.

Aging

Some degree of emphysema is common in the lungs of the older person, even a nonsmoker. Aging results in changes in the lung structure, the thoracic cage, and the respiratory muscles. As people age there is gradual loss of the elastic recoil of the lung. The lungs become more rounded and smaller. The number of functional alveoli decreases as a result of the loss of the alveolar supporting structures and loss of the intraalveolar septum. These changes are similar to those seen in the patient with emphysema. Clinically significant emphysema, however, is usually not caused by aging alone. Thinner alveolar walls contribute to loss of alveolar septal tissue and alveolar capillaries. With fewer capillaries available for gas exchange, arterial O_2 (PaO_2) levels decrease from 80 mm Hg at 20 years of age to 65 to 70 mm Hg by 70 years of age.

Thoracic cage changes result from osteoporosis and calcification of the costal cartilages. The thoracic cage becomes stiff and rigid, and the ribs are less mobile. The shape of the rib cage gradually changes because of the increased residual volume (RV), causing it to expand and become rounded. Decreased chest compliance and elastic recoil of the lungs caused by aging affects the mechanical aspects of ventilation and increases the work of breathing. Changes in the elasticity of the lungs reduce the ventilatory reserve, and ability to clear secretions decreases with age.

Pathophysiology

Chronic obstructive pulmonary disease (COPD) is characterized by chronic inflammation found in the airways, lung parenchyma (gas-exchanging surfaces of the lungs [respiratory bronchioles and alveoli]), and pulmonary vasculature. The pathogenesis of COPD is complex and involves many mechanisms. However, the primary process is inflammation. The inflammatory process starts with inhalation of noxious particles and gases (e.g. cigarette smoke, air pollution). The predominant inflammatory cells, macrophages and lymphocytes (primarily CD8 cells), increase and release inflammatory mediators, including leukotrienes, interleukins and tumor necrosis factor. These mediators cause damage to the lung tissue. Later, neutrophils infiltrate into the lungs and release more inflammatory mediators. The airways become inflamed, resulting in increased numbers of enlarged goblet cells. This results in excess mucus production (or chronic bronchitis). Peripheral airways (small bronchi and bronchioles with internal diameter < 2 mm) undergo repeated cycles of injury and repair of the airway walls with resultant structural remodeling. Increased collagen and scar tissue formation in the walls cause fibrosis (see Fig. 9.13).

Destruction of the lung parenchyma in COPD patients results in emphysema with significant loss of attachments, which could be likened to rubber bands connecting airways and keeping the airways open. With loss of attachments (rubber bands), the peripheral airways collapse. One type of emphysema, called centrilobular, involves dilation and destruction of the respiratory bronchioles and is the most commonly seen in upper lobes in mild disease. The pathologic changes may occur throughout the lungs in severe disease and the pulmonary bed may also be destroyed. The second type of emphysema involves destruction of the alveolar ducts, alveolar sacs, and respiratory bronchioles and is called *panlobular*. It is most prominent in the lower lobes and is seen with α_1-antitrypsin deficiency. Destruction of the lung parenchyma is thought to be due to an imbalance of proteinases/antiproteinases. This occurs as a consequence of inflammation, but there can be a genetic basis to the proteinase imbalance. Individuals have elastin, which provides the structural makeup of the connection tissue of the alveolar wall. In a healthy person, proteinases (elastase is the main component) in the parenchyma, function to break down the alveolar walls (elastin). Normally, proteinase inhibitors (called α_1-antitrypsin [AAT]) prevent this destructive process. In smokers, the numbers of neutrophils, macrophages, and other inflammatory cells are increased and with the inflammatory process overwhelm the body's normal AAT defense. Therefore, there is destruction of the basic elastin structure of the parenchyma. In addition, inflammatory cells in COPD release a variety of inflammatory mediators such as leukotrienes and interleukins. In the genetic form of emphysema there is a deficiency of AAT, and an imbalance of proteinases/antiproteinases occurs. As the disease progresses, these microscopic lesions may progress to bullae in the lung parenchyma or blebs in the visceral pleura. These anatomic changes can be likened to a balloon that has been blown up too many times. Bullae and blebs are areas with greatly reduced diffusion of gases as the alveolar capillary bed is destroyed.

In COPD, as the supporting structures of the lung are destroyed, there is no pull or traction on the walls of the bronchioles. Like air being blown into a paper bag, air goes into the lungs easily but is unable to come out on its own; it remains in the lung. Thus the bronchioles tend to collapse (especially on expiration) and air is trapped in the distal alveoli. This trapped air in the lungs gives the patient the typical barrel-chested appearance. In COPD the lungs can be inflated easily but can only partially deflate.

Pulmonary vascular changes can begin early in the disease. Inflammatory cells infiltrate the smooth muscle of the blood vessels causing thickening as the disease advances. Because of the loss of alveolar walls and the capillaries surrounding them, the amount of surface area that is available for diffusion of O_2 decreases. The patient with COPD compensates for this problem by increasing the respiratory rate to increase alveolar ventilation. Typically, the patient does not have difficulty with hypoxemia at rest until late in the disease. However, hypoxemia may develop during exercise, and the patient may benefit from supplemental O_2. Air can move into the lungs, thus there is ventilation. However, because of the anatomic changes noted previously, perfusion of gases is affected, and thus there is a ventilation/perfusion imbalance. Hypercapnia and respiratory acidosis do not develop until late in the disease process. In severe cases, collagen deposition in the vessels along with emphysematous destruction of the capillary bed occurs, leading to pulmonary hypertension and cor pumonale; the prognosis is poor.

These changes in the lungs result in the following characteristic disease manifestations: mucus hypersecretion, dysfunction of the cilia, airflow limitation and hyperinflation of the lungs, gas exchange abnormalities, pulmonary hypertension, and cor pulmonale (Fig. 9.29). Mucus hypersecretion and dysfunction of cilia lead to chronic cough and sputum production. Inability to expire air (largely irreversible) is the main smaller airways and is due to remodeling. Because of the loss of alveolar walls and attachments, the elastic recoil of the lung is decreased. Recoil is also affected by the influx of inflammatory cells and exudates in the bronchi together with hyperinflation of the lungs.

The COPD has been shown to have systemic effects with inflammation (oxidative stress and inflammatory cells) and skeletal muscle wasting. Cigarette smoking begins the process of inflammation via oxidative stress, but inflammation appears to be sustained years after smoking ceases. This mechanism is being investigated. These effects limit the exercise abilities of the patient and worsen the prognosis.

Clinically, it is common to find a combination of emphysema and chronic bronchitis in the same person, often with one condition predominating. Patients with COPD may also have asthma, and if they experience poorly reversible airflow limitation, the symptoms may be indistinguishable from COPD, but clinically are treated as asthma. Pathologically, the types of inflammatory cells are quite different between COPD and asthma.

Clinical Manifestations

Clinical manifestations of COPD typically develop slowly around 50 years of age after 20 pack-years of cigarette smoking. A diagnosis of COPD should be considered in any patient who has symptoms of cough, sputum production, or dyspnea, and/or a history of exposure to risk factors for the disease. An intermittent cough, which is the earliest symptom, usually occurs in the morning with the expectation of small amounts of sticky mucus resulting from bouts of coughing. Patients usually seek medical help when they have an acute respiratory infection, with dyspnea being the main concern.

- COPD is characterized by chronic cough, sputum production, and increased work of breathing as well as dyspnea on exertion
- Weight loss is common
- Symptoms are specific to the disease.

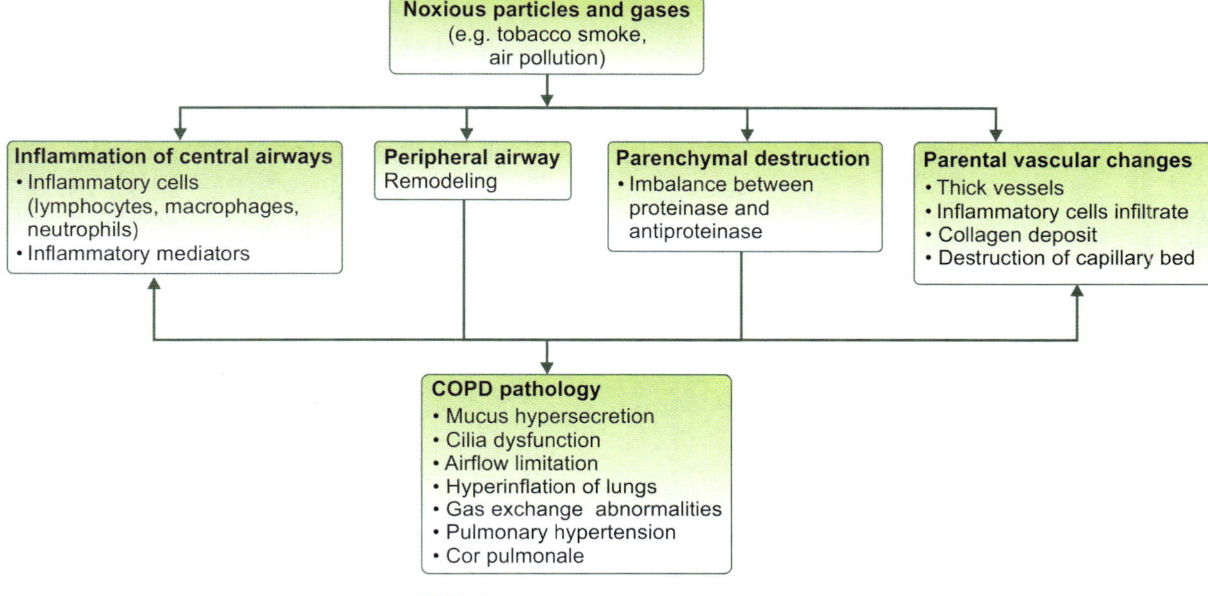

FIG. 9.29: Pathophysiology of COPD

See clinical manifestations under Asthma, Bronchiectasis, Bronchitis, and Emphysema.

Dyspnea is often progressive, and usually occurs with exertion. However, patients may dismiss the importance of this symptom as they rationalize, "I am just getting older". They change behaviors to avoid dyspnea, such as taking the elevator. Gradually, the dyspnea interferes with daily activities, such as carrying grocery bags, and they cannot walk as fast as their spouse or peers. Stages of COPD are listed in Box 9.14.

In late stages of COPD, dyspnea may be present at rest. As more alveoli become overdistended, increasing amounts of air are trapped. This causes a flattened diaphragm and an increased anter or-posterior diameter of the chest, forming the typical barrel chest. Effective abdominal breathing is decreased because of the flattened diaphragm from the overdistended lungs. The person becomes more of a chest breather, relying on the intercostal and accessory muscles. However, chest breathing is not efficient breathing.

The language that patients use to describe the dyspnea may be a key to determining that the etiology is respiratory rather than other causes such as heart failure. Patients with dyspnea because of COPD (compared to heart failure) often say, "My breath does not go out all the way". They may also use words such as "heaviness", "gasping", and "increased effort to breathe" to describe the dyspnea.

The cough initially may be intermittent. Later it is present every day, but is seldom present during the night. There are ranges in the amount of sputum produced. It is difficult to quantify the amount of sputum produced because many people swallow it, particularly women. In some people, the cough may be nonproductive.

Wheezing and chest tightness may be present, but may vary by time of the day or from day to day, especially in patients with more severe disease. The wheeze may arise from the laryngeal area, or wheezes may not be present on auscultation. Chest tightness, which often follows activity, may feel similar to muscular contraction.

During physical examination a prolonged expiratory phase of respiration, wheezes, or decreased breath sounds are noted in all lung fields. The patient may need to breathe louder than normal for auscultated breath sounds to be heard. The anterior-posterior diameter of the chest is increased (barrel chest) from the chronic air trapping. The patient may sit upright with arms supported on a fixed surface such as an overbed table (*tripod position*). The patient may naturally purse lips on expiration (pursed-lip breathing) inspiration. Edema in the ankles may be the only clue to right-sided heart involvement.

Over time, hypoxemia (PaO_2 < 60 mm Hg or O_2 saturation <88%) may develop with hypercapnia (Pa O_2 > 45 mm Hg) later in the disease. The bluish-red color of the skin results from polycythemia and cyanosis. Polycythemia develops as a result of increased production of red blood cells as the body attempts to compensate for chronic hypoxemia. Hemoglobin concentrations may reach 20 g/dL (200 g/L) or more. Cyanosis develops when there is at least 5 g/dL (50 g/L) or more of circulating unoxygenated hemoglobin.

As noted previously, it is sometimes quite difficult for the health care provider to distinguish COPD from asthma. However, there are some clinical features that are different.

Box 9.14 Stages of COPD

Stage I	Mild COPD. Mild airflow limitation, and sometimes, but not always, cough and sputum. Patient may not realize his lung function is abnormal
Stage II	Moderate COPD. Airflow limitation worsening; patient begins to feel short of breathe on exertion. Patient may seek medical help at this stage
Stage III	Severe COPD. Increasing airflow limitation and shortness of breath. Patient experiences decreased quality of life
Stage IV	Very severe COPD. Severe airflow limitation and significant reduction in quality of life; exacerbations may be life threatening

Classification of COPD

The COPD should be considered in any person with an exposure to risk factors such as cigarettes and/or environmental or occupational pollutants and/or chronic cough and dyspnea. The diagnosis is confirmed by spirometry. COPD can be classified as at risk, mild, moderate, severe, and very severe. The FEV_1/FEV <70% establishes the diagnosis of COPD, and severity of obstruction (as indicated by FEV_1) determines the stage of COPD. The management of COPD is primarily based on the patient's symptoms, but the staging provides a general guideline for the type of interventions.

Complications of COPD

Cor pulmonale: Cor pulmonale is hypertrophy of the right side of the heart, with or without heart failure, resulting from pulmonary hypertension. It is caused by diseases affecting the lungs or pulmonary blood vessels (Fig. 9.30). Cor pulmonale is a late manifestation of chronic pulmonary heart disease. The patient benefits most when a diagnosis of pulmonary heart disease can be made early so therapy can be instituted. In patients with severe COPD, 40 percent demonstrate cor pulmonale, and the prognosis is poor. In COPD, there may be an anatomic reduction of the pulmonary vascular bed as seen in emphysema with bullae. These patients would have increased pulmonary resistance.

Normally, the right ventricle and pulmonary circulatory system are low-pressure systems compared with the left ventricle and systemic circulation. When pulmonary hypertension develops, the pressures on the right side of the heart must increase to push blood into the lungs. Eventually, right-sided heart failure develops.

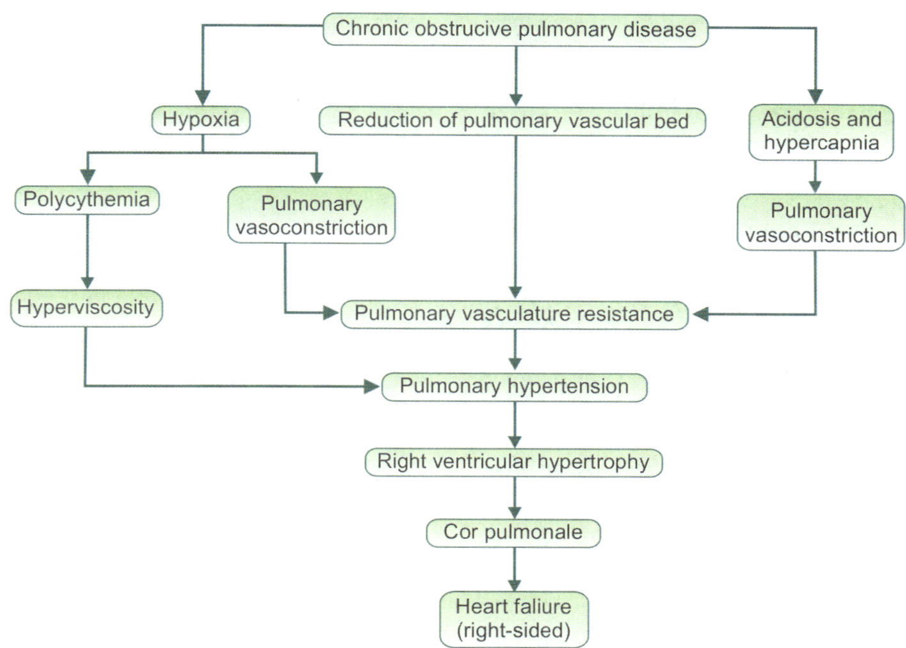

FIG. 9.30: The mechanisms involved in the pathophysiology of cor pulmonale secondary to chronic obstructive pulmonary disease

The clinical manifestations of chronic pulmonary heart disease and cor pulmonale are related to dilation and failure of the right ventricle with subsequent intravascular volume expansion and systemic venous congestion. Dyspnea is a usual symptom, and is associated with hypoxemia and hypercarbia. Lung sounds are normal or crackles may be heard in the bases of the lungs bilaterally. Heart sound changes include accentuation of the pulmonic component of the second heart sound, right-sided ventricular diastolic S3 gallop, and a loud pulmonic component of S2 along the left sternal border. ECG changes include increased P wave amplitude (P pulmonale), a tendency for right axis deviation, and incomplete right bundle branch block. Overt manifestations of right-sided heart failure may develop, which include distended neck veins (jugular venous distention), hepatomegaly with right upper quadrant tenderness, ascites, epigastric distress, peripheral edema, and weight gain.

Management of cor pulmonale includes continuous low-flow O_2. Long-term O_2 therapy improves survival of hypoxemic patients, especially when used >15 hours per day. Vasodilator therapy has not demonstrated sustained benefit and is not recommended on a routine basis. Although the use of digitalis is not indicated for right-sided heart failure, it may be used, but serum creatinie and blood urea nitrogen (BUN) are needed to monitor renal function as diuretics can cause volume depletion. Electrolytes must be monitored to assess for hypokalemia, which can predispose to dysrhythmias.

Exacerbations of COPD: Exacerbations of COPD are signaled by a change in the patients usual dyspnea, cough, and/or sputum that is different from the usual daily patterns. These flares require changes in management. Patients have an increase in dyspnea, sputum volume, and/or sputum purulence. They may also have nonspecific complaints of malaise, insomnia, fatigue, depression, confusion, decrease in exercise tolerance, increased wheezing, increased cough, or fever without other causes.

As the severity of COPD increases, exacerbations of COPD are associated with poorer outcomes. Exacerbations of COPD may be treated at home or in the hospital intermediate care unit or intensive care unit, depending on the severity. The primary causes of exacerbations of COPD are tracheobronchial infection and air pollution. Bacteria account for 33 to 75 percent of the cases of infection. The most common organisms causing exacerbations are *H. influenzae, M. catarrhalils*, and *S. pneumoniae*. Other causes of COPD exacerbations include viruses.

Medications used to decrease airway resistance during exacerbations of COPD are bronchodilators and oral systemic corticosteroids. If a patient has clinical signs of airway infection (e.g. increased volume and change in color of sputum and/or fever, especially in the severe stages of COPD with more than three to four exacerbations per year), antibiotic treatment is usually used. Therapies used to treat exacerbations of COPD in the hospital are similar to home management, except supplemental oxygen therapy titrated by ABG measurement may be used. Attempts are made to use noninvasive mechanical methods (e.g. intubation). Teaching the patient and family early recognition of signs and symptoms of exacerbations is important to promote early treatment to prevent hospitalization and possible respiratory failure.

Acute respiratory failure: Patients with severe COPD who have exacerbations are at risk for the development of respiratory failure. Frequently, COPD patients wait too long to contact their health care provider when they develop fever, increased cough and dyspnea, or other symptoms suggestive of exacerbation of cor pulmonale may also lead to acute respiratory failure. Discontinuing bronchondilator or corticosteroid medication may also precipitate respiratory failure. The use of β-adrenergic blockers (e.g. propranolol [Inderal]) may also exacerbate acute respiratory failure in the patient with a reversible component to the COPD However, cardioselective β-adrenergic blockers (e.g. atenolol, metoprolol) should not be withheld from patients with mild to moderate diseases because they do not produce clinically significant problems with respiration.

The indiscriminate use of sedatives, benzodiazepines and opioids, especially in the preoperative or postoperative patient who retains CO_2, may suppress the ventilatory drive and lead to respiratory failure. The person with COPD who retains CO_2 should be treated with low flow rates of O_2 with careful monitoring of ABGs to avoid hypercarbia to ensure that adequate oxygenation occurs and to monitor for acidosis. It has been thought that high flow rates of O_2 depress the respiratory center and that the patients respirations will diminish or cease. However, it is vital to provide adequate oxygen while assessing the ABGs, rather than not providing O_2 because of the fear of CO_2 narcosis.

Surgery or severe, painful illness involving the chest or abdominal organs may lead to splinting and ineffective ventilation and respiratory failure. To prevent postoperative pulmonary complications, careful preoperative screening, which includes pulmonary function tests and ABG assessment, is important in the patient with a heavy smoking history and/or COPD.

Peptic ulcer and gastroesophageal reflux disease: The incidence of peptic ulcer disease is increased in persons with COPD. The person for this occurrence is partly explained by hypersecretion of gastric acid resulting from increased arterial CO_2 and decreased arterial O_2 tension. This occurs only in patients who chronically retain CO_2. The ulcers are more commonly in the duodenum rather than stomach and do not cause pain. It is important to test gastric aspirates and feces for occult blood.

Gastroesophageal reflux disease (GERD), which may or may not be associated with a hiatal hernia, occurs frequently in patients with COPD and may aggravate respiratory symptoms. The reflux and accompanying heartburn may be aggravated or even precipitated by theophylline or β_2-adrenergic agonists. However, patients with severe COPD and GERD have also been found to have asymptomatic GERD.

Depression/anxiety: Patients with COPD experience many losses as the disease progresses over time. They can feel helpless with low self-esteem and unable to vent their emotions for fear of compromising their breathing. The reported prevalence of depression in COPD varies, but may be four times more frequent in COPD than in the general population. Anxiety can complicate respiratory compromise and may precipitate dyspnea and hyperventilation. When a person is exceptionally dyspneic, particularly if it occurs suddenly, the person becomes anxious and tries to breathe faster, thus affecting his or her oxygenation status. Proper screening for anxiety and depression by health care providers is needed for a proper diagnosis.

After diagnosis, treatment consists of cognitive and behavioral psychotherapy and/or pharmacotherapy. Selective serotonin reuptake inhibitors (SSRIs) are often used for both depression and anxiety. Buspirone, which is one medication used to treat anxiety, has few if any respiratory depression effects. Benzodiazepines are avoided because they may depress the respiratory drive and may be habit forming. The nurse should explore the psychologic realm of the patient's disease and the impact it has on the patient's quality of life. Providing sufficient time for nursing interventions during an acute exacerbation is important to help reduce anxiety. When the patient becomes anxious because of dyspnea, the use of pursed-lip breathing (discussed later in chapter) and short-acting bronchodilators may be appropriate.

Diagnostic Studies

The diagnosis of COPD is confirmed by pulmonary function tests. Goals of the diagnostic workup are to confirm the diagnosis of COPD via spirometry, evaluate the severity of the disease and determine the impact of the disease on the patient's quality of life. These factors enable the health care provider to design an individualized treatment plan. In addition to pulmonary function tests, other diagnostic studies are performed. Chest X-rays taken early in the disease are seldom diagnostic unless bullous disease is present. Patient may have significant airflow limitation as demonstrated by spirometry but not chronic cough. Most patients seek medical help because of dyspnea that starts affecting their daily activities. Later in the disease the findings presented in may be present.

A history and physical examination are extremely important in a diagnostic workup. Pulmonary function studies are useful in diagnosing and assessing the severity of COPD. Usually spirometry is ordered before and after bronchodilation. The most significant findings are related to increased resistance to expiratory airflow. Typical findings include the following:

- Reduced FEV_1, FEF25%-75% FEV_1/FVC ratio, diffusing capacity for carbon monoxide
- Increased residual volume, functional residual capacity (FRC).

When the FEV_1/FVC ratio is less than 70%, it suggests the presence of obstructive lung disease. The value of FEV_1 in milliliters can provide a guideline to determine the severity of the patients lung disease and the degree of disease progression.

The body mass index (BMI) and degree of dyspnea are useful in predicting outcomes, such as survival. Current practice guidelines recommend that the BMI and dyspnea be evaluated in all patients. BMI is obtained by dividing weight (in kilograms [kg]) by height (in square meter [m^2]). A BMI below 21 kg/m^2 is associated with an increase in mortality rate. Functional dyspnea can be assessed with the Medical Research Council Dyspnea Scale from level 0 (no trouble with breathlessness except with strenuous exercise) to level 4 (too breathless to leave the house or breathless when dressing or undressing).

ABGs are usually assessed in the severe stages and monitored in patients hospitalized with acute exacerbations. In the later stages of COPD, typical findings are low PaO_2, elevated PaO_2, decreased or low-normal pH, and increased bicarbonate (HCO_3) levels. In the early stages there may be normal or only slightly decreased PaO_2 and a normal PaO_2. A 6-minute walk to determine O_2 desaturation that occurs with exercise. An ECG may be normal or show signs indicative of right ventricular failure (e.g. low voltage, right-axis deviation, P-pulmonale). An echocardiogram or gated pool nuclear blood study can be used to evaluate right-sided ventricular and left ventricular function. Sputum for culture and sensitivity may be obtained if the patient is hospitalized for an acute exacerbation and has not responded to empiric therapy with antibiotics.

Management of COPD

The primary goals of care for the COPD patient are to (1) prevent disease progression, (2) relieve symptoms and improve exercise tolerance, (3) prevent and treat complications, (4) promote patient participation in care, (5) prevent and treat exacerbations, and (6) improve quality of life and reduce mortality risk. The majority of patients are treated as outpatients. They are hospitalized for exacerbations of COPD and potential complications when respiratory failure, pneumonia, and failure and/or cor pulmonale are also present. Environmental or occupational irritants should be evaluated for their possible negative effect and ways to control or avoid them should be determined. For example, aerosol hair sprays and smoke-filled rooms should be avoided. The patient with COPD is extremely susceptible to pulmonary infections. The patient with COPD should have a vaccination with influenza virus vaccine yearly and with pneumococcal vaccine. Pneumucoccal revaccination is recommended once if the patient is $\geq$ 65 years of age, the vaccination was $\geq$ 5 years previously, and the patient was $\leq$ 65 years of age at the time of the primary vaccination.

Exacerbations of COPD should be treated as soon as possible especially if the patient is in the severe stages of COPD. Often the best indication of the presence of a bacterial infection is the increasing quantity, viscosity, or purulence of sputum. Some patients are given a prescription for a 7- to 10-day supply of antibiotics and are instructed to begin taking them at the first signs of change is sputum. The most common antibiotics given for outpatients are macrolides (e.g. azithromycin [Zithromax]), doxycycline and newer cephalosporins (e.g. cefpodoxime [Vatnin]). Amoxicillin may be used, but patterns of antibiotic resistance are limiting its use. If the patient has failed prior antibiotic therapy or is hospitalized, common antibiotics are amoxicillin/clavulanate (Agumentin), or respiratory fluoroquinolones (e.g. levofloxacin [Levaquin]).

Medical Management

- Smoking cessation, if appropriate
- Bronchodilators, corticosteroids and other drugs
- Oxygen therapy, including nighttime oxygen
- Varied treatments specific to disease. See Medical Management under Asthma, Bronchiectasis, Bronchitis, and Emphysema
- Surgery: Bullectomy to reduce dyspnea; lung volume reduction to improve lobar elasticity and function; lung transplantation

The COD accentuates many of the physiologic changes associated with aging and is manifested in airway obstruction (in bronchitis) and excessive loss of elastic lung recoil (in emphysema). Additional changes in ventilation-perfusion ratios occur.

Smoking Cessation

Cessation of cigarette smoking in all stages of COPD is the single most effective and cost-effective intervention to reduce the risk of developing COPD and stop the progression of the disease. After discontinuation of smoking, the accelerated decline in pulmonary function slows and pulmonary function usually improves. Normally individuals after age 35 lose approximately 20 to 25 mL (as measured by FEV_1) of lung function per year as measured by spirometry. Persons with COPD who continue to smoke lose approximately 50 mL per year. With the cessation of smoking, the loss can fall to almost nonsmoking levels at 35 mL per year. Thus the sooner the smoker stops, the less pulmonary function is lost and the sooner the symptoms decrease, especially cough and sputum production.

Drug Therapy

Medications for COPD can reduce or abolish symptoms, increase the capacity to exercise, improve overall health and reduce the number and severity of exacerbations. Presently no drug modifies the decline of lung function with COPD. Bronchodilator drug therapy relaxes smooth muscles in the airway and improves the ventilation of the lungs, thus reducing the degree of breathlessness. Although patients with COPD do not respond as dramatically as those with asthma to bronchodilator therapy, a reduction in dyspnea and an increase in FEV_1 are usually achieved. The inhaled route of medication is preferred and given on a prn or regular basis. Medications are given in a stepwise fashion.

Bronchodilator medications commonly used are β_2-adrenergic agonists, anticholinergic agents, and methylxanthines. The choice of bronchodilator depends on the availability and the patient's response. However, when the patient has mild COPD or intermittent symptoms, a short-acting bronchodilator is used as needed. Short-acting bronchodilators increase exercise tolerance. Albuterol or ipratropium (Atrovent) may be used as single agents, but combining bronchodilators improves their effect and decreases the risk of adverse effects, compared with the use of a single agent. As a single agent, ipratropium (Atrovent) is superior to albuterol because the only side effect is usually dry mouth.

These two agents can be nebulized together (DuoNeb) or delivered by one MDI (Combivent).

As symptoms persist or moderate stages of COPD develop, a long-acting bronchodilator is used in addition to a short-acting bronchodilator. Salmeterol (Serevent) is a widely used long-acting β_2-adrenergic agonist and unlike in drug therapy for asthma, it can be used in COPD as monotherapy. Formoterol (Foradil) is another long-acting β_2-agonist.

Tiotropium (Spiriva), a long-acting anticholinergic, can be used for daily therapy of bronchosapsm, and dyspnea in COPD. Tiotropium also improves bronchodilation, results in less dyspnea, improves quality of life, and decreases the number of COPD exacerbations when compared with ipratropium (Atrovent). Tiotropium is the first inhaled drug for COPD to be dosed once a day.

The use of long-acting theophyline in the treatment of COPD is controversial because it interacts with many drugs. Although it has some action as a mild bronchodilator in the patient with partial reversibility of airflow obstruction, its main value may be to improve contractility of the diaphragm and decrease diaphragramatic fatigue.

Inhaled corticosteroid therapy may be beneficial for patients with moderate-to-severe COPD. However, inhaled corticosteroids (ICS) do not appear to help patients with mild COPD. ICS combined with long-acting β_2-adrenergic agonists (e.g. fluticasone/salmeterol [Advair]) are more effective than the single drug therapy. Oral corticosteroids should not be used for long-term therapy in COPD.

O_2 Therapy

O_2 therapy is frequently used in the treatment of COPD and other problems associated with hypoxemia. Long-term O_2 therapy (LTOT) improves survival, exercise capacity, cognitive performance, and sleep in hypoxemic patients. O_2 is a colorless, odorless, tasteless gas that constitutes 20.95 percent of the atmosphere. Administering supplemental O_2 raises the partial pressure of O_2 (PO_2) in inspired air. Used clinically it is considered a drug. For reimbursement purposes, it is considered durable medical equipment, which Medicare covers when certain clinical criteria are met (i.e. the patients O_2 saturation needs to be ≤ 88 percent, PaO_2 ≥ 55 mm Hg).

Indications for use: Goals for O_2 therapy are to reduce the work of breathing, maintain the PaO_2, and/or reduce the workload on the heart, keeping the SaO_2 > 90 percent during rest, sleep and exertion, or PaO_2 > 60 mm Hg. O_2 is usually administered to treat hypoxemia caused by (1) respiratory disorders such as COPD, pulmonary hypertension, cor pulmonlae, pneumonia, atelectasis, lung cancer, and pulmonary emboli; (2) cardiovascular disorders such as myocardial infarction, dysrhythmias, angina pectoris, and cardiogenic shock; and (3) central nervous system disorders such as overdose of opioids, head injury, and disordered sleep (sleep apnea).

Methods of administration: The goal of O_2 administration is to supply the patient with adequate O_2 to maximize the O_2-carrying ability of the blood. There are various methods of O_2 administration. The method selected depends on factors such as the fraction of inspired O_2 (FIO_2) required by the patient and delivered by the device, the mobility of the patient, humidification required, patient cooperation, comfort, cost, and available financial resources (Table 9.2).

O_2 delivery systems are classified as low- or high-flow systems. Most methods of O_2 administration are low-flow devices that deliver O_2 in concentrations that vary with the person's respiratory pattern. In contrast, the Venturi mask is a high-flow device that delivers fixed concentrations of O_2 independent of the patient's respiratory pattern. With the Venturi mask, O_2 is delivered to a small jet (Venturi device) in the center of a wide-based cone. Air is entrained (pulled through) openings in the cone as O_2 flows through the small jet. The mask has large vents through which exhaled air can escape. The degree of restriction or narrowness of the jet determines the amount of entrainment and dilution of pure O_2 with room air, and thus the concentration of O_2 delivered can be precise. Mechanical ventilators are another example of a high-flow O_2 delivery system. Because room air is mixed with O_2, in low-flow systems, the percentage of O_2 delivered to the patient is not as precise as with high-flow systems.

Humidification and nebulizers: O_2 obtained from cylinders or wall systems is dry. Dry O_2 has an irritating effect on mucous membranes and dries secretions. Therefore, it is important that O_2 be humidified when administered, wither by humidification or nebulization. A common device used for humidification when the patient has a catheter, cannula, or low-flow mask is a bubble through humidifier. It is a small jar filled with sterile distilled water that is attached to the O_2 source by means of a flow meter. O_2 passes into the jar, bubbles through the water, and then goes through tubing to the patient's catheter, cannula, or mask. The purpose of the bubble-through humidifier is to restore the humidity conditions of room air. However, the need for bubble-through humidifiers at flow rates between 1 and 4L per minute is dependent on patient preference (Table 9.2).

Another means of administering humidified O_2 is via a nebulizer. It delivers particulate water mist (aerosols) with nearly 100 percent humidity. The humidity can be raised by heating the water, which increases the ability of the gas to hold moisture. Heated (98.6°F [37°C]) and humidified (100 percent) gas is required when the upper airway is bypassed in acute

TABLE 9.2: Methods of oxygen administration

Advantages	Disadvantages	Nursing interventions
A. Low-flow delivery devices		
(i) *Nasal cannula*		
Most commonly used device. It is a safe and simple method that is relatively comfortable and acceptable. It is useful for a patient requiring low O_2 concentrations (e.g. those with chronic CO_2 retention). It allows patient to move about in bed. Patient can eat, talk or cough while wearing device	Cannula is difficult to maintain in position and can be easily dislodged. Patient must be alert and cooperative to keep cannula in proper place. High flow rates (>5 L/min) dry nasal membranes and may cause pain in frontal sinuses. Can irritate nares and skin around ears	Nasal cannula should be stabilized when caring for a restless patient. O_2 concentrations of 24 percent (at 1 L/min) to 44 percent (at 6 L/min) can be obtained. Amount of O_2 inhaled depends on room air and patients breathing pattern. Most patients with COPD can tolerate 2 L/min via cannula. May need to pad the cannula where it sits on the ears
(ii) *Simple face mask*		
O_2 can be given quickly for shock periods. Useful when transporting patients. O_2 concentrations of 35–50 percent can be achieved with flow rates of 6–12 L/min. Mask provides adequate humidification of inspired air	Lack of patient results in inadequate therapy. Mask may be uncomfortable because tight seal must be maintained between face and mask. Mask may produce pressure necrosis of the skin and confines heat radiating from the face about nose and mouth. It must be removed to eat or drink	Wash and dry under mask q2h. Mask must fit snugly. Nasal cannula may be provided while patient is eating. Watch for pressure necrosis at the top of ears from elastic straps (gauze or other padding may be used to alleviate this problem). Method requires at least 5 L/min flow to prevent accumulation of expired air in the mask
(iii) *Partial rebreathing mask*		
Mask is lightweight and easy to use. Reservoir bag conserves O_2. Useful for short-term (24 h) therapy for patients needing higher O_2 concentrations	Mask cannot be used with a high degree of humidity. Patient may find mask uncomfortable and refuse to wear it	Method is useful when blood O_2 concentrations must be raised. It is not recommended for patient with COPD and should never be used with a nebulizer. Bag should not be allowed to deflate during inspiration, so make sure the reservoir does not kink, which results in bag deflation
(iv) *Non-rebreathing mask*		
High concentration of O_2 can be delivered accurately. O_2 flows into bag and mask during inhalation. Valve prevents expired air from flowing back into bag. Good for short-term (24 h) therapy for patients needing higher O_2 concentrations	Mask cannot be used with a high degree of humidity. Patient may find mask uncomfortable and refuse to wear it	Mask should fit snugly. Flow rate must be sufficient to keep bag from collapsing during inspiration. Bag should not be allowed to deflate during inspiration. Make sure valves are open during expiration and closed during inflation to prevent drastic decrease in FIO_2. Monitor closely because patient may require intubation as the next step
(v) *Oxygen-conserving cannula*		
Cannula has a built-in reservoir that increases O_2 concentration delivered and allows patient to use lower flow, usually 30–50 percent, which increases comfort, lowers cost, and can be increased with activities. It can deliver up to 8 L/min of O_2. It is reportedly more comfortable than standard cannulas	Cannula cannot be cleaned: manufacturer recommends changing cannula every week. It is more expensive than standard cannulas and requires evaluation with ABGs and oximetry to determine correct flow for patient. Cannula is highly visible. Cannula heavy on ears	Method is generally indicated for patient requiring long-term O_2 therapy at home versus during hospitalization. It may be "moustache" or "pendant" type. May cause necroses over the tops of the ears; can be padded
(vi) *Transtracheal catheter*		
Catheter is less visible. Flow requirement may be reduced approximately 50–70 percent, which greatly increases amount of time available from portable source of O_2. Less nasal irritation occurs	Patient and family must learn entire program of care for tracheostoma and how to replace catheter. Procedure is invasive. Procedure and replacement add costs to O_2 therapy	Method may not be appropriate for patient with excessive mucus production from mucus plugging because the catheter may frequently become obstructed

Contd...

Contd...

Advantages	Disadvantages	Nursing interventions
(vii) *Face tent*		
Tent is ideal for providing moderate to high-density aerosol. O_2 concentration administered varies with O_2 flow rate	Amount of O_2 delivered is imprecise	Open plastic mask fits under chin. Temperature of aerosal must be checked to maintain at or near body temperature. It is rarely used
(viii) *Tracheostomy collar*		
Collar can deliver high humidity and O_2 via tracheostomy	Condensed fluid in tubing may drain into tracheostomy. Water traps are usually put in. Secretions collect inside collar and around tracheostomy. O_2 concentration is lost into atmosphere because collar does not fit tightly	Collar attaches to neck with elastic strap and should be removed and cleaned at least q4h to prevent aspiration of fluid and infection
(ix) *Tracheostomy T bar*		
Tight fit allows better O_2 and humidity delivery than tracheostomy collar	Condensed fluid in tubing may drain into tracheostomy. Water traps are usually put in	T bar must be removed for suctioning. Morch swivel may be used to eliminate the need for removal. It should be emptied as necessary
B. High-flow delivery devices		
Venturi mask		
Mask can deliver precise, high flow rates of O_2. Lightweight plastic, cone-shaped device is fitted to face. Masks are available for delivery of 24 percent, 28 percent, 31 percent, 35 percent, 40 percent and 50 percent O_2. Adaptors can be applied to increase humidification	Mask is uncomfortable and must be removed when patient eats. Patient can talk but voice may be muffled. Other disadvantages are the same as those discussed for the simple facemask	Entrainment device on mask must be changed to deliver higher concentrations of O_2. Method is especially helpful for administrating low, constant O_2 concentrations to patients with COPD. Air entrainment ports must not be occluded

care. however, patients with established tracheotomies do not always require 100 percent humidity. When nebulizers are used, large-size tubing should be employed to connect the device to a facemask or T bar. If small-size tubing is used, condensation can occlude the flow of O_2. Vapotherm can deliver high flows (15 to 20 L/min) of warm humidified air (either sterile air or O_2) to the patient through a nasal cannula or transtracheal cannula using technology to warm and saturate the gas stream.

Complications

Combustion: O_2 supports combustion and increases the rate of burning. This is why it is important that smoking be prohibited in the area in which O_2 is being used. A "No Smoking" sign should be prominently displayed on the patient's door. The patient should also be cautioned against smoking cigarettes with O_2 cannula in place.

CO_2 Narcosis: The two chemoreceptors in the respiratory center that control the drive to breathe respond to CO_2 and O_2. Normally, CO_2 accumulation is the major stimulant of the respiratory center. Over time some COPD patients develop a tolerance for high CO_2 levels (the respiratory center loses its sensitivity to the elevated CO_2 levels). Theoretically, for these individuals the "O_2 drive" to breathe is hypoxemia. Thus there has been concern regarding the dangers of administering O_2 to COPD patients and reducing their drive to breathe. This has been a pervasive myth but is not a serious threat. In fact, not providing adequate O_2 to these patients is much more detrimental. Although O_2 administration should be titrated to the lowest effective dose, many patients who have end-stage COPD require high flow rates and higher concentrations for survival. They may, in fact, exhibit higher than normal levels of CO_2 in their blood, but this is of little concern. What is important is careful, ongoing assessment when providing O_2 to these patients, monitoring both physical and cognitive effects of O_2.

It is critical to start O_2 at low flow rates until ABGs can be obtained. ABGs are used as a guide to determine what FIO_2 level is sufficient and can be tolerated. The patients mental status and vital signs should be assessed before starting O_2 therapy and frequently thereafter.

O_2 Toxicity: Pulmonary O_2 toxicity may result from prolonged exposure to a high level of O_2 (PaO_2). The development of O_2 toxicity is relatively rare, but is determined by patient tolerance, exposure time and effective dose. High concentrations of O_2 damage alveolar-capillary membranes inactivate pulmonary surfactant, cause interstitial and alveolar edema, and decrease compliance. These individuals develop acute respiratory distress syndrome (ARDS). Prevention of O_2 toxicity is important for the patient who is receiving O_2. The amount of O_2 administered should be just enough to maintain the PaO_2 within a normal or acceptable range for the patient. ABGs should be monitored frequently to evaluate the effectiveness of therapy and to guide the tapering of supplemental O_2. A safe limit of O_2 concentrations has not yet been established. All levels above 50% and used for

longer than 24 hours should be considered potentially toxic. Levels of 40% and below may be regarded as relatively nontoxic and may not result in development of significant O_2 toxicity if the exposure period is short.

Absorption atelectasis: Normally, nitrogen, which constitutes 79 percent of the air that is breathed, is not absorbed into the bloodstream. This prevents alveolar collapse. When high concentrations of O_2 are given, nitrogen is washed out of the alveoli and replaced with O_2. If airway obstruction occurs, the O_2 is absorbed into the bloodstream and the alveoli collapse. This process is called absorption atelectasis.

Infection: Infection can be a major hazard of O_2 administration. Head nebulizers present the highest risk. The constant use of humidity supports bacterial growth, with the common infecting organism being *Pseudomonas aeruginosa*. Disposable equipment that operates as a closed system should be used. There should be a hospital policy stating the required frequency of equipment changes based on the type of equipment used at that particular institution.

Chronic O_2 therapy at home: Improved survival occurs in patients with COPD who receive long-term O_2 therapy (LTOT) (> 15 hours/day) to treat hypoxemia. The improved prognosis results from preventing progression of the disease and subsequent cor pulmonale. The benefits of long-term O_2 therapy include improved mental acuity, lung mechanics, sleep, and exercise tolerance; decreased hematocrit; and reduced pulmonary hypertension. Some patients believe they will become "addicted" to O_2 and are very reluctant to use it. They need to be educated that it is not "addicting" and that it needs to be used for the prescribed times during the day because of the positive effects on the heart, lungs, and brain. The need for LTOT should be evaluated when the patient's condition has stabilized. The goal of O_2 therapy is to maintain SaO_2 > 90 percent during rest, sleep and exertion.

Short-term home O_2 therapy (1 to 30 days) may be indicated for the patient in whom hypoxemia persists after discharge from the hospital. For example, the patient with underlying COPD who develops a serious respiratory infection may continue to have clearing of the infection after completion of antibiotic therapy and discharge from the hospital. This patient may demonstrate continued hypoxemia for 4 to 6 weeks after discharge. It is important to measure the patient's oxygenation status by ABGs 30 to 90 days after an acute episode to determine if the O_2 is still warranted.

Patients whose disease is stable with a PaO_2 of 55 mm Hg or less (corresponding to an SaO_2 of 88 percent or less) should receive LTOT. A patient whose PaO_2 is between 55 and 60 mm Hg (SaO_2 89 percent and who exhibits signs of tissue hypoxia, such as cor pulmonale, erythorcytosis, peripheral edema from right-sided heart failure, or impaired mental status, should also receive LTOT. Desaturation only during exercise or sleep suggests consideration of O_2 therapy specifically under those conditions. Patients may receive O_2 only during exercise and/or sleep. The need for O_2 during these periods should be evaluated with a 6-minute walk test or overnight oximetry. Sleep disordered breathing may be seen in some of these patients, and they will require a full sleep study.

Periodic reevaluations are necessary for the patient who is using chronic supplemental O_2. Generally the recommendation is that the patient should be reevaluated every 30 to 90 days during the first year of therapy and annually after that, as long as the patient remains stable.

Nasal cannulas, either regular or the O_2-conserving type, are usually used to deliver O_2 from a central source in the home. The source may be a liver O_2 from a central source in the home. The source may be a liquid O_2 storage system, compressed O_2 in tanks, or an O_2 concentrator or extractor, depending on the patients home environment, insurance coverage, activity level, and proximity to an O_2 supply company. The patient can use extension tubing without adversely affecting the O_2 flow delivery to increase mobility in the home. Small, portable systems, such as liquid O_2 may be provided for the patient who remains active outside the home.

Home O_2 systems are usually rented from a company that sends a respiratory therapist to the patient's home. The therapist teaches the patient and family how to use the O_2 system, how to care for it, and how to recognize when the supply is running low and needs to be recorded. A patient and family teaching guide for the use of O_2 at home is presented.

The patient who uses home O_2 should be encouraged to remain active and to travel normally. If travel is by automobile, arrangement can be made for O_2 to be available at the destination point. O_2 supply companies can often assist in these arrangements. If a patient wishes to travel by bus, train, or airplane, the patient should inform the appropriate people when reservations are made that O_2 will be needed for travel. If there is a potential for the patient to become hypoxic, oxygen needs for flying can be determined via a hypoxia inhalation test or through a mathematical formula. Patients on LTOT should be instructed to increase the O_2 flow by 1 to 2 L/min during the flight. Those with resting PaO_2 of 70 mm Hg are likely to be safe to fly without O_2. However, they may become hypoxemic as PaO_2 may fall an average of 25 mm Hg. If patients have other comorbidities, such as certain cardiac disease or anemia, they may also become hypoxemic. Patients should be warned that walking along the aisles on an airplane cabins are pressurized to an elevation of 7,000 or 8,000 feet, the patient who uses supplemental O_2 should have it provided during flight. The airline's O_2 system must be used. Patients may not use their own O_2 system during must be used. Patients may not use their own O_2 system during flight because it is not properly pressurized. Airlines allow patients to bring their O_2 system to be carried in the reservoirs (liquid or tank) must be empty and the valves left open. Some patients may need to avoid prolonged exposure to high elevations during travel unless they are instructed by their health care provider regarding adjustments in their O_2 flow to attempt to compensate for attitude.

Surgical therapy for COPD: Three different surgical procedures have been used in sever COPD. One type of surgery is lung volume reduction therapy (LVRS). The goal of therapy is to reduce the size of the lungs by removing about 30 percent of the most diseased lung tissue so the remaining healthy lung tissue can perform better. The rationale for this type of surgery is that by reducing the size of the hyperinflated emphysematous lungs, there is decreased airway obstruction and increased room for the remaining normal alveoli to expand and function. The procedure reduces lung volume and improves lung and chest wall mechanics. There are different types of LVRS. In one approach a median sternotomy is performed and parts of each lung are removed and tissue reattached using a stapling device. Another approach is a video-assisted thoracoscopy that can be performed unilaterally or bilaterally. In this approach either a stapling or laser procedure can be done, or they can be done together. The most common postoperative complication is pneumonia. Another technique for LVRS is a minimally invasive technique via a bronchoscope. In certain patients LVRS has been shown to improve breathing, lung capacity and quality of life. However, it does not cure COPD. It is best used for patients with upper lobe emphysema. However, hospital costs of LVRS are high and it is still considered experimental.

The second surgical procedure is bullectomy. This procedure is used for patients with emphysematous COPD who have large bullae (>1 cm). The bullae are usually resected via thoracoscope. In certain patients this procedure has resulted in improved lung function and reduction in dyspnea.

The third surgical procedure is lung transplantation. COPD patients are the largest group of patient on waiting lists for lung transplantation. Although single-lung transplant is the most commonly used technique because of a shortage of donors, bilateral transplantation can be performed. In some cases LVRS is a bridge until transplantation. In appropriately selected patients with very advanced COPD, lung transplantation improves functional capacity and enhances quality of life. However, rejection and effects of immunosuppressive therapy remains an obstacle.

Respiratory and physical therapy: Respiratory therapy (RT) and physical therapy (PT) rehabilitation activities are performed by respiratory therapists or physical therapists depending on the institution. RT and/or PT activities include breathing retraining, effective cough techniques, and chest physiotherapy. RT is responsible for aerosol-nebulization therapy.

Breathing retraining: The patient with COPD develops an increased respiratory rate with a prolonged expiration to compensate for the obstruction to airflow resulting in dyspnea. In addition, the accessory muscles of breathing in the neck and upper part of the chest are used excessively to promote chest wall movement. These muscles are not designed for long-term use, and as a result the patient experiences increased fatigue. Breathing exercises may assist the patient during rest and activity (e.g. lifting, walking, stair climbing) by decreasing dyspnea, improving oxygenation, and slowing the respiratory rate. The main types of breathing exercises commonly taught are:

1. Pursed-lip breathing.
2. Diaphragmatic breathing.

The proposed rationale for using pursed-lip breathing (PLB) is to prolong exhalation and thereby prevent bronchiolar collapse and air trapping. Often instinctively patients will perform this technique. The patient should be taught PLB before, during, and after any causing dyspnea or tachypnea. The patient is taught to inhale slowly through the nose and then to exhale slowly through pursed lips, almost as if whistling. Exhalation should be at least three times as long as inhalation. It is helpful to have the nurse demonstrate the breathing exercises so the patient can imitate the action. The following techniques can be used to teach PLB:

1. Blow through a straw in a glass of water with the intent of forming small bubbles.
2. Blow at a lit candle enough to bend the flame without blowing it out.
3. Steadily blow a table-tennis ball across a table.
4. Blow a tissue held in the hand until it gently flaps.

Patients should be taught to use "just enough" positive pressure with the pursed lips because excessive resistance may increase the work of breathing. The issue of whether and how extensively PLB affects dyspnea is still questioned, but current evidence seems to support the use of PLB to improve the breathing of patients with COPD.

Diaphragmatic (abdominal) breathing focuses on using the diaphragm instead of the accessory muscles of the chest to:

1. Achieve maximum inhalation.
2. Slow the respiratory rate.

To date, evidence from controlled studies does not support the use of diaphragmatic breathing in patients with COPD patients. For patients with severe COPD, diaphragmatic breathing may result in hyperinflation because of increased fatigue and dyspnea and abdominal paradoxic breathing (the inward movement of the abdomen and the outward movement of the upper chest during inspiration) rather than with normal chest wall motion (the outward movement of the abdomen and upper chest simultaneously during inspiration).

The PLB slows the respiratory rate and is much easier to learn than diaphragmatic breathing. In the setting of extreme acute dyspnea when the patient is hospitalized for infection or heart failure, it is more important to focus on helping the patient slow the respiratory rate by using the principles of PLB.

The PLB is simple and easy to teach and learn. PLB should be practiced for 8 to 10 repetitions three or four times a day. PLB gives the patient more control over breathing, especially during exercise and periods of dyspnea.

Effective coughing: Many patients with COPD have developed ineffective coughing patterns that do not adequately clear their airways of sputum. In addition, they fear they may develop spastic coughing, resulting in increased dyspnea. Huff coughing is an effective technique that the patient can be easily taught. The main goals of effective coughing are to conserve energy, reduce fatigue and facilitate removal of secretions.

Chest physiotherapy: Chest physiotherapy (CPT) is indicated in the patient with:

1. Excessive bronchial secretions who has difficulty clearing secretions with expectorated sputum production greater than 25 mL per day.
2. Evidence or suggestion of retained secretions in the presence of an artificial airway.
3. Lobar atelectasis caused by or suspected of being caused by mucos plugging.

Chest physiotherapy consists of percussion, vibration, and postural drainage. Percussion and vibration are manual or mechanical techniques used to augment postural drainage. Postural drainage uses the principle of gravity to assist in bronchial drainage. Percussion and vibration are used after the patient has assumed a postural drainage position to assist in loosening the mobilized secretions. Percussion, vibration, and postural drainage may assist in bringing secretions into larger, more central airways. Effective coughing is then necessary to help raise these secretions. After each drainage position change, the patient should be given time to cough and deep breathe. These techniques are individualized based on the patient's pulmonary condition and response to the initial treatment. Sometimes, it takes several hours after CPT for secretions to be expectorated. It is important to evaluate CPT for both its effectiveness and relief of the patient's symptoms. CPT should be performed by an individual who has been properly trained. Complications associated with improperly performed CPT include fractured ribs, bruising, hypoxemia, and discomfort to the patient. CPT may not be beneficial and may be stressful for some patients. Some patients may develop hypoxemia and bronchospasms with CPT.

Percussion: Percussion is performed in the appropriate postural drainage with the hands in a cuplike position. The hands are cupped, and the fingers and thumbs are closed. The cupped hand should create an air pocket between the patient's chest and the hand. Both hands are cupped and used in an alternating rhythmic fashion. Percussion is accomplished with flexion and extension of the wrists. If it is performed correctly, a hollow sound should be heard. The air-cushion impact facilitates the movement of thick mucus. A thin towel should be placed over the area to be percussed, or the patient may choose to wear a T-shirt or hospital gown. The patients face should be in clear view when percussing in case a mucous plug occludes the airway and the patient is unable to speak. Percussion should not be performed over the kidneys, sternum, spinal cord, bony prominences, or may tender or painful area. Other contraindications to percussion include hemoptysis, carcinoma, and induced bronchospasm. Commercial devices that percuss are available if the patient lives alone and has no one to help with the therapy.

Vibration: Vibration is accomplished by tensing the hand and arm muscles repeatedly and pressing mildly with the flat of the hand on the affected area while the patient slowly exhales a deep breath. Isometric contractions of the arms and hands are also appropriate. The vibrations facilitate movement of secretions to larger airways. Mild vibration is tolerated better than percussion and can be used in situations where percussion may be contraindicated. Commercial vibrators are available for hospital and home use.

Postural drainage: The lungs are divided into five lobes, with three on the right side and two on the left side. There are 18 segments in the lungs, which can be drained by 18 positions. Figures 9.31 and 9.32 show the modified postural drainage positions most often used in clinical practice. The purpose of various positions in postural drainage is to drain each segment toward the larger airways. The postural drainage positions are determined by the areas of involved lung, which are assessed by chest X-rays, percussion, palpation, and auscultation. Aerosolized bronchodilators and hydration therapy are frequently administered before postural drainage. The chosen postural drainage position is maintained for 5 to 15 minutes or during percussion/vibration. The degree of slope can be obtained with pillows, blocks, books, or a tilt board.

The frequency and choice of postural drainage positions depend on the location of retained secretions and patient tolerance to dependent positions. A common order is two to four times a day. In acute situations, postural drainage may be performed as frequently as every 1 to 2 hours. The procedure should be planned to occur and be completed at least 1 hour before meals or 3 hours after meals.

If a patient has difficulty in assuming various positions, adaptations will be needed to reduce the angle or length of time of the procedure. A side-lying position can be used for the patient who cannot tolerate a head down position. There are also beds on the market that can rotate and percuss in various postural drainage positions. Some positions for postural drainage (e.g. Trendelenburg) should not be performed on the patient with trauma, hemoptysis, heart disease, or head injury, and in other situations where the patient's condition is not stable (Figs 9.31 and 9.32).

Flutter Mucus Clearance Device

The Flutter mucus clearance device is a handheld device that is shaped like a small, fat pipe. It provides expiratory pressure (PEP) treatment for patients with mucus-producing conditions. The Flutter has a mouthpiece, a high-density stainless steel ball, and a cone that holds the ball. When the patient exhales through the Flutter, the steel ball moves, which causes vibrations in the lungs and loosens mucus. It helps move mucus up through the airways to the mouth where the mucus can be expectorated.

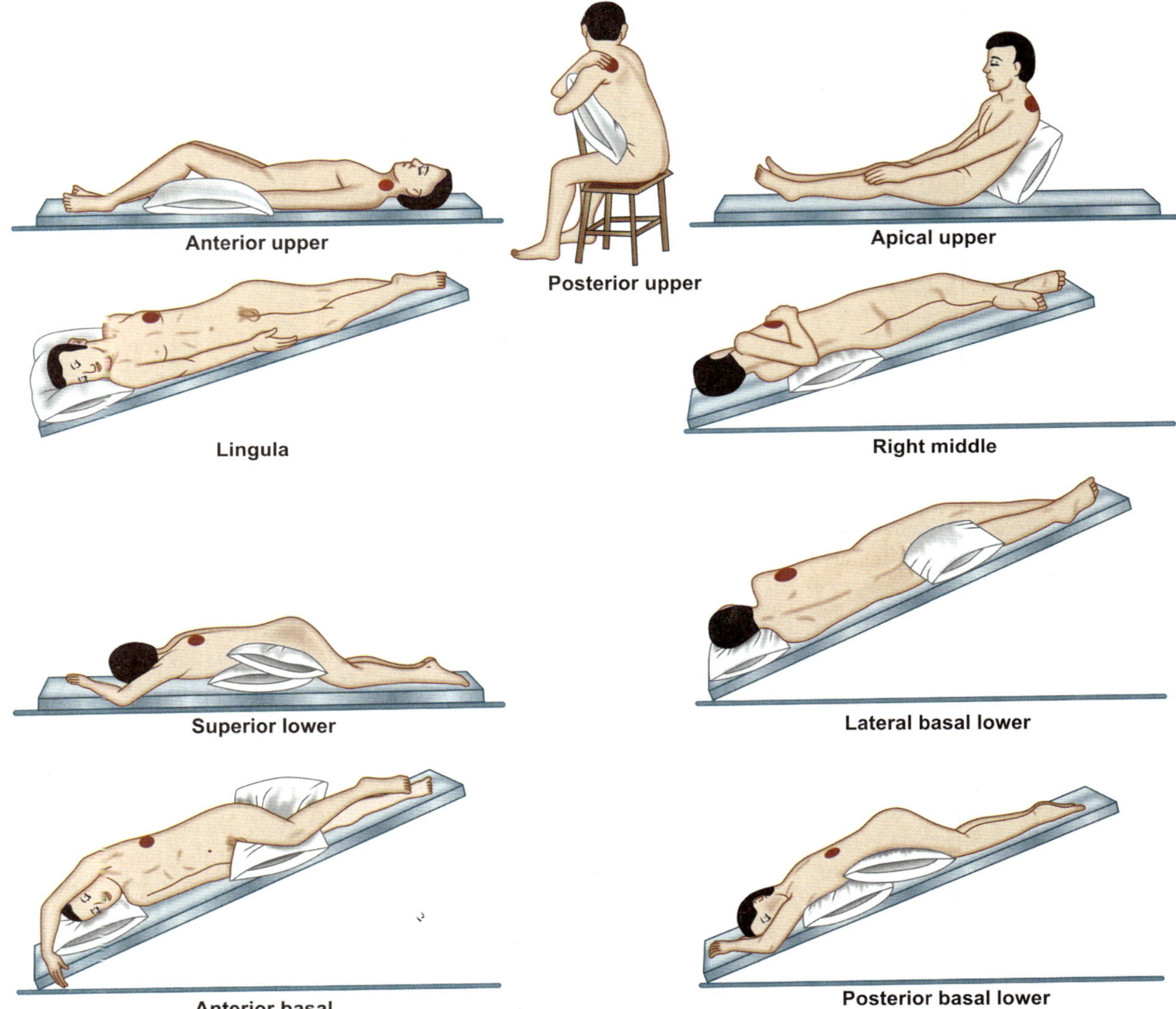

FIG. 9.31: Representative positions for postural drainage. Shaded areas in each drawing indicate the segment of the lung in which drainage is promoted

Although the Flutter valve is mostly used in patients with cystic fibrosis, it has been effectively used in patients with excessive secretions with COPD and bronchiectasis (Fig. 9.33).

High-Frequency Chest Compression (ThAIRapy Vest)

High-frequency chest compression uses an inflatable vest (ThAIRapy vest) with hoses connected to a high-frequency pulse generator. The pulse generator delivers air to the vest, which vibrates the chest. The high-frequency air waves clear all lobes of the lungs. The vest has been found to be more effective than conventional CPT in clearing mucus and it can be done without the aid of another person. The unit weighs only 30 lb and is quiet. It comes in its own suitcase and is portable.

Acapella

Acapella is a small handheld device that combines the benefits of both PEP therapy and airway vibrations of the Flutter valve to mobilize pulmonary secretions. It works by using oscillating vibrations that travel to the lung, shaking free mucus plugs that the patient can then cough up. It can be used in virtually any setting, as the patients are free to sit, stand or recline. It improves clearance of secretions, is easier to tolerate than CPT, takes less than half the time of conventional CPT sessions, and facilitates opening of airways.

Aerosol Nebulization Therapy

Medications for COPD patients are most often delivered via metered-dose or dry powder inhalers. This is the preferred

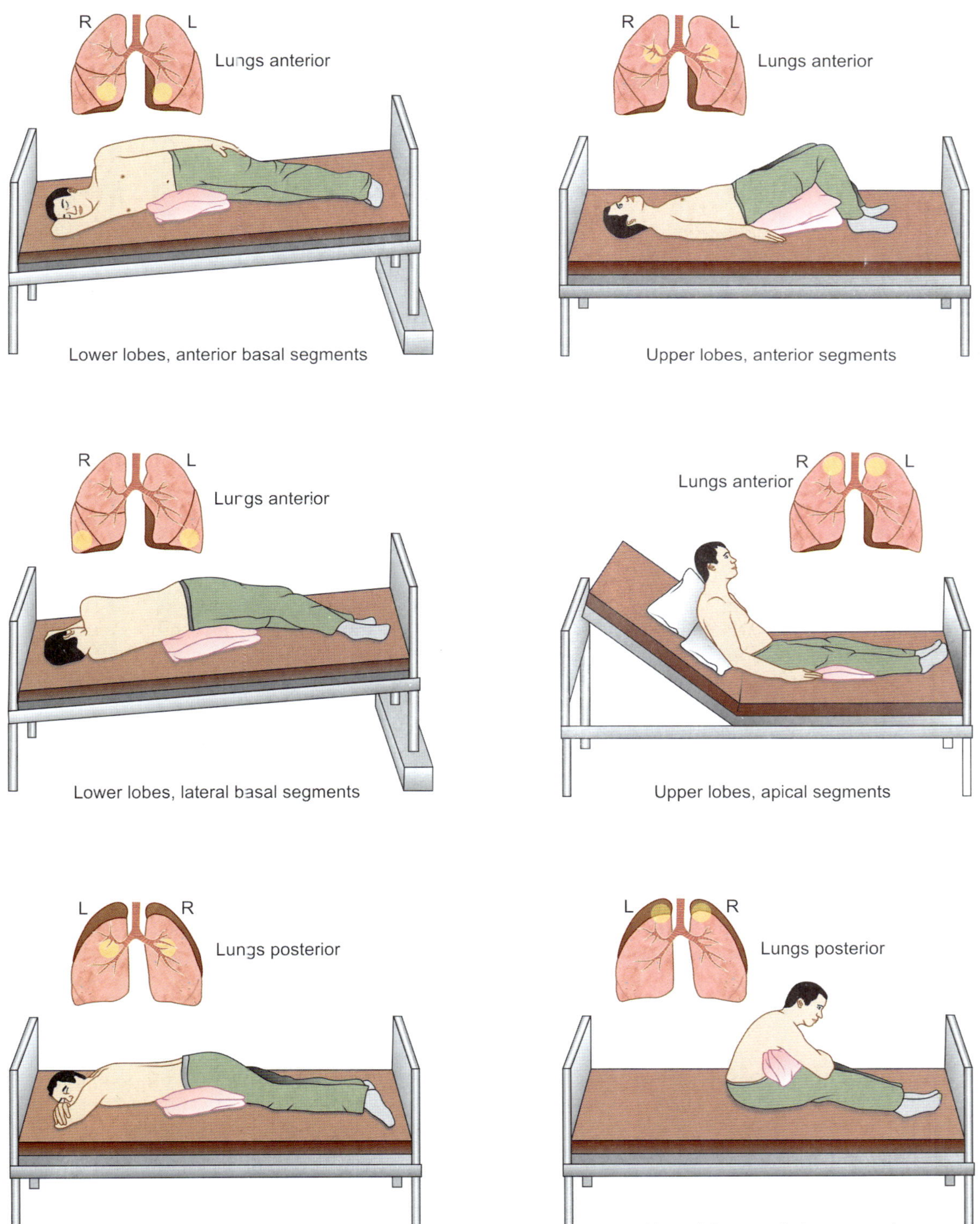

FIG. 9.32: Postural drainage positions and the areas of lungs drained by each position

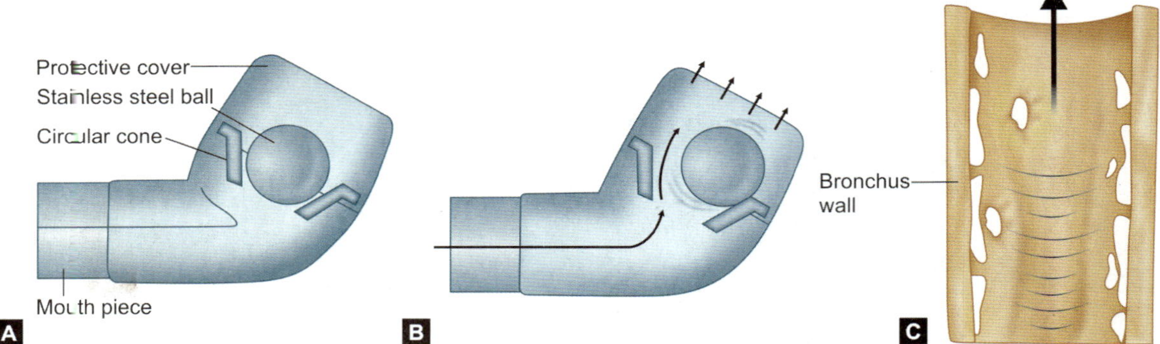

FIGS 9.33A TO C: Flutter mucus clearance device is a small handheld device that provides positive expiratory pressure (PEP) therapy. It is used to facilitate removal of mucus from the lungs. (A) It consists of a hard plastic, mouthpiece, a plastic perforated cover, and a high-density stainless steel ball resting in a circular cone; (B) The Flutter effects occur during expiration. Before exhalation, the steel ball blocks the conical canal of the Flutter. During exhalation, the position of the steel ball is the result of an equilibrium between the pressure of the exhaled air, the force of gravity on ball, and the angle of the cone where the contact with the ball occurs. As the steel ball rolls and moves up and down, it creates an opening and closing cycle that repeats itself many times throughout each exhalation. The net result is that vibrations occur in the airways resulting in the "fluttering" sensation; (C) These vibrations loosen mucus from the airway walls and facilitate their movement up the airways

delivery route, although devices that deliver a suspension of fine particles of liquid in a gas, called nebulizers, may also be used to deliver medications to the COPD patient. Nebulizers are usually powered by a compressed air or O_2 generator. At home the patient may have an air-powered compressor, in the hospital, wall O_2 or compressed air is used to power the nebulizer.

Aerosolized medication orders must include the medication, dose, diluent, and whether it is to be nebulized with O_2 or compressed air. Medication is nebulized or reduced to a fine spray, and depending on several factors, including droplet size, it can be inhaled into the patients tracheobronchial tree. The advantage to aerosol-nebulization therapy is that it is easy to use. Medications that are routinely nebulized include albuterol and ipratropium.

The patient is placed in an upright position that allows for most efficient breathing to ensure adequate penetration and deposition of the aerosolized medication. The patient must breathe slowly and deeply through the mouth and hold inspiration for 2 to 3 seconds. Deep diaphragmatic breathing helps ensure deposition of the medication. The patient is instructed to do normal breathing in between these large forced breaths to prevent alveolar hypoventilation and dizziness. After the treatment, the patient should be instructed to cough effectively. Postural drainage and CPT are ideally done after bronchodilator medications are given.

A disadvantage of nebulizer equipment use is the potential for bacterial growth. Because home nebulization is used for the patient with COPD, it is important for the health care professional in the hospital and home care setting to review cleaning procedures for home respiratory equipment with the patient. A frequently used, effective home-cleaning method is to wash the nebulizer daily in soap and water, rinse it with water, and soak it for 20 to 30 minutes in a 1:1 white vinegar-water solution followed by a water rinse and air drying. Commercial respiratory cleaning agents may also be used if directions are followed carefully. Cleaning the nebulizer in the top shelf of an automatic dishwater saves time, and the hot water destroys most organisms.

Nutritional Therapy

Weight loss and malnutrition are commonly seen in the patient with severe emphysematous COPD. The cause of this weight loss is not entirely known but is likely multifactorial. Eating becomes an effort because of dyspnea and O_2 desaturation, especially in the later stages COPD. Patients may require more caloric expenditure than calories ingested. A full stomach presses up on the flattened diaphragm, causing increased dyspnea and discomfort. It is difficult for some patient to eat and breathe at the same time; therefore inadequate amounts of food are eaten. Also large amounts of energy are expended to breathe and maintain even normal activities. Therefore, weight loss and muscle wasting are likely. Excessive weight loss is also related to increased energy inflammatory processes occurring in the lung, which may lead to a cachectic state.

The patient with COPD should try to keep body mass index (BMI) between 21 and 25 kg/m^2. Being either overweight or underweight can be problem with COPD. However, a reduced BMI or weight loss is associated with poor outcomes in acute exacerbations and increased morbidity and mortality rates in COPD patients.

To decrease dyspnea and conserve energy, the patient should rest for at least 30 minutes before eating, use a bronchodilator before meals, and select eat five to six small, frequent meals to avoid feelings of bloating and early satiety when eating. Liquid, blenderized, or commercial diets may be helpful. Foods that require a great deal of chewing should be avoided or served in another manner (e.g. grated, pureed). Cold foods may give less of a sense of fullness than hot foods. Exercises and treatments should be avoided for at least 1 hour before and after eating. The exertion involved in the preparation and eating of food is often fatiguing. The use of frozen foods and a microwave oven may help conserve the patient's energy in food preparation. The patients dentition should be assessed because broken, missing teeth or loose dentures make eating more difficult. Activity such as walking or getting out of bed during the day can stimulate the appetite and promote weight gain. Many patients with COPD have feelings of bloating and early satiety when eating. This sensation can be attributed to swallowing air while eating, side effects of medication (especially corticosteroids and theophylline), and the abnormal position of the diaphragm relative to the stomach in association with hyperinflation. Intestinal gas-forming foods should be avoided, such as cabbage, Brussels sprouts and beans.

Underweight patients with emphysematous COPD have a greater than normal nutritional requirement for protein and calories. They may need 25 to 45 kcal/kg and 1.2 to 1.9 g of protein per kilogram diet is recommended and can be divided into five or six small meals a day. High-protein, high-calorie nutritional supplements can be offered between meals. Ice cream added to these supplements can help increase calories. Drinking skim or 1 percent milk rather than whole milk may cause less mucus production. Nonprotein calories should be divided evenly between fat and carbohydrate while not overfeeding the patient. In most cases just getting the patients to eat adequate amounts of any foods can be difficult. The oral anabolic steroid, oxandrolone (Oxandrin), has shown promise in helping patients gain weight and improve muscle strength. Megestrol (Megace) has also been used to stimulate and increase appetite. If the patient has O_2 prescribed, use of supplemental O_2 by nasal cannulas while eating may also be beneficial, because eating expends energy. Fluid intake should be at least 3 L per day unless contraindicated for other medical conditions, such as heart or renal failure. Fluids should be taken between meals (rather than with them) to prevent excess stomach distension and to decrease pressure on the diaphragm. Sodium restriction may be indicated if there is accompanying heart failure.

Nursing Management

Assessment

Determining risk factors: Assess for risk factors such as cigarette, pipe, cigar or other kind of smoking or the passive inhalation of these products.

Obtaining health history: Obtain a history about current symptoms and previous disease manifestations:

- Duration of respiratory difficulty
- Dyspnea, shortness of breath, wheezing, exercise tolerance, fatigue
- Effect on eating and sleeping habits

Performing physical examination: Complete a thorough physical examination to obtain baseline data:

- Pulse, respiratory rate and rhythm
- Contraction of abdominal muscles during inspiration
- Use of accessory muscles to breathe; prolonged expiration
- Cyanosis, neck vein engorgement
- Peripheral edema
- Cough; color, amount and consistency of sputum
- Status of sensorium, increasing stupor, apprehension.

Diagnosis

Nursing Diagnoses

- Impaired gas exchange related to ventilation-perfusion inequality or inhalation to toxins
- Ineffective airway clearance related to bronchoconstriction, increased mucus production, ineffective cough and bronchopulmonary infection
- Ineffective breathing pattern related to shortness of breath, mucus, bronchoconstriction, and airway irritants
- Self-care deficit related to fatigue secondary to increased work of breathing and insufficient ventilation and oxygenation
- Activity intolerance due to fatigue, hypoxemia, and ineffective breathing patterns
- Ineffective coping related to less socialization, anxiety, depression, lower activity level and inability to work
- Deficient knowledge of self-care strategies to use at home.

Collaborative Problems/Potential Complications

- Respiratory insufficiency or failure
- Atelectasis
- Pneumonia and other pulmonary infection
- Pneumothorax
- Pulmonary hypertension.

Planning and Goals

Major goals of the patient include improved gas exchange, smoking cessation, improved breathing pattern, maximal self-management, improved activity tolerance, achievement of airway clearance, improved coping ability, improved health-related quality of life, and adherence to the therapeutic program and home care.

Objectives

- Demonstrates improved gas exchange
- Achieves maximal airway clearance
- Improves breathing pattern
- Maintains maximal level of self-care and physical functioning
- Achieves activity tolerance, and exercises and performs activities with less shortness of breath.

Nursing Diagnoses

Nursing diagnoses for the patient with CF include, but are not limited to, the following:

- Ineffective airway clearance related to abundant, thick bronchial mucus, weakness, and fatigue
- Ineffective breathing pattern related to bronchoconstriction, anxiety and airway obstruction
- Impaired gas exchange related to recurring lung infections
- Imbalanced nutrition: Less than body requirements related to dietary intolerances, intestinal gas and altered pancreatic enzyme production.

Planning

The overall goals are that the patient with CF will have:

- Adequate airway clearance
- Reduced risk factors associated with respiratory infections
- Adequate nutritional support to maintain appropriate BMI
- Ability to perform ADLs
- No complications related to CF
- Active participation in planning and implementing a therapeutic regimen.

Nursing Interventions

Improving Gas Exchange

- Monitor dyspnea and hypoxia
- Administer medications, and be alert for potential side effects
- Assess relief of bronchospasm through patient report of less dyspnea
- Monitor prescribed oxygen effectiveness with pulse oximetry or arterial blood gas (ABG) analysis.

Because hypoxemia is a stimulus for respiration in the patient with COPD, avoid depressing the respiratory drive when administering oxygen to correct hypoxemia.

Achieving Airway Clearance

- Encourage high fluid intake to liquefy secretions
- Instruct patient in directed or controlled coughing
- Provide chest physiotherapy with postural drainage and intermittent positive-pressure breathing (IPPB), when ordered
- Eliminate pulmonary irritants
- Instruct patient in effective breathing techniques
- Measure expiratory flow rates
- Teach breathing techniques to reduce respiratory rate and expel maximal air.

Preventing Bronchopulmonary infections

- Instruct patient to report signs of infection (e.g. fever; change in sputum color, character, consistency, or amount), and report any worsening of symptoms
- Advise patient to avoid outdoor exposure during high pollen counts or significant air pollution because these may increase bronchospasm. Also advise patient to avoid high temperatures and humidity as much as possible
- Encourage immunization against *Haemophilus influenzae* and *Streptococcus pneumoniae*. Also encourage yearly flu vaccination and pneumococcal vaccine every 5 to 7 years.

Improving Activity Tolerance

- Recommend the patient adopt a lifestyle of moderate activity, ideally in aclimate with minimal shift in temperature and humidity
- Encourage patient to avoid emotional disturbances and stressful situations
- Recommend strategies for smoking cessation and review progress with patient.

Promoting Home and Community-based Care

- Refer patient for home care as appropriate
- Demonstrate and supervise patient and family in performing all aspects of treatment regimen (e.g. metered-dose inhaler [MDI], IPPB, chest physiotherapy, and postural drainage), with return demonstration from patient before discharge.

Nursing Implementation

The nurse and other health professionals can assist young adults to gain independence by helping them assume responsibility for their care and for their vocational or school goals. An important issue that should be discussed is sexuality. Delayed or irregular menstruation is not uncommon. There may be delayed development of secondary sex characteristics such as breasts in girls. The person may use the illness to avoid certain events or relationships. The healthy person may hesitate to make friends with someone who is sick. Other crises and life transitions that must be dealt with in the young adult include building confidence and self-respect on the basis of achievements, persevering with employment goals, developing motivation to achieve, learning to cope with the treatment program, and adjusting to the need for dependence if health fails. Disclosing the CF diagnosis to friends, potential spouses, or employers may pose challenges emotionally and financially.

The issue of marrying and having children is difficult. Genetic counseling may be an appropriate suggestion for the couple considering having children. Most men with CF are sterile. Women with the disease may have difficulty becoming pregnant. In addition, any children produced will either be carriers of CF or have the disease. Another concern is the shortened life span of the parent with CF, and the parent's ability to care for the child must be taken into consideration.

Nursing care plan for COPD patient is listed in Table 9.3.

TABLE 9.3: Nursing care plan for the patient with chronic obstructive pulmonary disease in acute respiratory failure

Problems	Objectives	Nursing interventions	Rationales
Nursing Diagnosis # 1			
Airway clearance, ineffective, related to copious, thick, tenacious secretions	Patient will: • Be alert and oriented to person, place, time • Demonstrate deep breathing techniques and effective secretion-clearing cough • Minimize risk of aspiration Arterial blood gases will stabilize: • pH > 7.35 < 7.45 • PaO_2 > 60 mm Hg • $PaCO_2$ at level to maintain pH within acceptable range	• Perform a comprehensive respiratory assessment including: – Airway patency; rate, rhythm, and depth of breathing; chest and diaphragmatic excursion – Use of accessory muscles; presence of intercostal retraction – Auscultation of breath sounds • Monitor quality, quantity, color and consistency of sputum – Obtain sputum for culture and sensitivity on admission, and thereafter as dictated by patient's conditon – Assess secretions for state of hydration or need for mucolytic therapy – Monitor body temperature and white blood count profile • Institute prescribed bronchodilator therapy – Assess pulmonary function prior to and after bronchodilator therapy – Assist into semi-Fowler's position – Monitor for signs/symptoms of bronchodilator therapy toxicity (especially when theophylline or theophylline salts are used) ◆ Monitor theophylline level • Initiate chest physiotherapy techniques: – Postural drainage; percussion and vibration; deep breathing and coughing • Teach appropriate method of coughing – Avoid unnecessary or ineffective coughing • Institute pharyngeal and tracheobronchial suctioning as needed – Follow appropriate procedure for endotracheal suctioning • Instruct patient in use of incentive spirometry	• Major goal of airway management is to establish and/or maintain adequate alveolar ventilation – Baseline data are essential to evaluate effectiveness of therapeutic interventions – Increased work of breathing may be caused by small airway obstruction – May detect evidence of secretion accumulation, airway obstruction, atelectasis • Baseline data enable changes in sputum production and characteristics to be identified. Infection or other pulmonary insult may increase quantity of sputum production – Thinning of secretions facilitates mobilization and clearance – Early detection of an infectious or inflammatory process affords prompt intervention to minimize the effect of the insult on pulmonary and other body processes – Assists in determining effectiveness of therapy – Allows for best possible lung expansion – Theophylline and derivatives have a narrow therapeutic index • Loosens and dislodges secretions and enhances movement towards trachea from where they are accessible to removal by cough and/or suctioning • Achieve most effective cough with least amount of effort – May cause irritation of tracheo-bronchial tree • Suctioning is not without risks (hypoxemia, atelectasis, infection); it should be performed only as indicated. – Aseptic technique is essential to minimize risk of infection; oxygenation reduces risk of hypoxemia

Contd...

Contd...

Problems	Objectives	Nursing interventions	Rationales
		• Provide opportunity for rest periods – Schedule activities to avoid fatigue • Assure hydration state – Monitor intake and output; daily weight • Use a calm, reassuring approach – Anticipate needs for emotional support – Be accessible and offer explanations – Involve in decision-making regarding care when possible	• Increases vital capacity and helps to more evenly match ventilation with perfusion • Reduces oxygen demand; reduces fatigue • Adequate hydration moistens, loosens, and liquefies secretions • Assists to reduce anxiety – An informed patient is usually a cooperative patient – Allows patient to retain some control over his/her life
Nursing Diagnosis # 2			
Breathing pattern, ineffective, related to reduced maximum expiratory airflow (see Nursing Diagnosis # 11 below)	Patient will: 1. Demonstrate effective minute ventilation: Tidal volume (V_T) > 5–7 mL/kg Respiratory rate < 35/min (adult) 2. Achieve a vital capacity (V_C) > 12–15 mL/kg 3. Verbalize ease of breathing 4. Demonstrate pursed lip and diaphragmatic breathing 5. Exhibit breath sounds: – Audible throughout anterior/posterior chest. Reduced to absent adventitious sounds	• Assess respiratory function: – Rate, rhythm, depth, and pattern of breathing – Symmetry of chest wall and diaphragmatic excursion – Coordination of contraction of inspiratory and expiratory muscles – Use of accessory muscles – Auscultation of breath sounds – Pulmonary lung volumes: Total minute ventilation (V_E), tidal volume (V_T), respiratory rate (f), vital capacity (V_C). • Assist patient into position of comfort and to allow for best lung expansion – Low to semi-Fowler's position; unaffected side down in side-lying position – Provide table with pillow for patient to lean on • Teach breathing techniques: – Pursed-lip breathing – Diaphragmatic breathing – Avoid lying flat (supine) – Avoid hyperventilation – Controlled breathing: Slower, of increased depth; use abdominal muscles – Encourage hourly deep breathing in conjunction with chest physiotherapy techniques and bronchodilator therapy	– Reflect work of breathing: Increased work of breathing increases oxygen consumption and results in hypercapnia and physical fatigue/exhaustion – Effective ventilation requires synchronous movement of chest wall, diaphragm, and abdominal wall – Rapid, shallow respirations (tachypnea hyperventilation) move deadspace air, significantly reducing alveolar ventilation – Asymmetry of respiratory excursion may reflect underlying pathology (e.g. atelectasis, pneumothorax) – Ventilatory dyscoordination (a disordered sequence of the contraction of muscles of inspiration and expiration) may be an early but subtle clue as to the development of ARF – A minimal volume of ventilation is necessary to ensure adequate alveolar ventilation – Assessment of respiratory volumes allow close evaluation of effectiveness and efficiency of respiratory effort • Expansion of lungs facilitates more even distribution of ventilation; improves ventilation/perfusion matching – Reduces ventilation/perfusion mismatch – Increases expiratory airway resistance which functions to keep airways open longer to allow airflow and to reduce a trapping – Lifting of abdominal wall upward and onward allows for easier excursion of diaphragm by decreasing pressure within the abdomen – Causes abdominal contents to shift toward chest cavity, limiting diaphragmatic excursion; may predispose to atelectasis

Contd...

Contd...

Problems	Objectives	Nursing interventions	Rationales
			– May predispose to metabolic alkalosis and patient with chronic lung disease – Conscious control of breathing increased effectiveness of respiratory effort – Minimizes atelectasis; mobilizes section; improves ventilation
Nursing Diagnosis # 3			
Gas exchange, impaired, related to: 1. Alveolar hypoventilation 2. Ventilation/ perfusion mismatch 3. Diffusion impaired 4. Right-to-left shunting	Patient will: 1. Be alert and oriented to person, place, time 2. Demonstrate appropriate behavior 3. Maintain effective cardiovascular function: – Blood pressure within 10 mm Hg of baseline – Cardiac output ~5 liters/min – Without cyanosis if baseline "pink" – Lab values: Hematocrit Male: 45–52 percent Female: 37–48 percent Haemoglobin > 10–12 g/100 mL 4. Maintain optimal arterial blood gases: – pH 7.35–7.45 – PaO_2 > 60 mm Hg – $PaCO_2$ at level to preserve normal pH 5. Maintain alveolar-arterial gradient ($AaDO_2$): Within acceptable range based on FIO_2	• Perform neurologic examination including: – Mental status; level of consciousness; appropriateness of behavior – Deep tendon reflexes – Complaints of headache, dizziness, nervousness, restlessness • Avoid sedatives, narcotics, hypnotics, tranquilizers • Monitor vital signs including: – Blood pressure, heart rate – Respiratory rate; work of breathing – Evidence of distress; undue fatigue; secretion build-up • Monitor laboratory data: – Arterial blood gases: – Calculate alveolar-arterial gradient ($AaDO_2$) – Observe for decreasing PaO_2 and pH, and increasing $PaCO_2$; bicarbonate (HCO_3^-) is elevated. – Hematology profile: Hematocrit (Hct) – Hemoglobin (Hgb) • Administer prescribed oxygen concentration: – Use low-flow supplemental oxygen therapy ◆ 24–28% by Venturi mask ◆ 2–3 liters/min by nasal cannula. – Monitor arterial blood gases at regular intervals – Prevent complications related to precipitous decrease in $PaCO_2$. • Monitor criteria for acute respiratory failure – Additional considerations: Evidence of respiratory distress, "air hunger," secretion build up, undue fatigue • Intubate and initiate mechanial ventilation therapy when criteria for acute respiratory failure have been identified	• Hypercapnia may predispose to carbon dioxide narcosis with depression of central respiratory centers – Hypoxemia may predispose to cerebral tissue hypoxia • Depress central respiratory centers predisposing to alveolar hypoventilation with hypercapnia; may mask signs of significant carbon dioxide retention • Circulatory impairment will interfere with adequate gas exchange within lungs and at tissue levels: – Increased work of breathing increases oxygen consumption and demand; predisposes to tissue hypoxia – Most closely reflect effectiveness of gas exchange – Limitation of $AaDO_2$ is that it does not look at cardiopulmonary function as a whole – Patients with COPD will have a different range of normal than healthy individuals – Increased HCO_3^- reflects renal compensation (i.e. reabsorption of HCO_3^-) in response to decreased blood pH caused by hypercapnia – Sufficient red blood cells and hemoglobin are required for gas exchange to occur. In patients with long standing COPD, hematology should be monitored for polycythemia vera. • Alveolar hypoventilation and V/Q mismatch respond favorably to low-flow supplemental oxygen therapy – Overzealous oxygen therapy can wipe out hypoxic drive in patients with COPD – Reflect effectiveness of lungs in gas exchange – When ventilation has been interrupted (e.g. suctioning) or the FIO_2 has changed, blood sample for analysis should not be obtained for at least 20 minutes after therapy

Contd...

Contd...

Problems	Objectives	Nursing interventions	Rationales
			• Patients with COPD may experience difficult weaning from mechanical ventilatory therapy. Timely and aggressive implementation of respiratory support therapies (O_2 therapy, chest physiotherapy, treatment of underlying causes) may successfully prevent need for intubation and mechanical ventilation
Nursing Diagnosis # 4			
Cardiac output, alteration in: Decreased (diminished venous return) *Nursing Diagnosis #5* Tissue perfusion, alteration in: Cardiopulmonary	Patient will: 1. Maintain stable hemodynamics: – Blood pressure within 10 mm Hg baseline – Heart rate < 100 beats/min – Cardiac output ~5 liters/min – Central venous pressure (CVP) 0–8 mm Hg – Pulmonary capillary wedge pressure (PCWP) 8–12 mm Hg 2. Remain without: – Extreme weakness or fatigue – Peripheral (pedal) edema – Neck vein distention – Chest pain – Cardiac dysrhythmias 3. Maintain fluid and electrolyte balance: – Stable body weight – Balanced intake and output – Hourly urine output > 30 mL/h	• Perform ongoing cardiovascular assessment: – Continuous cardiac monitoring (establish baseline rate, rhythm, ectopy). – Continuous haemodynamic monitoring (establish baseline): CVP, PCWP – Heart sounds—loudness or intensity, splitting, extra heart sounds (S_3–S_4)? – Breath sounds—evidence of rales (crackles); altered pulmonary mechanics? – Fatigue, exhaustion? – Neck vein distention? Pedal edema? – Serial arterial blood gases • Implement fluid replacement therapy as prescribed. – Monitor hydration status: Daily weight, intake and output, urine specific gravity – Avoid fluid volume overload	– Cardiac tissue hypoxia may predispose to dysrhythmias – Offers significant data regarding cardiopulmonary function – Positive-pressure mechanical ventilation increases pressure within the thorax, which impedes venous return to the heart; decrease in venous return (preload) reduces cardiac output – Loud pulmonic sound or splitting is commonly seen in cor pulmonale; it is related to pulmonary hypertension due to long-standing hypoxemic state – In the patient with COPD, diminished breath sounds in a heretofore "noisy" chest may warn of hypoventilation with impending acute respiratory failure • Adequate fluid replacement therapy is essential to maintain blood volume and keep pulmonary secretions moist and easily mobilized – Long-standing pulmonary disease with pulmonary hypertension predisposes to right heart failure (cor pulmonale)
Nursing Diagnosis # 6			
Tissue perfusion, alteration in: Cerebral	Patient will: 1. Demonstrate appropriate behavior: – Oriented to person, place, time	• Assess ongoing neurologic function – Mental status, level of consciousness; behavior appropriate? • Assess fluid and electrolyte status. – Body weight – Intake and output (hourly urine output) – Serum electrolytes, BUN, creatinine • Maintain a quiet, relaxed milieu. – Use a calm, reassuring approach – Provide explanations of care – Provide frequent periods of rest and relaxation	• Compromised hemodynamics and hypoxemia predispose to cerebral hypoxemia with altered cerebral function • Reduced blood volume will further compromise venous return and cardiac output; blood volume may need to be expanded to minimize this effect – Reduced cardiac output may diminish renal perfusion, placing patient at risk of developing acute renal failure • Minimize fear and anxiety, which increases oxygen consumption and demand

Contd...

Contd...

Problems	Objectives	Nursing interventions	Rationales
		• Monitor for effects of drugs (e.g. theophylline) on cardiopulmonary function	– The work of breathing is often taxing; it is important to conserve patient's energy • Drug toxicity may further compromise cardiopulmonary function
Nursing Diagnosis # 7			
Fluid and electrolyte, alterations in	Patient will: 1. Maintain baseline body weight 2. Balance fluid intake with output 3. Have: – Good skin turgor – Absence of peripheral edema – Absence of rales (crackles) on auscultation – Stable vital signs 4. Stabilize in terms of serum electrolyte, BUN, creatinine, total protein within acceptable physiologic range	• Monitor hydration status: – Daily weight, intake and output, vital signs – Examine skin for signs of dehydration: Poor skin turgor; sunken eyeballs; dry, parched mucous membranes – Monitor mental status changes; lethargy; severe weakness; reduced urine output. – Examine for signs of overhydration: peripheral edema; hypertension; tachycardia; neck vein distention; elevated pulmonary hemodynamics; shortness of breath, dyspnea. • Monitor serum electrolytes, BUN, creatinine, total protein	• Patients receiving mechanical ventilation with humidified gas therapy are at risk to increase total body water. – Stress increases secretion of antidiuretic hormone (ADH) by posterior pitulitary gland, increasing water retention – Stress increases aldosterone secretion by adrenal cortex, which stimulates sodium reabsorption within the kidneys
Nursing Diagnosis # 8			
Acid-base balance, alteration in, related to overzealous oxygen therapy in the patient with long standing COPD	The patient's arterial blood gases will stabilize as follows: • pH 7.35–7.45 • PaO_2 > 60 mm Hg • $PaCO_2$, sufficiently reduced to maintain pH within acceptable range for the patient	• Administer oxygen therapy cautiously at prescribed concentration (FIO_2) – Closely monitor arterial blood gas values ◆ $PaCO_2$ must only be reduced to the level that "normalizes" pH	• In patients with long-standing COPD with chronic hypercapnia and consequent acidemia, the kidneys respond (compensate) by reabsorbing bicarbonate (HCO_3^-). This buffers the excess hydrogen ions associated with the hypercapnia and stabilizes the pH – Overzealous administration of oxygen can cause a precipitous fall in the $PaCO_2$, reducing hydrogenion concentration while leaving excess bicarbonate. The result is metabolic alkalemia, which, if sufficiently severe, can lead to serious cardiac dysrhythmias and seizures
Nursing Diagnosis # 9			
Nutrition, alteration in: Less than body requirements	Patient will: 1. Maintain body weight with 5% of baseline weight. 2. Maintain total serum proteins ~6.0–8.4 g/100 mL 3. Maintain laboratory data within acceptable range: BUN, serum creatinine, electrolytes, fasting blood sugar, serum albumin, hematology profile	• Arrange consultation with nutritionist and collaborate to perform nutrition assessment: General state of health; baseline body weight; nutritional history: Likes, dislikes, meal preparation, eating habits, cultural, religious considerations. – Lifestyle influences – Physiologic factors: Height, weight, triceps skinfold, mid-upper arm circumference	• Adequate nutritional intake is necessary to meet metabolic requirements to reverse acute respiratory failure – Nutritional deficiencies (especially in elderly) are often associated with chronic disease • Clinical semi-starvation leads to depression of the hypoxic ventilatory drive – Patients receiving mechanical ventilation therapy are highly stressed and require nutritional supplements to meet hypermetabolic needs

Contd...

Contd...

Problems	Objectives	Nursing interventions	Rationales
	4. Verbalize essentials of adequate diet	– Laboratory studies: Urinary/serum creatinine, BUN, fasting blood sugar, serum electrolytes, total protein (serum albumin), hematology profile • Maintain adequate nutrition with prescribed enteral and/or parenteral feedings – Special considerations – Avoid large glucose loads to meet caloric needs – Avoid hypophosphatemia – Avoid high amino acid loads • Place patient in optimal position during feedings (usually semi-Fowler's position) • Confirm placement of nasogastric tube in stomach before initiating feedings – Assess for protective reflexes (gag, cough, swallowing) • Provide frequent mouth care and other comfort measures • Monitor daily weight; fluid and intake • Assess bowel function: – Assess bowel sounds – Initiate bowel regimen, if indicated	– There is an obligate increase in carbon dioxide with increased glucose intake. Fat emulsions may be used to provide calories – In patients who are mechanically ventilated or who have reduced respiratory reserve, the increased carbon dioxide can lead to hypercapnia and may precipitate acute respiratory failure in the high risk patient – Reduced phosphate levels are associated with decreased energy levels, respiratory muscle weakness, and increased risk of infection – Increase O_2 consumption • Proper positioning and intact protective reflexes reduce risk of aspiration • Proper placement of nasogastric tube helps to prevent aspiration • May be esthetically pleasing to patient/family – Keep mucous membranes moist and intact – Maintains gastrointestinal smooth muscle tone; prevents constipation or impaction
Nursing Diagnosis #10			
Essential for	Patient will: 1. Maintain normal body temperature ~98.6°F (37°C) 2. Maintain white blood count at acceptable baseline level 3. Remain without evidence of acute infection: Redness, swelling, pain	• Identify patients at high-risk of developing an infection: Debilitated or elderly, chronic lung disease, multiple invasive lines, semistarvation state, immunosuppressed • Obtain baseline cultures: Sputum, urine, blood • Monitor the following parameters: – Body temperature – Hematology profile—evidence of leukocytosis; eosinophilia – Sputum for changes in color, quantity, consistency, odor; and ability of patient to handle secretions – Chest X-ray for pulmonary infiltrates • Institute vigorous chest physiotherapy and bronchial hygiene • Use aseptic technique for patient care: Tracheobronchial suctioning, care of invasive lines • Administer prescribed antibiotic therapy. – Monitor culture and sensitivity studies to assess response to therapy • Maintain nutrition	• Patients with COPD are especially at high risk due to: – Alteration in surfactant activity – Alterations in respiratory epithelium replication • Upon intubation, a baseline sputum specimen should be obtained – Use of artificial airway (endotracheal tube or tracheostomy) contaminates the tracheobronchial tree, which is usually considered to be sterile distal to the larynx • Early diagnosis with institution of timely and vigorous therapy (antibiotic) may help to minimize the impact of the infectious process on total body function • Secretion removal improves ventilation and reduces pooling of secretions, which may act as foci of infection • Reduces risks of infection

Contd...

Contd...

Problems	Objectives	Nursing interventions	Rationales
Nursing Diagnosis#11			
Pulmonary mechanics, alteration in, related to respiratory muscle atrophy (immobility, mechanical ventilation; see Nursing Diagnosis #2 above).	Patient will: 1. Perform deep breathing exercises. 2. Achieve maximum pulmonary function: – Tidal volume > 7 mL/kg – Vital capacity > 15 mL/kg – Maximal expiratory flow	• Teach deep breathing exercises – Instruct regarding the importance of deep-breathing exercises – Allow patient to demonstrate pulmonary exercises – Combine deep-breathing therapy with other chest physiotherapy maneuvers – Involve patient/family in decision-making (e.g. scheduling of exercise activities) – Encourage early ambulation (e.g. sitting up in chair) • Assess pulmonary volumes to determine effectiveness of therapy: Tidal volume, vital capacity	• Use of positive-pressure ventilation predisposes of atrophy of the respiratory musculature, which can present problems for weaning. – Improves pulmonary ventilation, mobilizes secretions, stimulates circulation – Teaching regarding pulmonary mechanics forms the foundation of patient's self-care after hospitalization – Patient should be allowed to learn one task before proceeding to the next. Always establish readiness to learn on the part of patient and family – The nature of chronic illness requires cooperation of all family members if exacerbations are to be prevented – Involvement in planning and decision-making enables patient/ family to begin to assume responsibility for their own lives
Nursing Diagnosis#12			
Skin integrity, impairment of, related to immobility, and altered nutritional status	Patient's skin will remain intact	• Establish routine for turning and repositioning • Assist with range-of-motion exercises to extremities – Provide support stockings to lower extremities – Assess extremities for calf tenderness – Measure circumference of thighs and calves daily • Provide special skin care to back and joints, and all pressure points – Establish regimen for: Skin inspection, skin care, decubitus care if necessary – Provide "egg-crate" or air mattress; sheep-skin; heel and ankle protectors – Apply local skin care	• Exercise maintains muscle tone and prevents muscle atrophy • Exercise stimulates circulation and prevents stasis – Immobility predisposes to thrombophlebitis • Maintains circulation to all areas; these patients frequently have a compromised body defense system and are at high risk of infection – It is essential to prevent skin breakdown – Pressure relief devices
Nursing Diagnosis#13			
Fear *Nursing Diagnosis#14* Knowledge deficit regarding chronic obstructive pulmonary disease	Patient/family will: 1. He ....verbalize fears and concerns 2. Identity strengths and coping capabilities 3. Verbalize knowledge regarding COPD 4. Verbalize intentions to make necessary adjustments in lifestyle 5. Demonstrate ability to carry out necessary interventions 6. Demonstrate self-confidence in their capabilities	• Assess knowledge regarding COPD and ex-... • Verbalize fears and concerns for patient and family • Help them to recognise and to express their feelings regarding disruption in their lifestyle – Encourage them to express fears regarding chronicity of disease: Necessity of oxygen therapy in the home setting; specific medication/ other therapies • Assess readiness to learn – Have patient/family assist in identifying needs and learning objectives • Assist family in problem-solving techniques – Help them identify family strengths and resources – Initiate referral to social services for necessary support: emotional, psychologic, financial, other	• Chronic lung disease is a "family disease" impacting every member to some degree • If the patient/family are to realize optimal function within the limitations of the disease, all family members should be involved in the educating and caring processes • Assists family in coping; increases self-confidence in their own capabilities – It is reassuring to have specific resources available to lend assistance and support

Teaching about Pulmonary Rehabilitation and Self-care

- Identify candidates for rehabilitation, and reinforce material learned in rehabilitation program
- Plan actions with patient to restore highest level of independent function and to improve quality of life; attend to both physiologic and emotional needs; help patient to accept realistic short-term and long-range goals
- Reinforce breathing exercises and retraining and exercise programs, and teach patient methods to alleviate symptoms. Instruct patient in activity pacing (avoiding activities requiring arm lifting and movement until after patient has been up and moving around for an hour or more)
- If prescribed, assist patient in learning inspiratory muscle training; breathing against resistance for 10 to 15 minutes every day, and increasing the resistance gradually. Then teach patient ways to coordinate diaphragmatic breathing with activities such as walking, bathing, bending and climbing stairs
- Encourage patient to begin gradually to bathe, dress and take short walks, resting as needed to avoid fatigue and excessive dyspnea, and to keep fluids readily available
- Educate patient about normal anatomy and physiology of the lung, pathophysiology and changes with COPD, medications and home oxygen therapy, nutrition, respiratory therapy treatments, symptom alleviation, smoking cessation, sexuality, coping with chronic disease, communicating with the health care team, and planning for the future (advance directives, living wills, informed decisions about health care alternatives)
- Assess nutritional and caloric needs and counsel patient about meal planning and nutritional supplementation
- If ordered, assist patient to adhere to the oxygen prescription by explaining the proper flow rate and required number of hours for oxygen use as well as the dangers of arbitrary changes in flow rates or duration of therapy. Reassure patient that oxygen is not "addictive," and explain the need to have regular evaluations of blood oxygenation by pulse oximetry of ABG analysis
- Inform patient that smoking with or near oxygen is extremely dangerous
- Teach proper use of bronchodilators, inhalers
- Teach coping measures (e.g. remaining active up to level of symptom tolerance; how to control symptoms to increase self-esteem, sense of mastery, and well-being; and use of support groups
- Arrange specific services for patient (e.g. respiratory therapy education, physical therapy for exercise and breathing retraining, and occupational therapy for conservation of energy during activities of daily living)
- Inform patient and family of resources (see also Table 9.3).
- Teaching is essential and should be tailored to the stage of COPD.

Monitoring and Managing Complications

- Assess patient for complications (respiratory insufficiency and failure, respiratory infection, and atelectasis). Teach proper use of bronchodilator medications to help prevent complications
- Monitor for cognitive changes, increasing dyspnea, tachypna and tachycardia
- Monitor pulse oximetry values and administer oxygen as prescribed
- Instruct patient and family about signs and symptoms of infection or other complications and to report changes in physical or cognitive status
- Emphasize that if condition worsens to the point of acute respiratory failure, intubation and mechanical ventilation will be necessary (Box 9.15).

Acute intervention for the patient with CF includes relief of bronchoconstriction, airway obstruction, and airflow limitation. Interventions include aggressive CPT, antibiotics, O_2 therapy, and corticosteroids in severe disease. Good nutrition is important to support the immune system. Advances in long-term vascular access (e.g. implanted ports) have made IV access and administration of medication much easier. This has also eased the transition for IV treatment at home.

Box 9.15 Caring for patients who are mechanically ventilated

- Introduce yourself to the patient each time you enter the room. Make sure he or she can see you
- Explain everything you are about to do
- Check ventilator settings regularly
- Give sedatives or antianxiety drugs as ordered. Request an order if necessary. Find out cause of unexplained anxiety (patient may be hypoxemic)
- Reassure the patient that anxiety is normal and that relaxing will help the ventilator to work with him or her
- Assess for comfort and reposition at regular intervals. Be careful not to pull on the ventilator tubing (pulling hurts)
- Suction quickly and smoothly, without jabbing. Avoid the use of saline with suctioning
- Provide good oral care, moistening the lips with a cool washcloth and water-based lubricant (patients get thirsty)
- Use restraints only as a last resort
- Take the time to communicate with the patient. Talk to him or her, and provide a magic slate or pen and paper so the patient can "talk" to you. Make sure the call light is within reach at all times
- Answer patient's call light ventilator alarms promptly.

CPT is the mainstay of intervention for ineffective airway clearance for these patients. Home management of cystic fibrosis includes an aggressive plan of postural drainage with percussion and vibration, use of mucus-clearing devices and techniques (discussed earlier in the chapter), aerosol-nebulization therapy, and breathing retraining. The patient is taught controlled coughing techniques, deep-breathing exercises, and progressive exercise conditioning such as a bicycling program.

The family and the person with CF have a great financial and emotional burden. The cost of drugs, special equipment, and health care is often a financial hardship. Because most CF patients live to childbearing age, family planning and genetic counseling are important. The burden of living with a chronic disease at a young age can be emotionally overwhelming. Community resources are often available to help the family. In addition, the Cystic Fibrosis Foundation can be of assistance. As the person continues toward and into adulthood, the nurse and other skilled health professionals should be available to help the patient and family cope with complications resulting from the disease.

BRONCHIECTASIS

Etiology

Bronchiectasis is characterized by permanent, abnormal dilation of one or more large bronchi. The pathophysiologic change that results in dilation is destruction of the elastic and muscular structures supporting the bronchial wall. The disease process results in a reduced ability to clear mucus from the lungs and decreased expiratory airflow. Thus, bronchiectasis is classified as an obstructive lung disease.

Pathophysiology

A variety of pathophysiologic processes can result in bronchiectasis. There can be primary disorders of structures in the bronchi (cartilage defects), diseases of mucus clearance (CF), infectious etiologies (severe childhood bronchial infections), and inflammatory diseases (ulcerative colitis). Bronchiectasis can cause generalized effects on the lungs, as seen with CF, or the pattern may be more localized in a segment of the lung. Most frequently infection is the primary reason for the continuing cycle of inflammation, airway damage, and remodeling. Bronchiectasis can follow a severe pneumonia, with a wide variety of infectious agents initiating bronchiectasis, including adenovirus, influenza virus, *S. aureus, Klebsiella*, and anaerobes. Infections cause the bronchial walls to weaken, and pockets of infection begin to form. When the walls of the bronchial system are injured, the mucociliary mechanism is damaged, allowing bacteria and mucus to accumulate within the pockets. The infection becomes worse and results in bronchiectasis.

Clinical Manifestations

The hallmark of bronchiectasis is persistent or recurrent cough with production of large amounts of purulent sputum that may exceed 500 mL/day. However, some patients with severe disease and upper lobe involvement may have no sputum production and little cough. The other manifestations of bronchiectasis are dyspnea, wheezing, pleuritic chest pain, and hemoptysis. On auscultation of the lungs, crackles are the most common finding, but wheezing is also found in about one third of the patients. Hemoptysis may occur during the frequent infections and it can be massive, thus necessitating immediate medical care.

Diagnostic Studies

An individual with a chronic productive cough with copious purulent sputum (which may be blood streaked) should be suspected of having bronchiectasis. Chest X-rays are usually done and may show some nonspecific abnormalities. High-resolution CT (HRCT) scan of the chest is the gold standard for diagnosing bronchiectasis. Bronchoscopy as a diagnostic tool is now largely obsolete with the advent of the noninvasive HRCT. Sputum may provide additional information regarding the severity of impairment and the presence of active infection. Patients are frequently colonized with *H. influenzae* or *P. aeruginosa*. Pulmonary function studies usually show an obstructive pattern including a decrease in FEV_1 and FEV_1/FVC.

Management

Bronchiectasis is difficult to treat. Therapy is aimed at treating acute flare-ups and preventing decline in lung function. Antibiotics are the mainstay of treatment and are often given empirically, but attempts are made to culture the sputum. Long-term suppressive therapy with antibiotics is reserved for those patients who have symptoms that recur a few days after stopping antibiotics. There has been some success with rotating antibiotics prophylactically to reduce exacerbation frequency to prevent antibiotic resistance. Antibiotics may be given orally, intravenously, or inhaled. Inhaled tobramycin is quite effective in patients with *P. aeruginosa*. Concurrent bronchodilator therapy is given to prevent bronchospasm. β_2 Agonists have been shown to stimulate mucoiliary clearance. Other forms of drug therapy may include mucolytic agents and anti-inflammatory agents such as ICS. Maintaining good hydration is important to liquefy secretions. Chest physiotherapy and other airway clearance techniques are important to facilitate expectoration of sputum. The individual should reduce exposure to excessive air pollutants and irritants, avoid cigarette smoking, and obtain pneumococcal and influenza vaccinations.

Surgical resection of parts of the lungs, although not used as often as previously, may be done if more conservative treatment is not effective. Surgical resection of an affected lobe or segment may be indicated for the patient with repeated bouts of pneumonia, hemoptysis, and disabling complications. Surgery is not advisable when there is diffuse or widespread involvement. For selected patients who are disabled in spite of maximal therapy, lung transplantation is an option.

Nursing Management of Bronchiectasis

The early detection and treatment of lower respiratory tract infections will help prevent complications such as bronchiectasis. Any obstructing lesion or foreign body should be removed promptly. Other measures to decrease the occurrence or progression of bronchiectasis include avoiding cigarette smoking and decreasing exposure to pollution and irritants.

An important nursing goal is to promote drainage and removal of bronchial mucus. Various airway clearance techniques can be effectively used to facilitate secretion removal. The patient should be taught effective deep-breathing exercises ways to cough. Chest physiotherapy with postural drainage should be done on affected parts of the lung. Some individuals require elevation of the foot of the bed by 4 to 6 inches airway vibration during the expiratory phase of breathing. Two to four 15-minutes sessions daily by a patient who has been properly trained can provide satisfactory mucus clearance. Positive expiratory resistance often used in conjunction with nebulized medications.

Administration of the prescribed medications is important. The patient needs to understand the importance of taking the prescribed regimen of drugs to obtain maximum effects or adverse effects that must be reported to the physician.

Rest is important to prevent overexertion. Bed rest may be indicated during the acute phase of the illness. Chilling and excess fatigue should be avoided.

Good nutrition is important and may be difficult to maintain because the patient is often anorexic. Oral hygiene to cleanse the mouth and remove dried sputum crusts may improve the patients appetite. Offering foods that are appealing may also increase the desire to eat. Adequate hydration to help liquefy secretions and thus make it easier to remove them is extremely important. Unless there are contraindications, such as renal disease, the patient should be instructed to drink at least 3 L of fluid daily. To accomplish this, the patient should be advised to increase fluid consumption from the baseline by increasing intake by one glass per day until the goal is reached. Generally the patient should be counseled to use low-sodium fluids to avoid systemic fluid detention.

Direct hydration of the respiratory system may also prove beneficial in the expectoration of secretions. Usually a bland aerosol with normal saline solution delivered by a jet-type nebulizer is used. Alternatively, hypertonic saline may be used for a more aggressive effect. At home a steamy shower can prove effective; extensive equipment that requires frequent cleaning is usually unnecessary. The patient and family should be taught to recognize significant clinical manifestations include increased sputum production, grossly bloody sputum, increasing dyspnea, fever, chills, and chest pain.

TABLE 9.4: Nursing care plan for the patient with adult respiratory distress syndrome in hypoxemic acute respiratory failure

Problems	Objectives	Nursing interventions	Rationales
Nursing Diagnosis #1			
Gas exchange, impaired, related to: 1. Right-to-left shunting 2. Ventilation/perfusion mismatch	Patient will: 1. Be alert and oriented to person, place, time 2. Demonstrate appropriate behavior 3. Maintain effective cardiovascular function: – Blood pressure within 10 mm Hg of baseline – Cardiac output ~5 liters/min – Without cyanosis if preexisting pulmonary function normal – Lab values: Hematocrit Male: 45–52 percent Female: 37–48 percent	• Perform neurologic assessment: – Mental status, level of consciousness. – Appropriate behavior – Protective and deep tendon reflexes • Monitor respiratory function: – Respiratory rate and pattern – Use of accessory muscles – Status of weakness and fatigue – Degree of chest wall excursion – Increase in fremitus? – Presence of dullness on percussion? – Breath sounds: ◆ Abnormal breath sounds ◆ Adventitious breath sounds • Assess cardiovascular function: – Heart rate. – Hemodynamic parameters: ◆ Systemic arterial pressure ◆ Pulmonary capillary wedge pressure ◆ Cardiac output – Evidence of cyanosis	• Hypoxemia may predispose to cerebral tissue hypoxia – Increased work of breathing fatigues the patient and predisposes to alveolar hypoventilation with hypercapnia and respiratory acidemia. – Consolidated lung tissue transmits vibrations better than airfilled lung spaces – Percussion over consolidated lung produces a "dull" sound – Bronchial breath sounds are often heard in areas of the lung that normally would reflect vesicular sounds; rales (crackles) may also be heard • Hemodynamic parameters reflect tissue perfusion • Administer prescribed humidified oxygen therapy – Late sign reflecting the desaturation of at least 5 g of hemoglobin; evidence of ventilation/perfusion mismatch and right-to-left shunt

Contd...

Contd...

Problems	Objectives	Nursing interventions	Rationales
	Hemoglobin Male: 13–18 g/100 mL Female: 12–16 g/100 mL 4. Maintain optimal arterial blood gases: pH 7.35–7.45 $PaO_2 > 60$ mm Hg $PaCO_2 \sim 35$-45 mm Hg 5. Alveolar-arterial oxygen gradient ($AaDO_2$):< 15 mm Hg on room air	– Cardiac dysrhythmias – Arterial blood gas values: pH • Monitor laboratory data: – Arterial blood gases pH PaO_2 significantly reduced < 60 mm Hg $PaCO_2$ reduced early < 35 mm Hg increased late > 45 mm Hg Calculate $AaDO_2$ – Hematology: Hematocrit, hemoglobin • Administer prescribed humidified oxygen therapy – Monitor for signs/symptoms of oxygen toxicity: Retrosternal chest pain; paresthesias in extremities; fatigue, lethargy, malaise, restlessness; anorexia, nausea, vomiting; dyspnea, coughing – Late symptomatology: Progressive respiratory distress; dyspnea, cyanosis; asphyxia; increasing $AaDO_2$; decreased compliance and lung volumes – Monitor serial arterial blood gas measurements • Implement positive end-expiratory pressure (PEEP) therapy in conjunction with mechanical ventilatory support – Dosage: Early non-cardiogenic pulmonary edema; 5–15 cm H_2O pressure; severe ARDS 15–30 cm H_2O pressure – Criteria used to determine effective PEEP level: Arterial blood gas analysis; mixed venous oxygen tension; lung compliance; hemodynamic parameters: pulmonary artery pressure; PCWP; cardiac output – PEEP is usually increased in increments 3–5 cm H_2O pressure until "best PEEP" is achieved – Monitor for complications of PEEP therapy: Reduction in venous return to the heart and cardiac output; reduction in cerebral perfusion—assess mental status – Barotrauma – Monitor fluid status	– Hypoxemia is commonly associated with myocardial irritability – A metabolic acidemia is often associated with decreased tissue perfusion; the consequent anerobic metabolism causes in rise in serum lactate levels with a progressive metabolic acidosis – Metabolic acidosis may depress myocardial function and predispose to dysrhythmias – Most closely reflect effectiveness of gas exchange – Extensive right-to-left shunting causes the hypoxemia to be refractory to oxygen therapy – Tachypnea and dyspnea cause carbon dioxide to be eliminated, predisposing to hypocapnia – Alveolar-arterial gradient < 250–300 mmHg with an FIO_2 of 100 percent; a classic hallmark of ARDS – Maintenance of normal physiologic levels of hemoglobin ensures maximal oxygen transport and release of oxygen to the tissues. Increased hemoglobin levels increase blood viscosity • Oxygenation is the mainstay of treatment of ARDS; a large right-to-left shunt predisposes to a hypoxemia refractory to administration of even high concentrations ($FIO_2 > 50\%$) of oxygen – Oxygen is administered in conjunction with mechanical ventilation and PEEP therapy – Precautions associated with oxygen therapy: ♦ Oxygen is a potent drug necessitating cautious use ♦ Oxygen concentration should be kept to a minimum to maintain $PaO_2 > 60$ mm Hg ♦ Duration of oxygen therapy should be kept to a minimum – Prolonged administration of high oxygen concentrations predisposes to oxygen toxicity – Use of an $FIO_2 > 50$ percent over a period of 6–30 h has been associated with oxygen toxicity. – Maintenance of a $PaO_2 > 60$ mm Hg can produce a hemoglobin saturation of ~90 percent

Contd...

Contd...

Problems	Objectives	Nursing interventions	Rationales
			– Signs and symptoms of oxygen toxicity are often subtle and may be easily overlooked: meticulous and thorough ongoing assessment and evaluation of patient's responses to therapy assist in determining effectiveness of therapy and prevention of complications – Frequent monitoring of arterial blood gases is a mandatory safety measure when an FIO_2 > 40 percent is used • PEEP therapy maintains airway opening pressure at end expiration above atmospheric pressure. This distending airway pressure increases lung volumes including FRC, it prevents airway collapse; it enhances gas exchange and oxygen transport; and it functions to reduce right-to-left shunting – Use of PEEP therapy increases PaO_2 without requiring an increase in FIO_2 – Lung compliance is determined by dividing the peak inspiratory pressure (PIP) into the tidal volume (V_T) – "Best PEEP" is achieved when the inherent "stiffness" of the lungs prevents further distention of air spaces; it is the level at which maximal benefit of PEEP is realised (i.e. PaO_2 > 60 mm Hg on FIO_2 50%) – Positive intrathoracic pressure generated by PEEP is applied to the great veins within the chest, reducing venous return to the right heart – Overdistention and rupture of alveoli are major complications of PEEP therapy – Overly vigorous administration of fluids may aggravate the pulmonary edema; the increased capillary hydrostate pressure favors movement of fluid into lung interstitium – Excessive fluid accumulation increases total lung water, causing an increase in ventilation/perfusion mismatching
Nursing Diagnosis #2			
Breathing pattern, ineffective: Tachypnea, hyperventilation	Patient will: 1. Achieve effective minute ventilation. – Tidal volume (V_T) > 5–7 mL/kg – Respiratory rate < 30/min 2. Achieve a vital capacity (V_C) > 12–15 mL/kg 3. Verbalize ease of breathing	• Assess respiratory function: – Rate, rhythm, depth, and pattern of breathing – Symmetry of chest wall and diaphragmatic excursion: Use of accessory muscles; flaring of nares. ◆ Monitor for fatigue, exhaustion – Lung compliance – Pulmonary lung volumes: ◆ Total minute ventilation (V_E) ◆ Tidal volume (V_T)	– Tachypnea is the compensatory mechanism for hypoxemia – Hyperventilatory effort is responsible for the hypocapnia observed during the edge course of the illness – Accumulation of fluid, edema, and secretions within the lungs, with lung consolidation, reduces lung compliance – Maximal respiratory effort is made to facilitate optimum ventilation

Contd...

Contd...

Problems	Objectives	Nursing interventions	Rationales
	– Breath sounds audible throughout anterior/posterior chest – Reduced to absent adventitious sounds	◆ Respiratory rate (f) ◆ Vital capacity (V_c) • Assist patient into position of comfort to allow for best lung expansion • Implement mechanical ventilation	– A minimal volume of ventilation is necessary to ensure adequate alveolar ventilation; this minimal volume of gas enlarge gas exchange to occur during the phase of the respiratory cycle when no new gas inspired (expiratory and end-expiration phases) • Expansion of lungs facilitates more even distribution of ventilation; increases ventilation/perfusion matching
Nursing Diagnosis #3			
Airway clearance, ineffective, related to increased tracheobronchial secretions	Patient will: 1. Be alert and oriented to person, place, time 2. Maintain effective alveolar ventilation: – Breath sounds audible throughout anterior/posterior chest – Reduced to absent adventitious sounds – Arterial blood gas values stabilized as follows: pH 7.35–7.45 PaO_2 > 60 mm Hg $PaCO_2$ 35–45 mm Hg	• Assess respiratory function with emphasis on status of pulmonary secretions and the patient's ability to handle secretions. – Presence of adventitious sounds ◆ Rales (crackles) wheezes • Assess fluid status. – Intake and output; daily weight • Implement chest physiotherapy and bronchial hygiene measures	• Patients with ARDS often have increased secretions, which impair adequate ventilation further compromising the hypoxemia • Excessive intrapulmonary accumulation fluid reduces compliance and further rales underlying right-to-left shunting ventilation/perfusion mismatching • Pooling of secretions within the tracheobronchial tree compromises ventilation predisposes to infection • In patients receiving PEEP therapy adapter should be used to maintain the reative and end-expiratory pressure • Even the slightest interruption of therapy can significantly increase the hypoxemia
Nursing Diagnosis #4			
Cardiac output, alteration in: Decreased (diminished) venous return	For specific patient outcomes related to these nursing diagnoses, see Table 9.3, Nursing Diagnosis #4, #5, and #6.	For specific nursing interventions and their rationales, See Table 9.3, Nursing Diagnoses #5 and #6.	
Nursing Diagnosis #5			
Tissue perfusion, alteration in: Cardiopulmonary			
Nursing Diagnosis #6			
Tissue perfusion, alteration in: Cerebral			
Nursing Diagnosis #7			
Fluid and electrolytes, alteration in	For specific patient outcomes related to this nursing diagnosis, see Table 9.3, Nursing Diagnosis #7	• Administer prescribed intravenous therapy	• Because of the alveolar-capillary ability defect in ARDS, the fluid of .... intravenous administration is cry rather than colloid. Colloids would be of intravascular space to equilibrate interstitial fluid

Contd...

Contd...

Problems	Objectives	Nursing interventions	Rationales
Nursing Diagnosis #8			
Acid-base balance, alteration in: Respiratory alkalosis (tachypnea, hyperventilation)	The patient's arterial blood gas values will stabilize as follows: pH 7.35–7.45 PaO_2 > 60 mm Hg $PaCO_2$ 35–45 mm Hg	• Assess for signs and symptoms of respiratory alkalemia: – Neurologic function: Light headedness, weakness, muscle cramps, twitching; paresthesias; hyperactive deep tendon reflexes, seizure activity; tetany – Cardiovascular function: Cardiac dysrhythmias – Serum calcium levels – Serial arterial blood gases • Implement supportive therapy to maintain adequate ventilation and optimal gas exchange – Increase tidal volume – Decrease respiratory rate – If mechanically ventilated, increase dead-space ventilation; decrease minute ventilation	• Respiratory failure in the patient is associated with tachypnea and hypoventilation as the body tries to compensation severe hypoxemia – Hyperventilation reduces $PaCO_2$ consequent rise in pH – A rise in pH reduces the serum concentration of freely ionized calcium by increase the calcium binding affinity of plasma proteins. The consequent hypocalcemia sufficiently severe, may predispose neuromuscular alterations – Increasing tidal volume and decreased respiratory rate decreases total minute ventilation; reduced ventilation enables the alveolar PCO_2 and, thus, the $PaCO_2$ return to an acceptable physiologic rate (35–45 mm Hg)
Nursing Diagnosis #9			
Nutrition, alteration in: Less than body requirements	For specific patient outcomes related to this nursing diagnosis, see Table 9.3, Nursing Diagnosis #9	For specific nursing interventions and their rationales, see chapter having NCP with similar nursing diagnosis	
Nursing Diagnosis #10			
Infection, potential for	For specific patient outcomes related to this nursing diagnosis, see Table 9.3, Nursing Diagnosis #10	For specific nursing interventions and their rationales, see chapter having NCP with similar nursing diagnosis	
Nursing Diagnosis #11			
Pulmonary mechanics, alterations in, related to respiratory muscle weakness and atrophy (immobility, mechanical ventilation)	Patient will: 1. Perform deep breathing exercises hourly 2. Achieve maximum pulmonary function: – Tidal volume >7–10 mL/kg – Vital capacity >15 mL/kg – Respiratory rate <30/min – Maximal expiratory flow	• Teach deep-breathing exercises: – Assess emotional and physiologic readiness for such teaching – Allow patient to demonstrate deep breathing exercises – Combine deep-breathing therapy with other chest physiotherapy maneuvers • Assess pulmonary volumes to determine effectiveness of therapy	• Use of positive-pressure ventilation for a prolonged period predisposes to atrophy of the respiratory musculature – Breathing exercises mobilize secretion improve ventilation, stimulate circulation and increase muscle tone
Nursing Diagnosis #12			
Skin integrity, impairment related to immobility	For specific patient outcomes related to this nursing diagnosis, see Table 9.3, Nursing Diagnosis #12	For specific nursing interventions and their rationales, see chapter having NCP with similar nursing diagnosis	

Contd...

Contd...

Problems	Objectives	Nursing interventions	Rationales
Nursing Diagnosis#13			
Coping, ineffective individual/family	Patient/family will: 1. Verbalize knowledge and understanding of the illness 2. Verbalize feelings as to what this potentially life-threatening illness means to each family member, individually and collectively 3. Verbalize strengths and coping capabilities 4. Identify family resources 5. Make decisions regarding matters of importance to patient and family	• Assess patient/family perceptions regarding a potentially life-threatening illness – Develop a trusting relationship with patient and family – Establish a caring rapport: Patient advocacy; accessible to patient/family – Encourage verbalization of perceptions, concerns, and feelings • Assist patient/family to identify past coping capabilities: – Emphasize strengths – Assist patient/family in defining areas requiring problem-solving and decision-making ◆ Support patient/family in this regard – Involve in decision-making regarding care ◆ Offer praise for accomplishments ◆ Encourage development of new coping mechanisms ◆ Assist patient/family to explore and identify options and the consequences of the options. Assist patient/family to implement chosen options • Initiate referrals to intrahospital and community resources for special needs: Psychiatric social worker, family pastor, home care	• Knowledge of patient and family perception of the illness assists in identifying coping capabilities and potential coping problem – A trusting, caring, supportive relation facilitates verbalization of concerns fears – A definitive, dependable support system insists patient/family to assume responsibility for decision-making – Unexpressed and unresolved fears and concerns may compromise ability to do effectively – Active participation in self-care assistant individual/ family to gain a new sense of dignity, self-worth, and self-esteem • Additional resources may assist patient potentially to gain increased awareness of self interactions among patient, family, the care providers, and environment

TABLE 9.5: Nursing care plan for the patient with pulmonary embolism

Problems	Objectives	Nursing interventions	Rationales
Nursing Diagnosis #1			
Anxiety, related to: 1. Sudden, acute respiratory insufficiency with disruption of lifestyle 2. Pain; hemoptysis 3. Knowledge deficit regarding illness and its prognosis 4. Intensive care setting	Patient will: 1. Verbalize feeling less anxious 2. Demonstrate a relaxed demeanor 3. Perform relaxation techniques with assistance 4. Verbalize familiarity with ICU routines and protocols	• Assess for signs/symptoms of anxiety: Restlessness, agitation, diaphoresis; tachypnea, sighing; tachycardia, palpitations; anorexia, nausea, diarrhea; presence of anxiety-related behaviors: nailbiting, insomnia, finger tapping; uncooperative or noncompliant behaviors; verbalization of fears and concerns • Examine the circumstances underlying the anxiety – Manipulate ICU environment to provide calm, restful periods • Assess patient/family coping behaviors and their effectiveness in dealing with current stressors – Provide positive reinforcement when desired response is achieved	• Thorough assessment assists in discerning underlying cause of anxiety and provides a basis for intervention *Examples:* (1) Relief of pain with medication often alleviates its anxiety-related symptomatology, (2) coping with the fear of dying with a listening ear and caring attitude may assist in reducing the patient's anxiety • Removal of precipitating factors may reduce anxiety – Reduction in stimuli is essential to assist patient/family to relax and avoid useless dissipation of compromised energy stores

Contd...

Contd...

Problems	Objectives	Nursing interventions	Rationales
		• Initiate interventions to reduce anxiety: – Relieve pain or other discomfort ◆ Medication for pain ◆ Comfort measures: Turning, positioning, mouth care, skin care, and so forth – Monitor effectiveness of ventilatory support and oxygen therapy if these therapies are indicated ◆ Serial arterial blood gas values – Listen attentively, encourage verbalization, provide a caring touch – Let patient know it's okay to feel anxious or to experience fear of dying – Remain with patient during periods of acute stress – Assess readiness to learn and implement the following when appropriate: ◆ Orient to environment, ICU equipment, routines, and staff ◆ Explain all procedures and activities involving the patient – Involve in decision-making regarding care when possible and appropriate – Help in establishing short-term goals that can be attained – Instruct in relaxation techniques	– Positive feedback nurtures self-confidence – Pain precipitates and/or aggravates anxiety – Inadequate gas exchange, hypoxemia and/or hypercapnia precipitate sympto-matology that contributes to the patient "sense of doom" – These nursing activities reassure the patient that he/she is not alone – Reassurance helps patient focus on his/her feelings, work them through, and, eventually, accept them – Readiness to learn facilitates meaningful learning and a sense of accomplishment – Knowing what to expect helps to reduce anxiety – Helps patient maintain some degree of control over his/her body and health care – Builds and reinforces self-confidence – Energy-release techniques allow an out for pent-up feelings; enable the patient have some control over anxiety
Nursing Diagnosis #2			
Gas exchange, impaired, related to: 1. Right-to-left shunting. 2. Ventilation/ perfusion mismatch.	For specific patient outcomes and related to these nursing diagnoses	For specific nursing interventions and their rationales pl. see chapters having NCP with similar nursing diagnosis	
Nursing Diagnosis #3			
Breathing pattern, ineffective, related to tachypnea, dyspnea			
Nursing Diagnosis #4			
Cardiac output, alteration in: Decreased, related to: 1. Pulmonary arterial hypertension 2. Right-sided congestive heart failure (cor pulmonale) 3. Decrease in left ventricular end-diastolic pressure (LVEDP)	Patient will: 1. Maintain stable hemody-namics: – Heart rate < 100 beats/min – CVP 0–8 mm Hg – Pulmonary artery pressure <25 mm Hg – PCWP 8–12 mm Hg – Cardiac output ~5 liters/min	• Assess for signs/symptoms of right-sided congestive heart failure: – Weight gain; fluid intake/output – Hemodynamic changes: ◆ Tachycardia (> 100 beats/min) ◆ Jugular neck vein distention ◆ Peripheral (dependent) edema ◆ CVP > 8–12 mm Hg ◆ Extra heart sounds; S_3, S_4; systolic murmur ◆ Fatigue; mottled appearance of skin, cool to touch; cyanosis of nailbeds	• The major hemodynamic disturbance associated with pulmonary embolism is pulmonary arterial hypertension (>25–30 mm) which may predispose to right ventricular failure – Hypoxemia, acidemia, and a reduced cross-sectional area of the pulmonary vascular bed all contribute to the development of pulmonary hypertension

Contd...

Contd...

Problems	Objectives	Nursing interventions	Rationales
4. Systemic arterial hypotension/ hypovolemic shock	– Systemic arterial blood pressure within 10 mm Hg of baseline	– Breath sounds may be clear and without adventitious sounds; or breath sounds may be diminished with localized rales (crackles) or wheezing. A pleural friction rub may be detected. Breathing pattern may reflect tachypnea, dyspnea – Hepatic involvement: ◆ Hepatomegaly, positive hepato-jugular reflex; abdominal distention; ascites – Gastrointestinal: Anorexia, nausea/ vomiting; abdominal distention – Oliguria – Mental status changes – Monitor diagnostic tests/studies: ◆ Laboratory studies: BUN, creatinine, hematocrit, serum albumin; electrolytes; arterial blood gases ◆ ECG may reflect signs of ischemia; dysrhythmias (atrial) ◆ Chest X-rays frequently reflect cardiomegaly, pleural effusion, and possibly, pulmonary edema (left-sided heart failure) • Administer prescribed medication regimen to treat cor pulmonale, a consequence of pulmonary hypertension – Vasopressor therapy (e.g. dopamine in the presence of heart failure and hypovolemic shock) – Cardiac glycosides (digoxin) ◆ Positive inotropic agent—improved contractility ◆ Negative chronotropic agent—reduced heart rate ◆ End result—improved cardiac output – Morphine ◆ Induces systemic venous vasodilation ◆ Reduces chest pain frequently associated with pulmonary embolism ◆ Decreases anxiety and helps to reduce the work of breathing ◆ Exerts a sedative effect, which assists in relaxing the patient – Diuretics (e.g. furosemide) – Vasodilator therapy may be initiated especially in the setting of left ventricular compromise – Anticoagulant therapy ◆ Heparin, coumadin derivatives ◆ Aspirin (antiplatelet agent)	– Right ventricular failure causes alteration in systemic hemodynamics; left ventricular failure alters pulmonary hemodynamics. Commonly, failure in one ventricle causes failure of the other – A massive pulmonary embolism with cor pulmonale may be characterized by dyspnea, cyanosis and hypovolemic shock • Serum sodium values reflect hydration status – Serum potassium needs to be carefully monitored especially during diuretic therapy • Therapies are directed toward decreasing myocardial oxygen consumption and demand – A pulmonary embolic epi- sode may reflexly trigger systemic peripheral arteriolar vasodilation with a consequent "relative" volume depletion, which, if severe, can cause hypotension or hypovolemic shock – Increased pooling of blood in the periphery reduces venous return to the right heart, which helps to decrease the work of the right ventricle – A reduction in total blood volume reduces venous return (preload) while also reducing systemic arterial blood pressure (after load). The end result is a decrease in myocardial work – Use of diuretics requires the maintenance of fluid volume – Vasodilators function to decrease preload and after-load and thus, decrease the work of the heart – Major focus of therapy in the patient experiencing a pulmonary embolic episode is to *prevent* recurrent embolization; anticoagulants function effectively in this capacity

Contd...

Contd...

Problems	Objectives	Nursing interventions	Rationales
Nursing Diagnosis #5			
Fluid volume, alteration	Patient will: 1. Maintain body weight within 5% of baseline 2. Balance fluid intake with output 3. Have: – Good skin turgor – Absence of peripheral edema – Absence of jugular vein distention – Absence of rales (crackles) on auscultation Serum electrolytes, BUN, creatinine, total protein, will stabilize within acceptable physiologic range	• Maintain fluid and electrolyte balance. – Administer prescribed fluid volume – Document intake and output, urine specific gravity – Record daily weight – Monitor electrolytes • Monitor hemodynamic parameters. – Systemic arterial blood pressure, CVP, pulmonary artery pressure, PCWP, cardiac output • Administer oxygen therapy as prescribed and monitor arterial blood gases to evaluate patient's response to therapy • Implement nursing measures to improve and/or maintain cardiac output – Manipulate environment to reduce stressors and promote rest and relaxation – Plan frequent rest periods – Maximize patient activities in accordance with the acuity of the illness – Place in high Fowler's position – Assist with frequent position changes – Provide special care to back and to skin over joints and pressure points – Assist with passive range-of-motion exercises	• Fluid therapy is directed towards reducing the work of the heart while still maintaining adequate tissue perfusion – Close monitoring of urine output helps to evaluate renal perfusion/ function; a reduc-tion in cardiac output may reduce renal perfusion, which is manifested clinically by a decrease in hourly urine output • These measures best reflect the patient's response to therapy, and insertion of a pulmonary artery flotation catheter is commonly indicated in the setting of massive pulmonary embolism • Hypoxemia in pulmonary embolism is a consequence of ventilation/perfusion mismatching and right-to-left shunting • A quiet, calm environment decreases anxiety and reduces sympathetic nervous system stimulation. The overall net effect is to reduce the work of the heart. – A reduction in cardiac work-load reduces myocardial oxygen consumption and demand – Nursing interventions are implemented to maximize circulation, prevent pooling or stasis of blood, maintain venous return and promote comfort – Facilitates breathing pressure on the diaphragm is reduced; less effort exerted - decrease in oxygen demand – Compromised circulation predisposes to tissue ischemia; statsis or pooling of blood predisposes to venous thrombosis; reduce venous return, which decreases cardiac output
Nursing Diagnosis #6			
Tissue perfusion alteration in, related to: 1. Thromboembolic disorder 2. Deep venous thrombosis 3. Pulmonary embolism	Patient will: 1. Remain without recurrent pulmonary embolism as reflected by: – Absence of pain – Stable vital signs (see Nursing Diagnosis #4 above) – Stable arterial blood gases (within acceptable physiologic range) pH 7.35–7.45 $PaCO_2$ 35–45 mm Hg PaO_2 > 60 mm Hg	• Assess for signs/symptoms of venous thrombosis: – Tenderness, warmth, pain, and peripheral (pitting) edema of lower extremities – Evidence of edema is best assessed and monitored by determining the circumference of the limb at a designated point using a tape measure – Skin color and temperature ◆ Observe extremities in both dependent and elevated positions – Bleeding/bruising tendency, petechiae, ecchymosis, hematuria, occult blood in stool	• Ninty-five per cent of all pulmonary emboli arise in the deep veins of the lower extremities – Edema is a characteristic manifestation when alteration in tissue perfusion is due to venous interference – In the presence of altered tissue perfusion or venous obstruction a bluish-red color of the skin may be observed – Temperature of skin is assessed by use of touch; usually warm temperatures in the lower extremities are commonly associated with venous thrombosis – Hypercoagulable state is often reflected by bleeding tendency

Contd...

Contd...

Problems	Objectives	Nursing interventions	Rationales
		– Complaints of pain: ◆ Pain associated with deep venous thrombosis may be described as heavy, aching, or cramping ◆ Pain associated with arterial insufficiency is characteristically sudden and sharp; the presence of cool skin temperatures suggests decreased arterial blood flow • Monitor for signs/symptoms indicative of extended or recurrent pulmonary embolism – Sudden occurrence of persistent or exacerbated chest and/or shoulder pain – Onset of respiratory difficulties: Tachypnea, dyspnea, cough with hemoptysis – Alterations in cardiopulmonary function: Tachycardia, hypotension, cyanosis – Neurologic findings: Restlessness, lethargy, confusion • Monitor laboratory data: – Arterial blood gas values – Hematologic studies: Complete blood count, hematocrit, hemoglobin. – Coagulation studies: aPTT; prothrombin time; clotting time. – Platelet count • Implement prescribed anticoagulant therapy • Implement measures to reduce the risk of recurrent pulmonary embolism – Maintain hydrated state as prescribed. – Apply antiembolic hose to both lower extremities; remove hose once per shift – Assist patient to perform active range-of-motion exercises; active/passive foot and leg exercises should be performed hourly unless otherwise contraindicated – Instruct patient to avoid positions that compromise blood flow in the extremities (e.g. gatch knees, pillow under knees, crossing of legs, prolonged sitting in one position) – Encourage deep breathing hourly – Caution patient to avoid activities that involve a Valsalva's maneuver (e.g. straining to defecate, breath holding)	– Pain occurs when there is an alteration in tissue perfusion • The presence of deep venous thrombosis places the patient at increased risk of pulmonary embolism – Dehydration increases blood viscosity. The consequent disturbed blood flow may predispose to endothelial injury within blood vessels, and/or a hypercoagulable state – Exercise enhances "skeletal-muscular pump," which functions to prevent pooling of blood in the lower extremities (venous stasis) and maintains venous return to the heart – If a thrombosis is suspected, the involved extremity should not be massaged or exercised to prevent possible dislodgement of thrombi with consequent pulmonary embolism – Positions that compromise blood flow can cause circulatory stasis – Expands lungs and minimizes areas of atelectasis – Such activities increase risk of dislodging thrombi

Contd...

Contd...

Problems	Objectives	Nursing interventions	Rationales
Nursing Diagnosis #7			
Comfort, alteration in: Pain associated with compromised pulmonary perfusion	Patient will: 1. Verbalize pain relief 2. Exhibit relaxed demeanor: – Relaxed facial expression and body posturing – Ease of breathing	• Determine how patient usually copes with pain – Pain tolerance – Willingness to discuss pain; or stoically "keeping it within" himself or herself – Willingness to use medication for pain • Assess for nonverbal clues as to the presence of pain (e.g. restlessness, or reluctance to move; tense facial features; clenched fists; diaphoresis; rapid, shallow breathing) • Assess complaints of pain including severity, location/radiation; influencing factors (e.g. what precipitates, aggravates, or ameliorates the pain; and associated signs and symptoms such as diaphoresis), pain duration and the quality of pain (e.g. sharp, dull, "knifelike) • Implement measures to alleviate pain: – Assist patient into comfortable position (e.g. high Fowler's) – Encourage deep breathing hourly – Teach/assist patient to splint chest with hands or pillow when coughing, deep breathing, or repositioning – Stay with patient until pain is relieved – Provide a listening ear and caring touch; encourage verbalization; explain procedures, routines, tests, and so forth – Refrain from non-essential activities – Provide comfort measures (e.g. position change, back care, reducing environmental stimuli) • Administer analgesic medication therapy as prescribed – Encourage to request medication when pain is first realized rather than waiting until it gets unbearable. – Evaluate effectiveness of pain medication in relieving the patient's pain	• To assist in comprehensive assessment – Upright position favors better lung expansion; improves alveolar ventilation – Minimizes atelectasis and improves distribution of ventilation – Splinting may help to reduce discomfort – Providing support can reduce anxiety and help the patient relax – Keeping the patient informed may help to alleviate anxieties, which may potentiate pain – Reducing patient's activities decreases oxygen consumption and demand – Comfort measures and touch therapy are often sufficient to alleviate pain – Pain medication administered early on may be more effective
Nursing Diagnosis #8			
Knowledge deficit, related to: 1. Thromboembolic disease 2. Follow-up care 3. Prevention	Patient/family will: 1. Identify risk factors of significance in thromboembolic disease 2. Identify activities that promote venous blood flow and reduce risks of venous thrombosis – Importance of individualized exercise program	Patient/family educatioan, for information essential to the patient/family's understanding of and compliance with, the prescribed therapeutic regimen	

Contd...

Contd...

Problems	Objectives	Nursing interventions	Rationales
	3. Explain the prescribed treatment regimen and the importance of complying with it: – Rationale for anticoagulant therapy – Medicatioan routine, dosage, and side effects – Signs/symptoms to report to healthcare provider – Measures to minimize risks of bleeding during anticoagulant therapy – Importance of follow-up care		

Procedure 9.1: Assisting with arterial puncture for blood gas analysis

Equipment:

- Commercially available blood gas kit

  or
- 2- or 3 mL syringe
- 23- or 25-gauge needle
- 0.5 mL sodium heparin (1:1,000)
- Stopper or cap
- Lidocaine
- Sterile germicide
- Cup or plastic bag with crushed ice
- Gloves.

Steps of procedure

Nursing action	Rationale
Preparatory phase	
1. Record patient's inspired oxygen concentration	1. Changes in inspired oxygen concentration alter the change in PaO_2. Degree of hypoxemia cannot be assessed without knowing the inspired oxygen concentration
2. Take patient's temperature, if not using a commercially available blood gas kit	2. May be taken into consideration when results are evaluated. Hyperthermia and hypothermia influence oxygen release from hemoglobin
3. Heparinize the 2 mL syringe a. Withdraw heparin into the syringe to wet the plunger and fill dead space in the needle	3. a. This action coats the interior of the syringe with heparin to prevent blood from clotting b. Air in the syringe may affect measurement of PaO2. Heparin in the syringe may affect measurement of the pH
Performance phase (by physician, nurse with special instruction)	
1. Wash hands	
2. Don gloves	

Contd...

Contd...

Nursing action	Rationale
3. Palpate the radial, brachial or femoral artery	3. The radial artery is the preferred site of puncture. Arterial puncture is performed on areas where a good pulse is palpable
4. If puncturing the radial artery, perform the Allen test In the conscious patient: a. Obliterate the radial and ulnar pulses simultaneously by pressing on both blood vessels at the wrist b. Ask patient to clench and unclench fist until blanching of skin occurs c. Release pressure on ulnar artery (while still compressing radial artery). Watch for return of skin color within 15 seconds *Note:* If the ulnar does not have sufficient blood flow to supply the entire hand, another artery should be used In the unconscious patient: a. Obliterate the radial and ulnar pulses simultaneously at the wrist b. Elevate patient's hand above heart and squeeze or compress hand until blanching occurs c. Lower patient's hand while still compressing the radial artery (release pressure on ulnar artery) and watch for return of skin color	4. The Allen test is a simple method for assessing collateral circulation in the hand. Ensures circulation if radial artery thrombosis occurs a. Impedes arterial blood flow into the hand b. Forces blood from the hand c. Documents that ulnar artery alone is capable of supplying blood to the hand, because radial artery is still occluded
5. For the radial side, place a small towel roll under the patient's wrist	5. To make the artery more accessible
6. Feel along the course of the radial artery the palpate for maximum pulsation with the middle and index fingers. Prepare the skin with germicide. The skin and subcutaneous tissues may be infiltrated with a local anesthetic agent (lidocaine)	6. The wrist should be stabilized to allow for better control of the needle
7. The needle is at a 45–60 degree angle to the skin surface and is advanced into the artery. Once the artery is punctured, arterial pressure will push up the hub of the syringe and a pulsating flow of blood will fill the syringe	7. The arterial pressure will cause the syringe to be filled within a few seconds
8. After blood is obtained, withdraw needle and apply firm pressure over the puncture with a dry sponge	8. Significant bleeding can occur because of pressure in the artery
9. Remove air bubbles from syringe and needle. Insert needle into rubber stopper	9. Immediate capping of the needle prevents room air from mixing with the blood specimen
10. Place the capped syringe in the container of ice	10. Icing the syringe will prevent a clinically significant loss of O_2
11. Maintain firm pressure on the puncture site for 5 minutes. If the patient is on anticoagulant medication, apply direct pressure dressing	11. Firm pressure on the puncture site prevents further bleeding and hematoma formation
12. For patients requiring serial monitoring of arterial blood, an arterial catheter (connected to a flush solution of heparinized saline) is inserted into the radial or femoral artery	12. All connections must be tight to avoid disconnection and rapid blood loss. The arterial line also allows for direct blood pressure monitoring in the critically-ill patient
Follow-up phase	
1. Send labeled, iced specimen to the laboratory immediately	1. Blood gas analysis should be done as soon as possible, because PaO_2 and pH can change rapidly
2. Palpate the pulse (distal to the puncture site, and assess for cold hand, numbness, tingling or discoloration	2. Hematoma and arterial thrombosis are complications following this procedure
3. Change ventilator settings, inspired oxygen concentration or type and setting of respiratory therapy equipment if indicated by the results	3. The PaO_2 results will determine whether to maintain, increase or decrease the $F1O_2$. The PaO_2 and pH results will detect if any changes are needed in tidal volume of rate of patient's ventilator

Procedure 9.2: Assisting with transtracheal aspiration

Equipment: Sterile transtracheal set:

- No. 14, no. 16 and no. 18 gauge needles
- Polyethylene catheter

- Syringe
- Skin preparation solutions
- Local anesthetic
- Sterile gloves, masks
- Specimen containers
- Atropine
- ECG monitoring equipment
- Endotracheal tube
- Suction apparatus with catheters
- Cardiac resuscitation equipment

Steps of procedure

Nursing action	Rationale
Preparatory phase	
1. Explain the procedure and give reassurance by skilled and empathetic attention to the patient's needs. Instruct the patient to breathe quietly and to remain still	1. Inform the patient that the procedure will cause coughing and that there will be an unpleasant sensation of breathe a foreign body in the lower airway
2. Administer supplemental oxygen, as directed during the procedure if the patient's arterial oxygen tension is below normal while the patient is breathing room air	2. This prevents worsening of hypoxemia
3. Extend the patient's neck and place a pillow under shoulders	3. This is the optimum position for cricothyroid puncture
Performance phase	
The cricothyroid membrane is identified by palpation	
1. The skin over the cricothyroid area is cleansed and the area is infiltrated with local anesthetic	1. The cricothyroid membrane is less vascular and offers more safety in preventing posterior wall puncture than other areas
2. A no. 14, 16, or 18 gauge needle is inserted through the cricothyroid membrane into the trachea, and a polyethylene catheter is threaded through the needle into the lower trachea. Caution the patient against swallowing or talking while the needle is introduced through the cricothyroid membrane	
3. The needle is withdrawn, leaving the catheter in place	3. The catheter's passage usually stimulates vigorous coughing
4. A syringe is attached to the catheter and secretions may be aspirated back into the syringe as the patient coughs. Request the patient to turn head while coughing	4. Sterile saline (2 to 5 mL) may be injected into catheter to reduce coughing if necessary
5. Air is removed from the syringe, and the syringe is capped or the sample is injected into an anaerobic transfer vial. The specimen is sent to the laboratory for immediate processing	5. This ensures anaerobic conditions cytologic, mycobacterial and other studies are carried out
6. The catheter is withdrawn and pressure is applied over the puncture site	6. Gentle firm pressure over the site for about 5 minutes helps prevent bleeding and reduces subcutaneous emphysema
Follow-up phase	
1. Instruct the patient to rest quietly for about an hour	
2. Observe for the following complications: Local bleeding, puncture of posterior tracheal wall, subcutaneous emphysema, vasovagal reactions, cardiac dysrhythmias	2. Assess for hoarseness after the procedure: This may be from a submucosal tracheal hematoma, which can cause suffocation, inform the patient that minor blood streaking of sputum almost always occurs after this procedure

Procedure 9.3: Assisting the patient undergoing thoracentesis

Equipment:

- Thoracentesis tray (if available)

  or
- Syringes, 5-, 20-, 50-mL
- Needles—no. 22, no. 26, no. 16 (7.5 cm long)

- Three-way stopcock and tubing
- Hemostat
- Biopsy needle
- Germicide solution
- Local anesthetic (e.g. lidocaine 1%)
- Sterile gauze sponges (4 × 4 and 2 × 2)
- Sterile towels and drape
- Sterile specimen containers
- Sterile gloves.

Steps of procedure

Nursing action	Rationale
Preparatory phase	
1. Ascertain in advance if chest X-ray and/or other tests have been prescribed and completed. These should be available at the bedside	1. Localization of pleural fluid is accomplished by physical examination, chest roentgenogram, ultrasound localization, or fluoroscopic localization

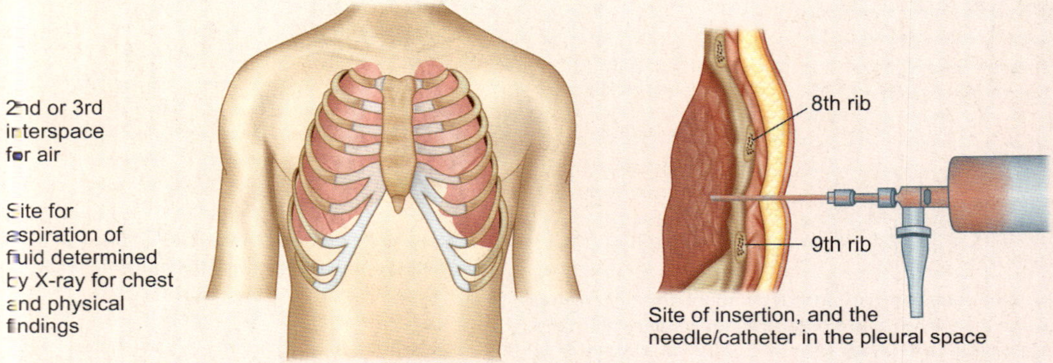

FIG. 9.34: Technique of thoracentesis

Nursing action	Rationale
2. See if consent form has been explained and signed	
3. Determine if the patient is allergic to local anesthetic agent to be used. Give sedation if prescribed	
4. Inform the patient about the procedure and indicate how he or she can be helpful. Explain: a. The nature of the procedure b. The importance of remaining immobile c. Pressure sensations to be experienced d. That no discomfort is anticipated after the procedure	4. An explanation helps orient the patient to the procedure, assists with coping and provides an opportunity to ask questions and verbalize anxiety
5. Make the patient comfortable with adequate supports. If possible, place upright (see accompanying figure and help patient maintain position during procedure	5. The upright position ensures that the diaphragm is most dependent and facilitates the removal of fluid that usually localizes at the base of the chest. A comfortable position helped reduce
6. Support and reassure the patient during the procedure a. Prepare the patient for sensations of cold from skin germicide and for pressure and sting from infiltration of local anesthetic agent b. Encourage the patient to refrain from coughing c. Be prepared to monitor patient's condition throughout the procedure	6. Discomfort by the patient can cause trauma to the visceral pleura with resultant trauma to the lung. A local anesthetic inhibits nerve conduction and is used to prevent pain during the procedure

Contd...

Contd...

Nursing action	Rationale
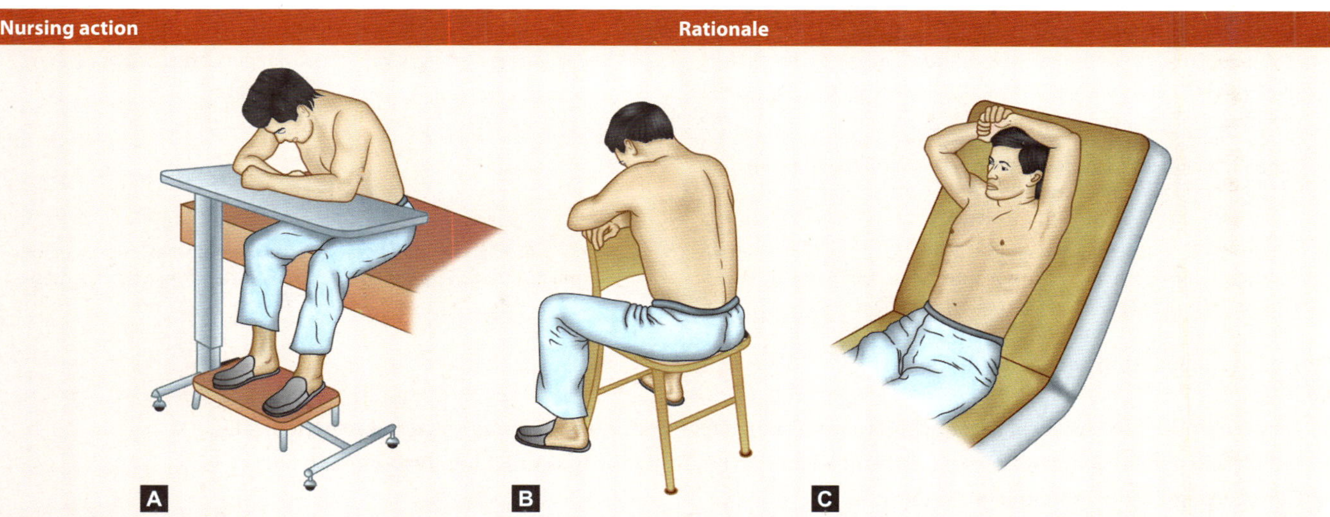 **FIGS 9.35A TO C:** Positioning the patient for a thoracentesis. The nurse assists the patient to one of three positions, and offers comfort and support throughout the procedure. (A) Sitting on the edge of the bed with head and arms on and over the bed table; (B) Straddling a chair with arms and head resting on the back of the chair; (C) Lying on unaffected side with the bed elevated 30 to 45 degrees	
Performance phase	
1. The site for aspiration is determined from chest X-rays, by percussion, or by fluoroscopic of ultrasound localization. If fluid is in the pleural cavity the thoracentesis site is determined by study of the chest X-ray and physical findings, with attention to the site of maximal dullness on percussion	1. If air is in the pleural cavity, the thoracentesis site is usually in the 2nd or 3rd intercostal space in the midclavicular line. Air rises in the thorax because the density of air is much less than the density of liquid
2. The procedure is done under aseptic conditions. After the skin is cleansed, the health care provider slowly injects a local anesthetic with a small-caliber needle into the intercostal space	2. An intradermal wheal is raised slowly, rapid intradermal injection causes pain. The parietal pleura is very sensitive and should be well infiltrated with anesthetic before the thoracentesis needle is passed through it
3. The thoracentesis needle is advanced with the syringe attached. When the pleural space is reached, suction may be applied with the syringe a. A 20 mL or 50 mL syringe with a three way adapter (stop-cock) is attached to the needle (one end of the adapter is attached to the needle and the other end to the tubing leading to a receptacle that receives the fluid being aspirated) b. If a considerable quantity of fluid is to be removed, the needle is held in place on the chest wall with a small hemostat c. A pleural biopsy may be performed	a. When a larger quantity of fluid is withdrawn, a three-way adapter serves to keep air from entering the pleural cavity. The amount of fluid removed depends on clinical status of the patient and absence of complications during the procedure b. The hemostat steadies the needle on the chest wall and prevents too deep a penetration of pleural space. Sudden pleuritic pain or shoulder pain may indicate that the visceral or diaphragmatic pleura are being irritated by the needle point
4. After the needle is withdrawn, pressure is applied over the puncture site and a small sterile dressing is fixed in place	4. This is done to prevent air entry into pleural space
Follow-up phase	
1. Place the patient on bedrest A chest X-ray is usually obtained after thoracentesis	1. Chest X-ray verifies that there is no pneumothorax
2. Record vital signs every 15 minutes for 1 hour	
3. Administer oxygen, as directed, if patient is suffering from cardiorespiratory disease	3. Pulmonary gas exchange may worsen after thoracentesis in patients with cardiorespiratory disease

Contd...

Contd...

Nursing action	Rationale
4. Record the total amount of fluid withdrawn and the nature of the fluid, its color and viscosity. If prescribed, prepare samples of fluid for laboratory evaluation (usually bacteriology, cell count and differential determinations of protein, glucose, LDH specific gravity). A small amount of heparin may be needed for several of the specimen containers to prevent coagulation. A specimen container with preservative may be needed if a pleural biopsy is to be obtained.	4. The fluid may be clear, serous bloody or purulent.
5. Evaluate the patient at intervals for increasing respiration's faintness, vertigo, tightness in the chest, uncontrollable cough blood-tinged mucus and rapid pulse and signs of hypoxemia.	5. Pneumothorax, tension pneumothorax, hemothorax, subcutaneous emphysema, or pyogenic infection may result from a thoracentesis.

Procedure 9.4: Endotracheal intubation

Equipment:

- Laryngoscope with curved or straight blade and working light source (check batteries and bulb periodically)
- Endotracheal tube with low pressure cuff and adapter to connect tube to ventilator or resuscitation bag
- Connect to guide the endotracheal tube
- Oral airway (assorted sizes) or bite block to keep patient from being into and occluding the endotracheal tube
- Adhesive tape or tube fixation system
- Sterile anaesthetic lubricant jelly (water-soluble)
- 10 mL syringe
- Suction source
- Suction catheter and tonsil suction
- Resuscitation bag and mask connected to oxygen source
- Sterile towel
- Gloves
- Goggles or other eye protection.

Steps of procedure

Nursing action	Rationale
Preparatory phase	
1. Assess the patient's heart rate, level of consciousness and respiratory status	1. Provide a baseline to estimate patient's tolerance of procedure
Performance phase	
1. Remove the patient's dental bridgework and plates	1. May interfere with insertion. Will not be able to remove easily from patient once in tubated
2. Remove headboard of bed (optional)	
3. Prepare equipment a. Patient may require ventilatory assistance during suction b. Assemble the laryngoscope. Make sure the light bulb is tightly attached and functional c. Select an endotracheal tube of the appropriate size (6.0 to 9.0 mm for average adult) d. Place the endotracheal tube on a sterile towel e. Inflate the cuff to make sure it assumes a symmetric shape and holds volume without leakage. Then deflate maximally f. Lubricate the distal end of the tube liberally with the sterile anesthetic water-soluble jelly	3. a. Ensure function of resuscitation bag with mask and procedure. Suction should be functional, because gagging and emesis may occur during procedure d. Although the tube will pass through the contaminated mouth or nose, the airway below the vocal cords is sterile, and efforts must be made to prevent iatrogenic contamination of the distal end of the tube and cuff. The proximal end of the tube may be handled, because it will reside in the upper airway e. Malfunction of the cuff must be ascertained before tube placement occurs f. Aids in insertion

Contd...

Contd...

Nursing action	Rationale

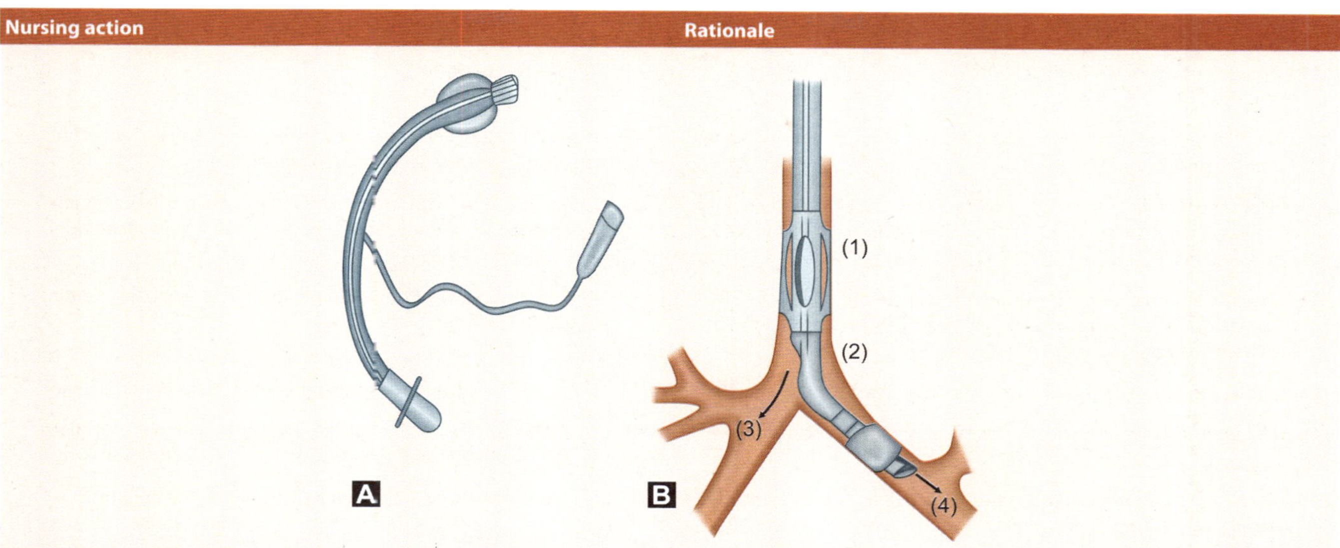

FIGS 9.36A AND B: (A) Single lumen endotracheal tube; (B) Double lumen endotracheal tube. When the double lumen tube is used, two cuffs are inflated. One cuff (1) is positioned in the tracks and the second cuff (2) in the left mainstem bronchus. After inflation, air flows through an opening below the tracheal cuff (3) to the right lung and through an opening below the bronchial cuff (4) to the left lung. This permits differential ventilation of both lungs, lavage of one lung, or selective inflation of either lung during thoracic surgery

Nursing action	Rationale
g. Insert the stylet into the tube (if oral intubation is planned). Nasal intubation does not employ use of the stylet	g. Stiffens the soft tube, allowing it to be more easily directed into the trachea
4. Aspirate stomach contents if nasogastric tube is in place	
5. If time allows, inform the patient of impending inability to talk and discuss alternate means of communication	5. Discuss alternate means of communication
6. If the patient is confused, it may be necessary to apply soft, wrist restraints	6. Restraint of the confused patient may be necessary to promote patient's safety and maintain sterile technique
7. Put-on goggles and gloves or other eye protection system	7. Prevent contact with patient's oral secretions
8. During oral intubation cervical is not injured, place patient's head in a position (i.e. extended at the junction of the neck and flexed at the junction of the spine and skull	8. Upper airway is open maximally in this position

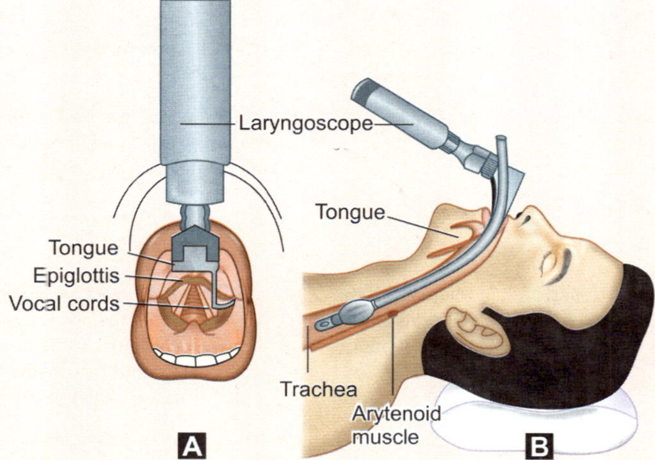

FIGS 9.37A AND B: Endotracheal intubation. (A) The primary glottic landmarks for tracheal intubation as visualized with proper placement of the laryngoscope; (B) Positioning the endotube

Contd...

Contd...

Nursing action	Rationale
9. Spray the back of the patient's with anesthetic spray if time is available	9. Will decrease gagging
10. Ventilate and oxygenate the patient with the resuscitation-bag and mask before	10. Preoxygenation decreases the likelihood of cardiac dysrhythmia or respiratory distress secondary to hypoxemia
11. Hold the handle of the laryngoscope in the left hand and hold the patient's mouth with the right hand by placing crossed fingers on the thumb	11. Leverage is improved by crossing the thumb and index fingers when opening of the patient's mouth (scissor-twist technique)
12. Insert the curved blade of the laryngoscope along the right side of the tongue to the left and use right thumb and index finger to pull patient's lower lip away from lower	12. Rolling the lip away from teeth prevents injury by being caught between teeth and blade
13. Lift laryngoscope forward to expose the epiglottis	13. Do not use teeth as a fulcrum, this could lead to dental damage
14. Lift laryngoscope upwards 45-degree angle to expose glottis	14. This stretches the hypoepiglottis ligament, folding the epiglottis upwards and exposing the glottis
15. As the epiglottis is lifted towards ceiling, the vertical opening of the vocal cords will come into view	15. Do not use wrist. Use shoulder and arm to lift the epiglottis
16. Once vocal cords are visualised into the right corner of the mouth and keeping vocal cords in constant view	16. Make sure you do not insert tube into esophagus; the esophageal mucosa is pink and the opening is horizontal rather than vertical
17. Gently push the tube through triangular space formed by the vocal cords and back wall of trachea	17. If the vocal cords are in spasm (closed), wait a few seconds before passing the tube
18. Stop insertion just after the tube cuff has disappeared from view beyond the cords	18. Advancing tube further may lead to its entry into a mainstem bronchus causing collapse of the unventilated lung
19. Withdraw laryngoscope while holding endotracheal tube in place. Disassemble mask from resuscitation bag, attach bag to ET tube, and ventilate the patient	
20. Inflate cuff with the minimal amount of air required to occlude the trachea.	20. Listen over the cuff area with a stethoscope. Occlusion occurs when no air leak is heard during ventilator inspiration or compression of the resuscitation bag
21. Insert bite block if necessary	21. This keeps patient from bitting down on the tube and obstructing the airway
22. Ascertain expansion of both sides of the chest by observation and auscultation of breath sounds	22. Observation and auscultation help in determining that tube remains in position and has not slipped into the right mainstem bronchus
23. Record distance from proximal end of tube to the point where the tube reaches the teeth	23. This will allow for detection of any later change in tube position
24. Secure tube to the patient's face with adhesive tape or apply a endotracheal tube stabilization device	24. The tube must be fixed securely to ensure that it will not commercially available be dislodged. Dislodgement of a tube with an inflated cuff may result in damage to the vocal cords
25. Obtain chest X-ray to verify tube position	
Follow-up phase	
1. Record tube type and size, cuff pressure, and patient tolerance of the procedure. Auscultate breath sounds every 2 hours or if signs and symptoms of respiratory distress occur. Assess ABGs after intubation if requested by the physician	1. ABGs may be prescribed to ensure adequacy of ventilation and oxygenation. Tube displacement may result in extubation (cuff above vocal cords), tube touching carina (causing paroxysmal coughing) or intubation of a mainstem bronchus (resulting in collapse of the unventilated lung)
2. Measure cuff pressure with manometer, adjust pressure. Make adjustment in tube placement on the basis of the chest X-ray results	2. The tube may be advanced or removed several centimeters for proper placement on the basis of the chest X-ray results

Contd...

Procedure 9.5: Assisting with tracheostomy insertion

Equipment:

- Tracheostomy tube (sizes 6.0 to 9.00 mm form most adults)
- Sterile instruments, hemostat, scalpel and blade, for suture material, scissors
- Sterile gown and drapes, gloves
- Cap and mask
- Antiseptic prepared solution
- Gauze sponges
- Shave prepared kit
- Sedation
- Local anesthetic and syringe
- Resuscitation bag and mask with oxygen source
- Suction source and catheters
- Syringe for cuff inflation
- Respiratory support available for post-tracheostomy (mechanial ventilation, tracheal oxygen mask, CPAP, T-piece)
- Goggles or other eye protection device.

Steps of procedure

Preparatory phase	
1. Monitor vital signs (heart rate, respiration, blood	1. Provide baseline for assessment of progress or pressure, temperature) before insertion complications
Tracheostomy Tube Placement	
Performance phase	
1. Explain the procedure to the patient. Discuss a communication system with the patient	1. Apprehension about inability to talk is usually a major concern of the tracheostomized patient
2. Obtain consent for operative procedure	
3. Shave neck region	3. Hair and beard may harbour micro-organisms. If beard is to be removed, inform the patient or family
4. Assemble equipment. Using aseptic technique, inflate tracheostomy cuff and evaluate for symmetry and volume leakage. Deflate maximally	4. Ensures that the cuff is functional before the insertion
5. Position the patient (supine with head extended, with a support under shoulders)	5. This position brings the trachea forward
6. Apply soft wrist restraints if patient is confused	6. Restraint of the confused patient may be necessary to ensure patient safety and preservation of aseptic
7. Give medication if ordered	
8. Position light source	
9. Assist with antiseptic preparation	
10. Assist with gowning and gloving	
11. Assist with sterile draping	
12. Put on goggles	12. Spraying of blood or airway secretions may occur during this procedure
13. During procedure monitor the patient's vital signs, suction as necessary, give medication as prescribed, and be prepared to administer emergency care.	13. Bradycardia may result from vagal stimulation due to tracheal manipulation or hypoxemia. Hypoxemia may also cardiac irritability
14. Immediately after the tube is inserted, inflate the cuff. The chest should be auscultated for the presence of bilateral breath sounds	14. Ensures ventilation of both lungs

Contd...

Contd...

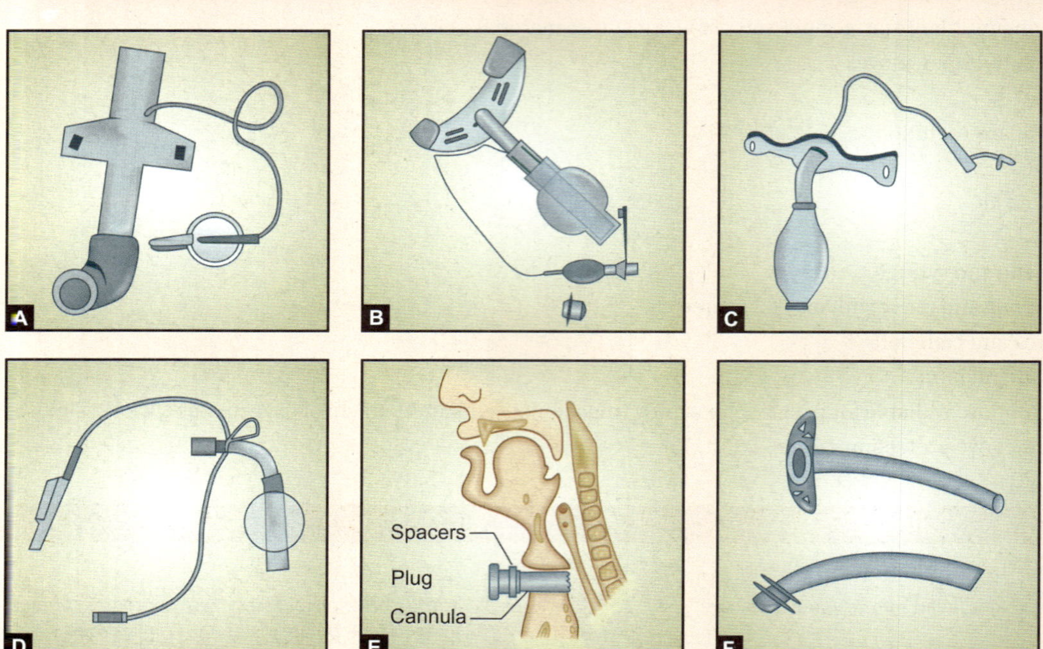

FIGS 9.38A TO F: Types of tracheostomy tubes. (A) Low pressure cuff (Shiley); (B) Fenestrated tube (Portex); (C) Polyurethane foam-filled cuff (FOME-Cuff); (D) Pitt speaking tube (National Catheter Corporation); (E) Tracheal button; (F) Silver tube

15. Secure the tracheostomy tube which will tapes or other securing device and apply dressing	
16. Apply appropriate respiratory assistive device (mechanical ventilation, tracheostomy, oxygen mask (Pap, T-piece adapter)	
17. Check the tracheostomy tube cuff pressure	17. Excessive cuff pressure may cause tracheal damage
18. "Tie sutures" or "stay sutures" of silk may have been placed through either side of the tracheal cartilage at the incision and brought out through the wound. Each is to be taped to the skin at a 45-degree angle laterally to the sternum	18. Should the tracheostomy tube become dislodged, the stay sutures may be grasped and used to spread the tracheal cartilage apart, facilitating placement of the new tube
Follow-up phase	
1. Assess vital signs and ventilatory status, note tube size used, physician performing procedure, type, dose, and route of medications given	1. Provides baseline
2. Obtain chest X-ray	2. Documents proper tube placement
3. Assess and chart condition of stoma a. Bleeding	3. a. Some bleeding around the stoma site is not uncommon for the first few hours. Monitor and inform the physician of any increase in bleeding. Clean site aseptically when necessary. Do not change tracheostomy ties for first 24 hours, because accidental dislodgement of the tube could result when the ties are loose, and tube reinsertion through the as yet unformed stoma may be difficult or impossible to accomplish
b. Swelling c. Subcutaneous air	c. When positive pressure respiratory assistive devices are used (mechanical ventilation, (CPAP) before the wound is healed, air may be forced into the subcutaneous fat layer. This can be seen as enlargement of the neck and facial tissues and felt as crepitus of "cracking" when the skin is depressed. Report immediately

Contd...

Contd...

4. An extra tube, obturator, and hemostat should be kept at the bedside. In the event of tube dislodgement, reinsertion of a new tube may be necessary. For emergency tube insertion a. Spread the wound with a hemostat or stay sutures b. Insert replacement tube (containing the obturator) at an angle c. Point cannula downward and insert the tube maximally d. Remove the obturator	4. The hemostat will open the airway and allow ventilation in the spontaneously-breathing patient. Avoid inserting the tube horizontally, because the tube may be forced against the back wall of the trachea

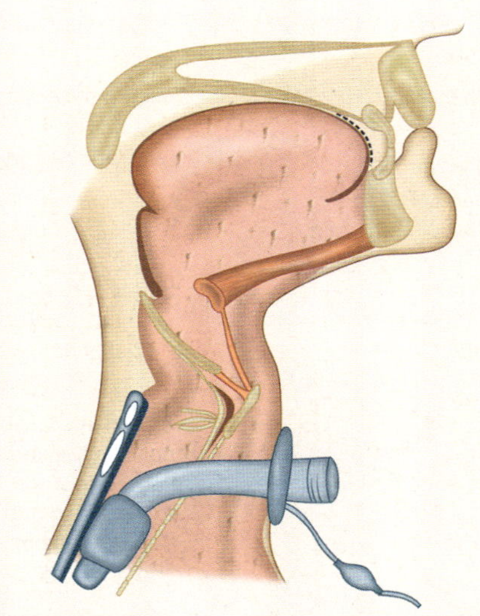

FIGURE 9.39: Tracheostomy tube placement

Procedure 9.6: Artificial airway cuff maintenance

Equipment:

- Suction catheter
- Tonsil suction
- Suction source
- 10 mL syringe
- Pressure manometer (mercury or aneroid)
- Manual resuscitation bag with reservoir, connected to 100 percent O_2 at 10 to 15 L/min
- Goggles or other eye protection device.

Steps of procedure

Nursing action	Rationale
Preparatory phase	
1. Note degree of air leakage around around cuff by listening over the cuff area with a stethoscope	1. Provides a baseline. Air leakage is heard as a crowing sound at peak, airway pressure
2. Auscultate breath sounds	2. Provides data baseline
Performance phase	
1. Explain procedure to the patient	1. Decrease the patient's anxiety and promotes cooperation
2. Put on goggles	2. Spraying of secretions may occur

Contd...

Contd...

Nursing action	Rationale
Deflating the cuff	
1. Suction the trachea, then the oral and nasal pharynx. Then replace the catheter with a second sterile suction catheter	1. Remove secretions collected above the cuff, which could the cuff, which could be aspirated into the lungs when the cuff is deflated. Do not reenter the trachea with the same catheter used for suctioning the mouth
2. Deflate the cuff slowly	2. The small test balloon at the end of the tube is inflated. A vacuum within the syringe is sensed when no more air can be aspirated
3. (Concomitant with step 2) Have patient cough, or the manually inflate the lungs with the resuscitation bag. Be ready to receive secretions in a tissue or aspirate with tonsil suction	3. Positive pressure in the air-ways may help force secretions upward and prevent aspiration of secretions
4. Suction through the tracheostomy or endotracheal tube	4. Secretions that may have been present above the inflated cuff and around the exterior tube have now seeped downward. Coughing reflex may be stimulated, helping to mobilize secretions
5. Provide adequate ventilation while the cuff is deflated a. If the patient does not require assisted ventilation, maintain humidified oxygen as directed b. If the patient requires assisted ventilation, provide manual ventilation via a resuscitation bag. Leave cuff deflated for as long as the tube repositioning requires, then reinflate	5. b. Monitor patient closely for tolerance. Loss of tidal volume or PEEP may promote hypoxemia and hypocarbia. Cuff should not be deflated for more than 30 to 45 seconds
Inflating a cuff 1. No leak technique a. Attach air-filled syringe to cuff injection port b. Slowly inject air until no air escapes from the patient's lungs around the cuff c. Note the amount of air injected to provide a seal	1. Air leakage will be heard when the intra-airway pressure is most positive (maximum peak airway pressure). For the spontaneously patient, air leakage will be heard on exhalation. For the patient on positive pressure ventilation, air leakage will be heard at maximum ventilator inspiration
2. Minimal leak technique (for mechanical ventilation) a. Attach air-filled syringe to cut off injection port b. Slowly inject air until no leak is heard at maximum peak airway pressure c. Slowly remove air from cuff until a small air leak is heard at maximum peak airway pressure d. Note amount of air injected	2. Inflates cuff at lowest possible pressure while still maintaining an adequate seal. Prevents tracheal necrosis from excessive or prolonged cuff pressure c. Adjustment in tidal volume setting may be necessary to compensate for the leak
3. Measurement of minimal occluding volume. Determination of minimal occluding volume and cuff inflation pressure. A stopcock is inserted into the cuff injection port. When the stopcock is opened to the manometer, cuff pressure is registered on the manometer. An aneroid manometer can also be used a. Inject sufficient air into the manometer tubing to raise the dial reading 1 cm H_2O above the zero reading b. Insert male part of three way stopcock into cuff injection port. One female port of stopcock holds the air filled syringe, and one port holds the pressure manometer c. Inject air into cuff until desired intracuff pressure is reached at maximum peak airway pressure d. Note amount of air needed to achieve the desired in-tracuff pressure e. Remove the stopcock from the injection port	 a. This "pressurizes" the tubing and prevents loss of air from the cuff to the tubing when the reading is taken c. Aneroid manometer measures cuff pressure in cm H_2P. A pressure of 20 to 25 cm H_2O is desired. Mercury manometer pressure should be 15 to 20 mm Hg pressure greater than upper limit may cause compression of tracheal vessels, resulting in decreased blood flow to tissue. Pressure less than lower limit may allow aspiration of gastric or oral secretions. e. Most injection ports have self-sealing valves. If not, a cap or closed stopcock may be left in the injection port (clamping of the inflation tubing is discouraged, because it may result in cracking or kinking of the line permanently

Contd...

Contd...

Nursing action	Rationale
Monitoring cuff pressure	
1. While the cuff is inflated, monitor cuff pressure every 4 hours. Maintain cuff pressure between 15 and 20 mm Hg or 20 and 25 cm H_2O	1. Excessive pressure will decrease blood flow to the tissue, resulting in tracheal necrosis, insufficient cuff pressure predisposes to aspiration
2. Document the amount of air required to maintain cuff pressure at this level	2. Establishes a baseline for evaluation of change in pressure
Inability to maintain a seal	
1. Assess the degree of leakage and length of time elapsed since volume was replenished	1. If an inflated cuff leaks air within 10 minutes, assessment cuff is necessary. Possibilities may be: a. Cuff positioned above the vocal cords (direct visualization necessary for repositioning) b. Incompetence of self-sealing valve on injection port c. Tracheal dilatation (requiring larger size tube) d. Cuff may be ruptured, requiring a new tube
2. Inflate the cuff to desired level	
3. Disconnect syringe (and manometer if used)	
4. Assess for leakage	
5. If leakage occurs place three way stopcock between syringe and close stopcock. Remove syringe and manometer (if used) leaving closed stopcock on port	5. Closed stopcock left in injection port acts as "plug" if selfsealing valve is incompetent.
6. If air enters tube or replacement may be consult with appropriate personnel	
Follow-up phase	
1. Note time and amount of air used for adequate seal, intercut and inability to achieve seal. Document intervention necessary to record or change tracheostomy tube to obtain a desired seal	
2. While the cuff is inflated, assess cuff-pressure every 4 hours. The cuff pressure manometer is useful for this	2. Leakage of air from the cuff or cuff injection port may occur. Assess the inflation status and adjust as needed

Procedure 9.7: Tracheostomy (routine)

Equipment:

- Assemble the equipment or obtain a prepackaged tracheostomy care kit
- Sterile towel
- Sterile gauze
- Sterile cotton
- Sterile gloves
- Hydrogen peroxide
- Sterile water
- Antiseptic solution and ointment (optional)
- Tracheostomy tie tapes or commercially available tracheostomy securing device.
- Goggles or other eye protection devices.

Steps of procedure

Nursing action	Rationale
Preparatory phase	
1. Assess area of stome before tracheostomy care (redness, swelling, character of secretions, presence of pure)	1. The presence of skin break-down or infection must be monitored. Culture of the site may be warranted by appearance of these signs

Contd...

Contd...

Nursing action	Rationale
Performance phase	
1. Suction the trachea and pharynx thoroughly before tracheostomy care	1. Removal of secretions before tracheostomy care keeps the area clean longer
2. Explain procedure to the patient	2. For cooperation of client
3. Wash hands neately	3. Prevent infection
4. Assemble equipment a. Place sterile towel on patient's chest under tracheostomy site b. Open four sterile sponges and pour hydrogen peroxide on them c. Open 2 gauze sponges and pour antiseptic d. Open 2 gauze sponges. Keep dry e. Open 2 gauze sponges and pour sterile water on them f. Place tracheostomy tube tapes on field g. Put on goggles and sterile gloves	4. a. Provides sterile field b. For removal of mucus and crust, which promotes bacterial growth c. May be applied to fresh stoma. Not necessary for clean, healed stoma g. Goggles prevent spraying of secretions into the nurse's eyes. Sterile gloves prevent contamination of the wound by nurse's hands and also protect the nurse's hands from infection

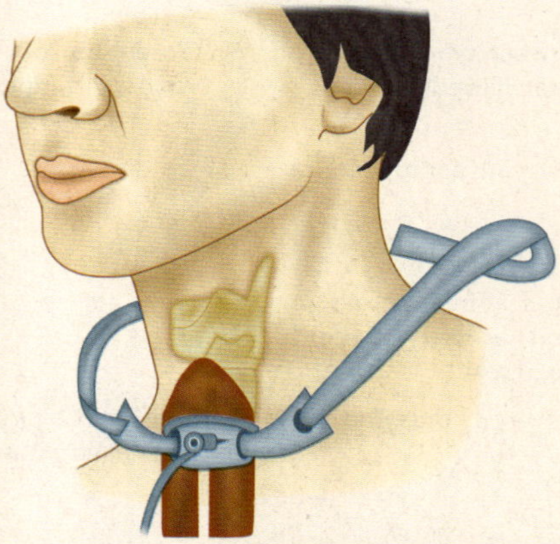

FIG. 9.40: Placement of tracheostomy tube tapes and elective gauze pad

Nursing action	Rationale
5. Clean the external end of the tracheostomy tube with 2 gauze sponges with hydrogen peroxide; discard sponges	5. Designate the hand you clean with as contaminated and reserve the other hand as sterile for handling sterile equipment
6. Clean the stoma area with 2 peroxide soaked gauze sponges. Make only a single sweep with each gauze sponge before discarding	6. Hydrogen peroxide may help loosen dry-crusted secretions
7. Loosen and remove crust with sterile cotton swabs	
8. Repeat step 6 using the sterile water-soaked gauze sponges	8. Ensures that all hydrogen peroxide is removed.
9. Repeat step 6 using dry sponges	9. Ensures dryness of the area. Wetness promotes infection and irritation
10. (Optional). An infected wound may be cleansed with gauze saturated with an antiseptic solution, then dried. A thin layer of antibiotic ointment may be applied to the stoma with a cotton swab	10. May help clear wound infection.
11. Change a disposable inner cannula, touching only the external portion, and lock it securely into place. If inner cannula is reusable remove it with your contaminated hand and clean it in hydrogen peroxide solution, using brush or pipe cleaners with your sterile hand. When clean, drop it into sterile saline solution and agitate to rinse thoroughly with your sterile hand. Tap it gently to dry it and replace it with your sterile hand	11. Because cannula is dirty when you remove it, use your contaminated hand. It is considered sterile once you clean it, so handle it with your sterile hand

Contd...

Contd...

Nursing action	Rationale
12. Change the tracheostomy tie tapes	12.
a. Cut soiled tape while holding the tube securely with other hand. Use care not to cut the pilot balloon tubing	a. Stabilization of the tube helps prevent accidental dislodgement and keeps due to tube manipulation at a minimum
b. Remove old tapes carefully	b. To prevent injury
c. Grasp slit end of clean tape and pull through opening on side of the tracheostomy tube	c. To prevent injury
d. Pull other end of tape securely through the slit end of the tape	d. To prevent injury
e. Repeat on the other side	e. To prevent injury
f. Tie the tapes at the side of the neck in a square knot. Alternate knot from side to side each time tapes are changed	f. To prevent irritation and rotate pressure site
g. Tape should be tight enough to keep tube securely in the stoma, but loose enough to permit two fingers to fit between the tapes and the neck	g. Excessive tightness of tapes will compress jugular veins, decrease blood circulation to the skin under the tape and result in discomfort for the patient
Note: If only one clinician is available, the stoma is new (less than 2 weeks), or the patient's condition is unstable, follow steps c through f before removing old tape. Two set(s) of ties will be in place at the same time. After completing step f, cut and remove the old tapes. Also a tracheostomy-securing device can be used instead of the tracheostomy ties.	
13. Place a gauze pad between the stoma site and the tracheostomy tube to absorb secretions and prevent irritation of the stoma according to institution policy (see accompanying figure). Many clinicians feel that gauze should not be used around the stoma. In their opinion, the dressing keeps the area moist and dark, promoting stomal infection. They believe the stoma should be left open to the air and the surrounding area kept dry. A dressing is used only if secretions are draining on to subclavian or neck IV sites or chest incisions	
Follow-up phase	
1. Document procedure performance observations of stoma (irritation redness, edema, subcutaneous air) and character of secretions (color, purulence). Report changes in stoma appearance or secretions	1. Provides a baseline
2. Cleaning of the fresh stoma should be performed every 8 hours, or more frequently if indicated by accumulation of secretions. Ties should be changed every 24 hours or more frequently if soiled or wet	2. The area must be kept clean and dry to prevent infection or irritation of tissues

Procedure 9.8: Insertion of a tracheostomy button

Equipment:

- Tracheostomy button kit (includes cannula, solid closure plug, spacers, universal adapter)
- Water-soluble lubricant
- Syringe for deflation of tracheostomy cuff
- Replacement tracheostomy tube.

Steps of procedure

Nursing action	Rationale
Preparatory phase	
1. Assess whether patient meets teria for use of tracheostomy button. Criteria include: able to be adequately oxygenated with nasal cannula or face mask; able to swallow and protect the airway; able to cough up secretions; and a non-infected, nonirritated tracheal stoma	1. If patient does not meet these criteria, use of tracheostomy tube as airway must be continued

Contd...

Contd...

Nursing action	Rationale
2. Determine vital signs, level of consciousness, SaO_2 of ABG	2. Provides baseline for future assessment
Performance phase	
1. Elevate the head of the bed 45 degrees, suction the airway, deflate the tracheostomy tube cuff and remove the tube	1. Protects against aspiration
2. Determine the distance from anterior tracheal wall to the outer edge of the stoma (skin surface) using a probe with a right angle bend (contained in the kit)	2. Insert the angled end of the probe into the stoma, pull gently until the probe touches the anterior wall, then mark the probe at the outer edge of the stoma (skin) surface
3. Compare the length of the tracheostomy button cannula with this measurement. If the cannula is too long, it can be sized to fit by adding spacers included into the kit	3. Spacer rings can be slipped over cannula to size it for individualised patient requirements
4. Coat the cannula with water-soluble lubricant. Ask the patient to relax and take several deep breaths. Insert the cannula into the stoma	4. The cannula should pass easily into the stoma. If insertion is difficult, recheck cannula size. Several sizes are available
5. Insert the closure plug into the cannula. Ties may be used to hold the button in place until the stoma closes round the button	5. A slight snap will be heard as the plug enters the cannula. The plug causes the proximal end of the cannula to flare, holding in place
6. Remove button two times a week, clean with antibacterial soap, and replace it	6. Periodic removal helps to keep tissue from granulating into distal portion of the cannula
Follow-up phase	
1. Observe immediate patient response and obtain SaO_2 or ABG after insertion. Report changes	1. Use of the button increases dead space, which may increase work of breathing or cause a decrease in SaO_2
2. Determine ability of patient to cough out secretions and swallow with button in place	2. Confirms patient will not retain secretions or be at risk for aspiration with use of this device

Procedure 9.9: Nasotracheal (NT) suctioning

Equipment:

- Assemble the following equipment or obtain a prepackaged kit
- Disposable curved-tipped suction catheter
- Sterile towel
- Sterile disposable gloves
- Sterile water
- Anesthetic water-soluble lubricant jelly
- Suction source at 80 to 120 mm Hg
- Resuscitation bag with face mask. Connect 100 percent O_2 source with flow of 10 L/min.

Steps of procedure

Nursing action	Rationale
Preparatory phase	
1. Monitor heart rate, respiratory rate, color, ease of respirations. If the patient is on monitor, continue monitoring heart rate or arterial blood pressure. Discontinue the suctioning and apply oxygen if heart rate decreases by 20 beats per minute or increases by 40 beats per minute. If blood pressure increases, or if cardiac dysrhythmia is noted	1. Suctioning may cause the occurrence of: a. Hypoxemia—initially resulting in tachycardia and increased blood pressure, and later causing cardiac ectopy, bradycardia, hypotension, and cyanosis b. Vagal stimulation resulting in bradycardia
Performance phase	
1. Ascertain that the suction apparatus is functional Place suction tubing within easy reach	1. The procedure must be done aseptically, because the catheter will be entering the trachea below the level of the vocal cords and introduction of bacteria is contraindicated

Contd...

Contd...

Nursing action	Rationale
2. Inform and instruct the patient regarding procedure a. At a certain interval, the patient will be requested to cough to open the lung passage, so the catheter will go into the lungs and not into the stomach. The patient will also be encouraged not to try to swallow, because this will also cause the catheter to enter the stomach b. The postoperative patient can splint the wound to make the coughing produced by NT suctioning less painful	2. A thorough explanation will decrease patient's anxiety and promote patient's cooperation
3. Place the patient in a semi-Fowler's or sitting position if possible	3. NT suctioning should follow chest physical therapy, postural drainage and/or ultrasonic nebulization therapy. The patient should not be suctioned after eating or after a tube feeding is given (unless absolutely necessary) to decrease the possibility of emesis and aspiration
4. Place sterile towel across the patient's chest. Squeeze small amount of sterile anesthetic water-soluble lubricant jelly on to the towel	
5. Open sterile pack containing curved tipped suction catheter	
6. Aseptically glove both hands. Designate one hand (usually the dominant one) as "sterile" and the other hand as "contaminated	6. The contaminated hand must also be gloved to ensure that not come in contact with the nurse's hand, possibly resulting in infection of the nurse
7. Grasp sterile catheter with sterile hand	
8. Lubricate catheter with the anesthetic jelly and pass the catheter into the nostril and back into the pharynx	8. If obstruction is met, do not for the catheter. Remove it and try the other nostril
9. Pass the catheter into the trachea. To do this, ask the patient to cough or say "ahh" If the patient is incapable of either, try to advance the catheter on inspiration. Asking the patient to stick out tongue or hold tongue extended with a gauze sponge, may also help to open the airway. If a protected amount of time is needed to position, the catheter in the trachea, stop and oxygenate the patient with face mask or the resuscitation bag-mask unit at intervals, if three < attempts to place the catheter are unsuccessful, request assistance	9. These maneuvers may add in opening the glottis and allowing passage of the catheter into the trachea. To evaluate proper placement, listen at the catheter end for air, or feel, for air movement against the cheek. An increase in intensity of breath sounds or more air movement against cheek indicates nearness to the larynx. Gagging or sudden lessening of sound means the catheter is in the hypopharynx. Draw back and advance again. The presence of the catheter in the trachea is indicated by: a. Sudden paroxysms of coughing b. Movement of air through the catheter c. Vigorous bubbling of air, when the distal end of the suction catheter is placed in a cup of sterile water d. Inability of the patient to speak
10. Specific positioning of catheter for deep bronchial suctioning: passage on the opposite side a. For left bronchial suctioning, turn the patient's head to the extreme right, chin up b. For right bronchial suctionteral pneumonia, atelectasis to the extreme left, chin up	10. Turning the patient's head to one side elevates the bronchial, making catheter insertion easier. Suctioning of a particular lung segment may be of value in patients with unilaing, turn the patient's head or collapse
Note: The value of turning the head as an aid to entering the right or left mainstem bronchi is not accepted by all clinicians.	
11. Never apply suction until catheter is in the trachea a. Once correct position is ascertained, apply suction and gently rotate catheter while pulling it slightly upward. Do not remove catheter fro the trachea	11. a. Because entry into the trachea is often difficult, less change in arterial oxygen may be leaving the catheter in the trachea than by repeated insertion attempts
12. Disconnect the catheter from the suctioning source after 5 to 10 seconds. Apply oxygen by placing a face-mask over the patient's nose, mouth and catheter and instruct the patient to breathe deeply	12. Ensure that adequate time is allowed to reoxygenate the patient as oxygen is removed, as well as secretions, during suctioning
13. Reconnect suction source. Repeat as necessary	13. Not more than three to four suction passes should be made per suction episode

Contd...

Contd...

Nursing action	Rationale
14. During the last suction pass, remove the catheter completely while applying suction and rotating the catheter gently. Apply oxygen when catheter is removed	14. Never leave the catheter in the trachea after the suction procedure is concluded, because the epiglottis is splinted open and aspiration may occur
Placement of nasotracheal tube for suctioning the tracheobronchial tree	
Follow-up phase	
1. Dispose of disposable equipment	
2. Measure heart rate and blood pressure. Record the patient's tolerance of procedure, type and amount of secretions removed and complications	2. Record any patient intolerance of procedure (changes in vital signs, bleeding, laryngospasm, upper airway noise)

Procedure 9.10 Sterile tracheobronchial suction by way of tracheostomy or endotracheal tube (spontaneous or mechanical ventilation)

Equipment:

- Assemble the following equipment or obtain a prepackaged suctioning kit
- Sterile suction catheters—No. 14 or 16 (adult) No. 8 or 10 (child). The outer diameter of the suction catheter should be no greater than one half of the inner diameter of the artificial airway
- Two sterile gloves
- Sterile towel
- Suction source at 80 to 120 mm Hg
- Sterile water
- Resuscitator bag with a reservoir connected to 100 percent oxygen source (if patient is on PEEP or CPAP, add positive end expiratory pressure (PEEP) valve to valve on resuscitation bag in an amount equal to that on the ventilator or CPAP device)
- Normal saire solution (in syringe or single-dose packet)
- Sterile cup for water
- Alcohol swabs
- Sterile water-soluble lubricant jelly
- Goggles or other eye protection device.

Steps of procedure

Nursing action	Rationale
Preparatory phase	
1. Monitor the heart rate and auscultate breath sounds. If the patient is monitored, continuously monitor heart rate and arterial blood pressure, progressing to blood pressure. If arterial blood gases are done routinely, know baseline values (it is important to establish a baseline because suctioning should be discontinued and oxygen applied or manual ventilation reinstituted if, during the suction procedure, the heart rate decreases by 20 beats per minute or increases by 40 beats per minute, blood pressure drops, or cardiac dysrhythmia is noted)	1. Suctioning may cause a. Hypoxemia, initially resulting in tachycardia and increased blood pressure, progressing to cardiac ectopy, bradycardia, hypotension and cyanosis b. Vagal stimulation which may result in bradycardia
Performance phase	
1. Instruct the patient how to "spling" surgical incision, because coughing will be induced during the procedure. Explain the importance of performing the suction procedure in an aseptic manner	
2. Assemble equipment. Check fun-function of suction and manual resuscitation bag connected to 100 percent O_2 source. Put on goggles	2. Make sure that all equipment is functional before sterile technique is instituted to prevent interruption once the procedure is begun. Use of 100 percent O_2 will help to prevent hypoxemia

Contd...

Contd...

Nursing action	Rationale
3. Wash hands properly	
4. Open sterile towel. Place in a biblike fashion on patient's chest. Open alcohol wipes and place on corner of towel. Place small amount of sterile water-soluble jelly on towel	
5. Open sterile gloves. Place on towel	
6. Open suction catheter package	
7. If the patient is on mechanical ventilation, test to make sure disconnection of ventilator attachment may be made with one hand	
8. Do not sterile gloves. Designate one hand as contaminated for disconnecting, bagging and working the suction control. Usually the dominant hand is kept sterile and will be used to thread the suction catheter	8. The hand designated as sterile must remain uncontaminated to organisms are not introduced into the lungs. The contaminated hand must also be from contacting the nurse's gloved to prevent sputum hand, possibly resulting in an infection of the nurse
9. Use the sterile hand to remove carefully the suction catheter from the package, curling the catheter around the gloved fingers	
10. Connect suction source to the suction fitting of the catheter with the contaminated hand	
11. Using the contaminated hand, disconnect the patient from the ventilator, CPAP device, or other oxygen source (place the ventilator connector on the sterile towel and flip a corner of the towel over the connection to prevent fluid from spraying into the area)	11. Prevents contamination of the connection
12. Ventilate and oxygenate the patient with the resuscitator bag compressing firmly and as completely as possible approximately four to five times (try to approximate the patient's tidal volume). The procedure is called "bagging" the patient, in the spontaneously breathing patient, coordinate manual ventilations with the patient's own inspiratory effort	12. Ventilation before suctioning helps prevent hypoxemia. When possible two nurses work as a team to suction. Attempting to ventilate against the patient's own respiratory efforts may result in high airway pressures predisposing the patient to barotrauma (lung injury due to pressure)
13. Lubricate the tip of the suction catheter. Gently insert suction catheter as far as possible into the artificial airway without applying suction. Most patients will cough when the catheter touches the carina	13. Suctioning on insertion would unnecessarily decrease oxygen in the airway
14. Withdraw catheter 2 to 3 cm and apply suction. Quickly rotate the catheter while it is being withdrawn	14. Failure to withdraw and rotate catheter may result in damage to tracheal mucosa. Release suction if a pulling sensation is felt
15. Limit suction time to not more than 10 seconds. Discontinue if heart rate decreases by 20 beats per minute or increases by 40 beats per minute, or if cardiac ectopy is observed	15. Sectioning removes oxygen as well as secretions and may also cause vagal stimulation
16. Bag patient between suction passes with approximately four to five manual ventilations	16. The oxygen removed by suctioning must be replenished before suctioning is attempted again
17. At this point, sterile normal saline may be instilled into the trachea by way of the artificial airway if secretions are tenacious a. Open prepackaged container and instill 3 to 5 mL normal saline into the artificial airway during spontaneous inspiration b. Bag vigorously and then suction	17. Some clinicians believe secretion removal may be facilitated with saline instillation. Others believe saline does not mix with mucus and that suctioning of the saline just instilled is the only effect produced by performing this step. It is now thought that the greatest benefit of instilling sterile normal saline is to initiate a cough a. Instillation of the saline during inspiration will prevent the saline from being blown back out of the tube b. Bagging stimulates cough and distributes saline to loosen secretions
18. Rinse catheter between suction passes by inserting tip in cup of sterile water and applying suction	
19. Continue making suction passes bagging the patient between passes, until the airways are clear of accumulated secretions. Not more than four suction passes should be made per suctioning episode	19. Repeated suctioning of a patient in a short time interval predisposes to hypoxemia, as well as being tiring and traumatic to the patient

Contd...

Contd...

Nursing action	Rationale
20. Give the patient four to five "sigh" breaths with the bag	20. Sighing is accomplished by dropping the bag slowly and completely with two hands to deliver approximately 1½ times the normal total volume to the patient, allowing for maximal lung expansion prevention of atelectasis
21. Return the patient to the ventilator or apply CPAP or other oxygen-delivery device	
22. Suction oral secretions from the oropharynx above the artificial airway cuff	
23. Clean elbow fitting of resuscitation bag with alcohol; cover with a sterile glove or 4 × 4	
Follow-up phase	
1. Note any change in vital signs patient's intolerance to the procedure. Record amount and consistency of secretions	1. Evaluate the effectiveness of procedure and patient response
2. Assess need for further suctioning at least every 2 hours, or more frequently if secretions are copious	
Note: A closed system for suctioning may be in place in the ventilator circuit that allows suctioning without removal from the ventilator. Teach caregivers to suction in the home situation using clean technique, rather than sterile. Wash hands well before suctioning and reuse catheter after rinsing it in warm water.	

Procedure 9.11: Teaching the patient breathing exercises

Steps of procedure

Nursing action	Rationale
Preparatory phase	
Instruct the patient as follows:	
Diaphragmatic breathing	
1. Place one hand on stomach just below the ribs and the other hand on the middle of the chest	1. This helps the patient become aware of the diaphragm and its function in breathing
2. Breathe in slowly and deeply through the nose, letting the abdomen protrude as far as it will. The abdomen enlarges during inspiration and decreases in size during expiration	2. Slow inhalation provides ventilation and hyperinflation of the lungs
3. Breathe out through pursed lips while contracting (tightening) the abdominal muscles. Press firmly inward and upward on the abdomen while breathing out	3. Contracting the abdominal muscles assists the diaphragm in rising to empty the lungs. The hand generates pressure, on the abdomen to facilitate more complete expiration
4. The chest should not move, attention is directed at the abdomen, not the chest	4. Contraction of the abdominal muscles should take place during expiration
5. Repeat for 1 minute (followed by a rest period of 2 minutes). Work up to 10 minutes, four times daily	
6. Learn to do diaphragmatic breathing while lying, then sitting, and ultimately standing and walking	6. Diaphragmatic breathing helps the patient breathe in a controlled manner during activities that produce dyspnea. If shortness of breach occurs, advise stopping the exercises until breathing pattern comes under control
Pursed-lip breathing	
1. Inhale through the nose	
2. Exhale slowly and evenly against pursed lips while contracting (tightening) the abdominal muscles (avoid exhaling forcefully)	2. Pursing the lips increases intrabronchial pressure (helps maintain the branch in an open position) as well as intra-alveolar pressure. The pursed lips maneuver also prolongs the expiratory phase of breathing, makes it easier to empty the air in the lungs, and promotes carbon dioxide elimination

Contd...

Contd...

Nursing action	Rationale
3. Sit in a chair. Fold arms across the abdomen a. Inhale through the nose b. Bend over and exhale slowly through pursed lips while counting up to 7	3. b. Leaning forward pushes the abdominal organs upward
4. While walking a. Inhale while walking two steps b. Exhale through pursed lips while walking four steps	4. Try any similar combinations according to breathing tolerance of patient
Lower side rib breathing	
1. Place hands on sides of lower ribs	
2. Inhale deeply and slowly while sides expand moving hands outward	
3. Exhale slowly through pursed lips and feel the hands and the ribs move inward	
4. Rest	
Lower back and ribs breathing	
1. Sit in a chair. Place hands behind back; hold flat against lower ribs	
2. Inhale deeply and slowly while rib cage expands backward; the hands will move outward	
3. Keep hands in place. Blow out slowly; hands will move in	
Segmental Breathing	
1. Place hands on sides of lower ribs	
2. Inhale deeply and slowly while concentrating on moving the right hand outward by expanding the right rib cage	
3. Ensure that the right hand moves outward more than the left hand	
4. Keeping hands in place, exhale slowly, and feel the right hand and ribs moving in	
5. Repeat concentrating on expanding left side more than the right side	
6. Rest	
Patient Education	
Instruct patient to:	
1. Always inhale through the nose. This permits filtration, humidification and warming of air	
2. Breathe slowly in a rhythmic and relaxed manner. This permits more complete exhalation and emptying of lungs; helps overcome anxiety associated with dyspnea and decreases oxygen requirement	
3. Avoid sudden exertion	
4. Practice in several positions; air distribution and pulmonary circulation vary according to position of the chest	

Procedure 9.12: Percussion (clapping) and vibration

Equipment:

- Pillows
- Tilt table
- Emesis basin
- Sputum cup
- Paper tissues.

Steps of procedure

Nursing action	Rationale
Performance phase	
1. Instruct the patient to use diaphragmatic breathing	1. Diaphragmatic breathing helps the patient relax and helps widen airways
2. Position the patient in prescribed postural drainage position/s. The spine should be straight to promote rib cage expansion	2. The patient is positioned according to the area of lung that is to be drained
3. Percuss (or clap) with cupped hands over the chest wall for 1 or 2 minutes from: a. The lower ribs to shoulders in the back b. The lower ribs to top of chest in the front	3. This action helps dislodge mucous plugs and mobilize secretions towards the main branch and trachea. The air trapped between the operator's hand and chest wall will produce a characteristic hollow sound
4. Avoid clapping over the spine, liver, kidneys, spleen, breast, scapula, clavicle or sternum	4. Percussion over these areas may cause injuries to the spine or internal organs
5. Instruct the patient to inhale slowly and deeply. Vibrate the chest wall as the patient exhales slowly through pursed lips a. Place one hand on top of the other over-affected area or place one hand on each side of the rib cage b. Tense the muscles of the hands and arms while applying moderate pressure downward and vibrate hands and arms c. Relieve pressure on the thorax as the patient inhales d. Encourage the patient to cough and using abdominal muscles, after three or four vibrations	5. This sets up a vibration that carries through the chest wall and helps free the mucus b. This maneuver is performed in the direction in which the ribs move on expiration d. Contracting the abdominal muscles while coughing increases cough effectiveness coughing aids in the movement and expulsion of secretions

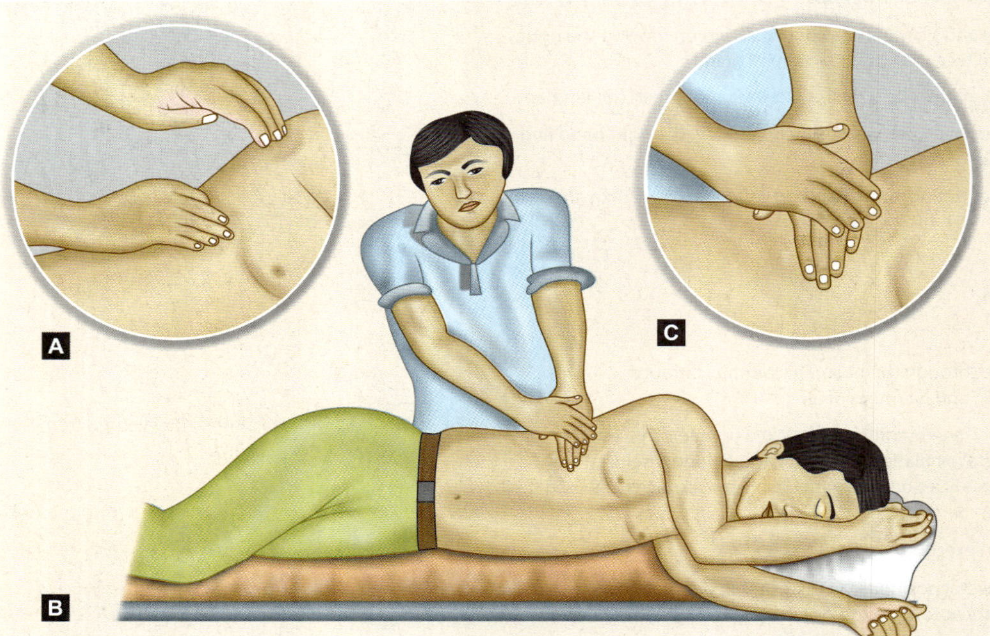

FIGS 9.41A TO C: Percussion and vibration. (A) Proper hand positioning for percussion; (B) Proper technique for vibration. Note that the wrists and elbows are kept stiff and the vibrating motion is produced by the shoulder muscles; (C) Proper hand position for vibration

Nursing action	Rationale
6. Allow the patient to rest for several minutes	
7. Listen with a stethoscope for changes in breath sounds	7. The appearance of crackles and rhonchi indicate movement of air around mucous in the bronchi
8. Repeat the percussion and vibration cycle according to the patient's tolerance and clinical response, usually 15 to 30 minutes	

Procedure 9.13: Administering nebulizer therapy
(Sidestream jet nebulizer)

Equipment:

- Air compressor
- Connection tubing
- Nebulizer
- Medication and saline solution.

Steps of procedure

Nursing action	Rationale
Preparatory phase	
1. Monitor the heart rate before and after the treatment for patients using bronchodilator drugs	1. Bronchodilators may cause cardia, palpitations, dizziness, nausea or nervousness
Performance phase	
1. Explain the procedure to the patient. This therapy depends on patient effort	1. Proper explanation of the procedure helps to ensure the patient's co-operation and effectiveness of the treatment
2. Place the patient in a comfortable sitting of semi-Flowler's position	2. Diaphragmatic excursion and lung compliance are greater in this position. This ensures maximal distribution and deposition of aerosalized particles to basilar area of the lungs
3. Add the prescribed amount of medication and saline to the nebulizer. Connect the tubing to the compressor and set the flow at 6 to 18 L/min	3. A fine mist from the device should be visible
4. Instruct the patient to exhale	
5. Tell the patient to take in a deep breath from the mouthpiece hold breath briefly, then exhale	5. This encourages optimal dispersion of the medication
6. Nose clips are sometimes used if the patient has difficulty breathing only through the mouth	
7. Observe expansion of chest to ascertain that patient is taking deep breaths	7. This will ensure medication is deposited below the level of the oropharynx
8. Instruct the patient to breathe slowly and deeply until all the medications is nebulized	8. Medication will usually be nebulized within 15 minutes at a flow of 6 to 8 L/min
9. On completion of the treatment encourage the patient to cough after several deep breaths	9. The medication may dilate airways, facilitating expectoration of secretions
Follow-up phase	
1. Record medication used and description of secretions	
2. Disassemble and clean nebulizer after each use. Keep this equipment in the patient's room. The equipment is changed every 24 hours	2. Each patient has own breathing circuit (nebulizer, tubing, and mouthpiece). Through proper cleaning, sterilization and storage of equipment, organisms can be prevented from entering the lungs
Nebulizer tubing and mouthpiece can be reused at home repeatedly. Recommend thorough rinsing with hot water after each use and periodic washing with liquid soap and hot water.	

Procedure 9.14: Administering oxygen by nasal cannula (Fig. 9.42)

Equipment:

- Oxygen source
- Plastic nasal cannula with connecting tubing (disposable)
- Humidifier filled with distilled water
- Flowmeter
- No smoking signs

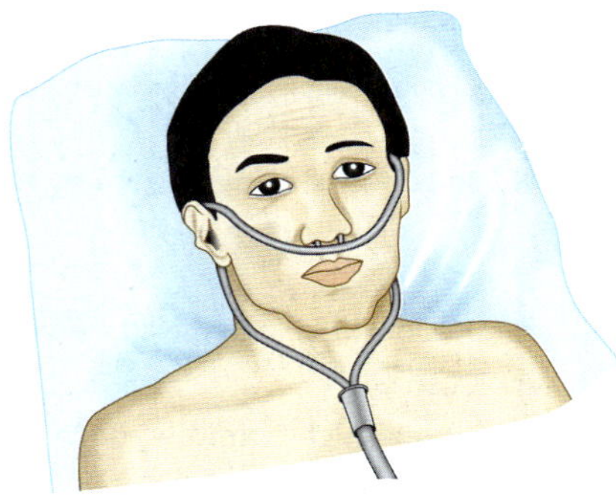

FIGURE 9.42: Nasal cannula for oxygen delivery

Steps of procedure

Nursing action	Rationale
Preparatory phase	
1. Determine current vital signs level of consciousness, and most recent ABG	1. Provides a baseline for future assessment. Nasal cannula oxygen administration is often used for patients prone to CO_2 retention. Oxygen may depress the hypoxic drive of these patients (evidenced by a decreased respiratory rate, altered mental status and further $PaCO_2$ elevation)
2.Assess rise of CO_2 retention with oxygen administration	2. If $PaCO_2$ is decreased or normal, the patient is not experiencing CO_2 retention and can use oxygen without fear of the above consequences
Performance phase	
1. Paste no smoking signs on the patient's door and in view of patients and visitors	
2. Show the nasal cannula to the patient and explain the procedure	
3. Make sure the humidifier is filled to the appropriate mark	3. Humidification may not be ordered if the flow rate is = 4 L/min
4. Attach the connecting tube from the nasal cannula to the humidifier outlet	
5. Set flow rate at prescribed liters/minute. Feel to determine if oxygen is flowing through the tips of the cannula Approximate oxygen concentrations delivered are: 1. L = 24 to 25 percent 2. L = 27 to 29 percent 3. L = 30 to 33 percent 4. L = 33 to 37 percent 5. L = 36 to 41 percent 6. L = 39 to 45 percent Patient's who require low constant concentrations of oxygen and whose breathing pattern varies greatly may need to use a venturi mask, particularly if they are carbon dioxide retainers	5. Because a nasal cannula is a low-flow system (patient tidal volume supplies part of the inspired gas), oxygen concentration will vary, depending on the patient's respiratory rate and tidal volume
6. Place the tips of the cannula in the patient's nose and adjust straps around ears for snug comfortable fit	6. Inspect skin behind ears periodically for irritation or breakdown Administering oxygen by nasal cannula. Patient's inspiration consists of a mixture of supplemental oxygen supplied via the nasal cannula and room air. Oxygen concentration is variable and depends on patient's tidal volume and ventilatory pattern
Follow-up phase	
1. Record flow rate used and immediate patient response	1. Note the patient's tolerance of treatment. Report any intolerance noted
2. Assess patient's condition ABG or SaO_2 and the functioning of equipment at regular intervals	2. Depression of hypoxic drive is most likely to occur within the first hours of oxygen use. Monitoring of SaO_2 with oximetry can be substituted for ABG if the patient is not retaining CaO_2
3. Determine patient comfort with oxygen use	3. Flow rates in excess of 4 L/min may cause irritation to the nasal and pharyngeal mucosa
Note: Avoid use of petroleum jelly to lubricate nares, because it may clog openings of cannula	

Procedure 9.15: Administering oxygen by simple face mask with/without aerosol (Fig. 9.43)

Equipment:

- Oxygen source
- Humidifier bottle with distilled water, if high humidity is desired
- Plastic aerosol mask
- Large-bore tubing (high humidity) or small-bore tubing
- Flowmeter
- No smoking signs
- For heated aerosol therapy humidifier heating element.

Steps of procedure

Nursing action	Rationale
Preparatory phase	
1. Determine current vital signs, level of consciousness, and SaO_2 or ABG, if patient is at risk for CO_2 retention	1. Because the aerosol face mask is a low-flow system (patient's tidal volume may supply part of inspired gas). Oxygen concentration will vary depending on the patient's respiratory rate and rhythm. Oxygen delivery may be inadequate for tachypneic patients (flow does not meet peak inspiratory demand) or excessive for patients with slow respirations
2. Assess viscosity and volume of sputum produced	2. Aerosol is given to assist in mobilizing retained secretions
Performance phase	
1. Paste no smoking signs on patient's door and in view of the patient and visitors	
2. Show the aerosol mask to the patient and explain the procedure	
3. Make sure that the humidifier is filled to the appropriate mark	3. If the humidifier bottle is not sufficiently full, less moisture will be delivered
4. Attach the large-bore tubing from the mask to the humidifier in the heating element, if used	
5. Set desired oxygen concentration of humidifier bottle and plug in the heating element, if used	5. The inspired oxygen concentration is determined by the humidifier setting. Usual concentrations are 35 to 50 percent
6. If the patient is tachypneic and concentration of 50 percent oxygen or greater is desired, two humidifiers and flow meters should be yoked together	6. The aerosol mask is a low-flow system. Yoking two humidifiers together doubles humidifier flow but does not change the inspired oxygen concentration

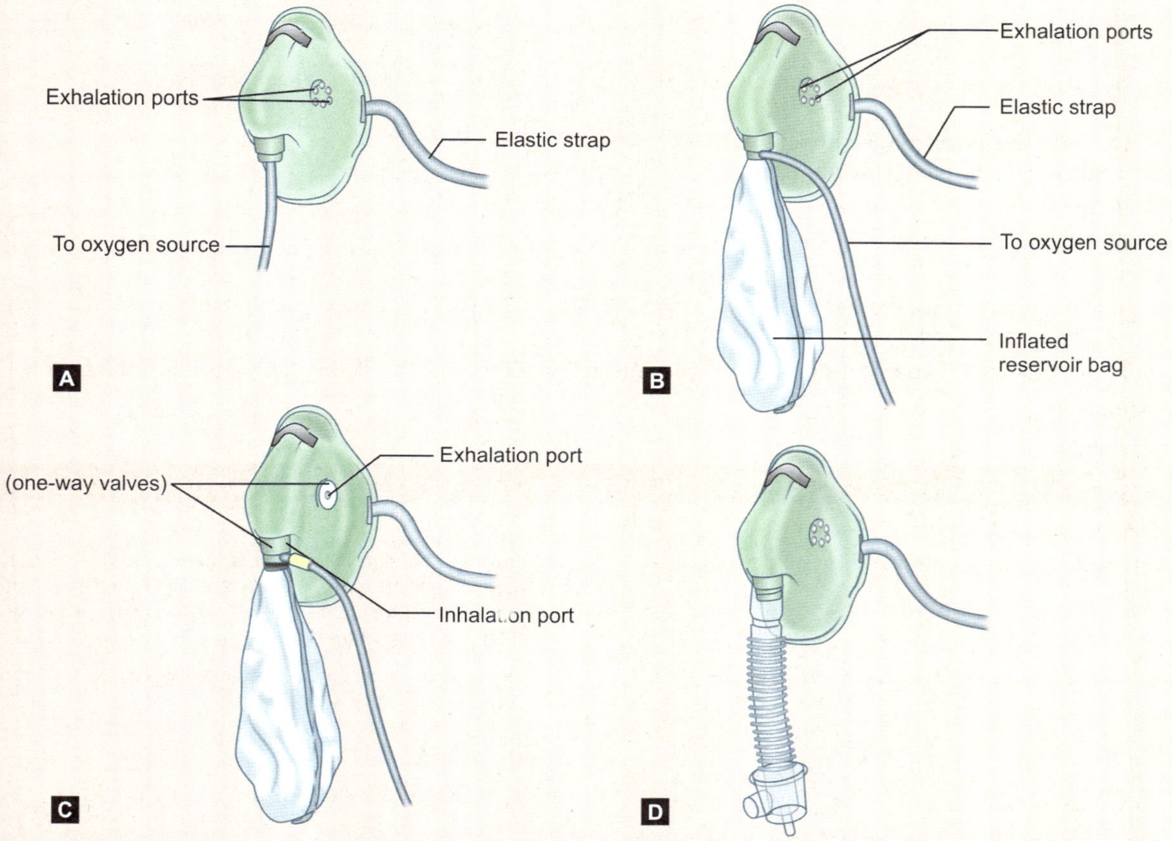

FIGS 9.43A TO D: Oxygen masks. (A) Simple mask; (B) Partial rebreather mask; (C) Nonrebreathing mask; (D) Venturi mask

Contd...

Contd...

Nursing action	Rationale
7. Adjust the flow rate until the desired mist is produced meet inspiratory demand and maintains a constant accurate concentration of oxygen	7. This ensures that the patient is receiving flow sufficient to (usually 10 to 12 L/min)
8. Apply the mask to the patient's face and adjust the straps so the mask fits securely	
9. Drain the tubing frequently by emptying condensate into a separate receptacle, not into the humidifier. If a heating element is used, the tubing will have to be drained more often	9. The tubing must be kept free of condensate allowed to accumulate in the delivery tube will block flow and alter oxygen concentration. If condensate is emptied into the humidifier, bacteria may be aerosolized into the lungs
10. If a heating element is used, check the temperature. The humidifier bottle should be warm, not hot to touch	10. Excessive temperatures can cause airway burns; patients with elevated temperature should be humidified with an unheated device
Simple face mask. Oxygen concentration varies with patient's tidal volume and respiratory rate	
Follow-up phase	
1. Record FiO_2 and immediate patient response. Note the patient's tolerance of treatment. Notify the physician if intolerance occurs	
2. Assess the patient's condition and the functioning of equipment at regular intervals	2. Assess the patient for change in mental status, diaphoresis, changes in blood pressure, and increasing heart and respiratory rates
3. If the patient's condition changes, assess SaO_2 or ABG	3. If the patient has a high air flow from the mask, may not be sufficient to meet inspiratory needs without pulling in room air. Room air will dilute the oxygen provided and lower the inspired oxygen concentration, resulting in hypoxemia. A change in mask or delivery system may be indicated
4. Record changes in volume and tenacity of sputum produced	4. Indicates effectiveness of humidification

Procedure 9.16: Administering oxygen by venturi mask

(High air flow oxygen entrainment (HAFOE)

Equipment:

- Oxygen source
- Flowmeter
- Venturi mask for correct concentration (24%, 28%, 31%, 35%, 40%, and 50%) or correct concentration adapter if interchangeable color-coded adapters are used
- If high humidity desired: Compressed air source and flowmeter humidifier with distilled water. Large bore tubing
- No smoking signs.

Steps of procedure

Nursing action	Rationale
Preparatory phase	
1. Determine current vital signs, level of consciousness, and most recent ABG	1. Provides a baseline for future assessment. Venturi masks are used for patients prone to CO_2 retention. Oxygen may depress the hypoxic drive of these patients (evidenced by a decreased respiratory rate, altered mental status and further $PaCO_2$ elevation)
2. Assess risk of CO_2 retention with oxygen administration	2. Risk is greater if the patient is experiencing an exacerbation of illness
Performance phase	
1. Paste no smoking signs on the door of the patient's room and in view of the patient and visitors	
2. Show the venturi mask to the patient and explain the procedure	

Contd...

Contd...

Nursing action	Rationale
3. Connect the mask diaphragm tubing to the oxygen source	
4. Turn on the oxygen flowmeter and adjust to the prescribed usually inscribed on the mask. Check to see that oxygen is flowing out the vent holes in the mask	4. To ensure the correct air/oxygen mix, oxygen must be set at the prescribed flow rate. Prescribed flow rates differ for different oxygen concentrations. Usually this information is printed on the mask or interchangeable color-coded source
5. Place venturi mask over the patient's nose and mouth and adjust flow	
6. Check entries are not obstructed by the patient's bearings	6. Proper mask function depends on mixing of sufficient amount of air and oxygen
7. If high air flow is used: a. Connect the humidifier to a compressed air source b. Attach the mask and connect the tubing to the at the base of the venturi mask	7. When a venturi mask is used with high humidity, both an oxygen source and compressed air source are required The compressed air source provides air for the air/ oxygen mix. Excessive oxygen would be inspired if both tubings were connected to an oxygen sources
Ventury mask constant concentrations of oxygen can be delivered	
Follow-up phase	
1. Record flow rate used and immediate patient response. Note the patient's tolerance of treatment. Report if intolerance occurs	1. Depression of hypoxic drive is most likely to occur within the first hours of oxygen use
2. If CO_2 retention is present, assess ABG every 30 minutes for 1 to 2 hours or until PaO_2 is > 50 mm Hg and the $PaCO_2$ is no longer increasing. Monitor pH. Report if the pH decreases below normal assessment value	2. A modest (5 to 10 mm Hg) increase in $PaCO_2$ may occur after initiation therapy. A decreasing pH indicates failure of compensatory mechanisms. Mechanical ventilation may be required
3. Determine patient comfort and oxygen use	
Venturi masks are best tolerated for relatively short periods because of their size and appearance. They also must be removed for eating and drinking. With improvement in patient condition, a nasal cannula may often be substituted.	

Procedure 9.17: Administering oxygen by partial rebreathing or nonrebreathing mask

Equipment:

- Oxygen source
- Plastic face mask with reservoir bag and tubing
- Humidifier with distilled water
- Flowmeter
- No smoking signs.

Steps of procedure

Nursing action	Rationale
Preparatory phase	
1. Determine current vital signs, level of consciousness	1. Provide a baseline for evaluating patient response. Typically used for short-term support of patients who require a high-inspired oxygen concentration
2. Determine most recent SaO_2 or ABG	
Performance phase	
1. Paste no smoking signs on the patients door and in view of the patient and visitors	
2. Fill humidifier with distilled water	2. If the humidifier is not sufficiently full, less moisture will be delivered
3. Attach tubing to outlet on humidifier	
4. Attach flowmeter	
5. Show the mask to the patient and explain the procedure	

Contd...

Contd...

Nursing action	Rationale
6. Flush the reservoir bag with oxygen to inflate the bag and adjust flowmeter to 6 to 10 L/min	6. Bag serves as reservoir, holding oxygen for patient inspiration
7. Place the mask on the patient's face	7. Be sure the mask fits snugly, because there must be an airtight seal between the mask and the patient's face
8. Adjust liter flow so the rebreathing bag will not collapse during the inspiratory cycle, even during the deep inspiration *Nursing focus* 1. Adjust the flow to prevent collapse of the bag, even during deep inspiration 2. A partial rebreathing mask does not have a one-way valve between the mask and reservoir bag, if the bag is allowed to collapse on inspiration, more exhaled air can enter the reservoir and the patient can inhale high concentrations of CO_2 3. A non-breathing mask will deliver a lower concentration of O_2 if the bag is allowed to collapse on inspiration. O_2 from the bag will be diluted by room air drawn in through the side holes of the mask	8. With a well-fitting rebreathing bag adjusted so that the patient's inhalation does not deflate the bag, inspired oxygen concentration of 60 to 90 per cent can be achieved. Some patients may require flow rates higher than 10 L/min to ensure that the bag does not collapse on inspiration
9. Stay with the patient for a time to make the patient comfortable and observe reactions	
10. Remove mask periodically (if the patient's condition permits) to dry the face around the mask. Powder skin and massage face around the mask	10. These actions reduce moisture accumulation under the mask. Massage of the face stimulates circulation and reduces pressure over the area
Follow-up phase	
1. Record the flow of air and immediate patient response. Note the patient's tolerance of treatment. Report if tolerance occurs	
2. Observe the patient for change of condition. Assess equipmentary malfunctioning and low water level in humidifier	2. Assess the patient for change in mental status diaphoresis, change in blood pressure, and increasing heart and respiratory rates

Procedure 9.1B: Administering oxygen by transtracheal catheter

Equipment:

- Oxygen source
- Transtracheal catheter with connecting tubing
- Flow-meter
- No smoking signs

Steps of procedure

Nursing action	Rationale
Preparatory phase	
1. Determine current vital signs level of consciousness and assess if patient is at risk for CO_2 retention	1. Provides a baseline for future assessment
2. Asses evidence of infection warmth, redness, swelling at infection site or temperature elevation	2. The transtracheal catheter provides a direct communication between the skin and trachea, if the insertion site is not kept clean and dry, infection can develop
3. Assess catheter patency, construction is indicated by a decreased SaO_2, whistling of the humidifier, high pressure of the delivery tubing, or stimulation of a cough	3. Mucus can form on the end of the catheter and restrict oxygen delivery. This increases pressure in the delivery tubing and humidifier. The mucus may touch the back of the trachea, stimulating a cough
Performance phase	
Stent phase	
1. Paste no smoking signs on the patient's door and in view of the patient and visitors.	

Contd...

Contd...

Nursing action	Rationale
2. Instruct the patient in purpose of stent	2. The stent is used to maintain a patient tract during the first week after catheter insertion. It facilitates breathing and al ows gradual adjustment to use of the catheter. It is not used for oxygen delivery
3. Teach that care of stent involve patient is at increased risk of cotton-tipped applicators and observation for signs of infection	3. Until the tract heals, the daily cleaning of the site with infection. Because the stent is open to the trachea, mucus, a 4×4 may be placed over that may be coughed from the stent
Immature tract (stent is removed and transtracheal catheter inserted)	
1. Instruct patient in cleaning and irrigation procedure. The patient should inject one half (1.5 mL) ampule of the sterile normal saline into the catheter, insert and remove the cleaning rod three times, and inject the remaining sterile normal saline two to three times a day (morning, noon and evening)	1. The catheter cannot be removed from the tract for cleaning until the tract completely heals (about 2 months). Cleaning in place helps to prevent mucus from forming on the end of the catheter and obstructing oxygen delivery
2. Teach the patient use of the staged cough technique (i.e. sit with feet on floor, pillow over abdomen, inhale three to four times in through the nose and out through the mouth, on the last exhalation cough while bending forward with pillow against abdomen)	2. Use of this cough technique helps to increase airflow during coughing. Higher air-flows help to dislodge any mucus that has formed on the outside of the catheter and cannot be removed by the cleaning technique
3. Instruct the patient to clean the insertion site daily with cotton-tipped applicators and report signs of infection	3. Mucus may form at the insertion site. Keeping the tract clean and dry decreases infection risk. Do not use hydrogen peroxide because it can dry mucous membrane
4. Teach the patient to place two small strips of transparent tape over the chain on either side of the catheter for the first 2 weeks of catheter use	4. This helps to keep the catheter in place during the night when the patient is sleeping. Serves as a second security system to keep the catheter from being inadvertently pulled from the tract during the initial adjustment phase
5. Instruct the patient to replace the nasal cannula and call for instruction if the catheter is displaced from the tract or if symptoms of subcutaneous emphysema develop (swelling insertion site, tight chain, change in voice)	5. If the catheter comes out of the tract before it is mature, reinsertion may be difficult. If the tract is not completely healed, O_2 may enter the tissues around the insertion site. The patient may need to return to the clinic for assistance in replacing the or catheter or delay in using it until the tract is fully healed
Mature tract (catheter is removed for cleaning)	
1. Instruct the patient in steps involved, in removing the tract for cleaning. Two catheters are used. The catheter in the tract is removed and replaced with a second catheter. The catheter removed from the tract is cleaned with antibacterial soap under warm running water, it then is air-dried and stored for reuse	1. The catheter should easily enter the tract. Practicing while looking in a mirror helps to develop skill in removing and reinserting the catheter. This step should be performed twice daily if a catheter with multiple side holes ($SCOOP_2$) is used. Removal daily, or less often, is necessary with a single end hole catheter ($SCOOP_1$)
2. Instruct the patient to report immediately signs of infection and difficulty replacing the catheter	2. These problems are less common with a mature tract, but can still occur
Follow-up phase	
1. Record flow rate of oxygen and patient response	1. Transtracheal oxygen delivery is more efficient. The same SaO_2 is typically maintained at one half of the former flow rate
2. Determine patient's ability to perform care independently	2. Repeat demonstration of care may be required before the patient masters selfcare skills
3. Ensure patient is able to demonstrate appropriate use of oxygen and attachment of oxygen to transtracheal catheter	
4. Discuss with patient signs and symptoms of oxygen toxicity and carbon dioxide retention	4. Too much carbon dioxide retention could lead to confusion, decreased level of carbon dioxide retention consciousness or somnolence

Procedure 9.19: Administering oxygen by continuous positive airway pressure (CPAP) mask

Equipment:

- Oxygen blender
- Flowmeter
- CPAP mask

- Valve for prescribed PEEP (2.5, 5, 5.7, 10 cm H_2O)
- Large bore tubing
- Nasogastric tube
- Sealing pad to accommodate nasogastric tube
- No smoking signs.

Steps of procedure

Nursing action	Rationale
Preparatory phase	
1. Assess the patient's level of consciousness and gag reflex	1. CPAP mask may lead to aspiration unless the patient is breathing spontaneously and is able to protect the airway
2. Determine current ABG	2. Document that patient meets criteria for use of this mask (normal or decreased $PaCO_2$) and provides baseline to evaluate whether therapy results in CO_2 retention
Please note that	
1. CPAP is used when patients have not responded to attempts to increase PaO_2 with other types of masks	
2. The patient will require frequent assessment to detect changes in respiratory status, cardiovascular status and level of consciousness	
3. If the patient's level of consciousness decreases or ABGs deteriorate, intubation may be necessary	
Performance Phase	
1. Paste 'no smoking' signs on the patient's door and in view of the patient and visitors	
2. Show the mask to the patient and explain the procedure	
3. Make sure humidifier is filled to the appropriate mark	
4. Insert nasogastric tube	With CPAP, the patient may swallow air, causing gastric distensions or emesis. Prophylactic nasogastric suction diminishes this risk
Note: Some clinicians do not believe a nasogastric tube is needed if the PEEP level is less than 10 cm H_2O.	
5. Attach nasogastric tube adapter	5. Use of adapter may increase air leak around the mask
6. Set desired concentration of oxygen blender and adjust flow rate so it is sufficient to meet the patient's inspiratory demand	6. O_2 blenders are devices that mix air and O_2 using a proportioning valve. Concentrations of 21 percent to 100 percent may be delivered depending on the model. Because the patient will be receiving all minute ventilation from this closed system, it is essential that the flow rate be adequate to meet changes in the patient's breathing pattern

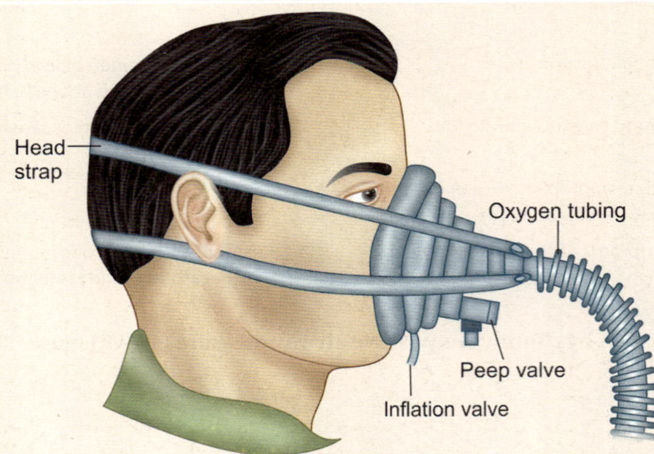

FIG. 9.44: Administering oxygen by face mask with continuous positive airway pressure (CPAP)

Contd...

Contd...

Nursing action	Rationale
7. Place the mask on the patient's face, adjust the head strap, and inflate the mask cushion to ensure a tight seal	7. To maintain CPAP, an airtight seal is required. Head straps and the inflatable cushion help to ensure that difficult areas, such as the nose and chin, are sealed with greater comfort to the patient
8. Organize care to remove the mask as infrequently as possible	8. If mask is removed (for coughing, suctioning) CPAP is not maintained and inspired oxygen concentration drop
Follow-up phase	
1. Assess ABGs, hemodynamic status, and level of consciousness frequently	1. Provides objective documentation of patient response, CPAP may increase work of breathing, resulting in patient's tiring and inability to maintain ventilation without intubation CPAP may also decrease venous return (PEEP effect), resulting in decreased cardiac output
2. Immediately report any increase in $PaCO_2$	2. An increase in $PaCO_2$ suggests hypoventilation, resulting from tiring of the patient or inadequate alveolar ventilation. Need for intubation and mechanical ventilation should be evaluated
3. Assess patency of nasogastric causing gastric distention	3. May become obstructed, tube at frequent intervals
4. Assess patient comfort and functioning of the equipment frequently	4. Tight fit of the mask may predispose to skin breakdown. System may develop leaks, resulting in air escaping between the patient's face and mask
5. Record patient's response. With improvement, oxygen therapy without positive airway pressure can be substituted. With deterioration intubation and mechanical ventilation may be required. Note the patient's tolerance of treatment. Report if intolerance occurs	5. Face mask CPAP is usually continued only for short periods (72 hours) because of patient tiring and the necessity to remove mask for suctioning and coughing

Procedure 9.20: Administering oxygen via endotracheal and tracheostomy tubes with a T-piece (BRIGGS) adapter

Equipment:

- Oxygen
- Oxygen blender
- Flowmeter
- Humidifier with distilled water (heating element may be used as described in aerosol masks)
- Large-bore tubing
- T-piece and reservoir tubing
- No smoking signs.

Steps of procedure

Nursing action	Rationale
Preparatory phase	
1. Assess patient's SaO_2, hemodynamic status, and level of consciousness frequently. If patient's condition changes, assess ABGs	1. Provide baseline to assess response
2. Assess viscosity and volume of sputum produced	2. Aerosol is given to assist in mobilizing retained secretions
Performance phase	
1. Paste no smoking signs on the patient's door and in view of the patient and visitors	1. Provides baseline to assess response
2. Show the T-tube to the patient and explain the procedure	
3. Make sure that the humidifier is filled to the appropriate mark	3. If humidifier is not sufficiently filled, less aerosol will be delivered
4. Attach the large-bore tubing from the T-tube to the humidifier outlet	

Contd...

Contd...

Nursing action	Rationale
5. Set desired oxygen concentration of O_2 blender or humidifier bottle and plug in heating element if used	5. O_2 blenders are devices that mix air and O_2 using a proportioning valve. Concentrations of 21 to 100 percent may be delivered at flows of 2 to 100 L/min, depending on the model. Used in situation when precise control is required
6. Adjust the flow rate until the desired mist is produced and meets the patient's inspiratory demand	6. The aerosol mist in the reservoir, tubing attached to the T-tube should not be completely withdrawn on patient inspiration. If mist is withdrawn (does not extend from reservoir tubing), on inspiration, room air may be inspired and O_2 concentration decreased
7. Drain the tubing frequently by emptying condensate into a separate receptacle, none into the humidifier, if a heating element is used the tubing will have to be drained more often	7. The tubing must be kept free of condensate allowed to accumulate in the delivery tube will block flow and alter oxygen concentration. If condensate is emptied into the himidifier, bacteria may be aerosolized into the lungs
8. If a heating element is used, check the temperature. The humidifier bottle should be warm, not hot, to touch	8. Excessive temperatures can cause airway burns, patients with elevated temperatures will be better humidified with an unheated device

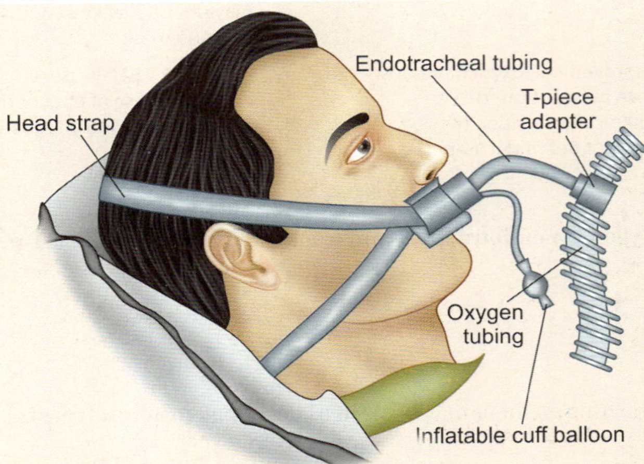

FIG. 9.45: Administering oxygen via endotracheal tube with a T-piece adapter. A T-piece adapter is attached to the endotracheal tube and large-bore tubing, which serves as a source of oxygen and humidity.

Nursing action	Rationale
Follow-up phase	
1. Record FiO_2 and immediate patient response. Note the patient's tolerance of treatment. Report if intolerance occurs	
2. Assess the patient's condition and the functioning of equipment at regular intervals	2. Assess the patient for change in mental status, diaphoresis, perspiration, changes in blood pressure, and increasing heart and respiratory rates
3. If the patient's condition changes, assess SaO_2 or ABGs and vital signs. Note changes suggesting increased work of breathing (diaphoresis, intercostal muscle retraction)	3. If the patient is being weaned, return to the ventilator if changes suggesting inability to tolerate spontaneous ventilation occur
4. Record changes in volume and city of sputum produced	4. Indicates effectiveness of humidification therapy

Procedure 9.21: Administering oxygen by manual resuscitation bag

Equipment:

- Oxygen source
- Resuscitation bag and mask

- Reservoir tubing or reservoir bag
- O_2 connecting tubing
- Nipple adapter to attach flowmeter to connecting tubing
- Flowmeter
- Gloves
- Goggles or other eye protection.

Steps of procedure

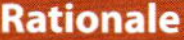

Nursing action	Rationale
Preparatory phase	
1. In cardiopulmonary arrest a. Follow steps to establish that a cardiopulmonary arrest has occurred If apneic, ventilate; palpate the carotid pulse; if absent	1. a. These steps are: Establish unresponsiveness, call for help, position the patient on a firm, flat surface, open the mouth and remove vomitus for debris. If visible; assess presence of respirations with the airway open; deliver chest compressions.
b. Use caution not to injure or increase injury to the cervical spine when opening the situations, the headtilt/chin-lift method can be used. These maneuvers lift the tongue off the back of the throat and, in some situations, may be all that is needed to restore breathing	b. If cervical spine injury is a potential, the modified jaw thrust should be used in other airway
2. In suctioning or transport situation. Assess patient's heart rate level of consciousness and respiratory status	2. Provides a baseline to stimulate patient's tolerance of procedure
Performance phase	
1. Attach connecting tubing from flowmeter and nipple adapter to resuscitation bag	1. A humidifier bottle is not used, because the high flow rates of oxygen required would force water into the cubing and clog it
2. Turn flowmeter to "flush" position	2. A high flow rate or "flush" position is necessary to meet the minute ventilation of the patient
3. Attach reservoir tubing or reservoir bag to resuscitation bag	3. A high inspired O_2 concentration is required. Without a reservoir inspired O_2 concentration will be low (28 to 56%) because inspired gas will be air/O_2 mix. With a reservoir, manual resuscitation bags can achieve a FiO_2 of > 96 at a flow rate of 15/L/min

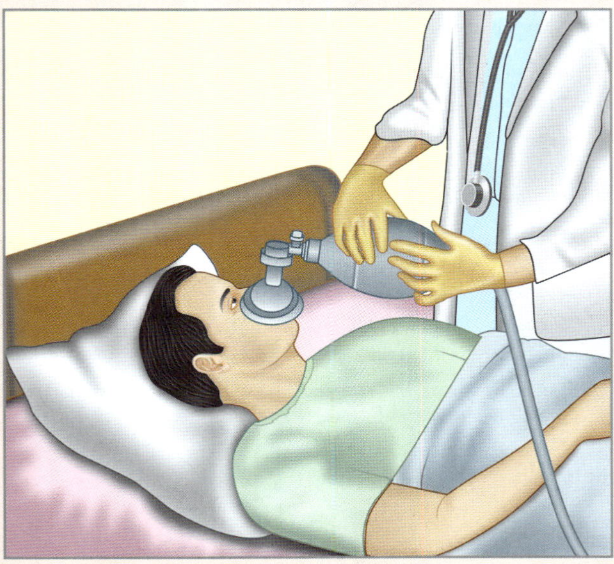

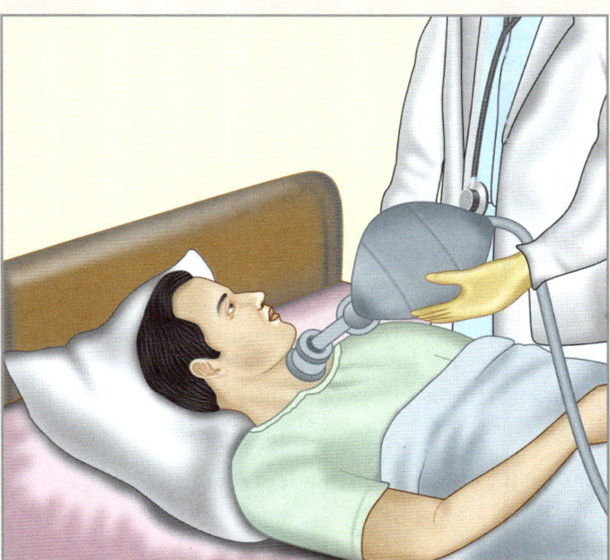

FIG. 9.46: Using a manual resuscitation bag, with mask (left), or connected to an artificial airway (right)

Contd...

Contd...

Nursing action	Rationale
Follow steps given below:	
1. If respirations are absent after the airway is open, insert an oropharyngeal airway and ventilate twice with slow, full breaths of 1 to 1.5 seconds each. Allow 2 seconds between breaths	1. The airway helps prevent obstruction from the tongue in an unconscious patient. If ventilation is difficult, confirm that airway is unobstructed. Airways are not appropriate in a conscious patient or patients with a gag reflex because stimulation of the propharynx could cause vomiting and aspiration
2. Breaths will have to be quickly interposed between cardiac compressions if the patient needs only respiratory assistance, watch for chest expansion listen with the stethoscope to ensure adequate ventilation	2. Squeeze resuscitation bag with sufficient force and at the rate necessary to maintain adequate minute ventilation
3. A rate of approximately 12 to 15 breaths per minute is used unless the patient is being given external cardiac compressions	3. Continue squeezing bag at appropriate interval until CPR is no longer required
Preoxygenation and suctioning	
1. If hyperinflation is being used with suctioning ventilate the patient before and after each suctioning pass including after the last suction pass	1. Hyperinflation before suctioning helps prevent hypoxemia. Hyperinflation after suctioning replaces O_2 removed during the procedure and helps to prevent atelectasis. The larger tidal volumes may also assist in mobilizing secretions and promote surfactant secretion
Transport	
1. If hyperinflation is used in transport, suction patient before disconnection for transport, monitor heart and respiratory rates and level of consciousness during procedure	1. Establishes a patient airway before patient is moved. Provides information for assessing tolerance of transport
2. Ventilate at rate of 12 to 15 breaths per minute	
Follow-up phase	
1. In cardiopulmonary arrest, verify return of spontaneous pulse and respirations initiate further support as needed	1. Establishes patient's need for definitive therapy (drugs, defibrillation, intensive care)
2. In suctioning or transport, return to previous support. Note patient tolerance of procedure. Report if tolerance occurs	2. Note SaO_2, heart rate, rate and ease of respirations, arterial blood pressure (if monitored), level of consciousness.

Procedure 9.22: Managing the patient requiring mechanical ventilation

Equipment:

- Artificial airway
- Mechanical ventilator
- Ventilation circuitry
- Humidifier
- See manufacturer's directions for specific machine.

Steps of procedure

Nursing action	Rationale
Preparatory phase	
1. Obtain baseline samples for serve as a guide in determining progress of therapy	1. Baseline measurements blood gas determinations (pH, PaO_2, $PaCO_2$, HCO_3) and chest X-ray
Performance phase	
1. Give a brief explanation to the patient	1. Emphasize that mechanical ventilation is a temporary measure. The patient should be prepared psychologically for weaning at the time if the ventilator is first used
2. Establish the airway by means of a cuffed endotracheal or tracheostomy tube	2. A closed system between the ventilator and patient's lower airway is necessary for positive pressure ventilation

Contd...

Contd...

Nursing action	Rationale
3. Prepare the ventilator (respiratory therapist does this in many institutions) a. Set up desired circuitry b. Connect oxygen and compressed air source c. Turn on power d. Set tidal volume (usually 10 to 15 mL/kg body weight) e. Set oxygen concentration f. Set ventilator sensitivity	3. d. Adjusted according to pH and $PaCO_2$ e. Adjusted according to PaO_2
g. Set rate at 12 to 14 breaths per minute (variable) h. Adjust flow rate (velocity of gas flow during inspiration). Usually set at 40 to 60 L/min. Is dependent on rate and tidal volume set to avoid inverse inspiratory expiratory (IE) ratio usual IE ratio is 1:2 i. Select mode of ventilation j. Check machine function—measure tidal volume, rate, IE, ratio, analyze oxygen, check all alarms	g. This setting approximates normal ventilation. These machines settings are subject to change according to the patient's condition and response, and the ventilator type being used h. The slower the flow, the lower will be the peak air way pressure resulting from set volume delivery. This results in lower intrathoracic pressure and less impedance of venous return. However, a flow that is too low for the rate selected may result in inverse inspiratory or expiratory ratios j. Ensures safe function
4. Couple the patient's airway to the ventilator	4. Be sure all connections are secure. Prevent ventilator tubing from pulling on artificial airway, possibly resulting in tube dislodgement or tracheal damage
5. Assess patient for adequate chest movement and fate. Do not depend on digital rate read-out of ventilator.Note peak airway pressure and PEEP. Adjust gas flow of necessary to provide safe IE ratio	5. Ensures proper function of equipment
6. Set airway pressure alarms according to patient's baseline a. High pressure alarm b. Low pressure alarm	6. a. High airway pressure or 'Pop off' pressure is set at about 20 cm H_2O above peak airway pressure. An alarm sounds if airway pressure selected is exceeded. Alarm activation indicates decreased lung compliance (worsening pulmonary disease), decreased lung volume (such as pneumothorax, tension pneumothorax, hemothorax, pleural effusion). Increased airway resistance (secretions, coughing, breathing out of phase with the ventilator), loss of patency of airway (mucus plug, airway spasm, biting or kinking of tube) b. Low airway pressure alarm set at 5 to 10 cm H_2O below peak airway pressure. Alarm activation indicates inability to build up airway pressure because of disconnection or leak, or inability to build up airway pressure because of insufficient gas flow to meet patient's inspiratory needs
7. Assess frequently for change in respiratory status via ABGs, pulse oximetry, spontaneous rate, use of accessory muscles, breath sounds, and vital signs. (Other means of assessing are through the use of exhaled carbon dioxide. If change is noted, notify appropriate personnel	
8. Monitor and troubleshoot alarm conditions. Ensure appropriate ventilation at all times	8. Priority is ventilation and oxygenation of the patient. In alarm conditions that cannot be immediately corrected, disconnect the patient from mechanical ventilation and manually ventilate with resuscitation bag
9. Positioning a. Turn patient from side to side every 2 hours or more frequently if possible b. Lateral turns are desirable from right semiprone to left semizone c. Sit the patient upright at regular interval if possible	9. Positioning a. For patients on long-term ventilation, this may result in sleep deprivation. Evolve a turning schedule best suited to a particular patient's condition c. Upright posture increases lung compliance

Contd...

Contd...

Nursing action	Rationale
Please note that: For patients in severe compromised respiratory state or who are unstable hemodynamically, consider use of specialty bed with rotational therapy. New versions may also have built in vibration and percussion as adjunct therapy options.	
10. Carry out passive range or motion exercises of all extremities for patients	
11. Assess for need of suctioning least every 2 hours	11. Patients with artificial airways on mechanical ventilation are unable to clear secretions on their own. Suctioning may help to clear secretions and stimulate the cough reflex
12. Assess breath sounds every 2 hours a. Listen with stethoscope to the chest from bottom to top on both sides b. Determine whether breath sounds are present or absent, normal or abnormal and whether a change has occurred c. Observe the patient's diaphragmatic excursions and use of accessory muscles of respiration	12. a. Auscultation of the chest is a means of assessing airway patency and ventilatory distribution, it also confirms the proper placement of the endotracheal or tracheostomy tube
13. Humidification. a. Check the water level in the humidification reservoir to ensure that the patient is never ventilated with dry gas. Empty the water the ordences in the delivery and exhalation tubing into a scarate receptacle not into the humidifier. Airways were hands after emptying fluid from ventilator circuit humidifier must be changed every 24 hours	13. a. Water condensing in the inspiratory tubing may cause increased resistance to gas flow. This may result in increased peak airway pressures. Warm, moist tubing is a perfect breeding area for bacteria. If this water is allowed to enter the humidifier, bacteria may be aerosolized into the lungs. Emptying the tubing also prevents introduction of water into the patient's airways
14. Assess airway pressure adequate intervals	14. Monitor for changes in compliance or onset of conditions that may cause airway pressure to increase or decrease
15. Measure delivered tidal volume and analyze oxygen concentration every 4 hours to more frequently if indicated	
16. Monitor cardiovascular function a. Monitor pulse rate and arterial blood pressure, intra-arterial pressure monitoring may be carried out b. Use Swan-Ganz catheter to monitor pulmonary capillary wedge pressure mixed venous oxygen, and cardiac output	16. Assess for depression a. Arterial catheterization for intra-arterial pressure monitoring also provides access for ABG samples b. Intermittent and continuous positive pressure ventilation may increase the pulmonary artery pressures and decrease cardiac output
17. Monitor for pulmonary injection a. Aspirate tracheal secretions into a sterile container and send to laboratory for culture and sensitivity testing. This is done immediately after endotracheal intubation and in some distances on an every other day basis b. Daily Gram's staining of secretions may also be done in some institutions c. Monitor for systemic signs and symptoms of pulmonary infection (pulmonary physical examination findings, increased heart rate, increased temperature, increased WBC count)	17. a. This technique allows for the earliest detection of infection or change in infecting organisms in the tracheobronchial tree
18. Evaluate need for sedation or to decrease anxiety, or to relax the patient to prevent "competing" with the ventilator. At times, pharmacologically-induced paralysis may be necessary to permit mechanical ventilation	18. Sedatives may be prescribed or muscle relaxants

Contd...

Contd...

Nursing action	Rationale
Please note the following:	
Never administer paralyzing agents until the patient is intubated and mechanical ventilation sedatives should be prescribed in conjunction with paralyzing agents	
19. Report intake and output precisely and obtain and accurate daily weight to monitor fluid balance	19. Positive fluid balance resulting in increase in body weight and interstitial pulmonary edema is a frequent problem in patient's requiring mechanical ventilation, prevention requires early recognition of fluid accumulation. An average adult who is dependent on parenteral nutrition can be expected to lose 0.25 kg (1/2 lb)/ day; therefore, constant body weight indicates positive fluid balance
20. Monitor nutritional status	20. Patients on mechanical ventilation require inflation of artificial airway cuffs at all times. Patients with tracheostomy tubes may eat, if capable, or may require enteral feeding tubes or parenteral nourishment. Patients with endotracheal tubes are to be NPO (the tube splints the epiglottis open) and must be entirely tube fed or parenterally nourished
21. Monitor GI function	21. Mechanically ventilated patients are at risk for development of stress ulcers
a. Test all stools and gastric drainage for occult blood	a. Stress may cause some patient's requiring mechanical ventilation to develop GI bleeding
b. Measure abdominal girth daily	b. Abdominal distention occurs frequently with respiratory failure and further hinders respiration by elevation of the diaphragm. Measurement of abdominal girth provides objective assessment of the degree of distention
22 Provide for care and communication needs of patient with an artificial airway	
23. Provide psychological support a. Assist with communication b. Orient to environment and function of mechanical ventilator c. Ensure that the patient has adequate rest and sleep	23. Mechanical ventilation may result in sleep deprivation and loss of touch with surroundings and reality
Follow-up phase	
1. Maintain a flowsheet to record ventilation patterns, ABGs, venous chemical determinations, hemoglobin and hematocrit, status of fluid balance, weight, and assessment of the patient's condition. Notify appropriate personnel of changes in the patient's condition	1. Establishes means of assessing effectiveness and progress of treatment
2. Change ventilator circuitry 24 hours, assess ventilator's function every 4 hours or more frequently if problem occurs	2. Prevents contamination of lower airways

Procedure 9.23: Weaning the patient from mechanical ventilation

Equipment:

- Varies according to technique used
- Briggs T-piece
- IMV or SIMV (set up in addition to ventilator or incorporated in ventilator and circuitry)
- Pressure support.

Steps of procedure

Nursing action	Rationale
Preparatory phase	
1. For weaning to be successful, the patient must be physiologically capable of maintaining spontaneous respirations. Assessments must ensure that— a. The underlying disease process is significantly reversed, as evidenced by pulmonary examination, ABGs, chest X-ray b. The patient can mechanically perform ventilation, should be able to generate a negative inspiratory force (NIF) – 20 cm H_2O have a vital capacity (VC) 10 to 15 mL/kg, have a resting minute ventilation (Ve) 10 L/min, and be able to double this, have a spontaneous respiratory fate of 25 breaths per minute, without significant tachycardia, not be hypotensive, have optimal hemoglobin for condition which have adequate nutritional status	1. Provides baseline, ensure that patient is capable of having adequate neuromuscular control to provide adequate ventilation
2. Assess for other factors, that cause respiratory insufficiency. a. Acid-base abnormality b. Nutritional depletion c. Electrolyte abnormality d. Fever e. Abnormal fluid balance f. Hyperglycemia	2. Weaning is difficult when these conditions are present
g. Infection h. Pain i. Sleep deprivation j. Decreased level of consciousness	
3. Assess psychological readness weaning	3. Patient must be physically and psychologically ready for weaning
Performance phase	
1. Ensure psychological preparation. Explain procedure and that weaning is not always successful on the initial attempt	1. Explaining procedure to patient will decrease patient anxiety and promote cooperation. The patient should not be discouraged if weaning is unsuccessful on the first attempt
2. Prepare appropriate equipment	
3. Position the patient in sitting or semi-Fowler's position	3. Increases lung compliance, decreases work of breathing
4. Pick optimal time of day, preferably early morning	4. The patient should be rested
5. Perform bronchial hygiene necessary to ensure that the patient is in best condition (postural drainage, suctioning) before weaning attempt	5. The patient should be in best pulmonary condition for weaning to be successful
T-piece weaning	
This system provides oxygen enrichment and humidity to a patient with an endotracheal or tracheostomy tube while allowing completely spontaneous respirations	
1. Discontinue mechanical ventilation and apply T-piece adapter	1. Stay with the patient during weaning time to decrease patient anxiety and monitor for tolerance of procedure
2. Monitor the patient for factors indicating need for reinstitution of mechanical ventilation a. Blood pressure increase of decrease greater than 20 mm Hg systolic or 10 mm Hg diastolic b. Heart rate increase of 20 beats/min or greater than 110 c. Respiratory rate increase greater than 10 breaths/min of rate greater than 30 d. Tidal volume less than 250 to 300 mL (in adults) e. Appearance of new cardiac ectopy or increase in base-line ectopy f. PaO_2 less than 60, $PaCO_2$ greater than 55, or pH less than 7.35 (may accept lower PaO_2 and pH 1 and higher $PaCO_2$ in patients with COPD)	2. Indicates intolerance of weaning procedure

Contd...

Contd...

Nursing action	Rationale
3. Increase time of ventilator with each weaning attempt as the patient's condition indicates. Evaluate for toleration before moving to the next increment	3. The patient will progress as he or she becomes mentally and physically, able to perform adequate spontaneous ventilation
4. Institute other techniques, helpful in encouraging weaning a. Mental stimulation b. Biofeedback c. Participation in care d. Provision of rewards e. Contact with successfully weaned patients	4. Provides motivation and positive feedback
5. When patient tolerates 40 to 60 minutes of continuous weaning, weaning increments can increase rapidly	
6. When the patient can maintain spontaneous ventilation throughout day, begin night weaning	
CPAP weaning	
1. The principles and techniques CPAP weaning are the same as for T-piece weaning on a T-piece	1. This weaning technique preferred for patient prone to atelectasis, when placed
2. The patient breathes with CPAP at low level (2.5 to 5 cm H_2O_2) rather than with the T-piece for periods that increase in length	
IMV or SIMV weaning (synchronised intermittent mandatory ventilation)	
1. Set ventilator to IMV or SIMV mode	
2. Set rate interval between machine the patient will breathe on	2. This determines the time delivered breaths during which own
3. If the patient is on continuous, flow IMV circuitry, observe reservoir bag to be sure that it remains mostly inflated during all phases of ventilation	3. The gas flows rate into the bag must be adequate to prevent the bag from collapsing during inspiration. Flow rates of 6 to 10 L/min are usually adequate
4. If gas for the patient's spontaneous breath is delivered via a demand valve regulator, ensure that machine sensitivity is at maximum setting	4. Aids in decreasing work of breathing necessary to open demand valve
5. Evaluate for tolerance of procedure. Monitor for factors indicating need for increase or decrease of mandatory respiratory rate (see step 3 of T-piece adaptor section above). In rapid weaning, changes may be made approximately every 20 to 30 minutes	5. If the patient does not tolerate the procedure, the $PaCO_2$ will rise and pH will fall
6. If $PaCO_2$ and pH levels remain stable, then continue to decrease mandatory rate as patient tolerates	6. May be done as frequently as every 20 to 30 minutes with ABG monitoring, pulse oximetry documentation of successful weaning
Pressure support	
1. May be beneficial adjunct to IMV or SIMV weaning	
2. The amount of pressure support (cm H_2O) provided to the airway is progressively decreased over-time, allowing the patient to increase role in supporting own spontaneous ventilation	
Follow-up phase	
1. Record at each weaning interval respiratory rate, FiO_2, ABG, pulse oximetry value, respiratory and ventilator rate (if IMV or SIMV), or length of time off ventilator if T-piece weaning	1. Provides record of procedure heart rate, blood pressure, and assessment of progress
Note: It is not within the scope of this manual to establish criteria for the use of one weaning modality as opposed to another.	

Procedure 9.24: Extubation

Equipment:

- Tonsil suction (surgical suction, instrument)
- 10 mL syringe
- Resuscitation bag and mask with oxygen flow
- Face mask connected to large bore tubing, humidifier, and oxygen source
- Suction catheter
- Suction source
- Gloves, goggles, or other eye protection devices.

Steps of procedure

Nursing action	Rationale
Preparatory phase	
1. Monitor heart rate, lung expansion, and breath sounds before extubation, record VI, VC, NIF	1. V1, VC and NIF are measured to assess respiratory muscle functions and adequacy of ventilation
2. Assess the patient for other signs of adequate muscle power a. Instruct the patient to tightly squeeze the index and middle fingers of your hand. Resistance to removel of your fingers from the patient's grasp must be demonstrated b. Ask the patient to lift head from the pillow and hold for 2 to 3 seconds	2. Adequate muscle strength is necessary to ensure maintenance of a patient airway
Please note the following	
Keep in mind that patient's underlying problems must be improved or resolved before extubation is considered. Patient should also be free from infection and malnutrition	
Performance phase	
1. Obtain orders for extubation and postextubation oxygen therapy is available and functioning at the bedsides	1. Do not attempt extubation until postextubation oxygen therapy
2. Explain the procedure to the patient a. Artificial airway will be removed b. Suctioning will occur before extubation c. Deep breath should be taken on command d. Instruction will be given to cough after extubation	2. Increases patient cooperation
3. Prepare necessary equipment. Have ready for use tonsil suction, suction catheter, 10 mL syringe, bag mask unit and oxygen via face mask	
4. Place patient in sitting or semi-Flowler's position (unless contraindicated)	4. Increased lung compliance and decreased work of breathing facilitates coughing
5. Put on goggle	5. Spraying of airway secretions may occur
6. Suction endotracheal tube	
7. Suction oropharyngeal airway above the endotracheal cuff as thoroughly as possible	7. Secretions not cleared from above the cuff will be aspirated when the cuff is deflated
8. Put on gloves, loosen type or endotracheal tube-securing device	
9. Extubate the patient a. Ask the patient to take as deep a breath as possible (if the patient is not following commands, give a deep breath with the resuscitation bag) b. At peak inspiration, deflate the cuff completely and pull the tube out in the direction of the curve (out and down-ward)	9. a. At peak inspiration, the traches and vocal cords will dilate, allowing a less traumatic tube removal
10. Once the tube is fully removed ask the patient to cough or exhale forcefully to remove secretions. Then suction the back of the patient's airway with the tonsil suction	10. Frequently, old blood is seen in the secretions of newly extubated patients. Monitor for the appearance of bright red blood due to trauma occurring during extubation

Contd...

Contd...

Nursing action	Rationale
11 Evaluate immediately for any signs of airway obstruction, stridor, or difficult breathing. If the patient develops any of the above problems, attempt to the resuscitation bag and mask and prepare for reintubation. (Nebulized treatments may be ordered to avoid having to reintubate patient)	11. Immediate complication: a. Laryngospasm may develop, causing obstruction of the airway b. Edema may develop at ventilate the patient with the cuff site. Signs of narrowing airway lumen are high-pitched crowing sounds, decreased air movement and respiratory distress
Follow-up phase	
1. Note patient tolerance of procedure, upper and lower airway sounds postextubation, description of secretions	1. Establishes a baseline to a assess improvement/development of complications
2. Observe patient closely postextubation for any signs and symptoms of airway obstruction or respiratory insufficiency	2. Tracheal or laryngeal edema develop postextubation (a possibility for up to 24 hours). Signs and symptoms include high pitched, crowing upper airway sounds and respiratory distress
3. Observe character of voice. Observe for worsening hoarseness or vocal cord paralysis	3. Hoarseness is a common postextubation complaint
Evaluation	
A. Respirations 24 shallow, lungs clear. ABGs within normal limits B. Blood pressure, CVP, and pulse stable C. Coughing and turning independently; reports reliefs of pain D. Performing active range of motion of affected arm and shoulder	

Procedure 9.25: Assisting the patient using an incentive spirometer

Equipment: According to the type of device used

Performing incentive spirometry

- The inspired air helps inflate the lungs. The ball or weight in the spirometer rises in response to the intensity of the intake of air. The higher the ball rises, the deeper the breath
- Assume a semi-Fowler's position or an upright position before initiating therapy
- Use diaphragmatic breathing
- Place the mouthpiece of the spirometer firmly in the mouth, breathe air in (inspire) through the mouth and hold the breath at the end of inspiration of about 3 seconds. Exhale slowly through the mouthpiece
- Coughing during and after each session in encouraged. Splint the incision when coughing postoperatively
- Perform the procedure approximately 10 times in succession, repeating the 10 breaths with the spirometer each hour during waking hours.

Steps of procedure

Nursing action	Rationale
Preparatory phase	
1. Measure the patient's normal VI and auscultate the chest	1. The patient's baseline is established
Performance phase	
1. Explain the procedure and its purpose to the patient	1. Optimal results are achieved when the patient is given pre-treatment instruction, pre-operative instruction is also beneficial for the surgical patient
2. Place the patient in a comfortable sitting or semi-Fowler's ever, if the patient is medically unable to be in this position, the exercise may be done in any position	2. Diaphragmatic excursion is greater in this position; low-position
3. For the postoperative patient, try as much as possible to avoid discomfort with the treatment administration. Try to co-ordinate treatment with administration of pain relief medications. Instruct and assist the patient with splinting of incision	3. More likely to have best results is in using incentive spirometry when patient suffers from as little pain as possible

Contd...

Contd...

Nursing action	Rationale
4. Set the incentive spirometer VI indicator at the desired goal the patient is to reach or exceed (500 mL, is often used to start). The V1 is set according to the manufacturer's instructions	4. The initial V1 may be prescribed, but the purpose of the device is to establish a base-line, V1 and provide insentive to achieve greater volumes progressively

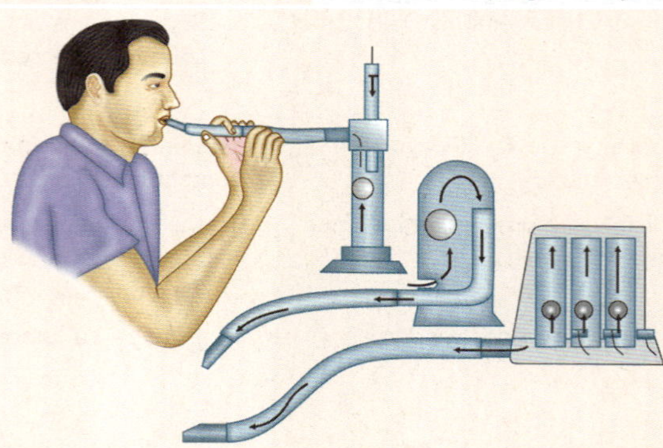

FIG. 9.47: Flow incentive spirometer. Patients are instructed to inhale briskly to elevate the balls and to keep them floating as long as possible. The volume inhaled is estimated and variable

Nursing action	Rationale
5. Demonstrate the technique to the patient	
6. Instruct the patient to exhale fully	
7. Tell the patient to take in a slow, easy deep breath from the mouthpiece	7. Nose clips are sometimes used if the patient has difficulty in breathing only through mouth. This will ensure full credit for each breath measured
8. When the desired goal is reached (lungs fully inflated), ask the patient to continue the inspiratory effort for 3 seconds, even though the patient may not actually be drawing in more air	8. Sustaining the inspiratory effort helps to open closed alveoli
9. Instruct the patient to remove the mouthpiece, relax and passively exhale, patient should take several normal breaths before attempting another one with the incentive spirometer	9. Usually one incentive breath per minute minimizes patient fatigue. No more that four to five maneuvers should be performed per minute to minimize hypocarbia
10. Continue to monitor the patient's spirometer breaths, periodically increasing the tidal volume as the patient tolerates	
11. At the conclusion of the treatment, encourage the patient to cough after a deep breath	11. The deep lung inflation may loosen secretions and enable the patient to expectorate them
12. Instruct the patient to take 10 sustained maximal inspiratory maneuvers per hour and note the volume on the spirometer	12. A total of 10 sustained maximal inspiratory maneuvers per hour during waking hours is a typical order. A counter on the incentive spirometer indicates the number of breaths the patient has taken
Flow incentive spirometer patients are instructed to inhale briskly to elevate the balls and to keep them floating as long as possible. The volume inhaled is estimated and variable	
Follow-up phase	
1. Auscultate the chest. Chart any improvement or variation, the volume of cough, description of any secretions expectorated	1. Note the effectiveness and patient tolerance of the treatment

Procedure 9.25: Assisting with chest tube insertion

Equipment:

- The thoracostomy tray
- Syringes
- Needles/trocar
- Basins skin germicide
- Sponges
- Scalps/sterile drape/gloves

- Suture material
- Local anesthetic
- Chest tube (appropriate size), connector
- Chest drainage system-connecting tubes and tubing.
- Collection bottles or commercial system, vacuum pump (if required)
- Two large clamps.

Steps of procedure

Nursing action	Rationale
Preparatory phase	
1. Assess patient for pneumothorax, hemothorax, presence of a respiratory distress	
2. Obtain a chest X-ray. Other means of localization of pleural fluid include ultrasound and/or fluoroscope localization	2. To evaluate extent of lung collapse or amount of bleeding in pleural space
3. Assemble drainage system	
4. Reassure the patient and explain the steps of the procedure. Tell the patient to expect a needle prick and a sensation of slight pressure during infiltration anesthesia	4. The patient can cope by remaining immobile and doing relaxed breathing during tube insertion
5. Position the patient as for an intercostal nerve block, or according to physician preference	5. The tube insertion site depends on the substance to be drained, the patient's mobility, and the presence/absence of coexisting conditions
Performance phase	
Needle or intracath technique:	
1. The skin is prepared and anesthetized using local anesthetic with a short 25 gauge needle A larger needle is used to infiltrate the subcutaneous tissue, intercostal muscles, and parietal pleura	1. The area is anesthetized to make tube insertion and manipulation relatively painless
2. An exploratory needle is inserted	2. To puncture the pleura and determine the presence of air/blood in the pleural cavity
3. The intracath catheter is inserted through the needle into the pleural space. The needle is removed, and the catheter is pushed several centimeters into the pleural space	
4. The catheter is taped to the skin	4. To prevent it from being pushed out of the chest during patient movement or lung expansion
5. The catheter is attached to a connector/tubing and attached to a drainage system (under water-seal or commercial system)	
Trocar technique for chest tube insertion	
A trocar catheter is used for the insertion of a large-bore tube for removal of a modest to large amount of air leak or for the evacuation of serious effusion	
1. A small incision is made over the prepared, anesthetized site. Blunt dissection (with a hemostat) through the muscle planes in the interspace to the parietal pleura is performed	1. To admit the diameter of the chest tube
2. The trocar is directed into the pleural space, the cannula is removed, and a chest tube is inserted into the pleural space and connected to a drainage system	2. There is a trocar catheter available equipped with an indwelling pointed rod for ease of insertion
Hemostat technique using a large bore chest tube	
A large bore chest tube is used to drain blood or thick effusions from the pleural space	
1. After skin preparation and anesthetic infiltration, an incision is made through the skin and subcutaneous tissue	1. The skin incision is usually made one interspace below proposed site of penetration of the intercostal muscles and pleura
2. A curved hemostat is inserted into the pleural cavity and the tissue is spread with the clamp	2. To make a tissue tract for the chest tube

Contd...

Contd...

Nursing action	Rationale
3. The tract is explored with an examining finger	3. Digital examination helps confirm the presence of the track and penetration of the pleural cavity
4. The tube is held by the hemostat and directed through the opening up over the ribs and into the pleural cavity	
5. The clamp is withdrawn and the chest tube is connected to a chest drainage system	5. The chest tube has multiple openings at the proximal and for drainage of air/blood
6. The tube is sutured in place and covered with a sterile dressing. Chest tube (tube thoracostomy) inserted via hemostat technique	
Follow-up phase	
1. Observe the drainage system for blood/air. Observe for fluctuation in the tube on respiration	1. If a hemothorax is draining through a thoracostomy tube into a bottle containing sterile normal saline, the blood is available for autotransfusion
2. Secure a follow-up chest X-ray	2. To confirm correct chest tube placement and re-expansion of the lung
3. Assess for bleeding, infection, leakage of air and fluid around the tube	

Procedure 9.27: Managing the patient with water-seal chest drainage (Fig. 9.48)

Equipment:

- Closed chest drainage system
- Holder for drainage system (if needed)
- Vacuum motor
- Sterile connector for emergency use.

Steps of procedure

Nursing action	Rationale
Performance phase	
1. Attach the drainage tube from the pleural space (the patient) to the tubing that leads to a long tube with end submerged in sterile normal saline	1. Water-seal drainage provides for the escape of air and fluid into a drainage bottle. The water acts as a seal and keeps the air from being drawn back into the pleural space
2. Check the tube connections periodically. Tape if necessary a. The tube should be approximately 2.5 cm (1 inch) below the water level b. The short tube is left open to the atmosphere	2. Tube connections are checked to ensure tight fit and patency of the tubes a. If the tube is submerged too deep below the water level, a higher intrapleural pressure is required to expel air b. Venting the short glass tube lets air escape from the bottle
3. Mark the original, fluid level with tape on the outside of the drainage bottle. Mark hourly/daily increments (date and time) at the drainage leve	3. The marking will show the amount of fluid loss and how fast fluid is collecting in the drainage bottle. It serves as a basis for blood replacement, if the fluid is blood. Grossly bloody drainage will appear in the bottle in the immediate postoperative period and, if excessive, may necessitate reoperation. Drainage usually declines progressively after the first 24 hours
4. Make sure that the tubing does not loop or interfere with the movements of the patient	4. Fluid collecting in the dependent segment of the tubing will decrease the negative pressure applied to the catheter, kinking looping or pressure on the drainage tubing can produce back pressure, thus, possibly forcing drainage back into the pleural space or impeding drainage from the pleural space

Contd...

Contd...

Nursing action	Rationale
5. Encourage the patient to assume a position of comfort. Encourage good body alignment. When the patient is in a lateral position, place a rolled towel under the tubing to protect it from the weight of the patient's body. Encourage the patient to change position frequently	5. The patient's position should be changed frequently to promote drainage and body kept in good alignment to prevent postural deformity and contractures. Proper positioning helps, breathing and promotes better air exchange. Pain medication may be indicated to enhance comfort and deep breathing
6. Put the arm and shoulder of the affected side through range of motion exercises several times daily. Some pain medication may be necessary	6. Exercise helps to avoid ankylosis of the shoulder and assist in lessening postoperative pain and discomfort
7. "Milk" the tubing in the direction of the drainage bottle as often as ordered (many institutions do not advocate milking because of the increased intrapleural pressure it causes	7. "Milking" the tubing prevents it from becoming plugged with clots of fibrin. Constant attention to maintaining the patency of the tube will facilitate prompt expansion of the lung and minimize complications
8. Make sure there is fluctuation ("tidaling") of the fluid level in the long glass tube	8. Fluctuation of the water level in the tube shows that there is effective communication between the pleural space and the drainage bottle, provides a valuable indication of the patency of the drainage system, and is a gauze of intrapleural pressure
9. Fluctuation of fluid in the tubing will stop when: a. The lung has re-expanded b. The tubing is obstructed by blood clots or fibrin c. A dependent loop develops (see step 4) d. Suction motor or wall suction is not operating properly	
10. Watch for leaks of air in the drainage system as indicated by constant bubbling in the water seal bottle a. Report excessive bubbling in the water-seal change immediately b. "Milking" of chest tubes in patients with air leaks should be done only if requested by surgeon	10. Leaking and trapping of air in the pleural space can result in tension pneumothorax
11. Observe and report immediately signs of rapid, shallow breathing, cyanosis, pressure in the chest, subcutaneous emphysema, or symptoms of hemorrhage	11. Many clinical conditions may cause these signs and symptoms, including tension pneumothorax, mediastinal shift, hemorrhage, severe incisional pain, pulmonary embolus, and cardiac tamponade. Surgical intervention may be necessary

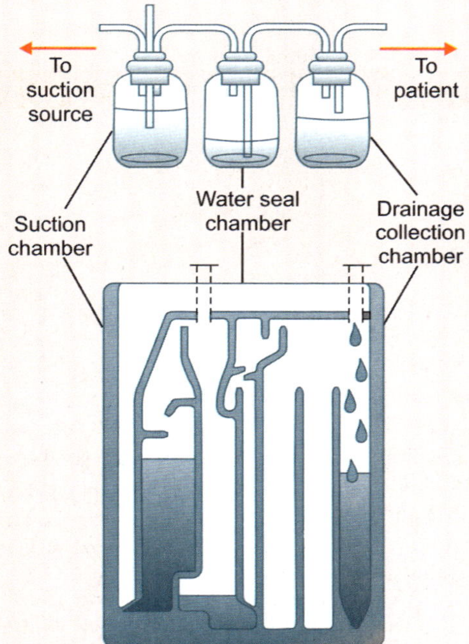

FIG. 9.48: Pleur-Evac chest drainage system

Contd...

Contd...

Nursing action	Rationale
12. Encourage the patient to breathe deeply and cough at frequent intervals. If there are signs of incisional pain, adequate pain medication is indicated	12. Deep breathing and coughing help to raise the intrapleural pressure, which allows emptying of any accumulation in the pleural space and removes secretions from the tracheobronchial tree so that the lung expands
13. If the patient had to be transported to another area, place the drainage bottle below the chest (as close to the floor as possible)	13. The drainage apparatus, must be kept at a level lower than the patient's chest to prevent backflow of fluid into the pleural space
14. If the tube becomes disconnected, cut off the contaminated tips of the chest tube and tubing. Insert a sterile connector in the chest tube and tubing, and reattach to the drainage system. Otherwise, do not clamp the chest tube during transport	
15. When assisting with removal of the tube a. Administer pain medication 30 minutes before removal of chest tube b. Instruct the patient to perform a gently Valsalva maneuver or to breathe quietly c. The chest tube is clamped and removed d. Simultaneously, a small bandage is applied and made airtight with petroleum gauze covered by a 4 × 4 inch gauze and thoroughly covered and sealed with tape	15. The chest tube is removed as directed when the lung is re-expanded (usually 24 hours to several days). During the tube removal, avoid a large sudden inspiratory effort, which may produce a pneumothorax
Follow-up phase	
1. Monitor patient's pulmonary status for signs and symptoms of decompensation	1. Patient could have reformation of pneumothorax upon removal

Procedure 9.28: Tuberculin skin test

Equipment:

- Purified protein derivative (PPD) tuberculin antigen, intermediate strength
- Tuberculin syringe
- Short 1.25 cm (½ inch) 26-94 27-gauze steal needle
- Alcohol sponge.

Steps of procedure

Nursing action	Rationale
Performance phase	
1. Determine if the patient has ever disease, immunosuppression by disease, drugs, or steroids	1. Any of these may cause had BCG vaccine, recent viral false readings
Performance phase	
1. Draw up PPD-tuberculin into tuberculin syringe	1. Follow the manufacturer's directions each 0.1 mL oz should contain 5 tuberculin units (TU of PD-tuberculin). Use the antigen immediately to avoid absorption to the plastic/glass syringe
2. Cleanse the skin of the inner aspect of forearm with alcohol. Allow to dry	
3. Stretch the skin taut	
4. Hold the tuberculin syringe close to the skin so the hub of the needle touches it as the needle is introduced, bevel up	4. This reduces the needle angle at the skin suites and facilitates the injection of tuberculin just between the surface of the skin
5. Inject the tuberculin into the superficial layer of the skin to form a wheal 6 to 10 mm in diameter	5. If no wheal appears (because the injection was made too deep) inject again at another site. East 5 cm (2 inches) away
Follow-up phase	
To read the test	
1. Read the test within 48 to 72 hours when the induration is most evident	1. Tuberculin skin tests are tests of delayed hypersensitivity

Contd...

Contd...

Nursing action	Rationale
2. Have a good light available. Flex the forearm slightly at the elbow	
3. Inspect for the presence of induration inspect from a side view against the light inspect by direct light	3. Induration refers to hardening or thickening of tissues
4. Palpate lightly rub the fingure across the injection site from the area of normal skin to the area of induration outline the diameter of induration	4. Erythema (redness) without induration is generally considered to be of no significance
5. Measure the maximum transverse diameter of induration (not erythema) in millimeters with a flexible ruler	5. The extent of induration is measured in two diameters and recorded
Interpretation	
1. Induration of 5 mm or more in diameter	1. Considered positive in: a. Persons with known HIV or unknown HIV but with risk factors for HIV b. Persons who have had recent contact with active tuberculosis c. Persons who have fibrotic changes or chest X-ray, consistent with healed TB
2. Induration of 10 mm or more in diameter	2. Considered positive in all persons who do not meet above criteria but who have other risk factors in tuberculosis, such as homelessness, alcoholism malnutrition, and health care work
3. Induration of 15 mm or more in diameter	3. Considered positive in persons who do not meet the above criteria

Procedure 9.29: Assisting with an intercostal nerve block

Equipment:

- Syringes, 10-mL Luer-Lok
- Needles No. 22 to 30 gauge
- Anesthetic solution (lidocaine, bupivacaine, procaine)
- Skin germicide, sterile gloves.

Steps of procedure

Nursing action	Rationale
Preparatory phase	
1. Inform the patient that he or she will experience the prick of the needle and a slight sensation of pressure	
2. Position the patient as directed. a. Have the patient sit up, bend forward and hug a pillow or b. Place the patient prone with pillow under chest or c. Have the patient on unaffected side with upper arm hanging over the side of the table	2. a. This posture moves the scapulae forward and out of the way b. The prone position helps immobilize the patient c. This pulls the scapula out of the way
3. Ask the patient to identify the site of pain	3. To determine which intercostal nerves are to be injected
Performance phase (by the physician)	
1. After the skin is prepared, the lower margin of the rib is palpated and a small skin wheal is raised, using a 25 to 30 gauge needle	1. This is infiltration anesthesia
2. Usually nerve blocks are done at the posterior angle of the ribs between the posterior axillary line and the spine.	2. The posterior angle is the most prominent and accessible, and an injection at this area produces a block of the entire distal nerve
3. A fine needle is advanced through the wheal and directed downward so it slips under the edge of the rib into the upper portion of the interspace	
4. The syringe (needle in place) is aspirated	4. To ensure that the needle has not punctured the lung or that an intercostal vessel has been entered

Contd...

Contd...

Nursing action	Rationale
5. The local anesthetic (usually 3–5 mL) is injected into the area	5. Usually the local anesthetic is injected above and below the painful rib to obtain complete relief of pain, as the sensory fields or intercostal nerves overlap
Follow-up phase	
1. Assess for relief of pain and less painful coughing	1. This is the expected outcome
2. Obtain a chest X-ray	2. To ensure that a pneumothorax has not occurred
3. Complications: a. Intravascular injection b. Puncture of the lung with pneumothorax c. Hypotension	

CHAPTER 10

Gastrointestinal Nursing

INTRODUCTION

The gastrointestinal (GI) system, also termed as the digestive system and alimentary canal, consists of the GI tract and its accessory organs (Fig. 10.1). The GI tract or alimentary canal is a hollow muscular tube that extends from mouth to the anus. Its principal function is to provide the body with fluid, nutrients and electrolyte. This is accomplished through the processes of ingestion (taking food), digestion (breakdown of food) and absorption (transfer of food products into circulation). Another main function of the GI system is the storage and final excretion of the solid waste products of digestion, i.e. elimination.

The GI system consists of the GI tract, and its associated organs and glands, which includes mouth, esophagus, stomach, small intestine, large intestine, rectum and anus. The associated organs are the liver, pancreas, and gallbladder. Proper functioning of the GI system is essential to the maintenance of proper nutrition and health. Psychological or emotional factors such as stress and anxiety influence GI functioning in many persons. Stress may be manifested as anorexia, epigastric and abdominal pain or diarrhea. However, GI problems should never be solely attributed to psychological factors. Organic and psychologically-based problem can exist independently or concurrently. Physical factors such as dietary intake, ingestion of alcohol, and cafeine-containing products, cigarette smoking and fatigue may affect GI function. Some organic diseases of the GI system such as peptic ulcer, ulcerative colitis may be aggravated by stress. These both physical and emotional factors affect the GI functions. So it is very essential for the nurses to understand the disorders of GI system, because they will come across such clients, and to provide proper nursing services.

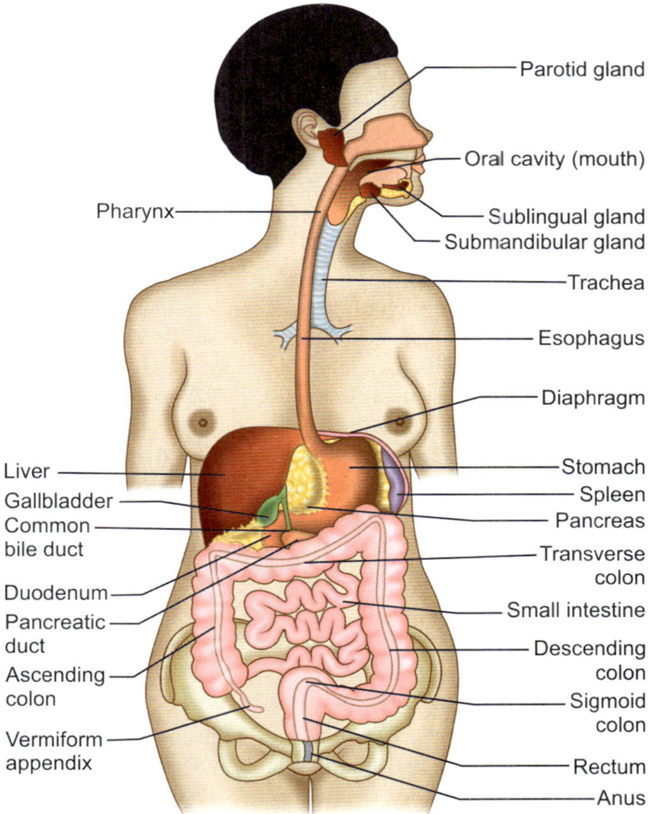

FIG. 10.1: Organs of the digestive system and associated structures

ASSESSMENT OF GASTROINTESTINAL SYSTEM

Assessment of GI system involves a detailed health history as well as a comprehensive physical examination of the oral cavity, abdomen, rectum and anus. And a review of the client's demographic data.

Demographic Data

A review of the patient's demographic data such as age, sex, culture, religion and occupation is helpful when assessing

GI system, because many GI disorders are associated with it. For example, many GI cancers occur more frequently in the elderly and in males, whereas others are more common in females. Sexual abuse may play role in GI problems in some women. Reproductive cycling in females contribute to other GI manifestations. Duodenal ulcers develop in younger adults, whereas gastric ulcers are more common in middle-aged and older adults.

Past Health History

The nurse collects data about previous hospitalizations, major illness, surgery, use of medications and allergies as a part of past health history.

- Informations should be gathered from the patients about the history or existence of the following diseases or problems related to GI functioning: Abdominal pain, gastritis, nausea, and vomiting, diarrhea, and constipation, hepatitis, colitis, peptic ulcer, abdominal distension, jaundice, anemia, hiatal hernia, gallbladder disease, dysphagia, heartburn, dyspepsia, changes in appetite, hematemesis, food intolerance, indigestion, excessive gas, bloating, melena, hemorrhoids, hernia, or rectal bleeding. In addition, nurse should ask whether the client currently has or previously had a change in bowel habits, GI bleeding, jaundice, ulcers, colitis, or unexplained weight loss or gain
- The health history should include an assessment of the patient's past and current use of medications, particularly in relation to liver problems. Because many chemicals and drugs are potentially hepatotoxic (e.g. alcohol, arsenic, carbon tetrachloride, gold compounds, mercury, phosphorous, anabolic steroids, halothane, isoniazid, propylthiouracil, sulfonamides, thiazide diuretics, methotrexate, acetaminophen). The nurse should ask the patient if laxatives or antacids are taken, including the kind and frequency. The use of prescription or over the counter appetite suppressant drug should be noted including name, duration, frequency and also any allergies to medication should be noted
- Information should be obtained about the hospitalization for any problems related to the GI system, including abdominal surgery, rectal surgery, reasons for surgery, postoperative course and possible blood transfusion, etc
- The nurse should also have the knowledge about the patient's health practices relted to GI system, such as maintenance of normal body weight, attention to proper dental care, maintenance of adequate nutrition and effective elimination habits and patient should be asked about exposure to hepatotoxic chemicals and exposure to hepatitis or parasitic infection. And also patient should be assessed in relation to certain habits like consumption of alcohol and cigarette smoking, which may delay healing of ulcers and lead to liver problems
- Thorough nutritional assessment is essential. The nurse should ask open-ended questions that will allow the patients to express beliefs and feelings about the diet. The nurse may need to ask the patient to do a 24 hours dietary recall to analyse the adequacy of diet and find out whether patient is taking adequate diet or not. The patient should be questioned about any changes in appetite food tolerance and weight. Anorexia and weight loss may indicate carcinoma. The nurse should ask the patient about allergies to any food and determine what GI symptoms show allergic response cause
- A detailed account of the patient's bowel elimination pattern should be elicited. The frequency, time of the day, and usual consistency of stool should be noted. The use of laxatives and enema, including type, frequency, and results should be documented. Any recent changes in bowel pattern should be investigated
- Activity and exercise may affect GI motility. Immobility is risk for constipation. So the patient's ambulatory status may be assessed to determine if the patient is capable of securing and preparing food. Any limitation in it should be noted
- The patient should be asked if GI symptoms affect sleep or rest. For example, a patient with a hiatal hernia may be awakened because of burning pain, sleep may be improved by elevating the head of the bed for such patients. Hunger can prevent sleep and should be relieved by a light, easily digested snack unless contraindicated. A patient often has bed time ritual that involves the use of a particular food or beverages, e.g. warm milk, herbal tea, etc. should be noted
- Cognitive-perceptual pattern, i.e. decrease in sensory adequacy can result in problems related to the acquisition, preparation and ingestion of food. For example, changes in taste or smell can affect appetite and eating pleasure. The nurse should assess the patient in this pattern to judge the effect of deficiencies on adequate nutritional intake and pain in another area that requires careful assessment related to its effect on GI system and nutrition. The possible effects of pain medication related to constitution, sedation and appetite suppressive should be assessed
- Self-perception and self-concept pattern should be assessed because many GI and nutritional problems can have a serious effect on the patient's self-perception, for example: (1) Overweight and underweight persons often have problems related to self-esteem and body image. (2) The altered physical changes often associated with liver disease can be problematic for the patient, e.g. jaundice, ascites
- It is important that the nurse should be aware of the role-relationship pattern of patient. For example, problem related to the GI system such as: Cirrhosis, alcoholism, hepatitis, ostomies, obesity and carcinoma can have a major impact on the patient's ability to maintain usual roles and relationships
- It is also important that nurse should ask sensitive questions to determine sexuality-reproductive pattern of the patient, changes related to sexuality and reproductive status on result from problems of the GI system. For example, obesity, jaundice, anorexia, could decrease the acceptance of a

potential sexual partner. Chronic alcoholism decreases meaningful sexual relationship. The presence of an ostomy could affect the patient's confidence related to sexual activity. Anorexia can affect the reproductive status of a female patient. Alcoholism can affect the reproductive status of both men and women

- The nurse should try to determine the coping stress tolerance pattern of the patient, because GI symptoms such as epigastric pain, nausea and diarrhea develop in many individuals in response to stressful or emotional situations. Some organic GI problems such as peptic ulcers are aggravated by stress. The nurse should also assess the value-belief pattern of the patients, i.e. the patient's spiritual and cultural belief regarding food and food preparations which helps for prescribing food and medication accordingly.

Physical Examination of GI System

The physical examination of the GI system include examination of the oral cavity, abdomen, anus and rectum. *Oral cavity:* Assessment of oral cavity involves inspection and palpation. The nurse puts on gloves, faces the client and begins by inspecting the lips. For observation of abnormalities of color, lesions, nodules and symmetry. The abnormalities of lips include pallor, or cyanosis, cracking ulcer, or fissure using a tonge blade. The nurse should inspect the buccal mucosa and not the color, any areas of pigmentation or any lesion. In assessing teeth and gums, nurse should look for caries, look teeth, abnormal shape and position of teeth, and swelling, bleeding, discoloration or inflammation of gingivae. Any distinctive breath odor should be noted. The pharynx should be inspected for any abnormalities. Abnormalities of mouth include thrush, leukoplakia, white plaques with red patches, cancer sore, etc.

The nurse should palpate any suspicious area in the mouth such as ulcer, nodules, indurations and areas of tenderness should be palpated. It should be noted that if patient having any dentures or partial appliances should be removed when examining the oral cavity.

Abdomen

To assess the patient's abdomen, have the client lie in a supine position with the arms at the sides. Bending the knees slightly helps to relax the abdomen muscles. Begin in the patient's right lower quadrants and proceed in clockwise manner. When assessing the abdomen, the nurse proceeds the following sequence: Inspection, auscultation, percussion and palpation. The sequence may vary according to situations.

I. *Inspection:* The nurse should inspect the abdomen for skin changes (color, texture, scars, striae, dilated veins, rashes and lesions), umbilicus (location and contour) symmetry, contour (flat, rounded, carved, concave, protuberant, distention), observable mass (hernias or other masses) and movement (pulsations and peristalsis).

II. *Auscultation* of the abdomen begins by listening with the diaphragm of the stethoscope, which provides information on bowel and vascular sounds. The stethoscope is lightly pressed on the abdominal wall in all four quadrants. Begin in the right lower quadrant at the ileocecal valve area because bowel sounds are normally present there. Normal bowel sounds occur 5 to 35 times per minute and sound like high-pitched clicks or gurgles. The nurse should listen for bowel sounds for 2 to 5 minutes. Bowel sounds cannot be described as absent until no sound is heard for 5 minutes in each quadrant. The frequency and intensity of the bowel sounds vary depending on the phase of digestion. Loud gurgles indicate hyperperistalsis termed as 'borborygoni (stomach growling). Terms used to describe bowel sounds include, present, absent, increased, decreased, high pitched, tinkling, gurgling and rushing.

    The nurse uses the bell of the stethoscope to auscultate vascular sounds. Three abnormal sounds should be listened for: A bruit, a venous hum, or a friction rub. The nurse listens over the aorta, renal arteries, and iliac arteries. A bruit is heard over the aorta which indicates presence of aortic aneurysm. A continuous venous hum heard in preumbilical area indicates engorged liver circulation. Friction rub indicates hepatic tumor or splenic infarction.

III. *Percussion* of the abdomen is to determine the size and location of the abdominal organs and to detect fluid, air and masses. The nurse uses percussion in all four quadrants and compare sounds. Normally, percussion sounds over the abdomen are tympanic (high-pitched loud or musical over gas) or dull (thud-like sounds over fluid or solid organs).

    To percuss the liver, the nurse should start below the umbilicus in the right midclavicular line and percuss lightly upward until dullness is heard, thus determining the lower border of liver dullness. After the lower border of the liver has been determined, the nurse should start the nipple line in the midclavicular line and percuss downward between ribs to the area of dullness indicating the upper border of the liver. The height or vertical space between two areas should be measured to determine the size of the liver. Dull sounds normally occur over the liver and spleen or a bladder filled with urine. Abnormal findings occur because of the presence of ascites or abnormal masses (Table 10.1).

    Interpretation of common finding of inspection
    - Scars on strials may be result of pregnancy, obesity, ascites, tumors edema, surgical procedure or healed burned areas
    - Engorged veins may be caused by obstruction of vena cava or portal vein and circulation from abdomen
    - Skin color observe for evidence of jaundice or inflammation (redness)
    - Visible peristalsis may be caused by pyrolic or intestinal obstruction; normally peristalsis not visible except the slow waves in thin persons

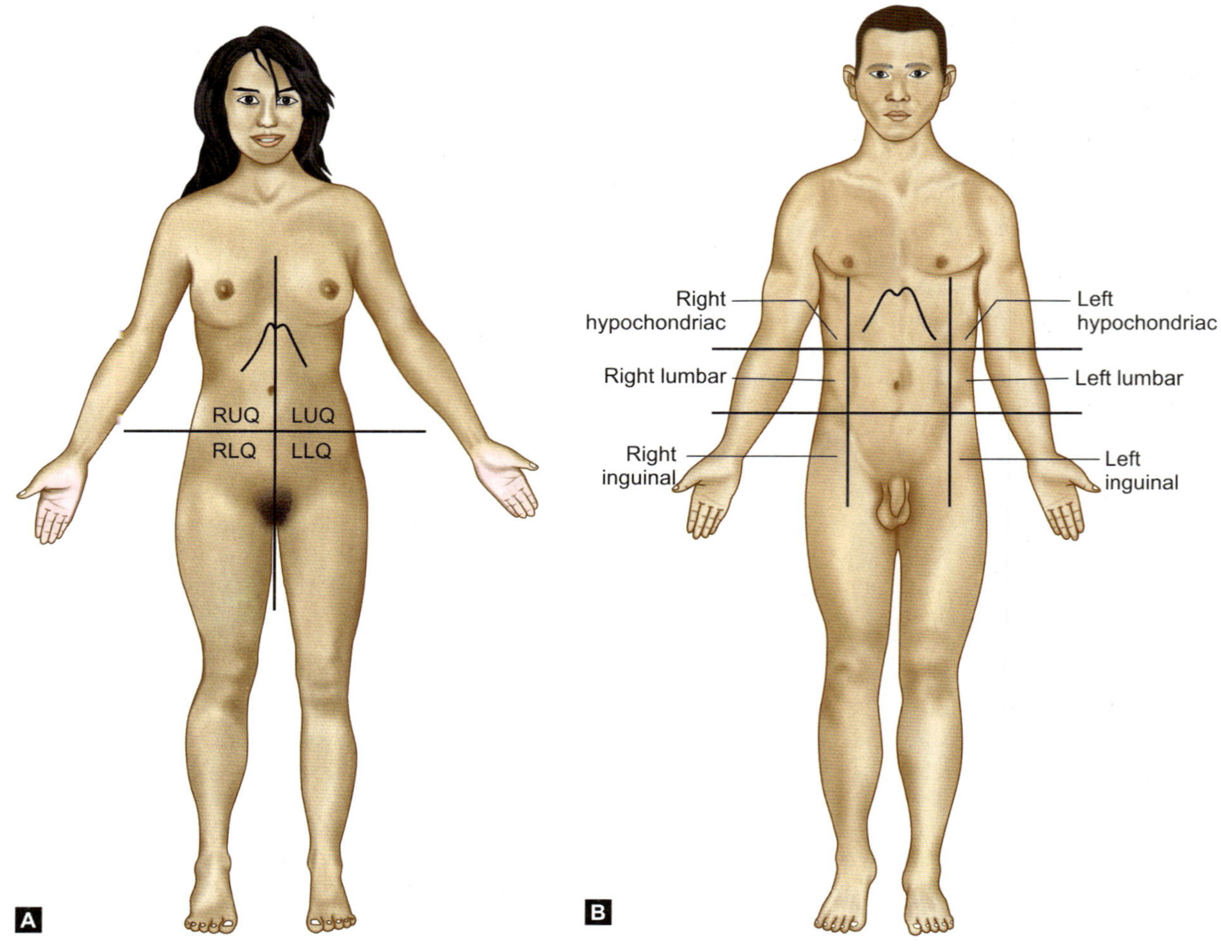

FIGS 10.2A AND B: (A) Abdominal quadrants; (B) Abdominal region

TABLE 10.1: Location of organs in each abdominal quadrant (Fig. 10.2)

• Right upper quadrant (RUQ) – Liver – Gallbladder – Duodenum – Right kidney – Hepatic flexure of colon	• Right lower quadrant (RLQ) – Cecum – Appendix – Right ovary and tube
• Left upper quadrant (LUQ) – Stomach, spleen – Left kidney, pancreas, – Splenic flexure of colon	• Left lower quadrant (LLQ) – Sigmoid colon – Left ovary and tube

– Visible pulsation normally slight pulsation of aorta is visible to epigastric region
– Visible masses and altered contour observe for hernia, distension of ascitis and obesity; instructing patient to cough may bring hernia 'bulge or elicit pain or discomfort in the abdomen, marked concavity may be caused by malnutrition
– Spider angioma appear on the upper portion of the body and blanch with pressure: Commonly result from liver disease.

Interpretation of common findings from auscultation

– Absence from sounds in 5 minutes may be due to peritonitis, paralytic ileus, pneumonia and hypokalemia
– Repeated, high-pitched sounds occurring at frequent intervals. Increased peristalsis heard in gastroenteritis, early pyloric obstruction, early intestinal obstruction and diarrhea
– Bruit presence of abnormal sounds (turbulence of blood flow through partially occluded or diseased aorta or renal artery)
– Hum and friction rub heard over liver and splenic areas, indicating an increased venous blood flow, possibly related to peritoneal inflammation.

IV. Palpation is of value in determining the outlines of the abdominal organs, determining the presence and characteristics of any abdominal masses, and identifying the presence of direct tenderness, guarding, rebound tenderness and muscular rigidity (Fig. 10.3).

Light palpation is used to detect tenderness or cutaneous hypersensitivity, muscular resistance, masses, and swelling. The nurse uses the pads of the fingertips with the finger together, and press gently, depressing the abdominal wall about 1 cm. All quadrants are palpated using smooth movement.

Deep palpation is used to delineate abdominal organs and masses. The palmar surface of the fingers should be used to press more deeply. Again all quadrants should be palpated. When palpating masses, the nurse should note the location, size, shape and presence of tenderness. The patient's facial expression should be observed during these maneuver, because it will give non-verbal cues of discomfort or pain (Fig. 10.4).

An alternate method for deep abdominal palpation is the two-hand method. One hand is placed on the top of the other. The fingers of the top hand apply pressure to the bottom hand. The fingers of the bottom hand feel for organs and masses.

To palpate nurse's left hand is placed behind the patient to support the right eleventh and twelth rib. The patient may relax on nurse's hand. The nurse should press the left hand forward and place the right hand on the patient's right abdomen lateral to the rectus muscle. The fingertips should be below the lower border of liver, dullness and pointed towards the right costal margin. The nurse should gently press in and up. The patient should take deep breath with the abdomen so that liver drops and is in a better position to be palpated. The nurse should try to feel the lower edge as it comes down to the fingertips. The liver edge should be firm, sharp and smooth. Any abnormality should be noted.

To palpate spleen, the nurse moves to the left side of the patient. The nurse places the left hand under the patient and supports and presses the patient's left lower rib cage forward. The right hand is placed below the left costal margin and pressed it in towards the spleen. The nurse should ask the patient to breathe deeply. The tip or edge of an enlarged spleen will be felt by the fingertips. The spleen is normally not palpable.

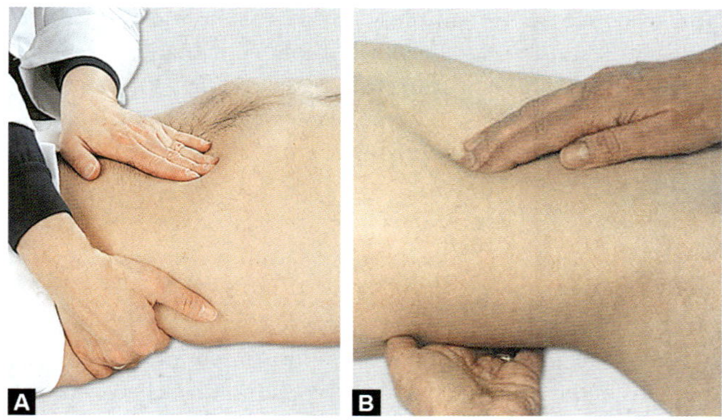

FIGS 10.3A AND B: (A) Technique for light palpation of the abdomen; (B) Technique for deep palpation

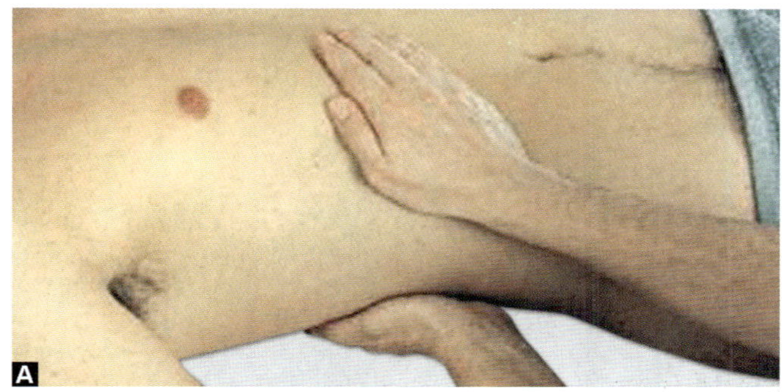

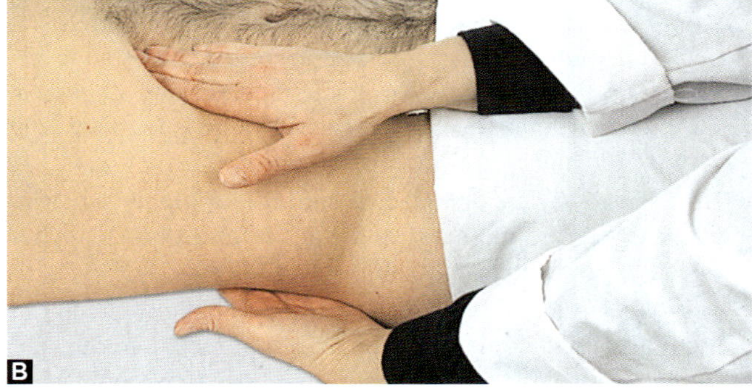

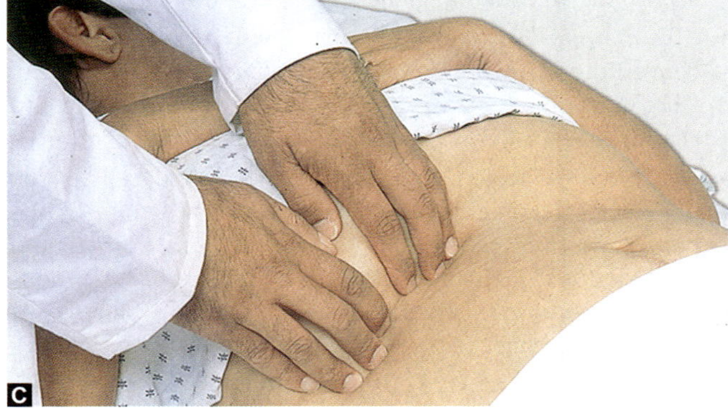

FIGS 10.4A TO C: (A) Technique for liver palpation; (B) Alternative technique; (C) Palpation of liver with fingers hooked over the costal region

Rectum and Anus

Examination of the anus and rectum is potentially embarrassing and uncomfortable for the patient. The nurse uses a gentle approach and a matter-of-fact manner. The client's position depends on the circumstances of the examination. A female client may be examined while in the lithotomy position immediately following assessment of the genitalia, in the Sim's position or in a dorsal recumbent position. A male client may be examined in the Sim's position or while standing and leaning across the examination table, a position which facilitates palpation of the prostate gland.

Clients are draped accordingly. For the digital examination of the rectum the gloved lubricated index finger is placed against the anus while the patient strains (Valsalva maneuver). Then as the sphincter relaxes, the finger is inserted. The finger is pointed towards the umbilicus. The nurse should try to get the patient to relax. The finger inserted into the rectum as far as possible, and all surfaces are palpated. Nodules, tenderness or any irregularities should be assessed. A sample of stool can be removed with the gloved finger and should be checked for occult blood. Abnormal findings may include pruritus ani, coccygeal or pilonidal sinus, tract openings, fistulas, fissures, external hemorrhoids, rectal prolapse and internal hemorrhoids, etc.

DIAGNOSTIC STUDIES IN GASTROINTESTINAL SYSTEM

Number of examinations and tests performed for diagnosis of problems of the GI system are both consuming and unpleasant. Several tests are intrusive procedures that are uncomfortable and embarrassing for the patient which results in added stress for the patient. It remains the nurse's responsibility to meet the educational and psychological needs of the patient by answering questions concerning the test procedure, rationale for its use and specific test preparation in a caring manner.

Laboratory Tests

Numerous tests may be used as a part of the evaluation of the GI biliary and exocrine pancreas function. The main blood and urine tests are as follows:

Blood Tests

- *Stomach gastrin test:* Gastrin is a gastric hormone that is a powerful stimulus for gastric acid secretion. Elevated levels are found in those with pernicious anemia and Zollinger-Ellison syndrome. The normal gastrin value is less than 200 dg/mL (200 mg/L)
- *Helicobacter pylori* detected in serum is a highly sensitive but less-specific indicator of an active infection. *H. pylori* infection predisposes to peptic ulcer disease
- *Total bilirubin test:* Bilirubin is exerted in the obstruction in the biliary tract contribute primarily to a rise in conjugated (direct) values. The normal value 0.1 to 1.0 mg/dL, conjugated 0.1–0.3 mg/dL, unconjugated 0.1–0.8 mg/dL
- *Alkaline phosphate*: It is found in many tissues with high concentration in bone, liver and biliary tract epithelium. Obstructive biliary tract disease and carcinoma may cause significant elevations. The normal value is 30–85 1U/mL
- *Amylase:* It is secreted normally by the acinar cells of the pancreas. Damage to these cells or obstruction of the pancreatic duct causes the enzyme to be absorbed into the blood is significant quantities. It is a sensitive yet non-specific test for pancreatic disease. The normal value is 80–150 Somogyl units
- *Lipase:* It is a pancreatic enzyme normally secreted into the duodenum. It appears in the blood when damage occurs to the acinar cells. It is a specific test for pancreatic disease. The normal value 0–110 units/L
- Calcium levels may be low in cases of severe pancreatitis or steatorrhea because calcium soaps are formed from the sequestration of calcium by fat necrosis. The normal value is 9.0–11.5 mg/dL
- Total protein of blood includes albumin and globulin. Although primarily a reflection of liver function, serum protein level is also a meausre of nutrition. Malnourished patients have greatly decreased levels of blood protein. The normal protein is 6.8 g/dL (Albumin 3.2–4.5 g/dL, Globulin 2.3–3.4 g/dL)
- *D-xylose absorption test:* D-xylose is a monosaccharide that is easily absorbed by the normal intestine but not metabolized by the body. D-xylose is administered orally and assists in the diagnosis of malabsorption. Normally blood levels of 25–40 mg/dL 2 hours after ingestion
- *Lactose tolerance test*: An oral dose of lactose is administered. In the absence of intestinal lactase, the lactose is neither broken down nor absorbed and plasma glucose levels do not rise. The test assists in the diagnosis of lactose intolerance. Normally rise in blood glucose level is more than 20 mg/dL
- *CEA test:* Carcinoembryonic antigen is a protein normally present in fetal gut tissue. It is typically elevated in persons with colorectal tumors. It is useful in determining prognosis and response to therapy. The normal value is less than 5 mg/mL.

Urine Tests

- *5-Hydroxyindoleacetic acid (5-HIAA):* Carcinoid tumors are serotin in secreting and are derived from neuroectoderm tissue, e.g. the appendix and intestine. These neurohormones are metabolized to 5-HIAA by the liver and excreted in urine. The normal value is 2–5 mg/2 h
- *Urine bilirubin:* Bilirubin is not normally excreted in the urine. Biliary structure, inflammation or stones may cause its presence
- *Urobilinogen:* A sensitive test for hepatic or biliary diseases. Decreased levels are seen in those with biliary obstruction and pancreatic cancer. In 24-hour collection, urobilinogen is 0.2–1.2 units and 0.05–2.5 mg
- *Urine amylase:* Normally 10–80 amylase units/hour. A rise in levels usually minimizes the rise in serum amylase. The level remains elevated for 7–10 days; however, which allows for retrospective diagnosis.

Stool Examination

Stool specimens are collected primarily for culture, determination of fat content and examination for the presence of ova, parasites, and fresh or occult blood. Stools to be analyzed for the presence of bacteria, i.e. *Salmonella, Shigella, Staphylococcus aureus*. Detection of occult blood in the stool is useful in identifying bleeding in the GI Tract. Occult blood may be identified by one of the three tests–guaiac test (hemoccult), benzidine, or orthotolidine (Occultest).

The color of the stool also indicates few clues for the following:

- Brown
  - Presence of fecal urobilinogen
- White
  - Barium
- Gray, tan (clay)
  - Lack of bile, biliary obstruction
- Black
  - Tarry—upper GI bleeding
  - Dry—rapid peristalsis with bile presence
- Green
  - Rapid peristalsis with bile presence.

Radiological Studies

Upper GI or Barium Swallow

It is an X-ray study with fluoroscopy with contrast medium. This is used to diagnose structural abnormalities of the esophagus, stomach and duodenal bulb. The nurse's responsibility in this procedure includes:

- Explain procedure to patient and that patient will need to drink contrast medium and assume various positions on X-ray table
- Keep patient NPO (nil per oral) for 8–12 hours before procedure
- Tell the patient to avoid smoking after midnight, the night before the study
- After X-ray test, take measures to prevent contrast medium impaction (fluids, laxatives)
- Tell patient that stool may be white up to 72 hours after test.

Small Bowel Series

In this contrast medium is ingested and flat film taken q20 minutes until medium reaches terminal ileum. Here the nurse's responsibilities are as stated in barium swallow.

These procedures are used to identify esophageal and stomach disorder such as strid varices, polyps, tumors, hiatal hernia and peptic ulcers.

Lower GI or Barium Enema

It is fluoroscopic X-ray examination of colon, used contrast medium, which is administered rectally (enema). Double contrast or air contrast barium enema is test of choice. Air is infused after barium is evacuated. The nurse's responsibility in barium enema includes:

- Before the procedure, administer laxatives and enema until colon is clear of stool evening before procedure
- Administer clear liquid diet evening before procedure
- Keep patient NPO for 8 hours before test
- Instruct patient about being given barium by enema
- Explain that cramping and urge to defecate may occur during procedure and that patient may be placed in various positions on tilt table
- After the procedure give fluids, laxatives or suppositories to assist in expelling barium
- And observe stool for passage of contrast medium.

This procedure identifies polyps, tumors and other lesion in colon.

Oral Cholecystogram (Gallbladder Series)

It is X-ray examination visualizes gallbladder (GB) after radiopaque dye such as iopanoic acid (Telepaque) has been ingested orally. It is used to determine the GB ability to concentrate and store dye and to observe the patency of the biliary duct system. It also may be used to detect gallstones, obstructions of the biliary tract and other GB disorders. In this procedure, the nurse's responsibilities will include:

- Assess patient for sensitivity to iodine (telepaque contains iodine)
- Administer radiopaque dye evening before test
- Give 6 tablets (3q) 1q 5 minutes
- Explain that patient may need 2 consecutive days of dye ingestion
- Keep patient NPO after ingestion of dye
- Observe for side effects of dye, such as nausea, vomiting, diarrhea
- May give fatty test meal after X-ray tet to check for GB emptying
- Assess patient's medication for possible contraindications, precautions or complications with the use of dye.

Cholangiography

Cholangiogram: The X-rays are used to visualize biliary duct system after IV injection of radiopaque dye, the nurse's responsibilities in the procedure will include:

- Keep patient NPO for 8 hours prior to procedure
- Assess sensitivity to iodine dye
- During injection of dye, assess for urticaria, extreme flushing and respiratory distress
- Assess patient's medications for possibly contraindication, complications, with the use of dye, percutaneous transhepatic cholangiogram. This is performed after local anesthesia. Liver is entered with long needles (under fluoroscopy) bile duct is entered, bile withdrawn and radiopaque dye injected. Fluoroscopy is used to determine filling of hepatic and biliary ducts. The nurse's responsibilities are:
  - Observe patient for signs of hemorrhage or bile leakage.
- Assess patient's medications for possible contraindications precautions or complications with the use of dye. Surgical

cholangiogram is performed during surgery on biliary structure such as gallbladder, contrast medium is injected into common bile duct. The nursing responsibilities are:

- Explain the patient that anesthetic will be used.

- Assess patient's medications for possible contraindications, precautions, or complications with the use of dye.

Ultrasound

This non-invasive procedure uses high frequency sound waves (ultrasound waves), which are passed into body structures and recorded as they are reflected (bounded). A conductive gel (lubricant jelly) is applied to the skin and a transducer is placed on the area. In these procedures, nurses should be aware that patient's bowel must be cleaned, because of the presence of solid material in GI tract causes change in reflected sounds and that ultrasound is not transmitted well through gas or air. Schedule test before upper GI or barium enema.

a. Abdominal ultrasound study detects abdominal masses (tumors and cysts) and is also used to assess ascitis.
b. Hepatobiliary ultrasound study detects subphrenic abscesses, cysts, tumors, cirrhosis and is used to visualize biliary ducts.
c. GB ultrasound study detects gallstones (high degree of accuracy) and can be used for a patient with jaundice, or allergic reaction to GB contrast media. The nurse's responsibilities include:
   - Administer clear liquids for 24 hours before examination
   - Give laxatives evening before and cleansing enema morning of examination
   - Keep patient NPO 8 hours prior to procedure.

Nuclear Imaging Scans

The purpose of nuclear imaging scans is to show size, shape, and position of organ. Functional disorders and structural defects may be identified. Radionuclide (radioactive isotope) is injected IV and a counter (scanning) device picks up radioactive emission, which is recorded on paper. Only tracer doses of radioactive isotopes are used. In these procedures, nurses use to:

- Tell patients that substances contain only traces of radioactivity and pose little to no danger
- Schedule no more than one radionuclide test on the same day
- Explain to patient need to lie flat during the scanning
   a. *Gastric emptying studies:* A radionuclide study is used to assess ability of stomach to empty solids or liquids. In solid emptying study, egg white containing $Tc^{99}m$ is eaten. In liquid emptying study, orange juice with $Tc^{99}m$ is drunk. Sequential images from gamma camera are recorded q2 minutes for up to 60 minutes. Study is used in patients with emptying disorders from peptic ulcer, ulcer surgery diabetes and gastric malignancy.
   b. *Liver and spleen scan:* Here patient is given LV injection of $Tc^{99}m$ and positioned under camera to record distribution of radioactivity in liver and spleen. In normal person, intensity of liver and spleen images is equal. Test is useful in detecting hepatomegaly hepatocellular diseases, hepatic malignancy and splenomegaly.

Computed Tomography (CT)

Computed tomography (CT) is a non-invasive radiological examination, which combines special X-ray machine used for CT (exposures at different depth) with computer. This study detects mainly biliary tract, liver and pancreatic disorders. Use of contrast medium accentuates density differences and helps detect biliary problems. In this procedure, nurses are used to explain procedures to patient and determine sensitivity to iodine if contrast material is used.

Magnetic Resonance Imaging (MRI)

MRI is a non-invasive procedure using radiofrequency waves and a magnetic field. This procedure is used to detect hepatic metastasis, sources of GI bleeding, and to stage colorectal cancer. The nurse's responsibilities in MRI includes:

- Keep patient NPO for 6 hours prior to procedure
- Explain procedure to patient
- This procedure contraindicated in patient with metal implants (e.g. pacemaker), or who is pregnant.

Endoscopic Examination

Endoscopy refers to the direct visualization of a body structure through a lighted instrument (scope). Most of the GI tract can be visualized by endoscopy, especially with the flexible fiberoptic scopes. The fiberscope is an instrument channel through which biopsy forceps and cytology brushes may be passed. Cameras may be attached and pictures taken. Endoscopy is frequently done in combination with the biopsy and cytologic studies. The major complication of GI endoscopy is perforations through the structure being scooped. All endoscopic procedures required informed, written consent.

Esophagogastroduodenoscopy (Fig. 10.5)

Esophagogastroduodenoscopy is a technique directly visualizes mucosal lining of esophagus, stomach and duodenum with flexible, fiberoptic endoscope. Tests may use video imaging to visualize stomach motility, inflammations, ulcerations, tumors, varices, or Mallory-Weiss tear may be detected. The nursing responsibility in this procedure includes:

- Keep patient NPO for 8 hours prior to the procedure
- Make sure signed consent is on chart
- Give preoperative medication if ordered (diazepam, midazolam, or meperidine)

- Explain to patient that local anesthetic may be sprayed on throat before insection of scope and that patient will be sedated during procedure
- After procedure, keep patient NPO until gag reflex returns
- Gently tickle back of throat to determine reflex
- Use warm saline gargles for relief of sore throat
- Check temperature q 15–30 minutes for 1–2 hours (sudden temperature spike is sign of perforation).

Colonoscopy

Study directly visualizes entire colon upto iliocecal valve with flexible fiberoptic scope. Patient's position is changed frequently during procedure to assist with advancement of scope to cecum.

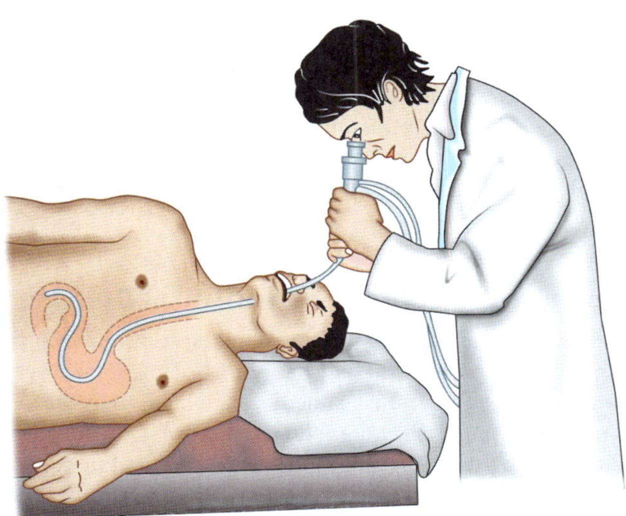

FIG. 10.5: Gastroscopy

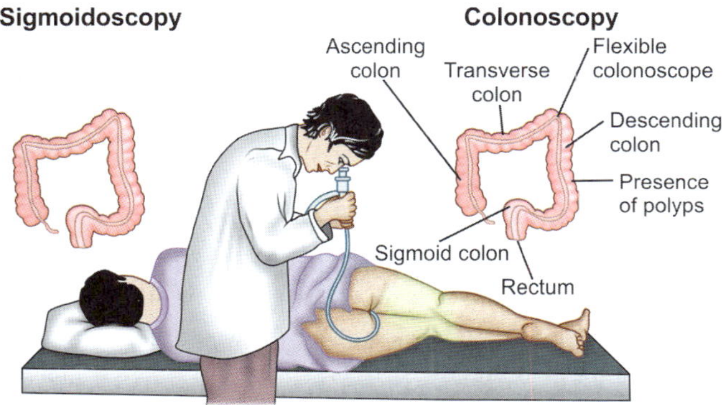

FIG. 10.6: Colonoscopy and flexible fiberoptic sigmoidoscopy. For the colonoscopy, the flexible scope is passed through the rectum and sigmoid colon into the descending, transverse, and ascending colon. For the flexible fiberoptic sigmoidoscopy, the flexible scope is advanced past the proximal sigmoid and then into the descending colon

Test is used to diagnose inflammatory bowel disease, detect tumors, and dilate strictures. Procedure allows for removal of colonic polyps without laparotomy. The nursing responsibilities in this procedure will include (Fig. 10.6):

- Before the procedure, keep patient on clear liquids 1–3 days
- Keep patient NPO for 8 hours prior to procedure
- Make sure signed consent is on chart
- Administer laxatives 1–3 days before and enema night before
- Explain to patient some information regarding insertion of scope as for sigmoidoscopy
- Explain to patient that sedation will be given
- Administer alternate preparation of 1 glass of golytely or colyte evening before (8 oz glass q 10 min)
- On morning of procedure, allow clear liquids
- After the procedure, be aware that patient may experience abdominal cramps caused by stimulation of peristalsis because the patient's bowel is constantly inflated with air during procedure
- Observe for rectal bleeding and signs of perforation (e.g. malaise, abdominal distentions).

Endoscopic Retrograde Cholangiopancreatography (ERCP) (Fig. 10.7)

In ERCP, fiberoptic endoscope is inserted through the oral cavity into descending duodenum, then common bile and pancreatic ducts are cannulated. Contrast medium is injected into ducts and allows for direct visualization of structures. Technique can also be used to retrieve a gallstone from distal GBD, dilate structures, biopsy tumors diagnose pseudocysts. In this procedure, the nursing responsibilities will include the following:

- Before the procedure, explain procedure to patient including patient's role
- Keep patient NPO 8 hours prior to procedure
- Ensure consent form is signed
- Administer sedation immediately before and during procedure
- Administer antibiotics if ordered

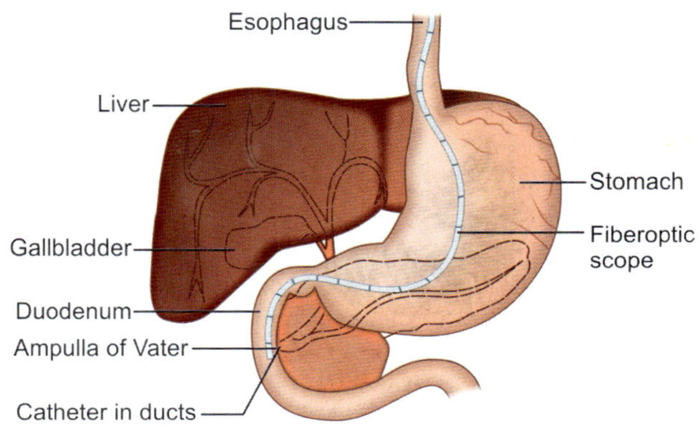

FIG. 10.7: Endoscopic retrograde cholangiopancreatography

- After the procedure, check vital signs
- Check for signs of perforation or infection
- Be aware that pancreatitis is most common complication
- Check for return of gag reflex.

Peritoneoscopy (Laparoscopy)

Peritoneal cavity and contents are visualized with laparoscope. Biospy specimen may also be taken. Double puncture peritoneoscope permits better visualization of abdominal cavity, especially liver. This technique can eliminate need for exploratory laparotomy in many patients. In this, following are the "nursing responsibilities".

- Make sure signed permit is on chart
- Keep patient NPO 8 hours before study
- Administer preoperative sedative medication
- Ensure that bladder and bowel are emptied
- Instruct patient that local anesthesia is used before scope insertion
- Observe for possible complications of bleeding and bowel perforation after the procedure.

Liver Biopsy

It is an invasive procedure; uses needle inserted between sixth and seventh or eighth and ninth intercostal spaces on the right side to obtain specimens of hepatic tissue. The nurse's responsibilities include:

- Check patient's coagulation status (PT, CT, BT) prior to procedure
- Ensure patient's blood is typed and cross matched
- Take vital signs as baseline data
- Explain holding breath after expiration when needle is inserted
- Ensure that informed consent has been signed
- After the procedure, check vital signs to detect internal bleeding, q 15 min × 2, q 30 min × 4, q 1 hour × 4
- Keep patient lying on right side for minimum 2 hours to splint puncture site
- Keep patient on bed in flat position for 12–14 hours
- Assess patient for complications such as bile peritonitis, shock pneumothorax.

PROBLEMS OF MOUTH

Ingestion is the process of taking food and fluids into the body via the GI tract. It begins in the mouth with mastication of food by teeth. Food then passes down the esophagus and into the stomach. It is important that sufficient nutrient is ingested to meet bodily requirements. Oral problems, such as poor dental health, infections and inflammation and cancer interfere with ingestion.

Dental Problems/Tooth and Gum Disorder

Tooth decay is by far the most common problem affecting the teeth termed as "dental caries". It is the result of a pathological process that causes the gradual destructions of the enamel and dentin of the teeth. Caries development starts when 'plaque' builds up and adheres to the teeth. Plaque is a gelatinous substance consisting of bacteria, saliva and epithelial cells.

Pathophysiology of Dental Decay

Dental plaque is a soft mass composed of proliferation bacteria in a matrix of polysaccharides and salivery glycoproteins. It adheres to the teeth and its both transparent and colorless. Acids produced by the bacteria slowly decalcify the inorganic tooth enamel. Food, particularly carbohydrates, stimulates bacterial acid production. Simple sugars have the greatest effect. The plaque begins to collect on the teeth within 2 hours of eating and the longer or more frequently carbohydrates are ingested, the longer it takes for the pH of the mouth returns to normal cavity formation is the visible clinical evidence of the progression of the decay process.

Pathophysiology of Periodontal Disease

The periodontium is the tissue surrounding and supporting the teeth. It is composed of the gingivae (gums), cementum, alveolar bone and the periodontal ligament, which helps to fix the tooth firmly in its bony socket. Periodontal disease is the major loss of tooth in adults. Gingivitis is the earliest form of periodontal disease, it is characterized by color alterations in the gums, swelling and easy bleeding. Inflammation causes gingivae to separate from the tooth surface. Pockets form in the gingivae that can collect bacteria, food particles and pus. As the process is gradually worsens over a period of time, the gum recedes, the alveolor bone is resorbed, and the teeth loosen. Bleeding of the gums with normal tooth brushing is a common early sign. There is usually no pain.

Etiology of Periodontal Disease

- Dental plaque, when dental plaque calcifies, it forms calculus, which is hard, tenacious mass on the crowns of teeth
- Malocclusion—faulty relationship between the teeth when the jaws are closed, margins of over-extended fillings, impacted food
- Systemic conditions such as:
  - Poorly, controlled diabetes mellitus
  - Thyroid diseases, pregnancy, HIV infections
  - Vitamins and nutritional deficiencies
  - Certain drugs, smoking also.

Management of Dental Problem

- Prevention is the most appropriate management of dental problem, which includes:
  - Widespread fluoridation of water supplies reduces dental decay. Fluoride makes tooth enamel more resistant to acids and is commonly added to drinking water in many localities. It is widely available in toothpastes, dental rinses and mouthwashes
  - Early treatment of periodontal disease consists of scaling and root planning
  - Scaling is the removal of calculus and root planning is the smoothening of root surfaces. Gingivectomy and gingivoplasty may be necessary.

Nursing Assessment

- The patient's mouth should be assessed for tooth caries, missing teeth displaced teeth and dental appliances.
- The face should be assessed for symmetry and the jaw should be palpated for lumps.
- The gingivae should be assessed for redness, pallor, bleeding, recession and ulcers.

Nursing Diagnosis

- Altered oral mucous membrane related to:
  - Caries, ineffective and hygienic, periodontal disease or ill-fitting dentine
- Altered nutrition less than body requirement related to inability to ingest adequate nutrients (ill-fitting dentures, displaced teeth, gingival discs, dental caries)
- Body image disturbance related to change in appearance of or unattractive teeth, difficulty with eating or Halitosis
- Non-compliance related to altered perception, lack of motivation, inadequate finance or lack of knowledge of consequence of non-compliance.

Planning

The objectives of the nursing management is:

- To decrease dental caries through improved oral hygiene
- Able to identify and reduce risk factors (caries and periodontium)
- To have a balanced diet intake.

Implementation

- Advise or assist in maintaining proper oral hygiene
- Advise and assist for regular periodic dental examination
- Reduce sugar intake and brush teeth after 30 minutes of eating sugar to reduce plaque formation
- Increase intake of vitamin C
- Advise use of fluoride content toothpaste
- Advise for fluoridation of drinking water in the community
- Referrals made for acute dental problem cases, such as:
  i. Local manifestation of pain that is caused by sensitivity to heat cold stimulation, dull and continuous pain, facial swelling, halitosis and bleeding or drainage of pus from the mouth.
  ii. Systematic manifestation of fever, nausea, vomiting and malaise.

Evaluation: Check the objective of care will be met or not.

ORAL INFECTIONS AND INFLAMMATION

Any of the structures of the mouth may develop infections when oral infections and inflammations are present, they can severely or seriously affect the ability of the patient to adequately and comfortably ingest food and fluids by mouth. These infections are inflammations; may be specific mouth disease or they may occur in the presence are inflammation may be specific mouth disease or they may occur in the presence of some systemic disease such as leukemia or vitamin deficiency.

Pathophysiology

The structure of the mouth causes many ulcerative diseases to have similar signs and symptoms. The mucus throughout the mouth is thin, and evolving vesicles and bullae break open rapidly into ulcers. The ulcers are typically further traumatized by the teeth and can become readily infected by the abundant oral flora. Many of the causative organisms are the same on those that cause common skin infections. The common inflammation and infections of the oral cavity are as follows. With this etiology, there comes clinical manifestation and treatment.

1. Gingivitis: Inflammation of the gingivae in the early form of periodontal disease. It may occur due to neglected oral hygiene, malocclusion, missing or irregular teeth, faulty dentistry, eating of soft rather than fibrous foods.

   The clinical manifestation include inflamed gingivae and interdental papillae, bleeding during toothbrushing, development of pus, formation of abscess with loosening teeth (periodontitis).

   Treatment include prevention through health teaching, dental care, gingival massage, professional cleaning of teeth, non-fibrous foods, conscientious brushing habits with flossing.
2. Vincent's angina (necrotizing ulcerative gingivitis, trench mouth): It is an acute bacterial infection of the gingivae, caused by a tremendous proliferation of normal mouth flora, such as spirochetes and fusiform bacilli. It is commonly triggered by poor oral hygiene, nutritional deficiencies (B and C vitamins), alcoholism, infections, or immunocompromise.

   The clinical manifestations are, painful bleeding gingivae, eroding necrotic lesions of interdental papillae, ulceration than bleed, increased saliva with metallic taste, fetid mouth odor, anorexia, fever and general malaise.

The nursing measure will include—advising the patient to take rest (physical and mental), avoidance of smoking and alcoholic beverages, advice soft nutritious diet, correct oral hygiene habits, topical application of antibiotics, mouth irrigations with H_2O_2 and saline solutions.

3. Oral candidiasis (monilasis or thrush) is caused by an increase in the level of *Candida albicans*, a yeast-like fungus is normally found in the skin, GI tract, vagina and oral cavity. Overgrowth of the organism may result from antibiotic depletion of normal flora (prolonged high dose of antibiotics) or immunosuppress from steroid therapy, chemotherapy or HIV infections.

   The clinical manifestations are pearly, bluish white (creamy white) "milk-curd" membranous lesions on mucosa of mouth and larynx, sore mouth, yeasty halitosis. The conditions is painful and if widespread, can interfere with oral nutrition. When mucosa bleeds, and ulcerates when patches are scraped off.

   Treatments include nystatin, or amphotericin B as oral suspension or buccal tablets, good oral hygiene. Oral nystatin, ketoconazole, clotrimazole; amphotericin for the immunocompromized person.

4. Herpes simplex stomatitis (cold sore, fever-blister): It is an externally common viral infection that produces characteristic blisters commonly called 'cold sore' or fever blister. It is caused by herpes simplex virus, type I or II, predisposing factors of upper respiratory infections, excessive exposure to sunlight, food allergies, emotional tensions, onset of menstruation.

   The virus is harboured in a dormant state by cells in the sensory nerve ganglia. Reactivation of the virus can occur with emotional stress, fever, exposure to cold or ultraviolet rays. The lesion appears most commonly on the mucus membranous border junction of the lips in the form of small vesicles, which then erupt and form painful, shallow ulcers. Vesicle formation may be single or clustered. Painful vesicles and ulceration of mouth, lips or edge of nose; may have prodromal itching or burning, fever, malaise, lymphadenopathy may occur.

   Treatment is palliative, which include mild antiseptic mouthwash. Application of spirits of camphor, corticosteroid cream, viscous lidocaine, removal or control of predisposing factors, topical or systemic antiviral agents, e.g. acyclovir (zovirax) in severe cases.

5. Aphthous stomatitis (cancer sore): It is a recurrent and chronic form of infection secondary to systemic disease, trauma, stress or unknown causes. It produces well-circumscribed ulcers on the soft tissues of the mouth, including lips, tongue, insides of the cheeks, pharynx and soft palate. Ulcers of the mouth and lips causing extreme pain, ulcers surrounded by erythematous base. Painful small ulceration on oral mucosa heals in 1 to 3 weeks.

   Treatment is palliative; includes mouthwashes, hydrocortisone, antibiotic ointment, fluocinonide (Lidex) ointment in orabase. Corticosterdoid (topical or systemic) tetracycline oral suspension for children.

6. Parotitis is an inflammation of the salivary or parotid glands. The viral inflammation known as "mumps" in children.

   Parotitis usually caused by *Staphylococcus* species, *Streptococcus* species, occasionally. Acute bacterial parotitis typically occurs in debilitated or elderly patients in whom dehydration, minimal oral intake, or medication have resulted in chronic dry mouth. Poor oral hygiene also causes parotitis. Acute parotitis occurs in postoperation patient called "surgical mumps".

   The clinical manifestations are: Pain in the glands with an abrupt onset, i.e. pain in area of gland and ear, absence of salivation, purulent exudate from duct of gland, fever and swelling.

   Treatment includes application of heat and cold, frequent oral hygiene, adequate hydration, broad spectrum antibiotics, occasionally needed. Nursing measures are mouthwashes, warm compresses, preventive measures such as chewing gum, sucking on hard candy (Lemon drops) adequate fluid intake.

7. Stomatitis is the inflammation of the mouth caused by trauma, pathogens, irritants (tobacco, alcohol) renal, liver and hematologic disorders, side effects of many cancer chemotherapeutic drugs.

The clinical manifestation is excessive salivation, halitosis, sore mouth.

Treatment includes, removal or treatment of cause, oral hygiene with soothing solutions, topical medication, soft, bland diet.

ORAL CANCER

Carcinoma of the oral cavity may occur on the lips or anywehre within the mouth which includes tongue, floor of the mouth, buccal mucosa, hard palate, soft palate, pharyngeal walls and tonsils.

Etiology

The development of oral cancer is clearly linked to a history of smoking and alcohol consumption and the risk increases strongly with heavy use. The exact cause of oral cancer is not clear, but there are number of predisposing factors, which includes:

- Constant over-exposure to ultraviolet radiation from the sun, for cancer lips
- Tobacco usage (smoking and chewing), i.e. pipe and cigarette smoking, snuff, chewing tobacco
- Chronic alcohol intake (excessive use of alcohol)

- Chronic irritation (jagged tooth, ill-fitting prosthesis, chemical or mechanical irritants)
- Ruddy fair complexion leads to lip cancer
- Syphilis, immunosuppression leads to lip cancer
- Recurrent herpetic lesions
- Poor oral hygiene
- Hot and spicy foods or drinks
- Malnutrition
- Cirrhosis of the liver
- Age over 45 years
- Family history of oral cancer.

Pathophysiology

The vast majority of oral cancer arise from the squamous cells, which line the surface, oral epithelium, epidermoid, basal cell and other carcinoma may arise. The majority of tumors arise on the lateral or ventral surfaces of the tongue, although rarely on the dorsal surface, and commonly go unnoticed by the patients. A single ulcer is the typical pattern. The tongue has an abundant vascular supply and lymphatic drainage channels, and spread of the cancer to adjacent structures may be rapid. Metastasis to the neck has already occurred in 60% of patients at the time of the diagnosis is made. The mortality rate is high, early metastasis is rare, although rapid extension to the mandible or floor of the mouth is possible. Tumors that involve the parotid gland are usually benign, although those arising submaxillary glands have a high rate of malignancy and tend to grow rapidly.

Clinical Manifestations

Many oral cancers are asymptomatic in the early stages. The premalignant lesions of the oral cavity are:

- Leukoplakia—is a potentially precancerous, yellow-white or grey white lesions may occur in any region of mouth also called "white patch" or "smoker's patch". Leukoplakia is the result of chronic irritation usually from the smoking and *Candida* infection.
- The patch becomes keratonical (hard and leathery) is sometimes described as hyperkeratosis.
- Erythroplasia—is a red, velvety-appearing patch that is often indicative of early squamous cell carcinoma occur on the mouth or tongue. These may turn to malignant.

Cancer of the lip usually appears as an indurated, painless ulcer on the lip. The first sign of carcinoma of tongue is ulcer or area of thickening. Soreness or pain of the tongue may occur, especially on eating hot or highly-seasoned foods. Cancer lesions are most likely to develop in the proximal half of the tongue. Later symptoms of cancer of the tongue include increased salivation, slurred speech, dysphagia, toothache, and earache.

Approximately 30% of oral cancer present with an asymptomatic neck mass. Anyhow, the common clinical manifestation of oral cancer are as follows:

- Masses in the mouth or neck
- Chronic ear pain
- Enlarged lymp nodes (cervical nodes are commonly affected)
- Discomfort or burning
- Ulcer on lateral or ventral surface of the tongue or elsewhere
- Dysphagia
- Visible lesions on lips or elsewhere
- Presence of erythroplasia (bright red, velvety leisions).

Diagnostic Study

- Biopsy of the suspected lesion with cytologic examination. It may be used to evaluate lymph nodes, leukoplakia or erythroplasia
- Ultrasonography is an excellent adjust to evaluate masses that are closed to the surface
- Computed tomography (CT) scans may be used to evaluate deeper, less definite masses
- Magnetic resonance imaging (MRI) is most useful in the effort to evaluate deep masses of the inconclusive structure.

Treatment

Treatment of oral cancer depends on the location and staging of the tumor. Early-stage cancer is usually treated by either radiation or surgery, depend upon the size and accessibility of the tumor. More invasive cancers may require both modalities and advanced cancers are treated palliatively.

Radiation Therapy for Oral Cancer

Early lesions are highly curable with radiation, if they are confined to the mucosa, and the use of radiation prevents widespread tissue destruction. Radiation may be delivered by external beam or through the insertion of needle. If both radiation and surgery are planned, the radiation therapy is usually administered after the surgery because irradiated tissue is more susceptible to infection and breakdown. Care of the patient with implanted radioactive needles in oral tissue includes the following:

- Implant care
  - Do not pull on the strings. Any movement could alter the placement or direction of the radiation or cause the needles to loosen
  - Check needles-patency several times each day
  - Monitor linens, bed areas and emesis basin, for needles that may dislodge
  - Ensure that a protective container is present in the room to contain any needles that might dislodge.

- Patient care
  - Be familiar with gentle oral hygiene q 2h while awake
  - Encourage the patient to avoid hot and cold foods and beverages as well as smoking
  - If the patient has dentures, encourage their removal at night, for comfort. Assess gums for irritations and bleeding whenever dentures are removed
  - Provide viscous lidocaine (xylocaine) solution or lozenges as needed, when oral discomfort interferes with nutrition
  - Provide the patient with an alternate means of communication, talking around implanted needles is usually difficult or impossible
  - Assist the patient to implement the mouth care regimen prescribed by the physician
  - The side effects of radiation therapy to the mouth and neck include mucositis, xerostomia, and dental decay should be reported and managed accordingly.

Surgical Management

Surgical management of oral cancers range from local excision of small tumors to expensive surgery for invasive tumors. Some examples are partial mandibulectomy, hemiglossectomy, resection of the buccal mucosa and floor of the mouth and radical neck dissection, etc. Chemotherapy and radiation therapy also may be used along with surgical measures wherever indicated in palliative purposes. Because of depression, alcohol or presurgery radiation treatment patient may be malnourished even before surgery and after the surgery also there may be chance to become malnourished. For which nurse must observe for tolerance of the feedings and adjust the amount, time and formula if nausea, vomiting, diarrhea or distension occurs. The patient usually instructed about the tube feedings. When the patient can swallow, small amount of water is given. Close observation for choking is essential. Suction may be necessary to prevent aspiration. While managing the patient undergoing for surgery for oral cancer, the nurse can follow the undermentioned guidelines for care.

- Preoperative
  - Clarify the patient's knowledge of changes expected after surgery
  - Explain expected postoperative measures including suctioning, nasogastric tube, etc.
  - Provide opportunities for the patient to begin to express feelings about changes in body image
- Postoperative.

Monitoring

- Assess facial movement for facial nerve damage (if parotid gland excised); ask the patient to raise the eyebrows, frown, smile, show the teeth, pucker the lips
- Assess the degree and character of drainage
  - Amount of drainage and presence of blood should be mentioned
  - Hemorrhage may occur with wide resection of tongue.

Maintaining an Adequate Airway

- Place the patient in sidelying position initially
- Place the patient in Fowler's position when fully alert
- Suction the mouth (except for loop surgery)
- Gauze wick may be used to direct salive into an emesis basin
- Maintain patency of drainage tubes if used.

Promoting Oral Hygiene and Comfort

- Clean involved areas of the mouth with a cotton applicator moistened with H_2O_2 and saline
- Mouth irrigations
  - Use sterile equipment
  - Use a solution of sterile water, diluted H_2O_2, normal saline, or sodium bicarbonate
  - Avoid commercial mouthwashes
  - Protect any dressings from getting wet
  - A catheter may be inserted along the side of the cheek and the solution injected with gentle pressure; a spray may also be used
  - Give analgesics as indicated (pain is not usually severe).

Promoting Nutrition

- Tube feedings will be used initially with hemiglossectomy
- Oral fluids: Place in back of throat with asepto syringe or feeding up with attached tubing
- Eating soft foods
  - Encourage the patient to feed self when possible
  - Teach the patient to drink clear water after all meals to cleanse the mouth
  - Avoid using a fork, which may traumatize new tissue
  - Avoid very hot or cold foods (hot foods may irritate new tissue whereas cold foods may cause facial pain or paralyze oral function).

Promoting Speech

- Limit patient's response intitially to yes or no, which can be answered by gestures
- When ability speech returns, encourage patient to speak slowly
- Listen carefully and validate communication before acting on requests
- Speak in a soft, clear voice
- Refer the patient to a speech therapist if needed.

Promoting Body Image

- Prepare all visitors for visible outcomes of surgery
- Include the family in all teaching
- Encourage the patient to ventilate feelings about changes
- Encourage socialization with others.

Nursing Management of Oral Cancer

Nursing Assessment

Subjective and objective data should be collected as follows:

The subjective data include:

- Important health information:
  - *Past health history:* Recurrent herpetic lesions, syphilis, exposure to sunlight
  - *Medications:* Use of immunosuppressants
  - *Surgical or other treatment:* Removal of prior tumors
- Functional health patterns:
  - Health perception—health management: Use of alcohol and tobacco, pipe smoking; poor oral hygiene
- Nutritional metabolic: Reduction in oral intake, weight loss, difficulty in chewing, increased salivation, intolerance to certain foods and temperatures of foods
- Cognitive-perceptual: Mouth or tongue soreness or pain, toothache earache, neck stiffness, dysphagia, difficulty in speaking.

The objective data includes:

- Integumentary: Indurated, painless ulcer on lips painless neckmasses
- Gastrointestinal: Areas of thickening or roughness, ulcers, leukoplakia, or erythroplasia on the tongue, increased salivation, drooling, slurred speech, foul breath odor.

Nursing Diagnosis

Nursing diagnosis for the patients with oral cancer may include the following:

Altered nutrition: Less than body requirement related to oral pain, difficulty in chewing and swallowing, surgical resection, and radiation therapy.

- Pain related to tumor and surgical radiation
- Anxiety related to diagnosis of cancer, uncertain future, potential for disfiguring surgery, recurrence bronchoscopy
- Ineffective individual coping related to body image change, smoking and alcohol cessation
- Altered health maintenance related to lack of knowledge of disease process and therapeutic regimen, and unavailability of support systems.

Planning

The objective of oral cancer patient will include that the patient will:

- Have a patent airway
- Be able to communicate
- Have adequate nutritional intake to promote healing
- Have relief of pain and discomfort.

Implementation

The nurse should take preventive measures such as:

- Teach clients to avoid excessive use of tobacco, alcohol, hot and spicy foods and drinks
- Encourage use of sunscreen during exposure to sunlight
- Screen smokers and drinkers of alcohol and teach them to stop smoking and to limit alcohol intake
- Ensure that client fix broken teeth and improperly-fitting dentures
- Teach persons at risk to observe for manifestation of cancer
- Ensure that client's tumor is excised and followed with chemotherapy and radiation as indicated
- Provide nutritional support with tube feedings or feedings through precaution endoscopic gastrostomy and gastrostomy tube.

Evaluation

The expected outcomes (objectives) that the patient with oral cancer will:

- Maintain airway
- Be able to communciate
- Have adequate nutritional intake
- Have relief of pain and discomfort.

NAUSEA AND VOMITING

Nausea and vomiting are the most common symptoms of GI diseases, which most often occur together but may occur independently. They are part of the body's protective mechanisms and are usually a response to chemical, bacterial, or viral insults to the body's integrity. They are present in a wide array of disorders and if persistent can lead to serious consequences.

Nausea is a feeling of discomfort in the epigastrium with a conscious desire to vomit. Anorexia usually accompanies nausea and is brought on by unpleasant stimulation involving any of the five senses. Generally, nausea occurs before vomiting and is characterized by contraction of the duodenum and by slowing of gastric motility and emptying.

Vomiting is the forceful ejection of partially digested food and secretions from the upper GI tract. It occurs when the gut becomes overly irritated, excited, or distended. It can be a protective mechanism to rid the body of spoiled or irritating foods and liquids. Immediately before the act of vomiting, the person becomes aware of the need to vomit. The autonomic nervous system is activated resulting in both parasympathetic and sympathetic nervous systems, stimulation sympathetic activation produces tachycardia, tachypnea and diaphoresis. Parasympathetic stimulation causes relaxation of lower esophageal sphincter, an increase in gastric motility and a pronounced increase in gastric motility and a pronounced increase in salivation.

Vomiting is a complex act that requires coordinated activities of several structures, closure of the glottis, deep inspiration with contraction of the diaphragm in the inspiratory position, closure of the glottis relaxation of the stomach and lower esophageal sphincter, and contraction of the abdominal muscles with increasing abdominal pressure. These stimulation activities force the stomach contents up through the esophagus into the pharynx and out of the mouth.

Etiology

Nausea and vomiting are the most common manifestations of the gastrointestinal disorders. They are also found in a wide variety of conditions that are unrelated in GI disease. These include:

- Pregnancy
- Infectious diseases
- CNS disorders (e.g. meningitis, CNS lesion)
- Cardiovascular problem (e.g. digitalis, antibiotics)
- Metabolic disorders (e.g. uremia, diabetic acidosis, etc.)
- Psychological factors (e.g. stress, fear, unpleasant nights and odors).

Pathophysiology

Nausea may be accompanied by weakness, hypersalivation, and diaphoresis. Gastric tone and peristalsis are typically slowed or absent. The neural pathways that control nausea are not well identified but probably are the same general pathways that control vomiting. The vomiting center is located in the medulla (brainstem) adjacent to the respiratory and salivary control centers and can be stimulated by the vagus nerve and sympathetic nervous system. Receptors can be found throughout the GI tract and internal organs that, when triggered by spasm or inflammation, can directly produce vomiting. Indirect stimulation can come from the chemoreceptor trigger zone (CTZ) which is located on the floor of the fourth ventricle and appears to act as an emetic chemoreceptor responding to chemical stimuli in the blood. A wide variety of medication and other substances can act on the CTZ in this manner. The CTZ also mediate the response to nonchemical stimuli such as radiation and motion sickness. There is a strong evidence that dopamine receptors in the CTZ play a role in mediating vomiting (Fig. 10.8).

When nausea and vomiting are prolonged, dehydration can rapidly occur. In addition to water, essential electrolytes, (e.g. potassium) are also lost. As vomiting persists, there may be severe electrolyte imbalances, loss of extracellular fluids (ECF) volume, decreased plasma volume and eventually circulatory failure. Metabolic alkosis can result from loss of gastric HCL. When contents from the small intestine are vomited. Weight loss is evident in a short time when vomiting is severe. The threat of aspiration is constant concern when vomiting is severe.

Nursing Management

Nursing Assessment

The nurse has to obtain the important health information, which include:

- Past health history: GI disorders, chronic indigestion, food allergies, pregnancy, infection, CNS disorders, recent travel, bulimia, metabolic disorders, cancer, cardiovascular disease, renal disease.
- Medications: Use of antiemetics, digitalis, opiates, ferrous sulfate aspirin, aminophylline, alcohol, antibiotics, general anesthesia, chemotherapy.
- Surgery of other treatment: Recent surgery.

And also functional health pattern like amount, frequency, character and color of vomitus, dry heaves, anorexia, weight loss, abdominal tenderness, weakness, fatigue, stress, fear, etc.

And also objective data include observing for lethargy, sunken eyeballs, pallor, dry mucous membrane, poor skin turgor, GI symptoms like amount frequency, character (e.g. projectile, or regurgitation) content (undigested food, bloody bile, feces) and color of vomitus (red, coffee ground, green-yellow) and decreased output of urine, concentrated urine to locate causes.

Nursing Diagnosis

- Selfcare deficiency related to fatigue and discomfort and prolonged nausea and vomitus

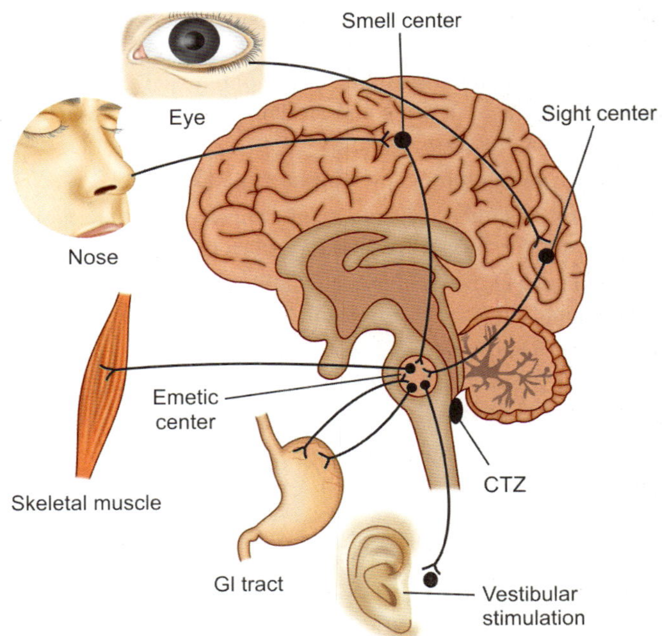

FIG. 10.8: Stimuli involved in the act of vomiting. CTZ, Chemoreceptor trigger zone: GI gastrointestinal

- Altered oral mucous membrane related to persistent vomiting and inadequate oral hygiene
- Vomiting related to multiple etiologies
- Fluid volume deficient related to prolonging
- Anxiety related to lack of knowledge of cause
- Altered nutrition less than body requirements.

Planning (Table 10.2)

The overall goals of the patient with nausea/vomiting will:

- Experience minimal or no nausea and vomiting
- Have normal electrolyte levels and hydration status
- Return to normal pattern of fluid balance and nutrition intake.

TABLE 10.2: Nursing care plan of patient with nausea and vomiting

Problem	Reason	Objective	Nursing intervention	Evaluation
Vomiting related to multiple etiologies	As manifested by episodes of nausea and vomiting	• Minimal or no nausea and vomiting • Verbalization of satisfaction with care	• Assess duration, frequency and nature of vomitus and aggravating and alleviating factors to plan appropriate action • Offer reassurance and explanations to increase patient cooperation • Remove visual stimuli and source of odors to avoid precipitating factors of nausea and vomiting • Provide mouth care; change soiled gown and linen to ensure patient comfort • Use diversional activities (if appropriate) to decrease awareness of nausea • Maintain quiet environment, restrict visitors and avoid unnecessary procedures to minimize triggering of vomiting • Administer antiemetics as ordered • Instruct patient to take several deep breaths, prevent sudden changes in position • Keep head of bed elevated to decrease stimulation of the vomiting center • Instruct patient to avoid foods and beverages that stimulate nausea and vomiting	
Fluid volume deficit related to • Prolonged vomiting • Inability to ingest, digest or absorb food and fluids	As manifested by decreased urine output and increased urine concentration, increased pulse rate, postural hypotension, decreased intake, decreased skin turgor, dry skin and mucous	No signs of dehydration	• Assess for signs of dehydration to plan appropriate care • Administer and monitor amount and type of IV fluids to maintain fluid and electrolyte balance • Administer antiemetic as prescribed • Provide small amounts of clear liquids when vomiting stops for maintaining hydration • Record amount and frequency of vomitus • Maintain accurate intake and output records • Weight daily in acute phase to accurately monitor fluid balance • Monitor lab results of serum sodium, potassium and chloride as indicators of electrolyte balance	
Anxiety related to • Lack of knowledge of the cause of it • Treatment plan and follow-up care	As manifested by verbalization of lack of knowledge apprehension	• Decrease in anxiety • Verbalization of understanding of causation factors and the repeutic interventions	• Explain rationale for plan of care and diagnosis tests to increase patient understanding to reduce anxiety • Instruct about relationships between nausea and vomiting and foods, medications, treatment regimens and psychosomal factors to elicit patient cooperation and avoiding potential causative factors	
Altered nutrition body requirement related to nausea and vomiting	As manifested by lack of interest in or aversion to food perceived or actual inability to ingest food weight loss	Gradual return to usual eating habits and weight	• Assess the patients interest in food, ability to ingest food, and weight to determine if a problem is present • Assure patient that appetite will return when nausea and vomiting are controlled • Maintain IV fluids or TPN until oral intake is possible, provide fluids, electrolytes, calories, and protein intake • Instruct patient to resume eating cautiously with bland, non-irritating foods	

Nursing Intervention

The patient with nausea and vomiting should be managed with following guidelines for:

Safety and Comfort

- Keep head of the bed elevated and emesis basin handy
- Protect airway with suction and positioning if patient is not alert
- Provide frequent mouth care
- Control sights and odors in room
- Reduce anxiety if possible
- Provide quiet or distraction on the basis of patient response
- Modify environmental stimuli (cool cloth, dim light) and evaluate response
- Provide ongoing patient support. Explore any strategies.

Diet Modification

- Maintain NPO if vomiting is severe
- Explore use of clear liquids:
  - Serve liquid cool or room temperature
  - Try effervescent drinks and evaluate effect
  - Avoid fatty foods
  - Avoid highly sweetened foods and milk products
  - Encourage adequate, fluids to prevent dehydration
  - Keep meals small, avoid overdistention.

Drugs/Medications

- Administer medication before vomiting occurs, if possible
- Evaluate the patient response to medication
- Maintain patient safety and assess for sedation or confusion.

Generally the drugs used for nausea and vomiting and their nursing intervention are as follows:

i. *Antihistamines* are believed to act on neurons in the vomiting center and in the vestibular pathways. They are effective in motion sickness and morning sickness management, but have little known effect in GI disorders. These drugs cause drowsiness and sedation. The nurse has to monitor drowsiness and sedation and instruct patient to use caution with all activities that require alertness. Driving may be hazardous, so should be avoided. The example of antihistamine are bucilizine hydrochloride, cyclizine hydrochloride, meclizine, promethazine (all generic names).

ii. *Antidopaminerics* are believed to act by antagonizing dopamine receptors in the CTZ. They also have antihistamine and anticholinergic effects. They are effective in managing mild symptoms and often first lane therapies. The examples of antidopamergics are prochlorperazine, ethylperazine, fluphenazine droperidol. The nursing measures in this therapy include:

   Monitor severity of drowsiness and sedation.

   Teach patient to avoid all hazardous activities and driving during use.

   Avoid alcohol and sun exposure.

iii. *Anticholinergics* reduce neuron transmission and are useful in the management of motion sickness and postoperative nausea. But the common side effects of dry mouth, urinary retention and drowsiness limit their use. During use, nurse should instruct patient to apply dry surfaces behind the ear. Use in advance anticipated need, e.g. scopalamine (Transderm-Scop).

iv. *Benzyamides* have complex action in both CNS and GI tract and useful in preventing vomiting associated with anesthetics and chemotherapeutic agents.

   Metadopramide stimulates gastric emptying.

   Domoperidone does not cross blood-brain barrier. Here nurse has to monitor side effects. Diarrhea and mild sedation.

v. *Serotonin antagonists* like ondansetron (Zofran) and Granisertron bind serotonin receptor sites along GI tract and afferent nerves. They are useful in controlling severe chemotherapy induced and postoperative vomiting.

vi. *Cannabis derivatives*: The antiemetic site of action is uncertain but the active ingredient in marijuana is often useful in controlling chemotherapy related nausea and vomiting. In such cases, the nurse has to instruct patient to alert on mood and behavioral changes. Drowsiness is common, so driving should be avoided. Avoid concurrent alcohol use while using this drug.

GASTROESOPHAGEAL REFLUX DISEASE

Gastroesophageal reflux diseases (GERD) is not a disease but a heterogeneous syndrome resulting from esophageal reflux. Most cases are attributed to the inappropriate relaxation of lower esophageal sphincter (LES) in response to unknown stimulus.

Etiology

The common cause of GERD is hiatal hernia, the presence of which displaces the LES into the thorax and number of environmental and physical factors have been identified that appear to influence the tone and contractility of the LES and these may play an etiological role in some cases of GERD. The pressure of the LES is lowered by fatty acids, chocolate, peppermint, cola, coffee and tea; nicotine, alcohol, drugs such as calcium channel blockers, the theophylline, and possible non-steroidal anti-inflammatory drugs (NSAIDs), elevated levels of estrogen and progesterone; and that conditions that elevate intra-abdominal pressure such as obesity, pregnancy or heavy lifting.

Pathophysiology (Fig. 10.9)

There are two zones of high pressure, one at each end of the esophagus, normally prevent the reflux of gastric contents. The zones maintain a constant pressure and relax only during swallowing. Although they are termed as LES, they are not really distinct anatomical structures. Esophageal reflux occurs when either gastric volume or intra-abdominal pressure is elevated or when LES tone is decreased. Periodic reflux occurs normally in most persons and is usually asymptomatic. The normal physiologic response to occasional reflux is immediate swallowing one or more rapid swallows induce peristaltic contractions to clear the reflux and neutralize the acid with bicarbonate-rich saliva. However, the esophagus has only a limited ability to withstand the damaging effects of acid reflux and GERD will develop when frequent episodes of reflux breakdown the mucosal barrier and initiate an inflammatory response.

The degree of esophageal inflammation related to the number, duration and acidity or alkalinity of the reflux episodes. The effectiveness and efficiency of esophageal clearance also are important. Esophageal clearance is particularly important at night when the swallowing rate and salivation decrease by two thirds and recumbent position interferes with clearance. An inflammed esophageal gradually loses its ability to clear reflexed material quickly and efficiently, and the duration of each episode gradually lengthens. Hyperemia and erosion occur in the face of chronic inflammation. Minor capillary bleeding is common, although frank bleeding is rare. Repeated episodes of inflammation and healing can gradually produce a change in the epithelial tissue, which makes it more resistant to acid. Overtime, fibrotic tissue changes can also result in esophageal stricture, which can progressively impair normal swallowing.

Clinical Manifestation

- Heartburn is caused by irritation of the esophagus by the gastric secretion. It is a burning, tight sensation that appears intermittently beneath the lower sternum and spreads upward to the throat or jaw. It occurs following ingestion of substances that decrease LES pressure. It is relieved with milk, alkaline substance or water
- Pulmonary symptoms including wheezing, hoarseness, coughing, (nocturnal cough), dyspnea are secondary to microaspiration of gastric contents into the pulmonary system
- Gastric symptoms including early satiety, prostating bloating, nausea and vomiting, are related to gastric stasis
- Regurgitation is effortless return of material from stomach into esophagus or mouth, oftenly described as hot, bitter or sour liquid coming into the throat or mouth. This taste is perceived in the pharynx
- Water brash a reflex, hypersecretion that does not have a bitter taste
- Frequent belching and flatulence and feeling of lump in the throat or food stopping
- Dysphagia difficulty in swallowing
- Odynophagia painfull swallowing
- Bleeching.

  In addition GERD patients may experience complication of respiratory system—bronchospasm, laryngospasm, circopharyngeal system and other complications include:
  - Esophageal stricture (due to repeated episodes)
  - Esophageal metaplasia (Barretts esophagus)
  - Pneumonia (due to aspiration of gastric contents to pulmonary system).

Management of GERD

Patients with GERD are rarely admitted to the acute care setting unless they require surgery or experience serious complications. The problem is self-managed in the outpatient setting. The goal of treatment is to decrease the incidence of reflux and eliminate the symptoms.

The diagnostic studies are performed to determine the causes are:

- Barium swallow for determining the protrusion of upper part of the stomach (gastric cardia)
- Radionuclide tests to detect reflux of gastric contents and the rate of esophageal clearance
- Esophagoscopy—to detect the incompetence of LES and the extent of inflammation, potential scarring and strictures
- Biopsy and cytologic tests to differentiate hiatal hernia, carcinoma and Barrett's esophagus

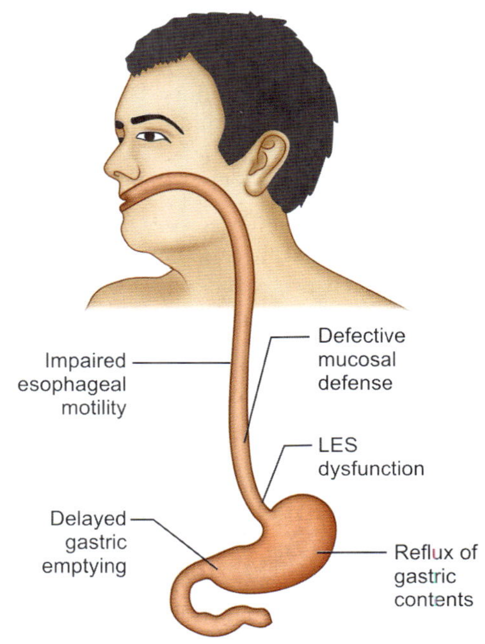

FIG. 10.9: Factors involved in the pathogenesis of gastro-esophageal reflux disease (GERD). LES, Lower esophageal sphincter

- Esophageal motility (manometry) studies to measure pressure in the esophagus and GES
- pH monitoring for presence of acid or alkaline.

  Pharmacologic management is focussed on improving LES function, increasing esophageal clearance, decreasing volume or acidity reflux, and protecting esophageal mucosa.
- Antacids are used to relieve heartburn by their neutralizing effect on hydrochloric acid (for example, Gelucil, Maalox, Mylanta).
- Antacids plus alginic acid (Gaviscon) are used to neutralize gastric acid and reacts with sodium bicarbonate and forms a viscous solution that floats to the surface of the gastric contents and coats the esophagus acting on mechanical barrier to reflux.

  When client is an antacid and alginic acid the nurse should evaluate the effectiveness of the drug, monitor frequency of use and monitor for constipation or diarrhea and assist patient to adjust product use as needed.

  Anti-secretory drugs, i.e. histamine (H_2) receptors are used to reduce the gastric acid secretion and supports tissue healing which include ranitidine, cimetidine, famotidine, nizaoidine. During use of these, the nurse should instruct patient to take drugs with meals if ordered at intervals, and monitor for common side effects, fatigue, headache, diarrhea.
- Prokinetic drugs are used to increase LES pressure and enhance gastrointestinal motility, which includes cisapride (propulsid). Here the nurse has to instruct patient to take drug no more than 15 minutes before eating and monitor levels of drugs that require useful titration.
- Proton pump inhabitors are used to inhabit enzyme system of gastric parietal cells and suppress gastric acid secretions by more than 90 percent. Here the nurse has to instruct patient to take the drug before meals and monitor for side effects, abdominal cramping, headache, diarrhea. For example, omeprazole lansoprazole are PP inhibitors.

Surgical management: Antireflux surgery is usually performed in patient with severe GERD who do not respond to aggressive medical management which includes:

- Nissen fundoplication
- Hill gastropexy
- Belseys fundoplication
- Antireflux prosthesis.

Nursing Management

The nurse by using nursing process, assesses the client on the basis of clinical manifestation stated above and take body weight, ascultate for signs for reflux aspirates and observe for hoarseness or wheezing-day or night.

The nursing diagnosis are made from analysis of patient's data. The diagnoses are not limited to pain and knowledge deficit. The objectives of nursing care will include reports, minimal or no episodes of heart burn and list diet and lifestyle changes. GERD is typically managed by using a combination of drug therapy, diet, and lifestyle modification and assisting surgical therapies if needed.

The nurse discusses the medication regimen with the patient and ensures that written information about the safe use and expected side effects of all medications is provided, and administer the ordered medication and observe for response and side effects. Antacids that contain aluminium tend to cause constipation, whereas those contain magnesium tend to cause diarrhea. Several of the antacids are combination of aluminium and magnesium designed to minimize these effects. If the patient is taking bethenechol (cholenergic) side effects to observe for urinary urgency, increased salivation, abdominal cramping with darrhea, nausea, vomiting and hypotension. Side effects of metadopramide (dopamine antogonist) a prokinetic drug includes restlessness, anxiety and insomnia. Side effects of sucralfate (acid-protective) include drowsiness, dizziness, nausea, vomiting, constipation, urticaria and rash.

When nursing the patient with GERD the nurse has to use the following. Diet and lifestyle modifications to manage the same:

- In relation to diet patient are encouraged to:
  - Eat 4–6 small meals daily
  - Follow a low-fat, adequate protein diet
  - Reduce intake of chocolate, tea and all foods and beverages that contain caffeine
  - Limit or eliminate alcohol intake
  - Eat slowly and chew food thoroughly
  - Avoid evening snacking and do not eat for 2–3 hours before bedtime
  - Remain upright for 1–2 hours after meals when possible and never eat in bed
  - Avoid any food that directly produces heart burn
  - Reduce over all body weight if indicated.
- The nurse has to promote lifestyle of the patient by encouraging to:
  - Eliminate or drastically reduce smoking
  - Avoid evening smoking and never smoke in bed
  - Avoid constrictive clothing over the abdomen
  - Avoid activities that involve straining, heavy lifting or working in a bent-over position
  - Elevate the head of the bed at least 6–8 inches for sleep using wooden blocks or a thick foam wedge
  - Never sleep flat in bed.
- For prevention of GERD, the nurse should use the following teaching guidelines for patient and family.
  - Explain the rationale for a high-protein, low-fat diet
  - Encourage the patient to eat small, frequent meals to prevent gastric distention
  - Explain the rationale for avoiding alcohol, smoking (causes an almost immediate, marked decrease in LES pressure) and beverage that contains caffeine
  - Instruct the patient not to lie down for 2 to 3 hours after eating, wear tight clothing around the waist, or bend over (especially after eating)

- Encourage the patient to sleep with head of bed elevated on 4–6 inch blocks (gravity fosters esophageal emptying)
- Teach regarding medication including rationale for their use and common side effects
- Discuss strategies for weight reduction if appropriate
- Encourage patient and family to share concerns about lifestyle changes and living with a chronic problem.

HIATAL HERNIA

Hiatal hernia is herniation of a portion of the stomach into the esophagus through an opening, or hiatus, in the diaphragm. It is also referred to as 'diaphragmatic hernia and esophageal hernia' (Fig. 10.10A).

Hiatal hernias are common in older adults and occur more frequently in women than in men. They are classified into two types: (1) Sliding hiatal hernia (2) Paraesophagical hiatal hernia.

- *In sliding.* The junction of the stomach and esophagus is above the hiatus of the diaphragm and a part of the stomach slides through the hiatal opening in the diaphragm. It "slides" into the thoracic cavity when the patient is supine and usually goes back into the abdominal cavity when the patient is standing upright (Fig. 10.10B).
- In paraesophageal or rolling, the esophagogastric junction remains in the normal position, but the fundus and the greater curvature of the stomach roll up through the diaphragm forming a pocket alongside the esophagus (Fig. 10.10C).

Etiology

The actual cause of hiatal hernia is unknown. Many factors contribute to the development of hiatal hernia. Structural changes, such as weakening of the muscles in the diaphragm around the esophagogastric opening are usually contributing factors. Factors that increase intra-abdominal pressure, including obesity, pregnancy, ascitis, tumors, tight corsets, intense physical exertions, and heavy lifting on a continued basis, may also predispose to development of a hiatal hernia. Other predisposing factors are increased age, trauma, poor nutrition, and forced recumbent position, as when a prolonged illness confines the person to bed. In some cases, congenital weakness is a contributing factor.

In a hiatal (hiatus) hernia, the opening in the diaphragm through which the esophagus passes becomes enlarged, and part of the upper stomach tends to move up into the lower portion of the thorax. There are two types of hernias: sliding and paraesophageal. With a type I, or sliding, hiatal hernia, the upper stomach and the gastroesophageal junction are displaced upward and slide in the out of the thorax; this occurs in about 90% of patient with esophageal hiatal hernias. The less frequent paraesophageal hernias are classified by extent of herniation (type II, III, or IV) and occur when all or part of the stomach pushes through the diaphragm next to the gastroesophageal junction (GED). Hiatal hernia occurs more often in women than men.

Pathophysiology

A hiatal hernia involves herniation of part of the stomach through weakness in the diaphragm. The resulting regurgitations and motor dysfunction cause the major manifestation of the hiatal hernia. With sliding hernias, the problems are rarely anatomical. The problems relate directly to the functional consequences of chronic reflux. Reflux occurs from the ongoing exposure of the LES to the low pressure environment of the thorax where sphincter function is significantly impaired.

Reflux is rarely a concern with rolling hernias, because the LES remains anchord below the diaphragm. However, the anatomical risks of volvulus, strangulation and obstructions are high. In addition, venous obstruction in the herniated portion of the stomach causes the mucosa to become engorged and to ooze. Slow bleeding leads to the development of iron deficiency anaemia, but significant bleeding is rare.

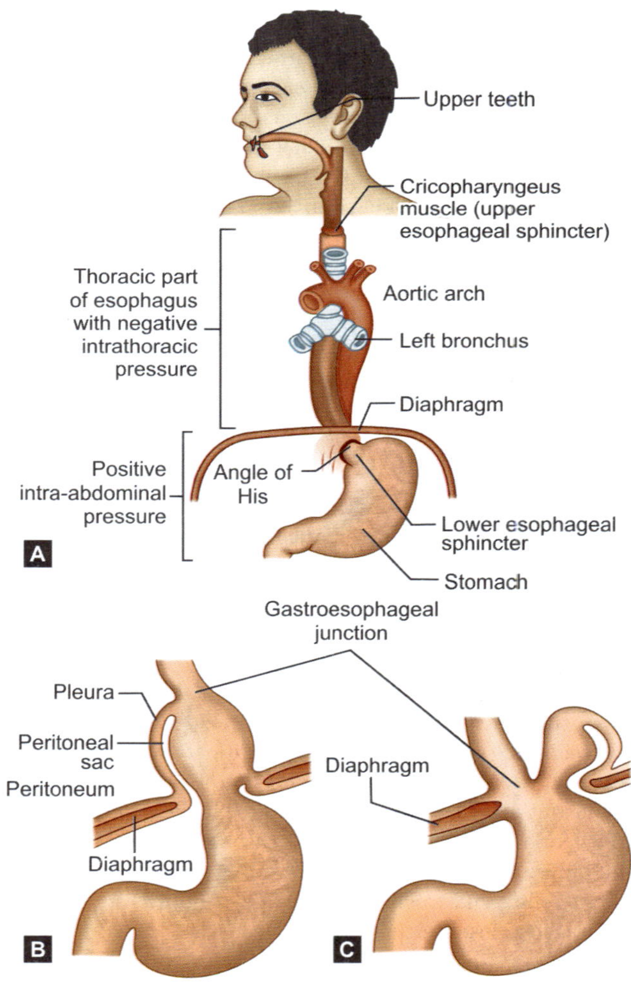

FIGS 10.10A TO C: (A) Normal esophagus; (B) Sliding hiatal hernia; (C) Rolling or paraesophageal hernia

Clinical Manifestation

Axial (Sliding) Hernia

- Heartburn, regurgitation and dysphagia; at least half of the cases are asymptomatic
- Often implicated in reflux.

Paraesophageal Hernia

- Sense of fullness after eating or may be asymptomatic
- Reflux does not usually occur
- Complications of hemorrhage, obstruction and strangulation possible.

Manifestation of hiatal hernia varies in kind and severity. In sliding hiatal hernia, clients may have heartburn 30 to 60 minutes after meals. In addition, reflux may result in substernal pain. The clients with a rolling hernia does not have manifestation of reflux but client may complain of a feeling of fullness after eating or have difficulty in breathing. Some clients experience chest pain similar to that of anginal pain. Pain is usually worse when the client assumes a recumbent position. Bending over may cause a severe burning pain which is usually relieved by sitting or standing. The other common factors of pain includes large meals, alcohol and smoking. Nocturnal attacks are common especially if the person has eaten before going to sleep.

The complication that may occur with hiatal hernia includes problems such as hemorrhage from erosion, stenosis, ulceration of the herniated portion of the stomach, strangulation of the hernia and regurgitation with tracheal aspiration. Severe chronic esophagitis may follow reflux problem.

Diagnostic Studies

A barium swallow is an important diagnostic measure that may show the protrusion of gastric mucosa through the esophageal hiatus in the patient with hiatal hernia. The other tests are similar that are performed in the GERD.

Management of Hiatal Hernia

Conservation therapy of hiatal hernia includes administration of antacids, and antisecretory agents, elimination of constricting garments, avoidance of lifting and straining, elimination of alcohol and smoking, and elevation of the head of the bed.

Elevation of the bed on 4 to 6 inch blocks assists gravity in maintaining the stomach in the abdominal cavity and also helps prevent reflux and tracheal aspiration. If obese, the client is encouraged to lose weight.

- Frequent, small feedings that easily pass through the esophagus are given
- Advise patient not to recline for 1 hour after eating (prevents reflux or hernia movement)
- Elevate head of bed on 4- to 8-inch blacks to prevent from sliding upward.
- Surgery is indicated in about 15% of patients
- Medical and surgical management of paraesophageal hernias is similar to that for gastroesophageal reflux antacids, histamine blockers, gastric acid pump inhibitors or prokinetic agents (metoclopramide [Reglan], cisapride [Propulsid]).

Surgical corrections of rolling hernias is mandatory because the risk of serous complications is significant. The objective of surgical interventions for hiatal hernia is to reduce reflux by enhancing the integrity of the LES. Surgical procedures are termed "Vulvoplastics or antireflux" procedures. There are three slightly varied procedures namely:

i. The Hill gastropexy,
ii. The Nissen fundoplications (Fig. 10.11), and
iii. The Belseys fundoplication.

The diet and activities of hiatal hernia are as discussed in GERD.

Major goals may include adequate nutritional intake, avoidance of respiratory compromise from aspiration, relief of pain, and increased knowledge level.

Nursing Interventions

Encouraging Adequate Nutritional Intake

- Instruct patient to eat a low-fat, high fiber diet
- Encourage patient to eat slowly and chew all food thoroguly
- Small, frequently feedings of nonirritating foods are recommended; sometimes drinking liquids with food help passage
- Prepare food in an appealing manner to help stimulate appetite; avoid irritants (tobacco, alcohol)

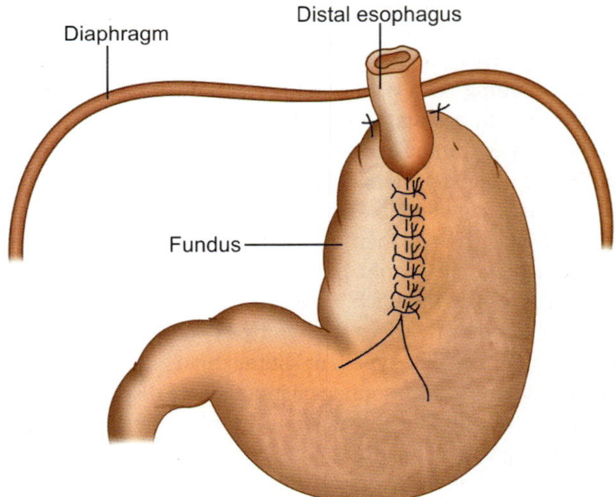

FIG. 10.11: Nissen fundoplication for repair of hiatal hernia. Fundus of stomach is wrapped around distal esophagus to itself

- Obtain a baseline weight, and record daily weight; assess nutrient intake.

Decreasing Risk of Aspiration

- If patient has difficulty swallowing or handling secretions keep him or her in at least a semi-Fowler's position
- Instruct patient in the use of oral suction to decrease risk aspiration.

Relieving Pain

- Teach patient to eat small meals frequently (6 to 8 daily)
- Instruct patient to avoid caffeine, tobacco, carbonated beverages, very hot or very cold beverages, and spicy foods
- Advise patient not to recline for 1 to 4 hours after eating to prevent reflux or movement of the hernia
- Advise patient to avoid any activities that put strain on the thoracic region and increase pain
- Elevate head of bed on 4- to 8-inch blocks; avoid tight clothes
- Advise patient not to use over-the-counter antacids because of possible rebound acidity
- Instruct in use of prescribed antacids or histamine antagonists.

Promoting Home and Community-based Care

Teaching Patients Self-Care

- Reassure patient and discuss all procedures and their purposes
- Give sufficient information for participation in care and diagnostic effort
- Prepare patient for surgery if required
- Help patient plan for needed physical psychological adjustments and follow-up care if condition is chronic
- Help in planning meals, using medications as prescribed, and resuming activity
- Teach patient and family to use special equipment (enteral or parenteral feeding advices, suction)
- Educate about nutritional requirements and how to measure the adequacy of nutrition (particularly in elderly and debilitated patients).

Continuing Care

- Arrange for home health care nursing support and assessment when indicated
- Teach patient to prepare blenderized or soft food if indicated
- Assist patient to adjust medication schedule to daily activities when possible
- Arrange for nutritionist, social worker, or hospice care when indicated.

Surgical Nursing Management of Hiatal Hernia

Preoperative teaching focus on instructing the patient in deep breathing, the correct use of an incentive spirometer and splinting the incision effectively, for coughing. The surgical approaches all involve the diaphragm and pulmonary hygiene is essential in preventing respiratory complications. Individuals who are overweight are encouraged to lose weight if possible before surgery and smokers are encouraged to significantly reduce or eliminate their use of tobacco. The nurse also teaches the patient about nasogastric tube that will be inserted during surgery with open procedures and planned time frame for restarting oral feedings.

Postoperative care focuses on concern related to prevention of respiratory complications, maintenance of fluid and electrolytic balance, and prevention of infection. If thoracic approach is used, a chest tube is inserted. Assessment and management related to closed chest drainage are important. After surgical intervention, there should be no symptoms of gastric reflux. The patient should be instructed to report symptoms such as heartburn and regurgitation. A normal diet can be resumed within 6 weeks. The patient should avoid foods that are causing gas problems and should try to prevent gastric distension. Food should be thoroughly chewed (Figs 10.12 and 10.13, Table 10.3).

ACHALASIA

Achalasia is a primary motility disorders of the esophagus are conditions in which the normal function of the esophagus is disturbed which problem may be primary in the esophagus or secondary to another systemic disease (neuromuscular disorders, i.e. cerebrovascular accident, multiple sclerosis, myasthenia grans, amyotrophic lateral sclerosis, myopathic cranial nerve disease or traum 5th, 9th, 10th). The classic motility disorder is a failure of the esophageal muscle to relax in synchrony, which can result in mechanical or functional obstruction of good passage. Failure to close adequately after swallowing can also occur, resulting in chronic reflux or regurgitation. Esophageal spasm is common component of motility disorder and the spasm is usually intense enough to mimic angina.

As stated above Achalasia is the predominant primary disorder in which the lower esophageal muscles and sphincter fail to relax appropriately in response to swallowing.

Etiology

The cause of the achalasia is unknown, although a familial link is possible. It usually develops in early or middle adulthood and

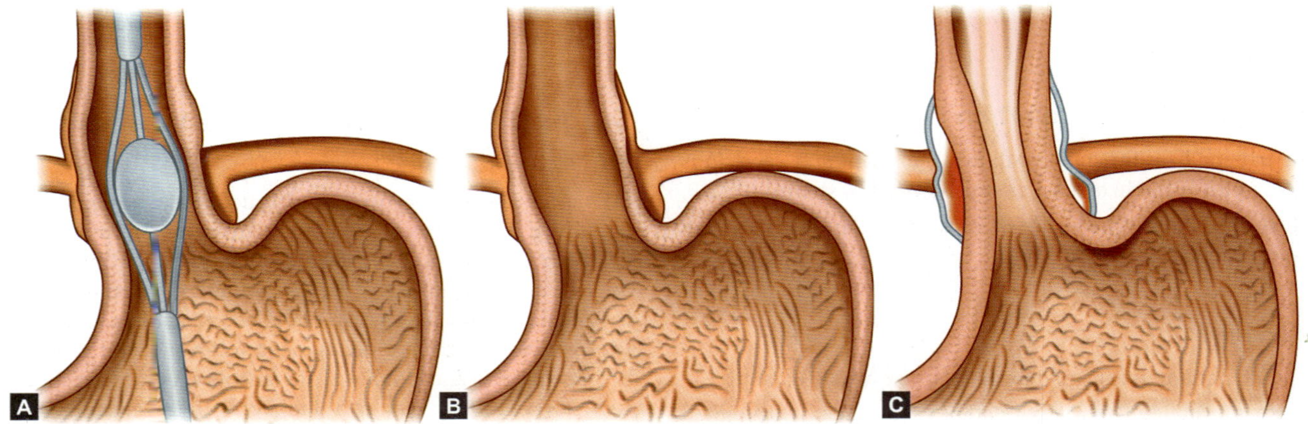

FIGS 10.12A TO C: Stretta procedure used to treat GERD. (A) Catheter positioned; (B) Multiple sites treated with radiofrequency energy; (C) Remodeling occurs with collagen formation

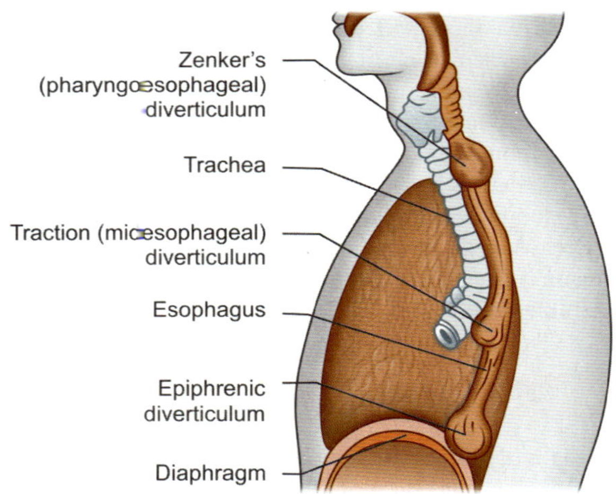

FIG. 10.13: Possible sites for the occurrence of esophageal diverticula. These hollow outpouchings may occur just above the upper esophageal sphincter (Zenker's, the most common type of pulsion diverticulum), near the midpoint of the esophagus (traction), and just above the lower esophageal sphincter (epiphrenic)

one-third of cases develop after age of 60 years and both sexes are affected equally.

Pathophysiology

Achalasia (cardiospasm) results from a neuromuscular defect that is localized in the inner circular muscle layer of the esophagus. Degeneration of ganglion cells causes both a failure of peristalsis and severe muscle spasm. Here the peristalsis of the lower third (smooth muscle) of the esophagus is absent.

Pressure in the LES is increased, along with incomplete relaxation of the LES. As the disease progresses, the portion of the esophagus around the constriction becomes dilated and the muscle walls hypertrophy. Obstruction of esophagus at or near the diaphragm occurs. Food and fluid accumulate in the lower esophagus. Although the severity of achalasia varies widely, the spasms may be so severe that little or no food can enter the stomach. In extreme cases, the esophagus may hold a liter or more food and fluid above the constricted area. The altered peristalsis is a result of impairment of the autonomic nervous system innervating the esophagus.

Chronic and progressively worsening dysphagia is the classic symptom and occurs more frequently with liquids. Spasm may be provoked by cold or hot liquids or foods and worsened by stress or overeating. Substernal chest pain (similar to pain of angina) occurs during or imemdiately after a meal. Halitosis and the inability to eructate are other symptoms. Another common symptom is regurgitation of sour tasting food and liquids especially when the patient is in horizontal position weight loss is typical. A foul mouth odor from retension of food and the esophagus may be a chronic problem.

Diagnostic Studies

The classic 'bird's beak narrowing plus dilation are readily observed with barium studies. Esophageal manometry reveals an elevated resting LES pressure, combined with diminished or absent peristaltic waves.

Management of Achalasia

Treatment of achalasia consists of dilation, surgery and use of drugs. All these therapies are directed at relieving the stasis caused by the increased LES pressure, non-relaxing LES and aperistaltic esophagus. The aim of management is to relieve

TABLE 10.3: Nursing care plan for client undergoing hiatal hernia repair

Problem	Reason	Objective	Nursing intervention	Evaluation
Ineffective airway clearance related to • Incisional pain, and • Limited mobility	Due to surgery	Maintains clear breath sounds effectively coughs up secretion	• Maintain head of bed in semi-Fowler's position (at least 30 degrees) (drugs diaphragm and lungs to facilitate ventilation) • Perform pulmonary assessment q2-4h (assess for atelectasis and retained secretions) • Monitor PCA pump or provide adequate narcotic analgesia (adequate pain control facilitates pulmohygiene and motility) • Supervise pulmonary hygiene q4-h – Incentives spirometry – Chest percussion and vibration – Deep breathing q1-2 hours (Prevents atelectasis and facilitates expulsion of secretions) • Assist with position changes and ambulation (It facilitates expulsion of secretion and prevent atelectasis) • Splint incisions for movement and position changes (facilitate ability to deeply breathe and cough)	
Impaired swallowing related to functional changes	Due to fundoplication surgery	Successfully progress from clear liquids to a normal diet without aspiration and discomfort	• Maintain initial NPO status and monitor patency of NG tube • Do not irrigate or reposition the NG tube (stomach must remain decompressed to prevent vomiting) • Report the incidence of any fresh blood in the drainage after 8 hours of postoperatively (fresh blood indicates incisional complication) • Offer frequent oral and nasal hygiene • Initiate feedings with 30 mL of clear liquids once peristalsis is reestablished • Evaluate presence and severity of dysphagia • Advance to multiple small feedings • Progress from liquids to solid as patient tolerates • Encourage thorough chewing of small food boluses • Teach patient to avoid air swallowing and gas bloat • Avoid carbonated beverages, using straws and gas-producing foods • Eat slowly and chew thoroughly • Always eat in sitting up position • Avoid overtalking while eating • Ambulate after meals	
Altered health maintenance related to lack of knowledge	Lack of knowledge concerning measures to prevent reflux	Correctly identifies dietary and lifestyle changes to reduce the incidence of reflux	• Provide patient with instructions about diet modifications: – Follow a low fat diet and avoid excessive tea, coffee, chocolate and other such foods – Strictly eliminate or limit alcohol intake – Eat 4–6 small meals daily – Eat slowly and chew food thoroughly – Remain upright 1–2 hours after meals – Never eat on bed – Avoid evening snacking – Reduce over 11 body weight – Avoid any food that induce heartburn – Discuss lifestyle modifications that can reduce incidence of reflux – Enroll in smoking cessation program – Avoid activities such as straining, lifting and stopping – Avoid constrictive clothing – Never sleep flat in bed – Elevate the head on a 6-inch foam wedge for sleep – Use antacids for occasional heartburn—report frequent or severe episodes	

symptoms. Symptomatic treatment consists of semi-soft bland diet, eating slowly and drinking fluid with meals and sleeping with the head elevated.

Esophageal dilation (bougienage) is an effective treatment measure for many patients. Pneumatic dilation of LES with a balloon-tipped dilator passed orally is usually used (Figs 10.14 and 10.15). The commonly used dilators for pneumatic dilation are the Mosherbag, the Tucker mercury dilator and Browne-McHardy dilator. They all depend on forcible expansion of a balloon in the LES. The forceful dilation does not restore normal esophageal motility, but it does provide for emptying of the esophagus into the stomach.

Surgical measures that may be necessary in the "Esophago-myotomy". In this procedure, the muscle fibers that enclose the narrowed area of the esophagus are divided. This allows the mucosa to pouch out through the division in the muscle layer to allow food to be swallowed without obstruction. Measure similar to this procedure is Heller's Myotomy (cardiomyotomy) which disrupts the LES in a similar manner and reduces LES pressure. An antireflux procedure is frequently done with myotomy. This procedure can be performed laparoscopically, reducing the potential for postoperative complications.

Various classes of medications are used in the treatment of achalasia include anticholenergics and calcium channel blockers (e.g. nifedipine procardia), but none of them proved to be effective. Analgesics may be needed when pain is severe. Recent studies indicated that botulinum toxin injection, which relaxes esophageal muscle, delivered endoscopically in the management of achalasia.

Health Education

The nurse works with the patient and family to explore diet and lifestyle modifications that will best control dysphagia, which is prominent in achalasia. Education begins with careful assessment of the scope and severity of dysphagia, which includes:

- Swallowing ability with liquids versus solids
- Response to foods of differing textures and temperature
- Variability of the dysphagia (intermittant or constant)
- Response to stress, fatigue and other activities
- Approaches used by the patient to manage the dysphagia and the degree of success.

The nurse encourages the person to experiment with various types and consistency of foods and meal sizes to evaluate their influence on swallowing. Small, frequent semi-soft meals, are usually best tolerated. Warm liquids are recommended, and extremes of temperature should be avoided because they usually worsen the spasm. The nurse also advises the patient to experiment with changing positions during eating. Some individuals can swallow more effectively if they arch their back. Use of the Valsalva, a maneuver (bearing down with a closed glottis) while swallowing may help proper food beyond the LES. Nocturnal reflux of retained food and fluid presents a significant risk for aspiration. The nurse should instruct the patients to sleep on a foam wedge or with the head of the bed elevated. And suitable advices also should be given to the patient who has undergone surgical procedures.

ESOPHAGEAL CARCINOMA

Carcinoma of the esophagus is unique in its geographic distribution. Both benign and malignant tumors occur in the esophagus. Benign tumors are usually leiomyomas, and

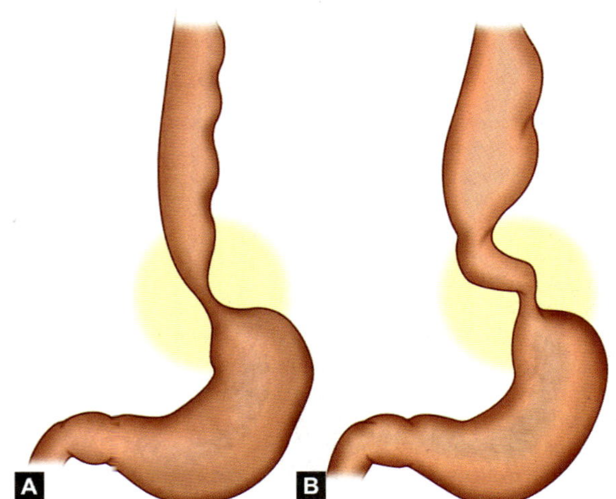

FIGS 10.14A AND B: Esophageal achalasia. (A) Early stage, showing tapering of lower esophagus; (B) Advance stage, showing dilated, tortuous esophagus

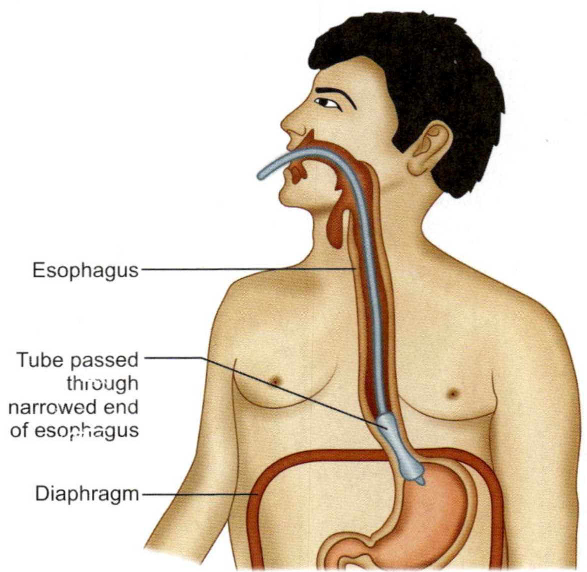

FIG. 10.15: Pneumatic dilation attempts to treat achalasia by maintaining an adequate lumen and decreasing lower esophageal sphincter (LES) tone

extremely rare and usually asymptomatic. They require no intervention unless symptoms necessitate local excision.

Malignant tumors of the esophagus are not common, but they assume increased importance because of their virulence.

Etiology

The cause of cancer of the esophagus is unknown. Possible predisposing factors are cigarette smoking, excessive alcohol intake chronic trauma, poor oral hygiene and spicy foods. The most important risk factors include exposure to asbestos and metal and low intake of fresh fruits and vegetables.

Pathophysiology

Tumors may develop any point along the length of the esophagus, but the majority occur in the middle and lower two-thirds of the esophagus. Squamous cell tumors have typically predominated. They tend to develop in the middle third and clearly related to the risk factors of smoking and alcohol use. Adenocarcinomas represent the remaining minority of tumors. These tend to develop in the lower third of the esophagus and may evolve from the Barret's epithelium. It is an acquired condition in which changes occur in response to acid irritation over a period of 1 to 2 years and its presence increases the risk of cancer.

Esophageal tumors of all types appear to emerge as a part of an initially slow process that begins with benign tissue changes. Local growth of the tumor is rapid, however, the early spread is common because of the rich lymphatic supply found in the esophagus. Tumors are characteristically intraluminal and ulcerating. With a tendency to encircle the esophageal wall, as well as extend upon down the length. The spread of cancer is by local invasion or through the blood stream or lymphatics. Neoplasm of the upper and middle esophagus may extend into the pulmonary system and those of the lower esophagus into the diaphragm, vertebral or heart.

The common clinical manifestation of esophageal cancer are as follows:

- Early disease is largely asymptomatic
- Gradually progressive dysphagia
- Odynophagia—typically steady, dull, substernal pain
- Regurgitation—foul breath, from retained food in esophagus
- Heartburn, anorexia, weight loss.

The onset of symptoms is usually late in relation to the extent of the tumor. Progressive dysphagia is the most common symptom and may be expressed as a substernal feeling as if food is not passing. Initially the dysphagia occurs only with meat, then soft foods and eventually with liquids. Pain develops late and it is described as occurring in the substernal, epigastric, or back areas and usually increases with swallowing. The pain may radiate to the neck, jaw, ears, and shoulders. If the tumor is in upper third of esophagus symptoms such as sore throat, choking and hoarseness may occur. Weight loss is fairly common. When esophageal stenosis is severe, regurgitation of blood-flecked esophageal contents is common.

The complication of the esophageal cancer will include the following:

- Hemorrhage may occur if the cancer erodes through the esophagus and into the aorta
- Esophageal perforation with fistula formation into the lung or trachea may develop
- Esophageal obstruction due to enlargement of the tumor.

Diagnostic Studies

- Barium swallow with fluoroscopy may demonstrate a narrowing of the esophagus at the site of tumor. Creater may be visible
- Esophagoscopy with biopsy is necessary to make a definitive diagnosis of carcinoma by identification of malignant cells
- Endoscopy—ultrasonography is also used to detect tumor invasion to muscle layer
- Bronchoscopic examination may be performed to detect malignant involvements of the trachea
- Computerized tomography scanning and magnetic resonance imaging are also used to assess the extent of disease.

Management

Treatment of esophageal cancer are based on the location and size of the tumor, degree of metastasis and the individual health status.

Non-surgical options are usually selected where the individual is unable or unwilling to undergo radical surgery. Surgery may not be performed if the patient is an older adult or in poor physical health. Palliative therapy consists of restoration of the swallowing function and maintenance of nutrition and hydration. Dilation, stent replacement or both can relieve obstruction. Laser therapy or vaporization with neodymium, yttrium aluminum-garnet (-Nd:YAG) by means of endoscopy may be used in combination with dilation. Dilation is done with various types of dilators (celestin tube) to relieve dysphagia and allows for improved nutrition. Placement of a stent or prosthesis may help when dilation is no longer effective. The prosthesis are composed of silicone rubber or nylon-reinforced latex tubes with distal and proximal cellars.

Radiation therapy is the treatment of choice for palliation. It reduces tumor size and gives consistent long-term symptom relief. But it may lead to debilitating stricture or stenosis because esophageal tissue is extremely sensitive to radiation. The best results of esophageal cancer treatment have been obtained by the surgery and radiation.

Radical surgery is the only definitive treatment of esophageal cancer. The types of surgical procedures that can be performed are:

- Esophagectomy: Removal of part or all of the esophagus with the use of a dacron graft to replace the resected pain
- Esophagogastrostomy: Resection of a portion of the esophagus and anastomosis of the remaining portion of the esophagus
- Esophagoenterostomy: Resection of a portion of the esophagus and anastomosis of a segment of colon to the remaining portion.

After surgery parenteral fluids are given. When fluids are allowed after bowel sounds have returned 30 to 60 mL water are given hourly with gradual progression to small, frequent, bland meals. The patient should be in an upright position to prevent regurgitation of the fluid. The patient is observed for signs of intolerance to the feeding or leakage of the feeding into the mediastinum. Symptom of leakage (pain, temperature, dyspnea) and food intolerance (vomiting and abdominal distension) should be monitored and suitable measures to be taken accordingly (Table 10.4).

GASTRITIS AND DYSPEPSIA

Gastritis, an inflammation of the gastric mucosa, is one of the most problems affecting the stomach. The terms gastritis and dyspepsia are used in a highly non-specific manner by both lay persons and health care professionals. Gastritis refers to a diffuse of localized response of the gastric mucosa to injury or infection. The dyspepsia refers to a symptom complex of fullness, heartburn, bloating and possibly nausea that is typically experienced after eating and may not be accompanied to any histological changes in the stomach or duodenum.

Dyspepsia Syndrome

Dyspepsia syndrome: It is a syndrome of chronic dyspepsia, one of the most common GI complaints encountered in primary practice. The person experiences persistent or recurrent discomfort centered in the upper abdomen. There is no evidence of structural or biochemical abnormality and the cause is unknown. Study findings to date indicate that individual with dyspepsia syndrome have:

- Normal rates of acid secretion
- Post-prondial hypomotility and delayed gastric emptying, and 25 to 50 percent cases. Cause is unknown
- Increased sensitivity of gastric distention, cause is unknown
- No identified link with life stress or personality profiles.

TABLE 10.4: Nursing care plan for the patient with cancer of the esophagus treated by surgery

Problem	Objective	Nursing intervention	Rationales
Nursing Diagnosis #1			
Alteration in cardiac output: Decreased, related to: 1. Altered hemodynamics associated with thoracic/abdominal surgery *Nursing Diagnosis #2* Alteration in tissue perfusion: Cardiopulmonary	Patient will: 1. Maintain presurgical cardiovascular function as manifested by: A. Stable hemodynamics. ◆ Blood pressure within 10 mm Hg of baseline ◆ Heart rate < 100 beats/minute ◆ Cardiac output ~5 liters/minute ◆ CVP: 0–8 mm Hg ◆ CWP: 8-12 mm Hg B. Absence of: Extreme weakness or fatigue, peripheral edema, neck vein distention or chest pain C. Absence of cardiac dysrhythmias 2. Maintain intact neurological status: – Mental status: Alert and oriented 3. Maintain fluid and electrolyte balance: – Stable body weight – Balanced intake and output – Hourly urine output >30 cc/h	• Perform ongoing cardiovascular assessment: – Continuous cardiac monitoring, Establish baseline rate, rhythm and ectopy – Continuous hemodynamic monitoring when indicated. Establish baseline CVP and PCWP measurements – Auscultate lungs q 4 h – Auscultate heart sounds—presence of S3 – Assess for fatigue, neck vein distention? Sacral edema? – Monitor arterial blood gases • Perform neurological assessment – Level of consciousness – Behavior • Assess fluid and electrolyte status. – Daily weight – Intake and output with hourly urine outputs – Serum electrolytes, BUN, creatinine	• Chest surgery may cause cardiac irritability. Many patients develop atrial fibrillation. This dysrhythmia may decrease cardiac output by 20–30 percent – Rales (crackles) are an indication of fluid overload – Diagnostic sign for congestive heart failure • Compromised hemodynamics and hypoxemia predispose to cerebral hypoxia with altered cerebral function • Reduced blood volume will further compromise venous return and cardiac output; blood volume may need to be expanded with use of colloids or fluids – Reduced cardiac output may diminish renal perfusion, placing-patient at risk of developing acute renal failure

Contd...

Contd...

Problem	Objective	Nursing intervention	Rationales
Nursing Diagnosis #3			
Impaired gas exchange, related to: 1. Pulmonary congestion associated with surgical manipulation of intrathoracic structures and altered by lymphatic drainage 2. Atelectasis	Patient will: 1. Maintain effective respiratory function: – Rate <25/minute – Rhythm eupneie – Breath sounds clear on auscultation – Mental status: Alert and oriented – Usual skin color – Arterial blood gases at baseline	• Monitor and report signs and symptoms of altered respiratory function: – Presence of rapid, shallow, or irregular respirations; dyspnea, orthopnea; use of accessory muscles – Presence of adventitious breath sounds on auscultation – Presence of restlessness, irritability, confusion, or somnolence – Presence of dusky red, mottled, or cyanotic skin color • Monitor arterial blood gas values and report abnormal results • Monitor pulse oximetry. Obtain ABGs for saturation of hemoglobin • Monitor hemoglobin/hematocrit • Implement measures to maintain adequate respiratory function: – Maintain semi-Fowler's position – Maintain prescribed O_2 therapy and monitor resposne – Encouage coughing and deep breathing q 1-2 h – Assist in turning q 2 h – Instruct to splint incision when coughing – Encourage use of pain medication as prescribed and monitor response	• Monitors the oxygen saturation of available hemoglobin • Anemia provokes tissue hypoxia – Due to extent of surgery, patient will "guard" incision, which leads to decreased lung expansion, atelectasis and poor gas exchange
Nursing Diagnosis #4			
Alteration in bowel elimination, related to: 1. Surgical trauma, stress and enteral tube feedings	Patient will: 1. Regain peristaltie activity and presurgical bowel function	• Maintain nasogastric tube to low suction. Irrigate with 30 cc normal saline solution q 4 h or as prescribed – Do not reposition or reinsert • Assess for presence of abdominal distention and auscultate for bowel sounds every shift • Inquire as to the presence or absence of flatulence – Encourage ambulation when indicated • Monitor daily intake and output, weight and electrolyte balance • Assess character and frequency of stool	• Maintains patency and prevents gastric distention which may cause stress to suture line and lead to an anastomotic leak – The tube is placed during surgery. Care must be taken to avoid harm to the anastomosis. Physician will determine benefit risk, and method of replacement • Distention may indicate malfunctioning NG and stress to the anastomosis • Bowel sounds indicate that the intestines have regained peristaltic activity • Fluid loss after gastrointestinal surgery may approach 2 liters or more. Fluid and electrolyte replacement may be required with the loss of large amounts of fluids • Diarrhea may result in wasting of Mg^{++} and Ca^{++}. Observe for muscle weakness or tetany

Contd...

Contd...

Problem	Objective	Nursing intervention	Rationales
Nursing Diagnosis #5			
Impairment of skin integrity, related to: 1. Surgical incision with potential for impaired wound healing due to: A. Preoperative radiation therapy B. Poor nutrition C. Infection 2. Irritation or breakdown related to: A. Contact of skin with wound drainage B. Stress from drainage tubes C. Use of tape	Patient will: 1. Experience normal healing of surgical wounds	• Position patient to reduce stress on suture lines • Maintain NG tube patency • Splint wounds while coughing • Change dressings frequently and perform aseptic wound care • Note type and amount of drainage. Obtain culture if indicated and monitor results • Note drainage tube sites. Provide anchoring tape to prevent tensions or "pulling" at insertion sites – Consider use of Montgomery straps • Monitor laboratory values for signs of anemia, decreased albumin levels, or an increased leukocyte count	• Prevents gastric distention • Equalizes pressure to the wounds. Reduces the possibility of dehiscence • Minimizes skin irritation from drainage and prevents nosocomial infections – Prevents skin abrasions due to frequent tape changes • Anemia will results in decreased oxygenation. Low albumin level: Indicates a decrease in the colloidal osmotic pressure, which will lead to edema and interference with healing. A leukocytosis may indicate an infectious process
Nursing Diagnosis #6			
Alteration in comfort level: Pain, related to: 1. Surgical procedure	Patient will: 1. Utilize measures effective in managing pain 2. Verbalize pain relief 3. Exhibit relaxed demeanor: – Relaxed facial expression and body posturing – Ease of breathing	• Determine pain "tolerance." Assess patient's willingness to use pain medication vs. stoic behavior • Assess for physical manifestations of pain – Restlessness, reluctance to move, guarding incision, clenched fist – Diaphoresis, rapid shallow breathing, tachycardia, hypertension • Assess complaints of pain including severity, location/radiation, duration, and quality (i.e. sharp, dull, knifelike) • Collaborate with physician and patient in titrating pain medication as needed • Suggest alternate position changes	• Many people fear they will become addicted to narcotics

Symptoms

- Epigastric discomfort or pain
- Feeling of fullness or flatulence
- Early satiety
- Bloating or nausea.

Treatment of Dyspepsia Syndrome

There is no approved drug treatment, but

- Histamine receptor antagonists may be used for ulcer-like pain
- Antacids may be used for occasional heartburn or bloating syndrome
- Prokinetic agents (Cispride) are helpful in many cases
- Diet and lifestyle changes are suggested will include:
  - Reducing dietary fat (it prolongs digestion, worsen bloating)
  - Avoiding foods that precipitate symptoms.

Gastritis may be acute or chronic and may be diffused or localized.

Acute Gastritis

Etiology (Box 10.1)

Acute gastritis is inflammation of the stomach mucosa lasting several hours to a few days. Dietary indiscretion is the usual cause (eating irritating food that is too highly seasoned or food that is infected). Other causes include excessive alcohol, aspirin, or other nonsteroidal anti-inflammatory drug (NSAID) use, bile reflux, or radiation therapy. A more severe form of acute gastritis is caused by strong acids or alkali, which may cause gastritis is caused by strong acids or alkali, which may cause the mucosa to become gangrenous or to perforate. Gastritis may also be the first sign of acute systemic infection. View of stomach (Fig. 10.16).

Chronic gastritis is a prolonged inflammation of the stomach that may be caused by either benign or malignant ulcers of the stomach or by bacteria such as *Helicobacter pylori.* Chronic gastritis may be associated with autoimmune diseases such as pernicious anemia and with dietary factors such as caffeine, drug use (e.g. NSAIDs, bisphosphonates, such as alendronate [Fosamax] or risedronate [Actonel]), alcohol, smoking, or reflux of intestinal contents into the stomach. It occurs in the fundus or body of the stomach. Superficial ulceration may occur and can lead to hemorrhage.

Acute gastritis is short-term inflammatory process that can be initiated by numerous factors such as excess alcohol ingestion, drug effects aspirin, NSAID, corticosteroids, etc.) severe physical stress or trauma, ingestion of caustic noxious substances, and bacterial contaminated water or food (*Staphylococcus, Salmonella* or staphylococci).

Box 10.1 Causes of gastritis

Diet
- Alcohol
- Spicy foods

Microorganisms
- *Helicobacter pylori*
- *Salmonella*

Medications
- Aspirin
- Nonsterioidal anti-inflammatory drugs
- Corticosteroids
- Digitalis
- Chemotherapy drugs

Stress
- Physiological
- Psychological

Trauma

Other factors
- Reflux of bile
- Smoking
- Radiation
- Nasogastric suctioning

Endoscopic procedures

Pathophysiology

Acute gastritis develops when the protective mechanism of the mucosa are overwhelmed by the presence of bacteria or irritating substances. In other words, gastritis occurs as the result of a breakdown in the normal gastric mucosal barrier. This mucosal barrier normally protects the stomach tissue from autodigestion by acid and the enzyme pepsia. When the barrier is broken, acid can diffuse back into the mucosa. This allows hydrochloric acid (HCl) to enter. The HCl acid stimulates the conversion of pepsinogen to pepsin and stimulates the release of histamine from mast cells. The combined results of these occurrences is tissue edema, disruption of capillary walls with loss of plasma into the gastric lumen and possible hemorrhage.

Regeneration of the gastric mucosa after injury is both prompt and efficient, however, and the disorder usually is self-limiting once the irritating agent is removed. The common symptoms of acute gastritis include anorexia, nausea, and vomiting, abdominal cramping or diarrhea, epigastric pain and fever. Painless GI bleeding, may occur and in persons using aspirin and NSAIDs.

Acute Gastritis

- Can be asymptomatic
- Abdominal discomfort with headache, lassitude, nausea, anorexia, vomiting and hiccupping
- Hemorrhage

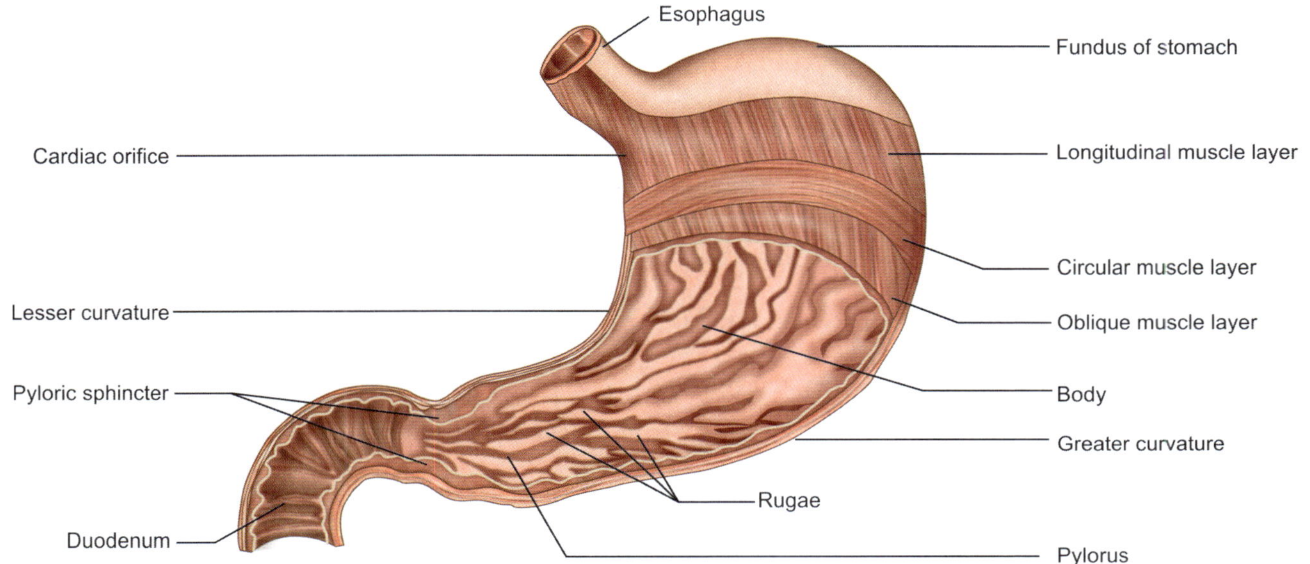

FIG. 10.16: Stomach anterior view partial section

- Colic and diarrhea resulting from irritating food that is not vomited but reaches the bowel
- Recovery in about 1 day, although appetite may be diminished for 2 to 3 days

Management

Acute gastritis cases are managed by removing the causative agent and supporting the patient while the mucosa heals itself. The person is usually put on nothing by mouth (NPO) status to support healing of the mucosa and then slowly advanced to liquids and a return to a normal diet. antacids and histamine 2 (H_2) receptor antagonists may be administered to reduce acid secretion and increase comfort. Temporary IV fluid and electrolyte replacement may be indicated in severe cases and the patient is monitored carefully for signs of bleeding.

The patient should refrain from alcohol and eating until symptoms subside. Then the patient can progress to a nonirritating diet. If symptoms persist, intravenous fluids may be necessary. If bleeding is present, management is similar to that of upper gastrointestinal tract hemorrhage.

If gastritis is due to ingestion of strong acids or alkali, dilute and neutralize the acid with common antacids (e.g. aluminum hydroxide); neutralize alkali with diluted lemon juice or diluted vinegar. If corrosion is extensive or severe, avoid emetics and lavage because of danger of perforation.

Supportive therapy may include nasogastric intubation, analgesic agents and sedative medications.

Emergency surgery may be required to remove gangrenous or perforated tissue; gastric resection (gastrojejunostomy) may be necessary to treat pyloric obstruction.

The nurse also should give health instruction to prevent bacterial food-borne illness and concerning safe good handling and preparation. The nurse will educate the individual and family to take general measures to prevent food-related illness as follows:

- Wash hands before handling food
- Do not thaw foods in the kitchen counter
- Keep meats, fish, poultry, mayonnaise and cream-filled food, refrigerated
- Wash hands and utensils after contact with raw meat or poultry
- Never leave perishable foods unrefrigerated for more than 2 hours less in hot weather
- Use a meat thermometer when cooking large pieces of meat especially pork
- Stuff poultry immediately before roasting (warm stuffing is a good medium for bacterial growth
- Avoid slow cooling of meat and poultry
- Freeze or refrigerate leftovers promptly
- Can low-acid food (foods other than tomatoes or fruits) under pressure to prevent botulism
- Discard any can that bulges.

CHRONIC GASTRITIS

Gastritis can occur from reflux of bile salts from the duodenum into the stomach as a result of anatomical changes following surgical procedures such as gastroduodenostomy and gastrojejunostomy. Prolonged vomiting may also cause reflux of bile salts, inflammation of the mucosal lining as a result of hypersecretion of HCl acid. The chronic gastritis can result from repeated episodes of acute gastritis.

Pathophysiology

Chronic gastritis is a separate clinical entity that can be further subdivided into type A and type B. Its presence is usually a sign of some underlying disease process.

- Type A is believed to be autoimmune in nature and involves all of the acid-secreting gastric tissue, particularly the tissue in the fundus. Circular antibodies are produced that attack the gastric parietal cells and eventually may cause pernicious anemia from loss of the intrinsic factor
- Type B is related to the presence of *Helicobacter pylori* (*H. pylori*). It primarily involves the antrum of the stomach. There is less reduction in the acid secretions, gastrin levels remain normal, and vitamin B_{12} absorption is rarely impaired. As the condition progresses, the mucosa increasingly atrophies, and acid secretion is reduced. The presence of *H. pylori* has been correlated with the presence of other gastric disorders including gastric and duodenal ulcer and gastric cancer.

The clinical manifestation of chronic gastitis are similar to those described for acute gastritis. In addition eventually the body's storage of cobalamin (B_{12}) in the liver is depleted and a deficiency state exists. Lack of this leads to important vitamins which is essential for the growth and development of RBC result in development of anemia, i.e. cobalamin deficiency anemia.

Diagnostic studies include endoscopic examination with biopsy. Breath, urine, serum or gastric tissue biopsy tests are available for the determination of *H. pylori*. CBC for presence of anemia, gastric analysis for presence of HCl acid and stool test for occult blood. Cytologic examination of carcinoma.

Management

Diet modification, rest, stress reduction, and pharmacotherapy are key treatment measures. If gastritis is related to *H. pylori* infection, treatment may include antibiotic therapy (e.g. tetracycline or amoxicillin) and bismuth salts (Pepto-Bismol).

The treatment of chronic gastritis focuses on evaluating and eliminating the specific cause (e.g. cessation of alcoholic intake abstinence from drugs), currently double and triple antibiotic combinations are used to eradicate infection with *H. pylori*.

Original triple therapy consists of tetracycline + metronidazole + bismuth sub-salicylate × 14 days. New triple therapy includes amoxicillin + clarithromycin + omeprazole) × 7 days.

For the patient with pernicious anemia, regular injection of cobalamin (vitamin B_{12}) are needed. An individualized bland diet and use of antacids are recommended.

Major goals include reducing anxiety, adequate nutritional intake, maintaining fluid balance, increasing awareness of dietary management and absent or minimal pain.

Nursing Intervention

Reducing Anxiety

- Carry out emergency measures for ingestion of acids or alkalies
- Offer supportive therapy to patient and family during treatment and after the ingested acid or alkali has been neutralized or diluted
- Prepare patient for additional diagnostic studies (endoscopy) or surgery
- Calmly listen to and answer questions as completely as possible; explain all procedures and treatments.

Promoting Optimal Nutrition

- Provide physical and emotional support for patients with acute gastritis
- Avoid foods and fluids by mouth for hours or days until acute symptoms subside
- Provide intravenous therapy as necessary and monitor serum electrolyte values daily
- Offer ice chips and clear liquids when symptoms subside
- Encourage patient to report any symptoms suggesting a repeat episode of gastritis as food is introduced
- Discourage caffeinated beverages (caffeine increases gastric activity and pepsin secretion)
- Discourage alcohol and cigarette smoking (nicotine inhibit neutralization of gastric acid in the duodenum). Instruct patient that nicotine increases muscular activity in the bowel, leading to nausea and vomiting (parasympathetic stimulation)
- Refer patient for alcohol counseling and smoking cessation when appropriate.

Providing Adequate Fluid Intake

- Monitor daily intake and output for dehydration (minimal intake of 1.5 L/day and urine output of 30 mL/h). Infuse intravenous fluids if prescribed
- Assess electrolyte values every 24 hours for fluid imbalance
- Be alert for indicators of hemorrhagic gastritis (hematemesis, tachycardia, hypotension), and notify physician.

Relieving Pain

- Instruct patient to avoid foods and beverages that may be irritating to the gastric mucosa
- Instruct patient in the use of medications to relieve chronic gastritis
- Asses pain and attainment of comfort through use of medications and avoidance of irritating substances.

Teaching Patients Self-Care

- Assess knowledge about gastritis and develop an individualized teaching plan that incorporates patients pattern of eating, daily caloric needs and food preferences
- Provide a list of substances to avoid (caffeine, nicotine, spicy foods, irritating or highly seasoned foods, alcohol); consult with nutritionist if indicated
- Educate about antibiotic agents, antacids, bismuth salts, sedative medications, or anticholinergic agents that may be prescribed
- Instruct patients with pernicious anemia about need for long-term vitamin B_{12} injections. Teach self-administration or arrange for patient to receive injections from health care provider.

UPPER GASTROINTESTINAL BLEEDING

Upper gastrointestinal bleeding is serious problem. The severity of bleeding depends on whether the origin is venous, capillary or arterial. The bleeding may be obvious or occult.

An obvious bleeding are (Box 10.2):

- Hematemesis refers to bloody vomitus appearing as fresh, bright red blood or 'coffee ground' appearance (dark, grain-digested blood)

Box 10.2 Overviews of gastric bleeding

Signs and symptoms	Occult blood in stool Hematemesis Melena Hypovolemic shock
Diagnostic test	Endoscopy Low hemoglobin and hematocrit
Therapeutic measures	Treat hypovolemic shock: NPO, IV fluids, oxygen therapy, NG tube Removal or ligation of bleeding area Medications to decrease gastric acid
Complications	Hypovolemic shock

- Melena refers to a black, tarry stools (often foul smelling) caused by digestion of blood in the GI tract. The black appearance is from the presence of iron
- Occult bleeding refers to small amount of blood in gastric secretions. Vomitus or stools not apparent by appearance detectable by guaiac test.

Bleeding from arterial source is profuse and the blood is bright red. It indicates that blood has not been contacted with gastric secretions. In contrast 'coffee ground' vomitus reveals that the blood and other contents have been in the stomach and have been changed by contact with gastric secretions. A massive upper GI bleeding is generally defiend as a loss of more than 1500 mL of blood of 25 percent of intravascular blood volume.

Etiology

The common causes of upper gastrointestinal bleeding includes:

- Drug induced: Some medications prescribed are self-administered and prolonged use causes bleeding which includes salicylates, corticosteroids, NSAIDs
- Chronic esophagitis, Mallory-Weiss tear or syndrome, or esophageal varices, leads to upper GI bleeding
- Peptic ulcer disease, stress ulcer, hemorrhagic gastritis, carcinoma polyps
- Systemic diseases such as blood dyscrasiasis, leukemia and uremia.

Management

As the nurse begins care of the patient admitted with upper GI bleeding, a thorough and accurate assessment is made by taking important health information including past health history (Table 10.5). Use of medication as mentioned in the etiology and observe for signs of fever, shock, etc. Sometimes, patient experiencing upper GI bleeding may not be able to provide specific information about the cause of bleeding until the immediate physical needs are met.

An immediate nursing assessment should be performed while getting the patient ready for initial treatment. The assessment should include the patient's level of consciousness, vital signs, appearance of neck veins, skin color and capillary refill. The abdomen should be checked for distension, guarding and peristalsis. Immediate determination of vital signs indicate whether the patient is in shock from blood loss and also provides a baseline blood pressure and pulse by which to monitor the progress of treatment. Signs and symptoms of shock include, low blood pressure, rapid, weak pulse increased thirst, cold, clammy skin and restlessness. Vital signs should be monitored every 15 to 30 minutes and concerned doctor should be informed of any significant changes. Treatment of shock should be initiated promptly.

The patient should be approached in a calm and assured manner to help decrease the level of anxiety. Once an infusion has been started, the IV Line must be maintained for fluid or blood replacement. An accurate intake and output record is

TABLE 10.5: Nursing care plan for the patient with acute upper gastrointestinal hemorrhage and hypovolemic, hemorrhagic shock

Problem	Objective	Nursing intervention	Rationales
Nursing Diagnosis #1			
Fluid volume deficit, actual, related to: 1. Acute blood loss hematemesis hematochezia 2. Gastric drainage (continuous)	Patient will: 1. Maintain an effective circulating blood volume and stable hemodynamic functions: – Heart rate (resting) <100 beats/min – Central venous pressure 0–8 mm Hg – Pulmonary artery pressure <25 mm Hg – Pulmonary capillary wedge pressure 8–12 mm Hg – Cardiac output ~5 liters/min – Systemic arterial blood pressure within 10 mm Hg of baseline, without orthostatic hypotension 2. Remain alert, and oriented to person, place and time without weakness and dizziness 3. Maintain urine output >30 mL/hour 4. Remain without signs of rebleeding: – No hematemesis; hematochezia – Gastric aspirate blood-free	• Assess for signs and symptoms of hypovolemic, hemorrhagic shock: – Observe for signs of acute or subacute hemorrhage; hematemesis, hematochezia; melena; abdominal distention, epigastric pain – Assess cardiovascular function: ◆ Hypotension (orthostatic) ◆ Resting pulse >100 beats/min. Characteristics–faint, rapid, thready ◆ Skin color-pallor, cyanosis; skin temperature; delayed capillary refill time (>3 sec) ◆ Signs of dehydration–poor skin turgor; weakness, fatigue ◆ Cardiac monitoring—rate and rhythm • Assess renal function: – Urine output > 30 mL/hour • Establish baseline abdominal assessment data: – Presence or absence of bowel sounds (timing and characteristics)	• A baseline assessment is necessary to establish the stage of shock initial compensatory, progressive or final, and emergent measures indicated; it serves as a measure of the patient's response to therapy – A drop in blood pressure of 10–15 mm Hg from supine to sitting position suggests blood loss of ~1 liter – Blood loss and enhanced peripheral vasoconstriction underlie diminished to absent pulses, coolness of the extremities, and pallor of conjunctiva, mucous membranes and nailbeds – Skin turgor is best assessed over forehead or sternum – Reflect effect of blood loss on cardiac function • Reduced circulating blood volume and hypotensive state compromises renal perfusion. The consequent reduction in glomerular filtration underlies the reduced urine output associated with hypovolemic shock

Contd...

Contd...

Problem	Objective	Nursing intervention	Rationales
	5. Maintain body weight within 5 percent of baseline 6. Balance intake with output 7. Exhibit good skin turgon moist mucous membranes; minimal thrist 8. Maintain laboratory parameters within acceptable physiological range: – Hematocrit 37–52 percent – Hemoglobin 12–18 g/100 mL – RBC and WBC counts – BUN, electrolytes, calcium	– Pain and tenderness (location, radiation, quality, severity, duration) – Hepatomegaly – Abdominal mass or bruit • Insert at least one, or more (if bleeding is massive) large gauge angiocatheters for rapid administration of blood and blood products, volume expanders, and fluids (Ringer's lactate, and normal saline) – Obtain blood samples for baseline laboratory data • Monitor Hct, Hgb; RBC, WBC counts; electrolytes, serum calcium; blood glucose levels – Monitor BUN and creatinine levels – Obtain blood samples for type and cross-match – Monitor prothrombin time, clotting factors, fibrin degradation products • Initiate aggressive infusion of electrolytes, and volume expanders until blood is ready for administration • Insert nasogastric tube: • Check for tube placement – Auscultate over the gastric area while injecting 50 mL air into the nasogastric tube • Assess gastric aspirate: – Presence of fresh blood, or a large amount of old blood (coffee-ground material) are indications for gastric lavage • Implement gastric lavage as prescribed – Maintain patency of tube by irrigation and repositioning if necessary • Maintain the patient NPO, and implement continuous gastric suction, as prescribed – Monitor amount and characteristics of gastric drainage • Maintain a strict intake and output – Include amount of fluid lavaged, and that removed via gastric suction – Document amount and characteristics of any emesis • Provide comfort measures: – Provide quiet, calm environment with frequent rest periods; minimize stimull	– Abdominal pain with muscle guarding and rebound tenderness is highly suggestive of peptic ulcer perforation, especially if preceded by an episode of severe abdominal pain, followed by sudden, but temporary relief, in patients at risk – Suggestive of elrrhosis with portal hypertension – Questionable abdominal aneurysm • A single peripheral intravenous catheter may not be sufficient to provide adequate blood replacement in a profusely bleeding patient – A central venous line or pulmonary artery catheter is indicated to closely monitor the patient's response to volume replacement • In patients bleeding profusely, there may be insufficient time for the blood volume to equilibrate. Thus, Hct and Hgb may not be reliable indicators of the patient's status. In such patients, changes in blood pressure and pulse are better indicators for replacement of blood and blood products. – Rapid fluid shifts during GI bleeding and subsequent infusion of blood, blood products and other fluids, require frequent assessment of serum electrolytes—sodium, potassium, chloride, bicarbonate, and serum calcium. The serum calcium level may become depressed after several units of anticoagulate (cltrate)-containing blood have been administered – Metabolism of blood by intestinal bacteria, coupled with compromised liver perfusion, causes the BUN level to rise ◆ A rising BUN in the presence of a normal creatinine is highly indicative of a massive upper GI bleed – Even in acute emergencies, there is usually sufficient time to type and cross-match blood for infusion properly. This reduces the incidence of blood incompatibility and transfusion reactions

Contd...

Contd...

Problem	Objective	Nursing intervention	Rationales
		– Provide mouth care with oral suctioning as necessary – Secure tube to patient's gown with adequate sluck – Lubricate nares; assess nares for pressure areas caused by nasogastric tube – Monitor body temperature ◆ Provide extra blankets if appropriate • Transfuse blood and blood products as prescribed – Consider unit procedure and protocols for: ◆ Administering blood therapy ◆ Monitoring patient's response to blood therapy ◆ Recognizing early signs of adverse effects and transfusion reactions ◆ Procedure to follow in the event of transfusion reaction • Insert Foley catheter to measure hourly urine output • Assist with insertion of hemodynamic pressure monitoring lines – Monitor hemodynamics: arterial, and pulmonary artery pressures-CVP, pulmonary artery and pulmonary capillary wedge pressures (PCWP); and cardiac output • Monitor hydration status during fluid replacement therapy – Assess respiratory function: Respiratory rate and rhythm; presence of adventitious sounds – Assess signs/symptoms of fluid overload – Monitor daily weight • Assist with insertion of Sengstaken-Blakemore tube in setting of persistent variceal bleeding	– Patients receiving massive fluid and blood replacement therapy are at risk of developing a dilutional coagulopathy; patients with profuse hemorrhaging are at high risk of developing consumptive coagulopathles (e.g. disseminated intravascular coagulation, DIC) • To decompress the stomach and assist (in conjunction with endoscopy) in determining site, amount, and rate of bleeding); to test gastric aspirate for blood, and pH; and to administer antacids, iced saline lavage (as prescribed) • Inadvertent placement of the nasogastric tube into the respiratory passage is always a potential complication of this procedure – A rush of air should be heard if the tube is properly placed • Removal of as much clot and intragastric material as possible is important; it assists in evaluating continuous bleeding; an empty stomach will allow the walls to collapse and may contribute to hemostasis • Irrigation with iced saline causes vasoconstriction of bleeding vessels; the efficacy of this treatment has yet to be substantiated – Use saline rather than water for lavage to minimize saline depletion via gastric mucosa • Continuous gastric suctioning enables close monitoring of bleeding; it minimizes the amount of blood passing into the intestine; where the action of the intestinal bacteria metabolizes blood to ammonia – To promote physical and mental rest; stimulation may provoke vomiting, bleeding – Aspiration is a potential complication – This prevents tugging on tube when patient moves, which can injured nose – Continuous Iced saline lavage can lower body temperature • Nursing care considerations, precautions, and summary of adverse reactions (respectively) in the administration of blood and blood products

Contd...

Contd...

Problem	Objective	Nursing intervention	Rationales
			• Hourly urine outputs assist in monitoring renal perfusion and function • Insertion of systemic arterial and pulmonary artery flotation (Swan-Ganz) catheters are indicated in the setting of massive upper GI hemorrhage, and massive blood and fluid replacement therapy – PCWP is a useful parameter for monitoring for fluid overload, a potential complication of massive, aggressive fluid replacement therapy – The detection of rales in previously clear lungs suggest possible overhydration – Should be maintained within 5 percent of baseline
Nursing Diagnosis #2			
Gas exchange impaired: Ventilation/perfusion imbalance, related to: 1. Reduced circulating volume and compromised hemodynamics	Patient will: 1. Be alert and oriented to person, place, time 2. Exhibit appropriate behavior 3. Maintain effective cardiovascular function: – Blood pressure within 10 mm Hg of baseline – Cardiac output:~5 liters/min 4. Maintain arterial blood gas parameters within acceptable physiological range: – pH 7.35–7.45 – $PaO_2 > 60$ mm Hg – $PaCO_2$ 35–45 mm Hg 5. Maintain hematologic values within acceptable range. – Hematocrit 37–52 percent – Hemoglobin 12–18 g/100 mL – Red blood cell count	• Perform neurological assessment – Mental status; orientation to person, place, time; level of consciousness; appropriateness of responses/behavior • Monitor cardiovascular function: – Cardiac dysrhythmias – Tachycardia; rapid, thready peripheral pulses. – Cyanosis • Monitor respiratory function: – Respiratory rate and pattern, breath sounds: normal and adventitious breath sounds – Arterial blood gases: pH, PaO_2, $PaCO_2$; alveolar-arterial gradient ($AaDO_2$) – Monitor hematologic profile: hematocrit, hemoglobin, red blood cell count • Administer prescribed humidified oxygen therapy – Monitor arterial blood gas and hematologic parameter as indicated – Provide frequent rest periods – Evaluate effectiveness of oxygen therapy: Assess neurological function and vital signs	• Hypoxemia coupled with hypovolemic shock can predispose to cerebral tissue hypoxia – Hypoxemia is commonly associated with myocardial irritability – Commonly associated with blood loss and consequent reduced circulating blood volume and peripheral vasoconstriction – Late sign reflecting desaturation of at least 5 g/100 mL of hemoglobin; commonly associated with ventilation/ perfusion mismatch and right to left shunting – Presence of rales (crackles) may be indicative of fluid overload – Most closely reflect effectiveness of gas exchange – Reflects hemoglobin oxygen-carrying capacity within blood; reduced hemoglobin levels can compromise oxygen delivery to tissues • Tissue hypoxia is a common consequence of hypovolemic, hemorrhagic shock due to depleted blood volume, and reduced number of RBCs – To reduce oxygen demand by tissues
Nursing Diagnosis #3			
Anxiety, related to: 1. Acute upper gastrointestinal hemorrhage (hematemesis)	Patient will: 1. Verbalize feeling less anxious 2. Demonstrate relaxed demeanor 3. Perform relaxation techniques with assistance	For specific nursing interventions and their rationales, please see related nursing diagnosis appeared in earlier or carring chapters	

Contd...

Contd...

Problem	Objective	Nursing intervention	Rationales
2. Abdominal pain 3. Transfusion therapy. 4. Intensive care setting	4. Verbalize familiarity with ICU routines and protocols		
Nursing Diagnosis #4			
Comfort, alteration in epigastric pain, related to: 1. Enhanced gastric acidity 2. Reflex muscle spasm	Patient will: 1. Verbalize pain relief 2. Exhibit relaxed demeanor: – Relaxed facial expression and body posturing Gastric aspirate: pH > 4.5	• Assess complaints of pain including: severity: location/ radiation; influencing factors (e.g. what precipitates, aggravates or ameliorates the pain?; what signs and symptoms are associated with the pain?) • Assess for nonverbal clues as to the presence of pain (e.g. restlessness, irritability, agitation, diaphoresis, tense facial features; rapid, shallow breathing) • Implement measures to reduce pain: – Administer the following medications as prescribed: ◆ Antacids ◆ Histamine, antagonist—cimetidine (Tagamet) or ranitidine (Zanatac) – Analgesics. ◆ Encourage patient to request medication when pain is first perceived, rather than waiting until it becomes severe ◆ Evaluate the effectiveness of medication in relieving patient's pain – Mild sedation • Determine how patient usually copes with pain or stress: – Pain tolerance – Willingness to discuss pain; or stoically "keeping it within" – Willingness to use medication for pain – Behavior used to reduce level of stress	• Use of the "SLIDT" tool assists in elicifing specific informatioan about the nature of the complaints – Antacids neutralize gastric acidity – Inhibit gastric acid secretion. The combination of antacids/ histamine antagonist therapy is more efficacious than either therapy alone in reducing the harmful effects of acid and pepsin on the bleeding lesion – It is absolutely essential to assist the patient to rest and relax, mentally and physically, to reduce danger of continued bleeding, or rebleeding • Details elicited at this time regarding patient/family attitudes about pain and stress may help lay the foundation for patient/family educatiaon in this regard
Nursing Diagnosis #5			
Nutritin, alteration in: Less than body requirements, related to: 1. Maintenance on NPO with continuous gastric suctioning	Patient will maintain: 1. Body weight within 5 percent of baseline 2. Total serum proteins 6.0–8.4 g/100 mL 3. Laboratory data within acceptable physiological range: – BUN, serum creatinine – Electrolytes, serum calcium – Blood glucose levels – Serum albumin 3.5–5.5 g/100 mL – Hematology profile 4. Triceps skinfold measurements within normal range	• Consult with nutritionist in assessing overall nutritional status; and signs and symptoms of malnutrition – Major considerations: General state of health—weakness; body weight; physiological factors—age, height, triceps skin fold; mid-upper arm circumference; food intolerance; allergies – Laboratory data: BUN, serum creatinine; fasting blood glucose; serum electrolytes, total protein (serum albumin); cholesterol; transfusion levels, hematology profile	• Catabolic state associated with critical illness rapidly depletes body stores of nutrients • The purpose of total parenteral nutrition (TPN) is to provide sufficient nutrients intravenously, to achieve anabolism, and to promote weight gain – Solution should be prepared in pharmacy under a laminar airflow unit to minimize danger of contamination – Helps to avoid air embolism upon insertion

Contd...

Contd...

Problem	Objective	Nursing intervention	Rationales
		• Maintain adequate nutrition with prescribed enteral and/or parenteral nutrition – Order prescribed feeding from pharmacy – Assist with placement of TPN central intravenous catheter. ◆ Explain purpose of parenteral therapy ◆ Explain procedure for insertion: - Use of Trendelenburg position and Valsalva maneuver. ◆ Apply dressing ◆ Prepare patient for chest X-ray ◆ Assess patient for signs and symptoms of respiratory distress: Dyspnea, decreased breath sounds; chest pain; hematoma formation ◆ Initiate prescribed parenteral feedings - Begin infusion at slow rate (60–80 mL/hour); increase infusion by 25 mL/day - Use flow control device or pump to administer feeding - Weight patient daily; record intake and output - Monitor serum glucose; monitor for signs of hyperglycemia (polyuria, glycosuria, elevated serum glucose) - Wean from TPN therapy slowly • Ongoing monitoring/maintenance: – Maintain catheter asepsis. Monitor body temperature at regular intervals and report any temperature elevation to physician, Follow unit protocol in obtaining specimens for culture and sensitivity – Never use TPN catheter for anything other than parenteral feedings – Provide catheter site care as per unit protocol	– To confirm correct placement of catheter and rule out potential pneumothorax – Pneumothorax, hemothorax, air embolism, and sepsis are major complications – Allows for physiological adjustments in pancreatic insulin secretion; helps to avoid glucose intolerance – This helps to prevent fluid or glucose overload – This avoids danger of hypoglycemic reaction as pancreatic secretion of insulin is allowed to decline accordingly – Consistent monitoring is necessary because there is no single febrile pattern associated with TPN sepsis. Temperature elevation may be low-grade, constant, or intermittent, or characterized by daily spiking – If catheter is used as a central access line in an emergency, it should not be resued for TPN – Cleansing of catheter site minimizes potential complications of sepsis, or mechanical disruption of catheter placement; it helps to preserve skin integrity at insertion site
Nursing Diagnosis #6 Infection, potential for, related to: 1. Invasive procedures 2. Malnutrition	Patient will: 1. Maintain body temperature within acceptable physiological range – ~98.6°F (37°C) 2. Maintain white blood count: – 5,000–10,000/mm^3	For specific nursing interventions and their rationales, see other chapters included similar nursing diagnosis in nursing care plan	

Contd...

Contd...

Problem	Objective	Nursing intervention	Rationales
	3. Remain without signs and symptoms of infection; urine free of infection		
Nursing Diagnosis# 7			
Sleep pattern disturbance, related to: 1. Frequent interruption for assessment and treatments 2. Intensive care environment and protocols 3. Psychologic stress	Patient will: 1. Verbalize underlying concerns regarding inability to sleep 2. Verbalize familiarity with ICU protocols and environmental stimuli 3. Assist in planning for undisturbed rest periods within the constraints of ongoing monitoring and essential patient care 4. Report a sense of well-being and restfulness	• Assess sleep pattern and difficulty sleeping: – Encourage patient to verbalize concerns regarding sleeplessness – Monitor the amount of time the patient is sleeping or napping ◆ Identify times and circumstances during which sleep seems most restful ◆ Identify factors particularly disturbing to the patient ◆ Observe for signs and symptoms of fatigue, restlessness, apprehension • Administer prescribed medications for pain and sedation – Monitor effectiveness of medications in relieving pain, and relaxing the patient • Provide comfort measures: – Include personal hygiene; back massage, position changes – Minimize room noise; dim lighting during rest periods (if possible); maintain comfortable room temperature • Assist patient to establish a pattern conducive to sleep – Explain ICU protocols and procedures – Encourage patient to verbalize feelings; provide an attentive, listening ear – Stay with patient at times that are especially stressful – Provide reassurance – Allow patient to make some decisions regarding his/her care (e.g. when to rest; or when to have visitors)	• To minimize bleeding and prevent rebleeding, it is essential to provide a clinical milieu that is as calm and quiet as possible, and conductive to patient rest and relaxation • Pain and anxiety undermine efforts to rest and relax • Comfort measures aid muscle relaxation – Understanding what to expect, and what is expected of the patient, may help to relieve concerns and apprehension – Demonstration of caring, concern, and acceptance may be reassuring to patient – Enables patient to assume responsibility for some aspects of overall care
Nursing Diagnosis #8			
Fear, related to: 1. Possibility of bleeding to death	Patient will: 1. Verbalize fear of dying 2. Verbalize knowledge of clinical status and proposed course of therapy 3. Demonstrate behaviors indicative of lessened fear (e.g. relaxed facies and posture)	• Assess degree of fear and patient's perceptions as to the reality of the possibility of dying – Encourage patient/family to discuss their perceptions and feelings regarding the patient's health status; to share subjective experiences – Observe nonverbal and verbal responses – Assess for accompanying changes in patient's physiological status ◆ Vital signs	• An episode of massive upper GI hemorrhage can be perceived by patient/family as an imminent threat that the patient is going to bleed to death – Recognize that sympathetic response to fear may actually aggravate bleeding, and needs to be minimized – These responses may assist patient/family to cope at least temporarily until patient/family have learned ways to reduce the threat

Contd...

Contd...

Problem	Objective	Nursing intervention	Rationales
		– Assess for accompanying changes in patient's psychological status ◆ Evidence of denial, anger, depression • Assist patient/family to deal with fear: – Stay with patient/family – Allow time for, and encourage expression of feelings and concerns – Assist patient/family to identify feelings – Clarify questions or misconceptions regarding illness or treatment • Assist patient/family to learn from this experience and to problem solve: – Identify strength of family members, individually and collectively – Acknowledge usefulness of fear, denial, anger, in coping – Promote honest and open communication between family members – Involve patient/family in problem-solving and decision-making • Referral to psychiatric liaison nurse and/or social worker as indicated, and/or requested by patient and/or family	• Recognize that fear can be a motivating factor for learning only if the arousal of fear is accompanied by steps/actions to reduce the threat – Assists patient/family in coping; this may help to increase self-confidence in their own capabilities • Patient/family may feel reassured that other resources are available to lend assistance and support

essential so that the patient's hydration status can be assessed. When the NG tube is inserted, the nurse pays her attention to keep it in proper position and observing the aspirate for blood. Care of nasogastric tube to be taken promptly.

Antacids are sometimes used after upper GI bleeding to reduce the acidity of gastric content. Anticipating the effect of prescribed preparations can be helped in providing better care. The expected outcomes of such bleeding cases will:

- Have no further GI bleeding
- Have the cause of the bleeding identified and treated
- Experience a return to a normal hemodynamic stage
- Experience minimal or no symptom of pain or anxiety.

For nursing care plan please refer Table 10.5.

PEPTIC ULCER DISEASE (PUD)

Peptic ulcer is an erosion of the gastrointestinal (GI) mucosa resulting from the digestive action of hydrochloric acid (HCl) and pepsin. Any portion of the GI tract that comes into contact with gastric secretions is susceptible to ulcer development, including the lower esophagus, stomach, duodenum and margin of gastrojejunal anastomosis after surgical procedure (Fig. 10.17).

Classification of PUD

Peptic ulcers can be classified as acute or chronic depending on the degree of mucosal involvement and gastric or duodenal according to the location.

i. The acute ulcer is associated with superficial erosion and minimal inflammation. It is of short duration and resolves quickly when the cause is identified and removed.
ii. A chronic ulcer is one of long duration, eroding through the muscular wall with the formation of fibrous tissue. It is present continuously for many months or intermittently throughout the person's life time. A chronic ulcer is at least four times as common as acute erosion.

Gastric and duodenal ulcer although defined as peptic ulcer are distinctly different in their aetiology and incidence, but generally treatment of all types of ulcer, is almost quite similar.

The differences between gastric and duodenal ulcers are given in Box 10.3.

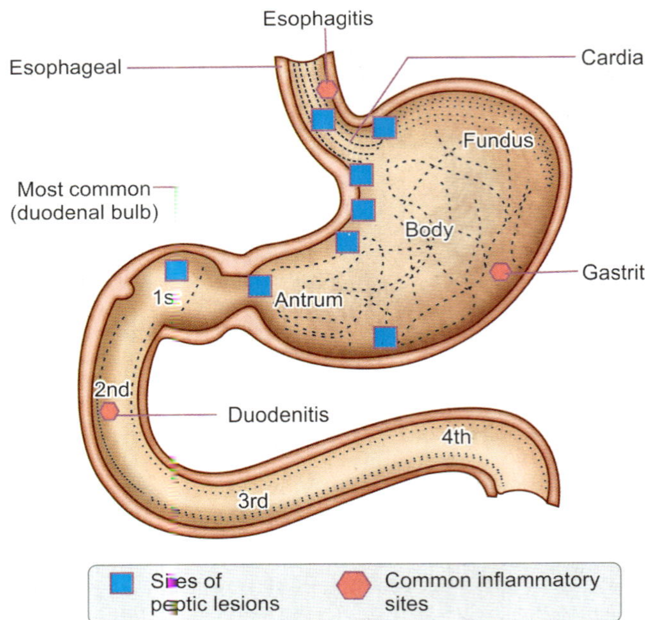

FIG. 10.17: The stomach is divided on the basis of its physiologic functions into two main portions. The proximal two-thirds, the fundic gland area, acts as a receptacle for ingested food and secretes acid and pepsin. The distal third, the pyloric gland area, mixes and propels food into the duodenum and produces the hormone gastrin. "Peptic" lesions may occur in the esophagus (esophagitis), stomach (gastritis), or duodenum (duodenitis)

Note: Peptic ulcer sites and common inflammatory sites (Fig. 10.17)

Etiology

Peptic ulcers were once believed to be the direct result of acid over secretion in response to stressful events. This assumption is reflected in the traditional treatment, approaches, which emphasized acid neutralization and acid reduction. Although it is true that ulcers will not develop in the absence of acid, it is increasingly apparent that the primary etiological factors relate to:

- Infection by the organism *Helicobacter pylori* (*H. pylori*) which produces a chronic gastritis
- The side effects of NSAIDs administration: These factors target the mucosal defenses of the stomach and duodenum and can eventually lead to ulceration. The other factors which are related to decreasing or increasing of gastrical secretions lead to peptic ulcer included in the difference between gastric and duodenal ulcer.

A peptic ulcer is an excavation formed in the mucosal wall of the stomach, pylorus, duodenum or esophagus. It is frequently referred to as a gastric, duodenal or esophageal ulcer, depending on its location. It is caused by the erosion of a circumscribed area of mucous membrane. Peptic ulcers are more likely to be in the duodenum than in the stomach. They tend to occur singly but there may be several present at one time. Chronic ulcers usually occur in the lesser curvature of the stomach, near the pylorus. Peptic ulcer has been associated with bacterial infection, such as *Helicobacter pylori* (present in 70% of patients with gastric ulcer and 95% of patients with duodenal ulcers, not associated with esophageal ulcers). The greatest frequency is noted in

Box 10.3 Differences between gastric ulcer and duodenal ulcer

Gastric ulcer	Duodenal ulcer
1. Lesion – Superficial; smooth margins round, oval, or cone shaped – Predominantly antrum, also in body and fundus of stomach	– Penetrating (associated with deformity of duodenal bulb from aling of recurrent ulcers – First 1–2 cm of duodenum
2. Gastric secretion incidence – Normal to decreased • Greater in women • Peak age fifth to sixth decade • More common in persons of lower socioeconomic status and in unskilled laborers • Increased with smoking, drug and alcohol use • Increased with incompetent pyloric sphincter • Increased with stress ulcers after severe burns, head trauma and major surgery	– Increased • Greater in men, but increasing in women in post menopausal • Peak age 35–45 years • Associated with psychologic stress • Increased with smoking, alcohol and drug use • Associated with other disease, e.g. COPD pancreatic disease hyperparathyroidism Zollinger-Ellison syndrome, chronic renal failure.
3. Clinical manifestations – Burning or gaseous pressure in high left epigastrium and back and upper abdomen – Pain 1–2 hour after meals; if penetrating ulcer, aggravation of discomfort with food – Occasional nausea and vomiting, weight loss	– Burning, cramping, pressure like pain across midepigastrium and upper abdomen; backpain with posterior ulcers – Pain 2–4 hours after meals and midmorning, midafternoon, middle of night, periodic and episodic – Pain relief with antacids and food; occasional nausea and vomiting
4. Recurrence rate complications – High – Hemorrhage, perforation outlet obstruction, intractability	– High – Hemorrhage, perforation obstruction

people between the ages of 40 and 60 years. After menopause, the incidence among women is almost equal to that in men. Predisposing factors include family history of peptic ulcer, blood type O, chronic use of nonsteroidal anti-inflammatory drugs (NSAIDs) alcohol ingestion, excessive smoking, and, possibly, high stress. Esophageal ulcers result from the backward flow of hydrochloric acid from the stomach into the esophagus.

Zollinger-Ellison syndrome (gastrinoma) is suspected when a patient presents with severe peptic ulcer or ulcer that is resistant to standard medical therapy. This syndrome involves extreme gastric hyperacidity (hypersecretion of astric juice) duodental ulcer, and gastrinomas (islet cell tumors, which are gastrin-secreting, benign or malignant tumors of the pancreas). About 90% of tumors are found in the gastic triangle. About one-third of gastrinomas are malignant. Diarrhea and steatorrhea (unabsorbed fat in the stool) may be evident. These patient may have coexistent parathyroid adenoms or hyperplasia and exhibit signs of hypercalcemia. The most frequent complaint epigastric pain. The presence of *H. pylori* is not a risk factor.

Stress ulcer (not to be confused with Cushing's or Curling's ulcers) is a term given to acute mucosal ulceration of the duodenum or gastric area that occurs after physiologically stressful even such as burns, shock severe sepsis (particularly in ventilator dependent post-traumatic or postsurgical patients), and multiple organ trauma. Fiberoptic endoscopy within 24 hours of injury shows shallow erosions of the stomach wall; by 72 hours, multiples gastric erosions are observed, and as the stressful condition continues, the ulcers spread. When the patient recovers; the lesions are reversed; this pattern is typical of stress ulceration.

Pathophysiology

The integrity of the gastric mucosa is maintained when a balance exists between the acid-secreting functions and mucosal protective functions of the stomach and duodenum. Peptic ulcers develop only in the presence of an acid environment. It has been well established that the patient with pernicious anemia and achlorhydria rarely has gastric ulcers. An excess of gastric acid may not be necessary for ulcer development. The typical person with gastric ulcer has normal to less than normal gastric acidity compared with person with a duodenal ulcer. However, some intraluminal acid does seen to be essential for gastric ulcer to occur (Figs 10.18 and 10.19).

The stomach is normally protected from autodigestion by gastric mucosal barrier. Under specific circumstances, the mucosal barrier can be impaired and back-diffusion of acid can occur. When the barrier is broken, HCl acid freely enters the mucosa and causes injury to the tissue, this results in cellular destruction and inflammation. Histamine is released from the damaged mucosa, resulting in vasodilation and increased capillary permeability. The release of histamine is then capable of stimulating further secretion of acid and pepsin. Variety of agents are known to destroy the mucosal barrier, by generating ammonia in the mucus layer. *H. pylori* may create a chromic inflammation. Ulcerogenic drugs inhibit synthesis of mucus, e.g. aspirin cause abnormal permeability, e.g. prostaglandin, decrease the rate of mucous renewal (Corticosteroids), and destroy the broncosal barrier (Cytotoxic drugs). When the mucosal barrier is disrupted, there is compensatory increase in blood flow. This phenomenon can occur in several ways (Box 10.4).

Clinical Manifestation

- Symptoms of duodenal ulcer (most common peptic ulcer) may last days, weeks, or months and may subside only to reappear without cause. Many patient have asymptomatic ulcers
- Dull, gnawing pain and a burning sensation in the mid epigastrium or in the back are characteristic
- Pain is relieved by eating or taking alkali; once the stomach has emptied or the alkali wears off, the pain returns

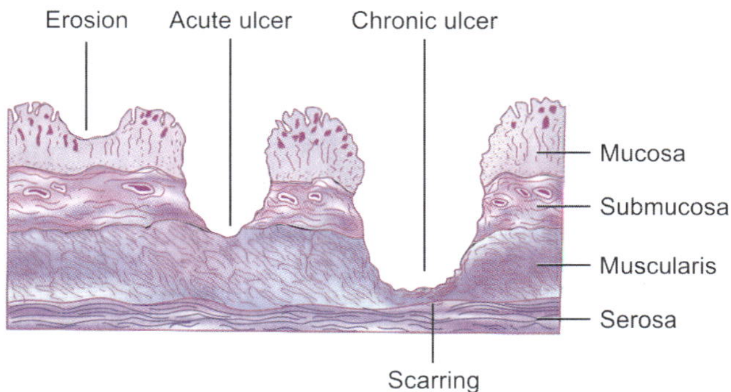

FIG. 10.18: Peptic ulcers, including and erosion, an acute ulcer, and a chronic ulcer, both the acute ulcer and the chronic ulcer may penetrate the entire wall of the stomach

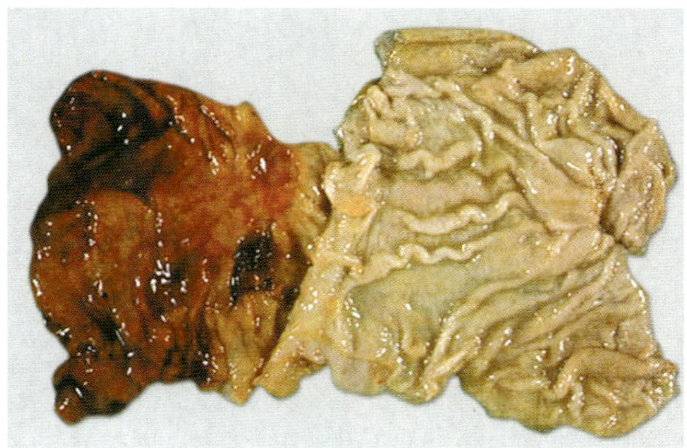

FIG. 10.19: Peptic ulcer of the duodenum

Box 10.4 An overview of peptic ulcer disease

Signs and symptoms	Gastric ulcer	Intermittent high left epigastric or upper abdominal burning or gnawing pain, increased 1–2 hours after meals or with food Variable pain pattern possible made worse by food Antacids ineffective Can lead to gastric cancer Patient may be malnourished Hematemesis more common than melena
	Duodenal ulcer	Intermittent midepigastric or upper abdominal burning or cramping pain, increased 2–4 hours after meals or in the middle of the night Relieved by food or antacids Patient usually well nourished Melena more common than hematemesis Anorexia Nausea and vomiting Bleeding (stomach secretions or stool positive for occult blood)
Diagnostic tests	*H. pylori*	Urea breath test IgG antibody detection test for *H. pylori* Biopsy Culture
	Peptic ulcer	Upper GI series (barium swallow) Esophagogastroduodenoscopy
Therapeutic measure	Antibiotics Proton pump inhibitors H_2 antagonists Bismuth subsalicylate Sucralfate (Carafate) Antacids Bland diet Avoiding irritants, such as smoking, caffeine, alcohol, trigger foods	
Complications	Bleeding Perforation Obstruction	

- Sharply localized tenderness is elicited by gentle pressure on the epigastrium or slightly right of the midline; some relief is obtained with local pressure to the epigastrium
- Other symptoms include pyrosis (heartburn) and a burning sensation in the esophagus and stomach, which moves up to the mouth, occasionally with sour eructation (burping)
- Vomiting is rare in uncomplicated duodenal ulcer; it may or may not be preceded by nausea and usually follows a bout of severe pain and bloating; it is relieved by ejection of the acid gastric contents
- Constipation or diarrhea may result from diet and medications
- Bleeding (15% of patients with gastric ulcers) and tarry stools may occur; a small portion of patients who bleed from an acute ulcer have no previous digestive complaints but develop symptoms later.

The clinical manifestation of gastric and duodenal ulcers may be completely symptomatic. Clinical manifestation associated with peptic ulcer disease are:

Duodenal ulcer	Gastric ulcer
1. Pain	
– Episodic in nature lasting 30 minutes to 2 hours	– Dull epigastric location near midline
– Epigastric location near midline, may radiate around costal border to back	– Early satiety
– Described as gnawing, burning aching	
– Occurs 1–3 hours after meals and at night (12–3 AM)	
– Often relieved by food or antacid	– Not usually relieved by food or antacid

In both there is common manifestation including dyspepsia, syndrome, anorexia, weight loss. The complication of peptic ulcer are hemorrhage, perforation, gastrointestinal obstruction.

Diagnostic Studies

The diagnostic measures used to determine the presence and location of peptic ulcers are:

• Complete blood count biopsy	• Fiberoptic endoscopy with
• Urinalysis study	• Upper GI barium-contrast
• Liver enzymes	• Gastric cytology
• *H. pylori* testing of breath, urine, blood, stool	

- Physical examination (epigastric tenderness, abdominal distention)
- Endoscopy (preferred, but upper gastrointestinal barium study may be done)
- Diagnostic tests include analysis of stool specimens for occult blood, gastric secretory studies, and biopsy and histology with culture to detect *H. pylori* (a breath test may also detect *H. pylori*).

Management

The goals of treatment are to eradicate *H. pylori* and manage gastric acidity.

- Stress reduction and rest are priority interventions. The patient needs to identify situations that are stressful or exhausting (e.g. rushed lifestyle and irregular schedules) and implement changes, such as establishing regular rest periods during the day in the acute phase of the disease. Biofeedback, hypnosis, or behavioral modification may also be useful
- Smoking cessation is strongly encouraged because smoking raises duodenal acidity and significantly inhibits ulcer repair. Support groups may be helpful
- Dietary modification may be helpful. Patients should eat whatever agrees with them; small, frequent meals are not necessary if antacids or histamine blockers are part of therapy. Oversecretion and hypermotility of the gastrointestinal tract can be minimized by avoiding extremes of temperature and overstimulation by meat extracts. Alcohol and caffeinated beverages such as coffee (including decaffeinated coffee, which stimulates acid secretion) should be avoided. Diets rich in milk and cream should be avoided also because they are potent acid stimulators. The patient is encouraged to eat three regular meals a day.

When the patient's clinical manifestations and health history suggest the diagnosis of a peptic ulcer and diagnostic studies confirm its presence, a medical regimen is instituted. The regimen consists of adequate rest, dietary modifications, medications, elimination of smoking and long-term follow-up care (Table 10.6).

TABLE 10.6: Nursing care plan for patient with peptic ulcer

Problem	Reason	Objective	Nursing intervention	Evaluation
Pain related to • Increased gastric secretion • Decreased mucosal protection • Ingestion of gastric irritants	As manifested by burning cramp-like pain in epigastrium and abdomen. • Pain onset 1–2 hours after meals with gastric ulcer • Pain onset 2–4 hours after meals	Verbalization of satisfaction with pain control	• Determine pain characteristics from verbal description and physical assessment data • Administer antacids, H_2 antagonists, PP inhibition, anticholenergic, protective agents on prescribed to reduce pain • Teach the patient to avoid smoking and ingesting spicy, hot or cold foods, coffee, tea and cold drinks and alcoholic beverages to prevent increasing acid production • Teach patients stress reduction as relaxation results in decrease acid products and reduction in pain	(Write the responses and progress of ulcers)
Ineffective management of therapeutic regimen related to • Lack of knowledge of management of peptic ulcer • Not following treatment plan • Unwillingness to modify lifestyles	As manifested by request question about home care, incorrect responses to questions about disease Noncompliance with medical regimen	Verbalization of plan to modify lifestyle and incorporate therapeutic regimen into lifestyle	• Explain ulcer disease process at patient level to faster understanding • Help patient to identify stressors and initiate modification in daily routine as stress causes hypersecretion of HCl and pepsin which can alter mucosal barrier • Discuss diet plan and assist with implementation at home and in work setting • Explain rationale for the elimination of alcohol, spicy foods, coffee, tea and cola from diets • Explain harmful effects of smoking which directly irritates gastric mucosa • Inform patient what to do if symptoms related to ulcer recur to ensure early initiation of treatment	
Pain related to acute exacerbation of disease process and inadequate comfort measures	As manifested by verbalization of increase in pain, non-verbal indication of pain, e.g. moaning, crying, doubling up	Expression of satisfaction with pain management	• Encourage bed rest or light activity to conserve energy and promote comfort • Provide quiet, relaxed environment and limit visitors to decrease stress and other factors that increase secretion • Administer medication as ordered to relieve pain	
Vomiting related to acute exacerbation of disease process	As manifested by increase in nausea and vomiting	Decrease in or absence of nausea and vomiting	• Maintain NPO status to prevent irritation of GI mucosa • Maintain NG tube to suction to keep stomach empty and remove any stimulus for HCl acid and pepsin secretion • Check vomitus or aspirate for occult blood to assess hemorrhage	

Contd...

Contd...

Problem	Reason	Objective	Nursing intervention	Evaluation
Potential for hemorrhage related to eroded mucus tissue		• Monitor for signs of hemorrhage • Carry out medical and nursing interventions if hemorrhage occurs	• Assess for evidence of hematemesis, bright red melena stool, abdominal pain or discomfort. Symptoms of shock to pain appropriate action • If ulcer is actively bleeding, observe NG tube aspirate or emesis for amount and color to assess degree of bleeding • Take vital signs every 15 to 30 minutes to determine hemodynamic status and an indication of shock • Maintain IV infusion line to provide ready access for blood and fluid replacement • If RBC infusion given, observe for transfusion reaction for appropriate action • Monitor hematocrit and hemoglobin as indicators for severity, fluid and blood replacement • Record intake and output to monitor fluid balance • Reassure patient and family to decrease anxiety • Remain calm and confident in plan of care to faster confidence in patient and family	
Potential for perforation of GI mucosa related to impaired mucosal tissue integrity		• Monitor signs of perforation • Report deviations from expected parameters • Carry out appropriate medical and nursing intervention	• Observe the manifestation of perforation to ensure early recognition and treatment: – Sudden severe abdominal pain – Rigid board-like abdomen – Pain to shoulder – Increasing distension – Decreasing bowel sounds • Monitor vital signs every 15 to 30 minutes as indicator of shock • Maintain NG tube to suction to provide continuous aspiration and gastric decompression to prevent further leakage of gastric fluid through perforation • Administer pain medication to promote comfort and reduce anxiety • Prepare patient for emergency diagnostic tests and possible surgical interventions to foster timely intervention	

- Adequate rest benefits the patient to elimination of stressors, help decrease the stimulus for overproduction of HCl acid
- Dietary modification may be necessary so that foods and beverages irritating to the patient can be avoided or eliminated (alcohol and caffeine contents). A bland diet consisting of six small meals may be suggested
- Smoking has an irritating effect on the mucosa, increases gastric motility and delays mucosal healing. So, it should be eliminated
- Medications have major role in the treatment of peptic ulcers (Box 10.5)
  - Antacids are weak bases that neutralize free hydrochloric acid to prevent irritation and permit mucosal healing
  - Histamine receptor antagonists inhibit HCl secretion by binding to the H_2 receptor on stomach cells and blocking, the release of histamine which is a secretogogue for HCl. Gastrict emptying is unaffected by their use, e.g. cimetidine, ranitidine, famotidine, nizatidine
  - Bosom pump inhibitors more effective than H_2 receptor antagonists, e.g. omeprazole, lansoprazole, pantaprazole
  - Mucosol protective agents, sucralfate, misoprostol
  - Antibiotic therapy is instituted for patients verified with *H. pylori.*

Nursing Interventions

Relieving Pain and Improving Nutrition

- Administer prescribed medications
- Avoid aspirin, which is an anticoagulant, and foods and beverages that contain acid-enhancing caffeine (colas, tea, coffee, chocolate)
- Encourage patient to eat regularly spaced meals in a relaxed atmosphere; obtain regular weights and encourage dietary modifications
- Encourage relaxation techniques, and assist patient to cope with stress and pain and to stop smoking.

Box 10.5 Treatment options for ***H. pylori*** infection

Type of therapy	Included in therapy	Examples to therapy options
Triple therapy	Two antibiotics + proton pump inhibitor	Amoxicillin (Amoxil) + clarithromycin (Biaxin) + omeprazole (Prilosec) Amoxicillin (Amoxil) + clarithromycin (Biaxin) + lansoprazole (Prevacid) (available as Prevpac)
Dual therapy	Antibiotic + proton pump inhibitor	Clarithromycin (Biaxin) + omeprazole (Prilosec) Amoxicillin (Amoxil) + lansoprazole (Prevacid)
Other therapy	Antibiotic + H_2 antagonist Two antibiotics + bismuth subsalicylate + H_2 antagonist	Clarithromycin (Biaxin) + H_2 antagonist Metronidazole (Flagyl) + tetracycline + bismuth subsalicylate (Pepto-Bismol) +H_2 antagonist

Reducing Anxiety

- Assess what patient wants to know about the disease, and evaluate level of anxiety; encourage patient to express fears openly and without criticism
- Explain diagnostic test; administer medications on schedule
- Reassure patient that nurses are always available to help with problems
- Interact in a relaxing manner, help in identifying stressors, and explain effective coping techniques and relaxation methods
- Encourage family to participate in care, and give emotional support.

Monitoring and Managing Complications

If hemorrhage is a concern;

- Assess for faintness or dizziness and nausea, before or with bleeding; test stool for occult or gross blood; monitor vital signs frequently (tachycardia, hypotension, and tachypnea)
- Monitor intake and output; insert and maintain an intravenous line for infusing fluid and blood
- Monitor laboratory values (hemoglobin and hematocrit)
- Insert and maintain a nasogastic tube and monitor drainage; provide lavage as ordered
- Treat hypovolemic shock as indicated.

If perforation and penetration are concerns:

- Note and report symptoms of penetration (back and epigastric pain not relieved by medications that were effective in the past)
- Note and report symptoms of perforation (sudden abdominal pain, referred pain to shoulders, vomiting and collapse, extremely tender and rigid abdomen, hypotension and tachycardia, or other signs of shock).

Promoting Home and Community-based Care

Teaching patients self-care

- Assist the patient in understanding the condition and factors that help or aggravate it
- Teach patient about prescribed medications, including name, dosage, frequency and possible side effects. Also identify medications such as aspirin that patient should avoid
- Instruct patient about particular foods that will upset the gastric mucosa, such as coffee, tea, colas and alcohol, which have acid-producing potential
- Encourage patient to eat regular meals in a relaxed setting and to avoid overeating
- Explain that smoking may interfere with ulcer healing patient to programs to assist with smoking cessation
- Help patient to reduce and manage stress by identifying sources of stress in family and work environments, by resting during the day if possible, and by using psychological couseling if desired
- Alert patient to signs and symptoms of complications that should be reported, including hemorrhage (cool skin, confusion, increased heart rate, labored breathing, blood in stool); perforation (severe abdominal pain, rigid and tender abdomen, vomiting, elevated temperature, increased heart rate); pyloric obstruction/gastric outlet obstruction (nausea, vomiting, distended abdomen, abdominal pain). To identify obstruction, insert and monitor nasogastric tube; more than 400 mL residual suggests obstruction.

Continuing Care

- Teach patient that follow-up supervision is necessary for about 1 year
- Tell patient that the ulcer could recur; advise patient to seek medical assistance if symptoms recur.

The nurse has to teach the following points for the patient and family members for self-care management to the patients with peptic ulcer disease.

1. Medication

- Know the dosage, administration, action and side effects of all drugs in use
- Take all the prescribed drugs, even when pain is relieved. It is essential to complete the full treatment
- Keep antacids available for use as needed, but do not take them at the same time as H_2 receptor antagonists. Antacids should be taken 1 to 3 hours after meals, at bed time and as needed for pain
- Avoid the use of over-the-counter H_2 receptor antagonists
- Use acetaminophen for routine pain relief during treatment if needed. Avoid the use of all NSAIDs including aspirin, ibuprofen
- If the treatment of arthritis or other chronic illness require the ongoing use of NSAIDs, explore the use of misoprostol with health care provider
- Know the symptoms of ulcer recurrence and report them promptly to the health care provider.

2. Diet

- Eat three balanced meals a day
- Eat between meal snacks if this helps control pain
- Avoid bed time snacking because it increases night time acid secretion
- Eat slowly and chew food thoroughly. Do not overeat
- Avoid any foods that increase discomfort
- Avoid the use of alcohol during treatment if possible. Never drink alcohol on an empty stomach.

3. Smoking

- Stop smoking if possible
- Explore community support for smoking cessation or use of nicotine withdrawal patches.

4. Stress Reduction

- Participate in recreation and hobbies that promote relaxation
- Participate in a moderate aerobic exercise program for promotion of well-being
- Provide for increased rest during healing

And explain the importance of reporting of any of the following:

- Increased nausea and/or vomiting
- Increase in epigastric pain
- Bloody emesis or tarry stools.

The nursing care plan of patient with peptic ulcer disease is listed in Table 10.6.

The nurse reviews with the patient and family, the signs and symptoms of complications to be reported. These complications include hemorrhage (cool skin, confusion, increased heart rate, labored breathing and blood in stools), penetration and perforation (severe pain, rigid and tendor abdomen, vomiting, elevates temperature, increased heart rate) and pyloric obstruction (nausea, vomiting, distended abdomen and abdominal pain).

Surgical Management of Peptic Ulcer

When the medical therapy has been tried and proved unsuccessful the surgery is indicated. The following criteria are used as general indication for surgical intervention.

- Intractibility: Failure of the ulcer to heal or recurrence of the ulcer after therapy
- History of hemorrhage or increased risk of bleeding during treatment
- Prepyloric or pyloric ulcers, both have high recurrence rates
- Concurrent conditions, such as severe burns, trauma, or sepsis
- Multiple ulcer sites
- Drug-induced ulcers, especially when withdrawal from the drug may put the person at risk
- Possible existence of a malignant ulcer
- Obstruction.

Usually the surgical procedure performed to treat ulcer disease are partial gastrectomy, vagotomy or pyloroplasty.

Partial gastrectomy with removal of the distal two-thirds of the stomach and anastomosis of the gastric stump to the duodenum is called "gastroduodenostomy" or Billroth's operation. Partial gastrectomy with removal of the distal two-thirds of the stomach and anastomosis of the gastric stump to the jejunum is called as "gastrojejunostomy" or Billroth's II operation. In both procedures the antrum and pylorus are removed, because the duodenum is bypassed. The Billroth's II operation is preferred to prevent recurrence of duodenal ulcers (Figs 10.20A to D).

Pain related to:

- Increased gastric secretion
- Decreased mucosal protection

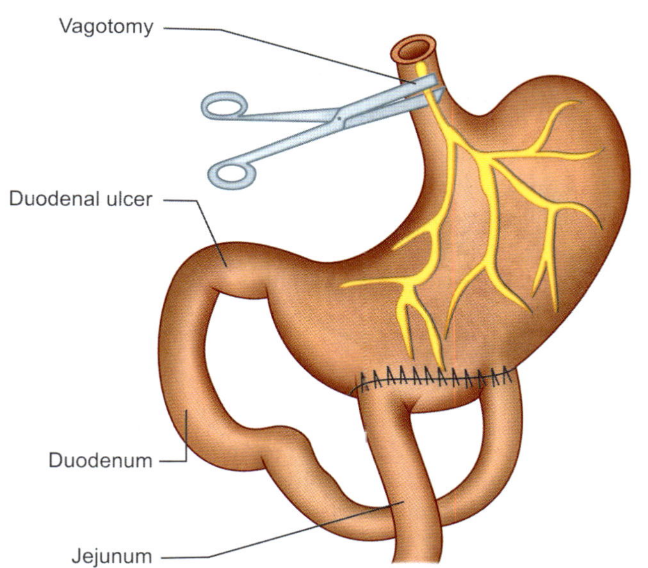

FIG. 10.20A: Gastrojejunostomy and vagotomy. The jejunum is anastomosed to the stomach to provide a second outlet of gastric contents. The severed vagus nerve reduces secretions and movements of the stomach (90% good results)

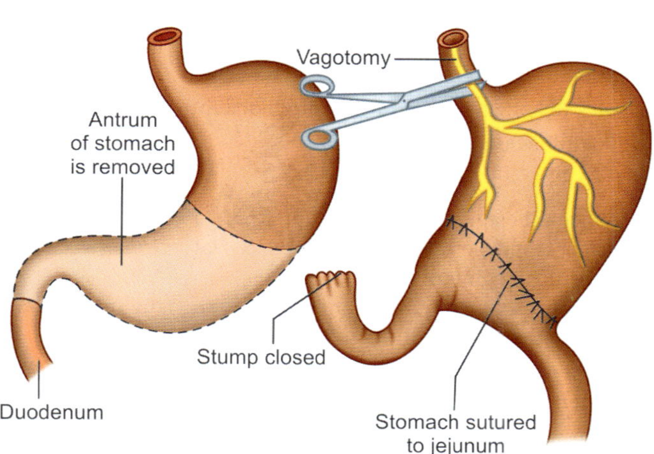

FIG. 10.20B: Antrectomy and vagotomy. The resected portion includes a small cuff of duodenum, the pylorus, and the antrum (about one half of the stomach). The stump of the duodenum is closed by suture, and the side of the jejunum is anastomosed to the cut end of the stomach

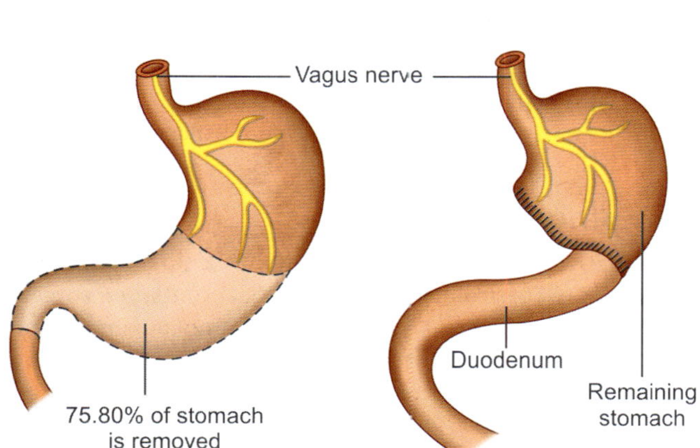

FIG. 10.20C: Subtotal gastrectomy. The resected portion includes a small cuff of the duodenum, the pylorus, and from two thirds to three quarters of the stomach. The duodenum or side of the jejunum is anastomosed to the remaining portion of the stomach

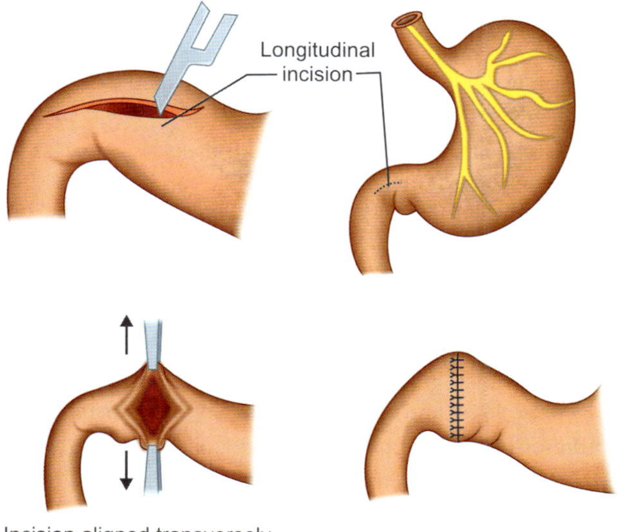

FIG. 10.20D: Vagotomy and pyloroplasty. A longitudinal incision is made in the pylorus, and it is closed transversely to permit the muscle to relax and to establish an enlarged outlet. This compensates for the impaired gastric emptying produced by vagotomy

- Ingestion of gastric irritants.
- As manifested by burning cramp-like pain in epigastrium and abdomen
- Pain onset 1–2 hours after meals with gastric ulcer.
- Pain onset 2–4 hours after meals.

Verbalization of satisfaction with pain control.

- Determine pain characteristics from verbal description and physical assessment data
- Administer antacids, H_2 antagonists, PP inhibition, anticholinergic, protective agents on prescribed to reduce pain

- Teach the patient to avoid smoking and ingesting spicy, hot or cold foods, coffee, tea, and cold drinks and alcoholic beverages to prevent increasing acid production
- Teach patients stress reduction as relaxation results in decrease acid products and reduction in pain.

Ineffective management of therapeutic regimen related to

- Lack of knowledge of management of peptic ulcer
- Not following treatment plan
- Unwillingness to modify lifestyles.

As manifested by request question about home care, incorrect responses to questions about disease. Noncompliance with medical regimen.

Verbalization of plan to modify lifestyle and incorporate therapeutic regimen into lifestyle.

- Explain ulcer disease process at patient level to faster understanding
- Help patient to identify stressors and initiate modification in daily routine as stress causes hypersecretion of HCl and pepsin which can alter mucosal barrier
- Discuss diet plan and assist with implementation at home and in work setting
- Explain rationale for the elimination of alcohol, spicy foods, coffee, tea and cola from diets
- Explain harmful effects of smoking which directly irritates gastric mucosa
- Inform patient what to do if symptoms related to ulcer recur to ensure early initiation of treatment.

Pain related to acute exacerbation of disease process and inadequate comfort measures.

As manifested by verbalization of increase in pain, non-verbal indication of pain, e.g. moaning, crying, doubling up.

Expression of satisfaction with pain management

- Encourage bed rest or light activity to conserve energy and promote comfort
- Provide quiet, relaxed environment and limit visitors to decrease stress and other factors that increase secretion
- Administer medication as ordered to relieve pain
  - Vomiting related to acute exacerbation of disease process
  - As manifested by increase in nausea and vomiting
  - Decrease in or absence of nausea and vomiting
- Maintain NPO status to prevent irritation of GI mucosa
- Maintain NG tube to suction to keep stomach empty and remove any stimulus for HCl acid and pepsin secretion
- Check vomitus or aspirate for occult blood to assess hemorrhage
- Potential for hemorrhage related to eroded mucus tissue
- Monitor for signs of hemorrhage
- Carry out medical and nursing interventions if hemorrhage occurs
- Assess for evidence of hematemesis, bright red melena stool, abdominal pain or discomfort. Symptoms of shock to pain appropriate action
- If ulcer is actively bleeding, observe NG tube aspirate or emesis for amount and color to assess degree of bleeding
- Take vital signs every 15 to 30 minutes to determine hemodynamic status and an indication of shock
- Maintain IV infusion line to provide ready access for blood and fluid replacement
- If RBC infusion given, observe for transfusion reaction for appropriate action.

  (Write the responses and progress of ulcers)

Vagotomy is the severing of the vagus nerve, either totally (truncal) or selectively at some point in its innervation to the stomach. In a truncal vagotomy the nerve is severed bilaterally in both the anterior and the posterior trunk.

Selective vagotomy consists of cutting the nerve at a particular branch of the vagus nerve, resulting in denervation of only a portion of the stomach, such as the antrum or the parietal cell mass.

Pyloroplasty consists of surgical enlargement of the sphincter to facilitate the easy passage of contents from the stomach. It is most commonly done after vagotomy or to enlarge an opening that has been constricted from scar tissue. A vagotomy causes decreased gastric motility. A pyloroplasty accompanying vagotomy increases gastric emptying.

The combination of a Billroth I or II operation with vagotomy has the advantage of eliminating the ulcer and the stimulus for acid secretion. Surgical removal of the antrum results in removal of the source of gastrin secretion. Vagotomy eliminates the stimulation of HCl acid and gastrin hormone secretion caused by vagal stimulation.

The postoperative complication of peptic ulcer surgery.

Dumping Syndrome

Dumping syndrome is the term used for a group of unpleasant vasomotor and gastrointestinal system that occurs after surgery. It is associated with meals having a hyperosmolar composition. The onset of symptoms occurs at the end of a meal or within 15 to 30 minutes after eating. The patient usually describes feeling of generalized weakness, sweating, palpitations and dizziness. These symptoms are attributed to the sudden decrease in plasma volume. The patients complain of abdominal cramps, borborygmi and the urge to defecate. In addition, diaphoresis, tachycardia, feeling of fullness or discomfort, nausea, diarrhea, may be present. These manifestations usually last for longer than an hour after meal.

For which, prevention is the key and its management which includes small frequent meals, moderate fat, high-protein diet, limited carbohydrates, no simple sugars, minimal liquids with meals, avoiding very hot or very cold foods and beverages, and rest on left side for 20–30 minutes after eating. Anticholinergic or antispasmodic medication are useful.

Postprandial Hypoglycemia

Postprandial hypoglycemia is considered a variant of the dumping syndrome, since it is the result of uncontrolled gastric emptying of a bolus of fluid high in carbohydrate into the small intestine. The bolus of fluid concentrated carbohydrate results in hypoglycemia and the release of excessive amounts of insulin into the circulation. The symptoms experienced are sweating, weakness, mental confusion, palpitations, tachycardia and anxiety.

The immediate ingestion of sugared fluids or candy relieves the hypoglycemic symptoms.

Bile Reflux Gastritis

Bile reflux gastritis occurs when surgery that involves the pylorus. Prolonged contact with bile damage, the gastric mucosa may cause bile reflux gastritis. The symptoms associated with epigastric distress that increases after meals. Vomiting relieved the distress but only temporarily. The administration of cholestyramine (Questran) either before or with meals are helpful to relieve bile reflux gastritis.

CANCER OF THE STOMACH

Cancer of the stomach is the most common malignant disease more prevalent among the lower economic class primarily living in urban areas. The male : female ratio is about 2:1. Gastric cancer is rare before the age of 40, and the incidence increases sharply with age. An overview of gastric cancer is given in Box 10.6.

Etiology

The cause of cancer of the stomach remains unknown yet it is highly erratic. Worldwide incidence pattern suggests the involvement of multiple environmental, genetic and possibly cultural factors. Diet and living conditions appear to be the most significant aspects in etiology and early life exposure is critical. The risk factors of gastric cancer will include the following.

- Diet high in smoked preserved foods which contain nitrites and nitrates
- Diet low in fresh fruits and vegetables
- High nitrate content in the soil and water
- Presence of chronic gastritis and achlorhydria.

Box 10.6 Cancer of stomach

Signs and symptoms	Rarely detected during early stages Symptoms often mistaken for peptic ulcer disease: indigestion, anorexia, pain, weight loss, nausea, vomiting, anemia Late symptoms include involvement of other organs such as the liver
Diagnostic test	X-ray studies Gastroscopy Gastric fluid analysis Serum gastrin levels
Therapeutic measures	Medical treatment not very effective Surgical treatment: Subtotal or total gastrectomy
Complications	Related to disease and surgery: Hemorrhage, acute gastric distention, nutritional problems

Pathophysiology

Gastric cancers are virtually all primary adenocarcinoma that are derived from the epithelium. They have been found traditionally in the pyloric and antral regions, particularly along the lesser curvature. There are numerous ways to classify gastric cancers, which manifest in a variety of forms. Histologically, the cancer is classified as diffused or intestinal. The intestinal form is associated with the presence of intestinal metaplasia in the stomach. The diffuse forms have believed to begin locally in the mucosa and exhibit a long latency.

Gastric cancers may spread directly through the stomach wall into adjacent tissues; to the lymphates, to the regional lymph nodes of the stomach; to the esophagus, spleen, pancreas and liver or through the bloodstream to the lungs or bones.

Involvement of regional lymph nodes occur early. Prognosis depends on the depth of invasion and extent of metastasis.

Gastric cancer has an insidious onset. It is accompanied by vague non-descript dyspeptic symptoms that overlap with multiple benign disorders, including non-ulcer dyspepsia and peptic ulcer.

The possible clinical manifestations of gastric cancer are:

- Dyspepsia: Early satiety, bloating, anorexia
- Epigastric pain or burning (usually mild and relieved by antacids)
- Mild nausea
- Weight loss (may be rapid and severe)
- Fatigue and weakness
- Change in the bowel habits; constipation or diarrhea
- Marked cachexia and a palpable mass in the abdomen.

Diagnostic Studies

- Biopsy
- Laboratory analysis of blood, stool, gastric secretion
- Endoscopy
- Blood chemistry studies
- Barium meal
- Carcinoembryonic antigen (CEA) test
- CT Scanning.

Management

When the diagnosis of gastric malignancy has been confirmed, the treatment of choice is surgical removal of the tumor. The

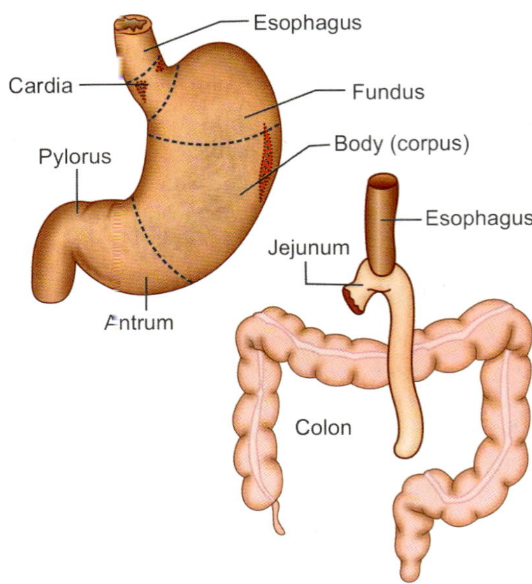

FIG. 10.21: Total gastrectomy for stomach cancer (total gastrectomy with esophagojejunostomy)

preoperative management of the patient with gastric cancer focuses on the correction of nutritional deficits, treatment of anemia, and replacement of blood volume.

The nursing care of the patient undergoing gastric surgery (a total gastrectomy for gastric cancer-total gastrectomy with esophagojejunostomy) are as follows (Fig. 10.21).

Preoperative Care

- Teach deep breathing exercises
- Explain special postoperative measures; nasogastric tube and parenteral fluids until peristalsis returns.

Postoperative Care

i. Promote pulmonary ventilation
   - Position patient in mid or high Fowler's position
   - Encourage patient to turn and breathe deep at least q2h (or more frequently until ambulating well); splint or support incision with hands or folded towel during coughing if needed to clear secretions
   - Provide adequate analgesics during first few days
   - Patient-controlled analgesia (PCA) is effective
   - Encourage ambulation
   - Provide good mouth care until oral fluids can be resumed.

ii. Promote nutrition
   - Measure NG drainage accurately, monitor for blood in drainage. Do not irrigate or reposition tube unless ordered
   - Monitor for signs of leakage of anastomosis (dyspnea, pain, fever) when oral fluids are resumed
   - Add food in small amounts at frequent intervals until well tolerated
   - Monitor for early satiety and regurgitation
   - If regurgitation occurs, tell patients to eat less food at a slower pace
   - Report signs of dumping syndrome to doctor (weakness, faintness, palpitations, diaphoresis, nausea and darrhea
   - Monitor weight.

iii. Provide patient/family education
   - Gradually increase amount of food each meal until able to eat 3 to 6 meals per day if possible
   - If discomfort occurs after eating, decrease size of meals and amount of fluids with meals; eat more slowly
   - Avoid eating simple carbohydrates and concentrated sweets
   - Avoid stress during and immediately after meals; plan a rest period after eating. Lie on left side
   - Elevate the head when lying down (if cardia of stomach removed)
   - Monitor weight regularly
   - Report signs of complications: Vomiting after meals, increasing feeling of abdominal fullness or weakness, hematemesis, tarry stools and persistent diarrhea.

IRRITABLE BOWEL SYNDROME (IBS)

Irritable bowel syndrome (IBS) is a symptom of complex characterized by intermittent and recurrent abdominal pain associated with an alteration in bowel function (diarrhea and constipation). Other symptoms commonly found include abdominal distention, excessive flatulence, urge to defecate, and sensation of incomplete evacuation.

Etiology

The cause is unknown. Much more common in women. Related to stress and excessive intake of food. Often linked to a history of physical or sexual abuse. Onset typically during late adolescence to mid-thirties. Most frequently encountered GI condition in medical practice.

Pathophysiology

Major findings are rarely present. Lab tests are typically normal but colon spasticity can be visualized by X-ray and endoscopy. Increased small bowel motility plus increased frequency and amplitude of large bowel contraction occurs. Symptom patterns include:

- Spastic colon: Colicky abdominal pain, periodic constipation and diarrhea
- Painless urgent diarrhea after meals.

Management

Treatment involves lifestyle modification and supportive care, i.e. diet modification includes avoiding rich fatty foods, gas producing foods, gastric stimulants (alcohol and smoking) using medication such as bulk forming, antispasmodic, antidiarrheal and motility agents. In addition, adequate rest, stress management and regular aerobic exercises are advised.

DIARRHEA

Diarrhea is a condition defined by an increased frequency of bowel movements (more than three per day), increased amount of stool (more than 200 g per day), and altered consistency (liquid stool). It is usually associated with urgency, perianal discomfort, incontinence, or a combination of these factors. Diarrhea can result from any condition that causes increased intestinal secretions, decreased mucosal absorption, or altered (increased) motility. A overview of diarrhea is given in Box 10.7.

Types of diarrhea include secretory, osmotic or mixed diarrhea. It can be acute (self-limiting and often associated with infection) or chronic (persists for a long period and may return sporadically). It is classified as secretory (high volume), osmotic (nonabsorbed particles), or mixed (includes inflammatory bowel disease). It can be caused by certain medications, tube feedings, metabolic and endocrine disorders, and viral and bacterial infections. Other causes are nutritional and malabsorptive disorders, anal sphincter deficit, Zollinger-Ellison syndrome, paralytic ileus, acquired immunodeficiency syndrome (AIDS), and intestinal obstruction.

Diarrhea is not a disease but a symptom. It is commonly used to denote an increase in stool frequency or volume and an increase in the looseness of stool. Diarrhea may be acute or chronic. Acute diarrhea, most commonly results from infection diarrhea is considered chronic when it persists for atleast 2 weeks or when it subsides and returns more than 2 to 4 weeks after the initial episode. Chronic diarrhea is usually related to changes in the GI tract, that alter the fluid and electrolyte balance.

Box 10.7 Overview of diarrhea

Signs and symptoms	Frequent, watery stools Abdominal cramping Distention Anorexia Intestinal rumbling
Diagnostic tests	History Laboratory examinations of stool
Therapeutic measures	Replacement of fluids and electrolytes Antidiarrheal medications Antimicrobials Lactinex

Etiology

Causes of diarrhea can be divided into the general classification of decreased fluid absorption, increased fluid secretion, motility disturbances or a combination of them. The causes of diarrhea are:

i. Decreased fluid absorption
   - Oral intake of poorly absorbable solutes (e.g. Laxatives)
   - Maldigestion and malabsorption
     - Mucosal damage: Tropical sprue, Crohn's disease, radiation injury, ulcerative colitis, ischemic bowel disease
     - Pancreatic insufficiency
     - Intestinal enzyme deficiency (e.g. Lactase)
     - Bile salt deficiency
     - Decreased surface area (e.g. intestinal resection).

ii. Increased fluid secretion
   - Infections: Bacterial endotoxin (e.g. cholera, *E.coli, Shigella, Salmonella, Staphylococcus, Clostridium, Campylobacter jejuni*)
     - Viral agents (Rotavirus, HIV)
     - Parasitic agents, *Giardia lamblia, Cryptosporidium, Trichinella*, hookworm)
     - Drugs: Laxatives, antibiotics, suspension or elixirs containing sorbitol (e.g. acetaminophen)
     - Hormonal: Vasoactive intestinal polypeptide (VIP) secretion from adenoma of the pancreas, gastrin secretion caused by Zollinger-Ellison syndrome, calcitonin secretion from carcinoma of thyroid
   - Tumor: Villus adenoma.

iii. Motility disorders
   - Irritable bowel syndrome
   - Diabetic enteropathy
   - Visceral scleroderma
   - Carcinoid syndrome
   - Vagotomy.

The risk factors of acute diarrhea are:

- Recent travel to developing nations
- Outdoor camping
- Ingestion of raw meat, seafood, or shellfish
- Eating at banquets, restaurants, picnics, or fast food centers
- Day care placement of employment
- Residence in institutions, nursing homes, prisons or mental institutions
- Prostitution
- Intravenous drug abuse.

Pathophysiology

Large-volume diarrhea is caused by hypersecretion of water and electrolytes by the intestinal mucosa. This secretion occurs in response to the osmotic pressure exerted by non-absorbed food particles in the chyme or from direct irritation of the mucosa. Peristalsis increased, and the transit time through the intestine is significantly decreased. Increased peristalsis may result from inflammation as mucosal cells hypersecrete water in the presence of infectious organisms. Diarrhea may be accompanied by severe abdominal cramping, tenesmus (persistent spasm) of the anal area, abdominal distension and borborygmus (loud bowel sounds).

Fluid and electrolyte imbalances can quickly result from diarrhea, depending on its severity. Mild diarrhea in adults can lead to losses of sodium and potassium (causing metabolic alkalosis). Severe diarrhea causes dehydration, hyponatremia, hypokalemia and metabolic acidosis (from the loss of large amounts of bicarbonate). Malnourished or elderly persons tolerate severe diarrhea less well than do younger or well-nourished persons. Persistent diarrhea also readily leads to skin breakdown in the perianal region.

Clinical Manifestations

- Increased frequency and fluid content of stool
- Abdominal cramps, distention, intestinal rumbling (borborygmus), anorexia and thirst
- Painful spasmodic contractions of the anus and ineffectual straining (tenesmus) with each defecation.

Other symptoms, depending on the cause and severity and related to dehydration and fluid and electrolyte imbalanes, include:

- Watery stools, which may indicate small bowel disease
- Loose, semisolid stools, which are electrolyte with disorders of the colon
- Voluminous greasy stools, which suggest intestinal malaborption
- Mucus and pus in the stools, which denote inflammatory enteritis or colitis
- Oil droplets on the toilet water, which are diagnostic of pancreatic insufficiency
- Nocturnal diarrhea, which may be a manifestation of diabetic neuropathy.

Complications of diarrhea include cardiac dysrhythmias due to fluid and electrolyte (potassium) imbalance, urinary output less than 30 mL/h, muscle weakness, paresthesia, hypotension, anorexia, drowsiness (report if potassium level is less than 3 mEq/L [SI 3 mmol/L]), and death if imbalance become severe.

Bacterial or viral infection of the intestine may result in explosive water diarrhea, tenesmus (spasmotic contraction of anal sphincter with pain and persistent desire to defecate) and abdominal cramping pain, perianal skin irritation may also develop. Systemic manifestations include fever, nausea, vomiting and malaise, leukocytes blood and mucus may be present in the stool depending on the causative agent as given below:

i. Viral (Rotavirus Norwalk)

Onset is 18–24 hours and duration 24–48 hours shows signs and symptoms include explosive, water diarrhea, nausea, vomiting and abdominal cramps.

ii. Bacterial

- *Escherichia coli:* Onset 4 to 24 hours duration 3–4 days, signs and symptoms are four or five loose stools per day, nausea, malaise, low-grade fever
- Enterohemorrhagic *E.coli*: Onset 4–24 hours, duration 4–9 days signs and symptoms are bloody diarrhea, severe cramping, fever
- *Shigella:* Onset 24 hours duration 7 days, signs and symptoms are watery stool containing blood and mucus, tenesmus, urgency severe cramping and fever
- *Salmonella:* Onset 6–48 hours duration 2–5 days. Signs and symptoms are watery diarrhea, nausea, vomiting, abdominal cramps and fever
- *Campylobacter* species*:* Onset 24 hours duration less than 7 days. Signs and symptoms are profuse watery diarrhea, malaise, nausea abdominal cramps, low-grade fever
- *Clostridium perfringens:* Onset 8–12 hours duration 24 hours. Signs and symptoms are watery diarrhea, abdominal cramps, vomiting
- *Clostridium difficile:* Onset 4 days after start of antibiotics, duration 24 hours. It is associated with antibiotic treatment, symptoms range from mild, watery diarrhea to severe abdominal pain, fever, leukocytosis and leukocytes in stool.

All these are treated with proper antibiotics and antidiarrheal drugs.

iii. Parasitic

- *Entamoeba histolytica leads to amebiasis:* Onset 4-day duration weeks to months. Here ingested cyst releases active trophozite that invades and ulcerates intestinal mucosa. It can migrate to liver and cause abscesses. Clinical manifestations are: Abdominal cramping, frequent soft stools with blood and mucus (in severe cases watery stools), flatulence, distention fever, leukocytes in stool and reappearance of symptoms. It is treated by metronidazole for 5–10 days often in combination with other amebicides.
- *Giardia lamblia* leads to giardiasis. Here infested cyst releases active trophozoite that infects the small intestine and onset is 1–3 weeks and duration is a few days to 3 months shows sudden onset, malodorous, explosive, watery diarrhea, abdominal cramping and bloating, malabsorption in severe cases. Treatment self-limiting in 2–6 weeks but may recur. Quinacrine (Atabrin or flage for at least 2–10 cases).
- *Cryptosporidium* leads to cryptosporidiosis. The parasite is present in birds, fish, cattle, sheet and spread by person to

person contact and contaminated water. In which organism is ingested and primarily affects the small intestine. It can affect the entire GI tract in immunocompromised persons. It causes massive watery diarrhea, which exceeds 4 L/day, if persistent malabsorption may develop nausea and fatigue. Abdominal cramps, weight loss in AIDS for which no effective therapy is available. Supportive treatment, replacement of fluid and electrolyte.

- *Trichinella spiralis* causes trichinosis. It is due to ingestion of undercooked pork and pork products. In which larvae of round worms infect the meat and mature in the intestine. Larvae are then released into blood and lymphatics and pass into striated muscle of the host where they encyst. Early state symptoms include nausea, anorexia, cramping and diarrhea, muscle pain and fever develop in 2–8 weeks can involve jaw, eyes diaphragm and heart, for which only symptomatic treatment can be available. Use of mebendazole or thiabendazole is helpful.

Diagnostic Studies

Accurate diagnosis and management require a thorough history, physical examination and when indicated laboratory tests.

When cause is unknown: stool examination for infectious or parasitic organisms, bacterial toxins, blood, fat, and electrolytes, complete blood count, chemical profile, endoscopy, or barium enema.

Management

The management of diarrhea involves the prevention of fluid and electrolyte imbalance, controlling the symptoms and treating the underlying cause if possible (Table 10.7). Aggressive rehydration with oral replacement solutions is used if the person is alert and able to take oral fluids. Solutions such as the WHO solution, pedialyte, resol, and rehydralate are preferred to fruit juices, soda or even gatorade because they have balanced electrolyte composition plus glucose. Clear liquids are provided along with diets low in fiber but rich in sodium and glucose. Oral rehydration therapy with available standard ORS can be instituted.

- Primary medical management is directed at controlling symptoms, preventing complications, and eliminating or treating the underlying disease
- Certain medications (e.g. antibiotics, anti-inflammatory agents) may reduce the severity of diarrhea and the disease
- Increase oral fluid; oral glucose and electrolyte solution may be prescribed
- Antidiarrheals, such as diphenoxylate (Lomotil) and loperamide (Imodium), may be prescribed to decrease motility from a non-infectious source
- Antimicrobials are prescribed when the infectious agent has been identified or diarrhea is severe
- Intravenous therapy is used for rapid hydration in very young or elderly patients.

The use of antidiarrheal agents are variable. Common medication for treatment of acute diarrhea are:

i. Local Acting

- Bismuth sub-salicylate (Pepto Bismol) mechanism not known may bind bacterial toxin
- Kaolin and pectin (Kao pectate) which soothes the intestinal mucosa and increases absorption of water, nutrients and electrolytes.

These are in liquid form. So, shake well before using. Bismuth product may turn the stool black. No significant side effects with Kaolin and pectin.

ii. Systemic Acting Drugs

Include loperamide (imodium, tincture of opium (Paregoric), Diphenoxylate hydrochloride with atrophine (Lomotil). These drugs act systematically to reduce peristalsis and GI motility. Be aware that these drugs are part of the narcotic family; potential for addiction exists with paregoric. Loperamide has few side effects and no associated physical dependence. Lomotil has a low potential for dependency. So, monitor patient response, can enhance bacterial invasion and prolong excreation of the pathogen. Monitor for narcotic side effects-CNS depression or respiratory depression.

Nursing Management

Assessment

- Elicit a complete health history to identify character and pattern of diarrhea, and the following, any related sign and symptoms, current medication therapy, daily dietary patterns and intake, past related medical and surgical history, and recent exposure to an acute illness or travel to another geographic area
- Perform a complete physical assessment, paying special attention to auscultation (characteristic bowel sounds), palpation for abdominal tenderness, inspection of stool (obtain a sample for testing)
- Inspect mucous membranes and skin to determine hydration status, and assess blood pressure (postural hypotension)
- Inspect perianal skin for irritation
- Note intake and output and weight.

Nursing Diagnoses

- Diarrhea related to infection, ingestion of irritating foods, or disorder of the bowel

TABLE 10.7: Nursing care plan of patient with acute infectious diarrhea

Problem	Reason	Objective	Nursing intervention	Evaluation
1. Diarrhea related to acute infectious process	As manifested by frequent loose, watery stools	• Normal bowel elimination	• Monitor frequency, amounts, color, consistency of stools to determine severity and need for intervention • Record intake and output to monitor fluid balance • Follow hospital procedure for infection control precautions, use strict aseptic technique, while handling bedpan, linens or patient to prevent the spread of infection • Monitor vital signs 4th hourly as changes can indicate hypovolemia • Administer anti-infective and anti-diarrheal medication as ordered	
2. Fluid volume deficit related to excessive fluid loss and decreased fluid intake secondary to diarrhea	As manifested by dry skin and mucous membrane, poor skin turgor, hypotension, tachycardia, urine output, electrolye imbalance	• Normal vital signs and skin turgor • Moist mucous membrane • Urine output >0.5 mL/kg/h • Normal serum electrolytes	• Assess skin turgor changes, sunken eyes, rapid pulse and anorexia, as indicator of fluid volume deficit • Monitor intake and output • Monitor serum Na. K. level • Monitor vital signs 4th hourly • Weight patient daily to monitor fluid loss • Administer IV fluid as ordered • Assess dehydration, administer ORS. • Medicate with antidiarrheal drugs as ordered	
3. Impaired skin integrity related to perianal contact with diarrheal stools and inadequate perianal hygiene	As manifested by redness, irritation swelling, possible ulceration of skin pain during elimination	• No evidence of skin breakdown in perianal area	• Assess skin perianal area to plan appropriate interventions • Cleanse area with warm water each bowel movement rinse well and dry with a soft towel to prevent skin excoriation • Apply ointment (e.g. Alo, Zinc Oxide) to protect skin and promote healing • Use an anesthetic ointment or spray foam to decrease local discomfort	
4. Risk for infection transmission related to lack of knowledge about prevention of reinfection or transmission of infectious disease	–	• No recurrence of symptoms • Knowledgeable about disease process and preventive measures	• Teach the patient to be alert for recurrence of diarrhea, fever, and other presenting symptoms in family members • Assist patient in identifying factors that precipitated diarrhea to avoid cause of reinfection of self • Stress importance of seeking medical care where diarrhea and other symptoms present for early treatment	

- Risk for deficient fluid volume related to frequent passage of stools and insufficient fluid intake
- Anxiety related to frequent, uncontrolled elimination
- Risk for impaired skin integrity related to frequent, loose stools.

Collaborative Problems/Potential complications

- Dehydration
- Fluid and electrolyte imbalance
- Cardiac dysrhythmias.

Planning and Goals

Major goals include regaining normal bowel patterns, avoidance of fluid and electrolyte deficit, reduction of anxiety, maintenance of perianal skin integrity, and absence of complications.

Nursing Interventions

Controlling Diarrhea

- Encourage bed rest, liquids, and foods low in bulk until acute period subsides
- Recommend bland diet (semisolids to solids) when food intake is tolerated
- Encourage patient to limit intake of caffeine and carbonated beverage, and avoid very hot and cold foods because these increase intestinal motility
- Advise patient to restrict intake of milk products, fat, whole grain products, fresh fruits, and vegetables for several days
- Administer antidiarrheal drugs as prescribed.

Maintaining Fluid and Electrolyte Balance

- Assess for dehydration (decreased skin turgor, tachycardia, decreased pulse volume, decreased serum sodium, thirst)

- Administer intravenous fluids if ordered for rapid rehydration (in elderly patients or those with pre-existing gastrointestinal disturbance)
- Encourage oral fluid replacement in the form of water, juices, bouillon, and commercial preparations, such as Gatorade; give parenteral fluids as ordered
- Monitor serum electrolyte levels closely
- Report evidence of dysrhythmias or changes in level of consciousness immediately.

Reducing Anxiety

- Provide opportunity for patient to express fears or worry about being embarrassed by lack of control over bowel elimination
- Assist to identify any factors that precipitate diarrhea. Teach patient to be sensitive to body clues, use absorbent underwear, and take prescribed antianxiety medicaitns.

Providing Skin Care

- Instruct patient to follow a perianal care routine, such as wiping or patting the area dry after defecation, cleansing with mild soap and warm water, patting dry
- Apply lotion or ointment as a skin barrier; a skin sealant may be used
- Treat all patients with diarrhea as potentially infections; use gloves and standard precautions, as with all patients.

FECAL INCONTINENCE

Fecal incontinence or the involuntary passage of stool may be due to multiple causes.

Etiology

The causes for the fecal incontinence are:

i. Traumatic
   - Obstetric
   - Post-surgical
   - Hemorrhoidectomy
   - Anterior resection
   - Fistulectomy
   - Anorectal surgery
   - Spinal cord injury.

ii. Neurologic
   - Stroke
   - Tumor
   - Degenerative diseases
   - Iatrogenic drug intoxication
   - Multiple sclerosis
   - Diabetes mellitus
   - Dementia.

iii. Inflammatory
   - Infections
   - Trauma
   - Radiation.

iv. Other
   - Pelvic floor relaxation
   - Perineal descent
   - Loss of elasticity of rectum
   - Decreased sphincter tone (age relaxation)
   - Rectal prolapse
   - Focal impaction
   - Diarrhea
   - Medications.

Pathophysiology

Normally fecal contents pass from the sigmoid colon into the rectum, causing rectal distention. Sensory (stretch) receptors in the muscles surrounding the rectum provide the sensation of rectal filling. This causes a reflex relaxation of the internal anal sphincter and contraction of the external anal sphincter. Sensory receptors in the epithelium of the anal canal can usually distinguish among solid, liquid, and gas. The combination of contraction of the abdominal muscles, relaxation of the pelvic muscles, squatting (which straightens the anorectal angle) and voluntary relaxation of the external anal sphincter allows for elimination of feces.

Management

The diagnosis and effective management of fecal incontinence require a thorough health history and physical examinations with appropriate diagnostic studies (as per causes stated above.) The nurse should identify normal bowel habits and current symptoms, including frequency and nature of the stools. The nursing diagnosis of the patient with fecal incontinence are:

- Impaired skin integrity related to incontinence of stool and irritation in perianal area.
- Social isolation related to embarrassment and odor.
- Self-esteem disturbance related to inability to manage bowel evacuation independently.

The overall goal is that patient with fecal incontinence will have normal bowel control.

- Maintain perianal skin integrity and
- Not suffer any self-esteem problem.

Preventions and treatment of fecal incontinence may be managed by implementing a bowel-training program. The patient should be put on a bedpan, assisted to a bedside commode, or walked to the bathroom at a regular time daily to assist with re-establishment of bowel regularity. Bowel training is the major approach used with patients who have cognitive and neurological problems resulting from stroke or other chronic diseases. If a person can sit on a toilet, it may be possible to achieve automatic defecation when a pattern of consistent timing, familiar surroundings, and controlled diet and fluid intake can be achieved. This approach allows many patients to defecate predictable and remain continent throughout the day. Surgical correction is possible for small groups of patients whose incontinence is related to structural problems of the rectum and anus. Perianal pouching is an alternative in the management of fecal incontinence. Pouching provides skin protection and fecal containment as well as comfort and dignity. Since odor is a problem deodorant spray and room deodars can be used.

CONSTIPATION

The term 'constipation' refers to an abnormal infrequency of defecation or the passage of abnormally hard stools or both. It may be defined as a decrease of frequency of bowel movement from what is "normal" for the individual, hard, difficult-to-pass stools, a decrease in stool volume, and retention of feces in the rectum. An overview of constipation are given in Box 10.8.

Etiology

Constipation refers to an abnormal infrequency or irregularity of defecation, abnormal hardening of stools that makes their passage difficult and sometimes painful, decrease in stool volume, or prolonged retention of stool in the rectum. This type is referred to as colonic constipation. It can be caused by certain medications; rectal or anal disorders; obstruction; metabolic, neurologic, and neuromuscular condition; endocrine disorders; lead poisoning; connective tissue disorders; and a variety of disease conditions. Other causative factors include weakness, immobility, debility, fatigue, and inability to increase intra-abdomial pressure to pass stools. Constipation develops when people do not take the time to defecate or as the result of dietary habits (low consumption of fiber and inadequate fluid intake), lack of regular exercise, and a stress-filled life.

Box 10.8 A overview of constipation

Signs and symptoms	Abdominal distention Indigestion Rectal pressure Feeling of incomplete emptying Straining at stool Hard, dry stool Intestinal rumbling
Diagnostic test	History Physical examination
Therapeutic measures	High-fiber diet 2–3 L fluid daily Strengthening of abdominal muscles Exercise Bulk-forming agents Stool softeners

Perceived constipation is a subjective problem that occurs when an individual's bowel elimination pattern is not consistent with what he or she perceives as normal. Chronic laxative use contributes to this problem, particularly in elderly people.

Frequently constipation may be due to insufficient dietary fibers, inadequate fluid intake, medication use, and lack of exercise. It may be due to sociocultural beliefs. Chronic laxative abuse, and multiple organic causes as given further.

i. Colonic disorders
   - Luminal or extra-luminal obstructing lesions
   - Inflammatory strictures
   - Volvulus
   - Intussusception
   - Irritable bowel syndrome
   - Diverticular disease
   - Rectocele.

ii. Drug induced
   - Antacids (calcium and aluminium)
   - Antidepressants
   - Anticholinergics
   - Anticonvulsives
   - Antipsychotics
   - Antihypertensives
   - Barium sulfate
   - Iron supplements
   - Bismuth
   - Calcium supplements
   - Laxative abuse.

iii. Systemic disorders
   - Metabolic disorders: Diabetes mellitus, hypothyroidism, pregnancy, hypercalcemia, hyperparathyroidism
   - Collagen vascular disease: Scleroderma, amyloidosis
   - Neurogenic disorders:
     - Hirschsprung's megacolon
     - Neurofibromatosis
     - Autonomic neuropathy (psudo-obstruction)
     - Multiple sclerosis
     - Parkinson's disease
     - Spinal cord lesion or injury
     - Cerebrovascular accident.

Pathophysiology

Constipation may result from decreased motility of the colon or from retention of feces in the laser portion of the colon or rectum. Dietary fiber increases the water content of the stool, and colonic motility is enhanced through the bacterial degradation of the fiber.

The longer the feces remain in the colon, the greater the amount of water reabsorbed and the drier the stool becomes. The stool is then more difficult to expel. Occassionally constipation is not detrimental to health, but habitual constipation leads to decreased intestinal muscle tone, increased use of Valsalvas maneuver as the person bears down in the attempt to pass the hardened stool, and an increased incidence of hemorrhoids, in mass complication of chronic constipation. Diverticulosis is other complication.

Clinical Manifestations

- Abdomial distention, borborygmus (intestinal rumbling) pain, and pressure
- Decreased appetite, headache, fatigue, indigestion, sensation of incomplete emptying
- Straining at stool; elimination of small volume of hard, dry stool; fewer than three bowel movements per week
- Complications such as hypertension, hemorrhoids and fissures, fecal impaction and megacolon.

The clinical manifestation of constipation are:

- Hard, dry stool
- Increased flatulence
- Abdominal distention
- Nausea
- Decreased frequency of bowel movement
- Anorexia
- Headache
- Abdominal pain
- Palpable mass
- Straining
- Stool with blood
- Rectal pressure
- Urinary retention
- Tenesmus
- Dizziness.

Management of Constipation

Medical Management

Treatment should be aimed at the underlying cause of constipation.

- Discontinue laxative abuse; increase fluid intake; include fiber in diet; try biofeedback, exercise routine to strengthen abdominal muscles
- If laxative is necessary, use bulk-forming agents, saline and osmotic agents, lubricants, stimulants, or fecal softeners
- Specific medication therapy to increase intrinsic motor function (e.g. cholinergies or cholinesterase inhibitors).

Nursing Management

Assessment

Use tact and respect with patient when talking about bowel habits and obtaining health history. Note the following:

- Onset and duration of constipation, current and past elimination patterns, patient's expectation of normal bowel elimination, food and fluid intake, lifestyle, stress level, and occupation
- Current medications, history of laxative or enema use and past medical and surgical history
- Report of any of the following: rectal pressure or fullness, abdominal pain, straining at defecation, and flatulence.

Nursing diagnoses

- Colonic constipation or fecal impaction related to health habits or effect of immobility on peristalsis
- Deficient knowledge about health maintenance practices to prevent constipation.

Planning

Major goals of the patient may include a regular pattern of bowel elimination, adequate intake of fluids and high-fiber foods, knowledge of methods to avoid constipation, relief of anxiety about bowel elimination patterns and absence of complications.

A thorough history and physical examination should be performed so that the underlying causes of constipation can be identified and treatment started. Usual diagnostic studies can be followed accordingly.

Most causes of constipation can be managed by/with the diet therapy including dietary fiber and fluid and an exercise program. Laxatives should always be used cautiously because with chronic overuse, they may become a cause of constipation. The common cathartic agents used in constipation are:

i. Bulk forming agents absorb water, increase bulk, thereby stimulating peristalsis in which polysaccharides and cellulose derivatives mix with intestinal fluids, swell and stimulate peristalsis, e.g. psyllium, methyl cellulose. During its use, ensure adequate fluid intake to prevent impaction or obstruction. Take separately from presribed drugs to avoid problems with absorption.

ii. Emollients are stool softeners and lubricants, which lubricate intestinal tract and soften feces, making hard stools easier to pass, do not affect peristalsis, e.g. Docusate sodium, Docusate calcium. These docusate salts act as a detergent in the intestine, reducing surface tension, which facilitates the incorporation of liquid and fat, softening the stool. The preparations lose effectiveness with long-term use. Discontinue if abdominal cramping occurs.

iii. Lubricants, i.e. mineral oils, soften fecal matter by lubricating the intestinal mucosa, facilitating easy stool passage. Excessive use interfere with absorption of fat soluble Vitamin ADE and K leading to deficiency. These mineral oils should not take with meals or drugs, because oils can impair absorption, swallow carefully to prevent lipid aspiration.

iv. Hyperosmalar laxatives like lactulose, polyethyline glysol, sorbitol, which nonabsorbable sugars are degraded by colonic bacteria and increase stool osmolarity. Fluid is drawn into the intestine, stimulating peristalsis. When these are used, adjust the dose and frequency of administration to control side effects and regulate defection. Monitor for fluid and electrolyte imbalance if response is severe.

v. Saline laxatives cause osmotic retention of fluid which distends the colon and increases peristalsis, e.g. magnesium citrate, magnesium sulfate, magnesium hydroxide. The liquids preparations are more effective than tablets. Take with full glass of water. Monitor for fluid and electrolyte imbalance if response is severe.

vi. Stimulants increase peristalsis by irritating colon wall and stimulating enteric nerves, e.g. cascara sagrada, senna, bisacodyl (Dulcolax), castor oil. Cramps and diarrhea can occur. Monitor for fluid and electrolyte imbalance if reaction is severe.

Nursing management should be based on the patient symptoms and the assessment of the patient. An important role of the nurse is teaching the patient the importance of dietary measures to prevent constipation. The following are teaching guidelines for the patient with constipation:

i. Eat dietary fiber
   - Eat 20 to 30 grams of fiber per day. Gradually increase amount of fiber eaten over 1 to 2 weeks. Fiber softens hard stools and add bulk to stool, promoting, evacuation
   - Food high in fiber: Raw vegetable and fruits, beans.

ii. Drink fluids
   - Drink 3 quarts per day. Drink water or fruit juice, avoid coffee, tea and cola.

iii. Exercise regularly
   - Walk, swim, or bike at least three times per week
   - Contract and relax abdominal muscles when standing or by doing sit-ups to strengthen muscles and prevent straining
   - Exercises stimulates bowel motility and moves stools through the intestine.

iv. Set a regular time to defecate

v. Do not delay defecations
   - Response to the urge to have bowel movement as soon as possible
   - Delaying defecation results in hard stools and decreased 'urge' to defecate
   - Water is absorbed from stool by the intestine over time
   - The intestine becomes less sensitive to the presence of stool in the rectum.

vi. Record your bowel eliminating time

   Develop a habit of recording when you have a bowel movement on your calender. Regular monitoring of bowel movement will assist in early problem identification.

vii. Avoid laxatives and enemas

   Do not overuse laxatives and enemas as they can actually cause constipation. The normal motility of the bowel is interrupted and bowel movements slow or stop.

Teaching Patients Self-Care

- Teach patient to assume normal position for defecation (semisquatting) when possible (assist patient to a bedside commode)
- Explain the physiology of defecation and emphasize heeding the urge to defecate
- Discuss normal variations in patterns of defecation
- Teach patient how to establish a bowel routine (e.g. after breakfast)
- Provide dietary information; suggest eating high-residue, high-fiber food, adding bran daily (introduce gradually), and increasing fluid intake (unless contraindicated)
- Detail the benefits of an exercise regimen, increased ambulation and abdominal muscle toning
- Describe abdominal toning exercises: Contracting abdomen muscles four times daily and leg to chest lifts 10 to 20 times daily
- Encourage patient confined to bed to perform range-of-motion exercises, turn frequently from side-to-side, and lie prone (if not contraindicated) for 30 minutes every 4 hours.

ACUTE ABDOMEN

The patient with an acute abdomen has an acute onset of abdominal pain requiring prompt decision-making. Many disorders must be ruled out before a diagnosis is confirmed. Common sites of pain are shown in Figure 10.22.

Etiology

Causes of an acute abdomen are varied as follows:

- Abdominal penetrating trauma
- Acute ischemic bowel
- Appendicitis
- Bowel obstruction with perforation or necrosis
- Cholecystitis
- Crohn's disease
- Diverticulosis with peritonitis
- Foreign body perforation
- Gastritis
- Gastroenteritis
- Mesenteric adenitis
- Pancreatitis

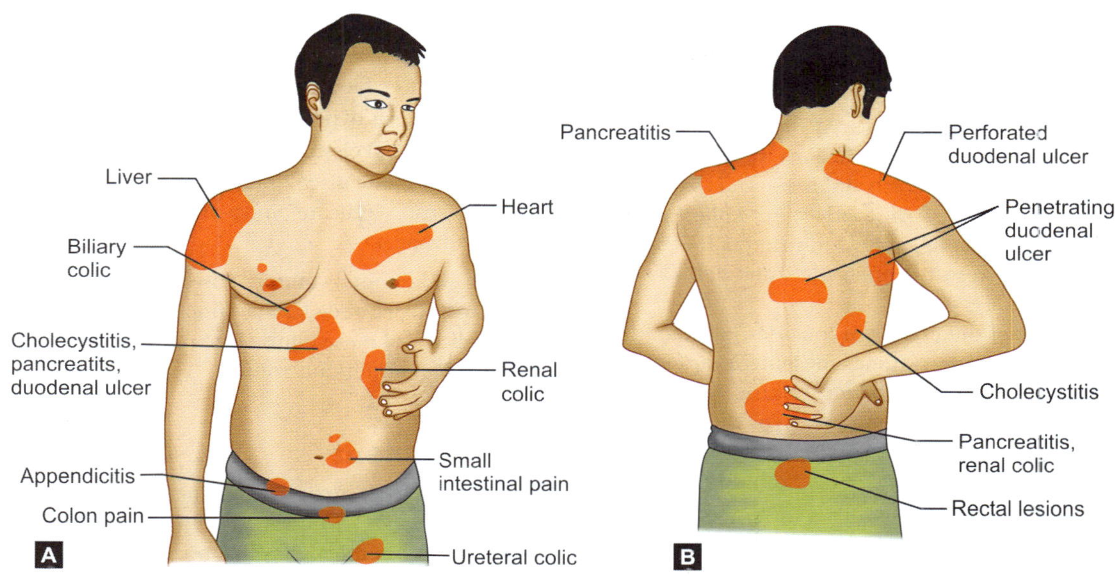

FIGS 10.22A AND B: Common sites of referred abdominal pain

- Pelvic inflammatory disease
- Perforated gastrointestinal malignancy
- Peritonitis
- Ruptured abdominal aneurysm
- Ruptured ectopic pregnancy
- Ruptured ovarian cyst
- Ulcerative colitis
- Uterine rupture
- Volvulus.

Clinical Manifestation

Pain is the most common presenting symptom. The patient also complains abdominal tenderness, vomiting, diarrhea, constipation, flatulence, fatigue, fever and increase in abdominal girth.

Management

Assessment begins with a complete history and physical examination including rectal and pelvic examination. CBC, urinalysis, abdominal X-ray, ECG, pregnancy test (for ladies) are also performed to get some clue for causes of acute abdomen. An assessment finding will include:

- Diffuse, localized, dull, burning or sharp, abdominal pain and tenderness
- Rebound tenderness
- Abdominal distention
- Abdominal rigidity
- Nausea, vomiting
- Diarrhea
- Hematemesis
- Melena.

In addition, signs and symptoms of hypovolemic shock:

- Decreased blood pressure
- Decreased pulse pressure
- Tachycardia
- Cool, clammy skin
- Decreased level of consciousness.

Acute abdomen requires an emergency management. The goal of which is to identify and treat the cause. Because many causes of which do not require surgery. An initial intervention will include:

- Ensure patent airway
- Administer oxygen via nasal cannula or nonbreather mask
- Establish IV access with large bore catheter and infuse warm normal saline or lactated Ringer's solution.

Insert additional large bore catheter if shock is present.

- Obtain blood for CBC; electrolytes
- Anticipate order for amylase, pregnancy test, clotting studies and type and crossmatch as appropriate
- Obtain urinalysis
- Insert nasogastric (NG) tube as needed
- Monitor vital signs, level of consciousness, O_2 saturation, intake and output
- Assess quality and amount of pain
- Anticipate surgical intervention
- Keep NPO.

ABDOMINAL TRAUMA

Injuries to the abdominal area most often occur as a result of blunt trauma or penetration injuries. (i) Blunt trauma usually occurs due to falls, motor vehicle collisions, pedestrian event, assault with blunt object, crash injuries and explosions. (ii) Penetrating injuries are due to stab, knife, gunshot wounds and other reasons. Regardless of whether it is blunt or penetration injury, the result is often the same damage to/or alteration of the internal organs.

Common injuries of the abdomen includes lacerated liver, ruptured spleen, pancreatic trauma, mesenteric artery tears, diaphragmatic rupture, urinary bladder rupture. These injuries may result in massive blood loss and hypovolemic shock. Surgery (laparotomy) is performed as early as possible to repair the damaged organs and to stop bleeding. Common sequelae of intra-abdominal trauma are peritonitis and massive infection, particularly when the bowel is perforated (Table 10.8).

Clinical Manifestation

The clinical manifestations of abdominal trauma are:

- Guarding and splinting of the abdominal wall
- A hard, distended abdomen (indicating intra-abdominal bleeding)
- Decreased or absent bowel sounds
- Contusions, abrasions or bruising over abdomen
- Abdominal pain
- Pain over the scapula caused by irritation of the phrenic nerve by free blood in the abdomen
- Hematemesis of hematuria and so
- Signs of hypovolemic shock
- An ecchymotic discoloration around the umbilicus (Cullen's sign) can indicate intra-abdominal or retroperitoneal hemorrhage.

Intra-abdominal injuries are often associated with rib fractures, feactured femur, fractured pelvis, and thoracic injury. If any of these injuries are present, the patient should be observed for abdominal trauma.

Management

Routine diagnostic procedures include CBC, urinalysis, X-ray of abdomen, CT scan and peritoneal lavage. For emergency management of the abdominal trauma focuses on establishing a patent airway, and adequate breathing fluid replacement and prevention of hypovolemic shock. The nursing intervention will include:

- Ensure patent airway
- Administer oxygen via non-breather mask
- Control external bleeding with direct pressure or sterile pressure dressing
- Establish IV access with large bore catheters and infuse warm normal saline or lactated Ringers solutions

TABLE 10.8: Nursing care plan for patient following laparotomy

Problem	Reason	Objective	Nursing intervention	Evaluation
1. Pain related to surgical incision and inadequate pain control measures	As manifested by complaints of pain, body posturing, unwillingness to move in bed or ambulate	Satisfactory level of pain control	• Assess for pain and give pain medications every 3 to 4 hours, as ordered for first 72 hours • Splint incision with pillow during coughing, deep breathing and moving to relieve pain while performing these activities • Position patient comfortable to relieve pain	
2. Nausea and vomiting related to decreased GI motility, GI distention and narcotics	As manifested by nausea, vomiting, lack of diminished bowel sounds. Abdominal distentions	• Relief of nausea, vomiting	• Administer antiemetic as ordered • Assess response to pain medication • Maintain patency of NG tube • Assess for bowel sounds and abdominal distention • Keep patient on NPO status until bowel sound returns • Limit unpleasant sights smells and stimuli to prevent initiate episodes of nausea and vomiting	
3. Constipation related to immobility, pain medication and G motility	As manifested by decreased or absent bowel sounds, abdomen pain, abdomen distention, inability to pass flatus or stool	• Normal bowel sounds within 72 hours • Soft-formed bowel movement within 4 days	• Assess abdomen for bowel sounds every shift to determine need for intervention • Administer cathartic as ordered if patient has not had bowel movement in 4 days • Encourage frequent position changes and ambulation as tolerated to increase peristalsis • Encourage increased fluid intake as tolerated to soften fecal material	

- Obtain blood for type and crossmatch and CBC
- Remove clothing
- Stabilize impaled objects with bulky dressing do not remove
- Cover protruding organs or tissue with sterile, saline dressing
- Insert indwelling urinary catherter if there is no blood at the meatus, pelvic fracture or boggy prostate
- Obtain urine for urinalysis
- Insert NG tube if no evidence of facial trauma
- Anticipate diagnostic peritonial lavage
- Monitor vital signs, level of consciousness, O_2 saturations and urine output
- Maintain patient's warmth using blankets, warm IV fluids or warm humidified oxygen.

Regardless of the mechanism of injury, physical evidence of abdominal trauma in a patient who is hemodynamically unstable mandates immediate laparotomy, for which routine preoperative procedure and postoperative intervention will be followed in addition to specific intervention.

APPENDICITIS

The appendix is a small, finger-like appendage attached to the cecum just below the ileocecal valve. Because it empties into the colon inefficiently and its lumen is small, it is prone to be coming obstructed and is vulnerable to infection (appendicitis). The obstructed appendix becomes inflamed and edematous and eventually fills with pus. It is the most common cause of acute inflammation in the right lower quadrant of the abdominal cavity and the most common cause of emergency abdominal surgery. Males are affected more than females, teenagers more frequently than adults; the highest incidence is in those between the ages of 10 and 30 years.

Appendicitis is an inflammation of the vermiform appendix, a narrow blind tube that extends from the inferior part of the cecum usually just below the ileocecal valve.

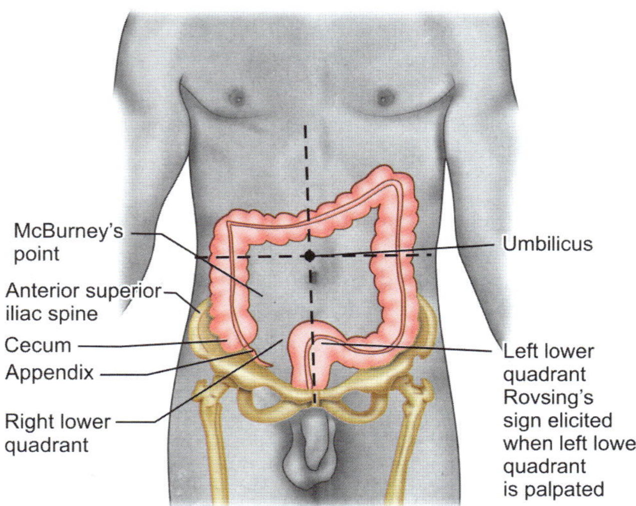

FIG. 10.23: When the appendix is inflamed, tenderness can be noted in the right lower quadrant at McBurney's point, which is between the umbilicus and the anterior superior iliac spine, Rovsing's sign is pain felt in the right lower quadrant after the left lower quadrant has been palpated

Etiology

The most common causes of appendicities are obstructions of the lumen by a fecalith (accumulated feces), foreign bodies, tumor of the cecum or appendix, or intramural thickening caused by lymphoid hyperplasia.

Pathophysiology

The inflammatory process of the appendicitis can involve all or part of the appendix. Intraluminal pressure increases, leading to occlusion of the capillaries and venules and vascular engorgement. Bacterial invasion follows and microabscesses may develop in the appendiceal wall or surrounding tissue, which, unless treated, can progress to gangrene and perforation within 24 to 36 hours. If the inflammatory process develops fairly, slowly the infection may be successfully be walled off in a local abscess. In more rapidly developing cases, the risk of rupture and acute peritonitis is quite high (Figs 10.23 to 10.25).

Clinical Manifestations

The clinical manifestations of appendicits is abdominal pain that comes in waves. The pain is persistent and continuous, eventually shifting to the right lower quadrant and localizing at McBurney's point (located half way between the umbilicus and the right iliac crest). It typically begins with periumbilical pain, followed by anorexia, nausea and vomiting. Further assessment of the patient reveals localized tenderness, rebound tenderness and muscle guarding. The patient usually prefers to lie still,

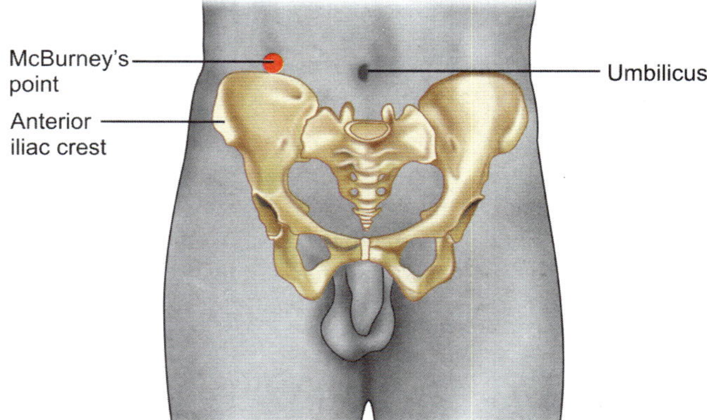

FIG. 10.24: Pain at McBurney's point is a symptom of appendicitis

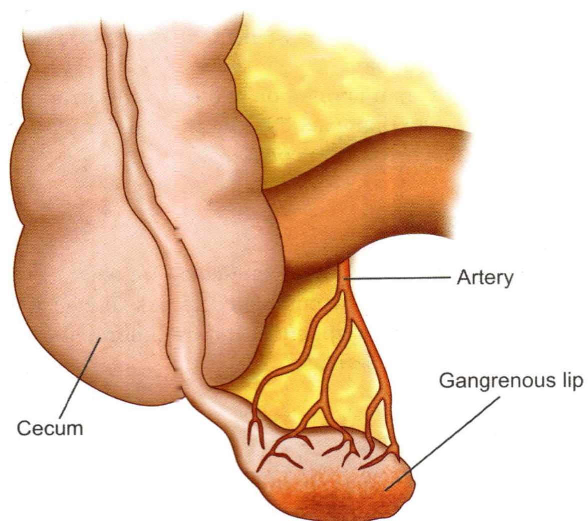

FIG. 10.25: In appendicitis the blood suppy of the appendix is impaired by inflammation and bacterial infection in the wall of the appendix, which may result in gangrene

often with right leg flexed. Low-grade fever may or may not be present, and coughing aggravates pain. Rovsing's sign may be elicited by palpation of the left lower quadrants, cauing pain to be felt in the right lower quadrant, complications of acute appendicities are performation, peritonitis and abscesses. In brief the symptoms includes:

- Lower right quadrant pain usually accompanied by low-grade fever, nausea, and sometimes vomiting
- At McBurney's point (located halfway between the umbilicus and the anterior spine of the ilium), local tenderness with pressure and some rigidity of the lower portion of the right rectus muscle
- Rebound tenderness may be present; location of appendix dictates amount of tenderness, muscle spasm and occurrence of constipation or diarrhea
- Rovsing's sign (elicited by palpating left lower quadrant, which paradoxically causes pain in right lower quardrant)
- If appendix ruptures, pain becomes more diffuse; abdominal distention develops from paralytic ileus, and condition worsens.

In the elderly, signs and symptoms of appendicitis may vary greatly. Signs may be very vague and suggestive of bowel obstruction of another process; some patients may experience no symptoms until the appendix ruptures. The incidence of perforated appendix is higher in the elderly because many of these people do not seek health care as quickly as younger people.

Management

The diagnosis of appendicits is made from the classic physical and laboratory indicators when they are present. The patient with abdominal pain is advised to see physician and to avoid self-treatment. Until then the patient is advised not to take anything by mouth (NPO) to ensure that stomach is empty in the event of surgery is needed. An icebag may be applied to the right lower quadrant to decrease the flow of blood to the area and impede the inflammatory process. Heat is never used because it may cause appendix to rupture.

Surgery is usually performed as soon as a diagnosis is made. Pre and postoperative nursing management is similar to that of patients after laparotomy or any surgical treatment. In addition, patient should be observed for evidence of peritonitis.

Medical Management

- Surgery (conventional or laparoscopic) is indicated if appendicitis is diagnosed and should be performed as soon as possible to decrease risk of perforation
- Administer antibiotics and intravenous fluids until surgery is performed
- Analgesic agents can be given after diagnosis is made.

Complications of appendectomy

- The major complication is preformation of the appendix, which can lead to peritonitis or an abscess
- Perforation generally occurs 24 hours after onset of pain; symptoms include fever (37.7°C [100°F] or greater), toxic appearance and continued pain or tenderness.

Nursing management

- Nursing goals include relieving pain, preventing fluid volume deficit, reducing anxiety, eliminating infection due to the potential or actual disruption of the gastrointestinal tract, maintaining skin integrity and attaining optimal nutrition
- Preoperatively, prepare patient for surgery, start intravenous line, administer antibiotic, and insert nasogastric tube (if evidence of paralytic ileus). Do not administer an enema or laxative (could cause perforation)
- Postoperatively, place patient in high Fowler's position, give narcotic analgesic as ordered, administer oral fluids when tolerated, give food as desired on day of surgery (if tolerated). If dehydrated before surgery, administer intravenous fluids
- If a drain is left in place at the area of the incision, monitor carefully for signs of intestinal obstruction, secondary hemorrhage or secondary abscesses (e.g. fever, tachycardia, and increased leukocyte count).

Teaching Patients Self-Care

- Teach patient and family to care for the wound and perform dressing changes and irrigations as prescribed
- Reinforce need for follow-up appointment with surgeon
- Discuss incision care and activity guidelines

- Refer for home care nursing as indicated to assist with care and continued monitoring of complications and wound healing.

PERITONITIS

Peritonitis involves either a local or generalized inflammation of the peritoneum, the membranous lining of the abdomen, that covers the viscera. Peritonitis may be primary or secondary, aseptic or septic and acute or chronic.

Peritonitis, inflammation of the peritoneum, is usually the result of bacterial infection, with the organisms coming from disease of the gastrointestinal tract, or, in women, the internal reproductive organs. It can also result from external sources, such as injury or trauma or an inflammation from an extraperitoneal organ, such as the kidney.

Etiology (Fig. 10.26)

Primary peritonitis usually caused by bacterial infection, bloodborne organism, genital tract organism and cirrhosis with ascitis. Whereas secondary peritonitis often results from trauma, surgical injury or chemical irritations, which includes ruptured appendix, perforated peptic ulcer, diverticulitis, pelvic inflammatory disease, urinary tract infections, or trauma bowel obstructions and surgical complications.

Peritonitis may appear in acute or chronic forms, and trauma or rupture of an organ containing chemical irritants or bacteria, which are released into peritoneal cavity, e.g. gastric ulcer perforations and ruptured ectopic pregnancy. Bacterial peritonitis can be caused by a traumatic injury (e.g. gunshot wound ruptured appendix) or it can be secondary to other diseases or conditions (e.g. pancreatitis, peritoneal dialysis).

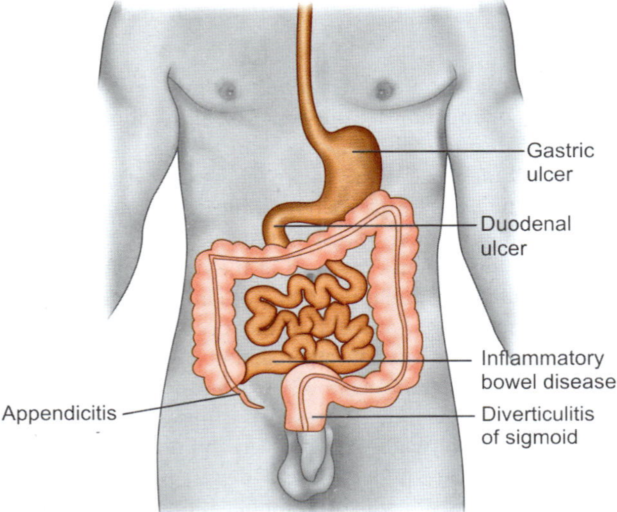

FIG. 10.26: Common gastrointestinal causes of peritonitis

Pathophysiology

Peritonitis is caused by leakage of contents from abdominal organs into the abdominal cavity, usually as a result of inflammation infection, ischemia, trauma or tumor perforation. The most common bacteria implicated are *Escherichia coli,* and *Klebsiella, Proteus,* and *Pseudomonas* species. Other common causes are appendicitis, perforated ulcer, diverticulitis and bowel perforation. Peritonitis may also be associated with abdominal surgical procedures and peritoneal dialysis. Sepsis is the major cause of death from peritonitis (shock, from sepsis or hypovolemia). Intestinal obstruction from bowel adhesions may develop.

The peritoneal lining serves as a semipermeable membrane lining that allows the flow of water and electrolytes between the blood stream and peritoneal cavity. When peritonitis occurs, fluid can shift into the abdominal cavity at a rate of 300 to 500 mL/h in response to acute inflammation. The inflammatory process also shunts extra blood to the inflammed areas of the bowel to contract the secondary bacterial infection and peristalsis typically ceases. The bowel increasingly becomes distended with gas and fluid. The circulatory fluid and electrolyte changes can rapidly become critical. Local reaction of the peritoneum include redness and inflammation and the production of large amounts of fluid that contains electrolytes and proteins. Hypovolemia, electrolyte imbalance, dehydration, and finally shock can develop. This loss of circulatory volume is proportional to the severity of peritoneal involvement. The fluid usually becomes purulent as the condition progresses and as the bacteria becomes more numerous. The bacteria also may enter the blood and cause septicemia.

Clinical Manifestation

Clinical features depend on the location and extent of inflammation.

- Diffuse pain becomes constant, localized and more intense near site of the process
- Pain is aggravated by movement
- Affected area of the abdomen becomes extremety tender and distended, and muscles become rigid
- Rebound tenderness and ileus may be present
- Temperature and pulse increase; leukocyte count is elevated
- Nausea and vomiting occur and peristalsis is diminished.

Abdominal pain is the most common symptom of peritonitis. A universal sign of peritonitis is tenderness over the involved area. Rebound tenderness, muscular rigidity and spasm are other major signs of irritation of the peritoneum. Abdominal distentions, or ascitis, fever, tachycardia, tachypnea, nausea, vomiting, altered bowel habits may also be present. These manifestations vary depending on severity and acuteness of the underlying cause. Complications of peritonitis include hypovlemic shock, septicemia, intra-abdominal abscess, formation, paralytic ileus, and organ failure.

Diagnostic Studies

- Leukocytes (elevated), complete blood count, hemoglobin hematocrit and serum electrolytes (altered potassium, sodium and chloride)
- Abdominal X-rays, computed tomography (CT) scan and peritoneal aspiration with culture and sensitivity studies
- Serum electrolytes
- Abdominal X-ray
- Abdominal paracentesis and culture of fluid
- CT scan or ultrasound and
- Peritonoscopy.

Management

The goal of management of peritonitis are to identify and eliminate the cause, combat infection and prevent complications. Patients with milder cases of peritonitis or those who are poor surgical risks may be managed non-surgically. Treatment consists of antibiotics, NG suction, analgesics and IV fluid administration.

Medical Management

- Fluid, colloid and electrolyte replacement with an isotonic solution is the major focus of medical management
- Analgesics are administered for pain, antiemetics are administered for nausea and vomiting
- Intestinal intubation and suction are used to relieve abdominal distention
- Oxygen therapy by nasal cannula or mask is instituted to improve ventilator function
- Occasionally, airway intubation and ventilator assistance are required
- Massive antibiotic therapy may be instituted (sepsis is the major cause of death)
- Surgical objectives include removal of infected material surgery is directed toward excision (appendix), resection (intestine), repair (perforation) or drainage (abscess).

Nursing Management

Pain Assessment

- Assess nature of pain, location in the abdomen and shifts of pain and location
- Assess vital signs, gastrointestinal function, fluid and electrolyte balance
- Monitor central venous and pulmonary artery pressures frequently
- Administer analgesic medication and position for comfort (e.g. on side with knees flexed to decrease tension on abdominal organs)
- Record intake and output and central venous pressure
- Administer and monitor intravenous fluids closely
- Observe and record character of any surgical drainage
- Observe for decrease in temperature and pulse rate, softening of the abdomen, return of peristaltic sound, and passage of flatus and bowel movements, which indicate peritonitis is subsiding
- Increase food and oral fluids gradually and decrease parenteral fluid intake when peritonitis subsides
- Observe and record character of drainage from post-operative wound drains if inserted; take care to avoid dislodging drains
- Postoperatively, prepare patient and family for discharge; teach care of incision and drains if still in place at discharge.

Patient who requires surgery need preoperative preparation as described earlier. Those patiens may need total parenteral nutrition (TPN) because of increased nutrition requirement. Postoperative nursing management is similar to that provided for any surgical patient who has undergone abdominal surgery.

DIVERTICULITIS

Diverticula are small outpouchings or herniation of the mucosal lining of the gastrointestinal track. Diverticulosis has been described as a disease of west because its higher incidence in developed countries. The incidence of the disease should wide geographic variation that are at least partly attributable to the quantity of non-absorbable dietary fiber. Low-fiber diets have been shown to increase intraluminal pressure in the bowel but aging also appears to change the composition of the bowel which decreases its tensile strength.

Etiology

A diverticulum is a sac-like outpouching or herniation of the lining of the bowel (the mucosa and submucosa) that protrudes through as weak portion of the muscle layer. Diverticula may occur anywhere along the gastrointestinal tract. Diverticulosis exists when multiple diverticula are present without inflammation or symptoms. Diverticulitis results when food and bacteria retained in the diverticulum produce infection and inflammation that can impede draining and lead to perforation or abscess. It may occur in aute attacks or persist as a chronic, smoldering infection. Diverticulitis is more common in the sigmoid colon. A congenital predisposition is likely when the disorder is present in those younger than 40 years of age. Diverticulosis is most common in people older than 60 years of age. A low intake of dietary fiber is considered a major predisposing factor. Complications of diverticulitis include fistulas, obstruction, peritonitis, abscess formation, and bleeding.

Pathophysiology

Diverticula tend to form at point in the colon wall where blood vessels penetrate the mucosal and muscular layers, creating points of relative weakness. The increased muscular contractions in the sigmoid colon that are generated to push stool in the rectum increase both the thickness of the muscle and the intraluminal pressure. The weaker connective tissue then herniates between the circular muscle and the intraluminal pressure, the weaker connective tissue then herniates between the circular muscle band and forms the diverticula.

Diverticulitis frequently develops in a single diverticulum in response to irritation initiated by trapped fecal material. Blood supply to the area decreases and bacteria proliferates in the obstructed diverticulum. Perforation of the dome may occur, which, if small is usually quickly and effectively walled off. Large perforation may progress to abscess formation or general peritonitis. Generalized inflammation can result in thickening and scarring of the bowel wall (Figs 10.27 and 10.28).

Clinical Manifestations

Usually diverticular disease is asymptomatic, but mild inflammation can trigger a nonspecific bowel dysfunction that resolves in a matter of hours or days. The clinical manifestations of diverticulitis reflect the inflammation of the diverticula or the developments of complication. Cramps lower left quadrant abdominal pain accompanied by low grade fever in classic sign.

Diverticulosis

- Frequently, no problematic symptoms are noted; constipation from spastic colon syndrome often precedes development
- Bowel irregularity and diarrhea
- Crampy pain in left lower quadrant
- Low-grade fever
- Nausea and anorexia and some bloating or abdominal distention.

Diverticulitis

- Narrowing of the large bowel with fibrotic stricture
- Cramps, narrow stools and increased constipation
- Occult bleeding
- Weakness, fatigue and anorexia
- Tenderness, a palpable mass, fever and leukocytes, which may indicate abscess development
- Abdominal pain, a rigid boardlike abdomen, loss of bowel sounds, and signs and symptoms of shock, which may indicate peritonitis
- Septicemia if condition remains untreated.

The pain is triggered by muscle spasms of the sigmoid colon and is acute and persistent in nature. Nausea, vomiting, and a feeling of bloating are also common. The inflammatory process also frequently involves the bladder and cause urinary symptoms. The development of abscess initiates the symptoms of localized peritonitis. Diverticular disease is one of the most common causes of GI bleeding. Meckel's diverticulum is a congenital abnormality in which a blind tube, similar in structure to the appendix is present, which is usually open into the distal ileum near the ileocecal valve. The tube may be attached to the umbilicus by a fibrous band (Fig. 10.29).

Management

The preliminary diagnosis of diverticulitis may be made from the history and presenting symptoms. CT scan, barium

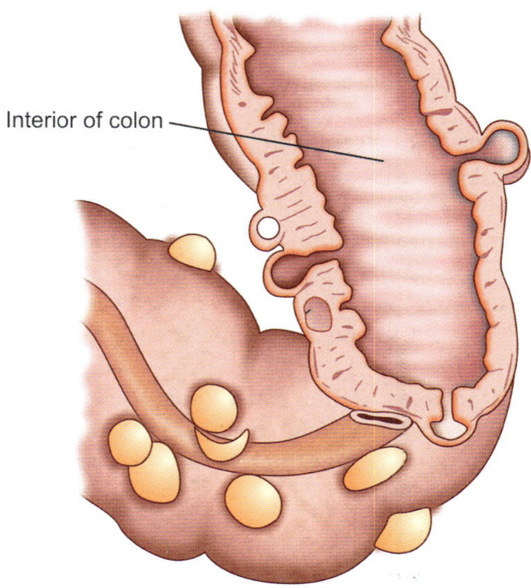

FIG. 10.27: Diverticula are outpouchings of the colon. When they become inflamed, the condition is diverticulitis. The inflammatory process can spread to the surrounding area in the intestine

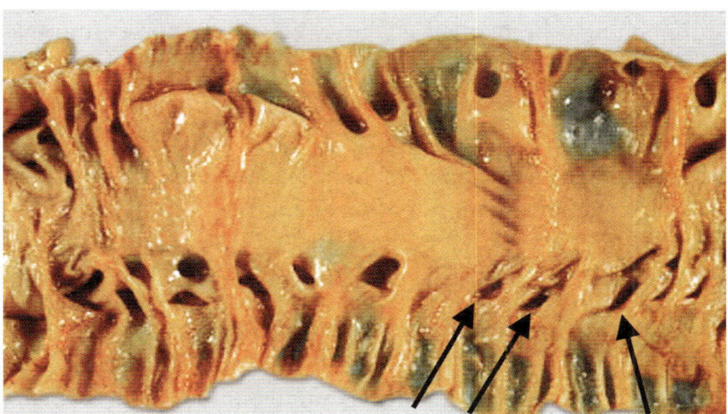

FIG. 10.28: In diverticular disease, the outpouches (arrows) of mucosa appear as slitlike opening from the mucosal surface of the open bowel

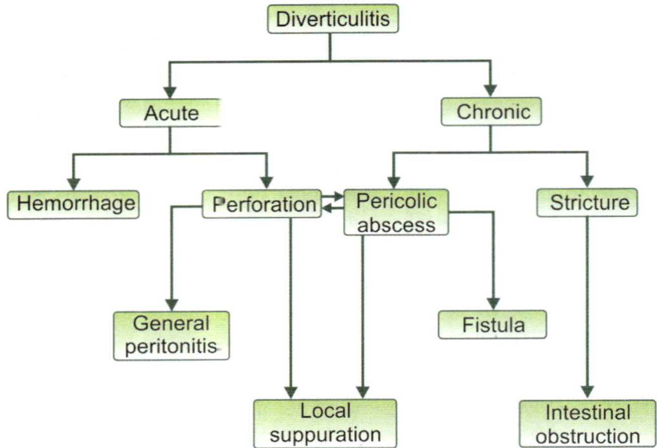

FIG. 10.29: Complications of diverticulitis

enema reveals presence of abscess and diverticular pouches respectively.

An episode of diverticulitis is managed by resting the bowel. Hospitalization may be required in acute episodes. The patient is given nothing by mouth and regimen of IV fluids, antibiotics, anticholinergic (Pro-Banthine) is started to reduce bowel spasm. Mild cases managed at home environment. Acute diverticulitis usually subsides with conservative medical management. However, surgical intervention may be needed to deal with complications.

The major goals of the patient may include attainment and maintenance of normal elimination, reduction in pain, improvement in gastrointestinal tissue perfusion and absence of potential complications.

Nursing Interventions

Maintaining Normal Elimination Patterns

- Increase fluid intake to 2 L/day within limits of patient's cardiac and renal reserve
- Promote foods that are soft but have increased fiber content
- Encourage individualized exercise program to improve abdominal muscle tone
- Review patient's routine to establish a set time for meals and defecation
- Encourage daily intake of bulk laxatives (e.g. Metamucil, stool softeners, or oil-retention enemas).

Relieving Pain

- Administer analgesic agents (usually opioid analgesics) for pain and antispasmodic medications
- Record and monitor intensity, duration and location of pain.

Monitoring and Managing Potential Complications

- Identify patients at risk
- Assess for indicators of perforation: Tender, rigid abdomen; elevated white blood cell count; elevated sedimentation rate; increased temperature; tachycardia and hypotension
- Perforation is a surgical emergency: Monitor vital signs and urine output, and administer intravenous fluids as ordered.

Nursing care during an acute episode is largely supportive and focussed on patient comfort. The nurse teaches rationale for bed rest and bowel rest and the role of their interventions play in bowel healing. The nurse monitors fluid and electrolytes balance and status of the pain. The patient is regularly assessed for complications. Asymptomatic diverticulosis is managed by prevention of constipation through the use of a high-fiber diet. Encourage mere fluid intake (2,500 mL to 3,000 mL/day). Diet modification may be made by allowing foods high in fiber with emphasis on cellulose and hemicellulose type (wheat, whole grain breads and cereals, peas, carrots, seedless grapes, lettuce, peaches, prunes) and avoiding foods containing nuts and seeds, or indigestible strings or threads (cucumbers, celery, tomatoes, cornpop, strawberries, raspberries, peanuts and seeds). The patient is also encouraged to avoid activities that increase intra-abdominal pressure. Weight loss may be recommended in the attempt to lower the baseline levels of intra-abdominal pressure.

INFLAMMATORY BOWEL DISEASE (IBD)

Inflammatory is an umbrella term used to describe conditions that are characterized by bowel inflammation. Crohn's disease and ulcerative colitis are the two major forms of IBD. They have distinctly different pathological characteristics but share among overlapping features. An overview of IBD (Box 10.9).

Box 10.9 Overview of inflammatory bowel disease

Signs and symptoms	Abdominal pain or cramping Wight loss Diarrhea Fluid and electrolyte imbalance Fissures, fistulas, abscesses Arthritis and skin lesions Inflammatory eye disorders
Diagnostic test	Abnormal liver function Endoscopy with biopsy Barium enema Laboratory examination Stool examination Absent bowel sounds
Therapeutic measures	Medications: anti-inflammatories, antidiarrheal, antibiotics, immunosuppressants, corticosteroids Surgery if necessary Avoidance of offending foods Elemental formula or TPN if required

Etiology

Exact cause is unknown. The passive causes include:

- An infectious agent (bacteria, virus)
- An autoimmune reaction from the presence of immune-related disorder
- Food allergies
- Heredity.

ULCERATIVE COLITIS

Ulcerative colitis is a recurrent ulcerative and inflammatory disease of the mucosal and submucosal layer of the colon and rectum. It is a serious disease, accompanied by systemic complications and a high mortality rate; eventually, 10% to 15% of the patients develop carcinoma of the colon. It is characterized by multiple ulcerations, diffuse inflammations, and desquamation of the colonic epithelium, with alternating periods of exacerbation and remission. Bleeding occurs from the ulceration and the mucosa becomes edematous and inflamed, with continuous lesions and abscesses. Ulcerative colitis most commonly affects Caucasian people, including people of Jewish heritage, and peaks in the third fifth decade of life.

Ulcerative colitis characterized by inflammation and ulceration of the colon and rectum. It may occur at any age but peaks between the ages of 15 and 25 years. There is a second, smaller peak onset between 50 and 80 years. It affects both sexes but has higher incidence in women.

Pathophysiology

The inflammation of ulcerative colitis is diffuse and involves the mucosa and submucosa. With alternate periods of exacerbations and remissions the disease is usually begun in the rectum and sigmoid colon and spreads up the colon in a continuous pattern. The mucosa of the colon is hyperemic and edematous in the affected area. Multiple abscesses develop in the crypts of the Lieberkühn (intestinal gland). As the disease advances the abscesses break through the crypts into the submucosa, leaving ulceration. These ulcerations also destroy the mucosal epithelium, causing bleeding and diarrhea. Losses of fluid and electrolytic occur because of the diseased mucosal surface area of absorption. Breakdown of cells results in protein loss through the stools. Areas of inflamed mucosa form pseudopolyps, tongue-like projection and the bowel lumen. Granulation tissue develops and the mucosa musculature becomes thickened, shortening in colon (Fig. 10.30).

Clinical Manifestations

- Predominant symptoms: diarrhea, abdominal pain, intermittent tenesmus, ineffective straining at stool, and rectal bleeding
- Pallor, if bleeding is severe

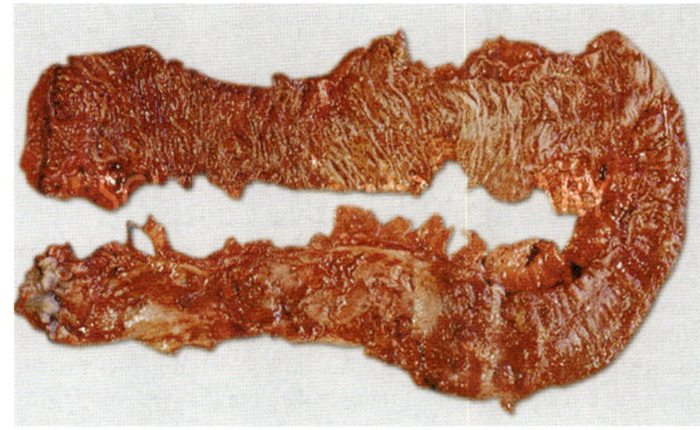

FIG. 10.30: Acute ulcerative colitis. Colitis with extensive mucosal ulceration involving the engine colon

- Anorexia, weight loss, fever, vomiting, dehydration, cramping, and feeling an urgent need to defecate (may report passing 10 to 20 liquid stools daily)
- Hypocalcemia and anemia
- Rebound tenderness in right lower quadrant
- Skin lesions eye lesions (uveitis), joint abnormalities and liver diseases
- Anorexia, nausea and weight loss
- Weakness and malaise
- Fever and leucocytosis (high fever and WBC more than 15000/mw suggest abscess)
- Iron deficiency anemia
- Profuse diarrhea (15–20 stool/day)
- Stools containing blood, mucus and possibly pus
- Abdominal cramping can be present before the bowel movements
- Loss of fluid, sodium, calcium, potassium and bicarbonate.

The complications of ulcerative colitis be classified into those that are intestinal and those that are extraintestinal. Intestinal include hemorrage, strictures perforation, toxic megacolon and colonic dilation. An extraintestinal complication of ulcerative colitis are:

- Joints involvement large joints, hips, ankles, wrists, elbows, peripheral arthritis, ankylosing, spondylitis, sacroiliitis and finger clubbing
- Skin—erythema nodosum, pyoderma gangrenosum
- Mouth—apthous ulcers
- Eye—conjunctivitis, uveitis, episcleritis
- Hepatocholelithiasis, fatty liver, cirrhosis, cholangitis
- Renal kidney stones, ureteral obstruction.

Diagnostic Studies

- Fiberoptic colonoscopy

- Sigmoidoscopy
- Barium enema
- CBC
- Stool for blood, culture and sensitivity.

Management of Ulcerative Colitis

Medical Management

Medical treatment for both regional enteritis and ulcerative colitis is aimed at reducing inflammation, suppressing inappropriate immune responses and providing rest for the diseased bowel so that healing may take place.

Nutritional Therapy

Initial therapy consists of diet and fluid management with oral fluids; low-residue, high-protein, high-calorie diets; supplemental vitamin therapy and iron replacement. Fluid and electrolyte balance may be corrected by intravenous therapy. Additional treatment measures include smoking cessation and avoiding foods that exacerbate symptoms, such as milk and cold foods. Parenteral nutrition (PN) may be provided as indicated.

Pharmacologic Therapy

- Sedative, antidiarrheal and antiperistaltic medications
- Sulfonamides: Sulfasalazine (Azulfidine) or sulfisoxaole (Gantrisin), which are effective for mild or moderate inflammation
- Antibiotics for secondary infections
- Adrenocorticotropic hormore (ACTH) and corticosteroids
- Aminosalicylates (topical and oral), including newer sulfa-free (mesalamine [Asacol, Pentasa])
- Immunomodulator agents (e.g. Imuran)

Psychotherapy

Psychotherapy is aimed at determining the factors that distress the patient, coping with these factors, and attempting to resolve.

The goals of treatment are to rest the bowel, control the inflammation, combat infection, correct malnutrition, alleviate stress and symptomatic relief using drug therapy. The common drugs used for IBD are:

i. Aminosalicylates (oral) are converted in colon to sulfapyridine and 5-amino salicylic acid, which may exert an anti-inflammatory effect, possibly through prostaglandin inhibition (e.g. azulfidine, olslazine, mesalamine). During this medications, nurse has to assess for allergy to sulfonamides or aspirins. Monitor for common side effects, anorexia, nausea, vomiting and headache and teach patients to take the drug in divided doses with full glass of fluid or with food. Maintain a liberal intake and report incidence of sit in rash or other adverse effects.

ii. Aminosalicylates (rectal) has same actions as stated in oral. Drugs used are mesalamine in suspension for retention enema and mesalamine suppository. Administer enema while patient is positioned on left side and teach patient to retain as long as possible.

iii. Corticosteroids (oral/IV) has potent systemic anti-inflammatory action, e.g. prednisolone/prednisone. During medication, teach patient to; take with food or fluid, monitor weight gain; assess for edema; Be alert to signs of infection and report promptly, discontinue drug. Maintain good personal hygiene and keep perianal area clean and dry.

iv. Corticosteroid (rectal) has same effect in oral or IV, e.g. hydrocortisone intrarectal foam (Cortifoam), retentive enema (cortenema). Budesonide enema has rapid presystemic metabolism minimizes absorption in addition to above actions. Hence, administer enema while patient is positioned on left side and teach patient to retain as long as possible. Other interventions as stated above, side effects should be less.

v. Immunosuppressive agents have potent systemic suppressors of immune response; may take 4–6 months for full effect, e.g. mercaptopurine (Purinethol), azathioprine (Imuran). During these medications, teach patient to report any signs of infection; be alert to easy bruising. Return for lab work as scheduled. Maintain liberal daily fluid intake with food or after meals. Another drug cyclosporine (Sandimmune) is oral solution. It may be mixed in glass and given with milk or orange juice at room temperature. Avoid refrigeration. Teach patient to monitor blood pressure; report hematuria or any change in urinary infection.

Surgical Management

When nonsurgical measures fail to relieve the severe symptoms of inflammatory bowel disease, surgery may be recommended (segmental, subtotal or total colectomy). A fecal diversion may be needed, such as ileostomy, continent ileal reservoir (Kock pouch), or ileoanal anastomosis. Strictureplasty or fecal diversions may be needed (e.g. ileal reservoir, ileoanal anastomosis). Proctocolectomy with ileostomy (excision of colon, rectum, and anus) may be performed if rectum is severely involved. A recently developed option may be intestinal transplantation, especially for children and young adults who have lost intestinal function because of the disease.

Surgical intervention may be selected for patients with incurable colitis whose disease cannot be satisfactorily controlled with standard medical management. This procedure is curative in nature and involves removal of the entire colon, i.e. Brook ileostomy, Dr Nils Kocks, continent ileostomy, ileoanal anastomosis, or ileorectostomy, ileoanal reservoir.

The drugs used are:

- Sulfasalazine
- Corticosteroids and
- Immunosuppressive agents (6-MP, azathioprine).

The dosage and the routes of administration depend on the severity of the illness and the area involved. The elemental diet and parenteral nutrition may be used. Parenteral nutrition for severe cases, small bowel fistulas, small bowel syndrome. It is given to promote healing and reduce complications. The elemental diet provides a high caloric, high nitrogen, fat free, no residue substrate that is absorbed in the proximal small bowel. Vitamin deficiency may develop. Vitamin B_{12} injection may be used.

Surgical intervention is avoided in Crohn's disease as much as possible because of recurrence of the disease process in same region is virtually inevitable.

The nurse should educate the patient and family to take care of the person with inflammatory bowel disease as given below.

Major goals may include normal bowel elimination, relief of abdominal pain and cramping, prevention of fluid volume deficit, optimal nutrition and weight, avoidance of fatigue, reduction of anxiety, effective coping, prevention of skin breakdown, knowledge and understanding of the disease process and therapeutic regimen and absence of complications.

Nursing Interventions

Maintaining Normal Elimination Patterns

- Determine if there is a relationship between diarrhea and certain foods, activities or emotional stress
- Identify any precipitating factors as well as stool frequency, consistency and amount
- Provide ready access to bathroom or bedpan; keep environments clean and odor-free
- Administer antidiarrheal agents as prescribed, and record frequency and consistency of stools after therapy has started
- Encourage bed rest to decrease peristalsis.

Relieving Pain

- Describe character of pain (dull, burning or cramp-like) and its onset, pattern, and medication relief
- Administer anticholinergic medications 30 minutes before meal to decrease intestinal motility
- Give analgesic agents as prescribed; reduce pain by position changes, local application of heat (as prescribed), diversional activities and prevention of fatigue.

Maintaining Fluid Balance

- Record intake and output, including wound or fistula drainage
- Monitor weight daily
- Assess for signs of fluid volume deficit: Dry skin and mucous membranes, decreased skin turgor, oliguria, exhaustion, decreased temperature, increased hematocrit
- Evaluate urine specific gravity, and note hypotension
- Encourage oral intake; monitor intravenous flow rate
- Initiate measures to decrease diarrhea: Dietary restrictions stress reduction and antidiarrheal agents.

Promoting Nutritional Measures

- Use PN when symptoms are severe
- Record fluid intake and output and daily weights during therapy; test for glucose daily
- Give feedings high in protein and low in fat and residue after PN therapy; note intolerance (e.g. vomiting, diarrhea distention)
- Provide small, frequent, low-residue feeding if oral foods are tolerated
- Restrict activities to conserve energy, reduce peristalsis and reduce calorie requirements.

Diet and Fluids

- Eat a high caloric and well-balanced diet
- Avoid any food that increases symptoms (e.g. fresh fruits, and vegetables, fatty foods, spicy foods and alcohol)
- Assess the effect of dairy products on disease symptoms and limit use if appropriate
- Take multivitamins/mineral supplements daily
- Ensure a liberal fluid intake—2,500–3,000 mL per day. Drink electrol or other commercial products if tolerated during flare-ups, to replace lost electrolytes
- Use salt liberally during disease flare-ups.

Elimination

- Take medication as prescribed
- Keep rectal area clean and dry; use analgesic rectal ointment or sitz baths for rectal discomfort
- Consult with physician about the appropriateness of antidiarrheal agents or bulk laxatives when diarrhea is present
- Monitor weight daily disease flare-ups.

Rest and Coping

- Maintain a regular sleep schedule
- Schedule daily activities to avoid fatigue, take rest periods as needed
- Use relaxation strategies when stress levels rise
- Discuss concern with family or support person
- Attend local IBD support group if available.

Promoting Rest and Activity Tolerance

- Recommend intermittent rest periods during the day, schedule or restrict activities to conserve energy and reduce metabolic rate
- Encourage activity within limits; advise bed rest with active or passive exercises for a patient who is febrile, has frequency stools or is bleeding.

Reducing Anxiety

- Establish rapport by being attentive and displaying a calm, confident manner
- Provide time for patient to ask questions and express feelings
- Note nonverbal indicators of anxiety (restlessness, tense facial expressions)
- Tailor information about impending surgery to patient's level of understanding and desire for detail.

Promoting Coping Skills

- Provide understanding and emotional support to patient who feels isolated, helpless and out of control
- Recognize that behavior may be affected by a number of factors unrelated to inherent emotional characteristics
- Support patient's attempts to deal with stresses
- Communicate that patient's feelings are understood; encourage patient to discuss any disturbing matters
- Use stress-reduction measures: Relaxation techniques, breathing exercises and biofeedback
- Refer for professional counseling as needed.

Preventing Skin Breakdown

- Examine skin, especially perianal skin
- Provide perianal care after each bowel movement
- Give immediate care to reddened or irritated areas over bony prominences
- Use pressure-relieving devices to avoid skin breakdown
- Consult with a wound care specialist or enterostomal therapist as indicated.

Monitoring and Managing Potential Complications

- Monitor serum electrolyte levels; administer replacements
- Report dysrhythmias or changes in level of consciousness
- Monitor rectal bleeding, and give blood and volume expanders
- Monitor blood pressure; obtain laboratory blood studies
- Monitor for indications of perforation; acute increase in abdominal pain, rigid abdomen, vomiting or hypotension
- Monitor for signs of obstruction and toxic megacolon: Abdominal distention, decreased or absent bowel sounds, changes in mental status, fever, tachycardia, hypotension, dehydration and electrolyte imbalance.

Promoting Home and Community-based Care

Teaching Patients Self-Care

- Assess need for additional information about medical management (medications, diet) and surgical interventions
- Provide information about nutritional management (bland low-residue, high-protein, high-calorie, and high-vitamin diet)
- Give rationale for using steroids and anti-inflammatory, antibacterial, antidiarrheal and antispasmodic agents
- Emphasize importance of taking medications as prescribed and not abruptly discontinuing regimen (especially steroids because serious medical problems may result)
- Explain procedure and preoperative and postoperative care if surgery is required. Review ileostomy care as necessary. Obtain information from the National Foundation of Ileitis and Colitis.

Continuing Care

- Refer for home care nurse if nutritional status is compromised and patient is receiving PN
- Explain that disease can be controlled and patient can lead a healthy life between exacerbations
- Encourage patient to rest as needed and modify activities according to energy levels during a flare-up. Advise patient to limit tasks that impose strain on the lower abdominal muscles and to sleep close to bathroom because of frequent diarrhea. Suggest room deodorizers for odor control
- Instruct about medications and the need to take them on schedule while at home. Recommend use of medication reminders (containers that separate pills according to day and time)
- Recommend low-residue, high-protein, high-calorie diet during an acute phase. Encourage patient to keep a record of foods that irritate bowel and to eliminate them from diet
- Recommend intake of eight glasses of water per day
- Provide support for prolonged nature of disease because it is a strain on family life and financial resources. Arrange of individual and family counseling as indicated
- Provide time for patient to express fears and frustrations.

CROHN'S DISEASE

Crohn's disease is a chronic, nonspecific inflammatory bowel disorder of unknown origin that can affect any part of the GI tract. It may occur at any age. But occurs most often between the age of 25 and 30 years. Both sexes are affected with slightly high incidence in women.

Pathophysiology

Crohn's disease can affect any part of the GI tract, but is most often seen in the terminal ileum, jejunum and colon. The infla-mmation involves all layers of the bowel wall (i.e. transmural). Area of involvements are usually discontinuous with segments of normal bowel occurring between diseased portions. Typically ulcerations are deep and longitudinal and penetrate between islands of inflammed edematous mucosa causing the classic cobblestone appearance. Thickening of bowel wall occurs as well as narrowing of the lumen with stricture development (Fig. 10.31). Abscesses or fistula tract, that communicates with other loops of bowel, skin, bladder, rectum or vagina may develop.

Clinical Manifestation

The manifestations depend largely on the anatomical site of involvement, extent of the disease process and presence or absence of complications. The onset of Crohn's disease is usually insidious. With non-specific complaints such as diarrhea, fatigue, abdominal pain, weight loss and fever. Fever diagnosis is difficult than ulcerative colitis. The principal symptoms are diarrhea and abdominal pain. Other manifestations include abdominal cramping, anal tenderness, abdominal distention, fever and fatigue. Extraintestinal manifestation such as arthritis, finger clubbing, may precede the onset of disease. As the disease progresses, there is weight loss, malnutrition, dehydration, electrolyte imbalances, anemia, increased peristalsis and pain around the umbilicus and right lower quadrant. The complications are fistulas, strictures, anal abscesses, perforation, toxic megacolon (Fig. 10.32).

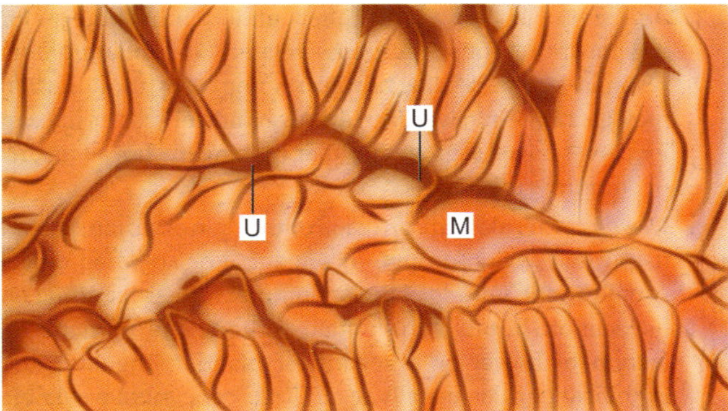

FIG. 10.31: Crohn's disease. The mucosa in Crohn's disease demonstrates a cobblestone pattern as a result of fissured ulcers (U) with intervening areas of edematous mucosa (M)

Diagnostic Studies

- Complete blood cell count
- Serum chemistries
- Stool for occult blood
- Barium enema of small and large intestine
- Procosigmoidoscope examination and
- Sigmoidoscopy and colonoscopy with biopsy.

Management

The goal of management is to control the inflammatory process, relieve symptoms, correct metabolic and nutritional problems and promote healing. Drug therapy and nutritional support are the mainstays of treatment (Table 10.9).

Health Maintenance

- Report signs requiring medical attention:
  - Change in pattern or severity of abdominal pain or diarrhea
  - Development of constipation
  - Change in stool character
  - Unusual discharge from rectum and
  - Fever
- Plan for regular follow-up care.

INTESTINAL OBSTRUCTION

Normal functioning of the small and large intestine depends on an open lumen for the movement of intestinal content, as well as adequate circulation and nervous innervation to sustain rhythmic peristalsis. Any factor or condition that either narrows the intestinal passage way or interfere with peristalsis can result in bowel obstruction. An overview of bowel obstruction (Box 10.10).

Intestinal obstruction occurs when intestinal contents cannot pass through the GI tract, and it requires prompt treatment. The obstruction may either be partial or complete.

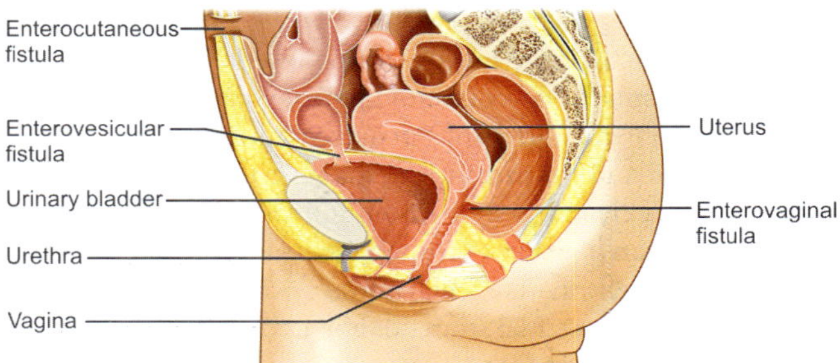

FIG. 10.32: Fistulas are a common complication of Crohn's disease

TABLE 10.9: Nursing care plan of patient with ulcerative colitis

Problem	Reason	Objective	Nursing intervention	Evaluation
1. Diarrhea related to irritated bowel; intestinal hyperactivity	As manifested by frequent diarrheal stools more than 10 per day	• Fewer firmer stool	• Monitor frequency and character of stools • Maintain food and fluid restrictions to rest bowel • Teach patient to avoid caffeine and food or fluids that are irritating to bowel • Rarely administer antidiarrheal medications, as they may precipitate colonic dilation	
2. Anxiety related to possible social embarassment. Unfamiliar environment, diagnostic test and treatment	As manifested by expression of concern about effect of disease on social relationships, questions about disease and treatment	• Less anxious feelings	• Monitor signs of anxiety • Encourage open discussions of feelings about diagnosis • Explain disease, treatments, diagnostic tests and medication • Provide privacy to reduce embarrassment	

In addition, NCP also incldue *problem* of altered nutritions; less than body requirements, impaired skin integrity, ineffective individual coping, ineffective management of the rapeutic regimen and hypovolemia and electrolyte imbalance can be looked for and proper nursing intervention be taken as stated earlier.

Box 10.10 Overview of bowel obstructs

Signs and symptoms	Abdominal pain Blood and mucus from rectum Feces and flatus cease Visible peristaltic waves in thin person Possible fecal vomiting Bowel sounds high pitched, tinkling or absent Abdominal distention Fluid and electrolyte imbalance
Diagnostic test	Abdominal X-ray examination CT scan CBC and electrolytes
Therapeutic measures	NPO status Frequent mouth care Nasogastric tube Fluid and electrolyte replacement Medication: Antibiotics, antiemetics, analgesics Surgery

Intestinal obstruction (mechanical or functional) occurs when blockage prevents the flow of contents through the intestinal tract. Large bowel obstruction results in an accumulation of intestinal contents, fluid and gas proximal to the obstruction. Obstruction in the colon can lead to severe distention and perforation unless gas and fluid can flow back through the ileal valve. Dehydration occurs more slowly than in small bowel obstruction. If the blood supply is cut off, intestinal strangulation and necrosis occur; this condition is lifethreatening.

Most bowel obstructions (85%) occur in the small intestine. Intestinal contents fluid and gas accumulate above the intestinal obstruction. Distention and retention reduce the absorption of fluids and stimulate gastric secretion. Reflux vomiting may also occur. Fluids and electrolytes are lost. Dehydration and acidosis develop because of water and sodium loss. With acute fluid losses, hypovolemic shock may occur. Increasing distention and pressure within the intestinal lumen cause a decrease in venous and arteriolar capillary pressure, resulting in edema, congestion, necrosis, and eventual rupture or perforation of the intestinal wall, with resultant peritonitis. Adhesions are the most common (60%) cause of obstruction. Other causes include hernias, neoplasms, intussusception, volvulus and paralytic ileus.

Etiology (Box 10.11)

The intestinal obstruction can be classified as mechanical and non-mechanical (Fig. 10.33).

The causes of mechanical obstruction are:

i. *Adhesions:* It may form after abdominal surgery for unknown reasons; perhaps related to inflammatory responses in the healing bowel. In some cases, the adhesion may become massive. The fibrous bands of scar tissue can loop over bowel segments, either causing the bowel to kink or compress the loop.
ii. *Hernias:* A hernia is a protrusion of an organ or structure from its normal cavity through a congenital or acquired defect usually in the muscle of the abdominal wall. Depending on its location, hernia may contain peritoneal uro-omentum, a loop of bowel or a section of bladder. Inguinal and umbilical hernias usually result from congenital weakness of the muscle, whereas incisional hernias for usually complications of surgery. Hernia can result in bowel obstruction if the abdominal wall defect through which the

Box 10.11 Mechanical causes of intestinal obstruction

Cause	Course of events	Result
Adhesions	Loops of intestine become adherent to areas that heal slowly or scar after abdominal surgery; occurs most commonly in small intestine	After surgery, adhesions produce a kinking of an intestinal loop
Intussusception	One part of the intestine slips into another part located below it (like a telescope shortening); occurs more commonly in infants than adults	The intestinal lumen becomes narrowed and blood supply becomes strangulated
Volvulus	Bowel twists and turns on itself and occludes the blood supply	Intestinal lumen becomes obstructed. Gas and fluid accumulate in the trapped bowel
Hernia	Protrusion of intestine through a weakened area in the abdominal muscle or wall	Intestinal flow may be completely obstructed. Blood flow to the area may be obstructed as well
Tumor	A tumor that exists within the wall of the intestine extends into the intestinal lumen, or a tumor outside the intestine cause pressure on the wall of the intestine. Most common type is colorectal adenocarcinoma	Intestinal lumen becomes partially obstructed; if the tumor is not removed, complete obstruction results

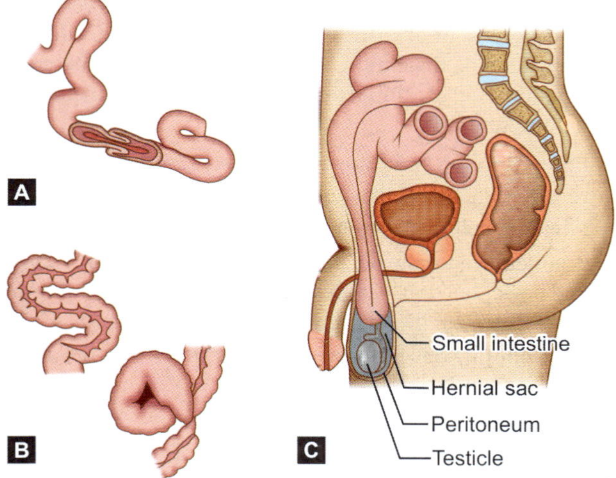

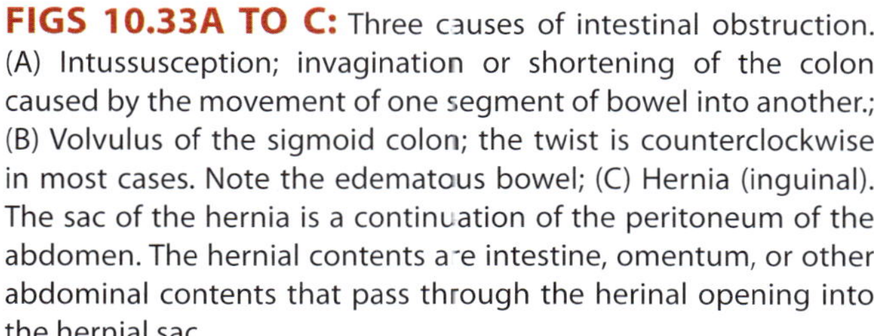

FIGS 10.33A TO C: Three causes of intestinal obstruction. (A) Intussusception; invagination or shortening of the colon caused by the movement of one segment of bowel into another.; (B) Volvulus of the sigmoid colon; the twist is counterclockwise in most cases. Note the edematous bowel; (C) Hernia (inguinal). The sac of the hernia is a continuation of the peritoneum of the abdomen. The hernial contents are intestine, omentum, or other abdominal contents that pass through the herinal opening into the hernial sac

hernia protrudes becomes so tight that the bowel segments become strangulated. The lumps or swellings may always be present or may have appeared suddenly after coughing, straining, lifting and other vigorous exertion.

iii. *Tumor:* Tumor mass will gradually restrict the internal tumors of the bowel as it enlarges. Eventually a fecal mass may be unable to pass through the constriction, leading to partial or complete obstruction.

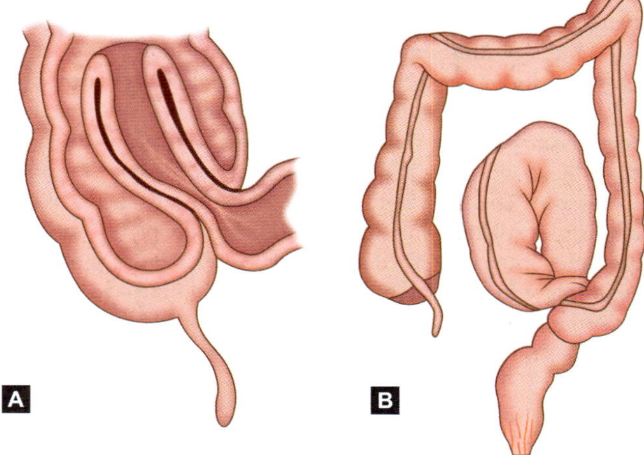

FIGS 10.34A AND B: Mechanical bowel obstructions. (A) Intussusception; (B) Volvulus

iv. *Volvulus:* A twisting of the bowel upon itself, usually at least a full 180°, obstructing the intestinal lumen both proximally or distally, is called 'Volvulus'. The acute obstruction can quickly result in bowel infarction and can be life-threatening as a result of necrosis, perforation and peritonitis.

v. *Intussusception:* Intussusception involves a telescoping of the bowel in itself. In invagination occurs with peristalsis and in the adult often is triggered by the presence of tumor mass. The bowel segment containing the mass is propelled by peristalsis and adjacent bowel segment. Constriction is immediate and strangulation of the trapped segment can develop (Fig. 10.34).

The other possible causes of mechanical obstruction will include fecal impaction, gallstones and stricture resulting from the diverticulitis and IBD.

The causes of nonmechanical obstruction may result from a neuromuscular or vascular disorder.

i. Paralytic ileus (or adynamic ileus) results from a lack of peristaltic activity, usually as a result of neurogenic impairment. Ileus is a common temporary problem after abdominal surgery particularly if the bowel has been extensively handled. Other causes of paralytic ileus include inflammatory responses (e.g. appendicitis, pancreatitis), electrolyte abnormalities, and thoracic and lumbar spinal fractures.
ii. Vascular distinctions are rare and are due to an interference with the blood supply to a position of the intestines. The common causes are emboli; and atherosclerosis of mesenteric arteries, thrombosis of the mesenteric arteries.

Pathophysiology

Intestinal obstruction triggers a series of GI tract events whose clinical manifestation depends largely on the location of the obstruction and the degree of circulatory compromise. Normally 6 to 8 liters of fluid enters the small bowel daily. Most of the fluid is absorbed before it reaches the colon. Approximately 75 percent of the intestinal gas is swallowed air. Bacterial metabolism produce methane and hydrogen gases fluid and intestinal content accumulates proximal to the intestinal obstruction. This causes distention and the distal bowel may collapse. The distention reduces the absorption of the fluids and stimulates intestinal secretion. As the fluid increases. So does the pressure in the lumen of the bowel. The incresaed pressure leads to an increase in capillary permeability and extravasation of fluids and electrolytes into the peritoneal cavity. Edema, congestion and necrosis from imparied blood supply and possible rupture of the bowel may occur. The retention of fluid in the intestine and peritoneal cavity can lead to a severe reduction in circulating blood volume and result in hypotension and hypovolemic shock.

Vascular compromise is the most serious aspect of obstruction. Bowel ischemia breaks down the normal barrier to bacteria and the stagnant and distended bowel becomes increasingly permeable to bacteria. Organism can enter the peritoneal cavity and lead to peritonitis. Bacteria are normally sparse in the small bowel but accumulated rapidly during obstruction. *E. coli, Klebsiella* prevalent and the release of toxins can result in septic shock. The ischemic process can progress to gangrene and perforation. Submucosal hemorrhage and sloughing can also be a source of substantial blood loss (Fig. 10.35 and Box 10.12).

Clinical Manifestation

The clinical manifestations of intestinal obstructions very based on the exact site of obstruction and include nausea, vomiting, abdominal pain, distention, inability to pass flatulence and constipation (fecal impaction secondary to constipation, colonar perforation).

Symptoms develop and progress relatively slowly:

- Constipation may be the only symptom for days (obstruction in sigmoid colon or rectum)
- Abdomen eventually becomes markedly distended, loops of large bowel become visible outlined through the abdominal wall, and patient has crampy lower abdominal pain
- Fecal vomiting develops; symptoms of shock may occur.

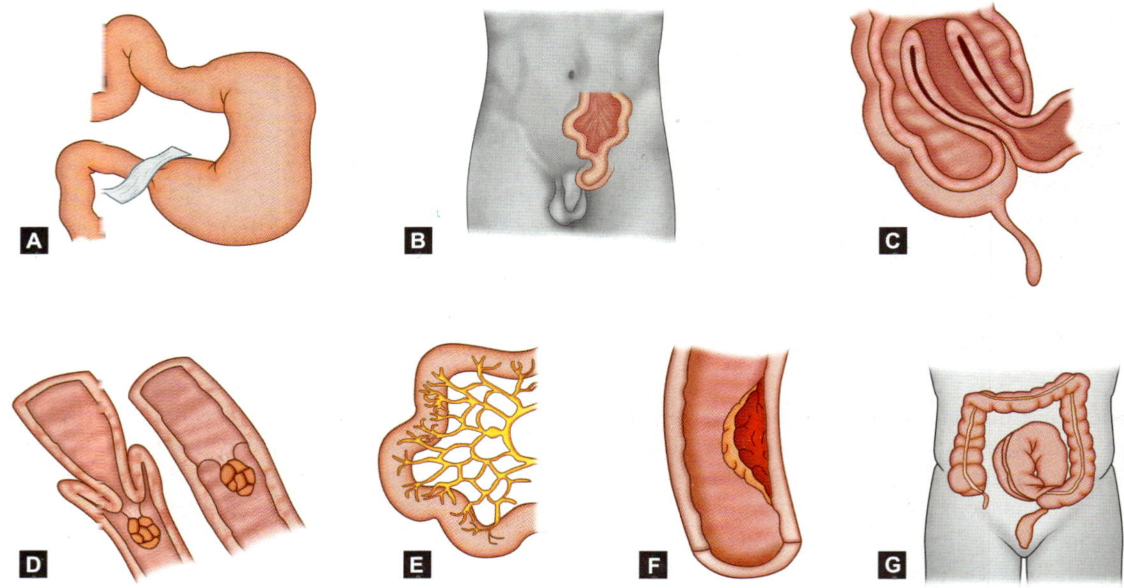

FIGS 10.35A TO G: Bowel obstruction. (A) Adhesions; (B) Strangulated inguinal hernia; (C) Ileocecal intussusception; (D) Intussusception from polyps; (E) Mesenteric occlusion; (F) Neoplasm; (G) Volvulus of the sigmoid colon

Box 10.12 Causes of nonmechanical obstruction

- Abdominal surgery and trauma
- Pneumonia
- Spinal injuries
- Hypokalemia
- Myocardial infection
- Peritonitis
- ascular insufficiency

In small bowel obstruction:

- Initial symptom is usually crampy pain that is wavelike and colicky. Patient may pass blood and mucus but not fecal matter of flatus. Vomiting occurs
- Peristaltic waves become extremely vigorous and assume a reverse direction, propelling intestinal contents toward the mouth, if the obstruction is complete
- If the obstruction is in the ileum, fecal vomiting takes place
- Dehydration results in intense thirst, drowsiness, generalized malaise and aching
- Tongue and mucous membranes become parched; abdomen becomes distended (the lower the obstruction in the gastrointestinal tract, the more marked the distention)
- If uncorrected, shock occurs due to dehydration and loss of plasma volume.

Obstruction located high in the small intestine produces rapid onset, sometimes projective vomiting with bile containing vomitus. Vomiting from more distal obstruction of the small intestine is more gradual in onset. The vomitus may be orange-brown and foul-smelling because of bacterial growth. Vomiting may be entirely absent in large bowel obstruction if the ileocecal valve is competent. Otherwise, the patient may eventually vomit feculent material.

Abdominal pain is fairly universal symptom. Simple obstruction produce cramy and poorly localized pain. Its onset parallels the initial increase in peristalsis that raises intraluminal pressure in an attempt to clear the obstruction. Frequent loud, high pitched bowel sounds are often heard on auscultation. The pain typically lessens as the obstructions worsen. Smooth muscle atony decreases peristalsis and bowel sounds are diminished. The pain associated with bowel strangulation is constant and severe vomitings usually relieve abdominal pain in high intestinal obstruction. Persistent, colicky abdominal pain is seen with lower intestinal obstruction.

Abdominal distention usualy develops slowly although constipation is common. Rising fever usually indicates the presence of dying bowel. Laboratory values typically reflect the progressive nature of the dehydration. There is decreased urine output, hemoconcentration, hypokalemia and hyponatremia.

Management

Intestinal obstruction is a potentially life-threatening condition. Assessment must begin with a detailed patient's history and physical examination. The type of location of obstruction usually causes characteristic symptoms. Symptoms plus radiologic studies (abnormal quantities of gas and/or fluid in bowel) and laboratory studies (electrolytes and complete blood count show dehydration and possible infection). The nurse should determine the location, duration, intensity and frequency of abdominal pain and whether abdominal tenderness or rigidity is present. Onset, frequency, color, odor and amount of vomitus should be recroded. Bowel function, including passage of flatus should be determined. This should auscultate for bowel sounds and document character and location, irrespective the abdomen for scars, palpable mass, and distention, and observe for muscle guarding and tenderness. The usual diagnosis measures taken are abdominal X-rays, barium enema, as these given, e.g. clues for locating obstruction. Laboratory tests are also helpful, CBC, serum-electrolyte, amylase, BUN. The nurse should prepare the patient for such measures.

Medical Management

For large bowel obstruction:

- Colonoscopy to untwist and decompress the bowel, if obstruction is high in the colon
- Cecostomy may be performed for patients who are poor surgical risks and urgently need relief from the obstruction
- Rectal tube to decompress an area that is lower in the bowel
- Usual treatment is surgical resection to remove the obstructing lesion; a temporary or permanent colostomy may be necessary; an ileoanal anastomosis may be performed if entire large colon must be removed.

For small bowel obstruction:

Decompression of the bowel may be achieved through a nasogastric or small bowel tube. However, when the bowel is completely obstructed, the possibility of strangulation warrants surgical intervention. Surgical treatment depends on the cause of obstruction (e.g. hernia repair). Before surgery, intravenous therapy is instituted to replace water, sodium, chloride and potassium.

Treatment is directed towards decompression of the intestine by removal of gas and fluid, correction and maintenance of fluid and electrolyte balance, and relief or removal of the obstruction. NG or intestinal tube may be used to decompress the bowel. NG tubes should be inserted before surgery to empty the stomach and relieve distention. They are also used instead of nasointestinal tubes to treat partial or complete small-bowel obstructions. Intestinal tubes such as the Center or Miller-Abbot or Dennis tubes are passed into the small intestine. They are 10 fect (9300 cm) long and mercury-weighed. The patient should be monitored closely for signs of dehydrations and electrolyte imbalance. A strict intake and output record should be maintained. All vomitus and tube drainage should be included. IV fluids should be administered. Serum electrolyte levels should be monitored. A patient with high obstruction is more likely to have metabolic alkalosis. A patient with low obstruction is at greater risk of metabolic acidosis. The patient is often restless and constantly changes position to relieve the pain. Analgesics may be with held until the obstruction is diagnosed because they may mask other signs and symptoms and decrease intestinal motility. The nurse should provide comfort measures to promote a restful environment, and keep distraction and visitors to a minimum. Nursing care of the patient after surgery for an intestinal obstruction is similar to the care of the patient after laparotomy.

Nursing Management

- Monitor symptoms indicating worsening intestinal obstruction
- Provide emotional support and comfort
- Administer intravenous fluids and electrolyte replacement
- Prepare patient for surgery if no response to medical treatment
- Provide preoperative teaching as patient's condition indicates
- Maintain the function of the nasogastric tube. Assess and measure nasogastric output. Assess for fluid and electrolyte imbalance
- Monitor nutritional status. Asses for improvement in bowel function (i.e. return of normal bowel sounds, decreased abdominal distention, improvement in abdominal pain and tenderness, passage of flatus or stool)
- Report discrepancies in intake and output, worsening of pain or abdominal distention, and increased nasogastric output
- If patients condition does not improve prepare him or her for surgery
- Provide postoperative nursing care similar to that for other abdominal surgeries.

COLORECTAL CANCER

Colorectal cancer has been widely spread by the turn of the last millennium. The causes of colorectal cancer remain unclear. Groups at high-risk of colorectal cancer have been identified are:

- Age (after 40 years) is a risk time for both men and women
- Colorectal polyps
- Chronic inflammatory bowel disease (history of ulcerative colitis)
- Family history of colerectal cancer or adenomas
- Previous history of colorectal cancer
- History of genital or breast cancer (woman)
- High caloric, high fat/or low-fiber diet
- Cigarette smoking
- Obesity (nature of the risk currently unknown)

Incidence of cancer is shown in Figure 10.36.

Pathophysiology

Adenocarcinoma is the most common type of colon cancer. Most colorectal cancers appear to arise from adenomatous polyps. All tumors tend to spread through the walls of the intestine and into the lymphatic system. Tumors commonly spread to the liver because the venous blood flow from the colorectal tumor is through the portal vein. Since the cancer of the colon may spread by direct extension or through the lymphatic or circulatory systems it may seed at distant point in the peritonium or at distant points in the colon. The liver and lungs are the major organs of metastasis.

An overview of colon cancer is given in Box 10.13.

Clinical Manifestation

The clinical manifestation of the colon cancer varies with the location of the tumor. There are usually no early symptoms and the disease is often diagnosed incidentally. Cancer in distal colon and rectum typically produces symphony related to partial obstruction. The lesions are more likely to be annular, and they grow circumferentially, encircling the colon wall. The lumen becomes narrow and constricted. Obstruction occurs when formed stool is unable to pass through the narrowed lumen.

- The patient may experience a change in bowel habits, a feeling of incomplete bowel emptying, or rectal bleeding. The clinical manifestation of bowel cancer are as follows (Figs 10.37 and 10.38):
  - Frequently a symptomatic and diagnosed incidentaly
  - Symptoms of partial bowel obstruction
    - Change in bowel habits, e.g. constipation or diarrhea and pencil or ribbon-shaped stool
    - Sensation of incomplete bowel emptying
    - Gas or bloating

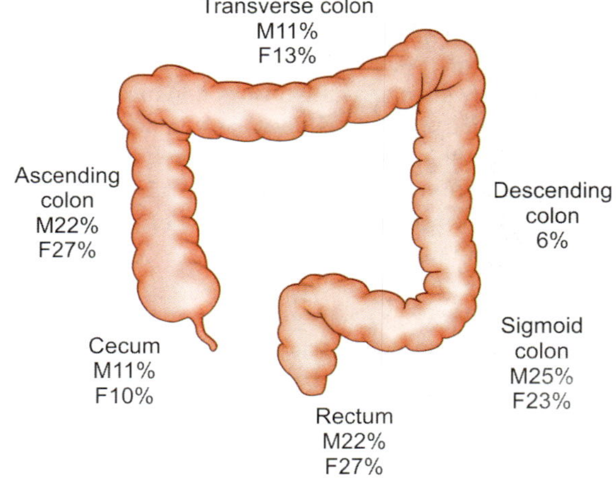

FIG. 10.36: Incidence of cancer. Approximately one half of all colon cancers occur in the rectosigmoid area. Percentages are listed for males (M) and females (F)

Box 10.13 Overview of colon cancer

Signs and symptoms	Change in bowel habits Blood or mucus in stools Abdominal or rectal pain Weight loss Anemia Obstruction
Diagnostic test	Colonoscopy with biopsy Sigmoidoscopy with biopsy Proctosigmoidoscopy Barium enema Abdominal and rectal examination Fecal occult blood
Therapeutic measures	Surgery, possibly colostomy Radiation Chemotherapy and/or radiation Medications: Analgesics TPN as needed Support and education

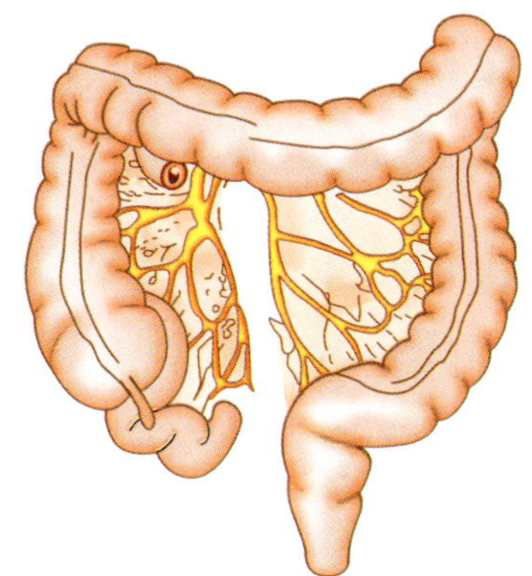

FIG. 10.37: Signs and symptoms of colorectal cancer by location of primary tumor

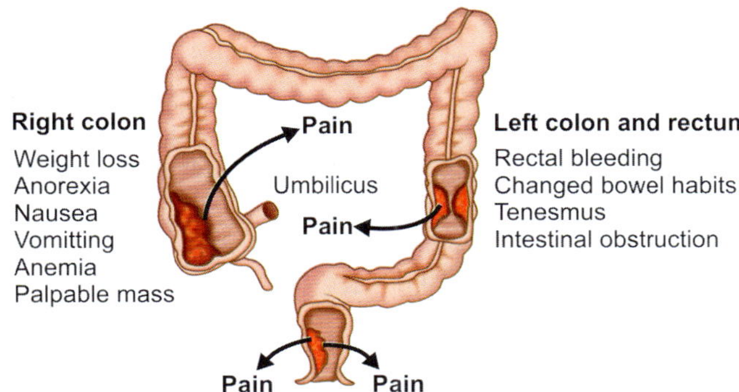

FIG. 10.38: Symptoms of carcinoma of the colon. Pain usually radiates toward the umbilicus of perianal area

- Occurs blood in the stool or rectal bleeding
- Weakness, fatigue, malaise, anorexia and anemia
- Weight loss usually accompany with metastasis
- Abdominal pain (usually accompanies in larger lesions).

Diagnostic test: Rectal examination, sigmoidoscopy, colonoscopy, barium enema, CBC, LFT, ocult blood test, CEA test, CT scan and ultrasound.

Management

Prognosis and treatment correlates with pathological staging of the disease. Several methods of staging currently being used are:

1. Duke's classification
2. TNM classification.

1. Duke staging system for colorectal cancer.
   - A – Negative nodes, limitations of lesion to mucosa.
   - B1 – Negative nodes, extension of lesion through mucosa but still within the bowel wall.
   - B2 – Negative nodes extention through entire bowel wall.
   - C1 – Positive nodes, limitation of lesion to bowel wall.
   - C2 – Positive nodes, extension of lesion through entire bowel wall.
   - D – Presence of distant unresectable metastasis.

This staging is used to establish the appropriates level of intervention and treatment.

The most recent classifications of colorectal cancer is the tumor, node, metastasis, (TNM) system which is based on pathologic assessment and includes data from the history and physical examination and presurgical and laboratory evaluation.

- T – Primary tumors
- T_x – Primary tumor can not be assessed
- T_0 – No evidence of primary tumour
- Tis – Carcinoma in situ
- T_1 – Tumor invades submucosa
- T_2 – Tumors invades muscularis propria
- T_3 – Tumor invades through the msculari propriat into the subserosa or into the non-peritonealized pericolic or perirectal tissue
- T_4 – Tumor perforates the visceral peritoneum or directly invades other organs or structures
- N – Regional lymph node involvement
- N_x – Regional lymph node cannot be assessed
- N_0 – No regional lymph node metastasis
- M_1 – Distinct metastasis.

After diagnosis has been confirmed, treatment may be initiated by radiation and chemotherapy.

Radiation may be used preoperatively or as a palliative measure for patients with advanced lesions. It is primary objective is to reduce tumor size and provide symptomatic relief.

Chemotherpay is recommended when a patient has a positive lymph node at the time of surgery or has metastatic disease. No drug is available that can cure malignant colon or rectal tumors.

Surgery is the only curative treatment of colorectal cancer. Success of surgery depends on resection of the tumor with an adequate margin of healthy bowel and resection of the regional lymph nodes. The usual surgical procedure includes:

i. Right hemicolectomy is performed when the cancer is located in the cecum, ascending colon, hepatic flexure, or transverse colon to the right of the middle artery. A portion of the terminal ileum, the appendix are removed, and an ileotransverse anastomosis is performed.

ii. A left hemicolectomy involves resection of the left transverse colon, the splenic flexure, the descending colon, the sigmoid colon and the upper portion of the rectum and abdominal-perineal resection, laparoscopy colectomy is also performed. Pre and postoperative care are similar to that of any laparotomy within specific activities is initiated accordingly (See Ostomy Surgery).

OSTOMY SURGERY

An ostomy is a surgical procedure in which an opening is made to allow the passage of intestinal contents from the bowel to an incision trauma. The stoma which is the opening on the surface of the abdomen is created when the intestine is brought through the abdominal wall and sutured to the skin. It may be permanent or temporary. Fecal matter is diverted through the stoma to the outside of the abdominal wall (Fig. 10.39).

- An ileostomy is opening from the ileum through the abdominal wall and is also referred to as a conventional or Brooke's ileostomy. It is most commonly used in surgical treatment of ulcerative colitis Crohn's disease and familial polyp. Types of ostomies (Figs 10.39 to 10.41)
- A cecostomy is an opening between the cecum and the abdominal wall. They are usually temporary most often used for fecal diversion before surgery or for palliation

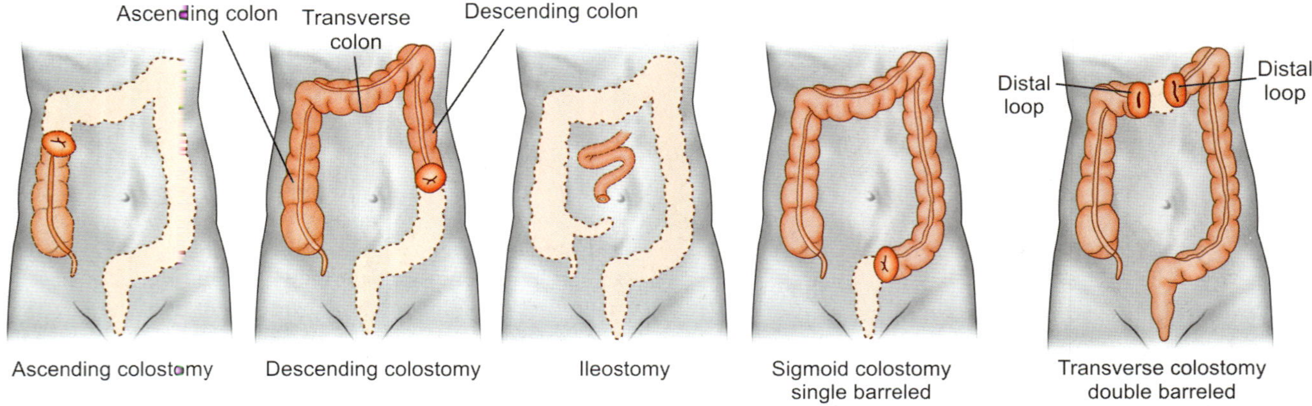

FIG. 10.39: Types of ostomies (See also Figures 10.40 and 10.41)

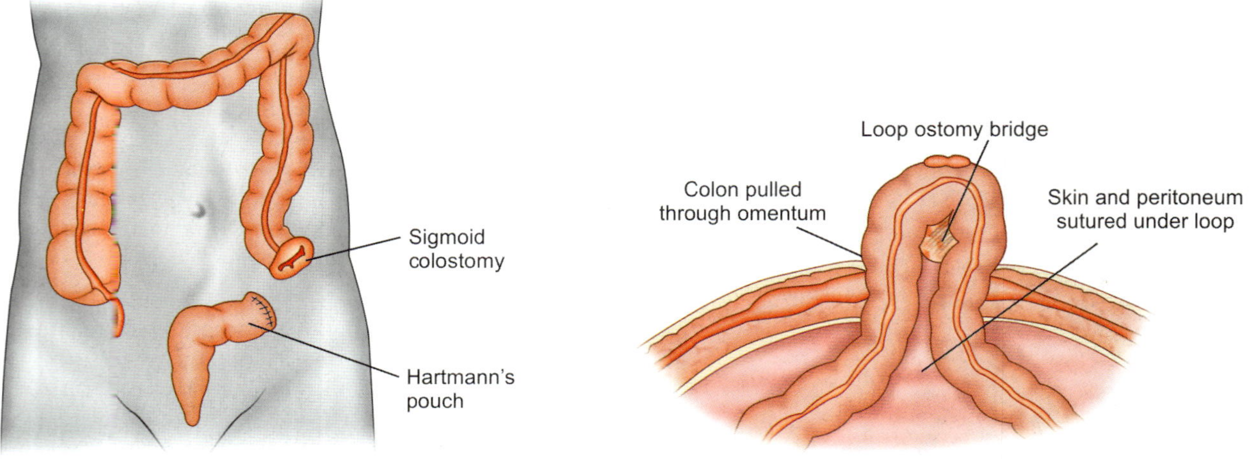

FIG. 10.40: Sigmoid colostomy. Distal bowel is oversewn and left in place to create Hartmann's pouch

FIG. 10.41: Loop colostomy

- A colostomy is an opening between the colon and abdominal wall. The proximal end of the colon is sutured to the skin. Temporary colostomy is usually performed to protect an end-to-end anastomosis after a bowel resection or in an emergency measure following bowel obstruction (e.g. malignant tumor), abdominal trauma (Gunshot wound) or a perforated diverticulum. Loop colostomy and double barrel colostomy are more commonly performed as temporary colostomy, but they may be permanent.

Preoperative Care

Preoperative care focuses on patient teaching. The nurse assesses the patient's knowledge and understanding of the proposed surgery and its outcomes. This inlcudes brief overview of GI tract structure and functioning and the nature of functioning of the ostomy. Emotional preparation for ostomy surgery is extremely important. The nurse encourages the pateint to verbalize feelings related to the radical change to body image and function. Validating the appropriateness of these concerns lays in the family for an effective working relationship with patient.

The patient may need to progress through the grieving process, and if the person is in the shock state, specific factual teaching may be ineffective. The nurse offers acceptance of all feelings and reinforces the importance of open communication.

The preparation phase may include nutritional support and possibly total parental nutrition (TPN), if the patient's nutritional state is inadequate for surgery. The patient should know what to except in the postoperative period. The nurse discusses the management of postoperative pain. The nature and apperance of all incisions and drains and the purpose of the NG tube and IV lines. Bowel cleansing is also performed and may include the use of enemas, laxatives and antibiotics to reduce intestinal bacterial flora.

Postoperative Care

Postoperative nursing care should focus on assessing the stoma protecting the skin, selecting the pouch, and assisting the patient to adapt psychologically to a changed body. In addition, maintenance of fluid and electrolyte balance, stoma monitoring and managing the wound are important. (Further please see nursing care plan of patient with colostomy/ileostomy (Table 10.10). Types of stomas are shown in Figure 10.42.

The following guidelines should be kept in mind while changing the ostomy pouch (Table 10.10).

i. Stoma measurement
   - Use the measuring guide and sample diameters and cut the ostomy appliances to fit pattern should be 1/8 to 1/4 inch larger than stoma
   - Use the same procedure to prepare the skin barrier.

   Note: The pouch opening is cut slightly larger than that of the skin barrier to prevent paper from cutting the stoma.

ii. Removing pouch
   - Empty drainable pouch to prevent spills
   - Disconnect pouch from skin wafer if two-piece system is used
   - Gently peel the wafer away from the skin beginning at the top.

iii. Skin care
   - Cleanse the skin with warm water and dry thoroughly. Use soap only stool adheres to skin. Rinse thoroughly with water
   - Assess peristomal skin and stoma carefully for signs of irritation or infection
   - Pat peristomal skin dry thoroughly.

iv. Applying new pouch
   - Center the pouch opening over the stoma. Ask patient to abdominal muscle to make application easier
   - Gently press into place and hold for at least 30 seconds to seal special emphasis will be on ostomy skin care as follows:
     - When a pouch seal leaks, the pouch should be immediately changed, not taped. Stool held against the skin quickly results in severe irritation
     - Pouches are removed gently, with one hand holding the skin in place to decrease pulling
     - The skin should be gently but thoroughly cleansed, rinsed and patted dry
     - Peristomal hair should be trimmed but not shaved to prevent folliculitis
     - A skin barrier should be used to protect the peristomal skin from liquid stools
     - A skin sealant should be used under all types
     - The patient should consult special nurse for specific care if available.

An ostomy irrigation is an enema given through the stoma to stimulate bowel emptying at a regular and convenient time for which the following guidelines are helpful:

- Assemble all equipment: Water container, irrigating sleeve and belt, skin care, items, new pouch system, ready for use
- Remove old pouch and dispose
- Clean the stoma and peristomal skin with water and assess
- Apply the irrigating sleeve and belt. Place open end of sleeve in toilet
- Fill irrigating container with 500 mL to 1000 mL of lukewarm tap water and suspend container at shoulder height
- Run water through the tubing to remove air
- Gently insert the irrigating cone into stoma, and slowly start the flow of water. Catheters are inserted no more than 2 to 4 inches. Do not fork. If cramping occurs, stop the irrigation and wait

TABLE 10.10: Nursing care plan of patient with a colostomy/ileostomy

Problem	Reason	Objective	Nursing intervention	Evaluation
1. Risk for impaired skin integriety related to irritation and lack of knowledge of skin	• Irritations from fecal drainage • Irritation of pouch	• Normal skin *integrity* • Intact pouch seal	• Have special nurse (ET Nurse) see before surgery to mark stoma site if possible • After surgery, assess peristoma skin for erythema with burning, itching, poorly fitting appliances with leakage, lack of adequate skin care and failure to use skin barrier • During pouch change, assess skin for signs of breakdown • Clean area with milk soap and water and dry thoroughly • Apply skin barrier to protect skin and to prevent direct contact to intestinal contents • Teach patient proper skin and pouch care • Plan home visit for outpatient for continued teaching • Empty pouch when it is one-third full prevent seal from leaking	
2. Body image disturbance related to presence of stoma, and malodor	As manifested by verbalization of embarrassment of shame due to stoma and odor	• Adjustment to altered body image • Satisfactory plan for control odor	• Assessment the patient attitude towards stoma • Instruct patient to measure for odor control, use of odor of pouch, pouch deodrant, and use of room deodrant when, pouch is opened/emptied • Teach patient to use loose clothing to conceal pouch • Discuss normal emotional response to stoma and encourage patient to express feeling • Encourage family members to be active in care • Provide patient with information on resources supporting ostomy patients • Prepare patient to do own stoma and pouch care	
3. Altered nutrition more than body requirement related to lack of knowledge of appropriate foods and decreased appetite	• As manifested by weight loss. Vitamin and mineral deficiency, inability to tolerate certain foods	• During intake to maintain weight at approved level	• Assess nutritional intake • Gradually introduce foods one at a time and begin with low-residue diet • Teach patient to chew food slowly and properly and make digestion earlier and prevent gas • Give list of foods to be avoided	
4. Altered sexuality pattern related to perceived loss of sexual appeal and possibility of accidental seepage of fecal material during sexual activity	• As manifested by verbalization of concern about intimate relation with spouse or significant others	• Confidence in ability to resume avoid sexual activity	• Assess patient's attitude about impact of ostomy on sexual functioning • Encourage discussion on meaning of sexuality to patient and his nears and dear in a non-threatening manner • Discuss way to avoid seepage and conceal stoma and/or pouch during intimate relation to avoid embarrassments	
5. Risk for fluid volume deficit related to excessive fluid loss	• Fluid loss from ileostomy or diarrhea with colostomy and inadequate oral intake	• Normal serum electrolytes • Normal vital signs • Good skin turger • Urine output more then 0.5 mL/kg/h	• Assess for signs of weakness, poor skin turgor sunken eyes, hypotension, tachycardia, hypokalemia, hyponatremia, oliguria • Record intaken and output and include ileostomy drainage to have an accurate record for replacement • Ensure fluid intake of at least 3,000 mL/day in the initial postoperative period • Instruct patient to maintain high fluid intake and increase it during hot weather, patient is perspiring excessively and during diarrheal episode • Monitor serum electrolyte • Instruct the patients on signs and symptoms of sodium, potassium and fluid deficit	

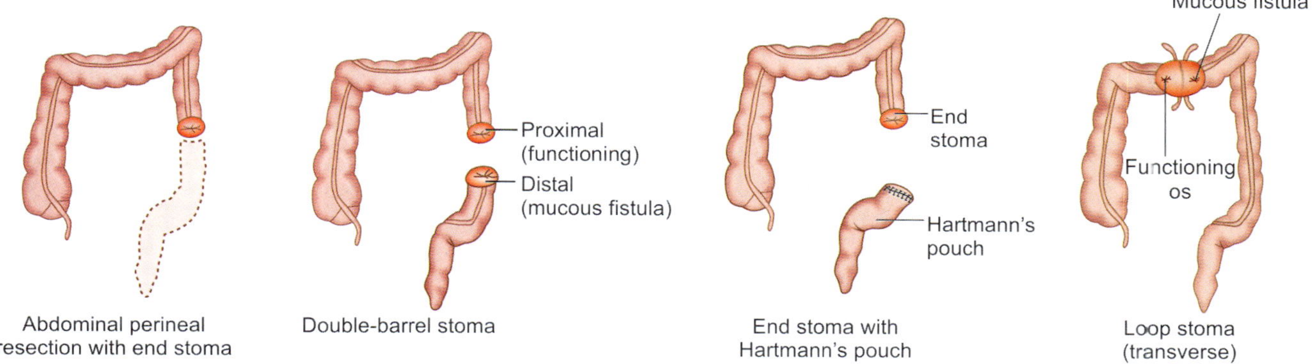

FIG. 10.42: Types of stoma

- Allow approximately 15 to 20 minutes for stool to empty
- Rinse sleeves, dry the bottom, roll it up and close off the end. Patient should go about regular activities for 30 to 45 minutes
- Remove sleeve, clean stoma and apply new pouch
- Clean and store the irrigating equipment.

ANORECTAL DISORDERS

A variety of common disorders can affect the perianal area. Persons who experience anorectal disorders typically seek medical care for symptoms such as pain, tenderness, itching or the development of rectal bleeding. Many of them will be treated on outpatient basis. They include hemorrhoid, fissure, abscesses, fistula, pilonideal sinus (Fig. 10.43).

Hemorrhoids are masses of dilated blood vessels that lie beneath the lining of the skin in the anal canal. They are dilated hemorrhoidal veins. They may be internal or external (Fig. 10.44). Internal occurring about the internal sphincter, external occurring outside the external sphincter. Symptoms of hemorrhoids include bleeding, pruritus, prolapse and pain are common in all age groups.

Hemorrhoids affect the person of all ages, but they typically cause more problems with increasing age. Pregnancy is common condition for initiating or aggravating hemorrhoids. Other conditions associated with the development of hemorrhoids include obesity, congestive heart failure and chronic liver disease which result in portal hypertension. These conditions are associated with persistent elevation in intra-abdominal pressure. Sedentary occupations that involve long period of sitting or standing also implicated though exact mechanism is unknown.

The diagnosis of hemorrhoids is done by inspection, digital examination, proctoscopy or examination with the flexible sigmoidoscopy.

Conservative management of hemorrhoids includes a high-fiber diet, bulk laxatives warm sitz baths, and gentle cleansing. A high fever diet and increased fluid intake prevent constipation

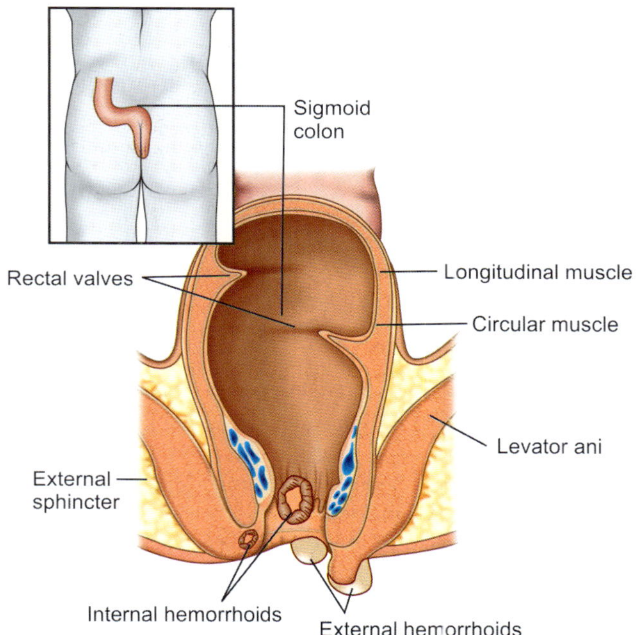

FIG. 10.43: Anatomic structures of the rectum and anus with external and internal hemorrhoids

and reduce straining, which allows engorgement of the veins to subside. Ointments such as Nupercaine, creams, suppositories and impregnated pads that contain anti-inflammatory agents, (hydrocortisone) or astrigent and anesthesia may be used to shrink the mucous membrane and relieve discomfort. Stool softeners may be ordered to keep the stool soft and sitz bath may be ordered to relieve pain.

Application of ice packs for few hours followed by warm packs may be used for thrombosed hemorrhoids. If severe pain, bleeding or thrombosis are present, more definitive treatment may be indicated. A variety of options have been used over time including sclerotherapy, cryotherapy, binocular diathermy, rubber band ligation and surgical hemorrhoidectomy.

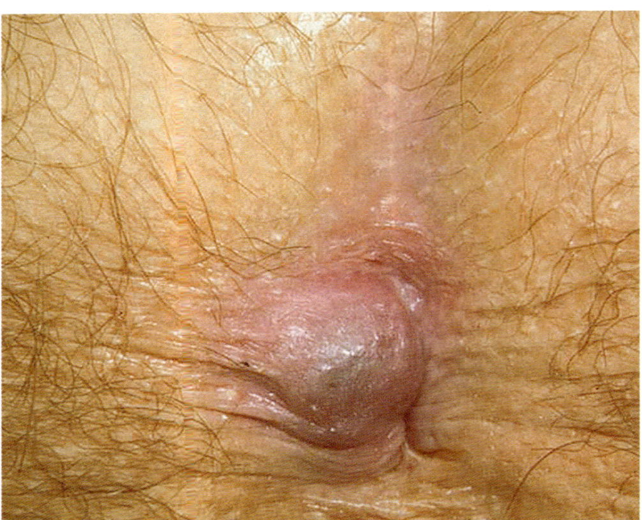

FIG. 10.44: Thrombosed external hemorrhoids

The following guidelines are helpful for persons undergoing anal/rectal surgery.

i. Preoperative care
   - Bowel preparation is standard, but an enema may not be prescribed if rectal pain is acute
   - Stool softeners may be given to promote a soft stool before surgery
ii. Postoperative care
   - Administer analgesics as prescribed, especially before initial defecation (considerable rectal discomfort may be present)
   - Provide emotional support before and after first defecation
   - Suggest side-lying position
   - Provide sitz baths as ordered (monitor for hypotension secondary to dilation of pelvic blood vessels in early postoperative period).
iii. Promotion of elimination
   - Administer prescribed stool softeners
   - Encourage patient to defectate as soon as the inclination occurs (prevents strictures and preserves normal anal lumen considerable anxiety is usually personal)
   - Monitor for hypotension, dizziness and faintness during first defecation
   - If an enema must be given, use small bore rectal tube.
iv. Patient teaching
   - Clean rectal area after each defecation until healing is complete (sitz bath is recommended)
   - Avoid constipation with a high-fiber diet, high-fluid intake, regular exercise and regular time for defecation
   - Use stool softeners until healing is complete
   - Seek medical consultation for rectal bleeding, suppurative drainage, continued pain on defecation, or continued constipation despite preventive measures.

Anal Fissure

An anal fissure or fissure in and around the anus is a skin ulcer or a crack in the lining of the anal wall that is caused by trauma or local infection. It is frequently associated with constipation and subsequent stretching of the anus from hard feces. The most common clinical manifestations are painful spasm of the anal sphincter and severe, burning pain during defecation. Some bleeding may occur and constipation resutls becasue of pain assocaited with bowel movements.

Conservative treatment consists of bowel regulations with mineral oil and stool softeners. Sitz bath and anal anesthetics suppositories (Anusol) are also ordered. Surgical treatment usually consists of excision of fissure. Postoperative care is similar to that of hemorrhoidectomy.

Anorectal Abscess

Anorectal abscesses are defined as undrained collections of perianal pus. They are due to perirectal infections in patient who have compromised local circulation or active inflammatory disease. The most common causative organism are *E. coli*, staphylococci and streptococci. Clinical manifestation includes local pain, swelling, foul-smelling, drainage, tenderness and elevated temperature and sepsis can occur (Fig. 10.45).

Surgical therapy consists of drainage of abscess of packing is used. It should be allowed to heal by granulation. The packing is changed every day and moist and hot compresses are applied to the area. Care must be taken to avoid soiling the dressing during urination and defecation. A low-residue diet is given. The patient may leave the hospital with area open. Teaching, should include wound care, the importance of sitz bath, thorough cleaning after bowel movement and periodic check-up.

Anorectal Fistula

An anorectal fistula is an abnormal tunnel leading out from the anus or rectum. It is a hollow tract leading through anal tissue from anorectal canal through skin near anus. It may extend to the outside the skin, vagina or buttocks. Anorectal fissures are complications of Crohn's disease. This condition often precedes an anorectal abscess (Fig. 10.45).

Feces may enter the fistula and cause an infection. There may be persistent, blood stained, purulent discharge or stool leakage from the fistula. The patient may have to wear a pad to prevent staining of clothes.

Surgical therapy involves a fistulotomy or a fistulectomy, Gauze packing is inserted and the wound is left to heal by granulation. Care is the same after hemorrhoidectomy.

Pilonidal Sinus (Fig. 10.46)

A pilonidal sinus is a small tract under the skin between the buttocks in the sacrococcygeal area. It is thought to be congenital

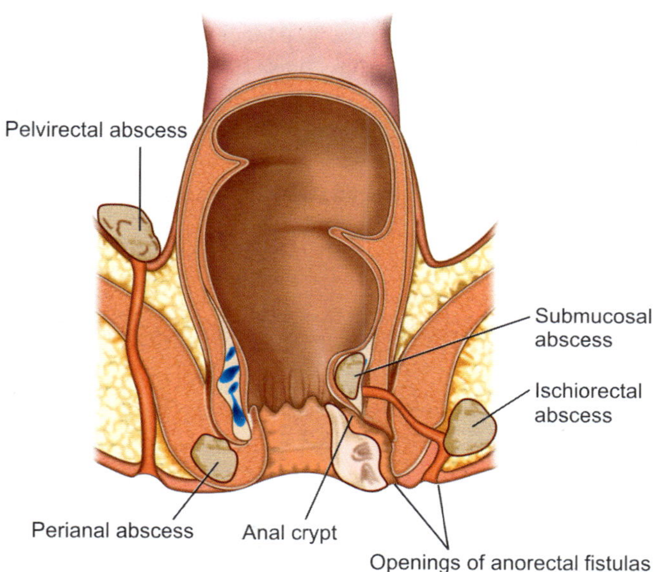

FIG. 10.45: Common sites of anorectal abscesses and fistula formation

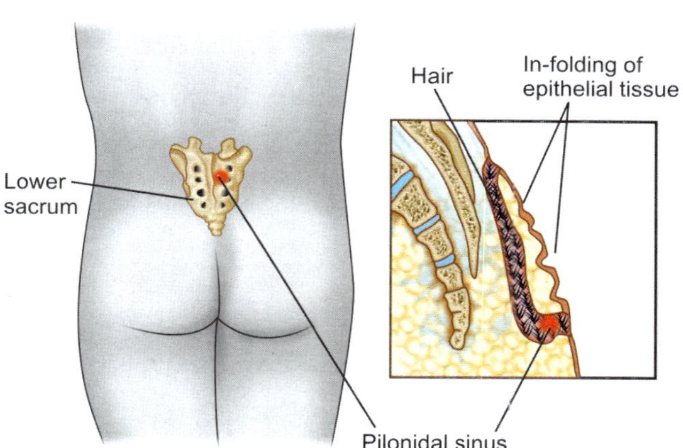

FIG. 10.46: (Left) Pilonidal sinus on lower sacrum about 5 cm (2 in) above the anus in the intergluteal cleft. (Right) Hair particles emerge from the sinus tract, and localized indentations (pits) can appear on the skin near the sinus openings.

origin. It may have several openings and is lined with epithelium and hair, thus the name pilonidal (a nest of hair).

The skin is moist and movement of the buttocks causes the short wiry hair to penetrate the skin. The irritated skin becomes infected and forms a pilonidal cyst or abscess. There are no symptoms unless there is an infection. If it becomes infested, the patient complains of pain and selling at the base of the spine.

A pilonidal sinus or cyst is found in the intergluteal cleft on the posterior surface of the lower sacrum. Current theories suggest that it results from local trauma, causing penetration of hairs into the epithelium and subcutaneous tissue. It may also be formed congenitally by an infolding of epithelial tissue beneath the skin, which may communicate with the skin surface through one or several small sinus openings. Hair frequently is seen protruding from these openings, and this gives the cyst its name, pilonidal (i.e. a nest of hair). The cysts rarely cause symptoms until adolescence or early adult life, when infection produces an irritating drainage of an abscess. Perspiration and friction easily irritate this area.

In the early stages of the inflammation, the infection may be controlled by antibiotic therapy, but after an abscess has formed, surgery is indicated. The abscess is incised and drained under local anesthesia. After the acute process resolves, further surgery is performed to excise the cyst and the secondary sinus tracts. The wound is allowed to heal by granulation. Absorptive dressing are placed in the wound to keep its edges separated while healing occurs.

The formed abscess requires incision and drainage. The wound may be closed or left open to heal by secondary intention. This wound is packed and sitz bath are ordered. Nursing care includes hot moist, heat application when an abscess is present. The patient is usualy more comfortable lying on the abdomen or side. The patient should be instructed to avoid contamination of dressing during urination or defecation and to avoid straining whenever possible.

Procedure 10.1: Assisting with a proctosigmoidoscopy

Equipment

- Fleet type enema used at least 1 hour before the sigmoidoscopy
- Oral laxative
- Water soluble lubricant
- Sigmoidoscopy
- Biposy forceps
- Culture swap
- Long applicator sticks
- Drapes or sheets
- Specimen bottles containing 10 percent Formalin culture tubes
- 4 × 4 gauze sponges
- Cytology brush
- Glass eyepiece to fit on scope during insufflation of air
- Disposable gloves for preliminary examination
- Suction machine
- Microscopic slides with fixative (cotton) or 95 percent ethyl alcohol
- Specimen labels

Nursing focus

1. Emergency resuscitation equipment needs to be available, because the vagus nerve is often stimulated and can tentiate a vagal reaction (pallor, diaphoresis, dizziness, weakness, unconsciousness, decrease in blood pressure, pulse rate, sometimes causing these vital signs to be unobtainable).
2. If giving enemas before the procedure, do not advance the tube too high into the colon, and administer the some slowly. If rectal bleeding or abdominal pain occur, stop at once and call the physician.

   Inform the health care provider of any known allergies and current medications; certain medications, such as anticoagulants, may be held before the test.

   Obtain prior X-rays and studies and send with the patient.

Steps of procedure

Nursing action	Rationale
Preparatory phase	
1. Record baseline vital signs. Leave the blood pressure cuff in place. An automatic blood pressure machine may be used, however, a manual cuff is preferred in the event the patient has a vagal reaction (see nursing alert above)	1. Monitoring of the blood pressure and pulse throughout the procedure will be necessary
2. Have the patient assume the knee-chest or Sim's lateral position	2. The position used depends on physician preference, patient condition, and nature of examining table (or bed)
a. Knee-chest position: 1. Knees are spread comfortable apart 2. Thighs are perpendicular to table 3. Feet are extended over the edge 4. Head is turned sideways to right (head shares pillow with chest) 5. Left arm is flexed to side of chest 6. Right arm may rest above head	a. This position permits the sigmoid to hang forward, diminishing the angle at the rectosigmoid junction
b. Sim's lateral position:	b. Used for elderly, ill, or arthritic patients or those who are reluc-tant to assume the knee-chest position.
1. Place, patient on left side with left leg partially flexed at hip and knee, right leg should be fully flexed	
2. Pelvis to be perpendicular to table	
3. Drape the patient so that only perineum is visible	3. A disposable large sheet with a circular opening is practical. This will minimize embarrassment
4. Explain to the patient to take slow deep breaths as the physician examines the rectum by digital examination	4. The physician is examining for tenderness, mucus, blood fistula, inflammation, ulceration and flexes. The digital examination also indicates the direction of the anal-canal, its patency, and the presence of any abnormality, if promotes anal relaxation and helps to lubricate the orifice
5. Warm sigmoidoscope in tap water or sterilizer to slightly above body temperature, lubricate tip of scope	5. A cold scope would cause discomfort and promote contraction rather than relaxation of perianal muscles. Water soluble lubricant permits easier passage of scope. It also minimizes the urge to defecate at tube insertion
6. Physician spreads buttocks and anal margins with left hand and inserts instrument with right hand (or vice versa). Have the patient breathe deeply	6. Keep instrument out of view of patient. Breathing slowly and deeply will help relax abdominal muscles and minimize cramping
7. Nurse encourages relaxation and explain each step in advance	7. Reassuring the patient promote relaxation
8. Physician may use a glass eye piece over viewing end of scope, an insufflation bulb and tubing are attached. A small quantity of air may be pumped into the bowel. Tell patient as the air moves down the bowel he may experience flatulence. This is normal	8. The purpose of inflating lower bowel with air is to expand the area viewed so that vision is not obstructed by mucosal folds and to facilitate passage into the sigmoid colon
9. Examination of the sigmoid, rectum and mucosa are done while the scope is being removed. If a rigid scope is used, passage of a large cotton swab through the scope may be done to remove blood, mucus and feces. If a flexible scope is used, only suction is necessary to clear the field. Turn suction to lowest setting initially	9. This clears the field of vision

Contd...

Contd...

Nursing action	Rationale
10. Passage of biopsy forceps, cytology brush, or culture swab through the scope is done to collect specimens	10. Specimens will be placed in 10 percent formalin and labelled. A specimen for cytology is placed in a container of 95 percent ethyl alcohol or affixed to a microscopic slide with slide fixative. Specimens for cultures will be sent in specimen tubes
11. Relay to the physician any expressions or complaints of pain by the patient	11. Tenderness and pain may be experienced by the patient with a history of abdominal surgery procedure may have to be terminated in order to risk perforation
Follow-up phase	
1. On withdrawal of scope, assist patient into gradually assuming a relaxed position	1. To promotes comfort
2. Wipe perianal area	2. Prevent soilage of garments
3. If disposable scope is used, rise and discard in proper receptable. Reusable scopes are properly cleaned with solution and water, per protocol. Sterilizable parts are sterilized before scope is stored	3. Prevents contamination and infection
4. Record the procedure, preparation of the patient, reaction of the patient, and patient's vital signs	
5. Label all specimens immediately and send to the laboratory	5. Minimize error, allow fresh samples for evaluation
6. Observe the patient for complications hemorrhage (increased pulse, decreased blood pressure, weakness, pallor, rectal bleeding and possible abdominal pain), perforation (sudden, severe abdominal pain), fever, malaise, changes in vital signs, bloody or mucoid rectal drainage, and possible abdominal distention	
7. Instruct the patient on these signs and symptoms and advise to notify health care provider immediately should they occur, ever after discharge	

Procedure 10.2: Administering an enema

Equipment

- Prepackaged enema or enema container
- Bedpan or commode
- Water-soluble jelly
- Basin
- Bath blanket
- Disposable gloves
- Washcloth and towel
- Water-proof pad
- Toilet tissue.

Steps of procedure

Nursing action	Rationale
Preparatory phase	
1. Assess the patient's bowel habits (last, BM, laxative usage, bowel patterns) and physical condition (hemorrhoids, mobility, external sphincter control)	1. Enema should not be given if there is a suspicion of appendicitis or bowel obstruction
2. Provide for privacy and explain procedure to patient	2. Provide comfort
Performance phase	
1. Wash hands	1. Promote hygiene
2. Place patient on left side with right knee fixed (Sims' position), place waterproof pad underneath patient and cover with bath blanket	2. Allow for enema solution to flow by gravity along the natural curve of the sigmoid colon and rectum
3. Place bedpan or bedside commode in position for patients who cannot ambulate to the toilet or who may have difficulty with sphincter control	3. Allow for easy accessibility
4. Remove plastic cover over tubing and lubricate tip of enema tubing 3–4 inches (7.5–10 cm) unless prepackaged (tip is already lubricated). Even prepackaged enema may need more lubricant	4. Prevent trauma and eases application
5. Apply disposable gloves	
6. Separate buttocks and locate rectum	

Contd...

Contd...

Nursing action	Rationale
7. Instruct patient that you will be inserting tubing and to take slow, deep breaths	7. Allows for patient relaxation and readiness
8. Insert tubing 3–4 inches for adult patients	8. Prevents tissue trauma of rectum
9. Slowly instill the solution using a clamp and the height of the container to adjust flow rate if using an enema bag and tubing for high enemas, raise enema container 12–18 inches, above anus; for low enemas, 12 inches. If using a prepackaged enema, slowly squeeze the container until all solution is instilled	9. Rapid infusion can cause colon distention and cramping container elevated past 12–18 inches, and controller on tubing not regulated contribute to rapid infusion
10. Lower container or clamp tubing if patient complains of cramping	
11. Withdraw rectal tubing after all enemas solution has been instilled or until clear (usually not more than three enemas)	11. "Until clear" means until results do not contain fecal matter and are clear
12. Instruct patient to hold solution as long as possible and that a feeling of distention may be felt	12. Promotes better results
13. Discard supplies in the appropriate trash receptacle	13. Maintains hygiene, minimizes patient embarrassment
14. Assist patient on the bedpan or to the bedside commode or toilet when urge to defecate occurs	
15. Observe enema return for amount, fecal content. Instruct patient not to flush toilet until the nurse has seen the results	
Note Enemas should not be given routinely to treat constipation because they disrupt normal defecation reflexes and the patient becomes dependent.	
Follow-up phase	
1. Document the type of enema given volume and results on the appropriate chart forms	
2. Assess and document presence or absence of abdominal distention after enema was given	
3. Assist the patient with washing perineum and rectal area, if indicated, may also need a clean gown or linen change	

NASOGASTRIC/NASOINTESTINAL INTUBATION

Nasogastric intubation refers to the insertion of a tube through the nasopharynx into the stomach. See procedure 10.3.

Nasointestinal intubation is performed by inserting a small bore-weighted tube that is carried via peristalsis into the duodenum or jejunum. It is primarily used for administering feedings and maintaining nutritional intake. See procedure 10.4; nasointestinal intubation.

Purposes of Nasogastric Intubation

1. Remove fluids and gas from stomach (decompression).
2. Prevent or relieve nausea and vomiting after surgery or traumatic events by decompressing the stomach.
3. Determine the amount of pressure and motor activity in the GI tract (diagnostic studies).
4. Irrigate the stomach for active bleeding or poisoning.
5. Treat mechanical obstruction.
6. Administer medications and feeding (gavage) directly into the GI tract.
7. Obtain a specimen of gastric contents for laboratory studies when pyloric or intestinal obstruction is suspected.

Procedure 10.3: Nasogastric intubation and removal

Equipment

- Nasogastric tube is usually single lumen (Levin) or double lumen (Salem), sump tube
- Water soluble lubricant
- Suction equipment
- Clamp for tubing
- Towel, tissues, and emesis basin
- Glass of water and straw
- Tincture of benzoin
- Hypoallergenic tape 1/2" and 1" bio-occlusive transparent dressing irrigating set with 20 mL syringe of a 50 mL catheter-tip syringe.
- Stethoscope
- Tongue blade
- Penlight
- Disposable gloves
- Normal saline

Follow-up equipment
Insertion procedure

- Lip pomade
- Mouth hygiene materials.

Preparatory phase

1. Ask the patient if he or she has ever had nasal surgery, trauma, or a deviated septum.
2. Explain procedure to the patient and tell how mouth breathing, panting and swallowing will help in passing the tube.
3. Place the patient in a sitting or high Fowler's position, place a towel across chest.
4. Determine with the patient what sign he or she might use, such as raising the index finger, to indicate "Wait a few moments" because of gagging or discomfort.
5. Remove dentures, place emesis basin and tissues within the patient's reach.
6. Inspect the tube for defects, look for partially closed holes or rough edges.
7. Place rubber tubing in ice-chilled water for a few minutes to make the tube firmer. Plastic tubing may already be firm enough, if too stiff, dip in warm water.
8. Determine the length of the tube needed to reach the stomach by placing the end of the tube at the tip of the patient's nose. Then extend it to the earlobe and down to the xiphoid process. Mark this distance with hypoallergenic tape (measurement range for the average-size adult is 55–66 cm (22–26 in).
9. Have the patient blow nose to clear nostrils.
10. Inspect the nostrils with a penlight, observing for any obstruction, occlude each nostril and have the patient breathe. This will help determine which nostril is more patient.
11. Wash your hands. Put on disposable gloves.

General Procedures/Treatment Modalities

1. Mark the nasoglastric tube at a point 50 cm from the distal tip; call this point 'A'.
2. Have the patient sit in a neutral position with head facing forward place the distal tip of the tubing at the tip of the patient's nose (N), extend tube to the tragus (tip) of his ear (E), and then extend the tube straight down to the tip of his xiphoid (X). Mark this point 'B' on the tubing.
3. To locate point C on the tube, find the midpoint between points A and B. The nasogastric tube is passed to point C to the ensure obtimum placement in the stomach.

Figures 10.47 to 10.50 and steps (1, 2, 3) indicate how far a nasogastric tube is passed for optimal placement in the stomach.

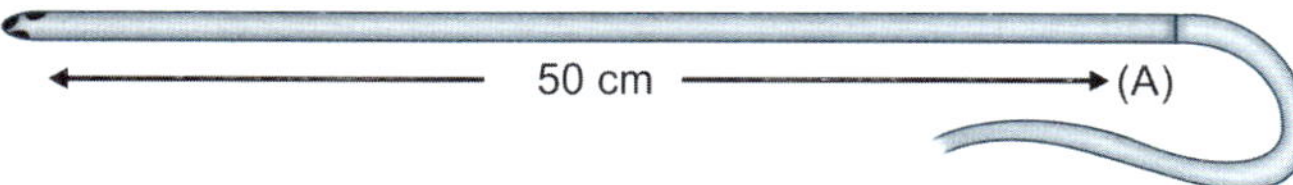

FIG. 10.47: Mark the nasogastric tube at a point 50 cm from the distal tip; call this point 'A'

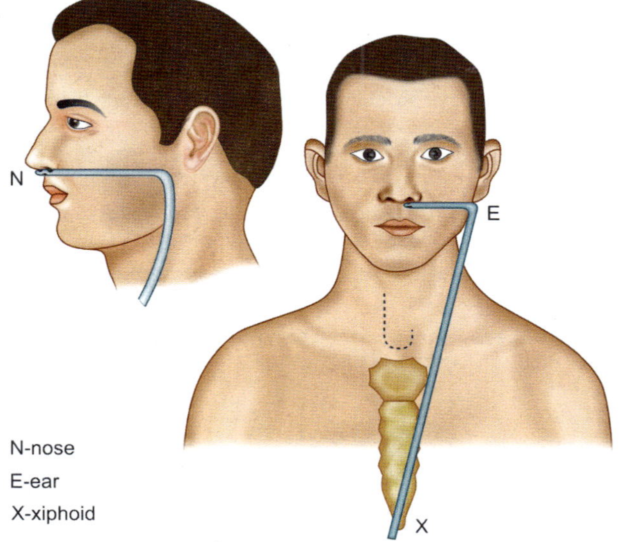

FIG. 10.48: Have the patient sit in a neutral position with head facing forward. Place the distal tip of the tubing at the tip of the patient's nose (N); extend tube to the tragus tip of his ear (E), and then extend the tube straight down to the tip of his xiphoid (X). Mark this point 'B' on the tubing

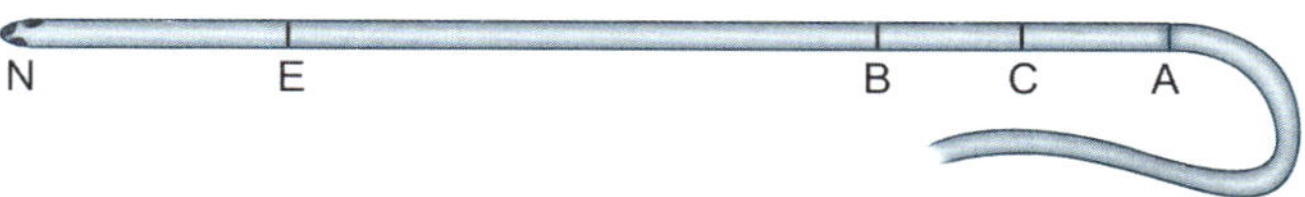

FIG. 10.49: To locate point C on the tube, find the midpoint between points A and B. The nasogastric tube is passed to point C to ensure optimum placement in the stomach

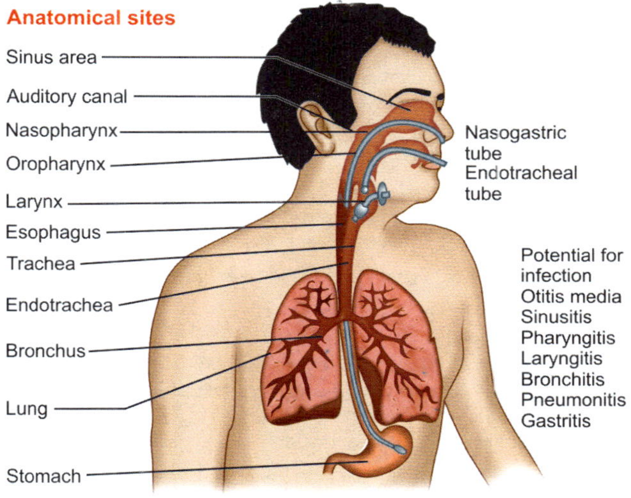

FIG. 10.50: All along the upper respiratory tract and upper digestive system, there is the potential for abnormal areas of colonization (infection) when various tubes are in place (i.e. tracheostomy, nasogastric or endotracheal tube). In addition, there is the potential for aspiration of secretions that may cause bronchitis and/or pneumonitis

Steps of procedure

Nursing action	Rationale
1. Coil the first 7–10 cm (3–4 in) of the tube around your fingers	1. This curves tubing and facilitates tube passage
2. Lubricate the coiled portion of the tube with water soluble lubricant. Avoid occluding the tube's holes with lubricant	2. Lubrication reduces friction between the mucous membranes and tube and prevents injury to the nasal passages. Using a water soluble lubricant prevents oil aspiration pneumonia if the tube accidently slips into trachea
3. Tilt back the patients head before inserting tube into nostril and gently pass tube into the posterior nasopharynx, directing downward and backward the ear	3. Passage of the tube is facilitated by following the natural contours of the body. The slower the advancement of the tube at this point, the lesser likelihood of putting pressure on the torbinates, which could cause pain and bleeding
4. When tube reaches the pharynx, the patient may gag; allow patient to rest for a few moments	4. Gag reflex is triggered by the presence of the tube
5. Have the patient tilt head slightly forward offer several sips of water sipped through a straw or permit patient to suck on ice chips, unless contraindicated. Advance tube as patient swallows	5. Flexed head position partially occludes the airway and the tube is less likely to enter trachea, swallowing closes the epiglottis over the trachea and facilitates passage of tube into the esophagus. Actually, once the tube passes the cricopharyngeal sphincter into the esophagus, it can be slowly and steadily advanced even if the patient does not swallow
6. Gently rotate the tube 180 degrees to redirect the curve	6. This prevents the tube from entering the patient's mouth
7. Continue to advance tube gently each time the patient swallows	
8. If obstruction appears to prevent tube from passing, do not use force. Rotating tube gently may help, if unsuccessful, remove tube and try other nostril	8. Avoid discomfort and trauma to patient
9. If there are signs of distress such as gasping, coughing or cyanosis, immediately remove tube	9. May have entered the trachea
10. Continue to advance the tube when the patient swallows until the tape mark reaches the patient's nostril	10. This is the reference point where the tube was measured
11. To check whether the tube is in the stomach a. Ask the patient to talk b. Use the tongue blade and penlight to examine the patient's mouth-especially an unconscious patient c. Attach a syringe to the end of the NG tube. Place a stetho- scope over the left upper quadrant of the abdomen and inject 10–20 cc of air while auscultating the abdomen d. Aspirate contents of stomach with a 50 mL catheter tip syringe. If stomach contents cannot be aspirated, place the patient on left side and advance the tube 2.5–5 cm (1–2 in) and try again	11. a. If the patient cannot talk, the tube may be coiled in throat or passed through vocal cards b. If the patient is choking or has difficulty in breathing the tube has probably entered the trachea c. Air can be detected by a "Whooshing" sound entering stomach rather than the bronchus. If bel-ching occurs, the tube is probably in the esophagus d. Aspirated stomach contents indicate that the tube is in the stomach e. X-rays may be done to confirm tube placement
12. After tube is passed and the correct placement is confirmed, attach the tube to suction or clamp the tube	12. Clamping can be done using a clamp, plastic plug, of folding the tube over and slipping the bend into the tube end
13. Apply tincture of benzoin to the area where the tape is placed	13. This helps make the tube adhere, especially with diaphoretic patients
14. Anchor tube with: a. Hypoallergenic tape; split lengthwise and only half way attach unsplit end of tape to nose and cross split ends around tubing. Apply another piece of tape to bridge of nose b. Bio-occlusive transparent dressing where it exits the nose	14. Prevents the patient's vision from being distrubed; prevents tubing from rubbing against nasal mucosa. This will ensure tape being secure
15. Anchor the tubing to the patient's gown. Use a rubber band to make a slip-knot to anchor the tubing to the patient's gown. Secure the rubber band to the patient's gown using a safety pin	15. To permit mobility of patient. This prevents tugging of the tube when the patient moves
16. Clamp the tube until the purpose for inserting the tube takes place	16. See Rationale 12
17. Attach the tube to suction equipment of prescribed	

Contd...

Contd...

Nursing action	Rationale
18. Assure the patient that most discomfort he or she feels will lessen as he or she gets used to the tube	
19. Irrigate the tube at regular intervals with small volumes of prescribed fluid a. If the tube is a Salem sump, it will require periodic placing of 10–20 mL of air through the vent port (blue port) b. Check the tube patency by placing the vent port next to your ear	19. Please Note: All enteric tubes must be irrigated with small volumes of fluid and at regular intervals to ensure patency a. A soft hissing sound is heard if the tube is patient b. If the port hangs downward and the tube backs up stomach contents will spill over the patient
20. Cleanse nares and provide mouth care every shift	20. To promote patient comfort and decrease risk of infection
21. Apply petrolatum to nostrils as needed and assess for skin irritation or breakdown	21. To keep tissue soft and prevent crusting and skin breakdown
22. Keep head of bed elevated at least 30 degrees	22. To minimize gastroesophageal reflux
23. Record the time, type and size of tube inserted. Document placement checks after each assessment, along with amount, color, consistency of drainage	23. To ensure proper tube and placement at all times, and assist in evaluation of tube effectiveness

Note

If the patient has a nasal condition that prevents insertion through the nose, the tube is passed through the mouth. Remove denture, slide the tube over the tongue, and proceed the same way as a nasal intubation. Make sure to coil the end of the tube and direct it downward at the pharynx.

Feeding tubes are more successfully declogged when intervention is initiated immediately after the obstruction is noted and if the obstruction is close to the proximal tube opening.

Other Nursing Patient Care Considerations

1. If the patient is unconscious, advance the tube between respirations to make sure it does not enter the tracheas. You will need to stroke the unconscious patient's neck to facilitate passage of the tube down the esophagus.
2. Watch for cyanosis while passing the tube in an unconscious patient, cyanosis indicates the tube has entered the trachea.
3. Never place the end of the tube in a container of fluid while checking for placement. If the tube is in the trachea the patient could inhale the water.
4. Do not tape the tube to the forehead; it can cause necrosis of the nostril.
5. a. Sucralfate (Carafate) may be ordered after NG tube insertion to provide a protective barrier against gastric acid, pepsin and bile. After administering carafate, clamp tube for half on hour, then unclamp and reconnect to suction (if ordered).
   b. Clotrimazole (Mycelex) may be ordered as prophylactic treatment for *Candida albicans*.
6. Pain or vomiting after the tube is inserted indicates tube obstruction or incorrect placement.
7. The air vent on the Salem sump tube should not be used for irrigation.
8. If the air vent (Salem sump tube) is draining fluid or is not drawing air, instill 20 cc of air through the vent.
9. Irrigate the NG tube every 2 hours unless otherwise ordered.
10. If the NG tube is not draining, the nurse should reposition tube by advancing or withdrawing it slightly (with a physician order). After repositioning, always check for placement.
11. Recognize the complications when the tube is inside for prolonged periods; nasal erosion, sinusitis, esophagitis, esophagus, tracheal fistula, gastric ulceration, and pulmonary and oral infections.

    All along the upper respiratory tract and upper digestive system, there is the potential for abnormal areas of colonization (infection) when various tubes are in place. (i.e. tracheostomy, nasogastric or endotracheal tube). In addition, there is the potential for aspiration of secretions that may cause bronchitis and/or pneumonitis.
12. Notify the health care provider of any continuous problems.

Removal Procedure

Preparatory phase

1. Be certain that gastric or small bowel drainage is not excessive in volume.
2. Ensure by ausculation that audible peristalsis is present.
3. Determine whether the patient is passing flatus, this indicates peristalsis.
4. There is a physician's order for removal.

Removing Nasogastric Tubing

Steps of Procedure

Nursing action	Rationale
1. Place a towel across the patient's chest and inform him or her that the tube is to be withdrawn	1. No doubt, the patient will be happy to have progressed to this stage
2. Apply disposable gloves	2. Provides protection from contaminated body fluids
3. Turn off suction, disconnect and clamp tube	3. Prevents fluids from leaking from tube
4. Remove the tape from the patient's nose	
5. Instruct the patient to take a deep breath and hold it	5. This maneuver closes the epiglottis
6. Slowly but evenly withdraw tubing and cover it with a towel as it emerges (as the tube reaches the nasopharynx, you can pull quickly)	6. Covering the tubing helps dispel patient's nausea
7. Provide the patient with materials for oral care and lubricant for nasal dryness	7. Mouthwash and a nasal lubricant will be appreciated for the patient
8. Dispose of equipment in appropriate receptacle	
9. Document time of tube removal and the patient's reaction	
10. Document tube removal and color, consistency, and amount of drainage in suction canister	
11. Continue to monitor the patient for signs of GI difficulties	11. Recurrence of nausea or vomiting may require reinsertion of nasogastric tubing, changes in vital signs may suggest infection

Procedure 10.4: Nasointestinal intubation (Fig. 10.51)

Small Bore-Feeding Tubes

Equipment

- Type of tube ordered by health care provider
- 30 cc or 60 cc Luer-Lok or tip syringe
- Water soluble lubricant
- Tape, rubber band, clamp and safety pin
- Glass of water
- Stethoscope.

Nursing focus

All tubes and endoscopes should be routinely pre-tested for patency and function before passage.

Maintaining tube function is an ongoing responsibility of the nurse, patient, and primary caregiver. To ensure patency and to decrease the chance of bacterial growth, crusting, or occlusion of the tube, at least 30 to 50 mL of water or normal saline is administered in each of the following instances:

- Before and after each dose of medication and tube feeding

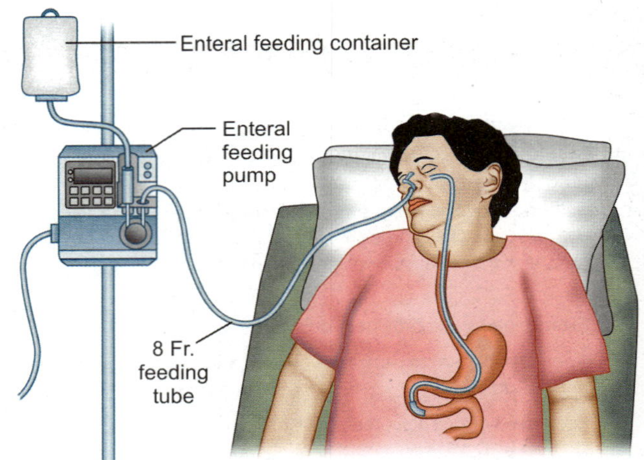

FIG. 10.51: Nasoenteric tube feeding by continuous controlled pump. The head of the bed should be elevated to prevent aspiration

- After checking for gastric residuals and gastric pH
- Every 4 to 6 hours with continuous feedings
- If the tube feeding is discontinued or interrupted for any reason
- When the tube is not being used, where a minimum of twice-daily flushing is recommended.

Any water or normal saline used to irrigate these tubes must be recorded as fluid intake. One study suggests that tap water may injure the small bowel and supports the practice of flushing postpyloric nasoduodenal or jejunostomy tubes with normal saline.

Providing medications by tube

When different types of medications are prescribed, a bolus method is used for administration that is compatible with the medication's preparation. The tube is flushed with 30 to 50 mL of water after medication administration, and this is recorded as intake. Medications should not be mixed with the feeding formula. When small-bore feeding tubes for continuous infusion are irrigated after administration of medications, a 30 mL or larger syringe is used because the pressure generated by smaller syringes could rupture the tube.

Administering medications through postpyloric enteric tubes may adversely affect their absorption; therefore, this should be avoided if possible.

Steps of procedure

Nursing action	Rationale
1. Tube preparation.	
a. Do not ice plastic tubes	a. Become too stiff to work with
b. Inject 10 cc of water into the tube	b. Aidee in insertion
c. Insert guidewire or stylet into tube, making sure it is positioned snugly against tube	c. Prevent trauma
d. Dip weighted tip into glass of water	d. Activate lubricant

Nursing action	Rationale
2. Similar to passing a short nasogastric tube and taping to patient	
3. After the tube enters the stomach, it passes by peristalsis and gravity into the small intestine a. Change patient's position from Fowler's to a position in which the patient is leaning forward	3. This will assist in advancing the tubing to and through the pylorus; tilting to the right is helpful
4. Obtain an X-ray of the abdomen after tube insertion	4. Confirm placement
5. Stylet should remain in place until position is confirmed	

Nursing/Patient Care Considerations

1. Beware of risk of aspiration in an unconscious patient.
2. Instruct patient on complications associated with tube feedings, such as nausea, vomiting and diarrhea.

Be alert for the following assessment findings:

- Tube placement, patient's position (head of bed elevated 30 to 45 degrees), and formula flow rate
- Patient's ability to tolerate the formula; observe for fullness, bloating, distention, nausea, vomiting, and stool pattern
- Clinical responses, as noted in laboratory findings (blood urea nitrogen, serum protein, prealbumin, electrolytes, renal function, hemoglobin, hematocrit)
- Signs of dehydration (dry mucous membranes, thirst decreased urine output)
- Amount of formula actually taken in by the patient
- Elevated blood glucose level, decreased urinary output, sudden weight gain, and periorbital or dependent edema
- Infection control practices: replace any formula administered by an open system every 4 hours with fresh formula; change tube feeding container and tubing every 24 to 72 hours
- Residual volume before each feeding or, in the case of continuous feedings, every 4 hours; return the aspirate to the stomach
- Intake and output
- Weekly weights
- Recommendations made on dietitian consult.

Although a residual volume of 200 mL or greater is generally considered a cause for concern in patients at high risk for aspiration, feedings do not necessarily need to be withheld in all patients.

Procedure 10.5: Changing a two-piece drainable fecal pouching system

Equipment:

- Duplicate wafer and pouch
- Tail closure
- Washcloth and towel
- Mid non-oily soap (optional)
- Accessory products prescribed for patient.

Steps of procedure

Nursing action	Rationale
Preparatory phase	
1. Explain the details of this activity	1. Encourages patient understanding and participation to learn selfcare
2. Gather equipment and place within easy reach	2. Minimizes distractions and fasters organization
3. Have the patient assume a relaxed position and provide privacy. The best position may be sitting, reclining, or standing	3. Patient must see stoma site to learn care
Performance phase	
1. To remove pouching system a. Wear nonsterile gloves b. Push down gently on skin while lifting up on the wafer (ostomy adhesive remover may be used) c. Discard soiled pouch and wafer in odorproof plastic bag. Save tail closure for reuse	a. Maintain universal precautions b. Minimize skin trauma c. Removes room odor and maintains universal precautions
2. To cleanse skin: a. Use toilet tissue to remove feces from stoma and skin if needed b. Cleanse stoma and peristomal skin with soft cloth and water, soap optional. The patient may shower with or without pouching system in place. Clip or shave peristomal hair if appropriate	a. Stoma may function during the change b. Minimizes skin breakdown and promotes hygiene

Contd...

Contd...

Nursing action	Rationale
c. Rinse and dry skin throughly after cleansing. It is normal for the stoma to bleed slightly during cleansing and drying	c. Removes residue, which may interfere with adhesion of wafer
3. To apply wafer.	
a. Use measuring guide or stomal pattern to determine stoma size	a. This step is omitted when stomal shrinkage is complete about 2 months postop
b. Trace correct size pattern on-to back of wafer and cut to nearly stoma size. It is acceptable to cut 1/16–1/8 in larger than stoma	b. Avoids wafer rubbing stoma, omit this step if the wafer is precut
c. Apply a line of skin barrier paste around stoma or on lip of wafer opening. Allow to set according to manufacturers instructions (other barrier may be used in place of paste, such as strips or washer, because some patients are allergie to the alcohol in paste)	c. Extra skin protection is imperative for ileostomy and right sided colostomy. A left sided colostomy may not need secondary barrier because formed stool is less harmful to skin, paste acts as "Caul King" to prevent undermining of feces
d. Remove paper backing(s) from the wafer, center opening over stoma, and press wafer down onto peristomal skin	d. Ensures adherence
4. Snap pouch onto the flange of the wafer according to manufacturer's directions (Fig. 10.52)	4. If attached properly, there will be no leakage or odor

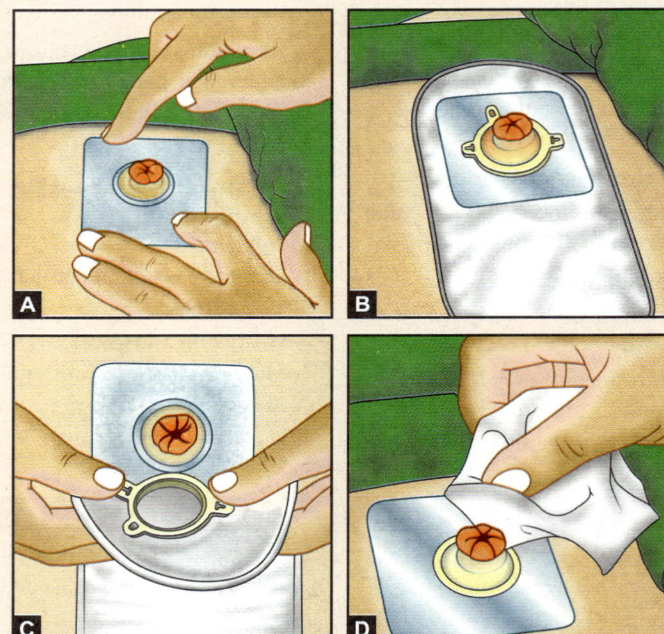

FIGS 10.52A TO D: (A) A wafer with flange (1 1/2", 1 3/4", 2 1/4", 2 3/4", 4") is applied after cleaning and drying of peristomal skin; (B) A transparent or opaque drainable pouch is positioned over stoma at desired angle; (C) Pouch may be removed without removal of wafer; (D) Stoma may be assessed without removing wafer (Adapted by permission from Convatec, A Bristol-Myers, Squibb Company)

Nursing action	Rationale
5. Apply till closure to pouch tail	5. Proper closure controls odor
Follow-up phase	
1. Dispose of plastic bag with waste materials	
2. Clean drainable pouch with soap and water, if appropriate Drainable pouches may be reused several times	2. Controls odor, reduces cost
3. A commercial deodorant can be placed in the pouch to reduce odor	
4. Gas can be released from the pouch by releasing the tail closure or by snapping off an area on the pouch flange. Never make a pinhole in the pouch to release gas	4. Destroys the odorproof seal

Procedure 10.6: Irrigating a colostomy

Equipment

1. Reservoir for irrigating fluids, irrigator bag or enema bag if irrigator bag not available.
2. Irrigating fluid 500–1,500 mL lukewarm water or other solution prescribed by health care provider (volume is titrated based on patient tolerance and results, average amount is 1,000 mL).
3. Irrigating tip cone tip or soft rubber catheter 22 or 24 with shield to prevent backflow of irigating solution. (Use only if cone not available. The cone is the preferred method to avoid possibility of bowel perforation).
4. Irrigation sleeve (long large capacity bag with opening at top to insert cone or catheter into stoma) available in different styles snap-on, self-adhering to skin, or held in place by belt.
5. Large tail closure.
6. Water-soluble lubricant.

Steps of procedure

Nursing action	Rationale
Preparatory phase	
1. Explain the details of the procedure to the patient and answer any questions 2. Select a consistent time, free from distractions. If the patient is learning to irrigate for bowel control, choose the time of day that will best fit into the patient's lifestyle 3. Have the patient sit in front of the commode on chair or on the commode itself providing privacy and comfort 4. Hang irrigating reservoir with prescribed solution so that the bottom of the reservoir is approximately at the level of the patient's shoulder and above the stoma	
Performance phase	
1. Remove pouch or covering from stoma and apply irrigation sleeve, directing the open tail into the commode	1. Allows wafer and feces to flow directly into commode
2. Open tubing clamp on the irrigating reservoir to release a small amount of solution into the commode	2. Removes air from the setup: avoids air from being introduced into the colon, which can cause crampy pain
3. Lubricate the tip of the cone/catheter and gently insert into the stoma. Insert catheter no more than 3 inch. Hold cone/shield gently, but firmly against stoma to prevent backflow of water	3. Prevents intestinal perforation and irritation of mucous membranes
4. If catheter does not advance easily, allow water to flow slowly while advancing catheter. Never force catheter. Dilating the stoma with lubricated gloved pinky finger may be necessary to direct cone/catheter properly	4. Slow rate relaxes bowel to facilitate passage of catheter
5. Allow water to enter colon slowly over a 5–10 minute period. If cramping occurs, slow flow rate or clamp tubing to allow cramping to subside, removed cone/catheter to release contents	5. Cramping may occur from too rapid flow, cold water excess solution, or colon ready to function
6. Hold cone/shield in place 10 seconds after water is instilled, then gently remove cone/catheter from stoma	6. Discourages premature evacuation of fluid
7. As feces and water flows down sleeve, periodically rinse sleeve with water. Allow 10–15 minutes for most of the returns, then dry sleeve tail and apply tail closure	7. Esophageal disorders
8. Leave sleeve in place for approximately 20 more minutes while patient gets up and moves around	8. Ambulation stimulates peristalsis and completion of irrigation return
9. When returns are complete, clean stomal area with mild soap and water pat dry; reapply pouch or covering over stoma.	9. Cleanliness and dryness promote comfort
Follow-up phase	
1. Clean equipment with soap and water, dry and store in well ventilated area	1. This will control odor and mildew prolonging the life of equipment
2. If applicable, the patient should use a pouch until the colostomy is sufficiently controlled	2. It may take several months to establish control. The patient can then use minipouch stoma cap, or gauze covering as desired

Other Nursing/Patient Care Considerations

1. It is a patient preference whether colostomy irrigations are attempted for control irrigation may occur every day or every other day depending on bowel pattern. It usually takes 1-2 months to establish control, patients with a preoperative history of regular, formed bowel movements are more likely to realize success.
2. Disadvantages to the colostomy irrigation approach for control include (a) It is a time-consuming procedure requiring consistency which may not fit into a patient's lifestyle. (b) Bowel dependency can occur with the irrigation as the stimulus for evacuation of bowel movements.
3. Only a patient with a descending or sigmoid colostomy is an irrigation candidate for fecal control. A colostomy more proximal than descending has too liquid and higher volume of fecal output to be managed through irrigation.

Community-based Care Points

If a patient discontinues colostomy irrigations, after months or years of performance, due to illness, hospitalization, or preference, a bulk of laxative or other stimulant may be routinely necessary to maintain regular bowel function.

Procedure 10.7: Teaching the patient with dysphagia how to swallow

Equipment

- Suction
- Face mask
- Glass with straw.
- Oxygen
- Selected foods

Steps of procedure

Nursing action	Rationale
Preparation	
1. Explain to the patient about your plan to work with him or her in developing an effective swallow	1. The patient's co-operation, concentration, and directed participation are essential to the success of the learning experience
2. Ensure that emergency equipment is available at the bedside- suction, oxygen and face mask	2. For use in the event that the patient chokes, vomits or aspirates
3. Place the patient in an upright sitting position in a chair or support with pillows in high-Fowler's position if unable to get out of bed for about 20 minutes before and 45–60 minutes after meals	3. This will allow time to adjust and relax in this position before meals; allows gravity to assist the swallowing procedure during meals, helps prevent reflux or regurgitation after meals
4. Provide mouth care before meals. Suction the patient of secretions are present. If the patient's mouth is dry, provide a lemon wedge or pickle to suck on	4. This will increase patient's ability to taste and enjoy the sensation of eating
5. Prepare an environment that is pleasant, peaceful, and without interruptions. Remove distracters, such as TV and radio	5. Patient must be able to concentrate on the process of swallowing in a relaxed manner
Food and fluid selection	
6. Food should be chosen that hold some shape, most enough to prevent crumbling but dry enough to hold a bolus shape casseroles, custards, scrambled eggs	6. Foods that crumble may be aspirated when they false apart foods that are too moist may be drooled through the lids
7. Mugs and glasses with spouts or a straw should be used for liquids	7. These utensils help prevent liquids from leaking out of corners of patient's mouth
8. Avoid sticky foods, peanut butter, chocolate, milk and ice cream	8. These foods stimulate thick mucos and will make swallowing more difficult
9. Dry foods can be moistened with margarine, gravy, or broths, If liquids are a problem, juices can be thickened with sherbets	9. Foods need to be of a consistency that will hold a bolus form until swallowed
10. Avoid tepid or room temperature foods	10. Hot and cold foods are thought to be maximally stimulate receptors that activate swallowing mechanism
Instructions during meals	
11. Have patient position head in the midline and forward, chin pointed toward chest	11. Improve ability to consciously swallow without food falling down the posterior pharynx. Support patient's forehead with a hand if the patient lacks neck control
12. Instruct the patient to smell the food before each bite, hold each bite for a few seconds; hold lips together firmly; concentrate on swallowing; then swallow	12. Concentrating on each step before swallowing will increase the effectiveness of the swallow

Contd...

Contd...

Nursing action	Rationale
13. If the patient has an increase in saliva during the meal, instruct the patient to collect the saliva with the tongue and consciously swallow it between bites throughout the meal	13. This will help prevent aspiration of saliva between mouthfuls
14. If the patient complains of a dry mouth during meals, instruct the patient to move the tongue in a circular form against the insides of the cheeks	14. This will help stimulate salivation
15. Caution the patient against talking during the meal or with the mouth full of food	15. Talking or laughing during eating is a common cause of airway obstruction
Follow-up care	
16. Provide mouth care after meals	16. Food particles may collect in the mouth or cheeks
17. Record the amount of intake, the patient's taste and food preferences, progress, and any special tactics that were effective in helping the swallowing process	17. Progress notes will assist in moving toward self care
18. Encourage family members to participate in the patient's feeding program	18. This will help provide continuity on discharge

Feeding the patient with an affected side of the mouth (facial paralysis, hemiplegia)

1. Turn the patient to the unaffected side.	1. This helps prevent food from falling down the weaker/paralyzed part of the oral cavity, a possible cause of aspiration.
2. Place food on the unaffected side of mouth rather than in the middle of the mouth.	2. Permits food to be managed more effectively.
3. Encourage the patient to form a bolus by moving the food around the mouth with the tongue.	3. This assists in placing food in a proper position for swallowing rather than permitting food to collect near the cheek.

CHAPTER

11

Hepatobiliary Pancreatic Nursing

INTRODUCTION

Hepatobiliary pancreatic nursing refers to the nursing care of the disorders of liver and pancreas. In this chapter, different disorder related to liver and pancreas and then nursing management discussed. See liver gallbladder pancreas and duodenum (Fig. 11.1).

JAUNDICE

Jaundice, a yellowish discoloration of body tissues, resulting from an alteration in normal bilirubin metabolism or flow of bile into the hepatic or biliary duct systems. It is a symptom which results when the concentration of bilirubin level has to be approximately three times normal level (2 to 3 mg) for jaundice

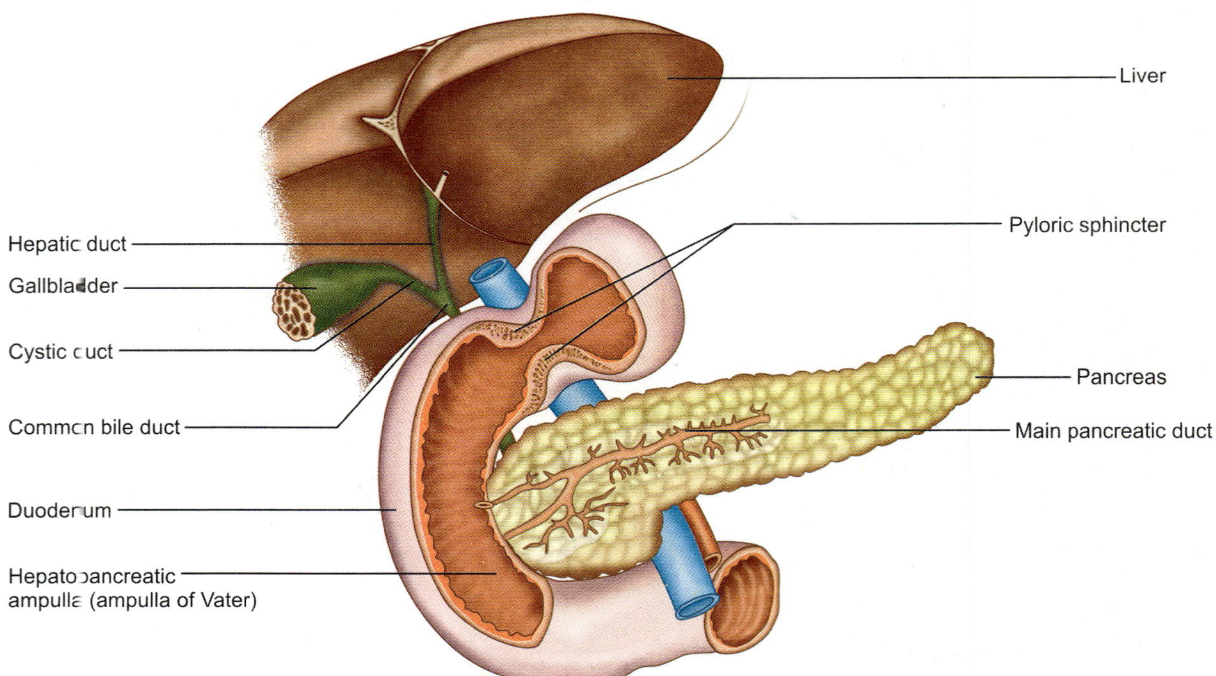

FIG. 11.1: The liver, gallbladder, pancreas and duodenum

to occur. The three types of jaundice are classified in hemolytic, hepatocellular and obstructive.

1. Hemolytic jaundice (prehepatic) is due to an increased breakdown of red blood cells which produces an increased amount of unconjugated bilirubin in the blood. The liver is unable to handle this increased load. Causes of this type include blood transfusion reaction, sickle cells crisis and hemolytic anemia.
2. Hepatocellular jaundice (hepatic) results from the liver's altered ability to take up bilirubin from the blood or to conjugate or excrete it. Both unconjugated and conjugated bilirubin serum levels increase. Because conjugated bilirubin is water soluble; it is excreted in the urine. The most common cause of this type are hepatitis, cirrhosis, and hepatocarcinoma.
3. Obstructive jaundice (posthepatic) is due to impeded or obstructed flow of bile through the liver or biliary duct system. The obstruction may be intrahepatic or extrahepatic. Intrahepatic obstructions are due to swelling or fibrosis of the liver's caliculi and bile ducts. This can be caused by damage from liver tumors, hepatitis or cirrhosis. Causes of extrahepatic obstructions include common bile duct obstruction from a stone, sclerosing cholangitis and carcinoma of the head of the pancreas. Here moderate elevation is both conjugated and unconjugated bilirubin and urine bilirubin.

Jaundice is a major problem in patients with diffuse hepatocellular disorder, which includes hepatitis, cirrhosis and hepatic carcinoma.

HEPATITIS

Hepatitis is an inflammation of the liver. Although the term hepatitis is most often used in conjunction with viral hepatitis, the disease can also be caused by the bacteria or toxic injury to the liver. Although some differences exist in the pathological and clinical phenomena of viral, bacterial, and toxic hepatitis, the clinical management of the person with any of these types of hepatitis is quite similar.

Toxic Hepatitis

Since liver has a primary role in the metabolism of foreign substances, many agents including drugs, alcohol, industrial toxins and persons can cause toxic hepatities. Many health care workers are concerned about hepatic injury caused by adverse drug reactions from the drugs they handle.

Etiology

The agents that produce hepatic injury are categorized into two major groups. Predictable (intrinsic) hepatotoxins and non-predictable (idiosyncratic) hepatotoxins.

i. Predictable hepatotoxic agents cause toxic hepatitis with predictable regularity and produce injury in a high percentage of persons exposed to them. Occurrence of toxic hepatitis is dose dependent. The predictable hepatotoxins are further divided into two subgroups—direct or indirect.
   - The direct predictable hepatotoxin agents have direct effect on hepatic cells and organelles, producing structural changes that lead to metabolic defects. For example:
     - Carbon tetrachloride and other chlorinated hydrocarbon (industrial toxin)
     - Yellow phosphorous (industrial toxin)
     - Mushroom poisoning (plant toxin).
   - The indirect predictable hepatotoxins are mostly; Drugs such as ethanol, tetracycline, methotrexate, L-asparaginase, puromycin, 6-mercaptopurine, acetaminophen, mithramycin, urethane, halothane, cholecystographic dyes, rifamycin B. These are agents which first interfere with normal metabolic function and this alteration in metabolic function produces structural change.

ii. Non-predictable hepatotoxic agents produce hepatic injury only in unusually susceptible persons and in only a small percentage of persons exposed to them. Occurrence is not dose-dependent. These drugs such as phenytoin, PAS, INH, chlorpromazine and androgens and anabolic steroids, chlorpropamide, imipramine, methyldopa, monoamine oxidase (MAO) inhibitors, oral contraceptives, sulfonamides, allopurinol, clindamycin, erythromycin, esters, nitrofurantoin, oxacillin and estrogen steroid.

Pathophysiology

The morphological changes produced in the liver by the toxin vary, depending on the specific hepatotoxin. For example, carbon tetrachloride, tetracycline, and ethanol cause fatty infiltration and/or necrosis, oral contraceptives, cholecystographic dyes and chlorpromazine produces cholestasis and portal inflammation. The alterations may result in only minimal manifestations of altered liver function such as slightly-elevated serum enzymes or major manifestation associated with terminal liver failure.

Clinical Manifestation

Early manifestation includes anorexia, nausea, vomiting, lethargy, elevated ALT and AST levels. Later manifestations are icterus, hepatomegaly, hepatic tenderness, dark urine, elevated serum bilirubin level and urine bilirubin level.

Management

Proper attention is focussed on identifying the toxic agents and removing or eliminating it. Gastric lavage, and cleansing of the bowel may be indicated to remove the hepatotoxins from the intestinal tract. There are specific treatments for particular hepatotoxins (Follow as prescribed). In most instances of toxic hepatitis, medical treatment is supportive and focussed on particular manifestation such as treatment of cirrhosis, portal-systemic encephalopathy or accompanying renal failure. Nursing care includes maintaining fluid and electrolyte balance, promoting a well-balanced diet, when food and fluids are allowed, and promoting rest and treating complications.

Nurses also should teach patient's family to use only prescribed medication with precaution to the liver injury. For prevention of hepatitis teach the following:

- Encourage proper community and home sanitation
- Encourage conscientious individual hygiene
- Instruct patients regarding safe practices for preparing and dispensing food
- Support effective health supervision of schools, dormitories, extended care facilities, barracks and camps
- Promote community health education programs
- Facilitate mandatory reporting of viral hepatitis to local health departments
- Recommend vaccination for all children 1 year of age and older
- Recommend vaccination for travelers to developing countries, illegal drug users (injection and noninjection drug users), men who have sex with men, and people with chronic liver disease, and recipients (e.g. hemophiliacs) of pooled plasma products
- Promote vaccination to interrupt community-wide outbreaks.

The dietary management of drug related viral hepatitis is as follows:

- Recommend small, frequent meals
- Provide intake of 2000 to 3000 kcal/d during acute illness
- Although early studies indicate that a high-protein, high-calorie diet may be beneficial, advise patient not to force food and to restrict fat intake
- Carefully monitor fluid balance
- If anorexia and nausea and vomiting persist enteral feeding may be necessary
- Instruct patient to abstain from alcohol during acute illness and for at least 6 months after recovery
- Advise patient to avoid substances (medications, herbs, illicit drugs and toxins) that may affect liver function.

Viral Hepatitis

Viral hepatitis is by far the most important liver infections. The term viral hepatitis is used to refer to several clinically similar but etiologically and epidemiologically distinct infections.

Etiology

Viral hepatitis can be caused by one of the five major viruses A, B, C, D and E, i.e. HAV, HBV, HCV, HDV, HEV. Two other forms of hepatitis—hepatitis F and hepatitis G have been identified but occur rarely.

- HAV is a RNA virus transmitted through feco-oral route. Incubation period is 15–50 days (average 28 days). Crowded condition, poor personal hygiene, poor sanitation, contaminated food, milk water and shell-fish, persons with subclinical infections, infected food handlers, and sexual contacts are the sources of infection and spread of disease. Most infections during 2 weeks before onset of symptoms; infectious until 1–2 weeks after symptoms start.
- HBV is a DNA virus that is transmitted by percutaneous (IV drug use, accidental needle-stick punctures or permucosal exposure to infective blood, blood products, or per mucosal exposure to infectious blood, blood products or other body fluids (semen, vaginal secretions, saliva). Perinatal transmission is also possible. The source and spread of disease are caused by contaminated needle, syringes and blood products, sexual activities with infected partners and asymptomatic carriers, e.g. Tattoo/body piercing bite, most infections before and after symptoms appear for 4–6-months in carriers it continues through patients' lifetime, incubation period is 45–18 days.
- HCV is RNA virus that is primarily transmitted percutaneously. Thus, the major risk factor for infection is direct percutaneous exposure such as injecting drugs, transfusion of blood products, hemodialysis, tattooing, high-risk sexual behavior, organ transplantation and exposure to blood and blood products by health workers. Less frequent routes are sexual and perinatal.
- HDV also called delta virus, is defective RNA virus that cannot survive on its own. So it can cause infections only together with HBV; routes of transmission same as for HBV. Blood is infectious at all stages of HDV infections. Incubation period is 2–26 weeks. Chronic carriers of HBV are always at risk.
- HEV is an RNA virus, that is transmitted by the fecal-oral route. The most common mode of transmission is drinking contaminated water.
- HGV is an RNA virus which is found in some blood donors and can be transmitted by transfusion. It frequently coexists with other hepatitis virus, e.g. HCV.

The risk factors for hepatitis B are:

- Frequent exposure to blood, blood products, or other body fluids
- Health care workers: Hemodialysis staff, oncology and chemotherapy nurses, personnel at risk for needle-sticks, operating room staff, respiratory therapists, surgeons, dentists
- Hemodialysis
- Male homosexual and bisexual activity
- IV/injection drug use
- Close contact with carrier of HBV
- Travel to or residence in area with uncertain sanitary conditions

- Multiple sexual partners
- Recent history of sexually transmitted disease
- Receipt of blood or blood products (e.g. clotting factor concentrate).

A combined hepatitis A and B vaccine (Twinrix) is available for vaccination of people 18 years of age and older with indications for both hepatitis A and B vaccination. Vaccination consists for three doses, given on the same schedule as that used for single-antigen hepatitis B vaccine.

Pathophysiology

Viral hepatitis causes diffuse inflammatory infiltrations of hepatic tissue with mononuclear cells and local spotty or single cell necrosis. The liver cells may be very swollen. With typical viral hepatitis, there is no collapse of lobules, no loss of lobular architecture, and minimal or no fibrosis. Inflammation degeneration and regeneration occur simultaneously, distorting the normal lobular pattern and creating pressure within and around the portal vein areas and obstructing the bile channels. These changes are associated with elevated serum transaminase levels, prolonged prothrombin time and slightly elevated bilirubin level. The outcome of viral hepatitis is affected by such factors as the following:

- Virulence of the virus
- Amount of hepatic damage sustained
- Natural individual barriers to damage and disease of the liver such as immune status, nutritional status, and overall health of the individual. Most patients recover normal level functions but the disease can progress to atypical life-threatening variants
- Fulminant viral hepatitis—sudden, severe, degenerated and atrophy of liver, resulting in hepatic failure
- Subacute viral hepatitis—severe, but slower degeneration of livers
- Confluent hepatic necrosis—submassive or massive destruction of substantial groups of adjacent cell with necrosis of portions of a lobule (submassive) or entire lobule (massive), can result in chronic active disease or cirrhosis but most patients will recover.

Clinical Manifestations

The clinical manifestation of viral hepatitis may be classified into three phases: (1) Preicteric or prodromal phase, (2) Icteric phase, (3) Posticteric phase or convalescent phase:

Preicteric	Icteric	Posticteric
Anorexia	Jaundice	Malaise
Nausea, vomiting	Pruritis	Easy fatigability
Right upper quadrant discomfort	Dark urine	Hepatomegaly
Constipation or diarrhea	Bilirubinuria	
Decreased sense of taste and smell	White stool	
Malaise	Fatigue	
Headache	Continual hepatomegaly with tenderness	
Fever	Weight loss	
Arthralgia		
Urticaria		
Hepatomegaly		
Splenomegaly		
Weight loss		

Complications that can occur include chronic persistent hepatitis, chronic active hepatitis, fulminant viral hepatitis and cirrhosis of the liver.

Diagnostic Studies

- Liver function studies
- Hepatitis serology
  - HGs Ag
  - Anti-HBs
  - Anti-HBs-IgH and IgG
  - Anti-HAV Igh and IgG
  - Anti-HCV.

Management

There is no specific treatment or therapy for viral hepatitis. Most patients can be managed at home. Emphasis on measures to rest the body and assist the liver in regenerating needs to be stressed. Adequate nutrients and rest seem to be more beneficial for healing and liver cell (hepatocyte) regeneration. Rest reduced the metabolic demands on the liver and promotes cell generation. The degree of rest depends on the severity of symptoms. Dietary emphasis is on a well-balanced diet that the patient can tolerate. A low fat, high carbohydrate diet may be better tolerated. Protein and sodium are restricted. Alcohol should be avoided.

Vitamin K is given if the prothrombin time is prolonged. Antihistamines are given for pruritis associated with jaundice, and antiemetics are given for nausea. Most patients of hepatitis are not hospitalized. Those requiring hospitalization include persons with serum bilirubin concentration 10 mg or greater than 10 times normal. In persons with fulminating hepatitis, hospitalization and bed rest are indicated. Unnecessary medication including sedatives are discontinued. Coagulation defects may be treated with administration of fresh frozen plasma. The patient's intake and output is carefully monitored, and intravenous fluid continuously. Electrolytes administered in vomiting and diarrhea may cause electrolyte imbalance, particularly hypokalemia.

Hepatitis A vaccine and immunoglobulins are used in the prevention of viral hepatitis. Hepatitis B vaccine and immunoglobulin is the first line of defence against hepatitis B.

The possible nursing diagnosis of viral hepatitis are:

- Fatigue related to imbalance between energy level and demand, decreased rest, feeling of malaise
- Activity intolerance related to fatigue, weakness
- Fluid volume deficit related to vomiting, sweating, decreased intake, increased temperature
- Infection (risk for) related to length of infectivity through blood and body fluids
- Nutrition, altered related to anorexia, inadequate intake, increased metabolic needs
- Pain related to arthralgia, pruritis, headache, abdominal tenderness
- Health maintenance, altered related to lack of knowledge, indifference to "safe sex" practice and needle
- Skin integrity related to jaundice, pruritis, scratching
- Injury related to altered clothing or prothrombin time.

Management usually occurs in the home unless symptoms are severe. Therefore, the nurse assists the patient and family is coping with the temporary disability and fatigue that are common in hepatitis and instructs them to seek additional health care if the symptoms persist or worsen. The patient and family also need specific guidelines about diet, rest, follow-up blood work, and the importance of avoiding alcohol, as well as sanitation and hygiene measure (particularly hand washing) to prevent spread of the disease to other family members.

Preventive Measures for Viral Hepatitis

All patients with hepatitis require precautions to prevent spread of virus. For patients with hepatitis A virus (HAV), the following transmission based precautions are necessary:

- Proper handwashing by patient and staff
- Wearing gloves when handling feces and urine
- Wearing a glove when soiling of uniform is likely
- Cleansing the toilet daily and use private toilet
- Having a private room (only if patient cannot take care of self regarding proper disposal of urine and feces)
- Proper cleansing, bagging and labelling of contaminated items such as bed linens and bedpan
- Discarding contaminated items such as rectal thermometer.

For the patients with HBV, transmission-based precautions are used and include the following:

- Good handwashing by patient and staff
- Wearing gloves when handling blood and body fluids
- Wearing gown, goggles and/or mask when splattering of blood and body fluid is likely
- Proper cleansing, bagging and labelling of contaminated equipments and linens
- Proper disposing of needles or any items exposed to the patient's blood or body fluids
- Careful labeling of blood specimen and protect personnel working with them
- Avoiding contamination of open cuts and mucus membranes with patient's blood and body fluids
- Teaching patients to avoid sexual contact until results of liver function tests have returned to normal.

Similar precaution is to be followed in other hepatitis. At times, the nurse in the hospital and particularly nurse in the community are also involved in identifying patient's contacts who will require prophylactic therapy.

CIRRHOSIS OF LIVER

Cirrhosis of the liver is the term applied to chronic disease of the liver characterized by diffuse inflammation and fibrosis resulting in drastic structural changes and significant loss of liver function in which extensive degeneration and destruction of the liver parenchymal cells. The liver cells attempt to regenerate but the regenerative process is disorganized, resulting in abnormal blood vessels and bile duct relationships from the fibrosis. The overgrowth of new and fibrous connective tissue distorts lever's normal lobular structure resulting in lobules of irregular size and shape with impeded vascular flow. Cirrhosis may be insidious and prolonged course.

Etiology and Pathophysiology

Cirrhosis is a chronic disease characterized by replacement of normal liver tissue with diffuse fibrosis that disrupts the structure and function of the liver. Cirrhosis, or scarring of the liver, is divided into three types: alcoholic, most frequently due to chronic alcoholism and the most common type of cirrhosis; postnecrotic, a late result of a previous acute viral hepatitis; and biliary, a result of chronic biliary obstruction and infection (least common type of cirrhosis).

Cirrhosis of the liver can be classified in various ways. The major types of cirrhosis based on pathological classification are:

i. Alcoholic previously called "Laennec's, cirrhosis" also called portal or nutritional cirrhosis is usually associated with alcohol abuse or malnutrition. The first change in the liver from excessive alcohol intake is an accumulation of fat in the liver cells. Uncomplicated fatty changes in the liver are potentially reversible if the person stops drinking alcohol. If the alcohol abuse continues, widespread scar formation occurs in the liver (Fig. 11.2).

ii. Postnecrotic cirrhosis is a complication of viral toxic or idiopathic (autoimmune) hepatitis due to massive necrosis from hepatotoxins. Broad bands of scar tissue from within liver.

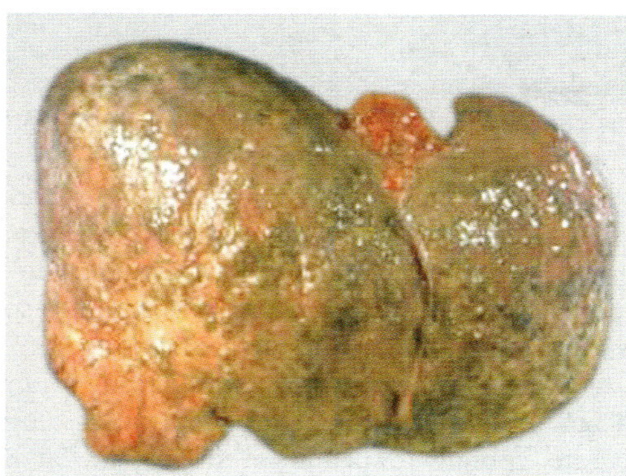

FIG. 11.2: Cirrhosis that developed secondary to alcoholism. The characteristic diffuse nodularity of the surface is due to the combination of regeneration and scarring of the liver

iii. Biliary cirrhosis is associated with inflammation of intrahepatic bile-ductules resulting in biliary obstruction in liver and common bile duct. Cholangitis (destruction of the intrahepatic bile ducts) of unknown etiology may occur. There is chronic impairment of bile drainage occurs. Liver is first large, then becomes firm and nodular, Jaundice is a major symptom. Pruritis, hypercholesterolemia, cholestasis (blockage of bile flow) and malabsorption are common manifestation due to diffuse fibrosis of liver.

iv. Cardiac cirrhosis results from long-standing, severe, right-sided heart failure in patient with cor pulmonale, constrictive pericarditis and tricuspid insufficiency.

v. Nonspecific metabolic cirrhosis are due to metabolic problems, infectious diseases, infiltrative diseases and GI diseases in which portal and liver fibrosis may develop, liver is enlarged and firm.

Clinical Manifestation

- Compensated cirrhosis: Usually found secondary to routine physical examination; vague symptoms (Fig. 11.3)
- Decompensated cirrhosis: Symptoms of decreased protein, clotting factors, and other substances and of portal hypertension
- Liver enlargement early in the course (fatty liver); later in course, liver size decreases from scar tissue
- Portal obstruction and ascites: Chronic dyspepsia, constipation or diarrhea, splenomegaly; spider telangiectasia may be observed
- Gastrointestinal varices: Distended abdominal blood vessels; varices or hemorrhoids; hematemesis; profuse hemorrhage, from the stomach; and esophageal varices in about 25% of patients
- Edema, jaundice, fever
- Vitamin deficiency (A, C and K) and anemia

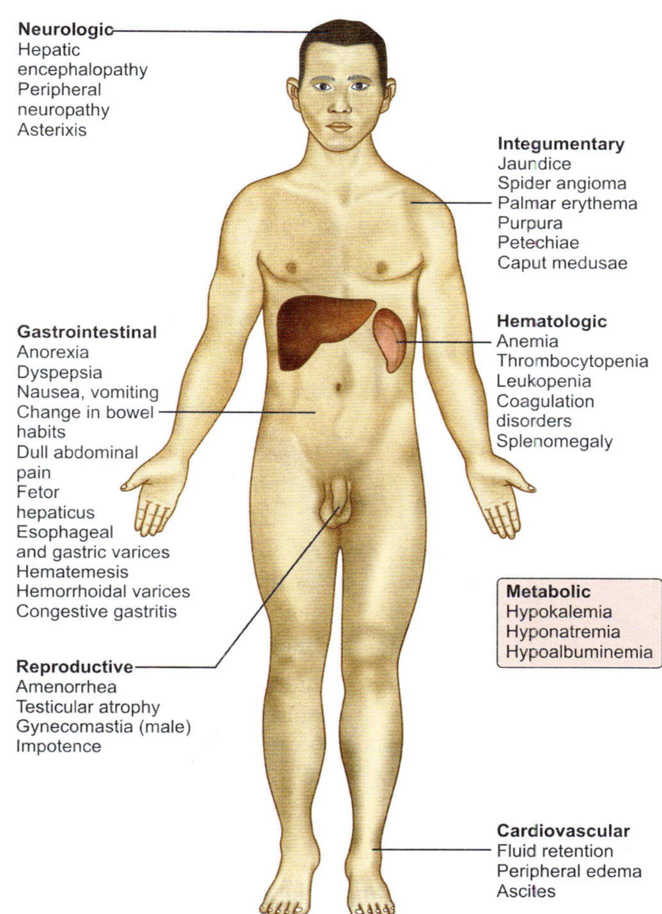

FIG. 11.3: Systemic clinical manifestations of liver cirrhosis

- Mental deterioration with impending hepatic encephalopathy and hepatic coma.

The onset of cirrhosis is usually insidious. GI disturbances are common, early symptoms include anorexia, dyspepsia, flatulence, nausea and vomiting and change in bowel habits (constipation or diarrhea) due to altered metabolism of carbohydrate, fats and proteins. Pain may be due to swelling and stretching of the capsule and spasm of biliary ducts, other symptoms include, fever, lassitude, slight weightlessness and enlargement of liver and spleen. Liver may be palpable. Later symptoms may be severe and result from liver failure and portal hypertension, jaundice, peripheral, edema, and ascites develop gradually. Other late symptoms are as follows:

Gastrointestinal
- Anorexia
- Dyspepsia
- Nausea
- Vomiting
- Change in bowel habits

Hematologic
- Anemia
- Thrombocytopenia
- Leukopenia
- Coagulation disorder
- Splenomegaly.

- Dull abdominal pain
- Factor hepatitis
- Esophageal and gastric varices
- Hematemesis
- Hemorrhoidal varices
- Congestive gastritis.

Endocrine disturbance/ metabolic

- Potassium deficiency
- Hyponatremia
- Hypoalbuminemia.

Cardiovascular

- Fluid retention
- Peripheral edema
- Ascites.

Integumentary/ skin lesions

- Jaundice
- Spider angioma
- Palmar erythema
- Purpura
- Petechiae
- Caput medusae

Neurologic

- Hepatic encephalopathy
- Peripheral neuropathy
- Asterixis
- Amenorrhea
- Testicular atrophy
- Gynecomastia
- Impotence.

The major complications of cirrhosis of liver are portal hypertension with resultant esophageal varices, peripheral edema and ascites, hepatic encephalopathy (coma) and hepatorenal syndrome.

Diagnostic Studies

Liver function tests (e.g. serum alkaline phosphatase, AST [SGOT], ALT SGPT], GGT, and bilirubin), prothrombin time, ABGs, laparoscopy, in conjunction with biopsy:

- Ultrasound scanning
- Computed tomography (CT) scan
- Magnetic resonance imaging (MRI)
- Radioisotopic liver scans
- Liver function studies
  - Alkaline phosphatase
  - Aspartate aminotransferase (AST)
  - Alanine aminotransferase (ALT)
  - Serum glutamic pyruvic transaminase (SGPT)
  - Y-glutamyl transferase
- Liver biopsy (percutaneous needle)
- Esophagogastroduodenoscopy
- Angiography
- Liver scan
- Serum electrolyte
- Prothrombin time
- Serum albumin
- CBC
- Stool for occult blood
- Upper GI barium swallow.

Management

Although there is no specific therapy for cirrhosis, certain measures can be taken to promote liver cell regeneration and prevent or treat complications.

Rest is significant in reducing metabolic demands of the liver and allowing for recovery of liver cells. At various times, during the progress of cirrhosis the rest may have to take the form of complete bed rest. Avoidance of alcohol and aspirin and administration of B-complex vitamin are helpful.

For ascetics, sodium restriction, diuretics and fluid removal are indicated. Administration of 3000-calories high carbohydrate, protein (depends on stage), low-fat diet, low sodium diet are advised. The diuretics used for ascetics are spironolactone (aldactone), amiloride (Midamor) triamterene (Dyrenium), Furosemide (Lasix). In some cases, paracentesis, or peritoneovenous shunts are indicated (Figs 11.4 and 11.5).

For esophageal varices β-adrenergic blockers, vasopressin are used. And endoscopic sclerotherapy or ligation, balloon tamponade, somatostatin, surgical shunting procedures, transjugular intrahepatic portosystemic shunt may be indicated accordingly (Table 11.1).

For hepatic encephalopathy, sterilization of GI tract with antibiotics, and levodopa are used.

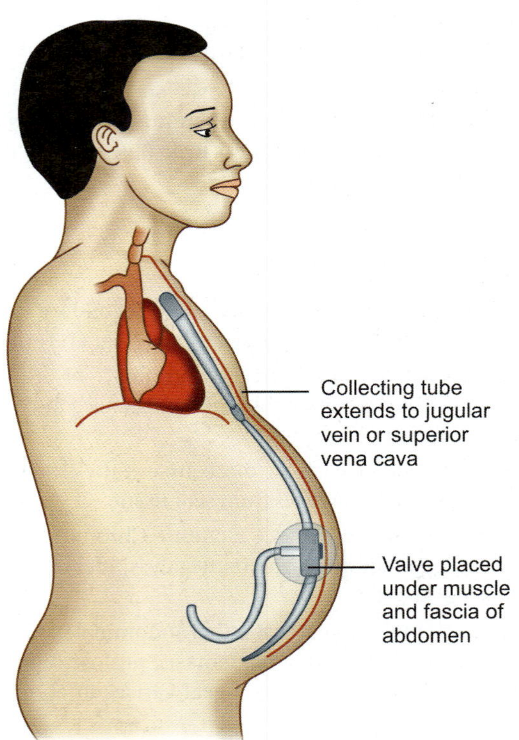

FIG. 11.4: Peritoneovenous shunt

Medical Management

Medical management is based on presenting symptoms.

- Treatment includes antacids, vitamins, balanced diet, and nutritional supplements; potassium-sparing diuretics (for ascites); avoidance of alcohol.
- Colchicine may increase the length of survival in patients with mild to moderate cirrhosis.

Nursing Management: The Patient with Hepatic Cirrhosis

Assessment

- Focus on dietary intake, nutritional status, onset of symptoms, history of precipitating factors, including long-term alcohol abuse, exposure to toxic agents, medications (Box 11.1)

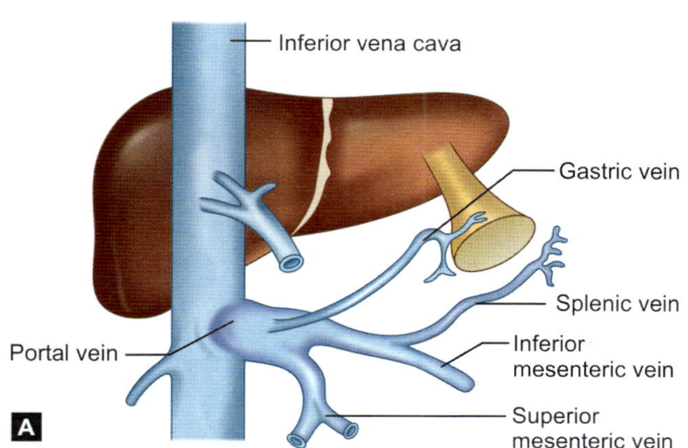

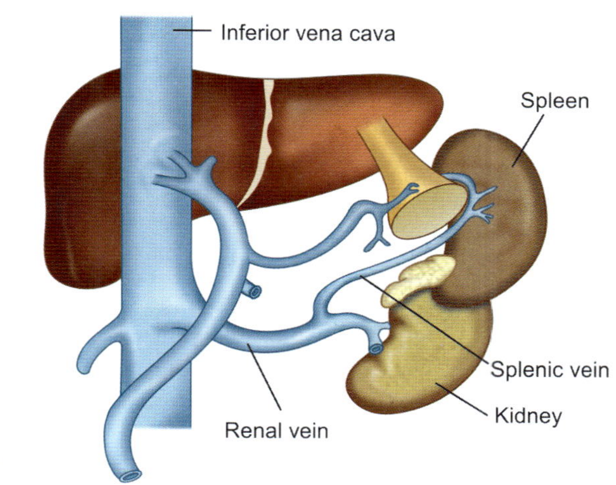

FIGS 11.5A AND B: Portosystemic shunts. (A) Portacaval shunt. The portal vein is anastomosed to the inferior vena cava, diverting blood from the portal vein to the systemic circulation; (B) Distal splenorenal shunt. The splenic vein is anastomosed to the renal vein. The portal venous flow remains intact while esophageal varices are selectively decompressed. (The short gastric veins are decompressed.) The spleen conducts blood from the high pressure of the esophageal and gastric varices to the low-pressure renal vein

TABLE 11.1: Nursing care plan for patient with cirrhosis of liver

Problem	Reason	Objective	Nursing intervention
Fatigue related to muscle wasting blood loss	Featuring potential anemia	No, fatigue or reduced fatigue	• Ensure or maintain bed rest in acute phase • Encourage increased activity gradually after acute phase • Restrict visitors • Make sure that patient is getting balanced prescribed diet
Altered nutrition more than body requirement related to anorexia, impaired utilization and storage of nutrients, nausea vomiting	As manifest by lack of interest in food, aversion to eating, inadequate food intake	• Adequate intake of food • Maintenance of normal body weight	• Monitor weight to evaluate nitrogen balance • Provide oral care before meals to remove foul taste and improve taste • Administer antiemetics as ordered • Provide small, frequent meals with nourishment • Determine food preferences and allow these whenever possible
Impaired skin integrity related to edema, ascites pruritis	As manifested by complaints of itching, areas of excoriation from scratching, taut, shining skin over edematous areas of skin breakdown	• Maintain skin integrity • No pruritus	• Restrict sodium intake and fluids to reduce edema • Administer prescribed diuretics • Monitor intake and output • Assess location and extent of edema by weighing, taking daily measurement of extremities and abdominal girth • Provide meticulous skin care • Reposition patient at least with the intervals of two hours • Elevate edematous area to promote venous drainage • Have patient use special mattresses to reduce skin breakdown • Clip patient's nails short and keep clean • Administer antipruritic medication as ordered • Provide diversions and distractions

Contd...

Contd...

Problem	Reason	Objective	Nursing intervention
Ineffective breathing pattern related to pressure on diaphragm and reduced-lung volume. Secondary to ascites	As manifested by dyspnea, cyanosis, changes in pulse, respn. depth or pattern	• Able to breathe with minimized difficulty	• Place the patient in semi-Fowler's or Fowler's position. Support the arms and chest with pillows • Auscultate chest for crakes to identifying fluid in lungs • Assess respiratory rate and rhythm to know dyspnea
Risk injury related to diminished perception secondary to peripheral neuropathy	Peripheral neuropathy	No injury due to decreased perception	• Assess numbness and tingling of lower extremities, decrease sensation in lower extremities • Prevent excess stimulation or trauma to extremities • Do not use restrictive bed-lining • Instruct patient to avoid tight clothing • Use care with heat and cold application • Assist with ambulation

Note: There may be problems of liver activity intolerance, risk for infection, ineffective airway clearance, potential for hepatic encephalopathy and take nursing measures accordingly.

- Assess mental status through interview and interaction with patient; note orientation to time, place, person
- Note relationships with family, friends, and coworkers regarding incapacitation secondary to alcohol abuse and cirrhosis
- Note abdominal distention and bloating, gastrointestinal bleeding, bruising and weight changes
- Document exposure to toxic agents, such as hepatotoxic medications or illicit drugs.

Nursing Diagnoses

- Activity intolerance related to fatigue, general debility, muscle wasting and discomfort
- Imbalanced nutrition: Less than body requirements, related to chronic gastritis, decreased gastrointestinal motility and anorexia
- Impaired skin integrity related to compromised immunologic status, edema and poor nutrition
- Risk for injury and bleeding related to altered clotting mechanisms.

Collaborative Problems/Potential Complications

- Bleeding and hemorrhage
- Hepatic encephalopathy
- Fluid volume excess.

Planning

Goals may include independence in activities, improved nutritional status, improved skin integrity, decreased potential for injury, improved mental status and absence of complications.

Box 11.1 Assessing for cirrhosis

Be alert for the following signs and symptoms:

Compensated
- Intermittent mild fever
- Vascular spiders
- Palmar erythema (reddened palms)
- Unexplained epistaxis
- Ankle edema
- Vague morning indigestion
- Flatulent dyspepsia
- Abdominal pain
- Firm, enlarged liver
- Splenomegaly

Decompensated
- Ascites
- Jaundice
- Weakness
- Muscle wasting
- Weight loss
- Continuous mild fever
- Clubbing of fingers
- Purpura (due to decreased platelet count)
- Spontaneous bruising
- Epistaxis
- Hypotension
- Spare body hair
- White nails
- Gonadal atrophy

Objectives

- Demonstrates ability to participate in activities
- Increase nutritional intake; avoids skin breakdown and other injuries.

Nursing assessment will include eliciting complete history focussing on recent history of fever, infected weakness, fatigue, changes in the sclera, edema, itching, muscle wasting, use of alcohol, change in appetite, weight loss, anorexia, nausea, vomiting, indigestion, flatulence, abdominal tenderness, change in the movement of bowel and bladder, sexuality (erectile dysfunction decreased libido or changes in menstrual pattern assessing vital signs), other manifestation and the need for nursing management see NCP of patient with cirrhosis of liver.

Nursing Interventions

Providing Rest

- Position bed for maximal respiratory efficiency; provide oxygen if needed
- Initiate efforts to prevent respiratory, circulatory and vascular disturbances
- Encourage patient to increase activity gradually and plan rest with activity and mild exercise.

Improving Nutritional Status

- Provide a nutritious, high-protein diet supplemented by B-complex vitamins and others, including A, C, and K and folic acid if there is no indication of impending coma
- Provide small, frequent meals, consider patient preferences, and encourage patient to eat; provide protein supplements, if indicated
- Provide nutrients by feeding tube total parenteral nutrition (PN)
- Provide patients who have fatty stools (steatorrhea) with water-soluble forms of fat-soluble vitamins A, D and E, and give folic acid and iron to prevent anemia
- Provide a low-protein diet temporarily if patient shows signs of impending or advancing coma; restore protein intake to moderate (1 to 1.5/kg) when patient's condition permits.

Providing Skin Care

- Change position frequently
- Avoid using irritating soaps and adhesive tape
- Provide lotion to soothe irritated skin; take measures to prevent patient from scratching the skin.

Reducing Risk of Injury

- Use padded side rails if patient becomes agitated or restless
- Orient to time, place and procedures to minimize agitation
- Instruct patient to ask for assistance to get out of bed
- Provide safety measures to prevent injury or cuts (electric razor, soft toothbrush)
- Apply pressure to venipuncture sites to minimize bleeding.

The usual nursing intervention of cirrhosis is supporting respiration (by using Fowler's position), controlling fatigue (with bedrest), maintaining fluid and electrolyte balance (IV or oral fluid if no restriction) helping the patient to avoid alcohol, preventing infection, preventing bleeding and falls, promoting nutrition, controlling pruritis, promoting positive self-esteem. The factors which are supposed to monitor in the person with cirrhosis are:

- Monitor urine and stool for blood
- Check up patient's body daily for purpura, hematoma and petechiae
- Check mouth especially gums, carefully for signs of bleeding
- Check vital signs at least every 4 hours
- Monitor prothrombin time, portal thromboplastin, and thrombocyte count frequently.

Following are the guidelines for decreasing the risk of bleeding:

- Avoid all intramuscular and subcutaneous injections if possible
- Use the smaller-gauge needle possible while giving an injection
- Apply pressure to injection site and venous puncture sites for at least 5 minutes and arterial punctures for 10 minutes
- Give vitamin K as ordered
- Use or instruct patient to use a soft bristle tooth brush or cotton swabs for oral hygiene
- Instruct patient to avoid foods (e.g. spicy, hot or raw) that can traumatize esophageal varices
- Provide assistance to avoid falling
- Make sure that room is free of clutters, that floors are dry, and shoes or slippers are worn to avoid injuries.

Monitoring and Managing Complications

Preventing bleeding due to decreased production of prothrombin and monitoring or hepatic encephalopathy are the primary concerns.

- Observe for melena, and check stools for blood
- Take precautionary measures (e.g. use padded side rails, apply pressure to injection site for long period of time and avoid sharp objects)
- Use appropriate dietary modification and stool softeners to prevent straining during defections
- Monitor closely for gastrointestinal bleeding
- Keep equipment to treat hemorrhage from esophageal varices readily available: intravenous fluids, medication Sengstaken-Blakemore tube
- Monitor closely to identify early evidence of condition
- Explain event and treatment if complication noted. Patient may need to be treated in ICU.

Promoting Home and Community-based Care

Prepare for discharge by providing dietary instruction, including exclusion of alcohol.

- Refer at alcoholics anonymous if indicated
- Continue sodium restriction; stress avoidance of raw shellfish
- Provide written instructions, teaching, support, and reinforcement to patient and family
- Encourage rest and probably a change in lifestyle (adequate well-balanced diet and elimination of alcohol)
- Instruct family about symptoms of impending encephalopathy and possibility of bleeding tendencies and infection
- Refer patient to home care nurse, and assist in transition from hospital to home.

PROBLEMS OF GALLBLADDER

The biliary system is affected by stones and obstructions, inflammation and infection. The most common disorders of the biliary system is cholelithiasis (stone in the gallbladder).

CHOLELITHIASIS

In cholelithiasis calculi (gallstones) usually form in the gall bladder from solid constituents of bile and vary greatly in size shape and composition. There are two major types of gallstones—pigment stones, which contain an excess of unconjugated pigments in the bile, and cholesterol stones (the more common form), which result from bile supersaturated with cholesterol due to increased synthesis of cholesterol and decreased synthesis of bile acids that dissolve cholesterol. Risk factors for pigment stones include cirrhosis, hemolysis, and infections of the biliary tree. These stones cannot be dissolved and must be removed surgically. Risk factors for cholesterol stones include gender (women have a four times higher incidence than men); use of oral contraceptives, estrogens, and clofibrate; age (usually older than 40 years); multiparous status; and obesity. There is also an increased risk related to diabetes, gastrointestinal disease, T-tube fistula, and ileal resection or bypass.

Gallstones can occur at anywhere in the biliary tree. The cholelithiasis refer to stone formation in the gallbladder. Either acute or chronic inflammation termed as "cholecystitis" can result precipitated by the presence of stones. When stones form in or migrate to the common bile duct the condition is termed as choledocholelithiasis.

Fatigue related to muscle wasting blood loss.

Featuring potential anemia.

No, fatigue or reduced fatigue.

- Ensure or maintain bed rest in acute phase
- Encourage increased activity gradually after acute phase
- Restrict visitors
- Make sure that patient is getting balanced prescribed diet.

  Altered nutrition more than body requirement related to anorexia, impaired utilization and storage of nutrients, nausea vomiting.

  As manifested by lack of interest in food, aversion to eating, inadequate food intake.

- Adequate intake of food
- Maintenance of normal body weight
- Monitor weight to evaluate nitrogen balance
- Provide oral care before meals to remove foul taste and improve taste
- Administer antiemetics as ordered
- Provide small, frequent meals with nourishment
- Determine food preferences and allow these whenever possible.

Impaired skin integrity related to edema, ascites, pruritis.

As manifested by complaints of itching, areas of excoriation from scratching, taut, shining skin over edematous areas of skin breakdown.

- Maintain skin integrity
- No pruritus
- Restrict sodium intake and fluids to reduce edema
- Administer prescribed diuretics
- Monitor intake and output
- Assess location and extent of edema by weighing, taking daily measurement of extremities and abdominal girth
- Provide meticulous skin care
- Reposition patient at least with the intervals of 2 hours
- Elevate edematous area to promote venous drainage
- Have patient use special mattresses to reduce skin breakdown
- Clip patient's nails short and keep clean
- Administer antipruritic medication as ordered
- Provide diversions and distractions.

Ineffective breathing pattern related to pressure on diaphragm and reduced-lung volume secondary to ascites.

As manifested by dyspnea, cyanosis, changes in pulse, respiration depth or pattern.

- Able to breathe with minimized difficulty
- Place the patient in semi-Fowler's or Fowler's position. Support the arms and chest with pillows
- Auscultate chest for crakes to identifying fluid in lungs
- Assess respiratory rate and rhythm to know dyspnea.

Risk injury related to diminished perception secondary to peripheral neuropathy.

No injury due to decreased perception.

- Assess numbness and tingling of lower extremities, decrease sensation in lower extremities
- Prevent excess stimulation or trauma to extremities

- Do not use restrictive bedlining
- Instruct patient to avoid tight clothing
- Use care with heat and cold application
- Assist with ambulation.

Note: There may be problems of liver activity intolerance, risk for infection, ineffective airway clearance, potential for herpetic encephalitis and take nursing measures accordingly.

Etiology

Cholecystitis is most commonly associated with stones. When it occurs in the absence of stones it is thought to be caused by bacteria reaching gallbladder via the vascular or lymphatic route or chemical irritant in the bile. *E. coli,* streptococci, and *Salmonellae* are common bacteria. Other causative factors include adhesions, neoplasms, extensive fasting, frequent weight fluctuations, anesthesia and narcotics.

The actual cause of cholelithiasis is unknown. It develops when the valeric that keeps cholesterol, bile salts and calcium in solutions is altered so that precipitation of these substances occurs. Conditions that upset this balance include infection and disturbance in the metabolism of cholesterol. A high percentage of gallstones are precipitated of cholesterol. Other components of bile that precipitates into stone are bile salts, bilirubin, calcium and proteins. Stones sometimes are mixed. The risk factors for cholesterol gallstones are obesity, middle age, pregnancy, multiparity, use of oral contraceptives, rapid weight loss, diseases of the ileum and hypercholesterolemia (Box 11.2).

Pathophysiology

Cholecystitis, an acute complication of cholelithiasis, is an acute infection of the gallbladder. Most patients with cholecystitis have gallstones (calculous cholecystitis). A gallstone obstructs bile outflow and bile in the gallbladder initiates a chemical reaction, resulting in edema, compromise of the vascular supply and gangrene. In the absence of gallstones, cholecystitis (acalculous) may occur after surgery, severe trauma, or burns, or with torsion cystic duct obstruction, multiple blood transfusions, and primary bacterial infections of the gallbladder. Infection causes pain, tenderness, and rigidity of the upper right abdomen and is associated with nausea and vomiting and the usual signs of inflammation. Purulent fluid inside the gallbladder indicates an empyema of the gallbladder.

Box 11.2 Risk factors for cholelithiasis

- Obesity
- Women, especially those who have had multiple pregnancies or who are of Native American of US Southwestern Hispanic ethnicity
- Frequent changes in weight
- Rapid weight loos (leads to rapid development of gallstones and high risk of symptomatic disease)
- Treatment with high-dose estrogen (e.g. in prostate cancer)
- Low-dose estrogen therapy—a small increase in the risk of gallstones
- Ileal resection or disease
- Cystic fibrosis
- Diabetes mellitus

Bile is primarily composed of water plus conjugated bilirubin, organic and inorganic ions, small amounts of proteins and three lipids bile salts, lecithin and cholesterol. When the balance of these three lipids remain intact, cholesterol is held in solution. If the balance is upset cholesterol can be precipitated. Cholesterol gallstone formation is enhanced by the production of a mucin glycoprotein, which traps cholesterol particles. Supersaturation of the bile with cholesterol also impairs gallbladder mobility and contributes to status.

Cholesterol stones are hard, white or yellow-brown in color, radiolucent and can be quite large up to 4 cm. Black-pigmented stones form as the result of an increase of unconjugated bilirubin and calcium with a corresponding decrease in bile salts. Gallbladder motility may also be impaired. Brown stones develop in the intra and extrahepatic ducts and are usually preceded by bacterial invasion.

Clinical Manifestations

Manifestation of cholecystitis varies from indigestion and moderate to severe pain, fever and jaundice. Initial symptoms of acute cholecystitis include indigestion and pain and tenderness in the right upper quadrant (RUQ), which may be referred to the right shoulder and scapula. The pain may be accompanied by anorexia, nausea and possibly vomiting, restlessness and diaphoresis. Manifestation of inflammation are such as leukocytosis and fever.

- They may be silent, producing no pain and only mild gastrointestinal symptoms
- They may be acute or chronic with epigastric distress (fullness, abdominal distention, and vague upper right quadrant pain) after a high-fat meal
- If the cystic duct is obstructed, the gallbladder becomes distended and eventually infected; fever and palpable abdominal mass; biliary colic with excruciating upper right abdominal pain, radiating to back or right shoulder with nausea and vomiting several hours after a heavy meal; restlessness and constant or colicky pain
- Jaundice, accompanied by marked itching, with obstruction of the common bile duct, in a small percentage of patients
- Very dark urine; clay-colored stool
- Deficiencies of vitamin A, D, E, and K (fat-soluble vitamins gallstone continues to obstruct the duct).

Physical findings include RUQ tenderness and abdominal rigidity. Symptoms of chronic cholecystitis include history of fat intolerance, dyspepsia, heart burn and flatulence.

Cholelithiasis may produce severe symptom or none at all. The severity of symptoms depends on whether the stones are stationary or mobile and whether obstruction is present. The clinical manifestations caused by obstructed blood flow are:

- Obstructive jaundice due to no bile flow into duodenum
- Dark amber urine which forms when shaken are due to soluble bilirubin in urine
- No urobilirubin in urine due to no bilirubin reaching small intestine to be converted to urobilirubin
- Clay-colored stools urobilirubin
- Pruritus due to deposition of bile salts in skin tissues
- Intolerance for fatty foods—no bile in small intestine for fat digestion
- Bleeding tendencies—lack or decreased absorption of vitamin K resulting in decreased production of prothrombins
- Steatorrhea—No bile salts in duodenum, preventing fat emulsion and digestion
- Biliary colic—murphy sign—i.e. pain colicy and more flow steady. Complications of cholecystitis include subphrenic abscess, pancreatitis, cholangitis (inflammation of bile ducts), biliary cirrhosis, fistulas, and rupture of gallbladder which can produce bile peritonitis.

Diagnostic Study

It includes:

- Abdominal radiography, ultrasonography or cholecystography, radionuclide imaging, or cholescintigraphy
- Endoscopic retrograde cholangiopancreatography (ERCP)
- Percutaneous transhepatic cholangiography (PTC)
- Ultrasound
- Cholecystogram or IV cholangiogram
- Liver function studies
- WBC counts
- Serum bilirubin.

Management

During an acute episode of cholecystitis the focus of treatment is on control of pain, control of possible infection with antibiotics and maintenance of fluid and electrolyte balance. Treatment is mainly supportive and symptomatic. Conservative therapy includes:

- IV fluids
- NPO with NG tube later progressing to low fat diets
- Antiemetic to prevent nausea and vomiting
- Analgesics to relieve pain (i.e. meperidine) as prescribed
- Administration of fat soluble vitamins (A B E/C)
- Anticholinergic to decrease secretions which prevents biliary contraction
- Antispasmodic counteracts smooth muscle spasm
- Hydrocholeretic drugs—Dehydrocholic acid, florantyrone (Zanchol)
- Antibiotics
- ETCEP with sphincterotomy (papillotomy)
- Cholesterol solvents
- Extracorporeal shock-wave lithotripsy (ESWL)

The dissolution therapy includes:

- Ursodeoxycholic acid (UDCA)
- Ursodil
- Chenodeoxycholic acid (CDCA)
- Any medication prescribed by the physician.

Medical Management

Major objectives of medical therapy are to reduce the incidence of acute episodes of gallbladder pain and cholecystitis by supportive and dietary management and, if possible, to remove the cause by pharmacotherapy, endoscopic procedures, or surgical intervention.

- Infusion of a solvent into the gallbladder to dissolve gallstones
- Stone removal using an instrument with a basket or by ERCP endoscope
- Extracorporeal shock-wave lithotripsy (repeated shock waves directed at the gallbladder or common bile duct to fragment the stones), intracorporeal shock-wave lithotripsy (fragmentation by ultrasound, pulsed laser, or hydraulic lithotripsy applied through an endoscope directly to the stones)

Supportive and Dietary Management

- Achieve remission with rest, intravenous fluids, nasogastric suction, analgesia and antibiotics
- Diet immediately after an episode is usually low-fat liquids with high protein and carbohydrates followed by solid soft foods as tolerated, avoiding eggs, fatty rich foods, gas-forming vegetables and alcohol.

Pharmacologic Therapy

- Analgesic agents such as meperidine may be required; avoid morphine because it increase spasm of the sphincter of Oddi
- Ursodeoxycholic acid and chenodeoxycholic acid (chenodiol or CDCA) are effective in dissolving primarily cholesterol stones
- Long-term follow-up and monitoring of liver enzymes.

Surgical Management

Goal of surgery is to relieve persistent symptoms, remove the cause of colic, and treat acute cholecystitis.

- Surgical intervention for disease of the biliary tract is the most common operation performed in the elderly
- Biliary disease may be accompanied or preceded by symptoms of septic shock: oliguria, hypotension, mental changes, tachycardia and tachypnea

- Mortality from serious complications is high. Risk of complications and shorter hospital stays make it essential that older patients and their family members receive specific information about signs and symptoms of complications and measures to prevent them
- Cholecystectomy is usually well tolerated and carries a low risk if expert assessment and care are provided before, during and after surgery.

Surgical intervention for cholelithiasis is frequently indicated and may consider any one of the several procedures as follows:

- Cholecystectomy
  - Removal of gallbladder
- Cholecystostomy
  - Incision of gallbladder for removal of stones
- Choledocholithotomy
  - Incision to common bile duct for removal of stones
- Cholecystogastrostomy
  - Anastomosis between stomach and gallbladder
- Cholecystoduodenostomy
  - Anastomosis between gallbladder and duodenum to relieve obstruction to distal end of common bile duct.
- Laparoscopic cholecystectomy (Fig. 11.6)
  - Removal of gallbladder via laparoscopy using a dissecting laser.

Nursing Management

The nurse has to follow the undermentioned guidelines for the patient undergoing open cholecystectomy in addition to general guidelines.

Assessment

- Assess health history: Note history of smoking or prior respiratory problems
- Assess respiratory status: Note shallow respirations, persistent cough, or ineffective or adventitious breath sounds
- Evaluate nutritional status (dietary history, general examination and laboratory study results).

Nursing Diagnosis

- Acute pain and discomfort related to surgical incision
- Impaired gas exchange related to high abdominal surgical incision
- Impaired skin integrity related to altered biliary drainage after surgical incision
- Imbalanced nutrition related to inadequate bile secretion
- Deficient knowledge about self-care activities related to incisional care, dietary modifications (if needed), medication, reportable signs or symptoms (fever, bleeding, vomiting).

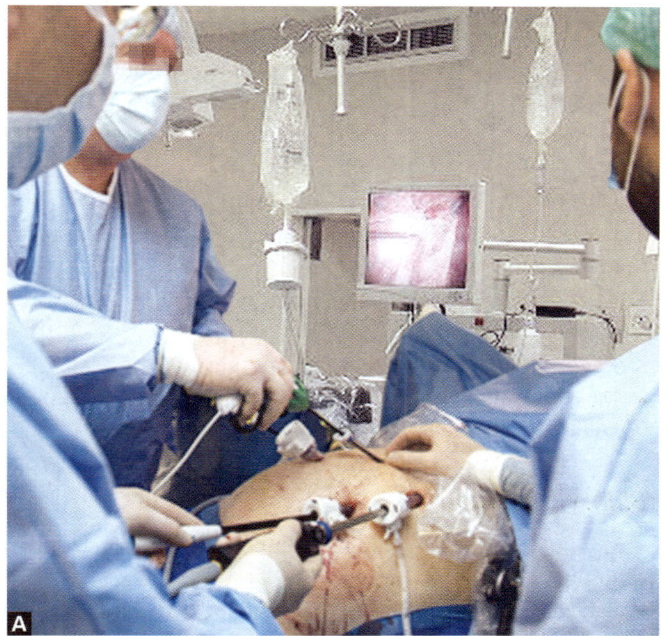

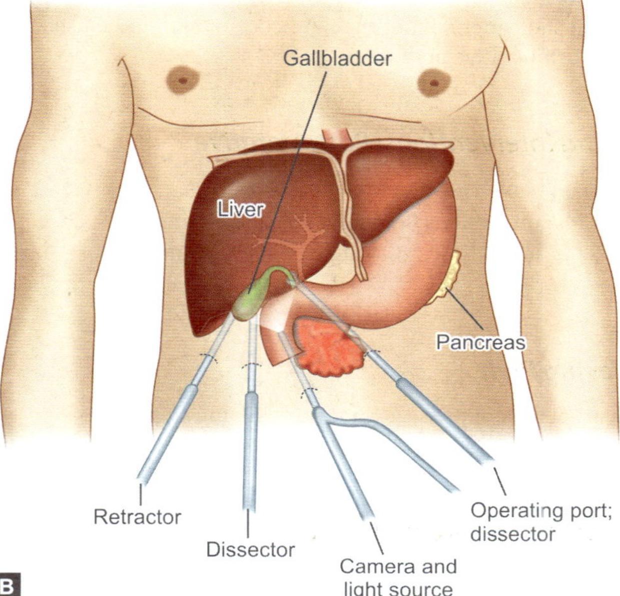

FIGS 11.6A AND B: (A) In laparoscopic cholecystectomy, the surgeon makes four small incisions (less than one half inch each) in the abdomen; (B) and inserts a laparoscope with a miniature camera through the umbilical incision. The camera apparatus displays the gallbladder and adjacent tissues on a screen, allowing the surgeon to visualize the sections of the organ for removal

Collaborative problems/Potential Complications

- Bleeding
- Gastrointestinal symptoms.

Planning

Goals include relief of pain, adequate ventilation, intact skin and improved biliary drainage, optimal nutritional intake, understanding of self-care routines and absence of complications. The objectives:

- Reports decrease in pain
- Demonstrates appropriate respiratory function
- Exhibits normal skin integrity around biliary drainage sites
- Obtains relief of dietary intolerance
- Are free of complications.

Preoperative care

- Patient with complete preoperative preparations at home before their arrival on the day of surgery. The nurse will verify that the patient has had NPO and completed any required bowel preparation. Preoperative teaching includes
  - Teach patient the importance of frequent breathing and use of incentive spirometer because the high incision and RUQ pain predispose the patient to atelectasis and right lower lobe pneumonia
- Explain the types of biliary drainage tubes which are anticipated if any
- Teach the patient about the pain control plan to be used in the postoperative period.

Nursing Interventions: Postoperative

- Place patient in low Fowler's position
- Provide intravenous fluids and nasogastric suction
- Provide water and other fluids and soft diet, after bowel sounds return.

Relieving Pain

- Instruct patient to use a pillow to splint incision
- Administer analgesic agents as ordered.

Improving Respiratory Status

- Remind patient to expand lungs fully and to cough hourly to prevent atelectasis; promote early ambulation
- Monitor elderly and obese patients most closely for respiratory problems.

Improving Nutritional Status

Advise patient at time of discharge to maintain a nutrition's diet and avoid excessive fats; fat restriction is usually lifted in 4 to 6 weeks.

Postoperative Care

- Place the patient in low-Fowler's position, assist to change position frequently
- Urge patient to deep by breathe at regular intervals (every 1 to 2 hours) and to cough if secretions are present until ambulating well. Assist patient to effectively splint the incision. Encourage use of incentive spirometer
- Give analgesics fairly liberally for the first 2 to 3 days
- Use patient-controlled analgesia if possible. Meperidine has been the drug of choice because it is believed to minimize spasms in the bile ducts, but morphine is being used with increasing frequency
- Maintain a dry, intact dressing, usually a drain is inserted near the stump of the cyst duct; Some serous fluid drainage is normal initially
- Encourage progressive ambulation when permitted
- Increase diet gradually to be regular with fat content as tolerated (appetite and fat tolerance may be diminished if there is external biliary drainage).

Promoting Skin Care and Biliary Drainage

- Connect tubes to drainage receptacle and secure tubing to avoid kinking (elevate above abdomen)
- Place drainage bag in patient's pocket when ambulating
- Observe for indications of infection, leakage of bile, obstruction of bile drainage, clay-colored stool, and change in vital signs
- Observe for Jaundice (check the sclera)
- Note and report right upper quadrant pain, nausea and vomiting
- Change dressing frequently, using ointment to protect skin from irritation
- Keep careful record of intake and output
- Measure bile collected every 24 hours; document amount color, and character of drainage.

Biliary Drainage

- Connect any biliary drainage tubes to be closed gravity drainage
- Attach sufficient tubing so the patient can move without restriction
- Explain to patient the importance of avoiding kinks, clamping or pulling of the tube

- Monitor the amount and color of drainage frequently, measure and record drainage at least every shift
- Report any signs of peritonitis (abdominal pain, rigidity or fever) to the concerned doctor
- Monitor color of urine and stools; stools will be grayish-white if the bile is flowing out a drainage tube, but the normal color should gradually reappear as external drainage diminishes and disappears.

Monitoring and Managing Complications

- Bleeding: Assess periodically for increased tenderness and rigidity of abdomen and report; instruct patient and family to report change in color of stool. Monitor vital signs closely. Inspect incision for bleeding
- Gastrointestinal symptoms: Assess for loss of appetite, vomiting, pain distention of abdomen, and temperature elevation; report promptly and instruct patient and family to report symptoms promptly; provide written reinforcement of verbal instructions.

Promoting Home and Community-based Care

Teaching patients self-care:

- Instruct patient, verbally and in writing, about care of drainage tubes and to report to physician promptly changes in amount or characteristics of drainage
- Teach about medications and their actions
- Instruct patient to report to physician symptoms of jaundice, dark urine, pale stools, pruritus, or signs of inflammation and infection (e.g. pain or fever after laparoscopy)
- Provide written and verbal instructions to patient and family about management of postoperative pain and about signs and symptoms of intra-abdominal complications that should be reported (loss of appetite, vomiting, pain, distention of abdomen and temperature elevation)
- Refer for home care during the first 24 to 48 hours because of drowsiness
- Emphasize importance of keeping follow-up appointments.

PRIMARY SCLEROSING CHOLANGITIS (PSC)

Inflammation and scarring of the biliary tree occur more commonly as a result of gallstones and bile duct infection. Parasites are most common source of infections. When no cause for the bile duct injury can be found, the process is called idiopathic or primary sclerosing cholangitis. It has closest link with inflammatory bowel disease.

Pathophysiology

The PSC causes changes in and around the large bile ducts from inflammation obstruction and intra and extrahepatic fibrosis. Strictures can usually be found in multiple locations. These strictures are short and diffusely distributed and alternate with normal or dilated segments of the ducts to create a bead-like appearance in X-ray. It is unusual for the gallbladder or cystic ducts to be involved.

Clinical Manifestation

Many patients are symptomatic in early stages. Others are seen with combination of fatigue, fever, jaundice, abdominal pain and weight loss. Persistent severe pruritus can be a particularly difficult aspect of the disease. Patient may experience recurrent attacks of cholangitis.

Diagnostic studies of other liver and biliary disorders.

Management

Drug therapy aimed at reducing biliary tree inflammation and preventing the scarring that leads to obstruction. The drug ursodeoxycholic acid has shown promise. Surgical procedures other than transplant have been effective for diffuse disease. Endoscopic treatment to remove stones, relieve obstruction, dilate ducts, and place stout tubes in ongoing but primarily in the form of clinical trials.

The uncertain nature of PSC is one of its most difficult characteristics. Patients are instructed about the disease and its possible outcome and are prepared for the possibility of the eventual need for liver transplant. Persistent jaundice may negatively affect body image, and chronic severe pruritus may be a daily nightmare. Some patients are responding to cholestyramine resin (drug), which theoretically binds the itching triggering elements in the bile. The nurse also suggests that patient experiments with common intervention that may lessen his/her itching. A low fat diet is recommended to patient who develops problems with diarrhea or steatorrhea and the fat restriction usually promptly corrects the problems. Fat-soluble vitamin replacement is often needed.

The following strategies to control pruritus are helpful:

- Avoid irritating clothing (wool or restrictive clothing)
- Use tepid water for bathing rather than hot
  - Experiment with nonirritating soaps and detergents
  - Pat skin dry after bathing or showering; do not rub
- Apply emollient creams and lotions to dry skin regularly
- Avoid activities that increase body temperature or cause sweating
- Experiment with treatments such as oatmeal baths
- Keep the fingernails short and consider use of cotton gloves at night to minimize skin damage from scratching
- Use antipruritic medications as ordered.

ACUTE PANCREATITIS

Acute pancreatitis is an acute inflammatory process of the pancreas. The degree of inflammation varies from mild edema to severe hemorrhage necrosis.

Pancreatitis (inflammation of the pancreas) is a serious disorder that can range in severity from a relatively mild, self-limiting disorder to a rapidly fatal disease that does not respond to any treatment.

Acute pancreatitis is commonly described as an autodigestion of this organ by the exocrine enzymes it produces, principally trypsin. Common cause of acute episodes are biliary tract disease and long-term alcohol use; 5% of patients with gallstones develop pancreatitis. Less common forms include bacterial or viral infection, with pancreatitis as a complication. Many disease processes and conditions have been associated with an increased incidence of hypercalcemia, and hyperlipidemia. Up to 20% of cases are idiopathic, and there is a small incidence of hereditary pancreatitis.

Mortality is high because of shock , anoxia, hypotension, or fluid and electrolyte imbalances. Complete recovery may occur, or the condition may become chronic.

Etiology

Acute pancreatitis is most common in middle-aged men and women, but affects more men than women. Many factors can cause injury to the pancreas. The primary etiological factors are biliary tract disease and alcoholism. The other less common causes are:

- Acute pancreatitis include trauma (postsurgical, abnormal)
- Viral infections (mumps, coxsackie virus B)
- Pancreating duodenum ulcer
- Abscesses
- Cystic fibrosis
- Kaposi's sarcoma
- Certain drugs (corticosteroids, thiazide diuretics, oral contraceptives sulfonamide and NSAIDs)
- Metabolic disorders (hyperlipidemia, renal failure)
- After surgical procedure (of pancreas, stomach, duodenum and biliary tract)
- After ERCP
- Idiopathic.

Pathophysiology

The most common pathogenic mechanism is believed to be autodigestion of the pancreas. The two major pathological varieties of acute pancreatitis are (1) acute intestinal form and (2) acute hemorrhagic form. Although either can be fatal, intestinal form is often a milder form. The defining characteristics of acute intestinal pancreatitis is a diffusely swollen and inflamed pancreas, which retains its anatomical features. There are minimal or no area of hemorrhage or necrosis in gland. The interstitial spaces become grossly swollen by extracellular edema and the ducts may contain purulent material. The acute hemorrhage disease presents with a different picture. The gland readily shows acute inflammation, hemorrhage, and marked tissue necrosis. Extensive fat necrosis is present in patients with fulminant disease not just in the pancreas but throughout the abdominal and thoracic cavities and subcutaneous tissues. Necrosis of vessel can cause significant loss of blood and abscesses and infections form in areas of walled-off necrotic tissue. Systemic complications such as fat emboli, hypotension, shock and fluid overload are common.

The etiologic factors cause injury to pancreatic cells or activation of the pancreatic enzymes in the pancreas. Trypsinogen is an inactive proteolytic enzyme produced by pancreas. Activation to pancreatic enzymes before they reach the duodenum has long been recognized as a major component of the disease process. Enzyme activation overwhelms all of the normal protective mechanisms of the pancreas and initiates a massive attack on the pancreatic tissues. Pancreatic autodigestion is initiated. Other systemic effects of the activated enzymes include:

- Activation of complement and kinin-producing increased vascular permeability and vasodilation
- Increased stickiness of the inflammatory leucocytes with formation of emboli, which plug the microvasculature
- Initiation of consumptive coagulopathy, leading to disseminated intravascular coagulation
- Increased permeability causing massive movement of fluids which leads to circulatory insufficiency
- Release of myocardial-depressant factor, which further compromises cardiac function
- Activation of the renin-angiotensin network, which impairs renal function in conjunction with circulatory insufficiency.

Clinical Manifestations

Severe abdominal pain is the major symptom.

- Pain the mid-epigastrium may be accompanied by abdominal distention, a poorly defined palpable abdominal mass, and decreased peristalsis
- Frequently acute in onset (24 to 48 hours after a heavy meal or alcohol ingestion); may be more severe after meals and unrelieved by antacids
- Patient appears acutely ill
- Abdominal guarding; rigid or boardlike abdomen
- Soft abdomen in the absence of peritonitis

- Ecchymosis in the flank or around the umbilicus, which may indicate severe hemorrhagic pancreatitis
- Nausea and vomiting fever jaundice, mental confusion, agitation
- Hypotension related to hypovolemia and shock
- Acute renal failure common
- May develop tachycardia, cyanosis and cold, clammy skin
- Respiratory distress and hypoxia
- Dyspnea
- Tachypnea
- Abnormal blood gas values
- Diffuse pulmonary infiltrates
- Myocardial depression, hypocalcemia, hyperglycemia and disseminated intravascular coagulation (DIC).

Pain

- Steady and severe in nature, excruciating in fulminant cases
- Located in the epigastric or umbilical region, may radiate to the back
- Worsened by lying supine; may be lessened by flexed knee, curved back positioning.

Vomiting

- Varies in severity but is usually protracted
- Worsened by ingestion of food or fluid
- Does not relive the pain
- Usually accompanied by nausea.

Fever

- Rarely exceeds 39°C.

Abdominal Findings

- Rigidity, tenderness, guarding
- Distension
- Decreased or absent peristalsis.

Additional Features of Fulminant Disease

- Symptoms of hypovolemic shock
- Oliguria; acute tubular necrosis
- Ascites
- Jaundice
- Respiratory failure
- Grey Turner's sign (bluish discoloration along the flanks)
- Cullen's sign (bluish discoloration around the umbilicus).

(These signs indicate the accumulation of blood in these areas and represent the presence of hemorrhagic pancreatitis).

The significant local complications of acute pancreatitis are pseudocyst and abscess. The main systemic complication as pulmonary (pleural effusion, atelectasis and pneumonia) and tetany and hypotension hypovolemia, hypoalbuminemia, leukocytosis, ARDS, GI bleeding, pseudocyst, hyperglycemia, hypocalcemia and hyperlipidemia.

Diagnostic Studies

The primary diagnostic tests are serum amylase, lipase and urinary amylase level. Usually there is elevation. The secondary tests are blood glucose, (hyperglycemic due to impaired carbohydrate metabolism due to E-cell damage and release of glucagon). Serum calcium (hypocalcemia) and serum triglycerides (hyperlipidemia) and also CTS, ERCEP.

Management

The main objective of the management of acute pancreatitis are: Relief of pain; prevention and alleviation of shock; reduction of pancreatic secretions, control of fluid and electrolyte imbalance, prevention and treatment of infections and removal of precipitatory cause for which the measures to be taken according to the following:

- Administer meparidine (analgesics) to relieve pain
- NPO with NG tube to suction and reduce secretions
- Cimetidine or ranitidine IV
- Administer antibiotics as prescribed
- Lactated Ringer's solution for fluid and electrolyte valency and bed rest and proper diet, good oral hygiene should be maintained and take measures to treat complications accordingly and teach patients to avoid alcohol.

The major goals of the patient include relief of pain and discomfort, improved fluid and nutritional status, improved respiratory function and absence of complications. For nursing care plan see Table 11.2.

Nursing interventions

Relieving Pain and Discomfort

- Administer morphine as ordered. This is the drug of choice
- Withhold oral fluids to decrease formation and secretion of secretin
- Use nasogastric suctioning to remove gastric secretions and relieve abdominal distention; avoid tension on tube and use water-soluble lubricant around nares; give frequent oral hygiene

TABLE 11.2: Nursing care plan for the patient with severe acute pancreatitis

Problem	Objective	Nursing interventions	Rationales
Nursing Diagnosis #1			
Tissue perfusion, alteration in related to hypovolemic shock.	Patient will: 1. Maintain stable hemodynamics: – Blood pressure within 10 mm Hg of baseline – Heart rate < 100 beats/min – Central venous pressure 0–8 mm Hg – Pulmonary capillary wedge pressure 8–12 mm Hg – Cardiac output ~5 liters/min – Skin warm with usual color 2. Demonstrate alert mental status, appropriate behavior and neurological function: – Oriented to person, place, time – Cranial nerves intact – Deep tendon reflexes brisk 3. Maintain renal function: – Urine output >30 mL/h – Balanced intake and output – BUN, serum creatinine within acceptable physiological range	• Perform ongoing cardiovascular assessment: – Continuous cardiac monitoring. ◆ Establish baseline rate, rhythm, ectopy – Continuous hemodynamic pressure monitoring: ◆ Establish baseline values: Central venous pressure, pulmonary capillary wedge pressure – Assess peripheral pulses: Rate, rhythm, quality – Assess skin temperature, moisture, color, turgor • Assess ongoing neurological function: Mental status; level of consciousness; behavior—appropriate?; cranial nerves; deep tendon reflexes • Monitor renal function: Hourly urine output; intake and output – Daily weight	• Establishing baseline data assists in evaluating subsequent responses to therapy – Cardiac tissue hypoxia may predispose to dysrhythmias – Offers significant data regarding cardiopulmonary status; affords trending, i.e. frequent serial measurements; trending more accurately reflects changes occurring in patient's condition and the patient's response to therapeutic measures – Presence of cool, moist skin with pallor or cyanosis reflects compensatory peripheral vasoconstriction response to permit blood to be shunted to vital organs • Compromised hemodynamics (hypotension) and hypoxemia predispose to cerebral hypoxia, reflected by alterations in cerebral function, level of consciousness, responsiveness of cranial nerves, and deep tendon reflexes • Reduction in urine output suggests decreased renal perfusion commonly associated with hypovolemic shock. Acute renal failure is a major complication of acute pancreatitis – Most closely reflects hydration status
Nursing Diagnosis #2			
Fluid volume deficit (intravascular): actual, related to: 1. Hemorrhage 2. Third-spacing (pancreatic ascites) A. Hypoalbuminemia 3. Dehydration A. NPO B. Nasogastric suctioning C. Vomiting	Patient will: 1. Achieve resolution of edema/ascites: – Body weight within 5% of baseline – Abdominal girth at baseline measurement	• Assess gastrointestinal function: – Abdominal assessment: Abdomen—soft, rigid; rebound tenderness; presence of Cullen or Grey-Turner signs; abdominal girth – Nausea/vomiting/constipation, hematemesis, melena	• Compensatory vasoconstriction of splanchnic circulation (sympathetic response), may result in decreased peristalsis, and ischemia of the gastric and intestinal mucosa – Cullen sign; Bluish umbilicus or family blue discoloration of skin associated with hemoperitoneum from any cause – Grey-Turner sign: Ecchymoses on abdomen and flanks possibly associated with infiltration of extraperitoneal tissues with blood
Nursing Diagnosis #3			
Electrolyte balance, alteration in related to: 1. Diuretic therapy 2. Acid-base imbalance	Patient will: 1. Restore/maintain laboratory parameters within acceptable physiological range: – Serum osmolality 285–295 mOsm/kg – Serum sodium>135 <148 mEq/liter	• Assess for signs and symptoms of electrolyte imbalance: – Hypokalemia—cardiac dysrhythmias; hypotension; weakness; fatigue; nausea, vomiting; lethargy, muscle weakness; paresthesias, hyporeflexia	• Acute pancreatitis usually predisposes to electrolyte imbalance. Nasogastric suctioning, vomiting, diarrhea and extravasation of fluid account for much of the loss of sodium, potassium, and chloride

Contd...

Contd...

Problem	Objective	Nursing interventions	Rationales
	– Serum potassium 3.5–5.5 mEq/liter – Serum albumin 3.5–5.5 g/100 mL – Hematocrit 37–52 percent – Hemoglobin 12–18 g/100 mL – CBC – Urine electrolytes and specific gravity	– Hyponatremia—nausea, vomiting, headache, lethargy, confusion, seizures, coma – Hypocalcemia—tremors, paresthesias, tetany laryngospasm, convulsions, positive Chvostek's and Trousseau's signs – Hypochloremia: Alkalemia. • Implement prescribed measures to re-establish and maintain normovolemia and electrolyte balance – Administer blood products and intravenous fluids – Replace serum albumin – Monitor for signs of circulatory overload: Generalized (dependent) edema, weight gain, increased blood pressure, bounding pulses; signs of pulmonary congestion—dyspnea, rales (crackles), elevation of central venous and pulmonary artery pressures; neck vein distention – Monitor for signs of hypovolemia: Hypotension, tachycardia, decreased central venous and pulmonary artery pressures; decreased urine output, increase in urine-specific gravity; signs of dehydration—elevated body temperature, poor skin turgor, sunken eyeballs, and dryness of mucous membranes – Administer prescribed inotropic and vasopressor therapy ◆ Dopamine hydrochloride – Replace serum electrolytes – Sodium ◆ Hyponatremia/hypernatremia: Monitor hydration status, monitor serum/urine sodium levels – Potassium ◆ Hypokalemia/hyperkalemia: Monitor ECG for dysrhythmias, monitor arterial blood gases (acid-base status), monitor serum potassium levels – Calcium ◆ Hypocalcemia – Monitor ECG for dysrhythmias – Monitor total serum protein and serum albumin levels – Chloride	– It is important to establish baseline blood chemistry values so that replacement therapy may be guided by serial studies, which should include total protein and serum osmolality in addition to electrolytes – To reverse hypovolemia/hypotension. Re-establishing intravascular volume improves circulation, tissue perfusion and oxygenation. Replace fluid losses associated with NPO, vomiting, and nasogastric suctioning – Irrigating and inflammatory effects of acute pancreatitis on the pancreatic parenchyma and surrounding tissues cause extravasation of fluids, electrolytes, and protein into the interstitium and peritoneal cavity (third-spacing) – Loss of plasma proteins from the intravascular space disrupts colloidal osmotic pressure, predisposing to even greater fluid loss with interstitial edema and ascites – Fluid overload is a complication of aggressive fluid volume replacement – Increases cardiac output by increasing preload (venous return) and cardiac contractility; enhances tissue perfusion – Hyponatremia is a frequent occurrence in acute pancreatitis – A decrease in total body sodium predisposes to hypovolemia – Intravenous replacement of sodium needs to be carefully monitored to prevent sodium excess (hypernatremia) with consequent fluid overload – Potassium, an intracellular ion, is closely associated with acid-base balance – Acidemia—hydrogen ions are driven into cells in exchange for potassium; this increases serum potassium levels – Alkalemia—hydrogen ions move out of cells in exchange for potassium; this decreases serum potassium levels – This reciprocal relationship between potassium and hydrogen ions also occurs in the distal tubules, necessitating that kidney function be closely monitored

Contd...

Contd...

Problem	Objective	Nursing interventions	Rationales
		◆ Hypochloremia: monitor acid-base status, monitor serum chloride	– Deposition of calcium into areas of fatty necrosis occurs frequently in acute pancreatitis and requires close monitoring of serum calcium levels. Calcium replacement therapy requires careful administration to prevent complications – Patent intravenous line needs to be maintained because tissue sloughing and necrosis can occur with extravasation of calcium preparations – Potentiation of digitalis effect by calcium can occur in patients receiving digitalis; this can predispose to digitalis toxicity. Continuous ECG monitoring is essential – Calcium is highly bound to serum proteins; alkalemia increases percent calcium bound to protein, thus reducing fraction of ionized calcium – Chloride is necessary for gastric production of HCl; it plays a major role in acid-base balance – Hypochloremia is associated with vomiting, and nasogastric suctioning; it predisposes to metabolic alkalosis
Nursing Diagnosis #4			
Breathing pattern, Ineffective, related to: 1. Hypoventilation associated with severe abdominal pain 2. Atelectasis 3. Pleural effusion *Nursing Diagnosis #5* Airway clearance, ineffective, related to: 1. Cough suppression and failure to deep breathe because of severe abdominal pain 2. Immobility	Patient will: 1. Demonstrate effective minute ventilation: – Tidal volume (Vt) >5–7 mL/kg – Respiratory rate < 25–30 per min 2. Achieve vital capacity (Vc) > 12–15 mL/kg 3. Verbalize ease of breathing 4. Demonstrate deep-breathing techniques and effective secretion-clearing cough 5. Maintain arterial blood gases within acceptable physiological range: – PaO_2 > 60 mm Hg – $PaCO_2$ 35–45 mm Hg – pH > 7.35 < 7.45 – Base excess +2/-2 6. Maintain appropriate responses on respiratory examination: – Tactile fremitus present on palpation – Resonance throughout lung fields on percussion – Vesicular breath sounds throughout peripheral lung fields on auscultation	• Assess respiratory function: – Rate, rhythm, depth and pattern of breathing – Symmetry of chest wall and diaphragmatic excursion – Use of accessory muscles – Auscultation of breath sounds – Pulmonary lung volumes: Total minute ventilation; tidal volume, respiratory rate; vital capacity – Assess quantity, quality, color, odor and consistency of sputum – Assess arterial blood gases • Implement measures to improve respiratory function: – Administer prescribed medication for abdominal pain and monitor response – Meperidine is drug of choice – Perform measures to reduce anxiety: ◆ Encourage verbalization of fears and concerns ◆ Provide a caring touch and listening ear ◆ Provide explanations and feedback regarding care and health status ◆ Identify patient/family coping strengths and resources	– Abdominal pain causes splinting and hypoventilation; hypoventilation predisposes to hypercapnia and atelectasis; atelectasis predisposes to ventilation/perfusion inequality ◆ Abdominal pain predisposes to cough suppression and immobility; pooling of secretions predisposes to pneumonia – Relief of pain encourages patient to breathe more deeply and to cough more vigorously – Meperidine causes less spasm of Oddi's sphincter than does morphine – A reduction in the level of anxiety or stress may help to reduce the level of pain, and facilitate breathing – Help to improve ventilation and oxygenation, and prevent atelectasis and pooling of secretions – Nasogastric suction helps to reduce gastric distention

Contd...

Contd...

Problem	Objective	Nursing interventions	Rationales
	7. Demonstrate an absence of atelectasis and pleural effusion	– Perform measures to facilitate chest wall expansion and diaphragmatic excursion: ◆ Minimize abdominal distention associated with gastrointestinal gas and fluid accumulation – Maintain proper placement and patency of nasogastric tube – Encourage frequent position changes ◆ Maintain patient in semi to high-Fowler's position unless contraindicated – Encourage patient to expel flatus whenever the urge arises – Monitor for signs and symptoms of pleural effusion: Shortness of breath; pleuritic pain; splinting to reduce chest excursion; dullness on percussion; and diminished to absent breath sounds over the affected area on auscultation – Perform measures to minimize pancreatic secretory activity – Administer anticholinergic drugs cautiously, if prescribed – Prepare patient and assist with thoracentesis – Prepare patient and assist with paracentesis (*Nursing Diagnosis* #1) – Implement prescribed respiratory support therapy – Oxygen therapy – Intermittent positive pressure breathing (IPPB)	– Patient is inclined to assume a position of greatest pain relief and to remain in that position. Coughing, deep breathing, and position changes may best be performed following administration of analgesics – Deep breathing and position changes may stimulate peristalsis and flatulence – The pancreas is stimulated by gastric juice in the duodenum; a patent nasogastric tube with suction reduces delivery of HCl to duodenum – Blocking parasympathetic stimulation (via vagus) decreases amount of gastric HCl secretion; use of anticholinergics in a patient with paralytic ileus may actually worsen the patient's condition by suppressing pancreatic secretion and allowing enzymes to accumulate within the pancreas – Decompression of pleural effusion facilitates greater lung expansion – Decompression of peritoneal fluid increases diaphragmatic excursion
Nursing Diagnosis #6			
Comfort, alteration in: Acute pain	Patient will: 1. Verbalize relief of pain 2. Exhibit relaxed demeanor: – Relaxed facial expression and body posturing – Ease of breathing 3. Identify effective pain relief and coping mechanisms	• Implement measures to reduce pancreatic stimulation – Maintain the patient NPO – Maintain patency of nasogastric tube with continuous nasogastric suction ◆ Confirm tube placement every 2 hours – Administer prescribed medications: ◆ Meperidine is usual analgesic of choice. Evaluate the effectiveness of the prescribed analgesic ◆ Anticholinergics, papaverine ◆ Provide frequent oral care ◆ Monitor urine output. – Provide frequent comfort measures: ◆ Mouth care; position changes; time periods of quiet and sleep; spending more time with patient	• Stimulation of inflamed pancreatic acinar cells aggravate pain – Pain and anxiety increase pancreatic secretory activity via enhanced parasympathetic stimulation – It is necessary to minimize gastric secretions as they stimulate secretion of the hormones secretin and cholecystokinin, both of which stimulate pancreatic secretion. – Nasogastric suction also relieves nausea, vomiting, and intestinal distention – Morphine is avoided because it causes a greater degree of spasm of the sphincter of Oddi than does meperidine – These drugs function to relax smooth muscle which may help to reduce pain – Anticholinergic drugs suppress salivary secretion; oral mucous membranes become dry

Contd...

Contd...

Problem	Objective	Nursing interventions	Rationales
		◆ Provide a listening ear – Involve patient/family in quiet recreational activities – Minimize visitors – Instruct family members, friends not to take food into the patient's room	– Urinary retention and paralytic ileus are also associated with anticholinergic therapy – This may help to distract the patient from thoughts of food and to avoid parasympathetic stimulation associated with the cephalic phase of digestive activity – Increased activity may aggravate pain – Sight of food can stimulate pancreatic secretory activity (cephalic phase of digestion)
Nursing Diagnosis #7			
Nutrition, alteration in, less than body requirements (malnutrition), related to: 1. Nausea and vomiting 2. NPO status 3. Malabsorption (altered fat metabolism) 4. Altered carbohydrate and protein metabolism A. Hypoglycemia B. Hypoalbuminemia	Patient will: 1. Maintain body weight within 5% of baseline 2. Maintain serum albumin within physiological range: – 3.5–5.0 g/100 mL 3. Demonstrate unimpaired integrity of skin and mucous membranes 4. Verbalize feeling of increased strength 5. Triceps skinfold within acceptable range 6. Laboratory parameters within acceptable range: – Hematology profile – Cholesterol – BUN, creatinine	Refer to Table nutritional support of the critically Ill patient, for details related to treatment and prevention of malnutrition	
Nursing Diagnosis #8			
Oral mucous membranes, alteration in, related to: 1. Altered fluid and electrolyte imbalance (dehydration) 2. Mouth breathing with nasogastric tube 3. Reduced salivation associated with dehydration and medication regimen (e.g. narcotics, anticholinergics)	Patient will: 1. Maintain integrity of mucous membranes: – Mucous membranes moist – Lips without cracking or fissures	• Assess and monitor status of mucous membranes: Monitor daily weight, intake and output; monitor dietary intake • Implement measures to prevent drying and cracking of mucous membranes: – Maintain hydration – Provide frequent oral hygiene, rinsing mouth frequently – Keep lips well lubricated – Assess lips, mouth and pharynx for lesions, fissures, or bleeding • Implement measures to treat drying and cracking or oral membranes: Apply topical ointment to keep mucous membranes moist	• When nutritional intake is less than body requirements, the patient becomes at risk of infections, and healing capabilities become compromised – Adequate hydration is necessary to keep mucous membranes moist – Prevent cracking and fissure formation – Ongoing assessment assists in determining changes in the mucosa, and the effectiveness of therapy
Nursing Diagnosis #9			
Infection, potential for, related to: 1. Malnutrition 2. Invasive procedures 3. Peritonitis associated with autodigestion of adjacent tissues by pancreatic juices	Patient will: 1. Maintain body temperature within acceptable physiological range ~98.6°F 2. Maintain white blood count: ~5000–10,000/mm³ 3. Remain without signs and symptoms of infection: Pain, erythema, edema, increased temperature (peripheral sites)	• Monitor • Check for WBC visual signs • Administer antibiotics as orderd • Provide nourishments as prescribed • Observe for complications	

Contd...

Contd...

Problem	Objective	Nursing interventions	Rationales
Nursing Diagnosis #10			
Knowledge deficit regarding: 1. Convalescence and follow-up care 2. Impact on lifestyle – Alcoholism – Stress	Patient will: 1. Verbalize importance of strict adherence to prescribe dietary regimen: – Total abstinence from alcohol – High carbohydrate and protein diet; low-fat intake 2. Verbalize alternatives in pain relief: – Medication therapy – Relaxation exercises 3. Identify effective coping mechanisms in stress management	• Establish a trusting rapport with patient and family members – Verbalize fears and concerns for patient and family • Assess patient/family baseline knowledge and readiness to learn – Encourage patient/family to assist in identifying needs and learning objectives • Assist patient/family in problem-solving techniques – Help to identify family strengths and weaknesses • Determine appropriate teaching strategies to facilitate learning: – Encourage open discussions regarding illness and impact on family lifestyle ◆ Consider role of alcohol in lifestyle if appropriate • Initiate health teaching concerned with the following: "Diet management: Emphasis importance of strict adherence to prescribed diet; abstinence from alcohol and high-fat intake – Consider who in the family is responsible for meal preparation – Pain management: Advise patient as to alternatives in pain relief: Medication therapy; surgery; relaxation exercises, recreational therapy ◆ Support patient/family in their decision ◆ Include the following in teaching: Purpose, action(s), dosage, frequency and route of administration and drug interactions for prescribed medications – Management of stress: Assist patient/family to: Identify sources of stress; identify effective and ineffective coping mechanisms and their usefulness; assist patient/family to become in touch with their feelings, and to communicate these feelings to each other • Initiate referrals to appropriate resources: – Nutritionist – Social worker – Psychiatric liaison nurse – Other	• An environment of mutual respect and trust can enhance the learning process. Often a long convalescence follows recovery from acute pancreatitis. Discharge planning should begin as early as possible – While the patient may be too ill initially to participate in learning, involvement of family members in the patient's overall care may impact on the progress made by patient and family members alike towards level of health and well-being desired • An informed patient/family can participate in care and make necessary adjustments in lifestyle – Assisting patient/family to cope increases self-confidence in their own capabilities • Learning should occur at a rate that is meaningful to participants – It is essential for the family member who cooks to appreciate the patient's diet and its preparation – Effective stress management may be helpful in reducing pain • Successful recovery of all members of the family from the stress of acute illness, and continued health maintenance requires timely and ongoing support. No one lives in a vacuum

- Maintain patient on bed rest to decrease metabolic rate and reduce secretion of pancreatic enzymes; report increased pain (may be pancreatic hemorrhage or inadequate analgesic dosage)
- Provide explanations about treatment; patient may have clouded sensorium from pain fluid imbalances and hypoxemia.

Improving Nutritional Status

- Monitor laboratory test results, daily weights and anthropometric measures
- Assess nutritional status and increased metabolic requirements (note increased body temperature, restlessness, increased physical activity) and fluid lost through diarrhea
- Provide mouth care; patient should receive nothing by mouth during an attack
- Administer fluids, electrolytes, and parenteral nutrition (PN) as prescribed
- Monitor serum glucose level every 4 to 6 hours and give insulin as prescribed
- Introduce oral feedings gradually as symptoms subside
- Avoid heavy meals, alcoholic beverage, excessive use of coffee, and spicy foods.

Improving Respiratory Function

- Maintain patient in semi-Fowler's position to decreased pressure on diaphragm
- Change position frequently to prevent atelectasis and pooling of respiratory secretions
- Administer anticholinergic medications to decrease gastric and pancreatic secretions; dry respiratory tract secretions
- Assess respiratory status frequently (pulse oximetry, artery blood gas values) and teach patient techniques of cough and deep breathing.

Providing Wound Care

- Assess the wound, drainage sites and skin carefully for signs of infections, inflammation, and breakdown
- Carry out wound care as prescribed, and take precautions to protect intact skin from contract with drainage; consult with an enterostomal therapist as needed to identify appropriate skin care devices and protocols
- Turn patient every 2 hours; use of specially beds may be indicated to prevent skin breakdown. Surgical wound may be irrigated and repacked every 2 to 3 days.

Monitoring and Managing Complications

Fluid and electrolyte disturbances

- Assess fluid and electrolyte status by noting skin turgor and moistness of mucous membranes
- Weight daily; measure all fluid intake and output
- Assess for factors that may affect fluid and electrolyte status fever, fluid loss through diarrhea, vomiting, nasogastric suctioning, or wound drainage
- Observe for ascites, and measure abdominal girth
- Administer intravenous fluids, electrolytes, blood, and albumin to maintain volume and prevent or treat shock
- Assist patient to turn and change positions every 2 hours
- Report decreased blood pressure, reduced urine output and low serum calcium and magnesium.

Pancreatic Necrosis

- Transfer patient to intensive care unit for close monitoring
- Administer fluids, medications and blood products
- Assist with supportive management, such as mechanical ventilation.

Multiple Organs Dysfunction Syndrome

- Monitor patient closely for early signs of neurologic, cardiovascular, renal, and respiratory dysfunction
- Prepare for rapid changes in patient status, treatment, and therapies; respond quickly
- Inform family of status and progress of patient; allow time with patient.

Promoting Home and Community-Based Care

Teaching patients self-care:

- Provide patient and family with facts and explanations of the acute phase of illness; provide necessary repetition and reinforcement. Offer printed teaching materials
- Reinforce the need for a low-fat diet, avoidance of heavy meals, and avoidance of alcohol
- Provide additional explanations on dietary modifications if biliary tract disease is the cause.

Continuing Care

- Assess the home situation and reinforce teaching
- Refer for home care (often indicated)

- Provide information about resources and support groups, particularly if alcohol is the cause of acute pancreatitis
- Permit patient and family to air questions and concerns, and provide education and emotional support.

CHRONIC PANCREATITIS

Chronic pancreatitis is progressive destruction of the pancreas with fibrotic replacement of pancreatic tissue structure and calcification may also occur in the pancreas.

Chronic pancreatitis is an inflammatory disorder characterized by progressive anatomic and functional destruction of the pancreas. Cells are replaced by fibrous tissue with repeated attacks on pancreatitis. The end result is mechanical obstruction of the pancreatic and common bile ducts and duodenum. In addition the secreting cells of the pancreas become inflamed and destruction ensues. Alcohol consumption in Western societies and malnutrition worldwide are the major causes. Among alcoholics, the incidence of pancreatitis is 50 times the rate in the nondrinking population.

Etiology

Chronic pancreatic may follow acute pancreatitis. The two major types are chronic-obstructive pancreatitis and chronic-calcifying pancreatitis. Chronic obstructive pancreatitis is associated with biliary disease. The most common cause is inflammation of the sphincter of oddi associated with cholelithiasis. It could also be casued by cancer or the ampulla of vater, or caner of the duodenum or pancreas. In chronic calcifying pancreatitis, there are inflammation and sclerosis mainly in the head of the pancreas and around the pancreatic duct. It is associated with alcohol. These are also called "alcohol-induced pancreatitis".

Pathophysiology

The basic pathological change of chronic pancreatitis is destruction of the exocrine parenchymas and replacements with fibrous tissue. This process is associated with varying degrees of duct dilation. Scarring and fibrotic changes may occur throughout the pancreas or be limited to the selected areas. Calcium salts may be deposited in both the ducts and the parenchyma, usually in areas of fat necrosis. Ductal obstructions occur secondarily. The factors which influence the solubility on the calcium-rich pancreatic secretions are not well-identified. As the process becomes increasingly severe the islets of Langerhans are also involved and destroyed.

Clinical Manifestation

As with acute pancreatitis, a major manifestation of the chronic pancreatic is abdominal pain.

- Recurring attacks of severe, upper abdominal and back pain accompanied by vomiting; narcotics may not provide relief
- There may be continuous severe pain or dull, nagging constant pain
- Risk of addiction to opiates is high because of the severe pain
- Weight loss is a major problem
- Altered digestion (malabsorption) of foods (proteins and fats) results in frequent, frothy, and foul-smelling stools with a high fat content (steatorrhea)
- As disease progresses, calcification of the gland may occur and calcium stones may form within the ducts.

The patient may have episodes of acute pain, but it is usually chronic (recurrent attack at intervals of months or years). The attacks may become more and more frequent until they are almost constant, or they may diminish as the pancreatic fibrosis develops. The pain is located in the same area as in the acute pancreatitis, but it is usually described as heavy, gnawing feeling and sometimes a burning and cramp like. The pain is not relieved by food or antacids. The other manifestations are pancreatic insufficiency including malabsorption with weight loss, constipation, mild jaundice with dark urine, steatorrhea and diabetes mellitus. The steatorrhea may become severe with voluminous, foul, fatty stools. Urine and stools may be frothy. Some abdominal tenderness may be present.

Diagnosis: Diagnostic studies as in acute pancreatitis.

Management

- Endoscopic retrograde cholangiopancreatography (ERCP) is the most useful study
- A glucose tolerance test evaluates pancreatic islet cell function.

Medical Management

Treatment is directed toward preventing and managing acute attacks.

- Pain and discomfort are relieved with analgesics
- Patient should avoid alcohol and foods that produce abdominal pain and discomfort. No other treatment will relieve pain if patient continues to consume alcohol
- Diabetes mellitus resulting from dysfunction of pancreatic islet cells is treated with diet, insulin, or oral hypoglycemic agents. Patient and family are taught the hazard of severe hypoglycemia related to alcohol use
- Pancreatic enzyme replacement therapy is instituted for malabsorption and steatorrhea
- Surgery is done to relieve abdominal pain and discomfort, restore drainage of pancreatic secretions, and reduce frequency of attacks (pancreaticojejunostomy) (Fig. 11.7).

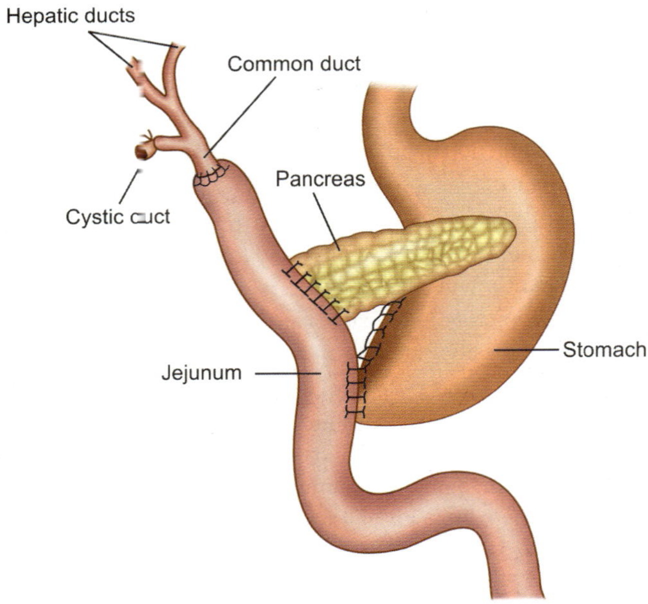

FIG. 11.7: Whipple procedure or radical pancreaticoduodenectomy. This surgical procedure involves resection of the proximal pancreas, adjoining duodenum, distal portion of the stomach, and distal portion of the common bile duct. An anastomosis of the pancreatic duct, common bile duct, and stomach to the jejunum is done

- Morbidity and mortality after surgical procedures are high because of patient's poor physical condition before surgery and concomitant occurrence of cirrhosis.

Nursing Management

When the patient with chronic pancreatitis is experiencing an acute attack, the therapy is identical as that for acute pancreatitis. At other times, the focus is on prevention of further attacks, relief of pain, and control of pancreatic exocrine and endocrine insufficiency. It sometimes takes large, frequent doses of analgesics to relieve pain. And diet, pancreatic enzyme replacement, and control of diabetes are measures used to control pancreatic insufficiency. The diet is a bland, low-fat, high-carbohydrate and high protein diet. The patient does not tolerate fatty, rich and stimulating foods and these should be avoided to decrease pancreatic secretions and demands on the pancreas. Alcohol must be totally eliminated. Antacids and anticholinergic drugs may be given to decrease HCl acid. Where stimulus pancreatic is active, i.e. cimetidine and ranitidine pancreatic enzymes such as pancreatin, pancrelipase are used to replace enzymes. For diabetes insulin is giving as per instruction of the medical doctors. When pseudocysts or obstruction develops, surgery may be indicated and treated accordingly. Nursing care plan of hepatic failure and hepatc encephalopathies is listed in Table 11.3

TABLE 11.3: Care plan for the patient with hepatic failure and hepatic encephalopathy

Problem	Objective	Nursing interventions	Rationales
Nursing Diagnosis #1			
Fluid volume deficit (intravascular, actual), related to: 1. Ascites and anasarca (third spacing) A. Hypoalbuminemia B. Portal hypertension C. Hyperaldosteronism (secondary) D. Capillary fragility/increased permeability	Patient will: 1. Maintain stable hemodynamics: – Heart rate (resting) <100 beats/min – Central venous pressure 0-8 mm Hg – Pulmonary artery pressure <25 mm Hg – Pulmonary capillary wedge pressure 8–12 mm Hg – Cardiac output ~5 liters/min – Systemic arterial blood pressure within 10 mm Hg of baseline	• Assess for signs and symptoms of hypovolemia: – Assess cardiovascular function: ◆ Heart rate (resting) ◆ Hypotension (orthostatic) ◆ Skin color—pallor, mottled appearance; cyanosis; cool to touch; peripheral edema (anasarca) ◆ Assess for ascites—abdominal assessment: - Inspect for bulging of flanks or a protruding, misplaced umbilicus; skin tautness; new striae - Percuss for shifting dullness - Palpate for fluid wave	• Establish baseline assessment data with which to evaluate the patient's response to therapy. – An increase in heart rate reflects a compensatory response to maintain cardiac output – A decrease in blood pressure of more than 10–15 mm Hg from a supine to sitting position reflects a reduced circulatory (intravascular) volume – Compensatory peripheral vasoconstriction shunts blood from skin and nonvital organs to the heart and brain

Contd...

Contd...

Problem	Objective	Nursing interventions	Rationales
2. Bleeding A. Bleeding varices (hematemesis) B. Erosive gastritis C. Coagulopathy *Nursing Diagnosis #2* Electrolyte balance, alteration in: hypokalemia, related to: 1. Diuretic therapy 2. Hyperaldosteronism (sodium retention)	2. Maintain baseline mental and neurological status; deep tendon reflexes brisk 3. Achieve resolution of ascites and anasarca. – Body weight within 5% of baseline – Abdominal girth at baseline measurement – Functioning peritoneovenous shunt (if inserted) 4. Balance intake and output 5. Maintain urine output >30 mL/hour 6. Maintain laboratory parameter as follows: – Serum osmolality 285–295 mOsm/kg – Serum sodium > 135 and < 148 mEq/liter – Serum potassium 3.5–5.5 mEq/liter – Serum albumin 3.5–5.5 g/100 mL – Haematocrit 37–52 per cent – Hemoglobin 12–18 g/100 mL – RBC count > 4.7–5.9 million/mm³ – Platelet count > 150,000 mm³	• Measure abdominal girth daily using markings indicated on abdomen • Determine body weight • Assess serum albumin levels – Cardiac monitoring – Hemodynamic pressure monitoring parameters: Central venous pressure; pulmonary artery pressure; pulmonary capillary wedge pressure: cardiac output; arterial pressure monitoring – Assess neurological function: Mental status, orientation; thought processes; motor responses; deep tendon reflexes – Assess renal function: Intake and output; hourly urine output; monitor creatinine and BUN	– Ascites results from a combination of low intravascular colloidal osmotic pressure (hypoalbuminemia), portal hypertension, overproduction of hepatic lymph, and secondary retention of sodium and water • When forces favoring movement of fluid from the intravascular space into the interstitium (portal hypertension) exceed forces favoring movement of fluid in the opposite direction (e.g. decreased intravascular colloidal osmotic pressure), fluid accumulates. When the capacity of the lymphatic system to return fluid to the circulating blood is exceeded, ascites results. Of central importance to the formation of ascites is renal sodium and water retention – Measurement of abdominal girth assists in evaluating the status of the ascites. Markings made on the abdomen help to assure that repeated measurements are made at the same circumference; measure with patient in same position. Clinical findings of ascites are usually demonstrable after more than 1500 mL of ascites fluid has accumulated – Daily measurement of body weight most closely reflects total body fluid volume – Serum albumin is largely responsible for maintaining serum colloidal osmotic pressure – Cardiac dysrhythmias may occur in response to ischaemia or electrolyte imbalance – Monitoring of these parameters is indicated in the setting of hypovolemic shock, hemodynamic instability, and during massive fluid, albumin, and blood replacement, to monitor patient's response to therapy and prevent fluid overload – See *Nursing Diagnosis #7*, Thought processes, alteration in (below)

Contd...

Contd...

Problem	Objective	Nursing interventions	Rationales
		– Assess for signs and symptoms of electrolyte imbalance: Hypokalemia—general malaise, fatigue, anorexia, nausea, vomiting, diarrhea; abdominal cramps; muscle weakness hyporeflexia; cardiac dysrhythmias – Monitor serum electrolytes • Implement prescribed measures to re-establish normovolemia: – Maintain fluid restriction (~1000–1500 mL/day) – Maintain sodium restriction (200–500 mg/day) ◆ Avoid use of saline for intravenous therapy gastric lavage or other irrigation – Administer diuretic therapy with necessary potassium replacement therapy – Furosemide, thiazide diuretics – Spironolactone therapy – Administer inotropic agents and vasopressors (e.g. low-dose dopamine) – Administer protein supplementation – Administer salt-poor albumin intravenously • Assist with abdominal paracentesis: – Key nursing considerations: ◆ Have patient urinate prior to procedure ◆ Provide necessary explanations ◆ Position appropriately and as comfortably as possible ◆ Note that fluid removal should not exceed 1–1.5 liters ◆ Removal of fluid should be done slowly ◆ Monitor vital signs pre-, peri- and post-paracentesis ◆ Measure abdominal girth pre- and post- paracentesis, and daily thereafter ◆ Assess insertion site; monitor for complications of hypotension, bleeding, protein depletion, and infection • Implement ongoing monitoring: – Cardiovascular status: ◆ Monitor heart rate, pulses, blood pressure, hemodynamic parameters	– Hypovolemia can cause a decrease in renal perfusion; patients with hepatic failure are at risk of developing hepatorenal failure. Renal function is best monitored by serum creatinine; BUN may be altered by GI bleeding and impaired liver function – Excessive sodium reabsorption and retention associated with increased aldosterone secretion, and diuretic therapy can predispose to hypokalemia and metabolic alkalemia • Therapeutic goal is to gradually mobilize fluid back into the intravascular compartment and prevent further third-spacing – To decrease ascites and generalized edema – To reduce fluid retention as ascites and anasarca, and enhance mobilization of excessive fluids from the tissues – Controlled diuresis decreases water load with consequent reduction in ascites and edema. It minimizes the risk of renal failure – Require monitoring of serum potassium with concomitant potassium replacement therapy – A potassium-sparing diuretic, it inhibits the action of aldosterone on the distal tubular cells, thereby increasing excretion of sodium chloride and water, while retaining potassium – To increase cardiac output and maintain effective renal perfusion – To restore intravascular colloidal osmotic pressure to within acceptable physiological range; and enhance movement of ascitic and edema fluid into the intravascular space, promoting diuresis – Replaces albumin levels, restores intravascular volume and maintains renal perfusion. Monitor for fluid overload • In patients with severe ascites, paracentesis may be necessary to relieve dyspnea and compromised respiratory excursion, and/or urinary frequency – Reduces risk of nicking bladder with needle – May help patient to relax

Contd...

Contd...

Problem	Objective	Nursing interventions	Rationales
		– Respiratory status – Monitor respiratory rate and pattern; respiratory excursion, breath sounds (normal and adventitious) ◆ Monitor arterial blood gases – Renal status: Assess urine output (hourly); BUN, creatinine – Assess fluid and electrolyte status: Accurate intake and output; daily weight; daily measurement of abdominal girth – Serum studies: Electrolytes; protein (albumin/globulin ratio); osmolality, glucose – Urine studies: Electrolytes, specific gravity • Assist in preparation of patient for peritoneovenous shunt (e.g. LeVeen and Denver shunts): – Monitor for effectiveness of shunt post-surgery – Maintain bedrest as indicated – Enhance flow through shunt using abdominal binder and teaching patient to perform breathing exercises – Monitor for complications: hemodilution; congestive heart failure; gastrointestinal bleeding: leakage of ascitic fluid from incision site; infection, sepsis, coagulopathy (DIC); shunt occlusion/malfunction	– Sufficient quantity of fluid is removed to decrease intra-abdominal pressure; altered hemodynamics including hypotension and shock can be precipitated by the removal of too large a volume of fluid – Assists in assessing possible intra-abdominal bleeding – Assists in assessing for further fluid accumulation • Assists in evaluating the patient's response to therapy; reduces risk of complications – Patients with cirrhosis, ascites and bleeding potential are at high risk of complications – Respiratory embarrassment caused by ascites can lead to pulmonary complications; e.g. compromised alveolar ventilation with CO_2 retention (CO_2 narcosis may cause hepatic encephalopathy); and pneumonia – Assists in evaluating effectiveness of ventilation; and acid-base balance – Assists in evaluating the patient's response to therapy • This procedure may be indicated for the treatment of intractable ascites. It allows ascitic fluid to flow from the peritoneal cavity through a catheter tunneled under subcutaneous tissues, into the jugular vein or superior vena cava. The patient's own breathing triggers the shunt: On inspiration, the diaphragm descends, increasing intra-abdominal pressure while reducing intrathoracic pressures. This difference in pressure allows the fluid to flow from the peritoneal cavity into the thoracic veins
Nursing Diagnosis #3			
Breathing pattern, Ineffective, related to: 1. Ascites (abdominal distention) 2. Weakened, debilitated state	Patient will: 1. Maintain baseline mental status 2. Maintain effective respiratory function: – Respiratory rate <25–30/min – Tidal volume (Vr) >5–7 mL/kg – Vital capacity (Vc) > 12–15 mL/kg	• Assess respiratory function: Assess specific parameters—rate, pattern, depth of breathing; symmetry of chest wall and diaphragmatic excursion – Assess use of accessory muscles; breath sounds, evidence of adventitious sounds (rales, wheezes); dyspnea, tachypnea, orthopnea – Assess effectiveness of cough; sputum production – Assess pulmonary volume/capacity; tidal volume (Vr); vital capacity (Vc) – Monitor arterial blood gases: PaO_2, $PaCO_2$ pH	• Ascites causes pressure on diaphragm, limiting respiratory excursion and contributing to decreased alveolar ventilation, and atelectasis. The end result is hypoxemia – Weakened, debilitated status may compromise patient's respiratory effort, reducing alveolar ventilation and predisposing to hypoxemia – Accumulation of fluids and secretions reduces ventilation and predisposes to infection – Reflect effectiveness of ventilation and gas exchange

Contd...

Contd...

Problem	Objective	Nursing interventions	Rationales
		• Assess tissue perfusion and oxygenation – Assess cerebral function: mental status—restlessness, apprehension, confusion; drowsiness – Assess cardiovascular function: evidence of cyanosis—lips, mucous membranes, nail-beds; vital signs—heart rate, blood pressure, peripheral pulses, cardiac dysrhythmias – Assess fluid status: Intake and output; body weight – Laboratory data: Hematocrit, hemoglobin, serum electrolytes; BUN; serum osmolality • Assist patient to semi-Fowler's position	• These signs and symptoms may be reflective of hypoxemia and tissue hypoxia • This position allows for maximal respiratory excursion and lung expansion. Adequate lung expansion facilitates more even distribution of ventilation; it enhances ventilation/ perfusion matching
Nursing Diagnosis #4			
Airway clearance, ineffective, related to: 1. Compromised cough reflex 2. Immobility with decreased mobilization of secretions	Patient will: 1. Verbalize ease of breathing: – Breath sounds audible throughout anterior and posterior chest – Reduced to absent adventitious sounds 2. Maintain arterial gases: – pH 7.35–7.45 – PaO_2 > 60 mm Hg – $PaCO_2$ 35–45 mm Hg	• Monitor quality, quantity color, odor consistency of sputum – Obtain sputum for culture as indicated – Assess secretions for state of hydration – Monitor body temperature, sputum production, and white blood count profile – Obtain baseline cultures: Sputum, urine, blood, wounds, IV sites when changed • Initiate chest physiotherapy—bronchial hygiene (as appropriate) – Encourage coughing and deep breathing: use incentive spirometry if appropriate – Turn and position every 2 hours ♦ Position so as to minimize risk of aspiration, especially in lethargic or semi-comatose patient – Provide necessary pharyngeal and tracheal suctioning if patient is unable to handle pulmonary secretions • Consider endotracheal intubation and mechanical ventilation in the following settings: – Hypoxemia: PaO_2 < 60 mm Hg on FIO_2 > 40 percent – Cerebral edema, as a complication of fulminant hepatic failure – High risk of aspiration (e.g. patient unable to handle secretions; absent or compromised gag reflex) • Administer prescribed oxygen therapy – Humidify inspired oxygen	– Maintaining hydration keeps secretions thin and easily mobilized – Early detection of an infectious or inflammatory process affords prompt intervention to minimize the effect of the insult on pulmonary and other organ functions • These activities help to loosen and dislodge secretions and facilitate movement towards trachea from where they are accessible to removal via cough and/or suctioning – Turning and deep breathing assist to mobilize secretions, enhance ventilation and prevent areas of atelectasis – Tissue hypoxia predisposes to lactic acidosis – Carbon dioxide retention ($PaCO_2$ > 45 mm Hg) may precipitate cerebral vasodilation and aggravate existing cerebral edema • Assists in relieving hypoxemia – Humidification liquefies secretions • Adequate hydration moistens, loosens, and liquefies secretions

Contd...

Contd...

Problem	Objective	Nursing interventions	Rationales
		• Maintain hydrated state – Monitor intake and output; weigh daily	
Nursing Diagnosis #5			
Potential for infection: pneumonia, related to: 1. Prolonged immobility 2. Compromised cough reflex 3. Compromised immune response	Patient will: 1. Remain without signs/ symptoms of pulmonary infection: – Body temperature 98.6°F – WBC at baseline – Lungs resonant to percussion – Vesicular breath sounds over peripheral lung fields 2. Demonstrate effective cough	• Monitor patient's environment for potential sources of infection – Visitors, staff, other patients • Administer prescribed antibiotic therapy: – Obtain necessary cultures prior to initiation of antibiotic therapy	• Depression of immune response associated with liver disease places patient at increased risk of infection
Nursing Diagnosis #6			
Acid-base balance, alteration in: Metabolic alkalemia, related to: 1. Hypokalemia 2. Diuretic therapy 3. Nausea/vomiting or continuous nasogastric decompression (suctioning) 4. Secondary hyper-aldosteronism 5. Poor nutrition	Patient will: 1. Maintain serum electrolyte levels: – Sodium > 135 < 148 mEq/ liter – Potassium 3.5–5.5 mEq/ liter – Chloride 100–106 mEq/ liter 2. Maintain serum pH 7.35–7.45 (arterial blood gas) 3. Maintain serum ammonia within acceptable physiological range: 80–110 µg/100 mL.	• Monitor laboratory data: – Serum electrolytes. ◆ Sodium, potassium, chloride – Arterial blood gas—pH – Serum ammonia levels – Blood urea nitrogen • Administer prescribed potassium replacement therapy • Administer spironolactone therapy • Titrate dietary protein intake	• Patients with cirrhosis have depleted stores of potassium related to nausea, vomiting, poor nutrition, diuretic usage, and secondary hyperaldosteronism. Hypokalemia contributes to metabolic alkalemia – Alkalemia shifts the ammonia-ammonium ion dissociation equilibrium in favor of ammonia: $NH_3 + H^+ - NH_4^+$ ↑ pH – Ammonia easily crosses blood-brain barrier; high ammonia levels in the setting of liver disease are associated with hepatic encephalopathy – It is necessary to titrate patient's protein intake so as to keep serum ammonia and BUN at acceptable levels – In hepatic failure the liver is unable to convert ammonia, a by-product of protein metabolism, to urea for elimination • Use of furosemide and thiazide diuretics should be accompanied by potassium therapy • This drug is a potassium-sparing diuretic • Excess dietary protein is an excellent substrate for the generation of NH_3.
Nursing Diagnosis #7			
Thought process, alteration in, related to: 1. Hepatic encephalopathy associated with high serum ammonia levels caused by the inability of the liver to convert ammonia to urea	Patient will: 1. Maintain baseline mental status: – Level of consciousness: arousable; oriented to person, place and time. – Mentation: memory intact; able to concentrate; performs simple calculations; demonstrates abstract reasoning	• Assess for signs and symptoms of hepatic encephalopathy – Mental status: Level of consciousness; arousable; comatose – Mentation: Memory lapses, shortened attention span; confusion; ability to perform simple calculations; abstract reasoning	• Signs and symptoms of hepatic encephalopathy are categorized into stages; familiarity with the stages of hepatic coma assists in bedside assessment, and in evaluation of response to therapy • Establishing a baseline and ongoing monitoring is essential to determine the clinical course and the patient's response to therapy

Contd...

Contd...

Problem	Objective	Nursing interventions	Rationales
	– Usual personality – Appropriate behavior 2. Maintain baseline neurological function: – Able to write name and draw simple figures/ numbers – Speech intact, without slurring – Absence of asterixis; deep tendon reflexes brisk – Without seizure activity 3. Maintain serum ammonia levels within acceptable range	– Behavior: Appropriate or inappropriate. ◆ Agitation, combativeness; incoherent; drowsiness, lethargy – Personality changes – Neurological status: Status of speech—evidence of slurring; asterixis; tremors; deep coma—unarousable, unresponsive to painful stimuli; pupillary responses, oculocephalic reflexes, decorticate/decerebrate posturing: Hyperactive deep tendon reflexes, bilateral Babinski sign – Electroencephalogram (EEG) • Monitor serum ammonia levels • Implement anti-ammonia regimen: – Initiate and/or assist with measures to prevent or control bleeding – Initiate gastric decompression with iced gastric lavage (as prescribed) – Assist with insertion of Sengstaken-Blakemore tube – Assist with selective angiography with continuous vasopressin (pitressin) infusion (as prescribed) – Assist with sclerotherapy – Initiate prescribed therapy to reduce gastric acidity: ◆ Combination of parenteral ranitidine or cimetidine (histamine, antagonists) and antacid therapy via nasogastric tube – Serial monitoring of gastric pH – Cautiously administer blood replacement therapy: Packed RBCs should be administered in conjunction with massive blood replacement with stored whole blood ◆ Monitor hematology profile, prothrombin time, clotting factors – Implement nursing measures to prevent/control bleeding • Initiate lactulose (cephalic) therapy. – Initial dosage: 30–45 mL/hourly (orally or via nasogastric tube) until first bowel movement – Maintenance dose: 30–45 mL 3–4 times daily. Overdose can cause diarrhea – Monitor serial serum glucose	– Family and friends may assist in establishing baseline data – There is a characteristic but not pathogenic slowing of EEG. These changes may precede clinical deterioration, but are not usually present early in the course • Increase in circulating serum ammonia levels predisposes to hepatic encephalopathy as ammonia is toxic to cerebral tissues. However, hepatic encephalopathy can occur in the absence of elevated ammonia levels, and mechanisms of toxicity remain undefined – Possible toxic effects of ammonia on cerebral tissues include: Alteration in cerebral energy metabolism; disruption of resting membrane potentials; and altered neurotransmission – Blood in the gastrointestinal tract is metabolized by intestinal bacteria with the production of ammonia. In liver disease, with intrahepatic and portal hypertension, ammonia absorbed from gut bypasses liver and enters the systemic circulation. Ammonia easily traverses the blood-brain barrier – Evacuates blood and allows assessment of the extent of bleeding – Inserted to control esophageal and variceal bleeding – This therapy may be prescribed for patients with uncontrollable bleeding who are poor surgical risks – Gastric acidity plays a key role in the pathogenesis of upper gastrointestinal bleeding – Ideally gastric pH should be maintained at > 4.5 – Stored whole blood is deficient in some clotting factors and can predispose to dilutional coagulopathy – See *Nursing Diagnosis #10*, Injury, potential for: bleeding diathesis (below) • Lactulose, in conjunction with the action of intestinal bacteria, creates an acidic milieu within the colon that favors conversion of ammonia to ammonium, which is speedily evacuated by the cathartic action of lactulose ↓pH $NH_3 + H^+ - NH_4^+$

Contd...

Contd...

Problem	Objective	Nursing interventions	Rationales
		• Initiate antibiotic therapy: – Aminoglycosides used: Neomycin (most commonly) and Kanamycin – Avoid use with other aminoglycosides, or other nephrotoxic or ototoxic drugs – Contraindicated in the setting or renal insufficiency and hepatorenal failure – Monitor renal function: BUN, creatinine, urine output (hourly); intake and output • Avoid constipation – Lactulose is a good cathartic – Administer stool softeners as prescribed • Restrict or eliminate protein dietary intake – Administer high carbohydrate diet (~1400 calories); or intravenous infusion of 10% glucose – Provide potassium supplements ◆ Cautious use of diuretic therapy – Maintain fluid and electrolyte balance • Prevent hepatotoxicity: – Avoid use of sedatives, hypnotics and other drugs normally metabolized by the liver, or containing ammonia – Review patient's entire drug regimen: ◆ Dosage may need to be revised in presence of hepatocellular failure ◆ Potential for adverse drug reactions and toxicity should be monitored ◆ Assess effect of newly prescribed drugs on neurological function • Implement nursing interventions in caring for the patient with hepatic encephalopathy: – Monitor neurologic function hourly (if in coma) – Monitor serial laboratory studies: Serum ammonia; BUN, creatinine, electrolytes • Implement specific measures: – Maintain safe environment: Remove hazardous objects from bedside; use padded rails; keep rails in up position; provide close supervision; initiate seizure precautions	– Lactulose contains galactose and glucose; it may elevate glucose levels; use with caution with diabetes; contraindicated in patients requiring a low-galactose diet • Antibiotics reduce intestinal bacterial flora, thereby reducing bacterial ammonia production. Note: Lactulose and neomycin should not be administered concurrently. Lactulose requires bacteria for its action; neomycin destroys intestinal bacteria flora – The nephrotoxic and ototoxic effects may be potentiated – Approximately 1–3 percent of drug is absorbed; in the presence of renal failure, the drug can accumulate, predisposing to nephrotoxicity and ototoxicity • Intestinal bacteria have a longer exposure and greater bulk to convert to ammonia • To reduce ammonia production and consequent increase in serum ammonia levels – Glucose provides the primary source of energy for cerebral tissues; prevents gluconeogenesis (protein catabolism) – Hypokalemia predisposes to metabolic alkalemia which favors the conversion of ammonium to ammonia $NH_3 + H^+ - NH_4^+$ $\downarrow K^+$ – Refer to *Nursing Diagnosis #1* above • Compromised hepatocellular function may cause accumulation of drug; some drugs may be toxic to the liver. Such drugs, or combination of drugs, may precipitate or aggravate encephalopathy or mask signs of developing coma – Specific parameters are listed under nursing interventions at the beginning of *Nursing Diagnosis #7*, in the section on assessing for signs and symptoms of hepatic encephalopathy, neurological status – A confused, agitated, or unreliable patient is at greater risk of injury (e.g. falling out of bed) – This affords continuity of care, and facilitates very close monitoring of the patient's response to therapy

Contd...

Contd...

Problem	Objective	Nursing interventions	Rationales
		– Reorient patient to person, place, time – Explain procedures clearly – Obtain feedback from family and friends regarding mental status, personality and behavior – Plan for same staff members to care for the patient (if possible) – Provide comfort measures: Oral hygiene, back care, gentle passive range of motion exercises – Plan for undisturbed rest periods – Use calm, reassuring approach: Anticipate patient/family needs for support; be accessible; offer directions and explanations; allow patient/family to verbalize fears and concerns – Involve patient/family in decision-making process regarding care when possible	– Relaxes tired muscles; a caring touch may help to relieve anxiety and apprehension – All efforts should be directed towards keeping the patient relaxed and quiet to prevent bleeding or rebleeding – Enables patient/family to assume some control and responsibility for their well-being
Nursing Diagnosis #8			
Nutrition, alteration in, less than body requirements, related to: 1. Malnutrition associated with insufficient dietary protein intake 2. Avitaminosis associated with impaired absorption of fat-soluble vitamins 3. Vitamin B_{12} deficiency associated with liver disease 4. Anorexia, nausea/vomiting, weakness and fatigue associated with elevated serum ammonia levels	Patient will: 1. Maintain stable body weight within 5 percent of baseline 2. Maintain the following laboratory parameters within acceptable physiologic range: – Total serum protein; serum albumin – Serum ammonia levels – Serum cholesterol; fasting serum glucose – Hematology profile – Vitamin B_{12}, folate – Transferrin levels 3. Verbalize an increase in strength and improved appetite	• Collaborate with nutritionist to perform comprehensive nutritional assessment. – Assess the following parameters: Total serum protein; serum albumin; fasting serum glucose; serum cholesterol; hematology profile, vitamin B_{12}, folate; transferrin levels; body weight (dry), height; skin-fold measurements – Assess for anorexia, nausea, vomiting, diarrhea, dyspepsia • Implement nutritional plan: – Acute phase (hepatic encephalopathy) dietary requirements include: ◆ Restriction of protein, sodium and fluid - Protein 20–60 g/day - Sodium 250–500 g/day - Fluids ~ 1000 mL/day – High carbohydrate intake – Vitamin supplementation: ◆ Fat-soluble vitamins: A, D, E, and K ◆ Folate B_9 (parenterally) ◆ Vitamin B_{12} (parenterally) ◆ Thiamine (vitamin B_1) (parenterally) – Minerals and trace elements supplementation – Methods of dietary intake: – Oral: Provide mouth care; pleasant environment; assist to comfortable position	• Assists in determining basic caloric requirements sufficient to meet the energy needs of the body, while limiting protein to that amount which the liver can effectively metabolize • Goal of diet therapy is to reduce dietary protein so that a minimum of protein will remain in the gastrointestinal tract for conversion to ammonia – The degree of protein restriction will depend upon patient's level of consciousness and clinical status – Except in advanced coma, it is seldom necessary to reduce daily protein intake to less than 20 g. Further reduction of protein offers little benefit because of consequent catabolism of endogenous proteins – Sodium restriction is necessary because of sodium and water retention associated with secondary hyperaldosteronism – Degree of fluid restriction depends on degree of third-spacing (ascites and anasarca) – Glucose prevents hypoglycemia and breakdown of energy reserves – Hepatocellular dysfunction alters bilirubin metabolism and bile synthesis; inadequate bile secretion impairs absorption of fat, and fat-soluble vitamins – Hepatic stores depleted in liver disease

Contd...

Contd...

Problem	Objective	Nursing interventions	Rationales
		◆ Minimize nausea/vomiting; eliminate noxious stimuli ◆ Offer frequent smaller meals; avoid fatigue; plan rest period prior to meal-time ◆ Consider patient's preference for food choices ◆ Encourage visit by family at meal times if patient desires so – Enteral feedings ◆ Assess gag reflex prior to feeding ◆ Confirm tube placement in stomach prior to feeding ◆ Assess for signs of gastrointestinal intolerance of feeding (e.g. nausea, vomiting, abdominal distention, hyperactive bowel sounds) – Total parenteral nutrition ◆ Provides for nutritional needs including: Hypertonic glucose ◆ Amino acids; high concentration branched chain amino acids; low concentration aromatic amino acids ◆ Electrolytes; minerals, vitamins, trace elements; lipid therapy (when indicated) – Document: Type of feeding, amount; how tolerated by patient; adverse effects, if any – Monitor: Weight, intake and output; laboratory data (see "Assess the following parameters" under nursing interventions at the beginning of *Nursing Diagnosis #8)*	– Used to correct anorexia, and neuritis associated with alcoholism (Wernicke-Korsakoff's syndrome) – Large meals may precipitate nausea – Enteral approach to feeding may be necessary for patients unable to ingest food normally; bleeding varices necessitate enteral feedings – To avoid pulmonary aspiration – If adequate intake of nutrients is impossible via oral or enteral feedings, total parenteral nutrition may be indicated – Amino acid imbalance may predispose to synthesis of false neurotransmitters that may be responsible for neurologic changes seen in hepatic encephalopathy. Aromatic amino acids are precursors to false neurotransmitters (e.g. octopamine)
Nursing Diagnosis #9			
Tissue perfusion, alteration in, hepatorenal syndrome, related to: 1. Hypovolemia associated with ascites (third-spacing) 2. Renal arteriolar vasoconstriction	Patient will: 1. Maintain adequate hemodynamics: – Systemic arterial blood pressure within 10 mm Hg of baseline 2. Maintain adequate renal function: – Urine output > 30 mL/hour – Urine specific gravity: 1.010–1.025 – BUN, serum creatinine, urinary sodium within acceptable range	• Assess for signs and symptoms of hepatorenal syndrome: – Specific features: Oliguria (urine output < 30 mL/h); azotemia; specific gravity > 1.015; low urinary sodium; increasing ascites; peripheral edema; weight gain; rising BUN, serum creatinine; hyperphosphatemia; hyperkalemia	• Hepatorenal syndrome describes development of progressive functional renal failure in the setting of advanced liver disease

Contd...

Contd...

Problem	Objective	Nursing interventions	Rationales
	3. Maintain body weight within 5 percent of baseline	• Implement prescribed measures to re-establish normovolemia: – Specific measures: Restrict fluids and sodium; administer prescribed diuretic therapy and potassium replacement therapy; administer inotropic agent/ vasopressor (e.g. low-dose dopamine); administer protein supplementation – Assist with abdominal paracentesis (if indicated) • Monitor patient's response to therapy • Prepare for dialysis if indicated	
Nursing Diagnosis #10			
Injury, potential for, bleeding diathesis, related to: 1. Massive blood transfusion for treatment of bleeding varices (dilutional coagulopathy) 2. Decreased synthesis of clotting factors related to impaired hepatocellular function, and impaired vitamin K absorption 3. Thrombocytopenia associated with splenomegaly (portal hypertension)	Patient will: 1. Maintain stable vital signs: – Systemic arterial pressure within 10 mmHg of baseline – Heart rate (resting) < 100 beats/min – Respiratory < 25–30/min 2. Maintain baseline mental status: – Level of consciousness; mentation intact 3. Maintain stable hematologic profile: – Hematocrit; Hemoglobin, platelets 4. Maintain stable coagulation profile 5. Remain without signs of bleeding: – No petechiae, ecchymosis – No hematuria; no occult blood in stool, vomitus, gastric drainage – No unusual joint pain/ swelling 6. Maintain stable abdominal girth	• Assess for signs/symptoms of bleeding: – Vital signs: Blood pressure (orthostatic), heart rate, peripheral pulses; respiratory rate – Physical signs: petechiae, ecchymosis; gingival bleeding; epistaxis; hematemesis, melena, hematochezia expanding abdominal girth; unusual joint swelling; hematuria; oozing from wounds, venipuncture and invasive sites – Neurological signs: Headache, dizziness, confusion, lethargy; deep tendon reflexes – Hematologic profile: Hematocrit, hemoglobin, platelet count – Coagulation profile: Prothrombin time; activated partial thromboplastin time; platelet count; bleeding time • Implement measures to prevent or minimize bleeding: – Specific measures: Use smallest gauge needle possible for venipuncture and subcutaneous injection – Avoid intramuscular injections; apply firm, prolonged pressure to venipuncture and injection sites – Avoid activities with the potential to cause bleeding: Avoid use of straight razor, use electric razor; avoid gingival bleeding associated with vigorous tooth brushing; pad bedrails for confused, restless or agitated patients; provide close supervision	• Increased risk of bleeding in hepatic failure is associated with reduced hepatocellular synthesis of clotting factors (including vitamin K dependent factors II, VII, IX, X) and reduced inactivation of activated clotting factors. – In the setting of profuse bleeding with massive blood transfusions, bleeding may be associated with dilutional coagulation. – Minimizes tissue trauma – There is a greater tendency to bleed with intramuscular injections – Necessary for synthesis of clotting factors A, D, E, K – Necessary for absorption of vitamin K – Stored whole blood lacks some of the clotting factors; citrate, used as a blood preservative (anticoagulant) may not be metabolized by hepatocytes – To maintain hemodynamic parameters and hematologic profile within acceptable limits – Maximizes arterial blood oxygenation – To determine presence of upper gastrointestinal bleeding, and the extent of bleeding – For specific nursing care considerations of patients with a Sengstaken-Blakemore tube – Profuse hemorrhage can be a frightening experience for patient and family

Contd...

Contd...

Problem	Objective	Nursing interventions	Rationales
		• Administer prescribed therapy to improve hemostasis – Vitamin K (parenterally) – Bile salts – Administration of fresh, frozen plasma or packed red blood cells • Consider the following if bleeding occurs: – Apply firm, prolonged pressure to bleeding site if possible – Administer fluids and blood products as prescribed – Administer prescribed oxygen therapy – Maintain gastric decompression – Initiate iced gastric lavage (as prescribed) – Prepare to assist with insertion of Sengstaken-Blakemore tube; if tube is in place, assess its position, balloon inflation, and catheter patency – Provide reassurance and support to patient and family – Monitor vital signs, neurological status, hourly urine output	
Nursing Diagnosis #11			
Skin integrity, impairment of, potential, related to: 1. Increased skin fragility associated with generalized edema (anasarca and ascites) 2. Malnutrition 3. Immobility associated with stupor and edema 4. Pruritus associated with hyperbilirubinemia	Patient will: 1. Maintain skin intact, no breaks, lesions, irritation or infection; good skin turgor	• Assess skin, especially reddened areas over bony prominences where skin is thin – Assess generalized edema, especially dependent areas (e.g. sacrum, extremities) • Initiate measures to prevent skin breakdown – Mobilize extracellular fluid accumulation, especially in dependent areas ◆ Turn patient at least every 2 hours; administer backrubs – Provide supportive measures and pressure-relief device: ◆ Utilize alternating pressure or egg carton mattress; provide sheepskin; change linen frequently – Keep skin well lubricated. If pruritus is present, apply calamine lotion with 1% phenol, or use cholestyramine or cool baking soda bath (as prescribed) – Assist with range of motion exercises. Handle limbs gently Apply support stockings – Assist with personal hygiene ◆ Provide oral hygiene frequently, especially when a nasogastric tube or Sengstaken-Blakemore tube is in place	– Promotes circulation and relieves muscle tension; helps to prevent decubiti: ◆ If reddened areas at pressure points do not blanch within less than 30 minutes, avoid using the position except for shorter periods at less frequent intervals. – Exercise promotes circulation and prevents venostasis, a contributing factor to the development of a coagulopathy (e.g. disseminated intravascular coagulation, DIC) – To minimize trauma from scratching. Patient may need gloves or mittens at night while asleep

Contd...

Contd...

Problem	Objective	Nursing interventions	Rationales
		◆ Provide perineal care, keeping buttacks clean and dry restrict use of soap Keep nails trimmed and clean ◆ Instruct patient to apply firm pressure over pruritic areas rather than scratching	
Nursing Diagnosis #12			
Self-concept, disturbance in, related to: 1. Altered physical appearance associated with jaundice, ascites, alopecia, gynecomastia, and other changes associated with chronic liver disease	Patient will: 1. Express feelings about self 2. Participate in decision-making process regarding care 3. Initiate self-care activities	• Establish a trusting rapport and working relationship: – Spend time to get to know patient – Explain all procedures simply and clearly – Allow patient participation in procedures whenever possible. – Encourage patient to participate in decision-making process whenever appropriate ◆ Assess readiness for decision-making – Encourage patient to talk about the illness and how it impacts on self, family and others ◆ Explain that jaundice, edema, and ascites are usually temporary – Help patient to identify strengths, weaknesses, and coping capabilities ◆ Utilize time during direct patient care to involve patient in discussion of needs, priorities and how to cope ◆ Encourage patient to ventilate feelings; provide listening car and "sounding board" – Call attention to areas of improvement in the patient's condition – Offer immediate praise and feedback for patient's accomplishments no matter how small	• It is important to encourage/assist the patient to verbalize concerns, to acknowledge and cope with the illness, and to achieve independence in self-care – Emphasis is focused on assisting the patient/family to get in touch with their feelings, to identify them, and to begin to deal with them – It is important to assist the patient to acknowledge his/her perceptions, and how they differ from those of others, or from the actual situation – Praise helps to build self-confidence
Nursing Diagnosis #13			
Grieving, dysfunctional, related to: 1. End-stage liver disease 2. Altered appearance and lifestyle associated with chronic liver disease	Patient will: 1. Verbalize feelings about liver disease and how it impacts on patient/family 2. Demonstrate progress in dealing with stages of grieving at own pace 3. Participate in self-care activities and in decision-making process regarding care	• Assess patient's perception of liver disease and how it impacts on patient/family lifestyle • Identify the stage of grief being experienced by patient/family – Assist patient/family to acknowledge that grieving is a process and experiencing the stages of grief is most appropriate and necessary	• Stages of grief include denial, anger, bargaining, depression, and acceptance. – The nurse must be aware that not every stage is experienced or expressed by each individual; and some individuals will remain in one stage longer than others. In chronic disease, the grief may recur

Contd...

Contd...

Problem	Objective	Nursing interventions	Rationales
		♦ Assist patient to acknowledge bodily changes and consequent changes in lifestyle so that the process of grieving can begin • Assist patient/family to develop a plan for discharge and follow-up care – Be honest and forthright in discussing disease and its ramifications both with patient and family – Help patient and family to identify resources ♦ Assist with referrals to counseling services and support groups	

Procedure 11.1: Assisting with Abdominal Paracentesis

Equipment

- Sterile paracentesis tray and gloves
- Local anesthetic
- Drape or cotton blankets
- Collection bottle (vacuum bottle)
- Skin preparation tray with antiseptic
- Specimen bottles and laboratory forms.

Steps of procedure

Nursing action	Rationale
Preparatory phase	
1. Explain procedure to the patient	1. This may reduce the patient's fear and anxiety
2. Record the patient's vital signs	2. Provides baseline values for later comparison
3. Have the patient void before treatment is begun. See that consent form has been signed	3. This will lessen the danger of accidentally piercing the bladder with the needle or trocar
4. Keep the patient in Fowler's position with back, arms, and feet supported (sitting on the side of the bed is a frequently used position)	4. The patient is more comfortable and a steady position can be maintained
5. Drape the patient with sheet exposing abdomen	5. Minimizes exposure of patient and keeps patient warm
Performance phase	
1. Assist in preparing skin with antiseptic solution	1. This is considered a minor surgical procedure, requiring aseptic precautions
2. Open sterile tray and package of sterile gloves; provide anesthetic solution	2. Preliminary indications of shock must be watched for keeping emergency drugs available
3. Have collection bottle and tubing available	3. Drainage is usually limited to 1–2 L to relieve acute symptoms and minimize risk of hypovolemia and shock
4. Assess pulse and respiratory status frequently during procedure; watch for pallor, cyanosis, or syncope (faintness)	4. Elasticized adhesive patch is effective, serving as waterproof adhering dressing
5. Physician administers local anesthesia and introduces needle or trocar	
6. Needle or trocar is connected to tubing and vacuum bottle or syringe, fluid is slowly drained from peritoneal cavity	

Contd...

Contd...

Nursing action	Rationale
7. Apply dressing when needle is withdrawn	
Follow-up phase	
1. Assist the patient to a comfortable position after treatment	
2. Record amount and characteristics of fluid removed, number of specimens sent to laboratory, the patient's condition during treatment	
3. Check blood pressure and vital signs every half an hour for 2 hours, every hour for 4 hours, and every 4 hours for 24 hours	3. Close observation will detect poor circulatory adjustment and possible development of shock
4. Usually, a dressing is sufficient, however, if the trocar wound appears large, the physician may close the incision with sutures	
5. Watch for leakage or scrotal edema after paracentesis	5. If seen, report at once

Procedure 11.2: Using balloon tamponade to control esophageal bleeding (Sengstaken-Blakemore tube method, minnesota tube method)

Equipment

- Esophageal balloon (Sengstaken-Blakemore or Minnesota)
- Basin with cracked ice
- Clamps for tubing
- Water soluble lubricant
- Syringe (50 mL with catheter tip)
- Towel and emesis basin
- Glass of water and straw
- Adhesive tape
- Device to apply traction (e.g. football helmet)
- Large scissors (for emergency deflation)
- Manometer (to measure balloon pressure).

Steps of procedure

1. Provide support and reassure the patient that this procedure will help to control bleeding.
2. Explain procedure to the patient and explain how breathing through the mouth and swallowing can help in passing the tube (Fig. 11.8).
3. Elevate head of bed slightly unless the patient is in shock.

Esophageal varices and their treatment by a compressing balloon tube (Sengstaken-Blakemore). (A) Dilated veins of the lower esophagus. (B) The tube is in place in the stomach and the lower esophagus but is not inflated. (C) Inflation of the tube causing compression of the veins. It may be necessary to pass an additional tube through the other nostril to aspirate.

Note: The Minnesota four-lumen esophagogastric tamponade tube has an additional outlet for aspiration of the esophagus.

Nursing action	Rationale
Preparatory phase	
1. Check balloons by trial inflation to detect leaks	1. This is best done under water because it is easier to see escaping air bubbles
2. Chill the tube, then lubricate it before the physician passes it via mouth or nose (preferable)	2. Chilling makes the tube more firm and lubrication lessens friction
3. Provide the patient with a few sips of water	3. This will help pass the tube more easily
4. After the tube has entered the stomach, verify its placement by irrigating the gastric tube with air while auscultating over the stomach	4. It is imperative to be certain that the tube is in the stomach so that the gastric tube is not treated in the esophagus
5. After obtaining an X-ray film of the lower chest and upper abdomen to verify placement in the stomach, inflate gastric balloon (200–250 mL) with air and gently pull tube back to seat balloon against gastroesophageal junction	5. This is to exert force against the cardia

Contd...

Contd...

Nursing action	Rationale
6. Clamp gastric balloon, mark tube location at nares	6. This prevents air leakage and tube migration. The mark on the tube allows for easy visualization of movement of the tube
7. Apply gentle traction to the balloon tube and secure it with a foam rubber cube at the nares or tape it to the faceguard of a football helmet	7. This prevents the tube from migrating with peristalsis and assists in exerting proper pressure
8. Attach Y connector to esophageal balloon opening attach syringe to one arm of the Y connector and manometer to the other. Inflate esophageal balloon to 25–35 mm Hg. Clamp esophageal balloon	8. Maintains enough pressure to tamponade bleeding while preventing esophageal necrosis
9. Apply suction to gastric aspiration opening irrigate at least hourly	9. Suctioning and irrigating the tube can remove old blood from the stomach and prevent hepatic encephalopathy allows, monitoring of bleeding status
10. (If using Sengstaken-Blakemore tube) Insert a nasogastric tube, positioning it above the esophageal balloon and attach to suction (If using a Minnesota tube) Attach fourth port, esophageal suction port, to suction	10. To Suction saliva accumulated above the esophageal balloon, which may be aspirated, and to check for bleeding above the esophageal balloon
11. Label each port	11. To prevent accidental deflation or irrigation
12. Tape scissors to head of bed	12. Airway occlusion may occur if the esophageal balloon is pulled into the hypopharynx. If this occurs, the esophageal balloon tube must be cut and removed immediately
Nursing responsibilities	
1. Maintain constant vigilance while balloons are inflated in the patient	
2. Keep balloon pressures at required level to control bleeding (clamp help to maintain pressure)	
3. Observe and record vital signs, monitor color and amount of nasogastric lavage fluid (subtracting lavage input) for evidence of bleeding	
4. Be alert for chest pain—may indicate injury or rupture of esophagus	
5. Irrigate suction tube as prescribed, observe and record nature and color of aspirated material	
6. Keep head of bed elevated to avoid gastric regurgitation and to diminish nausea and a sensation of gagging	
7. Maintain nutritional and electrolyte levels parenterally	
8. Maintain nasogastric suction or suction to esophageal suction port to aspirate any collected saliva	
9. Note nature of breathing; if counterweight pulls the tube into oropharynx, the patient may be asphyxiated	
Nursing focus Keep a pair of scissors leaped to the head of the bed in the event of acute respiratory distress, use the scissors to cut across tubing (to deflate both balloons) and remove tubing	
Note: This procedure should be reserved for patients who are known, without a doubt, to be bleeding from esophageal varices and in whom all forms of conservative therapy have failed	

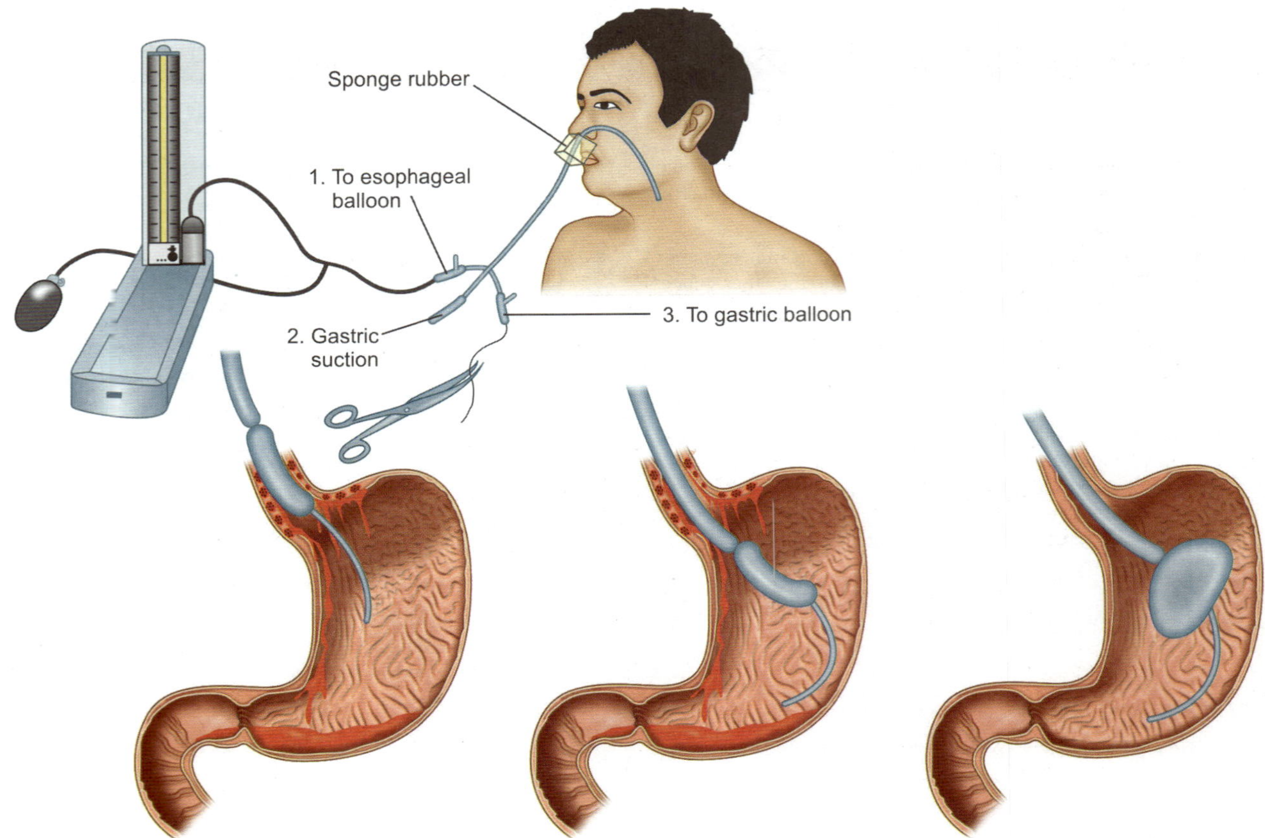

FIGS 11.8A TO C: Esophageal varices and their treatment by a compressing balloon tube (Sengstaken-Blakemore). (A) Dilated veins of the lower esophagus; (B) The tube is in place in the stomach and the lower esophagus but is not inflated; (C) Inflation of the tube causing compression of the veins. It may be necessary to pass an additional tube through the other nostril to aspirate. *Note*: The Minnesota four-lumen esophagogastric tamponade tube has an additional outlet for aspiration of the esophagus

ASSISTING WITH PERCUTANEOUS LIVER BIOPSY

Equipment

- Liver biopsy tray (contains needles, scalpel, specimen tubes, etc.)
- Sterile gloves
- Antiseptic solution
- Local anesthetic
- Sterile dressing
- Sphygmomanometer to monitor BP.

Implementation

Nursing interventions	Rationale
Preprocedure	
1. Ascertain that results of coagulation test (prothrombin time, partial thromboplastin time and platelet count) are available and that compatible donor blood is available	1. Many patient with liver disease have clotting defects and are at risk for bleeding

Contd...

Contd...

Nursing interventions	Rationale
2. Check for signed consent; confirm that informed consent has been provided	2. Ensures that the patient consents to this invasive procedure
3. Measure and record the patient pulse, respirations, and blood pressure immediately before biopsy	3. Prebiopsy values provide a basis on which to compare the patient's vital signs and evaluate status after the procedure
4. Describe to the patient in advance steps of the procedure; sensations expected after-effects anticipated; restrictions for activity and monitoring procedures to follow	4. Explanations allay fears and ensure cooperation
During procedure	
1. Support the patient during the procedure	1. Encouragement and support of the nurse enhance comfort and promote a sense of security
2. Expose the right side of the patient's upper abdomen (right hypochondriac)	2. The skin at the site of penetration will be cleansed and a local anesthetic will be infiltrated
3. Instruct the patient to inhale and exhale deeply several times, finally to exhale and to hold breath at the end of expiration. The physician promptly introduces the biopsy needle by way of the transthoracic (intercostal) or transabdominal (subcostal) route penetrates the liver, aspirates, and withdraws	3. Holding the breath immobilizes the chest wall and the diaphragm; penetration of the diaphragm thereby is avoided, and the risk of lacerating the liver is minimized
4. Instruct the patient to resume breathing	4. The patient often continuous holding his or her breath because of anxiety
FIG. 11.9: Site of percutaneous liver biopsy	
Post-procedure	
1. Immediately after the biopsy, assist the patient to turn on to the right side; place a pillow under the costal margin, and caution the patient to remain in this position, recumbent and immobile for several hours. Instruct the patient to avoid coughing or straining	1. In this position, the liver capsule at the site of penetration is compressed against the chest wall, and escape of blood or bile through the preformation is prevented
2. Measure and record the patient's pulse, respiratory rate, and blood pressure at 10 to 15 minutes intervals for the first hour then every 30 minutes for the next 1 to 2 hours or until the patient's condition stabilizes	2. Changes in vital signs may indicate bleeding severe hemorrhage or bile peritonitis, the most frequent complications of liver biopsy
3. If the patient is discharged after the procedure instruct the patient to avoid heavy lifting and strenuous activity for 1 week	3. Activity restriction reduces the risk of bleeding at the biopsy puncture site

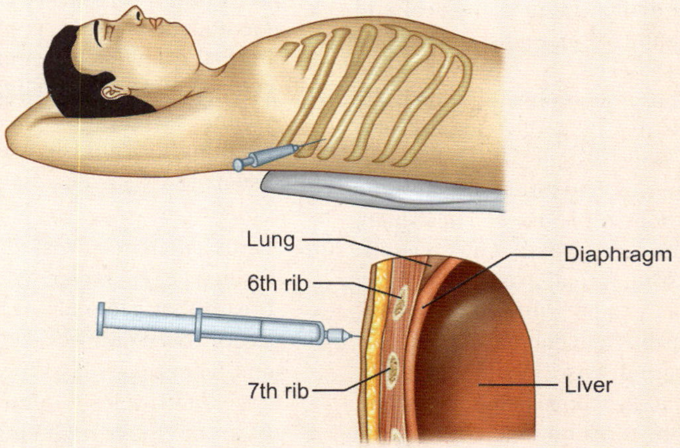

CHAPTER

12

Cardiovascular Nursing

CARDIOVASCULAR ASSESSMENT

Systematic cardiovascular assessment provides the nurse with baseline data useful in identifying the physiological and psychosocial needs of the patient and for planning appropriate nursing interventions to meet these needs.

A careful history and physical examination should help the nurse in differentiating symptoms that reflect a cardiovascular problem from problems of other body systems. Many illnesses affect the cardiovascular system directly or indirectly. The patient should be questioned about a history of chest pain, shortness of breath, alcoholism, or excessive drinking, anemia, rheumatic fever, streptococcal sore throat, congenital heart disease, stroke, syncope, hypertension, thrombophlebitis, intermittent claudications, varicosities and edema.

The classic symptoms of heart disease include dyspnea, chest pain, or discomfort, edema, syncope, palpitations and excessive fatigue. Cardiovascular function, which may be adequate at rest may be insufficient during exercise or exertion. Therefore, careful attention is directed to the effect of activity on the patient's symptoms.

i. Dyspnea

Dyspnea is an abnormally uncomfortable awareness of breathing, in which patient complains of shortness of breath. It is a subjective experience associated with anxiety and variety of disease processes.

- Exertional dyspnea: Dyspnea on exertion is a common symptom of cardiac dysfunctions. In the early stages of heart failure, dyspnea usually is provoked only by effort and is relieved promptly by rest. It is important to identify the amount of exertion necessary to produce dyspnea, because the lower the cardiac reserve (heart's ability to adjust and adapt to increased demands), lesser the effort is required to precipitate dyspnea.
- Orthopnea refers to dyspnea in the recumbent position. It is usually a symptom of more advanced heart failure that is exertional dyspnea. Patients insist that they require two or more pillows to sleep restfully. When the person assumes the recumbent position, gravitational forces redistribute blood from the lowest extremities and splanchnic bed increase venous return. The augmentation of intrathoracic blood volume elevates pulmonary venous and capillary pressures, resulting in a transient pulmonary congestion, orthopnea, usually is relieved in less than 5 minutes after the patient sits upright.
- Paroxysmal nocturnal dyspnea is also known as cardiac asthma, is characterized by severe attacks of shortness of breath that generally occur 2 to 5 hours after the onset of sleep. This condition is commonly associated with sweating and wheezing. Classically, the person awakens from sleep, arises and quickly opens with the perception of needing fresh air. These frightening attacks are precipitated by the same physiological mechanism that causes orthopnea. The diseased heart is unable to compensate for this increase in blood volume by pumping extra fluid into the circulatory system and pulmonary congestion results. Paroxysmal nocturnal dyspnea is relieved by sitting on the side of the bed or getting out of the bed. For relief of dyspnea, 20 minutes or more is needed. The cues to dyspnea are air hunger, especially after exertion, pillows or upright chair necessary for sleep.

ii. Chest Pain

Although pain or discomfort in the chest is one of the cardinal symptoms of cardiac disorder, chest pain can be precipitated by various conditions. For example, chest pain may be caused by anxiety, ischemia, heart disease, acute dissection of the aorta, acute pericardia, pulmonary disorders, (pleurisy and pulmonary embolism) esophageal spasm, or reflux, and peptic ulcer disease. The cues for chest pain-related heart disorders are indigestion, burning, numbness, tightness or pressure in mid-chest, epigastric or substernal pain, radiating to shoulder, neck, and arms.

iii. Syncope

Syncope is dyspnea as a generalized muscle weakness with an inability to stand upright, accompanied by loss of consciousness. The most common cause of syncope is decreased perfusion to the brain. Any condition that results in a sudden reduction of cardiac output (CO) and therefore reduced cerebral blood flow could potentially cause a syncopal episode. In patients with cardiovascular disorders, conditions such as orthostatic hypotension, hypovolemia, or variety of dysrhythmias may precipitate syncope.

iv. Palpitation

Palpitation is a common subjective phenomenon defined as an unpleasant awareness of the irregular heartbeat. It may be precipitated by a change in cardiac rate or rhythm, i.e. by an increase in myocardial contractility. Patient may experience sensation of heart in throat or skipped beat, racing heart, and dizziness. Patients may describe that heart beat as "pounding", "racing" or skipping. Palpitation that occurs either during or after strenuous activity are considered physiological. Palpitations that occur during mild exertion may suggest the presence of heart failure, anemia or thyrotoxicosis. Other non-cardiac factors may precipitate palpitation include, nervousness, heavy meals, lack of sleep and a large intake of Caffeine-containing beverage, alcohol or tobacco.

v. Fatigue

Fatigue refers to no energy, needs more rest than usual, normal activities result in tiring. Fatigue and lassitude have many causes, but it has direct consequence of heart failure. The exact physiological mechanism is not known. But probably, it is a consequence of an inadequate cardiac output. Such fatigue can occur during effort or at rest and generally worsens as the day progresses. Fatigue that occurs after mild exertion may indicate a low cardiac reserve if the heart is unable to meet even small increase in metabolic demand.

vi. Dizzy

Dizzy, light headedness: Dizzy with change of position; woozy, unstable and weak.

vii. Edema (Fluid Retention)

The cues for edema are: Weight gain, bloated feeling, swelling, tightening of clothing, shoes no longer fitting comfortably, marks or identification left from constricting garments.

viii. Tenderness in Calf of Legs

The cues for tenderness of calf of legs are—inability to bear weight, swelling of the involved extremity; inflamed warm skin over vein; distended, discolored, tortuous veins in calves of legs, ache in lower extremities after standing for short periods.

PHYSICAL EXAMINATION

Physical examination of the CVS includes the standard assessment techniques of inspection, palpation, percussion and auscultations.

1. Inspection

Inspection of the patient includes skin color, neck vein distention, respiration, pulsations and clubbing and capillary refill. The inspection of the skin color, hair distribution and venous blood flow provide information about arterial blood flow. A person's normal color depends on race, ethnic background and lifestyle and is an indication of adequate cardiac output (CO) and circulation. Pallor may indicate anemia, hypoxia, or peripheral vasoconstriction. Cyanosis (cerebral), a bluish discoloration of the skin is most easily observed by examining the earlobes, the oral mucosa at the base of the tongue, legs and the nail-beds. Peripheral cyanosis results from low CO and generally is accompanied by decreased skin temperature and mottling. In contrast to central cyanosis, no cyanosis of the tongue is present. Central cyanosis is caused by low arsenal oxygen saturation, (e.g. congenital heart defects). Skin color and the extremities also be assessed for noting any erythema or pigmentation changes as well as the shiny, or dry, scaly skin, which may indicate vascular disorders.

A general estimate of venous pressure can be obtained by observation of the neck veins. Normally, when a person is supine, the neck veins are distended. However, when the head of the bed is elevated to a 45 degree angle, the neck veins are collapsed. If jugular distention is present, assess the jugular venous pressure by measuring from the highest point of visible distention to the sternal angle. Measurements above 3 cm area considered elevated. The jugular veins reflect venous tone, blood volume and right atrial pressure. Therefore, distended neck veins suggest increased venous pressure, which may be caused by right-sided heart failure, circulatory volume load, superior vena caval obstructions or tricuspid valve regurgitation.

The rate and character of the patients' respirations are important to assess. Normally an adult breathes comfortably at a rate of 12 to 20 times per minute. Particular attention is paid to the case of difficulty in breathing and patient's general demeanor.

Inspection of the anterior chest is best accomplished with the patient lying supines, either flat or with the head slightly elevated. Observe the pericardium for the apical impulse, which is a pulsation of the chest wall caused by the forward thrusting of the left ventricle during systole. When visible, the apical impulse occupies the fourth or fifth intercostal space at or inside midclavicular line. The apical impulse was formerly known as the point of maximal impulse. The apical impulse is not always visible, but it is palpable in about half of adults.

The nails are assessed for clubbing and capillary refill. The exact cause is unknown. However, clubbing of the finger in the fistulas with right to left shunting. Capillary filling or blanching (whitening) is an indicator of peripheral circulation to the fingers and toes and can be tested in all nail-beds. The examiner presses a thumbnail against the edge of a patient's finger nails or toe nail and quickly releases it and notes the blanching response and observes for the returning color within 3 seconds.

2. Palpations

Palpations of the pulses in the neck and extremities also provides information on arterial blood flow. One method of evaluating arterial flow of the vascular system is to palpate the extremities simultaneously to determine skin temperature. A second method is to palpate the peripheral pulses, which are evaluated bilaterally on the basis of their absence or presence, rate, rhythm, amplitude, quality and equality. Each pulse, except the carotids should be palpated on the left and right sides simultaneously to evaluate the contralateral symmetry.

A scale may be used to document pulse volume or amplitude by rating on a scale of 0 to +4 as follows:

0	=	Absent
+	=	Palpable, but diminished
++	=	Normal or average
+++	=	Full and risk
++++	=	Full and bounding, often visible.

Several abnormalities may be detected during palpation of pulses:

- A hypokinetic (weak) pulse signifies a narrowed pulse pressure, that is decreased differences between systolic and diastolic pressure. It is usually produced by a low CO and is associated with often detected in such conditions as severe LVF, hypovolemia, or mitral and aortic valve stenosis.
- A hyperkinetic (bounding) pulse represents a widened pulse pressure. It is usually associated with increased left ventricular stroke volume and a decreased peripheral vascular resistance. This is found in hyperkinetic circulatory state caused by exercise, fever, anemia or hyperthyroidism.
- Pulsus alternans is a condition in which the heart beats regularly, but the pulses vary in amplitude. It is caused by an alternating left ventricular contractile force and usually indicates severe depression of myocardial infarction, pulsus alternans can be detected by palpation and accurately by auscultation.
- Pulsus paradoxus signifies a reduction in the amplitude of the arterial pulse during inspiration. Variation in pulse strength can be palpated and also readily detected by sphygmomanometry. Pulsus paradoxus is a result of decreased left ventricular stroke volume and the transmission of negative intrathoracic pressure to the aorta. It may occur in conditions such as cardiac tamponade and constrictive pericarditis and also COPD.

Edema is defined as an accumulation of fluid in the interstitial spaces. It may be localized to one particular body part, organ or tissue or that may be generalized distribution. An important indicator for cardiovascular function in the presence or absence of peripheral edema, especially in the feet, ankles, legs and the sacrum. This is caused by gravity flow or by interruption of the venous return to the heart as a result of constricting clothing or pressure on the veins of the lower extremities. Edema often disappears on elevation of the body part. In contrast, pitting edema does not disappear with elevation of the extremity of body part, and it may indicate fluid overload or pathological condition (e.g. congestive heart failure). Pitting edema is present if an indication is left in the skin after a thumb or finger has been used to apply gentle pressure.

3. Percussion

The borders of the right and left sides of the heart can be estimated by percussion. The use of percussion for detecting cardiac enlargement generally has been replaced by chest X-ray which is much more accurate. The nurse stands to the right of the recumbent patient and percusses along the curve of the rib in the fourth and the fifth intercostal spaces (ICS), starting at the midaxillary line. The percussion note over the heart is dull in comparison with the resonance over the lung and is recorded in relation to midclavicular line. Cardiac dullness is the characteristics of cardiac hypertrophy.

4. Auscultation

The movement of the cardiac valves creates some turbulence in the blood flow. The vibration of the blood causes normal heart sounds. These sounds can be heard through a stethoscope placed on the chest wall. The first heart sound (S_1) which is associated with the closure of the tricuspid and mitral valve (AV) has a soft "lubb" sound. S_1 is longer and lower pitched than the second heart sound (S_2). The second heart sound (S_2) which is associated with the closure of the aortic and pulmonic (semilunar) valve, has a sharp "dubb" sound. The first and second heart sounds together are referred to as "lub-dub". S1 corresponds to the beat of the carotid pulse. As stated earlier S_2 is caused mainly by the closure of the semilunar valves. S_2 is usually loudest at the base of the heart and is described as shorter, higher pitched and "snappier" than S_1. S_1 signals the beginning of systole, S_2 signals the beginning of diastole. The nurse should listen to the auscultatory areas in sequence with both the diaphragm and bell of the stethoscope.

The first and second heart sounds are heard best with diaphragm of the stethoscope because they are high-pitched.

Extra heart sounds (S_3 or S_4) if present, are heard best with the bell of the stethoscope because they are low-pitched. The nurse listens at the apical area with diaphragm of the stethoscope while simultaneously palpating the radial pulse. If fewer radial than apical pulse are counted, a pulse deficit is present. A patient with a pulse deficit should have the apical and radial pulse taken often to monitor this abnormality. A judgment about the rhythm (regular or irregular) is also made when listening at the apex.

Normally no sounds are heard between S_1 and S_2 during the periods of systole and diastole. Sounds that are heard during these periods probably represent abnormalities and should be described. An exception to this is normal splitting of S_2, which is best heard at the pulmonic area during inspiration. Splitting of this heart sound can be abnormal if S_1 is heard during expiration or if it is constant (fixed) during the respiratory cycle.

If an abnormal sound is heard, it should be documented. This description should include the timing (during systole or diastole), location (the site on the chest where it is heard the loudest), pitch (heard best with the diaphragm or bell of the stethoscope), position (heard best when the patient is recumbent, sitting, leaning forward, or in the left lateral decubitus position). Characteristic (harsh, musical, soft, short, long) and any abnormal findings (irregular cardiac rhythms or palpable chest wall heaves) associated with sound.

The abnormal sound, occurring during diastole and systole are classified as either murmurs or extra sound (S_3 and S_4). Murmurs are sounds produced by turbulent blood flow through the heart or the walls of large arteries. Most murmurs are the result of cardiac abnormalities, but some occur in normal cardiac structures. Murmurs are graded on six point scale of loudness and recorded as Roman numeral ratio, the numerator is intensity of the murmur and denominator is always VI which indicates the six point scale sued.

DIAGNOSTIC STUDIES OF CVS

A number of diagnostic procedures add to the information obtained from the history and physical examination of the cardiovascular system. These procedures are usually classified as noninvasive or invasive. If only needle insertion for withdrawal of blood or injection of dye is used these studies are usually considered noninvasive. Catheter insertion for angiography is considered as invasive procedure. Certain responsibilities of the nurse remains the same regardless of whether patient is to undergo invasive or noninvasive procedure. First, the nurse must see that the procedure is scheduled and that any necessary preliminaries (e.g. special diets or changes in medication) are completed. Appropriate safety measures, such as the use of bedside rails after administration of preprocedure medication or identification of patient allergies should be instituted. Comfort measures such as oral care before procedure are important. The nurse must also check to see to it that in obtaining consent the procedure should be explained skillfully, relieving the anxiety of patients and significant ones of the patient. These are the most common diagnostic measures to be carried out by nurses to assess the cardiovascular system and main nursing responsibility required for the same is presented as follows:

1. Chest X-ray

A radiograph of the chest may be taken to determine overall size and configuration of the heart in which patient is placed in two upright positions to examine the lung fields and size of the heart. The two common positions are anterior/posterior (AP) and left lateral. Normal heart size and contour for the individual age, sex and size are noted. Most abnormalities of heart size and calcification of the heart muscle, valves and great vessels can be detected with a standard posterior anterior and lateral view of the chest.

The nursing responsibilities include inquiring about the frequency of recent X-rays and possibility of pregnancy (of female). Provide lead shielding to the areas not being viewed, remove any jewellery or metal objects that may obstruct the view of the heart and lungs.

2. Cardiac Fluoroscopy

It facilitates the observation of the heart from varying view while the heart is in motion. Fluoroscopy can be used to detect ventricular aneurysms, monitor prosthetic valve movement, or assess the position of cardiac calcification during the cardiac cycle. Because of the radiational risk associated with fluoroscopy, most of them are not used in this procedure. Nursing responsibility is the same as for chest-X-rays.

3. Electrocardiogram (ECG)

The ECG is a graphic representation of the electrical forces produced within the heart. The ECG is an essential tool for cardiac evaluation, but it must be combined with other data sources for an accurate diagnosis. An ECG may be normal even in the presence of heart disease. Conversely, abnormal variance may be seen in the ECG of a normal heart. The ECG may be used for a variety of diagnostic purposes as given below:

- Tachycardia, bradycardia, dysrhythmia
- Sudden onset of dyspnea
- Pain occurring in the upper portion of the trunk and in the extremities
- Syncopical episodes
- Shock state or coma
- Preoperative status
- Postoperative hypertension
- Hypertension, murmurs, or cardiomegaly
- Artificial pacemaker function.

In taking ECG, electrodes are placed on the chest (Box 12.1, Figs 12.1 and 12.2) and extremities, allowing the ECG machine to record cardiac electrical activity from different views by

Box 12.1 Applying electrodes

The monitoring system requires an adequate electrical signal to analyze the patient's cardiac rhythm. When applying electrodes, the following recommendations should be followed to optimize skin adherence and conduction of the heart's electrical current.

- Debride the skin surface of dead cells with soap and water and dry well (or as recommended by the manufacturer)
- Clip (do not shave) hair from around the electrode site if needed
- If the patient is diaphoretic (sweaty), apply a small amount of benzoin to the skin, avoiding the area under the center of the electrode
- Connect the electrodes to the lead wires prior to placing them on the chest (connecting lead wires when electrodes are in place may be uncomfortable for some patients)
- Peel the backing off the electrode and check to make sure the center is moist with electrode gel
- Locate the appropriate lead placement and apply the electrode to the skin, securing it in place with light pressure
- Change the electrodes every 24 to 48 hours (or as recommended by the manufacturer), examine the skin for irritation, and apply the electrodes to different locations
- If the patient is sensitive to the electrodes, use hypoallergenic electrodes

using standard 12-lead ECG machine. ECG can detect rhythm of heart, site of pacemaker, conduction abnormalities, position of the heart, size of atria and ventricles and presence of injury.

The nurse has to inform the patient step-by-step procedure and assures of its safe, painless nature and comfortability.

Instruct the patient to avoid moving to decrease muscle motion artifact.

4. Ambulatory ECG Monitoring

i. Holter Monitoring

It is used to obtain a continuous graphic tracing of patient's ECG during daily activities, in which recording of ECG rhythm for 24–48 hours and then correlating rhythm changes with symptoms recorded in diary. Normal patient activity is encouraged to stimulate conditions that produce symptoms. Electrodes are placed on chest and a recorder is used to store information until it is recalled, printed and analyzed for any rhythm disturbance. It can be performed on an inpatient or outpatient basis (Fig. 12.2).

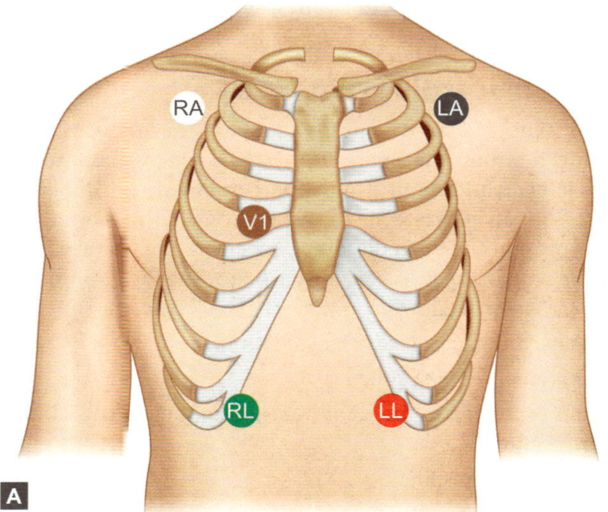

RA–Righ arm (white)
LA–Left arm (black)
RL–Right leg (green)
LL–Left leg (red)
V1–Chest or precordium (brown)

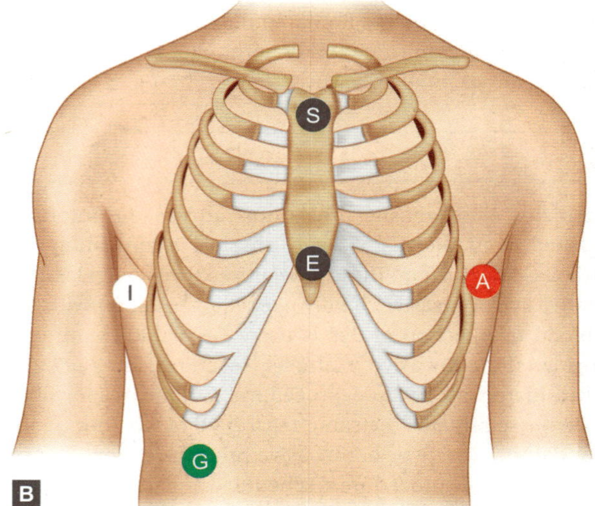

E–Lower sternum at 5th intercostal space ICS (black)
A–5th ICS at left midclavicular line (red)
S–Upper sternum (black)
I–5th ICS at right midclavicular line (white)
G–Ground any area (green)

FIGS 12.1A AND B: Electrode placement used in continuous electrocardiographic monitoring for (A) three-lead system, placement on RA, LA and LL; four-lead system, placement on RA, LA, RL, and LL; five-lead system, placement on RA, LA, RL, LL, and V1; and (B) EASI-derived 12-lead ECG system

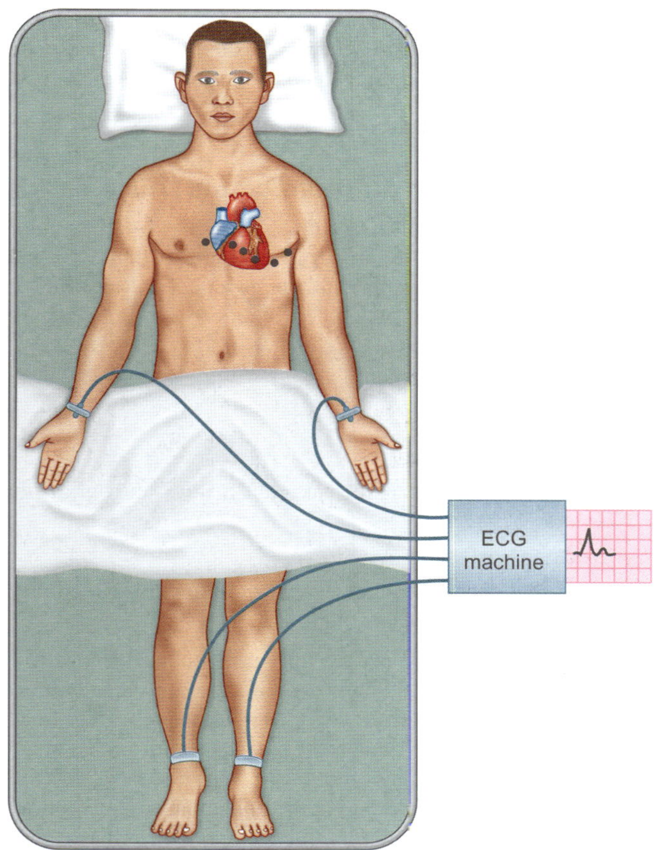

FIG. 12.2: Transmission of heart's impulse to a graphic display by ECG machine. The electrodes that are capable of conducting electrical activity from the heart to the ECG machine are placed at strategic positions on the extremities and chest precordium

In this procedure, nurse has to prepare skin and apply electrodes as leads. Explain importance of keeping an accurate diary of activities and symptoms. Tell the patient that no bath or shower can be taken during monitoring. Skin irritations may develop from electrodes. Take care of it.

ii. Stress Testing (ECG during Exercise)

It may be performed for a variety of reasons and often combined with ECG to obtain additional information about heart functions. Indications for performing a stress test are:

- Evaluation of the patient with symptoms suggestive of coronary artery disease
- Determination of the patient's physical work capacity and aerobic capacity
- Determination of the patient's functional capacity after a myocardial infarction and as an aid in planning and exercise rehabilitation program
- Evaluation of the exercise-induced dysrhythmias
- Evaluation of the symptom-free person older than 40 years of age who is at risk for coronary artery disease
- Evaluation of pharmacological intervention for dysrhythmias, angina or ischemia.

Various protocols are used to evaluate the effect of exercise tolerance on myocardial function. A common protocol uses 3 minutes, stages at speeds and elevation of the treadmill belt. Continued monitoring of vital signs and ECG rhythms or ischemic changes are important in the diagnosis of left ventricular function and coronary artery disease. An exercise bike may be used if the patient is unable to walk on the treadmill. Stress test is designed to progressively increasing myocardial oxygen demand. Some patients may experience untoward effects (ventricular tachycardia, change in systolic BP, chest pain, etc. So test may be terminated at any point of test.

Adequate preparation for stress testing is important. Although procedure is not painful. It can be fatiguing. Patient may become anxious because they will be exercising at a level that may produce symptoms such as dyspnea, palpitations and chest pain. The nurse may review the purposes and method of stress testing and encourage the patient to do the following:

- Avoid coffee, tea and alcohol on the day of test
- Avoid smoking and taking nitroglycerine during the 2 hours immediately before the test
- Wear comfortable, loose-fitting clothes (women should be advised to wear a brassiere for support)
- Wear sturdy, comfortable walking shoes
- Consult the physician about taking any medication before the test.

And the nurse should:

- Instruct the patient about procedure and application of lead placements
- Monitor vital signs and obtain 12-lead ECG before exercise, during each stage of exercise, and after exercise until all vital signs and ECG changes have returned to normal
- Monitor patient's symptoms throughout procedure.

iii. Transtelephonic Event Recorders

Allow more freedom than regular Holter Monitor. It records rhythm disturbances that are not frequent enough to be recorded in a 24-hour period. Some units have electrodes that are attached to the chest and have a loop of memory that captures the onset and end of an event. Other types are placed directly on patient's wrist, chest, or fingers have no loop memory, but records the patient's ECG in real time. Recordings are transmitted over the phone to a receiving unit, and the recordings are printed out for review. Tracings can then be erased and the unit can be reused.

The nurse has to instruct the patient in the use of equipment for recording and transmitting transient events. Teach the patient about skin preparation for lead placement or steady skin contact for units not requiring electrodes. This will ensure the reception of optimal ECG tracings for analysis.

5. Sonic Studies

i. Echocardiogram (M-mode-two-dimensional)

Echocardiography uses ultrasound to assess cardiac structure and mobility noninvasively. It is useful in the diagnosis of a variety of cardiac conditions as follows:

- Abnormal pericardial fluid
- Vulvar disorders including prosthetic valves
- Ventricular aneurysms
- Cardiac chamber size
- Stroke volume and cardiac outputs
- Some myocardial abnormalities, such as idiopathic hypertrophic subaortic stenosis (IHSS)
- Wall motion abnormalities.

In this, a small transducer is placed on the chest of the patient at the level of third or fourth intercostal space near the left lower sternal border. The transducer transmits high frequency sound waves then receives these waves back from the patient as they are reflected from different structures. The ultrasonic beam that is reflected back from the patient's heart produces "echoes" that are viewed as lines and spaces on an oscilloscope. These lines and spaces represent bone, cardiac chambers and valves, the septum and the muscle. A copy of echocardiogram is recorded on paper.

Here, the nursing responsibility is to place the patient in supine position on left side facing equipment. Instruct patient and family about procedure and sensations (pressure and mechanical movement from head of transducer). No contraindication to procedure exists.

ii. Stress Echocardiogram

It is the combination of exercise, treadmill test and echocardiogram. Resting images of the heart are taken with ultrasound and then the patient exercises. Postexercise images are taken immediately after exercise (which 1 minute of stopping exercises). Differences in left ventricular wall motion and thickening before and after exercise is evaluated. Here, the nurse has to instruct and prepare patient for exercise treadmill. Make the patient aware that ultrasound is not harmful and the importance of speed in returning to examination table for imaging after exercise. Contraindication includes any patient unable to reach peak exercise. Take precautions.

iii. Dobutamine Echocardiogram

It is used as a substitute for the exercise stress test in individual unable to walk on a treadmill. Dobutamine (a positive inotropic agent) is infused IV and dosage is increased in 5 minutes intervals while echocardiogram is performed to detect wall motion abnormalities in each stage. In this, nursing responsibilities include—starting IV infusion, administering dobutamine, monitoring vital signs before, during and after test until baseline is achieved. Monitor patient for signs and symptoms of distress during procedure.

iv. Transesophageal Echocardiogram (TEE)

Cardiac Doppler, color-flow imaging.

TEE allows high resolution ultrasonic imaging of the cardiac structure and great vessels via the esophagus. The clinical indications for TEE are:

- Mitral valve prosthetic dysfunction
- Mitral valve regurgitation
- Infective endocarditis
- Congenital heart disease
- Intracardiac thrombi (especially left atrium and left atrial appendage)
- Cardiac tumor
- Intraoperative assessment: Left ventricle functions, adequacy of valve repair and replacement.

This technique uses a probe with an ultrasound transducer at the tip is swallowed. This procedure can be performed at the bedside without contrast dye. It is performed under local anesthetic and sedation. Usually the physician controls the angle of and depth of esophagus with transducer. As it passes down the esophagus, it sends back clear images of heart size, wall motion, valvular abnormalities, and possible source of thrombi without interference from lungs or chest ribs. A contrast medium may be injected IV for evaluating direction of blood flow if an atrial or ventricular septal defect is suspected. Doppler ultrasound and color flow imaging can also be used concurrently.

In this procedure, nursing responsibility will include the following:

- Instruct patient to be NPO for at least 6 hours before test
- A tranquilizer will be given and throat locally anesthetized. So, if done as an outpatient, a designated driver is needed
- Monitor vital signs and oxygen saturation levels and perform suctioning continually during procedure
- Explain to patient the proper procedure for easy passage of transducer
- Assist patient to relax
- Patient may not eat or drink until gag reflex returns.

6. Scintigraphic Studies

Nuclear cardiological study involves IV injection of radioactive isotopes. Radioactive uptake is counted over the heart by scintillation camera. It supplies information about myocardial contractility, myocardial perfusion and acute cell injury. The common nuclear cardiological at:

i. Thallium 201 Scan

Thallium 201 is injected IV and used to evaluate blood flow in different parts of heart. Cold spots correlate with area of infarction. For stress testing, IV thallium is given 1 minute before the patient reaches maximum heart rate on bicycle or treadmill. Patient is then required to continue exercise for 1 minute to circulate the radioactive isotopes. Actual scanning is done within 5–10 minutes after exercise. A second testing scan performed 2–4 hours later and compared to postexercise scan. Instruct patient to eat only a light meal between scans.

ii. Dipyridamole Thallium Scan

As with thallium exercise test, dipyridamole (Persantine) is also injected. This drug acts as a powerful vasodilator and will increase blood flow to well-perfused coronary arteries. Scanning procedure is same as with thallium scan. In this, instruct the patient to hold all caffeine products for 12 hours before procedure.

iii. Technetium ^{99}m Sestamibi Scan

In this technetium ^{99}m sestamibi is injected IV and taken up area of MI, producing hot spots. Maximum results are produced when performed 1–6 days after suspected MI waiting period after injection is 1½–2 hours.

iv. Blood Pool Imaging

In this technetium ^{99}m per technetate injected intravenously. Single injection allows sequential evaluation of heart for several hours. Study is indicated for patient with recent MI or congestive heart failure, especially if not recovering well. It can be used to measure effectiveness of various cardiac medications and can be done at the patient's bedside.

v. Positron Emission Tomography (PET)

PET is a radionuclide-based imaging technique that uses short-lived radionuclides as tracers to report both perfusion and metabolic events. Here, uses two radionuclides. Nitrogen-13-ammonia is injected intravenously and scanned to evaluate myocardial perfusion. A second radioactive isotope. Fluoro-18-1deoxyglucose is then injected and scanned to show myocardial metabolic function. In the normal heart, both scans will match, but in an ischemic or damaged heart, they will differ. The patient may or may not be stressed. A baseline resting scan is usually obtained for comparison. Here the nurse has to:

- Instruct the procedure
- Explain that patient will be scanned by a machine and will need to stay still for a period of time
- Patient's glucose level must be between 6 and 140 mg/dL for accurate metabolic activity
- If exercise included as part of testing, patient will need to be NPO and refrain from tobacco and caffeine for 24 hours prior to test.

In general, in all studies related to IV injection of isotopes, nurse has the responsibility to:

- Explain procedure to patient
- Establish IV line for injection of isotopes
- Explain that isotopes used in small diagnostic and will lose most of its radioactivity in a few hours
- Patient's glucose level must be between 60 and 140 mg/dL, for accurate metabolic activity
- If exercise is included as a part of testing, patient will need to be NPO and refrain from tobacco and caffeine for 24 hours prior to test.

In general, in all studies related to IV injection of isotopes nurse has the responsibility to:

- Explain procedure to patient
- Establish IV line for injection of isotopes
- Explain that isotopes are used in small diagnostic quantities and will lose most of their radioactivity in a few hours
- Inform the patient that he or she will be lying down on back with arm extended overhead for period of time
- Repeated scans are performed within a few minutes to hours after the injection.

7. Magnetic Resonance Imaging (MRI)

It is a noninvasive imaging technique which obtains information about cardiac tissue integrity, aneurysms, ejection factions, cardiac output, and patency of proximal coronary arteries. It does not involve ionizing radiations and is an extremely safe procedure. It provides images in multiple planes with uniformly good resolution. It has limited use in critical care patients, because of access and equipment problem. It cannot be used in persons with any implanted metallic devices. In this procedure, the nurses will explain the procedure to patient, inform the patient that the small diameter of the cylinder along with loud nose of the procedure may cease panic or anxiety. Antianxiety medications and music may be recommended.

8. Blood Studies

The important blood studies are followed in diagnosis are:

- Creatine kinase (CK)
- CK-MB fraction
- AST (SGOT)
- (Myoglobin)
- Troponin
- Lactic dehydrogenase (LOH)
- Serum lipids—cholesterol, triglycerides, lipoproteins.
- Drug levels—digoxin, quinidine, inderal (propranolol).

9. Cardiac Catheterization

It is an extremely valuable diagnosis tool used for obtaining detailed information about the structures and functions of the cardiac chambers, valves and coronary arteries. This diagnostic study involves insertion of catheter in the heart. Information can be obtained about O_2 saturation and pressure readings within chambers. Dye can be injected to assist in examining structure and motion of heart. Procedure is done by insertion of catheter into a vein for right-sided heart or an artery for left-sided heart.

The nursing responsibilities before procedure are:

- Obtain written permission
- Withhold food and fluids for 6–18 hours before procedure
- Give sedation if ordered
- Inform patient about use of local anesthesia, insertion of catheter and feeling of warmth and fluttering sensation of heart as catheter is passed
- Note that patient may be instructed to cough or take a deep breathing when catheter is inserted
- See that the patient is monitored by ECG throughout procedure.

After the procedure, nurse has the responsibility to:

- Assess circulation to extremity used for catheter insertion
- Check peripheral pulses, color and sensation of extremity, every 15 minutes for 1 hour and then with decreasing frequency
- Observe injection site for swelling and bleeding
- Place sand bag over arterial site if indicated
- Monitor vital signs
- Assess for abnormal heart rate, arrhythmias and signs of pulmonary emboli (respiratory difficulty)
- In addition to above diagnostic tests, the following should also be performed
- Coronary angiography
- Intracoronary ultrasound
- Hemodynamic monitoring
- Electrophysiology study
- Peripheral arteriography and venography
- Digital subtraction angiography and general routine blood tests, urinalysis, etc.

HYPERTENSION

Hypertension is defined as a consistent constant elevation of the systolic or diastolic pressure above 140/90 mm Hg. It is sustained deviation of blood pressure (BP). In adults, hypertension exists when systolic blood pressure (SBP) is equal to or greater than 140 mm Hg or diastolic blood pressure (DBP) is equal to or greater than 90 mm Hg for extended periods of time. The diagnosis of hypertension requires that elevated readings be present on at least three occasions during several weeks.

High blood pressure (HBP) means that the heart is working harder than normal, putting both the heart and the blood vessels under strain. HBP may contribute to myocardial infarctions, cerebrovascular accidents, (CVA), renal failure and atherosclerosis. Hypertension causes no symptoms to motivate a person to seek treatment. When symptoms do occur, they signify either secondary causes of hypertension or effects of sustained elevation of BP on target organs (coronary artery disease, left ventricular hypertrophy, cerebrovascular disease, peripheral vascular disease, or renal insufficiency).

Etiology

Hypertension is defined as a systolic blood pressure above 140 mm Hg or a diastolic pressure above 90 mm Hg, based on two or more measurements. Hypertension can be classified as follows:

- Normal: Systolic < 120 mm Hg; diastolic < 80 mm Hg
- Prehypertension: Systolic 120 to 139 mm Hg; diastolic 80 to 89 mm Hg
- Stage 1: Systolic 140 to 159 mm Hg; diastolic 90 to 99 mm Hg
- Stage 2: Systolic ≥ 160 mm Hg; diastolic ≥ 100 mm Hg.

Hypertension is a major risk factor for atherosclerotic cardiovascular disease, heart failure, stroke and kidney failure. Hypertension carries the risk for premature morbidity or mortality, which increase as systolic and diastolic pressure rise. Prolonged blood pressure elevation damages blood vessels in target organs heart, kidneys, brain and eyes).

The etiology of hypertension can be classified as either primary (essential) or secondary.

Primary (essential) hypertension accounts for more than 90 percent of all cases and has no known cause, although it is theorized that genetic factor, hormonal changes, and alterations in sympathetic tone all may play a role in its development.

In the adult population with hypertension, between 90% and 95 percent have essential (primary) hypertension, which has no identifiable medical cause; it appears to be a multifactorial, polygenic condition. For high blood pressure to occur, an increase in peripheral resistance and/or cardiac output must occur secondary to increased sympathetic stimulation, increased renal sodium reabsorption, increased renin-angiotensin-aldosterone system activity, decreased vasodilation of the arterioles, or resistance to insulin action.

On occasion, hypertension appears abruptly and severely and takes a "malignant" course that cause rapid deterioration, signalling an emergency state known as hypertensive crisis or hypertensive urgency.

Hypertensive crisis or hypertensive emergency, exists when an elevated blood pressure level must be lowered immediately (not necessarily to less than 140/90 mm Hg) to halt or prevent target organ damage. Hypertensive urgency exists when blood pressure must be lowered within a few hours. Hypertensive crisis requires prompt treatment in an intensive care setting because of the risk for serious organ damage. The medication regimen (e.g. nitroprusside, nicardipine hydrochloride) requires extremely close hemodynamic monitoring. Vital signs should be checked as often as every 5 minutes.

Although the exact cause is unknown, several contributing factors including increased SNS activity, overproduction of sodium retaining hormones and vasoconstrictors, increased sodium intake, more than ideal body weight, diabetes mellitus and excessive alcohol intake. The identified risk factors in primary hypertension are as follows:

- *Age:* Blood pressure rises progressively with advancing or increasing age—elevated BP is present in approximately 50 percent of people over 65 years of age, and with onset usually between the ages of 30 and 50 years
- *Sex:* Hypertension is more prevalent in men and young adulthood and early middle age. After the age of 55, hypertension is more prevalent in women
- *Race:* Incidence of HBP is twice as great in African-Americans as in Caucasians
- *Family history:* Level of BP is strongly familial. Risk of hypertension increases for those with a close relatives having hypertension
- *Obesity:* Weight gain is associated with increased frequency of hypertension. The risk is greater with central abdominal obesity
- *Smoking:* Smoking greatly increases the risk of cardiovascular disease. Nicotine constricts blood vessels. Hypertensives who smoke are at even greater risk
- *High salt diet:* Sodium causes water retention, increasing blood volume. Excessive dietary sodium intake can contribute to hypertension in some patients, and decreases the efficacy of certain antihypertensive medication
- *Elevated serum lipids:* Elevated levels of cholesterol and triglycerides are primary risk factors in atherosclerosis. Narrowing of arteries increases blood pressure. Hyperlipidemia is more common in hypertensives
- *Alcohol:* Alcohol increases plasma catecholamines. Excessive alcohol intake is strongly associated with hypertension. Hypertensives should limit their daily intake of ethanol to 1 Oz
- *Sedentary lifestyles:* Regular physical activity can help control weight and reduce cardiovascular risk. Physical activity may decrease
- *Diabetes mellitus:* Hypertension is more common in diabetics. Where hypertension and diabetes coexist, complications are more severe
- *Socioeconomic status:* Hypertension is more prevalent in low socioeconomic groups and among the less educated
- *Emotional stress:* Stress stimulates sympathetic nerve systems. People exposed to repeated stress may develop hypertension more frequently than others. People who become hypertensive may respond differently to stress from those who do not become hypertensive. Emotional disturbances, obesity, excessive alcohol intake and overstimulation with coffee, tobacco and stimulatory drugs play a role. Hypertension is strongly familial. Hypertension affects more women than men, but African-American men are less able to tolerate the disease.

Secondary Hypertension

Secondary hypertension is characterized by elevations in blood pressure with a specific cause, such as arterial disease, renal disease, certain medications, tumors and pregnancy. Hypertension can also be acute, a sign of an underlying condition that causes a change in peripheral resistance or cardiac output.

It develops as a consequence of a particular underlying disease or condition. It is elevated BP with a specific cause that often can be identified and corrected. This type of hypertension accounts for less than 5 percent of hypertension in adults but more than 80 percent of hypertension in children. If a person below the age of 20 or over the age of 50 suddenly develops hypertension, if it is severe, a secondary cause should be suspected. Clinical findings suggest that secondary hypertension include unprovoked hypokalemia, abdominal bruit, variable pressure with tachycardia, sweating and tremor, or family history of renal diseases. Causes of secondary hypertension include the following:

- Coarctation or congenital narrowing of the aorta
- Renal disease such as renal artery stenosis parenchymal disease (Glomerulonephritis, renal failure) and renovascular disease
- Endocrine disorders such as pheochromocytoma (excessive secretion of catecholamines). Cushing syndrome (blood volume), hyperaldosteronism, primary aldosteronism (increase in aldosterone causing sodium and water retention and increase blood volume)
- Neurologic disorders such as brain tumor, quadriplegia and head injury
- Sleep apnea
- Medications such as sympathetic stimulants (including cocaine) monoamine oxidase inhibitors taken with tyramine containing foods, estrogen replacement therapy, oral contraceptive pills, and nonsteroidal anti-inflammatory drugs (NSAIDs)
- Pregnancy-induced hypertension: Cause is unknown, generalized vasospasm may be a contributing factor.

Pathophysiology

Blood pressure is the force exerted by the blood against the walls of the blood vessels and must be adequate to maintain tissue perfusion during activity and rest. The maintenance of normal BP and tissue perfusion requires the integration of both systemic factors and local peripheral vascular effects. Arterial BP (ABP) is primarily a function of cardiac output (CO) and systemic vascular resistance (SVR). The relationship is summarized by following equation:

$$ABP = CO \times SVR$$

Cardiac output (CO) is the total blood flow through the systemic or pulmonary circulation per minute. CO can be described as the stroke volume amount of blood pumped out of the left ventricle per beat (approximately 70 mL) multiplied by the heart rate (HR) for 1 minute. Systemic vascular resistance (SVR) is the force opposing the movement of blood within the blood vessels. Radius of the small arteries and arterioles is the principal factor determining vascular resistance. A small change in the radius of the arterioles create a major change in the SVR. If SVR is increased and CO remains constant or increases ABP will increase.

The mechanism that regulates BP can affect either CO or SVR or both. Regulation of BP is a complex process involving nervous, cardiovascular, renal and endocrine functions. BP is regulated by both short-term (seconds to hours) and long-term (days to weeks mechanisms). Short-term mechanisms including autonomic nervous system and vascular endothelium, one active within a few seconds. Long-term mechanisms include renal and hormonal process that regulates arteriolar resistance and blood volume.

The regulation of blood pressure is a complex process involving renal control of sodium and water retention and nervous system control of vascular tone. The two primary regulatory factors are blood flow and peripheral vascular resistance refers to size of the peripheral blood vessels. The more constricted the vessel, the greater the resistance to flow and the more dilated the vessel, the lesser is resistance. As peripheral vessels become more constricted, the blood pressure becomes more elevated. Dilation and constriction of the peripheral blood vessels are controlled by primarily by the SNS in stimulated, catecholamines such as epinephrine and norepinephrine are released. These chemical causes increased vasoconstriction, increased cardiac output, and increased strength of ventricular contraction. Likewise, when the renin-angiotensin system is activated, angiotensin causes vasoconstriction of the blood vessels. Long-term vasoconstriction of renal vessels causes permanent renal damage and may lead to kidney failure. Other important organs such as the brain and heart also suffer long-term damage from untreated hypertension. An overview of hypertension is given in Box 12.2.

Clinical Manifestation

- Physical examination may reveal no abnormality other than high blood pressure
- Changes in the retinas with hemorrhages (cotton-wool spots from small infarcts), exudates, narrowed arterioles and papilledema may be seen in severe hypertension
- Symptoms usually indicate vascular damage related to organ system served by involved vessels
- Coronary artery disease with angina or myocardial infarction is the most common sequelae

Box 12.2 Overview of hypertension

Signs and symptoms	Often none Increased blood pressure Headache, bloody nose, severe anxiety, or shortness of breath
Diagnosis	Prehypertension is greater than systolic or 120 mm Hg and diastolic of 80 mm Hg. Hypertension is an average blood pressure, using two or more reading on different dates, greater than a systolic of 139 mm Hg and diastolic of 89 mm Hg
Therapeutic measures	Lifestyle modification Medications
Complications	Heart failure, myocardial infarction, stroke, renal failure

- Left ventricular hypertrophy may occur; left heart failure ensues
- Pathologic changes may occur in the kidney (nocturia and increased blood urea nitrogen [BUN] and creatinine levels)
- Cerebrovascular involvement may occur (stroke or transient ischemic attack [i.e. temporary hemiplegia, sudden falls, dizziness, weakness, or alterations in vision or speech]).

Hypertension is called the "Silent Killer", because it is a disease that usually occurs without any symptoms. It is frequently asymptomatic until it becomes severe and target organ disease has occurred. A patient with severe hypertension may experience a variety of symptoms secondary to effects on blood vessels in the various organs and tissues or to the increased work load of the heart. These secondary symptoms include fatigue, reduced activity tolerance, dizziness, palpitations, angina and dyspnea. The most advanced disease may produce symptoms such as early morning headache, blurred vision, and spontaneous nose-bleed, and depression. However, these symptoms are not more frequent in people with hypertension than in the general population.

The most common complications of hypertension are target organ disease occurring in the heart (hypertensive heart disease), brain (cerebrovascular disease), peripheral vasculature (peripheral vascular disease), kidney (nephrosclerosis) and eyes (retinal damages).

Diagnostic Studies

- History and physical examination, including retinal examination; laboratory studies for organ damage, including urinalysis, blood chemistry (sodium, potassium creatinine, fasting glucose, total and high-density lipoprotein); electrocardiogram (EDG); and echocardiography to assess left ventricular hypertrophy

- Special studies: Intravenous pyelography, renal arteriography, split renal function studies, renin levels, 24 hours urine protein, creatinine clearance.

The initial diagnosis of hypertension is made on the basis of two or more elevated blood pressure readings, supine and sitting, obtained on at least two separate occasions. If the first two readings differ more than 5 mm Hg additional readings should be obtained. Postural changes in BP and pulse should be measured in older adults, people taking antihypertensive drugs and when orthostatic hypertension is suspected.

Specific diagnostic test will be ordered to rule out an underlying cause or evaluate the extent of organ damage. A comprehensive physical examination is performed, including careful evaluation of blood vessels of the retina and as typically supplemented with laboratory tests, that will evaluate the neurological, cardiovascular and renal system for evidence of target organ damage. The laboratory studies that are performed in a person with sustained hypertension, routine urinalysis, BUN and serum creatinine levels are used to screen for renal involvement.

Measurement of serum electrolytes, especially potassium levels is important to detect hyperaldosteronism. Fasting blood glucose level (diabetes) serum cholesterol and triglyceride level provide information about additional risk factors that predispose to atherosclerosis. Complete blood count, serum chemistry, ECG to know cardiac status.

Management

The goal of any treatment program is to prevent death and complications by achieving and maintaining an arterial blood pressure below 140/90 mm Hg (130/80 mm Hg for people with diabetes mellitus or proteinuria > 1 g/24 hours), whenever possible.

- Nonpharmacologic approaches include weight reduction; restriction of alcohol, sodium, tobacco; regular exercise and relaxation. A DASH (Dietary Approach to Stop Hypertension) diet high in fruit and vegetables and low in dairy products has been shown to lower elevated pressures
- Select a drug class that has the greatest effectiveness, fewest side effects, and best chance of acceptance by patient. Two classes of drugs are available as first-line therapy—diuretics and beta blockers
- Promote compliance by avoiding complicated drug schedules.

The management of hypertension does not involve any specific treatment but management is usually improved when the patient is able to make targeted lifestyle adjustment that support the drug therapy. Two important measures are abstaining from smoking and stress reduction management. Smoking has a direct vasoconstrictive effect on the blood vessels and should be given up it at all possible costs. The role of stress is less clear but the use of relaxation and stress management strategies are often helpful in blood pressure control.

Box 12.3 Lifestyle modifications for hypertension

- Stop smoking
- Limit alcohol intake
- Decrease amount of salt intake
- Obtain daily allowances of potassium and calcium
- Reduce dietary saturated fat and cholesterol
- Lose weight
- Get regular aerobic exercise such as walking for 30 minutes
- Get adequate sleep (more than 5 hours)

Lifestyle modifications should be used in all hypertensive patients either as definitive or adjunctive therapy. These modifications directed toward reducing BP and overall cardiovascular risk. Modifications include (Box 12.3):

1. Dietary changes
2. Limitation of alcohol intake
3. Regular physical activity
4. Avoidance of tobacco use (smoking and chewing).

Based on assigned risk group, lifestyle modifications are usually continued up to 1 year before drug therapy is used. Patients with hypertension are encouraged to develop a pattern of regular aerobic exercise, which may help control their hypertension and also contributes to weight loss and reduces cardiac risk factors. Patients are cautioned to avoid strenuous exercises, particularly activities involve heavy-lifting or the Valsalva's maneuver. Weightlifting should be avoided and sustained moderate exertion is preferable to bursts of efforts.

Drug Therapy

This is the primary treatment of essential hypertension. The drug currently available for treating hypertension have two main actions—reduction of ever and volume of circulating blood. The drugs used in the treatment of hypertension include diuretics, adrenergic (sympathetic) inhibitors, vasodilators, angiotensin inhibitors and calcium channel blockers. The details of medications used for hypertension are as follows:

A. Diuretics

1. Thiazide/Thiazide-like Diuretics

Thiazide/Thiazide-like diuretics blocks or inhibits sodium reabsorption in the distal convoluted tubule, in the portion of ascending tubule; Water exerted with sodium, producing decreased volume. They will be increased in Na^+ and Cl. Initial decrease in ECF and sustained decrease in SVR lowers BP moderately in 2 to 4 weeks. The technical terms used for these drugs are bendroflumethiazide, benzthiazide, chlorothiazide, cyclothiazide, hydrochlorothiazide, (Esidrex), hydroflumethiazide indapamide, methyl chlorothiazide, metalazine, polythiazide, quinethazone and trichlormethiazide, Thiazides are ineffective in renal failure.

The side effects of thiazides are:

- Fluid and electrolyte imbalances:
  Volume depletion, hypocalcemia, hyponatremia, hypercalcemia, hyperuricemia, metabolic alkalosis
- CNS effects: Vertigo, headache, weakness
- GI effects, anorexia, nausea, vomiting, diarrhea, constipation and pancreatitis
- Sexual problems: Impotence and decreased libido
- Blood dyscrasias and dermatologic effects; photosensitivity and skin rash
- Decreased glucose tolerance.

During this treatment nurses have to monitor the following:

1. Check vital signs before administering in early days of treatment
2. Monitor laboratory value of electrolytes, particularly potassium
3. Monitor patient weight
4. Teach patients to:
   - Take drug early in the day
   - Maintain liberal fluid intake
   - Take drug with food if GI upsets occur
   - Eat potassium-rich diet (e.g. fruits, legumes, whole grains, cereals and potato)
   - Expect an increased frequency and volume of urination
   - Report the incidence of muscle weakness, cramping, fatigue and nausea
   - Change positions slowly.

2. Loop Diuretics

It blocks sodium and water reabsorption in medullary portion of ascending tubule, cause rapid volume depletion. The drugs used are bumetanide, ethacrynic acid, furosemide (Lasix). The side effects are fluid and electrolyte imbalance as with thiazides except hypercalcemia, ototoxicity (hearing impairment, deafness, vertigo) that is usually reversible. Metabolic effects including hyperuricemia, hyperglycemia, increased LDL cholesterol and triglycerides with decreased HDL cholesterol. Nursing intervention are as same as with thiazides, but potassium loss can be severe. So, nurse has to monitor:

- Daily weight to assess response to treatment
- Laboratory values for increase in uric acid and glucose BUN.

3. Potassium Sparing Diuretics

It inhibits aldosterone; sodium excreted in exchange of potassium. The drugs are amiloride, spironolactone and triamterene. The side effects are hyperkalemia, nausea, vomiting, diarrhea, headache, leg cramps and dizziness. Nursing intervention includes:

- Monitor laboratory value for potassium excess
- Weigh patient daily
- Teach patient to:
  - Expect an increased volume of urine
  - Avoid potassium-rich foods
  - Report any incidence of drowsiness or GI side effects.

B. Adrenergic Inhibitors

1. Centrally Acting Alpha Blockers

These activate central receptors that suppress vasomotor and cardiac centers causing decrease in peripheral resistance. They reduce sympathetic outflow from CNS and peripheral sympathetic tone produces vasodilation and decreases SVR and BP. Commonly used are clonidine, guanabenz, guanfacine, methyldopa (Aldomet). The side effects of these drugs are—dry mouth, sedation, impotence, nausea, dizziness, sleep disturbance, nightmares, restlessness, and depression. There is symptomatic bradycardia in patient with conduction disorder. In this, nursing intervention includes:

- Change position slowly
- Teach patient to:
  - Change position slowly
  - Avoid hot baths, steam rooms, saunas
  - Use gum or hard candies to counteract dry mouth
  - Be cautious in driving or operating machinery if drowsiness or sedation occurs.
  - Report any decline in sexual responsiveness.

2. Peripheral Acting Adrenergic Antagonists

It depletes catecholamine, in peripheral sympathetic postganglionic fibers and blocks norepinephrine release from adrenergic nerve endings. Usually used are guanadrel, guanethidine (ismelin) rauwolfia, serpentina, reserpine (texpasil). The side effects include marked orthostatic hypertension, diarrhea, cramps bradycardia, retrograde or delayed ejaculation, sodium and water retention sedation and inability to concentrate, depression, nasal stuffiness with reserpine. The nursing intervention is as with the above (1) drug and report incidence of edema in hands and feet.

3. Beta-adrenergic Blockers

Beta-adrenergic blockers block beta-adrenergic receptors of sympathetic nervous system, decreasing heart rate and blood pressure. Please note that beta blockers should not be used in patients with asthma. COPD, CHF and heart block. Use with caution in diabetes and peripheral vascular disease. Commonly used beta-blockers are acebutolol, atenolol, betaxolol, carteolol, metoprolol, nadolol, penbutolol, pindolol, propranolol, timolol and esmolol (IV). The side effects of these drugs are bronchospasm, atrioventricular conduction block, impaired peripheral circulation, nightmares, depression, weakness, reduced exercise capability. It can be included in exacerbate symptom of ischemic heart disease. The nursing intervention includes:

- Establish baseline vital signs and laboratory values before treatment
- Check blood pressure and pulse before administration
- Teach patients to:
  - Change position slowly
  - Take drug as prescribed

- Avoid abruptly discontinuing the use
- Report any decline in sexual responsiveness
- Report incidence of fatigue, drowsiness, difficulty in breathing
- Be alert to the signs of hypoglycemia if diabetic drug masks the symptoms.

4. Combined Alpha and Beta-adrenergic Blockers

Labetalol is a common drug used as combined one. Action and nursing actions are as same as beta blockers.

C. Vasodilators

Vasodilators such as diazoxide, hydralazine, minoxidil, nitroglycerin (tridil) dilate peripheral blood vessels by directly relaxing vascular smooth muscle. These are usually used in combination with other antihypertensives as they increase sodium and fluid retention and cause reflex cardiac stimulation.

Diazoxide direct arterial vasodilation reduces SVR and BP. It is used intravenously for hypertensive crisis in hospitalized patients. It should be administered only into peripheral veins. The side effects include reflex sympathetic activation producing increased HR, CO and salt and water retention. Hyperglycemia is especially in type 2 diabetes.

Hydralazine has same effect as diazoxide; it should be given IV in hypertensive crisis in hospitalized patients. Also use two oral doses per day. The side effects are headache, nausea, flushing, palpitation bradycardia, angina, hemolytic anemia, vasculitis and rapidly progressive glomerulonephritis.

Minoxidil (Loniten) used in severe hypertension associated with renal failure. It may cause reflex tachycardia, fluid retention and ECG changes and tridol administered intravenously in case of hypertensive crisis with myocardial ischemia.

The nursing intervention during the use of vasodilator in hypertension clients are as follows:

- Check BP and pulse before each dose. Palpitation and tachycardia are common during first week of therapy
- Teach patients to:
  - Change in position slowly because dizziness is common
  - Avoid hot baths, steam rooms, saunas
  - Take drug with meals
  - Be prepared for nasal congestion and excess lacrimation
  - Report incidence of constipation or peripheral edema.

D. Angiotensin Inhibitors

1. ACE (Angiotensin Converting Enzyme) Inhibitors

These inhibit conversion of angiotensin I to angiotensin II, thus blocking the release of aldosterone, thereby reducing sodium and water retention. The commonly used are benazepril, captopril, cilazapril, enalapril, fosinopril, lisinopril, moexipril, perindopril, ramipril, quinapril, trandolapril, enalapril (injectable). The side effects are hypotension, loss of taste, cough, hyperkalemia, acute renal failure, skin rash angioneurotic edema. The nursing interventions are:

- Monitor for first-dose syncope in patients with CHF
- Monitor renal function through lab work and potassium levels
- Check BP before administering
- Teach patient to change position slowly, report any incidence of fatigue, skin rash, impaired taste and chronic cough.

2. Angiotensin II Receptor Antagonist

It selectively blocks the binding angiotensin I to the angiotensin II receptors found in many tissues and vascular smooth muscle, which blocks its vasoconstrictive and aldosterone-secreting effects. The commonly used are candesartan, irbesartan, losartan, tasosartan, valsartan. The side effects are hyperkalemia and decreased renal function. These drugs prevent action of angiotensin II and produce vasodilative and increasing salt and water excretion. The nursing intervention are as in ACE inhibitors.

E. Calcium Channel Blockers

Calcium channel blockers inhibit influx of calcium into muscle cells; act on vascular smooth muscles (primary arteries) to reduce spasms and promote vasodilation. Here it blocks movement of extracellular calcium into cells causing peripheral vasodilation and decreased SVR. The commonly used calcium channel blockers are amlodipine, diltiazem, felodipine, isradipine, mibefradil, nicardipine, nifedipine, nisoldipine, verapamil (isoptin) and verapamil SR. The side effects are nausea, headache, dizziness, peripheral edema, reflex tachycardia. Reflex disease in HR (with diltiazem), constipation (with verapamil). The nursing interventions include:

- Check vital signs before administering (bradycardia is common)
- Monitor renal and liver function tests
- Teach patient to take drugs before meals, change positions slowly, report any incidence of peripheral edema, fatigue and headache.

In addition to the above, the patient and family especially the members who prepare the meals should be educated about sodium-restricted diet.

NURSING MANAGEMENT

Assessment

- Assess blood pressure at frequent intervals; know baseline level. Note changes in pressure that would require a change in medication. See Box 12.4 for measuring BP
- Note the apical and peripheral pulse rate, rhythm and character

Box 12.4 Taking accurate blood pressure measurements

- Use auscultatory method with properly calibrated and validated blood pressure instrument
- Seat patient quietly for at least 5 minutes in a chair (not on examination table) with feet on the floor and arm supported at heart level
- Use appropriate-sized cuff in which cuff bladder encircles at least 80% of arm
- Take at least two blood pressure measurements
- Systolic blood pressure = first of two more sounds heard
- Diastolic blood pressure = disappearance of sounds
- Provide patients, verbally and in writing, their specific BP reading

- Assess symptoms such as nosebleeds; angina pain shortness of breath; alteration in vision, speech or balance (vertigo); headaches or nocturia
- Assess extent to which hypertension has affected patient personally, socially or financially.

Diagnosis

Nursing Diagnoses

- Deficient knowledge regarding the relationship between the treatment regimen and control of the disease process
- Noncompliance related to side effects of prescribed therapy.

Collaborative problems/Potential Complications

- Retinal hemorrhage
- Heart failure
- Renal insufficiency and failure
- Cerebrovascular accident (CVA)
- Transient ischemic attack (TIA)
- Myocardial infarction
- Left ventricular hypertrophy.

Planning and Goals

The major goals of the patient include understanding the disease process and its treatment, compliance with the self-care program and absence of complication:

- Maintains adequate tissue perfusion
- Complies with self-care program
- Experiences no complications.

Nursing Intervention

Increasing Knowledge

- Emphasize the concept of controlling hypertension (with lifestyle changes and medications) rather than curing it
- Arrange a consultation with a dietitian to help patient plan weight loss
- Obtain patient education materials from the American Heart Association
- Advise patient to limit alcohol intake and avoid use of tobacco.

Monitoring and Managing Potential Complications

- Assess all body system when patient returns for follow-up care
- Question patient about blurred vision, spots, or diminished visual acuity
- Report any significant findings promptly to determine whether additional studies or changes in medications are required.

Gerontologic Considerations

Isolated systolic hypertension is common in older adults as a result of age-related changes. Compliance with the therapeutic program is even more difficult for elderly people because medication therapy must be continuous, may be complicated, and may be expensive for a person on a fixed income.

- Promote monotherapy (treatment with a single agent) if appropriate to simplify the medication regimen and make it less expensive. The dosage of medication is often half that needed in younger patients
- Make sure that patient understands the medication regimen, can read the instructions, can open the container, and is prepared to adjust to postural hypotensive effects of antihypertensive medications (change position slowly, use supportive devices)
- Include the family in the teaching program so that they understand the patient's needs, support adherence to the therapeutic program, and know when to seek guidance from health professionals
- Encourage return to the outpatient setting for follow-up care
- Asses all body systems to detect evidence of vascular damage to vital organs, such as eyes (blurred vision, spots in front of eyes, diminished visual acuity), heart, nervous system, and kidneys.

Promoting Home and Community-Based Care

Teaching patients self-care

- Support patient and promote adherence to therapy in a cost-effective manner; collaborate with patient to set goals
- Reinforce the importance of taking medication as prescribed, scheduling regular follow-up appointments, maintaining dietary restrictions of sodium and fat, increasing fruits and vegetable and controlling weight
- Support patient in planning lifestyle changes, including an exercise program with regular physical activity
- Encourage counseling, education and weight control; cessation of smoking; and stress self-help groups of family and patient

- The patient and caregivers should be cautioned that antihypertensive medications can cause hypotension. Low blood pressure or postural hypotension should be reported immediately. The elderly have impaired cardiovascular reflexes and thus are more sensitive to the extracellular volume depletion caused by diuretics and to the sympathetic inhibition caused by adrenergic antagonists. The nurse teaches patients to change positions slowly when moving from a lying or sitting position to a standing position. The nurse also counsels elderly patients to use supportive devices such as handrails and walkers as necessary to prevent falls that could result from dizziness.

Promoting Compliance with Self-Care Program

- Encourage active participation of patient in the program, including self-monitoring of blood pressure and diet for increased compliance
- Encourage patient to abstain from alcohol because alcohol may have a synergistic effect with medication
- Discourage use of tobacco and nicotine products
- Give patient written information regarding expected effects and side effects of medications
- Teach patient and family how to measure blood pressure as follows.

Equipment

For the patient at home

- Automatic or semiautomatic device with digital display of readings.

For the caregiver

- Mercury sphygmomanometer, recently calibrated aneroid manometer, or validated electronic device
- Cuff.

Instructions for the patient

- Avoid smoking cigarettes or drinking caffeine for 30 minutes before BP is measured
- Sit quietly for 5 minutes before the measurement
- Sit comfortably with the forearm supported at heart level on a firm surface, with both feet on the ground; avoid talking while the measurement is being taken.

Instructions for the Caregiver

- Select the size of the cuff based on the size of the patient. (The cuff size should have a bladder width of at least 40 percent of limb circumference and length at least 80 percent of limb circumference.) The average adult cuff is 12 to 14 cm wide and 30 cm long. Using a cuff that is too small will give a higher BP measurement, and using a cuff that is too large results in a lower BP measurement compared to one taken with a properly sized cuff
- Routinely calibrate the sphygmomanometer
- Wrap the cuff firmly around the arm. Center the cuff bladder directly over the brachial artery
- Position the patient's arm at the level of the heart
- Palpate the systolic pressure before auscultating. This technique helps to detect the presence of an auscultatory gap more readily
- Ask the patient to sit quietly while the BP is measured because the BP can increase when the patient is engaged in conversation
- Initially, record BP results of both arms and take subsequent measurements from the arm with the higher BP. Normally, the BP should vary by no more than 5 mm Hg between arms
- Record the site where the BP was measured and the position of the patient (e.g. right arm)
- Inform the patient of his or her BP value and what it means. Emphasize the need for periodic reassessment, and encourage patients who measure BP at home to keep a written record of readings.

Interpretation

Assessment is based on the average of at least two readings (if two readings differ by more than 5 mm Hg, additional readings are taken and an average reading is calculated from the results.)

Continuing Care

- Reinforce importance of regular follow-up care
- Obtain patient history and perform physical examination at each clinic visit
- Assess for medication-related problems (orthostatic hypotension).

The primary nursing responsibilities for long-term management of hypertension are to assist the patient in reducing BP and complying with the treatment plan. Nursing actions include patient and family education, detection and reporting of adverse treatment effects, compliance assessments, enhancement and evaluation of therapeutic effectiveness. Patient education includes diet therapy, drug therapy, physical activity, home monitoring of BP (if appropriate) and avoidance of tobacco (if applicable). When presenting information to the patient or family, the nurse should do the following:

- Provide the numerical value of the patient's BP and explain that it exceeds normal limits
- Inform the patient that hypertension usually asymptomatic and symptoms do not reliably indicate BP levels
- Explain that long-term follow-up and therapy are necessary
- Explain that therapy will not cure but should control hypertension
- Tell the patient that controlled hypertension is usually compatible with an excellent prognosis and a normal lifestyle
- Explain to the patient about dangers of uncontrolled hypertension
- Be specific about the names, actions, dosages and side effects of prescribed medication

- Tell the patient to plan regular and convenient times for taking medications
- Tell the patient not to discontinue drugs abruptly because withdrawal may cause a severe hypertensive reaction
- Tell the patient not to double upon doses when a dose is missed
- Instruct the patient that if BP increases, not to take an increased medication dosage before consulting a health care provider
- Tell the patient not to take a medication belonging to someone else
- Make aware the patient that side effects of medication often diminish with the passage of time
- Tell the patient to consult the health care provider about changing drugs or dosage if impotence or other sexual problems develop
- Tell the patient to supplement diet with foods high in potassium (e.g. citrus fruits, and green leafy vegetables) if he/she is taking potassium-losing diuretics
- Tell the patient to avoid hot baths, excessive amounts of alcohol, and strenuous exercises within 3 hours of taking medication that promote vasodilation
- Explain to decrease orthostatic hypotension, the patient should arise slowly from bed, sit on side of bed for a few minutes, stand slowly, not stand still for a long time, do leg exercises to increase venous return, sleep with head of bed raised or on pillows, and lie or sit down when dizziness occurs.

CORONARY ARTERY DISEASE (CAD)

Coronary artery disease is a type of blood vessel disorder that is included in the general category of atherosclerosis. The term atherosclerosis is derived from two Greek words. 'Athero' meaning 'Fatty Mish' and 'Skleros' meaning "Hard". This word-combination indicates that atherosclerosis begins as soft deposits of fat, that hardens with age. Atherosclerosis is often referred to as 'hardening of the arteries' (Fig. 12.3). Although this condition can occur in any artery in the body, the atheromas (fatty deposits) have a preference for the coronary arteries. Patients with CAD often seek health care after experiencing angina or myocardial infarction (MI). Vascular diseases such as dysrhythmia, heart failure, and cardiomyopathy. All nurses need to be familiar with the management of coronary artery diseases.

Etiology

Atherosclerosis is the major cause of coronary artery diseases. It is characterized by a focal deposit of cholesterol and lipids, primarily within the wall of the artery. Many risk factors have been associated with CAD are:

- *Age and gender:* Incidence of CAD occurs in men between 35 to 45 years age. After the age of 65 incidence of men and women equalizes; although there is evidence suggesting that more women are being seen with CAD earlier because of increased stress, increased smoking, presence of hypertension and use of birth control pills. For both decrease in elasticity of arteries with age. Estrogen in females lowers serum cholesterol.

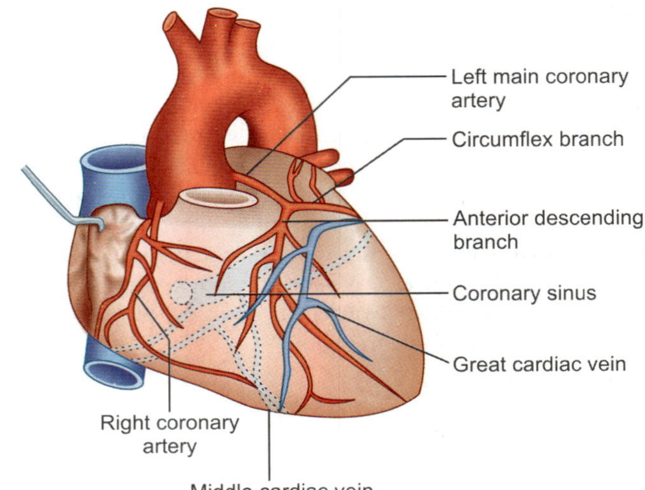

FIG. 12.3: Diagram of the coronary arteries arising from the aorta and encircling the heart. Some of the coronary veins are also shown

- *Heredity:* Genetic predisposition is an important factor in the occurrence of CAD, but exact mechanism is not yet known.
- *Diabetes:* Incidence of CAD is two-three times more in diabetes. This may be due to elevated levels of circulating insulin helps to form atheroma and damaged arterial intima and insulin also modifies lipid metabolisms.
- *Hypertension:* Hypertension affects the ability of blood vessels to constrict or dilate. Decreased elasticity of blood vessels, tearing affect on arteries, and increased resistance of ejection of ventricular volume may lead to CAD.
- Smoking and tobacco use.

The unifying factor promoting CAD is nicotine. Nicotine has the following physiological effects and may cause CAD:

- Decreased high-density lipoproteins (HDL)
- Displacement of oxygen from hemoglobin
- Increased catecholamine in response to nicotine, increasing heart rate and blood pressure
- Increased platelet adhesiveness
- Accelerates atheroma formation
- Accelerates atheroma formation
- Coronary spasm
- Sedentary lifestyle.

This alters lipid metabolism and decrease in HDLS. Physical inactivity may lead to CAD.

- *Diet:* Dietary intake of more cholesterol and fat, provides more substance for lesion formation. Hypercholesterolemia, familial hyperlipidemia, increased levels of low density lipoproteins and increasing atherogenesis.

- *Obesity:* Obese persons are more prone to diabetes, hypertension and hyperlipidemias. In addition, they often demonstrate other behaviors such as sedentary lifestyles, that are known as risk factors for CAD.
- *Stress and behavior pattern:* Catecholamine, released during stress response, increases platelet aggregation and may also precipitate vasospasm. It was generally agreed that individuals with type 'A' behavior had a higher incidence of CAD than individuals who were more relaxed. The type 'A' personality characters include the following:
  - Perfectionistic
  - Always tense
  - Competitive
  - Unduly irritable
  - Aggressive
  - Obsessed with number of sale made, articles written
  - Constantly time-oriented
  - Patients seen, forms completed
  - Has hurry sickness
  - Never says 'no'
  - Holds in feelings
  - Compulsive
  - Never has leisure time
  - Impatient
  - Never takes a relaxing vacation or day offs.

Nursing care plan for CAD given in Table 12.1.

There are three major clinical manifestations in coronary artery disease, which include angina pectoris, acute myocardial infarction and hidden cardiac death. They are stages of the continuum and CAD. The detailed description of these three are as follows:

TABLE 12.1: Nursing care plan of coronary artery disease (CAD)

Problem	Reason	Objectives	Nursing intervention	Evaluation
1. Pain related to imbalance of O_2 supply	(Write subjective and objective data highlighting related key points)	Pain will be reduced.	• Determine the intensity of the patient's angina • Observe the other signs and symptoms – Diaphoresis – Shortness of breath – Protective body posture – Dusky facial color – Changes in level of consciousness – Place the patient in comfortable position • Administer oxygen if prescribed • Obtain blood pressure, AHR respiration • Obtain a 12-lead ECG as directed • Administer antianginal medication as prescribed • Report findings to physician • Note duration of anginal pain episode • Take vital signs until pain relief • Monitor progression of stable angina to unstable angina • Determine the level of activity that precipitated anginal episode • Identify specific activities patient may engage in, that are below the level at which pain occurs • Reinforce the importance of notifying nursing staff whenever angina pain is experienced	Patient verbalizes relief of pain
2. Decreased cardiac output related to reduced preload after load in	"	Improving cardiac output	• Monitor patient response to drug therapy – Take BP and HR in sitting and lying positions – Recheck vital signs as indicated – Note patient's complaints for headache and dizziness – Administer analgesics as prescribed – Encourage supine position for dizziness • Institute continuous ECG monitoring as directed • Evaluate the development of heart failure (When beta-blockers-calcium channel blocker advised) – Obtain serial weights – Auscultate lung fields for crackles – Monitor the presence of edema • Be sure to remove previous nitrate patch or paste before applying new paste or pad (prevents hypotension) • Be alert to adverse reaction related to abrupt discontinuation of beta-blockers and others • Report all untoward drug effects to physician	Blood pressure and heart status are stable

Contd...

Contd...

Problem	Reason	Objectives	Nursing intervention	Evaluation
3. Anxiety related to chest pain and others	"	Alleviation of anxiety	• Explain to the patient and family, reasons for hospitalization, diagnostic tests and therapies • Encourage the patient to verbalize fears and concerns regarding illness, by good listening • Answer the patient's questions with concise explanations • Explain to the patient the importance of anxiety reduction to assist in angina • Teach relaxation techniques • Discuss measure to be taken when angina episode occurs	Patient verbalizes lessening anxiety ability to cope
4. Knowledge deficit related to coronary artery disease	Patient and family do not have proper knowledge of CAD	Educate the patient and family regarding CAD	• Instruct the patient and family about CAD (anatomy and physiology and heart warning signals of angina) • Identify suitable activity level to prevent angina: – normal activities do not produce discomfort to chest – Avoid activities known to cause angina – Rest after meals – Try to avoid cold weather – Reduce weight if necessary • Instruct about appropriate use of medications and side effects: – Carry nitroglycerine at all times – Demonstrate how to administer nitroglycerin – Place nitroglycerin under the tongue – Teach side effects of other medications Constipation: Verapamil Ankle edema: Nifedipine Heart failure: Beta or calcium blockers Dizziness: Vasodilators	

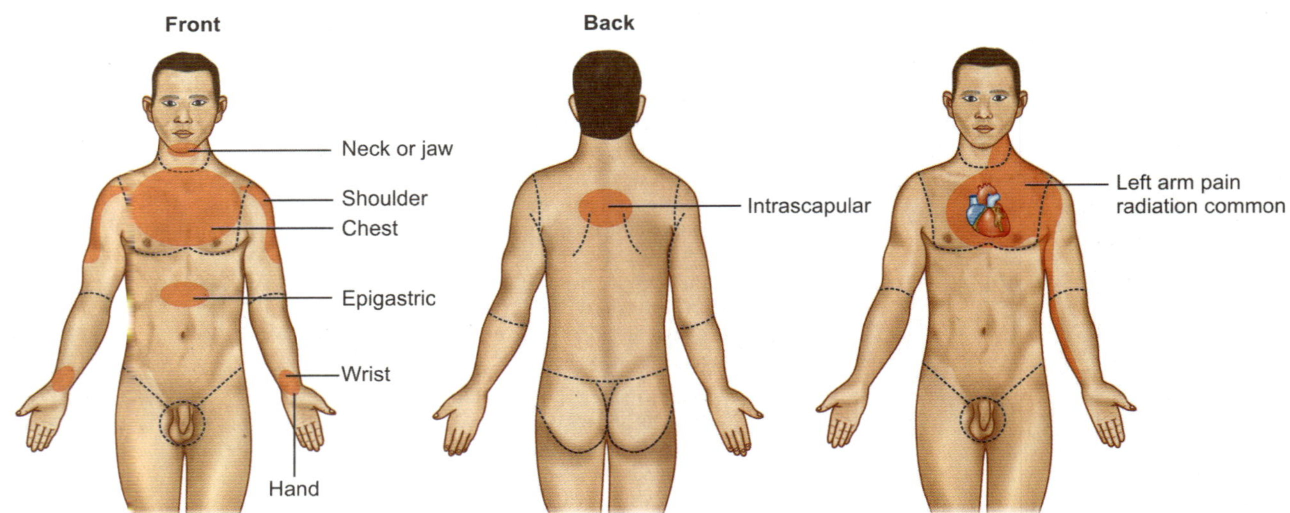

FIG. 12.4: Common locations of anginal pain, which may vary in combination and intensity

ANGINA PECTORIS

Angina pectoris is a clinical syndrome characterized by paroxysms of pain or a feeling of pressure in the anterior chest. The cause is insufficient coronary blood flow, resulting in an inadequate supply of oxygen to meet the myocardial demand. Angina is usually a result of atherosclerotic heart disease and is associated with a significant obstruction of a major coronary artery. Factor affecting anginal pain are physical exertion, exposure to cold, eating a heavy meal, stress, or any emotion-provoking situation that increase myocardial workload. Atypical angina is not associated with the above and may occur at rest. Diabetic neuropathy can interfere with neuroreceptors, thus dulling the patients perception of pain. Common locations of anginal (Fig. 12.4).

Angina pectoris is literally translated as pain (angina) in the chest (pectoris). Myocardial ischemia is expressed symptomatically as angina. More specifically, angina pectoris is transient chest pain caused by myocardial ischemia. It usually lasts for only few minutes (3 to 5 minutes), and commonly subsides when the precipitating factor (usual exertion) is relieved. Typical exertional angina should not persist longer than 20 minutes after rest and administration of nitroglycerin.

Etiology

Myocardial ischemia develops when the demand for myocardial oxygen exceeds the ability of the coronary arteries to supply it. The below given are the primary reasons for insufficient blood flow in narrowing of coronary arteries by atherosclerosis. Extracardiac factors may precipitate myocardial ischemia and anginal pain. They include:

- Physical exertion: Increases the heart rate (HR) Increasing heart rate decreases the time the heart spends in diastole, which is the time of greatest coronary blood flow. Walking outdoors is the most common form of the exertions that produce an attack. Isometric exertions of the arms as on raking leaves, painting or lifting heavy objects also causes exertional angina.
- Strong emotions stimulate the sympathetic nervous system and increase the work of the heart. This results in an increase in HR, BP and myocardial contractility.
- Consumption of heavy meal (especially if the person exerts afterwards) can increase the work of the heart. During the digestive process, blood is diverted to the GI system, causing a low flow rate in the coronary arteries.
- Temperature extremes may be either hot or cold, which increases the workload of the heart (blood vessels constrict in response to the cold climate; blood vessels dilate and blood pools in the skin in response to a hot stimulus). Cold weather also causes increased metabolism to maintain internal temperature regulation.
- Cigarette smoking causes vasoconstriction and an increased HR because of nicotine stimulation of the catecholamine release. It also diminishes available oxygen by increasing level of carbon monoxide.
- Sexual activity increases the workload and sympathetic stimulation. In a person with severe CAD, the resulting extra workload of the heart may precipitate angina.
- Stimulants, such as cocaine, cause increased HR and subsequent myocardial demand. Stimulation of catecholamine release is the precipitating factor.
- Circadian rhythm have been related to the occurrence of the stable angina, unstable angina, MI and cardiac death. These manifestations of CAD tend to occur in the early morning after awakening.

Pathophysiology

Coronary artery disease refers to the development and progression of plaque accumulation in the coronary arteries. This process has three stages along the continuum viz. stable angina, unstable angina and myocardial infarction.

Normally the endothelium of the coronary artery allows for unrestricted blood flow to the myocardium. Any kind of trauma or irritant can disrupt this protective endothelium. The body's response to injury is a complex interplay of chemical mediators designed to protect the area. Endothelial injury causes the release of thromboxane, which minimizes the extent of injury through local vasoconstriction and by stimulating platelet aggregation. The intima releases prostacyclin in response to the effects of thromboxane. Prostacyclin works to restore equilibrium through local vasodilation and by opposing platelet aggregation. With repeated injury, the deteriorated intima cannot produce enough prostacyclin and platelet aggregation forces predominate.

Platelets and accumulating monocytes release powerful growth factors into the arterial wall. These factors stimulate the proliferation and migration of medial smooth muscle cells into the intima. This structural changes cause an increased permeability of the vessel wall to the cholesterol. The accumulation of cholesterol produces a fatty streak that protrudes into the lumen of the artery. Smooth muscle cells and fibrous tissue form a fibrous cap over the fatty streak. The fatty streak continues to grow, invading both the intima and media. Involvement of the media affects the ability of the vessel wall to vasodilation and vasoconstriction. The artery may continue to maintain the supply of oxygen and nutrients to the myocardium as long as the blockage is less than 70 percent of the arterial lumen. Concomitant conditions such as anemia, smoking and hypovolemia further compromise the delivery of oxygen to the myocardium.

The presence of risk factors accelerate atherogenesis, thereby decreasing oxygen supply. Risk factors can also increase the myocardium's demands for oxygen. The demand of the myocardium for oxygen can be met only by an adequate blood supply. As long as supply is greater than or equal to demand, aerobic metabolism occurs. When demand is greater than that of supply, the myocardium must switch to anaerobic metabolism for nourishments. Anaerobic metabolism produces lactic acid which is believed to be responsible for ischemic anginal pain. The pain is the most common initial symptom of CAD. With stable angina the patient is usually experiencing a known threshold beyond which myocardial oxygen demand exceeds supply. Myocardial oxygen demand increases with any condition causing an increase in heart rate, an increase in resistance to ejecting blood volume, and an increase in myocardial size.

When atherosclerosis progresses beyond 70 percent, pressure within the lesion (plaque) can increase to the point of plaque rupture. Rupture of the fibrous cap exposes the inner plaque to the circulating blood. In an effort to heal, collagen accumulates, smooth muscle cells proliferate and clotting factors are activated. Aggregating platelets activate the coagulation system immediately to seal the rupture. With plaque disruptions stable angina becomes unstable angina.

Risk factors like nicotine from tobacco use increases platelet adhesion and increases the potential for clotting at the site of disruption. Catecholamines released during the stress response also increase platelet aggregation. The third stage that occurs is complete obstruction of the coronary artery with a fibrous cloth called coronary thrombosis or acute MI.

Clinical Manifestation

The following may occur with stable angina, unstable angina or acute MI:

- Chest pain or anginal equivalent (jaw pain, left arm pain)
- Non-verbal indicators of pain: Clutch, rib, stroke and the chest
- Increase or decrease in heart rate
- Dysrhythmias
- Increase or decrease in blood pressure
- Angina that occurs with predictable level of exertion (in stable angina)
- Angina not necessarily associated with activity and ST depression (or unstable angina)
- Pain varies from a feeling of indigestion to a choking or heavy sensation in the upper chest to agonizing pain. The patient with diabetes mellitus may not experience severe pain with angina
- Angina is accompanied by severe apprehension and feeling impending death
- The pain is usually retrosternal, deep in the chest behind the upper or middle third of the sternum
- Discomfort is poorly localized and may radiate to the neck, jaw, shoulders, and inner aspect of the upper arms (usually the left arm)
- Patient feels a tightness, heavy choking, or strangling sensation with a viselike, insistent quality. Shortness of breath, pallor, diaphoresis, dizziness, light-headedness, nausea, and vomiting may be noted (called angina-like signs if noted alone; may represent myocardial infarction)
- Angina is accompanied by a feeling of weakness or numbness in the arms, wrists, and hands
- An important characteristic of angina pain is that it subsides when the precipitating cause is removed with nitroglycerin.

In addition to the unique feature of myocardial infarction which includes:

- Angina not relieved by rest or nitroglycerin therapy
- Associated with symptoms: Dizziness, dyspnea, nausea, vomiting feeling of impending doom
- Altered neurological status, if decreased output
- Rales, if decreased contractility creates left ventricular function
- Presence of S_3 or S_4 gallop
- Diminished pulses
- Pallor
- ECG ST elevation, Q-waves, J-wave abnormalities
- Elevated ESR.

Management

When a patient has a history indicating coronary artery disease, thorough physical examination should be carried out and physician may order several diagnostic studies, which the nurse has to promptly attend and assist.

Medical Management

The goals of medical management are to decrease the oxygen demands of the myocardium and to increase the oxygen supply through pharmacologic therapy and risk factor control

Evaluation of clinical manifestations of pain and patient history

- Electrocardiogram changes (12-lead ECG), stress testing, blood tests
- Echocardiogram, nuclear scan, or invasive procedures such as cardiac catheterization and coronary artery angiography.

The elderly person who experiences angina may not exhibit the typical pain profile because of age-related changes in neuroreceptors. In older patients, pain may be sensed in the jaw or fainting may occur. Advise patient to recognize feelings of weakness as an indication for rest or taking prescribed medications. During exposure to cold temperature, elderly patients may experience anginal symptoms more quickly than younger people. Encourage these patients to wear warm clothing as appropriate.

Frequently, therapy includes a combination of medicine and surgery. Surgically, the goals of management include revascularization of the blood supply to the myocardium.

- Coronary artery bypass surgery or minimally invasive direct coronary artery bypass (MIDCAB)
- Percutaneous transluminal coronary angioplasty (PTCA) or percutaneous transluminal myocardial revascularization (PTMR)
- Application of intracoronary stents and atherectomy to enhance blood flow
- Lasers to vaporize plaques
- Percutaneous coronary endarterectomy to extract obstruction.

Pharmacologic Therapy

- Nitrates, the mainstay of therapy (nitroglycerin) (Box 12.5)
- Beta-adrenergic blockers (metoprolol [Toprol])
- Calcium ion antagonists and calcium-channel blockers (amlodipine [Norvasc] and diltiazem [Cardizem])
- Antiplatelet and anticoagulant medications (aspirin, clopidogrel [Plavix], ticlopidine [Ticlid], or heparin)
- Oxygen therapy.

Those studies include chest-X-ray, ECG, serum enzyme level (CK-LDH) cardiac troponin, serum lipid level. Exercise stress test. Nuclear imaging studies, position emission tomography (PET), coronary angiographic studies and echocardiography.

(CK = Creatine kinase, LDH = Lactic dehydrogenase.)

Box 12.5 Key points for using sublingual nitroglycerin

- Carry nitroglycerin (NTG) at all times
- Keep NTG tightly sealed in the original container and protected from heat, light, and moisture
- Replace NTG at least every 6 months for maximum effect, or every 3 to 4 months if carried in a pocket next to body heat
- Take NTG before an activity known to cause chest pain
- Sit or lie down when taking NTG, if possible
- Take one NTG tablet and repeat every 5 minutes up to three doses if pain is not relieved. If pain is unrelieved after one dose and other symptoms of myocardial infarction are present, call 911 for emergency medical care
- Tingling should be felt under the tongue for emergency medical care
- NTG may cause a headache initially. Aspirin may relieve it
- NTG may cause light-headedness. Rise slowly to prevent falls

Nursing assessment made on the basis of present subjective and objective data. Nursing diagnosis for the patient with angina may include chest pain, anxiety, decreased cardiac output, activity intolerances related to myocardial ischemia. The main nursing objectives for the patient with angina are pain assessment, evaluation of treatment and reinforcement of appropriate therapy. Because chest pain may be caused by many factors other than ischemia (e.g. pericarditis, valvular disease, pulmonary artery stenosis, MI congestive cardio-myopathy). It is important to have a clear understanding of the patient's chest pain.

The nurse should determine whether breathing in or out of changing positions makes the patient's chest pain better or worse. Anginal pain does not vary with body positions or respiration. In contrast, the pain is deep or superficial, mild or intense, diffuse or localized. Cardiac pain usually is deep or intense and diffuse. The patient may rub the entire chest to explain as to where the pain is occurring. If the nurse is present during anginal attack, the following measures should be taken:

- Administration of oxygen
- Determination of vital signs
- 12-lead ECG
- Prompt pain relief Ist with a nitrate followed by narcotic analgesic if needed
- Physical assessment of the chest
- Comfortable positioning of the patient.

The patient will more likely appear distressed and have pale, cool, clammy skin. The blood pressure and heart rate will probably be elevated and an atrial gallop (S_4) sound may be heard. If a ventricular gallop (S_3) is heard, it may indicate LV decompensation. A murmur may be heard during an angina attack secondary to ischemia of a papillary muscle. The murmur is likely to be transient and abates with the cessation of symptoms. Supportive and realistic assurance and a calm, soothing manner help reduce the patient's anxiety.

The patient should be instructed in the proper use of nitroglycerin tablets. Nitrates decrease myocardial oxygen demand by vesodilate (decrease preload), peripherally vasodilated (decrease afterload), increase myocardial oxygen supply and coronary vasodilate. Nitroglycerin should be easily accessible to the patient at all times. However, patients should be taught not to carry nitroglycerin in their pockets because heat from the body can cause loss of potency of the tablet. For protection from degradation. It should be kept in a tightly closed dark glass bottle. The patient should be instructed to place a nitroglycerin tablet beneath the tongue and allow it to dissolve. This should cause a fizzing or slightly warm feeling locally. The patient should be warned that heart rate may increase and pounding headache, dizziness or flush may occur. The patient should be cautioned against quickly rising to standing position, because postural hypertension may occur after nitroglycerin ingestion. If pain has not been relieved after 5 minutes ask him/her to repeat the dose, but not to exceed three tablets. If pain persists after three doses, the patient should be referred to seek immediate proper medical attention.

The patient should be reassured that a long, productive life is possible even with angina. The patient should be educated regarding coronary artery disease and angina, precipitating factors, risk factors and medication. Educating the patient and family about diet that are low in sodium and reduced in saturated fat may be appropriate. Maintaining ideal body weight is important in controlling angina because weight above the level increase myocardial workload, and may cause pain. Several small meals in place of three meals per day may be suggested. Application of topical nitrates over the chest may be taught to patient.

NURSING MANAGEMENT

Assessment

Observe and record facts about pain (location, description and intensity) and patient activities that precede and precipitate attacks of anginal pain (from patient history).

Nursing Diagnoses

- Ineffective cardiac tissue perfusion secondary to coronary artery disease as evidenced by chest pain (or equivalent symptoms)
- Death anxiety
- Deficient knowledge about underlying disease and methods for avoiding complications
- Noncompliance, ineffective therapeutic regimen management or noncompliance related to nonacceptance of necessary lifestyle changes.

Potential Complications

Potential complication of angina include myocardial infarction and its complication; acute pulmonary edema, heart failure, cardiogenic shock, dysrhythmias and cardiac arrest, myocardial rupture, pericardial effusion and cardiac tamponade.

Planning

Goals may include pain relief and absence of return of pain, reduction of anxiety, awareness of the underlying nature of the disorder, understanding of the prescribed care, adherence to the self-care program, and absence of complications.

Objectives

- Report pain is relieved promptly
- Report and demonstrate less anxiety
- Understand ways to avoid complications and demonstrates freedom from complications
- Complies with self-care program.

Nursing diagnosis will be made thorough nursing assessment by asking the patient to describe the angina attack (when, where, how often, how long and other associative symptoms and signs), family history, previous history and their habits, etc. The main nursing diagnosis which needs nursing interventions are:

- Pain related to an imbalance in O_2 supply and demand
- Decreased cardiac output related to reduced preload, overload, contractility and HR secondary to the hemodynamic effects of drugs
- Anxiety related to chest pain, uncertain prognosis and threatening environment.
  In addition, control of angina pectoris is achieved through the:
  - Review information on low-fat/low cholesterol diet with patient
  - Inform patient of available cardiac rehabilitation programs, that offer structured classes on exercise, smoking cessation and weight control
  - Avoid excessive caffeine intake (coffee, cola drinks) that can increase the heart rate and produce angina
  - Avoid the use of alcohol or drink only in moderation
  - Avoid use of 'diet pills', nasal decongestants or any over the counter medication that can increase the HR or stimulate HBP.

Nursing Interventions

An overall goal of ongoing intervention is to design a logical program of prevention using data collected during the nursing assessment.

Preventing Pain

- Teach patient to understand the symptom complex and avoid activities known to cause angina pain as given below:
  - Sudden or excessive exertion
  - Exposure to cold
  - Tobacco use
  - Heavy meals
  - Excessive weight
  - Some over-the-counter drugs, such as diet pills, nasal decongestant, or drugs that increase heart rate and blood pressure
- Direct patient to stop all activities and sit or rest in bed in a semi-Fowler's position if chest pain is sensed
- If patient has frequent pain or pain with minimal activity, discuss ways to alternate rest and activity periods
- Assess pain and vital signs, noting respiratory distress, and ST segment on ECG
- Administer nitroglycerin (up to 3 doses) and oxygen.

Reducing Anxiety

- Explore implications that the diagnosis has for patient
- Provide essential information about the illness and methods of preventing progression. Explain importance of following prescribed directives for the ambulatory patient at home
- Explore various stress reduction methods with patient (e.g. music therapy).

Teaching Patients Self-Care

- Educate patient about basic nature of the illness
- Furnish facts needed to reorganize living habits in order to reduce the frequency and severity of angina attacks, to delay underlying disease, and to protect against other complications
- Collaborate on a self-care program with patient, family, or friends
- Plan activities to minimize angina episodes
- Teach patient that any pain unrelieved within 30 minutes by the usual methods should be treated at the closest emergency center. Patient should call 911 for assistance.

MYOCARDIAL INFARCTION

Myocardial infarction occurs when ischemic intracellular changes become irreversible and necrosis results. Angina as a result of ischemia causes reversible cellular injury, and infarction in the result of sustained ischemia causing irreversible cellular death. Area of ischemia is shown in Figure 12.5.

Myocardial infarction (MI) refers to the process by which myocardial tissue is destroyed in regions of the heart that are deprived of an adequate blood supply because of reduced coronary blood flow. The cause is usually a critical narrowing of a coronary artery due to atherosclerosis or complete occlusion of an artery due to embolus or thrombus. Decreased coronary blood may also result from vasospasm of a coronary artery,

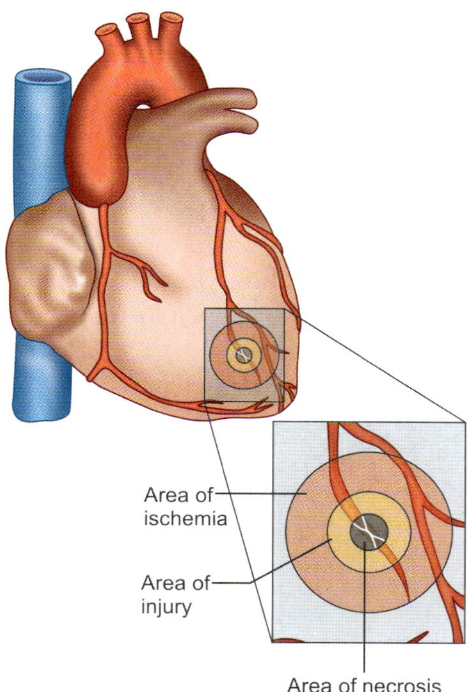

FIG. 12.5: Myocardial infarction. Areas of ischemia, injury, and necrosis caused by a blockage in the left anterior coronary artery

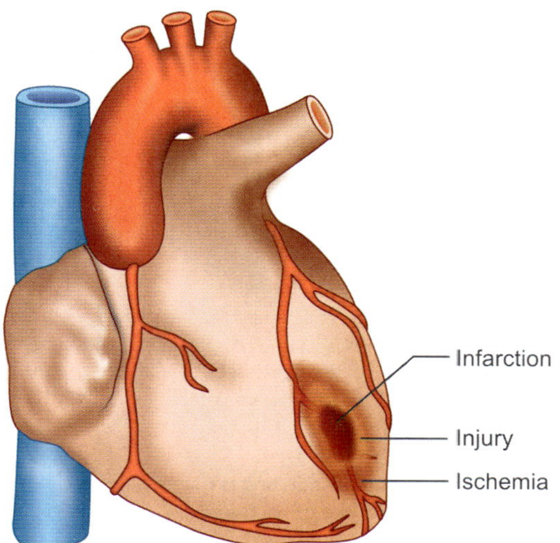

FIG. 12.6: Different degrees of damage occur to the heart muscle after a myocardial infarction. The diagram shows the zones of necrosis, injury, and ischemia

decreased oxygen supply (e.g. shock and hemorrhage), or increased demand for oxygen (e.g. tachycardia, thyrotoxicosis, or ingest of cocaine). In each case, there is a profound imbalance between myocardial oxygen supply and demand. An MI may be defined by the type, the location of the injury to the heart muscle (ventricular wall) or by the point in time in the process of infarction (acute, evolving, old).

Pathophysiology

Cardiac cells can withstand ischemia condition for approximately 20 minutes before cellular death (necrosis) begins. Contractile function of the heart stops in the area of myocardial necrosis. The degree of altered function depends on the area of the heart involved the LV. A transmural MI occurs when the entire thickness of the myocardium in a region involved. A subendocardial MI (non-transmural) exists when the damage has not penetrated through the entire thickness of the myocardial wall (Fig. 12.6). Infarction is described as the area of occurrence, as anterior, inferior, lateral, or posterior wall infarctions, common combination and anterolateral or anteroseptal MI. An inferior MI also called diaphragmatic MI. The location and area of the infarct correlates with the part of the coronary circulation involved. The degree of pre-established collateral circulation also determines the severity of infarction. The clot extends into lumens, completely obstructs lumen. Complete obstruction of the coronary artery with the fibrous clot is termed as coronary thrombosis or coronary occlusion. Coronary occlusion creates a rapid series of physiological events. The first of these events is immediate myocardial ischemia distal to the occlusion. Ischemia alters the integrity and permeability of the myocardial cell membranes to vital electrolytes. This instability depresses myocardial contractility and predisposes the patients to sudden death from dysrhythmias.

The body responses to cell death is inflammatory process within 24 hours, leukocytes infiltrate the area. Enzymes are released from the dead cardiac cells and important diagnostic indicators of MI. An overview of myocardial infarction is given in Box 12.6.

Clinical Manifestation

- Chest pain that occurs suddenly and continues despite rest and medication is the primary presenting symptom. ECG may be abnormal or normal (Figs 12.7 and 12.8)
- In many cases, the signs and symptoms cannot be distinguished from those of unstable angina
- Pain may radiate to the jaw, neck, shoulders and arm (usually left)
- Pain may be accompanied by cool skin, pallor, clammy diaphoresis, tachycardia, and tachypnea if stimulation of the sympathetic nervous system occurs

Box 12.6 An overview of MI

Signs and symptoms	*Classic* Crushing, viselike chest pain with radiation to arm, shoulder, neck, jaw, or back Shortness of breath Dizziness Nausea Sweating *Atypical* Absence of chest pain Fatigue Cramping in chest Anxiety Feeling of impending doom Falling *More common in Women* Epigastric or abdominal pain Chest discomfort, pressure, burning Arm, shoulder, neck, jaw, or back pain Discomfort/pain between shoulder blades Shortness of breath Fatigue Indigestion or gas pain Nausea or vomiting
Diagnostic tests	ECG Serum cardiac troponin I or T Serum myoglobin Serum CK-MB CBC Serum magnesium and potassium Vital signs, oxygen saturation, intake and output
Therapeutic measures	Medications Oxygen Morphine sulfate Nitrates Fab four cardiac medications: aspirin, statin, ACEI, beta blocker Platelet aggregation inhibitors Thrombolytics Anticoagulants Antidysrhythmics Vasodilators Percutaneous coronary interventions and stents Myocardial revascularization-CABG Fluid restriction Daily weights Bed rest with bedside commode/bathroom privileges Low-sodium diet advanced to diet as tolerated; no caffeine Cardiac rehabilitation
Complications	Dysrhythmias Heart failure Cardiogenic shock Valvular insufficiency

- Patients with diabetes mellitus may not experience severe pain because the neuropathy that accompanies diabetes can interfere with neuroreceptors, dulling the pain

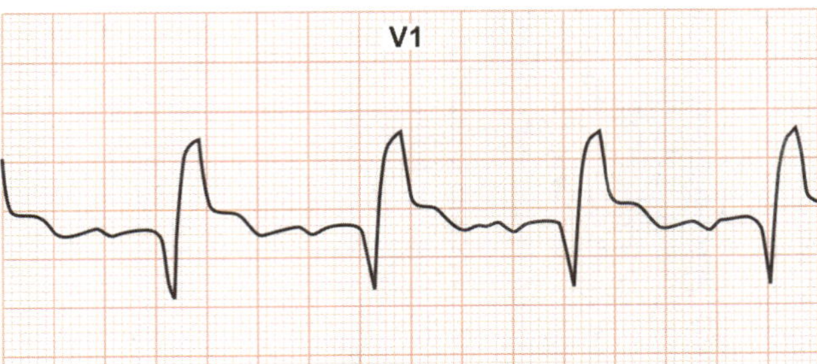

FIG. 12.7: Abnormal Q wave

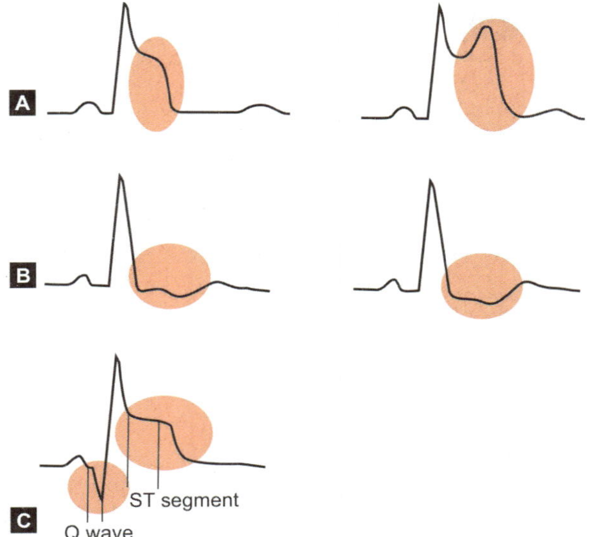

FIGS 12.8A TO C: ECG changes during myocardial infarction. (A) Injury: ST-segment elevation; (B) Ischemia: ST-segment inversion; (C) Necrosis: Large Q wave and ST-segment elevation

- Chest pain very severe immobilizing chest pain not relieved by rest or nitrate administration is the hallmark of MI. This pain is usually described as a heaviness, tightness or constrictions. Common locations are substernal or retrosternal, radiating to the neck, jaw and arms or to the back. It may occur when patient is active, or at rest, awake or during sleep and it commonly occurs at early morning hours. It lasts for 20 minutes or more
- Nausea and vomiting as a result of vasovagal reflexes initiated from the area of the infarcted myocardium
- Sympathetic nervous system stimulation is increased due to release of increased catecholamine (norepinephrine) and epinephrine leads to ashen cool and clammy skin (cold sweats)
- Fever: The temperature may increase up to 38°C.
- Cardiac vascular manifestation includes elevated BP and HR. Later, BP may drop as decreased cardiac output, urinary output may be decreased. Crackles may be noted in the lungs.

Later hepatic engorgement and peripheral edema occurs which indicates cardiac failure.

In addition, following complications may develop:
- Arrhythmias (abnormal wave)
- Congestive heart failure
- Cardiogenic shock
- Papillary muscle dysfunction
- Ventricular aneurysm
- Pericarditis
- Dressler's syndrome
- Right ventricular infarction
- Pulmonary embolism.

Management

Common diagnostic parameters used to determine whether a person has sustained an acute MI include: (1) The patient's history of pain. Risk factors and health history; (2) 12-lead ECG. Consistent with acute MI. (ST-T wave elevated by greater than 1 mm or more in two continuous leads and (3) Serious measurement of myocardial serum enzyme and comparison of the pain with angina as given below:

Angina	Myocardial infarction
1. Precipitating factors – Stress, either physiologic (exertion or psychology) – Digestion of heavy meal – Valsalva's maneuver during micturition or defecation – Extremity of weather – Hot baths or showers – Sexual excitation	Precipitating factors – Exertion or rest – Physical or emotional stress – Often no precipitation factors are associated with angina
2. Location – Midanterior chest – Substernal – Abdominal with radiation to neck, back arms, fingers – Diffuse, nor easily located	– Midanterior chest – Substernal – Diffuse – Radiation to neck and jaw or down left arm or both arms to fingers
3. Description – Deep sensation of tightness or squeezing feeling – Mild to moderate in severity or pressure – Similar attack each time – Twinges or dullness in thoracic arc	– Severe pressure, squeezing or heaviness with a crushing oppressive quality – Report of such severe pain that the patient would rather than experience pain again – Residual 'soreness' of several days following MI
4. Onset and duration – Gradual or sudden onset – Usual duration of 15 minutes or less (usually less than 30 minutes) – Relief by nitroglycerin	– Sudden onset – Duration of 30 minutes to 2 hours – No relief from rest or nitroglycerin
5. Associated clinical manifestations: – Apprehension – Dyspnea – Diaphoresis – Nausea – Desire to void – Belching	– Apprehension – Nausea and vomiting – Dyspnea – Diaphoresis – Extreme fatigue – Dizziness or faintness (after abatement of pain)

Acute nursing interventions for patient with MI are best done in a specialized unit (ICCU). Such nursing includes the initial ICCU stay for 1 to 2 days and the rest of hospitalization for 4 to 6 days. Priorities for nursing intervention in the initial stage of recovery after MI includes pain assessment and relief, physiologic monitoring, promotion of rest and comfort, alleviation of stress and anxiety and understanding of the patient's emotional and behavioral reactions. In initial stages, of emergency management, the nursing responsibility includes:
- Ensure patent airway
- Administer oxygen by nasal cannula or non-rebreather mask
- Insert two IV catheters
- Obtain 12-lead ECG
- Determine location of pain—assess severity using pain scale (0–10)
- Medicate for pain as ordered (e.g. morphine, nitroglycerin)
- Identify underlying rhythm
- Obtain cardiac enzyme levels
- Assess need for thrombolytic therapy as appropriate
- Administer aspirin and beta-adrenergic blockers for cardiac-related chest pain unless contraindicated.

Ongoing monitoring by nurses include the following:
- Monitor vital signs, level of consciousness, cardiac rhythm, and O_2 saturation
- Monitor pain and remedicate as needed
- Reassure patient
- Anticipate need for intubation if respiratory distress is evident
- Prepare for CPR, defibrillation, transcutaneous pacing, or cardioversion.

And nurses should keep in mind that common medication used for coronary artery disease and nursing intervenstion during their administration as follows:

1. Antiplatelet agents (aspirin, ticlopidine) inhibits platelet aggregation: Aspirin should be prescribed unless a true hypersensitivity reaction is present or the patient has a severe risk of bleeding.
2. Nitrates (isosorbide dinitrate, isosorbide mononitrate, nitroglycerin): Nitrate decreases myocardial oxygen by vasodilate, peripherally vasodilate, increase myocardial oxygen supply and coronary vasodilate. Patient should be lying or sitting with administration of sublingual nitrates. Intravenous nitroglycerin is titrated to relief of symptoms

or limiting side effects such as headache or systolic BP less than 90 mm Hg. IV preparations are usually replaced with oral or topical preparation when the patient has been symptom-free for 24 hours. Cautiously use with known aortic stenosis. Anticipate headache develop within 24 hours. A nitrate-free interval of 6 to 8 hours may improve responsiveness to therapy.

Topical nitrates must be cleaned from the skin surface before applying new dose. Appropriate areas of application include any hair-free area, preferably in noticeable areas when the initial dose is being determined. Application areas should be rotated. Gloves should be worn when applying topical preparation.

3. Beta blockers (atenolol, metoprolol, timolol, esmolol, propranolol): Beta blocker decreases myocardial oxygen demand by decreasing contractility, slow heart rate, slow impulse conduction, decreased BP. They also increase myocardial O_2 supply, slow heart rate, thereby increasing diastolic filling time and coronary perfusion and decreases incidence of morbidity and mortality after MI. IV Metoprolol is given in 5 mg increments over 1 to 2 minutes. Other beta blockers may be prescribed IV instead metoprolol. All IV preparations are followed by oral preparations after patient is stabilized. Monitor for atrioventricular block including PR interval, symptomatic bradycardia hypotension, left ventricular failure (rales, decrease CO) and bronchospasm. Beta 1 cardioselective agents are the profound drugs. Beta 2 agents should be avoided in patients with respiratory or peripheral vascular disease. Target heart rate for beta-blockade is 50 to 60 beats per minute.
4. Calcium channel blockers (amlodipine, diltiazem, verapamil, nifedipine) which decrease myocardial oxygen demand and increase in myocardial oxygen supply by inhibiting the influx of calcium through the slow calcium channels Heart rate decreases and conduction through the AV node slows (decreases demand indirectly increases supply). Inhibition of calcium influx into the arterial cell also promotes vasodilation of peripheral arteries (decreased demand) and coronary arteries (increased supply).

   They often prescribed when vasospasm is considered as the part of the pathology or if significant hypertension exists. Monitor for symptomatic bradycardia, prolonger PR intervals advanced heart blocks, hypotension, congestive heart failure and peripheral edema.
5. Heparin (intravenous) prevents propagation of established thrombus by rapidly inhibiting thrombin. Nursing intervention here includes that heparin PTTs should be measured 6 hours after any change in dose. Dose is weight based. Therapeutic levels should be maintained between 1.5 and 2.5 times patient's control. Hemoglobin, hematocrit, and platelets should be followed for heparin-induced thrombocytopenia. Recurrent ischemia, active bleeding and hypotension may signify subtherapeutic or supratherapeutic dosage should be evaluated immediately.
6. Thrombolytics (Streptokinase, tissue plasminogen activator). They are given in acute myocardial infarction to activate plasmin for lysis of obstructive clots specific, therefore, systemic lysis may occur. Patients must be carefully screened before administration of thrombolytic agents. The nurse monitors for reperfusion, reocclusion and bleeding complications with thrombolysis administration. Interventions are directed towards preventing bleeding complications.
7. Morphine sulfate blunts the deleterious consequences of sympathetic stimulation with pain, and vasodilates creating decreased preload. Here, nurse should establish baseline vital signs, level of consciousness and orientation. Monitor for hypotension, respiratory depression changes in level of consciousness. Doses are usually given in increments of 2 to 5 mg.
8. Oxygen increases arterial O_2 saturation. Monitor for adequate arterial oxygenation with finger pulse oximetry. Maintain saturation level by about 90%.
9. Cholesterol lowering agent (atorvastatin, lovastatin, pravastatin, simvastatin, gemfibrozil, nicotinic acid) they reduce the substance for lipid deposition in the coronary artery. Side effects vary with drug class. Insolence of side may limit the usefulness of certain medications. Lipid levels should be obtained at regular intervals to monitor for success in effecting charges. Patients must be educated that cholesterol-lowering agents do not substitute for dietary modification.
10. Angiotensin-converting enzyme inhibitor (captopril, enalapril, benazepril, lisinopril, fosinopril). They decrease afterload and preload, thereby decreasing the workload of the heart. This prevents remodeling of the left ventricle (remodeling refers to hypertrophy of the unaffected left ventricle to compensate for the infarcted area). Long-term consequences of remodeling are increased oxygen demand and heart failure. During their administration, nurse monitors for adverse affects: angioneurotic edema, cough, hypotension, hyperkalemia, pruritic rash, renal failure. First dose requires taking BP before and 30 minutes after administration. NPO (-Nil per orally) in coronary artery diseases may be treated with following procedures.
    - Intra-aortic balloon (IABP)
    - Percutaneous transluminal coronary angioplasty (PTCA)
    - Intracoronary stunting
    - Coronary artery bypass graft (CABP).

Health teaching for patients with coronary artery disease include use and storage of nitroglycerin in case of angina and guidelines for sexual activity after MI, risk factors, modification and resumption of activities.

1. Use and storage of nitroglycerin.
   - Sit or lie down at onset of angina/chest pain
   - Place tablet under the tongue and allow tablet to dissolve, do not chew
   - If pain not relieved within 5 minutes, take a second tablet. A third tablet can be used after an additional 5 minutes if pain persists. Continuing pain after 3 tablets and 15 minutes indicate need to receive immediate medical attention
   - Tablet will cause tingling sensation under the tongue
   - Rest for 15 to 20 minutes after taking nitroglycerin to avoid faintness
   - A tablet with the physician's permission may be taken 10 minutes before an activity known to trigger an anginal attack
   - Anticipate the occurrence of hypotension, tachycardia, and headache in response to the medication. Headache may persist for 15 to 20 minutes after administration
   - Keep a record of number of anginal attacks experienced, the number of tablets needed to obtain pain relief and precipitating factors if known
   - Carry tablets for immediate use if necessary. Do not pack in luggage when traveling
   - Keep tablets in tightly-closed original container. Tablets need to be protected from exposure to light and moisture
   - Tablet should be stored in a cool dry place
   - Check expiry date on prescription. Tablet should be discarded after 6 months once the bottle has been opened. Plan for replacement of supply.
2. Risk factor modification.
   - Provide specific instruction on smoking cessation, daily exercise and diet modification
   - Consider referral to a smoking cessation program or outpatient cardiac rehabilitation program
   - Encourage adherence to a diet low in calories saturated fats and cholesterol
   - Discuss the benefits of stress management techniques in decreasing negative effect on oxygen demand. Refer to individual or group counseling as needed.
3. Resumption of activities.
   - Provide specific instructions on activities that are permissible and those that should be avoided
   - Discuss resumption of driving and return to work
   - Discuss guidelines for resuming sexual relations (e.g. 2 weeks for low risk patients to 4 weeks for post-CABG patients) as given below:

During sex, your heart beats should be about 117 items a minute.

Stages of sexual response

Arousal: Flushed, breathing and heart rate increase, BP goes up slightly.

Plateau: Increase in respiration, BP and heart rate.

Orgasm: (15 to 20 seconds): Pulse may reach 150 beats per min. BP reaches 160/90.

Resolution: Return to resting state within second; angina or palpations are most likely to occur during resolution.

General guidelines for sexual activity in MI

- Sexual foreplay at a relaxed pace allows your heart rate and BP to increase more slowly
- Hugging, stroking, and touching are safe ways to get back in touch with your partner
- Talk with your partner. Express your feelings
- Extramarital affairs or sex with new partner may produce more stress
- Avoid positions for sex that require you to support yourself on your arms for a long time
- Have a sex in a pleasant, comfortable environment
- Do not take very hot or cold baths or showers before or after sex
- Be rested before sex
- Do not have sex after a heavy meal or drinking alcohol
- If you have any question about side effects of any drug, do not stop taking the drug, but talk to your health care provider
- Masturbation and manual or oral stimulation are not harmful to your heart. Anal intercourse may lead to an irregular heartbeat. Avoid this choice unless you clear it with your health care professional.

Treatment of MI

The treatment of MI is aimed at the following.

- Protection of ischemic and injured heart tissue to preserve muscle function
- Reduce the infarct size and prevent death
- Early restoration of coronary blood flow by innovation modalities,
- Use of pharmacologic agents to improve oxygen supply and demand, reduce and/or prevent dysrhythmias, and inhibit the progression of coronary artery disease
- Endogenous catecholamines release during pain imposes an increased workload on the heart muscle, thus causing an increase in oxygen demand.

Thus, the treatment modalities will include:

Use rapid transit to the hospital.

Obtain 12 lead electrocardiogram (ECG) to be read within 10 minutes.

Obtain laboratory blood specimens or cardiac biomarkers, including troponin.

Obtain other diagnostics to clarify the diagnosis.

Begin routing medical interventions:

- Supplemental oxygen
- Nitroglycerin
- Morphine
- Aspirin 162 to 325 mg

- Beta-blocker
- Angiotensin-converting enzyme inhibitor within 24 hours
- Anticoagulation with heparin and platelet inhibitors.

Evaluate for indications for reperfusion therapy:

- Percutaneous coronary intervention
- Thrombolytic therapy

Continue therapy as indicated

- Intravenous heparin, low-molecular-weight heparin, bivalirudin, or fondaparinux
- Clopidogrel (plavix)
- Glycoprotein IIb/IIIa inhibitor
- Bed rest for a minimum of 12 to 24 hours
- The patient should be admitted in ICU of the hospital
- The patient is given resuscitation if required and oxygen inhalation for respiratory distress. Good oxygen therapy improves oxygenation to ischemic heart muscle
- The patient is given analgesic to control pain. An opiate analgesic therapy includes:
  - Morphine is used to relieve pain, improve cardiac hemodynamics by reducing preload, and afterload, and to provide anxiety relief. Those who are allergic to morphine-meperidine may be given to avoid respiratory depressions
  - Nitroglycerin may be administered IV (severe cases) sublingual or paste, to promote venous (low-dose) and arterial (high-dose) relaxation as well as relaxation of coronary vessels and prevention of coronary spasm
  - Benzodiazepine (Diazepam) are also used with analgesics to reduce anxiety
- In addition following drugs will be used for MI:
  - Thrombolytic agents such as tissue plasminogen activator (activase), streptokinase (streptase), and urokinase (abbokinase) are used to re-establish blood flow in coronary vessels by dissolving obstructing thrombus through IV or intracoronary. During administration of thrombolytics following points to be kept in mind:

    Indications

    - Chest pain for longer than 20 minutes, unrelieved by nitroglycerin
    - ST-segment elevation in at least two leads that face the same area of the heart
    - Less than 6 hours from onset of pain.

    Absolute contraindications

    - Active bleeding
    - Known bleeding disorder
    - History of hemorrhagic stroke
    - History of intracranial vessel malformation
    - Recent major surgery or trauma
    - Uncontrolled hypertension
    - Pregnancy.

    Nursing considerations

    - Minimize the number of times the patient's skin is punctured
    - Avoid intramuscular injections
    - Draw blood for laboratory tests when starting the IV line
    - Start IV lines before thrombolytic therapy; designate one line to use for blood draws
    - Avoid continual use of noninvasive blood pressure cuff
    - Monitor for acute dysrhythmias and hypotension
    - Monitor for reperfusion: Resolution of angina or acute ST-segment changes
    - Check for signs and symptoms of bleeding: Decrease in hematocrit and hemoglobin values, decrease in blood pressure, increase in heart rate, oozing or bulging at invasive procedure sites, back pain, muscle weakness, changes in level of consciousness, complaints of headache
    - Treat major bleeding by discontinuing thrombolytic therapy and any anticoagulants; apply direct pressure and notify the physician immediately
    - Treat minor bleeding by applying direct pressure if accessible and appropriate; continue to monitor
  - Along with thrombolytic agents, anticoagulants are also useful for patients who are in situations like prolonged bedrest, pulmonary embolism, deep vein thrombosis, mural thrombi, cardiogenic shock and atrial fibrillation, e.g. Heparin by subcutaneously and every 8 hours
  - Beta-adrenergic blocking agents (e.g. metaoprolol as prescribed) are used for the purpose of limiting the extent of cardiac damage and to improve oxygen supply and demand, decrease sympathetic stimulation to the heart, promote blood flow in the small vessels of the heart, and antidysrhythmic effects
  - For control of arrhythmia, hypokalemia if present, is corrected, and the patient is given lignocaine (xylocaine) as prescribed. Lignocaine decreases ventricular irritability, which commonly occurs in postmyocardial infarction
  - Calcium channel blockers also may be used to improve the balance between oxygen supply and demand by decreasing heart rate, blood pressure and dilating coronary vessels
  - In cases of sinus bradycardia, hypotension or syncope, the patient is given atropine sulfate 0.3 mg by IV and repeated if necessary
  - If the hypotension is severe due to arrhythmias, treatment is with direct current shock. In cases of ventricular fibrillation, treatment given with direct current shock. If it fails cardiac massage, alternating with direct mouth-to-mouth resuscitation is given until defibrillator is available. The patient is also given IV infusion of 8.4 percent solution of sodium bicarbonate, 50–100 mL. Thereafter, lignocaine IV and follow-up as prescribed by the physician.

Nursing Management

- The patient is kept in rest with restriction of patients' physical activity and is advised to avoid alcohol and for abstinence from smoking (if they are in that habit). Once the acute phase is over, the patient can gradually increase physical activity and it is usually taking 6 weeks time to resume normal life
- In nursing assessment the nurse should gather information regarding patient's chest pain, its nature, intensity, onset and duration, location and radiation and also precipitating and aggravating factors (any maneuvers and medications alleviating pain)
  - And also observe other symptoms experienced associated with pain, i.e. diaphoresis, facial pallor, dyspnea, guarding behaviors, rigid posture, weakness, and confusion
  - And also previous health status, current medication, allergies, (opiate analgesics, iodine, shellfish) recent trauma or surgery, aspirin ingestion, peptic ulcers, fainting spells, drug and alcohol use and also any significant ones
- The probable nursing diagnoses will be:
  - Pain related to an imbalance in oxygen supply and demand
  - Anxiety related to chest pain, fear of death, threatening environment
  - Decreased cardiac output related to impaired contractility.
  - Activity intolerance related to insufficient oxygenation to perform ADL and deconditioning effects of bedrest.
  - Risk for injury (bleeding) related to dissolution of protective clot.
  - Altered tissue perfusion (Myocardial), related to coronary restenosis and extension of infarction.

Major goals of the patient include relief of symptoms of ischemia (chest pain, ST segment changes), absence of respiratory difficulties, adequate tissue perfusion, reduced anxiety, adherence to self-care program, and prevention or early recognition of complications.

The nursing care plan of MI is given in Table 12.2.

TABLE 12.2: Nursing care plan for the patient with an acute myocardial infarction

Problems	Objective	Nursing interventions	Rationales
Nursing Diagnosis #1			
Tissue perfusion, alteration in, related to: 1. Coronary artery occlusion resulting in decreased myocardial tissue perfusion 2. Ventricular dysfunction resulting in decreased perfusion to brain, kidneys, lungs and liver 3. Thromboembolism resulting from deep venous thrombosis or mural thrombi	Patient will: 1. Maintain hemodynamic stability: – BP within 10 mm Hg of baseline – HR 60–80/min – Absence of dysrhythmias – Cardiac output 4–8 L/min – Brisk capillary refill (within 2 seconds) – Urine output > 30 mL/h – Mental status: alert oriented 2. Remain without thromboembolic events or, if they occur, thromboembolism will resolve without significant sequelae – Extremities warm to touch; pulses palpable and equal bilaterally – Absence of positive Homan's sign – Circumference of extremities equal bilaterally	• Initiate rest-promoting activities: Bedrest until hemodynamically stable, quiet environment; limit visitors if needed to ensure patient rest • Allow bedside commode privileges if hemodynamically stable • If MI is uncomplicated, patient should be allowed out of bed to the chair for periods of 1–2 hours and should be allowed to use the commode instead of a bedpan from the time of admission • For patient with complicated MI, initiate activities to counteract effects of bedrest – Elevate head of bed when possible – Have patient turn frequently in bed – Teach footboard exercises (limit contraction durations to less than 10 seconds when performing these) – Apply anti-embolism stockings – Consult physician regarding initiation of mini-dose heparin (5,000 units subcutaneously q 8-12 h) • Allow to feed self if able and if patient desires • Assist with bathing the first day and as needed on subsequent days • Monitor for factors that may cause an increase in myocardial oxygen consumption and institute measures to correct these	• Rest decreases myocardial oxygen consumption • Use of bedside commode is associated with less stress than use of a bedpan • Prolonged bedrest is associated with many complications (fluid shifting, orthostatic intolerance, increased heart rate, progressive decalcification resulting in osteoporosis and urolithiasis, and thromboembolism). Early ambulation is the most effective means to combat these • Footboard exercises may decrease venous stasis. Contractions less than 10 seconds in duration cause no significant detrimental cardiovascular response • Self-feeding is less stressful for most patients • Bed bathing is associated with insignificant cardiovascular responses in terms of blood pressure, ECG, heart sounds, oxygen uptake • Hypotension, hypertension, increased heart rate, increased contractility, pain, fever, anemia, volume depletion, and psychological stress cause an increase in myocardial oxygen consumption and may increase infarct size • Pharmacologic measures to increase myocardial oxygen supply or to decrease demand may help to limit infarct size

Contd...

Contd...

Problems	Objective	Nursing interventions	Rationales
		• Administer pharmacologic therapy as ordered (nitrates, nitroprusside, beta-blockers, calcium channel blockers) to increase myocardial oxygen supply or decrease MVO_2 • Administer oxygen as prescribed – Monitor for possible negative effects of O_2 therapy including increased HR and systemic vascular resistance • Monitor for signs and symptoms of pulmonary embolus including tachypnea, tachycardia, shortness of breath anxiety, hypotension, deteriorating oxygenation, pulmonary artery pressure elevation, jugular venous distention • Monitor for signs of deep vein thrombosis: – Positive Homan's sign – Change in color, temperature, or girth of extremity – Presence of tenderness and/or cords	• Oxygen may have negative cardiovascular effects • Early detection and treatment of thromboembolic events may aid in more successful recovery
Nursing Diagnosis #2			
Alteration in cardiac output, related to: 1. Dysrhythmias conduction disturbances 2. Left ventricular dysfunction 3. Hypovolemia	Patient will: 1. Maintain electrophysiologic stability. – Absence of dysrhythmias – 12-lead ECG return to baseline 2. Maintain hemodynamic stability – HR 60–80/min – BP within 10 mm Hg of baseline 3. Be normovolemic. – Cardiac output 4–8 liters/min – Brisk capillary refill (2 seconds)	• Attach to cardiac monitor as soon as possible • Select best lead to monitor based on type of MI patient is having type of conduction disturbance, and needs of monitor, especially if a computerized dysrhythmia detection system is used. Multiple lead monitoring is preferable • Treat lethal dysrhythmias immediately (V-tach, V-fib, asystole) per unit protocols. Notify physician • Be aware of potential significance of warning dysrhythmias—VPBs > 6/ minute, R-on-T VPBs, coupling. • Notify physician and institute treatment of tachyarrhythmias and bradyarrhythmias as soon as possible • Check vital signs (BP, HR, PAP, CVP, CO) with any change in rhythm or conduction • Allow hot or cold beverages in small quantities if patient desires. Elevate head of bed during ingestion • Take oral temperature routinely; rectal temperature may be taken if necessary • Assess for signs and symptoms of left ventricular dysfunction. These include sinus tachycardia; dyspnea, orthopnea; pulmonary rales; S3 gallop, pulsus altern; jugular venous pressure elevation, positive hepatojugular reflex, peripheral or sacral edema; hypotension, elevated pulmonary capillary wedge pressure, elevated central venous pressure, decreased cardiac output and cardiac index	• Early detection of dysrhythmia allows for early treatment • Appropriate lead monitoring allows ECG changes (i.e. ST segment, T wave, PR or QRS interval prolongation) to be seen and treated properly • Prompt treatment of lethal dysrhythmias is more successful than delayed treatment • "Warning dysrhythmias" may precipitate episodes of V-tach, V-fib. These dysrhythmias may also occur without warning • Bradyarrhythmias and tachyarrhythmias may compromise CO, and increase myocardial oxygen consumption • Rhythm or conduction changes may be associated with hemodynamic compromise, particularly in a patient with marginal left ventricular function • Hot or cold beverages in small quantities (1 glass) consumed in a sitting position (at least semi-Fowler's) are not associated with dysrhythmias, ECG changes • Taking oral temperature is less stressful to the patient • Rectal route is not associated with vagal stimulation and thus may be used if necessary • Myocardial ischemia and/or infarct predisposes patient to left ventricular dysfunction • Degree of LV dysfunction is a major determinant of post-MI mortality

Contd...

Contd...

Problems	Objective	Nursing interventions	Rationales
		• Assess for signs of ventricular septal defect (VSD) including a holosystolic murmur heard best at the lower left sternal border; left-to-right shunting; signs of heart failure as above with the degree dependent on the size of the VSD • Assess patient for signs of hypovolemia. These include hypotension (BP may be increased initially); decreased central venous pressure; decreased pulmonary capillary wedge pressure; tachycardia; oliguria; decreased cardiac output and cardiac index	• Myocardial damage may result in a defect in the ventricular septal wall • Vomiting, severe diaphoresis, aggressive treatment with diuretics or nitrates may deplete intravascular volume
Nursing Diagnosis #3			
Alteration in comfort: Pain, related to: 1. Myocardial ischemia, necrosis 2. Extension of infarct 3. Pericarditis 4. Dressler's syndrome (late pericarditis)	Patient will: 1. Be pain free 2. Notify staff immediately of chest pain episodes 3. Maintain hemodynamic stability: – BP with 10 mm Hg of baseline – HR at rest: 60–80/minute without dysrhythmias – Mental status: Alert and oriented to person, place, and time – Urinary output greater than 30 mL/h	• Have patient describe pain, including location, radiation, associated symptoms (nausea, vomiting, diaphoresis, shortness of breath, palpitations), precipitating factors, quality, duration, relief mechanisms, association with movement, respiration or palpation • Administer nitrates and/or narcotic analgesia as needed and monitor response to therapy • Monitor vital signs before and per unit protocol after medication administration. Assess for hypotension, tachycardia, and respiratory depression. Assess for relief of pain • Obtain 12-lead ECG prior to medication administration, particularly if this is undiagnosed or new-onset chest pain, or recurrence of chest pain in a patient who has been pain free for 24 hours • Stay with patient until ischemic chest pain is relieved • Assess patient for pericarditis or Dressler's syndrome (depending on time interval after MI) if recurrent MI and infarct extension have been ruled out. Symptoms of pericarditis or Dressler's syndrome may include: – Chest pain increased by deep inspiration – Chest pain alleviated by leaning forward – Presence of a pericardial friction rub – ECG changes associated with pericarditis (diffuse or localized ST segment elevation, with upward concavity) – Atrial arrhythmias – Persistent fever > 101°F (38.3°C) – Symptoms of pleuritis, pericardial effusion, or tamponade – Response to aspirin or indomethacin – If patient is on anticoagulant medication, check with physician about continuation	• Description helps to determine-etiology of chest pain • Nitrates help to relieve pain by means of coronary vasodilatation and both preload and afterload reduction. Narcotics act centrally to relieve pain and also have some afterload reducing effects • Significant change in vital signs (BP decrease > 10 mm Hg and/or HR increase > 20 beats/min and/or respiratory rate < 10/min) may necessitate discontinuation of medication • Documentation of changes on a 12-lead ECG helps to make the diagnosis of cardiac chest pain (vs. other types of chest discomfort), and also helps to diagnose infarct extension, Prinzmetal's angina, or pericarditis • Presence of caring, supportive, knowledgeable nurse may reduce patient anxiety, which reduces stress response. This causes reduced circulating catecholamines (epinephrine), which help to increase the pain threshold, thereby reducing myocardial oxygen consumption • Either condition may occur following myocardial infarction, particularly following transmural MIs. Symptoms are similar. Time courses are somewhat similar and overlap does occur, sometimes making it difficult to distinguish between these two syndromes – Anticoagulants may precipitate cardiac tamponade

Contd...

Contd...

Problems	Objective	Nursing interventions	Rationales
Nursing Diagnosis #4			
Anxiety, related to: 1. Knowledge deficit regarding illness and its prognosis 2. Pain 3. Intensive care setting 4. Disruption of daily life activities, role and self-image changes, family concerns	Patient will: 1. Verbalize basic understanding of his/her illness 2. Verbalize feeling less anxious 3. Describe pain and verbalize when it is relieved 4. Verbalize familiarity with ICU routines and practices	• Assess level of understanding of disease process and readiness to learn – Provide patient with appropriate information on coronary artery disease and myocardial infarction when patient is ready – Reassure patient appropriately regarding prognosis – Initiate other anxiety-relieving measures; remain with patient during stressful periods or when patient needs to talk; encourage to verbalize fears and anxieties; listen attentively; explain all procedures and equipment involved in the patient's care; involve in decision-making whenever possible; instruct in relaxation techniques; limit nursing personnel caring for patient to increase continuity; orient patient and family to all ICU routines • Assess for signs and symptoms of anxiety: Restlessness, agitation, tachycardia, tachypnea, diaphoresis, crying, uncooperative or non-compliant behavior, verbalization of fears, concerns, inability to concentrate • Administer nitrates and/or narcotic medications until pain is relieved or until significant decrease in BP occurs ($< 90–100$ mm Hg) – Administer sedatives as needed. • Manipulate ICU environment to promote as much rest for patient as possible. • Assess family members' coping abilities • Support family members in dealing with their own as well as patient's needs • Encourage family members to avoid stressful and controversial issues at this time • Assess family members' level of knowledge and educate appropriately when they are ready • Allow family members to verbalize fear, concerns • Facilitate family visiting by individualizing visiting hours to patient and family needs • Assess need for spiritual counselor	• Fear and anxiety initiate the stress response. This causes increased catecholamine release, which causes increased myocardial oxygen consumption (MVO_2), as well as decreasing the pain threshold, which further increases MVO_2 – Presence of a caring supportive individual may help to increase patient's ability to cope – Knowing what to expect help to reduce anxiety – Maintaining some sense of control helps to reduce anxiety – Use of relaxation techniques helps to promote a sense of control over situation • Underlying cause of anxiety must be determined in order to provide appropriate intervention – Some behaviors may be helpful during the acute phase of an MI, as for example, denial • Pain precipitates and/or aggravates anxiety • Narcotics alleviate chest discomfort and also decrease anxiety and increase the patient's sense of well-being • Mild sedation helps to decrease anxiety and increase sense of well-being • Physical rest reduces myocardial oxygen consumption, promotes a sense of well-being and reduces anxiety • Family coping behaviors influence patient's coping abilities and may positively or negatively affect patient's level of anxiety • Family members' lack of knowledge may influence their level of anxiety and ultimately patient's anxiety level • Short artificially terminated visiting hours are arousing to patient's cardiovascular system and may increase anxiety and myocardial oxygen consumption • Spiritual support is helpful to some patients to decrease anxiety
Nursing Diagnosis #5			
Coping, potential intellective individual, related to: 1. Diagnosis and fear of death	Patient will: 1. Verbalize feelings of fear and depression	• Assess for symptoms of depression, including anorexia, insomnia, listlessness, crying, expression of feelings of hopelessness, lack of self-esteem	• Depression may interfere with patient's ability to deal realistically with situation and may compromise patient's recovery

Contd...

Contd...

Problems	Objective	Nursing interventions	Rationales
	2. Use denial (if he/she chooses) as a defense mechanism to control fear and anxiety but not to interfere with ultimate acceptance of prognosis and rehabilitation program	• Encourage to verbalize feelings • Assess use of denial as a defense mechanism; signs of this include explicit verbal denial, inappropriate cheerfulness, unrealistic non-compliance with medical regimen • Support appropriate use of denial by the patient • Monitor physiologic parameters (HR + BP) closely during conversations that deal with potentially stressful topics	• Denial is commonly used by patients after an MI to deal with the overwhelming anxiety associated with having an MI. Survival rate during the first few days of CCU care is higher in patients who effectively deny their illness • HR and rhythm changes may occur when patient engages in conversations about stressful topics (pain, symptoms before admission, concerns about death, the consequences of death for their dependents, the consequences of continued survival, the life problems that await them after discharge, the difficulties they had with compliance, and guilt about noncompliance and its contribution to their present illness)
Nursing Diagnosis #6			
Sexual patterns, potentially altered, related to: 1. Fear and lack of knowledge about sexual activity after a myocardial infarction	Patient and/or significant other will: 1. Feel comfortable expressing concerns about sexuality 2. Verbalize that sexual activity is a form of exercise 3. Be able to verbalize criteria for "safe sex" after an MI 4. Be able to verbalize practices to be avoided	• Answer patient's (or significant other's) questions regarding sex directly and honestly • Describe the following guidelines to patient: – Sex may be resumed when patient can climb 20 steps in 10 seconds without symptoms or when HR rises to 110–120 bpm without causing chest pain or shortness of breath – Encourage foreplay before intercourse – Inform patient that intercourse in a familiar place, with a familiar partner, and in a familiar position has very little risk • Describe the things to avoid: – Anal intercourse – Sex when fatigued or after a large meal or heavy alcohol intake – Sex in very hot or cold environment	• Patient who brings this up during ICU stay is obviously anxious about it. Answering questions directly and honestly should decrease anxiety – These activities are the metabolic equivalent of sexual intercourse and can be used as guidelines for when the patient is physically ready to resume sexual activities – Foreplay allows HR and BP to increase gradually – Familiarity with place, partner, and position is associated with less anxiety – Anal intercourse may precipitate vagal stimulation and bradycardia – These increase metabolism demands and workload on the heart – Same as above

Nursing Interventions

Relieving Chest Pain

- Administer vasodilator (e.g. nitroglycerin), anticoagulant (heparin) medications, and aspirin as prescribed to preserve heart muscle
- Provide thrombolytic therapy if patient clinically qualifies
- Administer analgesic agents (morphine sulfate)
- Administer oxygen in tandem with analgesia to ensure maximum relief of pain (inhalation of oxygen reduces pain associated with low levels of circulating oxygen)
- Assess vital signs, as long as patient is experiencing pain
- Assist patient to rest with back elevated or in cardiac chair to decrease chest discomfort and dyspnea.

Resolution of pain is the primary clinical indicator that myocardial oxygen demand and supply are in equilibrium.

Improving Respiratory Function

- Assess respiratory functions to detect early signs of complications
- Pay attention of fluid volume status to prevent overloading the heart and lungs
- Encourage patient to breathe deeply and change position often to prevent pooling of fluid in lung bases.

Promoting Adequate Tissue Perfusion

- Keep patient on bed or chair rest to reduce cardiac workload
- Check skin temperature and peripheral pulses frequently to determine adequate tissue perfusion
- Administer oxygen to enrich supply of circulating oxygen.

Reducing Anxiety

- Develop a trusting and caring relationship with patient
- Provide frequent and private opportunities to share concerns and fears
- Provide an atmosphere of acceptance to help patient know that his or her feelings are realistic and normal.

Monitoring and Managing Complications

Monitor closely for cardinal signs and symptoms that signal onset of complications.

Promoting Home and Community-based Care

Teaching Patients Self-Care

- Educate about the disease process.
- Work with patient to develop a plan to meet specific needs to enhance compliance.

To extend and improve the quality of life, a patient who has had an MI must adjust his or her lifestyle to promote heart-healthy living. With this in mind, the nurse and patient develop a program to help the patient achieve desired outcomes.

Lifestyle Recommendations During Convalescence and Healing

Adaptation to an MI is an ongoing process and usually inquires some modification of lifestyle. Instruct patients to make the following specific modifications:

- Avoid any activity that produces chest pain, extreme dyspnea, or undue fatigue
- Avoid extremes of heat and cold and walking against the wind
- Lose weight, if indicated
- Stop smoking and use of tobacco; avoid secondhand smoke
- Develop heart-healthy eating patterns and avoid large meals and hurrying while eating
- Modify meals to align with the Therapeutic Lifestyle Changes (TLC) or other recommended diet
- Adhere to medical regimen, especially in taking medications
- Follow recommendations that ensure blood pressure and blood glucose are in control
- Pursue activities that relieve and reduce stress.

Adoption of an Activity Program

Additionally, the patient needs to undertake a structured program of activity and exercise for long-term rehabilitation. Advise patients to:

- Engage in a regimen of physical conditioning with a gradual increase in activity duration and then a gradual increase in activity intensity
- Walk daily, increasing distance and time as prescribed
- Monitor pulse rate during physical activity
- Avoid physical exercise immediately after a meal
- Alternate activity with rest periods (some fatigue is normal and expected during convalescence)
- Participate in a daily program of exercise that develops into a program of regular exercise for a lifetime.

Managing Symptoms

The patient must learn to recognize and take appropriate action for recurrent symptoms. Make sure that patients know to do the following:

- Call 911 if chest pressure or pain (or prodromal symptoms) is not relieved in 15 minutes by nitroglycerin
- Contact the physician if any of the following occur: Shortness of breath, fainting, slow or rapid heartbeat, swelling of feet and ankles.

Preparing for Cardiac Rehabilitation

Goals of rehabilitation for the patient with MI are to extend and improve quality of life. The immediate objective are to limit the effects and progression of atherosclerosis, return patient to work and pre-illness lifestyle, enhance patients psychosocial and vocational status, and prevent another cardiac event.

- Encourage physical activity and physical conditioning
- Educate patient and family
- Provide counseling and behavioral interventions when necessary.

SHOCK

Shock is defined as a complex, life-threatening condition (or syndrome) characterized by inadequate blood flow to the tissues and cells of the body (Rice 1991). In other words, it is a failure of the circulatory system to maintain adequate perfusion of vital organs. Various disorders leading to inadequate tissue perfusion. This inadequate oxygenation results in anaerobic cellular metabolism and accumulated waste products in cells. If the condition is untreated, cell and organ death occurs.

Adequate blood flow to the cells and tissues require the following components.

- An adequate cardiac pump
- An effective vasculature or circulatory system and
- Adequate blood volume.

If one of these components is impaired, blood flow to the tissues will be threatened or compromised. Inadequate blood flow to the tissues results in inadequate oxygen and nutrients to the cells, cellular starvation, cell death, organ failure and

Box 12.7 Effect of shock on organs and organ systems

Organ or organ system	Effect
Lungs	Acute respiratory failure Acute respiratory distress syndrome
Renal system	Renal failure
Heart	Dysrhythmias Myocardial ischemia Myocardial depression
Liver	Abnormal clotting Decreased production of plasma proteins Elevated serum levels of ammonia, bilirubin and liver enzymes
Immune system	Depletion of defense components
Gastrointestinal system	Mucosal injury Paralytic ileus Pancreatitis Absorption of endotoxins and bacteria
Central nervous system	Ischemic damage, necrosis, brain death

eventual death if not treated. Thus, shock is a clinical syndrome resulting in decreased blood flow to body tissues, causing cellular dysfunction and eventual organ failure. Regardless of the cause of shock the end result is inadequate supply of oxygen and nutrients to body cells from impaired tissue perfusion.

Shock affects all body systems (Box 12.7). It may develop rapidly or slowly depending on the underlying cause. During shock the body struggle to survive, calling on all its homeostatic mechanisms to restore blood flow and tissue perfusion. Shock may occur as a complication of many disorders and therefore all patients have the potential to develop shock.

Shock is a complex clinical syndrome that may occur at any time and in any place. It is a life-threatening condition often requiring team action by many health care providers including nurses, physicians, laboratory technicians, etc.

Shock causes thousands of deaths and unknown number of permanent injuries every year. Because shock is potentially lethal, it is essential that nurses are able to identify clients at risk of developing shock, recognize the early assessment finding indicating shock, and initiate appropriate interventions before shock ensues. In order to recognize the development of shock, it is important for the nurses to understand the process taking place in the body.

Classification of Shock

There have been many attempts to classify shock, but none of these have been total satisfaction. Here, one classification suggested by many is that it is based on a consideration of defects in the three primary mechanisms responsible for adequate circulation:

i. Defect in vascular tone, i.e. distributive shock
ii. Defect in the ability of the heart to act as a pump, i.e. cardiogenic shock
iii. Defect in the intravascular volume, i.e. hypovolemic shock.

Distributive Shock

Distributive or vasogenic shock occurs when there is a maldistribution of the blood volume in the vasculature. It is due to changes in blood vessel tone, that increases the size of the vascular space without an increase in the circulating blood volume. This results in relative hypovolemia (total fluid volume remains the same but is redistributed). Vasogenic shock is further divided into three types, i.e. anaphylactic, neurogenic and septic shock.

i. Anaphylactic Shock

It is a severe hypersensitivity reaction resulting in massive systemic vasodilation. The precipitating factors of this anaphylactic shock will include drugs (penicillin), insect bites/stings, contrast media, blood transfusions, anesthetic agents, foods and vaccine. Anaphylactic shock is an acute and potentially life-threatening allergic reaction. It is an immediate hypersensitive reaction characterized by dilatation of arterioles and capillaries and increased capillary permeability causing microvascular leakage throughout the body. Anaphylactic shock can result in respiratory failure as a result of laryngeal edema or severe bronchospasm and circulatory failure resulting from vasodilatation.

ii. Neurogenic Shock

Neurogenic shock is an uncommon and often transitory disorder, is caused by massive vasodilatation as a result of loss of sympathetic vasoconstrictor tone in the vascular smooth muscle and impairment of autonomic function. The massive vasodilatation causes pooling of blood in the venous vasculature, decreased venous return to the heart, decreased cardiac output, and eventually inadequate tissue perfusion. Typically, the patient in neurogenic shock which develop hypotension and bradycardia. There are several precipitating factors that can lead to neurogenic shock, which includes injury and disease to the spinal cord; spinal anesthesia, deep general anesthesia or epidural block; and vasomotor center depression due to severe pain, drugs, hypoglycemia and emotional stress.

iii. Septic Shock

Septic shock, the most common type of circulatory shock, is caused by widespread infection. Gram-negative bacteria are the most common pathogens. Other infectious agents, such as gram-positive bacteria (increasingly) and viruses and fungi, can also cause septic shock.

Risk Factors

Conditions placing patients at risk for septic shock are immunosuppression, extremes of age (younger than 1 year and older than 65 years of age), alcoholism, malnourishment, extensive trauma or burns, chronic illness, diabetes, malignancy, and invasive procedure.

Pathophysiology

Microorganism invasion causes an immune response. This immune response activates biochemical mediators associated with an inflammatory response and produces a variety of effects leading to shock. The resulting increased capillary permeability, with and fluid loss from the capillaries and vasodilation, results in inadequate perfusion of oxygen and nutrients to the tissues and cells.

Septic shock is due to a release of vasoactive substances. It is more commonly caused by gram-negative bacteria, although many patients with septic shock never have positive blood culture. Septic shock can also occur secondary to staphylococcal, streptococcal, fungal and protozoal infections. The causes of septic shock will include:

- Infections e.g. urinary tract, respiratory tract, postabortion, postpartum, caused by invasive procedures, and indwelling lines and catheter
- Compromised patients including older adults, patients with chronic diseases (diabetes, cancer and AIDS), patients receiving immunosuppressive therapy, and malnourished or debilitated patients.

Clinical Manifestations

First Phase: Hyperdynamic or "Progressive" Phase

- High cardiac output with vasodilation
- Hyperthermia (febrile) with warm, flushed skin bounding pulses
- Heart and respiratory rates elevated
- Blood pressure may remain within normal limits
- Subtle changes in mental status
- Urinary output decreased or normal
- Gastrointestinal status compromised (e.g. decrease sounds, nausea, vomiting, or diarrhea).

Later Phase: Hypodynamic or "Irreversible" Phase

- Low cardiac output with vasoconstriction
- Decreased blood pressure
- Skin cool and pale
- Temperature normal or below normal
- Heart and respiratory rates rapid
- Anuria and multiple organ dysfunction progressing to failure.

Septic shock may be manifested by atypical or confusing clinical signs. Suspect septic shock in any elderly person who develop an unexplained acute confused state, tachypnea, or hypotension.

Medical Management

- Urine, blood, sputum, and wound drainage specimens collected to identify and eliminate the cause of infection
- Broad-spectrum antibiotic therapy begins immediately and potential routes of infection are eliminated (intravenous lines rerouted if necessary). Abscesses are drained and necrotic areas debrided.
- Fluid replacement is instituted and aggressive nutritional supplementation (high protein) is provided. Enteral feedings are preferred.
- Treatment with recombinant human activated protein C (APC), an antithrombotic, anti-inflammatory, and profibrinolytic agent proved to reduce mortality.

Nursing Management

- Identify patients at risk for sepsis and septic shock
- Carry out all invasive procedures with correct aseptic technique and follow with careful hand washing
- Monitor for signs of infection at intravenous lines, arterial and venous puncture sites, surgical incisions, trauma wounds, urinary catheters and pressure ulcers
- Reduce patient's temperature when ordered for temperatures above 104.8°F (40.8°C) or if the patient is uncomfortable by administering salicylates, ice bags, and hypothermia blankets; monitor closely for shivering
- Administer prescribed intravenous fluids and medications
- Monitor and report blood levels (antibiotic, blood urea nitrogen, creatinine, white blood count)
- Monitor hemodynamic status, fluid intake and output, and nutritional status
- Monitor daily weights and serum albumin levels to determine daily protein requirements.

Cardiogenic Shock

Cardiogenic shock often referred to as "Pump failure" occurs when heart can no longer pump blood efficiently to all parts of the body and when cardiac output is decreased. There is no decreased intravascular volume or vasodilatation of the vascular space. Cardiogenic shock is the usual result of left ventricular dysfunction. However, the right ventricle also may be involved. The ventricles are the pumping chambers of the heart and when either one fails, blood backs up into the systemic circulation. Left ventricular dysfunction causes blood to back up into pulmonary system causing pulmonary congestion and decreased cardiac output to the systemic circulation. A vicious cycle develops as the SVR increases in response to the decreased cardiac output. The failing heart has to pump harder against this higher systemic resistance.

Cardiogenic shock occurs when the heart has an impaired pumping ability, it may be of coronary or non-coronary origin. It is due to inadequate pumping action of the heart, because of primary cardiac muscle dysfunction or mechanical obstructions of blood flow caused by myocardial infarction (MI). Valvular insufficiency is due to disease or trauma, cardiac dysrhythmias, or an obstructive condition such as pericardial tamponade or pulmonary embolus, pericardial disease, tension pneumothorax, autovalvular damage and pulmonary embolism.

Hypovolemic Shock

In hypovolemic shock, the most common type of shock, a loss of effective circulating blood volume occurs. Hypovolemic shock is caused by external fluid losses form hemorrhage, internal fluid shifts (e.g. severe dehydration, severe edema, or ascites), and fluid losses from prolonged vomiting or diarrhea. Decreased blood volume results in decreased venous return, decreases stroke volume cardiac output, and decreased tissue perfusion.

- Fall in venous pressure, rise in peripheral resistance, tachycardia
- Cold, moist skin; pallor; thirst; diaphoresis
- Altered sensorium, oliguria, metabolic acidosis, tachypnea
- Most dependable criterion: Level of arterial blood pressure.

Medical Management

Goals of treatment are to restore intravascular volume, redistribute fluid volume, and correct the underlying cause. If the patient is hemorrhaging, bleeding is stopped by applying pressure or by surgery. Diarrhea and vomiting are treated with medications.

Fluid and Blood Replacement

- Dual IV lines are inserted to administer fluid, medications and/or blood
- Lactated Ringer's solution, colloids, and 0.9% sodium chloride solution (normal saline) are administered to restore intravascular volume
- Blood products are used only if other alternatives are unavailable or blood loos is extensive and rapid; autotransfusion methods may be considered for closed cavity hemorrhage.

Redistribution of Fluids

Patient is positioned properly to assist in fluid redistribution (modified Trendelenburg). Military antishock trouser (MAST) are used in extreme emergency situations when bleeding cannot be controlled.

Pharmacologic Therapy

The same medications are used that are given in cardiogenic shock. The type medication depends on the underlying cause.

Nursing Management

- Closely monitor patients at risk for fluid deficits (younger than 1 year or older than 65 years of age)
- Assist with fluid replacement before intravascular volume is depleted
- Ensure safe administration of prescribed fluids and medications and document effects
- Monitor and report signs of complications and effects of treatment. Monitor patient closely for adverse effects
- Monitor for cardiovascular overload and pulmonary edema hemodynamic pressure, vital signs, arterial blood gases, and fluid intake and output
- Reduce fear and anxiety about the need for oxygen mask by giving patient explanations and frequent reassurance.

Hypovolemic shock occurs when there is disease in the intravascular volume. It is due to inadequate circulating blood volume resulting from hemorrhage with actual blood loss, burns with a loss of plasma proteins and fluid shifts to dehydration with a loss of fluid volume. Hypovolemic shock is the most common type of shock and develops when the intravascular volume decreases to the point where compensatory mechanisms are unable to maintain organ and tissue perfusion. The precipitating factors of hypovolemic shock as already stated above, to be specific, are given below:

- External fluid losses are due to:
  - Hemorrhage (most common cause)
  - Burns
  - Excessive use of diuretics
  - Loss of GI fluid (vomiting, diarrhea, fistulas, nasogastric suctioning)
  - Diabetes insipidus
  - Diabetic ketoacidosis
  - Profound diaphoresis.
- Internal fluid shifts.
  - Pooling of blood in the interstitial spaces (ascitis, peritonitis and intestinal obstruction)
  - Internal bleeding (fracture of long bones, ruptured spleen, hemothorax, severe pancreatitis, femoral arterial puncture or catheters in patient on anticoagulant therapy).

Pathophysiology of Shock

Shock is a dynamic event in which several different processes may be occurring at the same time. In addition, patient may progress towards death or towards normal homeostatic functioning over widely varying time periods. The shock syndrome can be divided into four stages.

i. Initial stage
ii. Compensatory stage
iii. Progressive stage, and
iv. Irreversible or refractory stage.

Although there are no clear-cut divisions between the stages, in order to understand the pathophysiology of the shock syndrome, these stages are helpful in the management of shock by nurses.

1. Initial Stage

During the initial stage, there will be no clinical sign or symptoms, however, changes are occurring at the cellular level. When body cells lack an adequate blood supply and an adequate supply of oxygen, the ability to metabolize energy is impaired. Energy metabolism occurs within the cell where nutrients are chemically broken down and stored in the form of adenosine triphosphate (ATP). Cells use this stored energy to perform necessary functions such as active transport, muscular contraction and biochemical synthesis as well as specialized cellular function such as the conduction of electrical impulses. ATP can be synthesized aerobically or anaerobically. Aerobic metabolism yields far greater amounts of ATP per mole of glucose than aerobic metabolism and therefore, is a more efficient and effective means of producing energy. Additionally, anaerobic metabolism results in the accumulation of the toxic and product, lactic acid which must be removed from the cell and transported to the liver for conversion into glucose and glycogen.

In shock, the cells lack adequate blood supply and are deprived of oxygen and nutrients, therefore, they must produce energy through anaerobic metabolism. This results in low energy yields from nutrients and an acidotic intracellular environment. The cell swells and its membrane becomes more permeable allowing electrolytes and fluids to seep from and into the cell. The sodium-potassium pump becomes impaired. Cell structures (mitochondria and lysosomes) are damaged and death of the cell results.

2. Compensatory Stage

The compensatory stage is the reversible stage in which compensatory mechanisms are effective in maintaining adequate perfusion to the vital organs. In this stage, most of the metabolic needs of the body continue to be met. Here, regardless of the cause of shock, the body attempts to compensate for a decrease in tissue perfusion in a variety of ways. First, a decrease in arterial pressure causes a similar decrease in capillary hydrostatic pressure. When the hydrostatic pressure no longer exceeds the colloidal osmotic pressure, fluid moves from the interstitial space to the intravascular space. This process is sometimes called "auto-transfusion". It may add sufficient volume to the vascular space to maintain normal arterial pressure without the help of other compensatory mechanisms.

A reduction in mean arterial pressure will inhibit baroreceptor activity, resulting in stimulation of the vasomotor center in the medulla, causing activation of the sympathetic nervous system and release epinephrine. Stimulation of alpha adrenergic receptor causes selective peripheral vasoconstriction. Blood flow to the heart and brain is maintained, whereas the blood flow to the kidneys and skin is decreased. Beta-adrenergic receptors' stimulation causes a mild increase in heart rate and force of contraction, resulting in an increased cardiac output. This sympathetic stimulation causes dilatation of the coronary arteries, resulting in an increase in oxygen to the myocardium, which now has an increased oxygen demand as a result of increase in heart rate and contractility.

The decrease in the blood flow to the kidneys stimulates the release of rennin into the blood. In the bloodstream, renin activates angiotensinogen to produce angiotensin I, which then circulates to the lungs where it is converted to angiotensin II. Angiotensin is a strong vasoconstrictor resulting in arterial and venous constriction. The net result is increased venous return to the heart and an increase in blood pressure. Angiotensin also simultaneously stimulates the adrenal cortex to release aldosterone, which results in sodium reabsorption by the kidneys. The increased reabsorption raises the serum osmolarity and stimulates the release of ADH. The action of ADH results in increased water reabsorption by the kidneys, increased blood volume and increased venous return to the heart. Thus, venous return is increased by the combination of autotransfusion, vasoconstriction and hormonal changes. Increased venous return, as well as increased heart rate and myocardial contractility caused by beta-adrenergic receptor stimulation result in increased cardiac output, maintenance of blood pressure, and adequate tissue perfusion.

The clinical manifestation of the compensatory stage may be subtle and can be overlooked. One of the most reliable signs of this stage is the patient's level of consciousness. Subtle changes in sensorium, usually in the form of restlessness, irritability or apprehension are frequently observed and are primarily caused by hypoxia of brain cells. Sedation at this time is contraindicated because it will mask important neurologic signs. Pupil size may not be an accurate indicator of the degree of shock, because drugs such as atropine and morphine will cause dilatation or constriction of the pupil.

During this stage, the resting supine, blood pressure may be slightly elevated, slightly decreased or normal for the patient. For this reason, blood pressure may not be useful indicator at this stage. Orthostatic hypotension (a decrease in at least 15 mm Hg when a patient is raised from a flat position to an elevation of 90 degrees or standing) is significant and indicated absolute or relative volume depletion.

The heart rate in this stage is moderately increased. The pulse may be bounding or thready, depending on the stroke volume and the degree of peripheral vasoconstriction. Respirations increase in rate and depth in an attempt to compensate for tissue hypoxia, resulting in respiratory alkalosis. Urine output may begin to decrease because of reduced renal perfusion as a result of vasoconstriction. Because of extravascular volume, depletion, the patient complains thirst. In addition, thirst may be caused by decreased secretion of saliva secondary to peripheral vasoconstriction. Vasoconstriction in the skin will result in cool and pale extremities. An exception is septic shock, in which skin may be warm and dry. The body temperature at this stage will be slightly decreased except in septic shock, in which, it may be elevated. Bowel sounds will often be hypoactive because of decreased peristalsis as a result of reduced blood flow to the gastrointestinal system.

3. Progressive Stage

In this stage of shock, compensating mechanisms are becoming ineffective and may even be detrimental to the patient.

Aggressive management is necessary at this stage to reverse the shock stage.

When shock is not detected and the precipitating cause is not corrected during the earlier stages, a massive sympathetic nervous system occurs. Profound vasoconstriction of most vascular beds occurs with some peripheral vessels possibly becoming totally occluded. Renal ischemia leads to activation of the renin-angiotensin mechanism, causing even more pronounced vasoconstriction. Despite the attempt of the body to increase cardiac output by increasing the heart rate and myocardial contractility, there is a net decrease in cardiac output. The decreased cardiac output and profound vasoconstriction leads to tissue hypoxia which causes the cells to undergo anaerobic metabolism. A by-product of anaerobic cellular metabolic is lactic acid production. Metabolic acidosis results from the accumulation of lactic acid and impaired renal excretion of acids. As the shock stage progresses, the rise in the lactic acid level will often correlate with the severity of the shock state. Acidosis has a direct depressant effect on cardiac function by impairing calcium metabolism within myocardial cells.

Associated with the sympathetic nervous system response is the secretion of large amounts of catecholamines from the adrenal medulla. Catecholamines enhance the cellular metabolism of the brain and heart. Catecholamines also stimulate the liver to undergo glycogenolysis, releasing its glycogen stores in the form of glucose. In addition, the pancreatic release of insulin is suppressed. Therefore, the brain, which does not require insulin for glucose utilization, has large quantities of glucose available for metabolism.

The clinical manifestation of progressive stage of shock includes the patient demonstrates listlessness, apathy and confusion. In addition a decreased response to painful stimuli may be observed. When the blood pressure begins to fall, the patient is no longer in compensatory shock. Regardless of the previous blood pressure, a systolic pressure below 80 mm Hg should be regarded as a danger signal. It is important to remember that a hypertensive patient does not often initially display a pressure this low. A guide for determining hypotension is a reduction in blood pressure greater than 25 percent of the baseline for the patient. In addition to hypotension, a narrowed pulse pressure (difference between systolic and diastolic BP) is often present. This finding indicates decreased stroke volume from a decrease in systolic pressure and a normal or elevated diastolic pressure. Since cuff pressures are likely to be inaccurate during this stage of shock because of the severe peripheral vasoconstrictions, intra-arterial monitoring may be used to provide more reliable pressure readings.

Tachycardia is evident during this stage of shock, and the pulse is older adults and patients who are receiving beta-adrenergic blocking drugs may be an exception and show like heart rate change. Respirations increase in rate in an attempt to compensate for tissue hypoxic and metabolic acidosis. However, the respirations become more shallow as the patient begins to tire and weaken. Urine output decreases and fall below 0.5 mL/kg/h indicating inadequate renal perfusion, which can lead to renal failure. The lips and mucosa are dry, and the patient may continue to complain of thirst. The skin is cold, pale and clammy with slow capillary refill noted. There may be cyanosis caused by tissue hypoxia. Body temperature is usually subnormal.

4. Irreversible or Refractory Stage

Irreversible or refractory stage of shock is the stage during which compensatory mechanisms are either nonfunctioning or totally ineffective. Cellular necrosis and multiple organ dysfunction syndrome (MODS) may occur. Attempts to restore the blood pressure have failed and death is imminent.

As shock progresses, the sympathetic nervous system activity can no longer compensate to maintain homeostasis. Thus, one of the major compensatory mechanisms has failed. There is pooling and sludging of blood because of the lack of vasomotor tone. Thrombosis of small blood vessels also occurs. Tissue hypoxia resulting from peripheral vasoconstriction and decreased cardiac output makes it necessary for cells to metabolize anaerobically. The accumulation of lactic acid and other acid metabolites in the body's tissues contribute to cell death. The acid environment also causes increased capillary permeability, allows fluid and plasma proteins to leave the vascular space. Because the venous end of the capillaries remains constricted and the arterial end is dilated, blood pools in the capillary bed. This also causes further peripheral vasoconstrictions and a vicious cycle of decompensation ensues.

As shock progresses, hypotension and the resulting tachycardia decrease coronary blood flow leading to myocardial depression, which further decreases cardiac output. Cerebral ischemia occurs. The body cannot maintain vasoconstriction for long with the vicious cycle repeating itself. Consequently, failure of the medullary vasomotor center occurs, which results in loss of sympathetic tone. The result is respiratory or cardiac arrest and death.

The clinical manifestation of this stage includes all body systems, especially the cardiovascular system, show evidence of decompensation. The patient is usually unconscious and may be unresponsive to all stimuli. The systolic blood pressure continues to fall and may not respond to therapeutic measures to raise it. The diastolic pressure blood pressure falls toward zero. The heart rate becomes progressively slower. The pulse is weak, and a pulse deficit may be present. Cardiac dysrhythmias may develop because of an ischemic myocardium and increased serum potassium levels from the release of potassium from the dead cells.

Box 12.8 Overview of shock

Signs and symptoms	Tachycardia Tachypnea Hypotension Oliguria Cyanosis Altered mental state
Diagnostic test	Decreased hemoglobin Increased lactic acid Decreased hematocrit in hemorrhage Increased WBC in sepsis Decreased pH in metabolic acidosis
Therapeutic measures	Oxygen IV fluids Vasopressor medications Treat underlying cause
Complications	Acute respiratory distress syndrome (ARDS) Disseminated intravascular coagulation (DIC) Multiple organ dysfunction syndrome (MODS)

Because of the respiratory center depression, there are likely to be slow shallow respirations with an irregular rhythm and sometimes Cheyne-Stokes respirations. If the patient is in an ICU, intubation and mechanical ventilation will usually be used. Damage to the pulmonary endothelial cells increases capillary permeability and interstitial and alveolar edema and hemorrhage an impaired gas exchange may occur. The resulting hypoxemia and respiratory acidosis will further decrease tissue oxygen delivery.

Ischemia of the intestinal mucosa also increases permeability, allowing bacteria and their toxins to enter the bloodstream and causing sepsis. Renal ischemia may result in acute tubular necrosis with altered fluid and other metabolic disturbances. Urine output is minimal, and there may be a considerable in serum creatinine and BUN level, indicating some degree of acute renal failure.

The skin is cold and clammy, with a significant decrease in temperature (except in septic shock). Cyanosis may be present and is usually observed in the lips, mucous membranes and nail beds. However, it may be more obvious in the palms, soles and palpebral conjunctiva (inside the eyelids) of dark-skinned patients.

Infection, acute tubular necrosis, acute respiratory distress and disseminated intravascular coagulation are the common complications of shock. An overview of shock is given in Box 12.8.

Management of Shock

It is difficult to know when shock actually exists and when therapy should begin. Treatment should generally be instituted for shock whenever at least two of the following three conditions occur:

- Systolic BP 80 mm Hg or less
- Pulse pressure of 20 mm Hg or less
- Pulse rate of 120 or more.

Pulse pressure is calculated by subtracting diastolic BP from systolic BP. Normally pulse pressure is between 30 and 50 mm Hg.

Emergency Management

Emergency care of the patient in shock is important and may increase greatly the patient's chances of survival. For example, emergency management of hypovolemic shock is as follows:

The possible causes of hypovolemic shock are major traumas resulting in multiple or serious injuries that are associated with blood or fluid loss, esophageal varices, postoperative bleeding, etc.

The possible assessment findings are:

- Decreased level of consciousness
- Restlessness, anxiety and weakness
- Rapid, weak and thready pulse
- Hypotension
- Cool and clammy skin
- Tachypnea, dyspnea or shallow irregular respirations
- Extreme thirst
- Nausea, vomiting
- Chills
- Feeling of impending doom.

Nursing intervention will:

- Establish and maintain airway; anticipate need for intubation if respiratory distress is evident
- Administer high flow humidified oxygen (100%) by non-rebreather mask
- Maintain cervical spine precautions if indicated
- Monitor vital signs, level of consciousness and cardiac rhythm
- Establish IV access with two large gauge catheters and administer IV fluids
- Assess for external bleeding sites and apply pressure dressings. Use of pneumatic antishock garment (PASG) to control bleeding if indicated
- Assess for life-threatening injuries (e.g. hemothorax, cardiac tamponade liver laceration and pelvic fractures)
- Insert an indwelling catheter and nasogastric tube if indicated.

Therapeutic Management

Whenever possible, the patient should be treated in an ICU and should receive continuous ECG monitoring. A general goal is to keep the mean arterial BP greater than 60 mm Hg.

- *Establishment of patent airway:* Management of shock begins by ensuring that the patient has an adequate airway. Maintaining clients' airway is vital to the treatment of shock. In all types of shock, supplemental oxygen is administered to protect against hypoxemia. Oxygen can be delivered via nasal cannula, mask highflow nonrebreathing mask, endotracheal tube.
- *Fluid replacement:* In shock, various fluids are given to correct specific problems such as electrolyte or protein deficiencies or other defects of the blood, including acidosis and hyponatremia. However, in treating hypovolemic shock, the immediate result of therapy seems to depend less on the type of fluid administered for fluid replacement than on the amount of fluid administered. Because shock (except cardiogenic) almost always involves as a decreased effective circulating blood volume, the cornerstone of shock therapy is expansion of that volume by the IV administration of appropriate fluids either crystalloids, colloids or blood products or combinations. At least two large-gauge IV catheters should be inserted immediately before severe vasoconstriction access and intravenous access becomes difficult.

Crystalloids are electrolyte solutions that are either hypotonic, hypertonic or isotonic relative to plasma. However, in the critically-ill patient, approximately two-thirds of the volume will diffuse out of the vascular space because of the increased permeability and reduced oncotic pressure. Therefore, large amount of crystalloids are needed for adequate volume replacement. Because of the expansion of the interstitial space following large amounts of crystalloid administration, the development of systemic edema is common. The common crystalloids are 0.9 percent Saline. Ringer's lactate (Isotonic); hypertonic saline 3 percent, i.e. D5 NS (hypertonic) 45 percent NS, 33 percent NS D5W (hypotonic).

Colloids are primarily remaining in the intravascular space because of the size of the molecules. The osmotic pressure of these solutions draws fluid into the intravascular space expanding the intravascular volume. Colloids are extremely effective volume expanders. However, none is ideal. Each colloid has significant toxicities that must be considered. Colloids are used in the treatment of shock when plasma protein loss is excessive as in burn shock and peritonitis. If needed, packed cells are administered as soon as possible after they have been typed and crossmatched.

Pharmacologic Management

The primary purpose of drugs used in the treatment of shock is correction of the poor tissue perfusion. These drugs are administered intravenously. They are as follows:

1. Sympathomimetic drugs are drugs that mimic the action of the sympathetic nervous system. The effects of these drugs are mediated through action on the alpha-adrenergic, or beta-adrenergic receptors. The various drugs differ in their alpha and beta effects. Dobutamine, dopamine, epinephrine (adrenaline), isoproterenol, levarterenol, meteraminol, methoxamine, and phenylephrine are examples of sympathomimetic drugs. Many of them (epinephrine and norepinephrine) can cause peripheral. Vasoconstriction drugs are referred to as 'vasopressor drugs'.
2. Vasodilator: Some patients in shock show evidence of excessive vasoconstriction and poor perfusion in spite of volume replacement and normal high systemic pressures. An excessive constriction can reduce blood flow. In such cases vasodilators are used. The common vasodilators are nitroglycerin, sodium nitroprusside, phentolamine and morphine sulfate.
3. Corticosteroids have several effects that may assist the client in neurogenic shock after the spinal cord injury. IV corticosteroid therapy may be helpful in anaphylactic shock. Steroids may prevent the delayed symptoms that are thought to be caused by the release of chemical mediators. The common steroids used are dexamethasone, hydrocortisone and methylprednisolone. They inhibit inflammatory process, stabilizes lysosomal membranes, reduces capillary permeability, reduces release of chemical mediators in the septic process, and promotes sodium retention.
4. Antibiotics are essential when shock is due to infection. If septic shock, it is suspected that a blood specimen for culture and sensitivity is taken once and broad-spectrum antibiotics are started even though the specific infections organism is not identified.

Nutritional Management

During the acute phase of shock syndrome, the patient receives nothing by mouth because of gastrointestinal tract is not adequately perfused. As recovery begins, nutrition plays an important role in limiting morbidity. Since anorexia is almost universally present, parenteral or enteral feeding is often used. Enteral tube feeding via a feeding pump is commonly the initial method of supplying nutrition. Parenteral feeding is generally adopted only if tube feeding is contraindicated or if they fail to meet the patient's caloric requirements.

Nursing Management

In shock, patient's condition can change rapidly, frequent nursing assessment is essential. Documentations of progress and response to intervention needs to be concise, yet convey the patient's status minute by minute.

The first step in assessing a person in shock via general overview, giving attention as necessary to the ABCs (airways breathing and circulation). Once the airway is patent, air exchange is adequate, a pulse is present and cervical spine is immobilized (if it is trauma....). Perform rapid cursory initial head-to-toe physical assessment. The initial assessment goal is to identify major problems and gross abnormalities. Give further detailed attention to specific injuries or problems after shock is stabilized with the use of physical assessment skills, the nurse has to make following observations.

- Airway patency: Presence of noisy respirations and obstructions
- Breathing respiratory rate and efforts
- Respiratory pattern: Chest wall expansion; Chest wall bulges or deflates. Tachypnea, wheezing, crackles, absence of breath sounds, coughing (anaphylaxis) and choking
- Circulation: Pulse, blood pressure, skin color, and temperature. Tachycardia, hypotension, weak thready pulse, flat neck vein and fullness of jugular vein engorgement (JVE)
- Heart sounds: Abnormal heart sounds and dysrhythmias
- Level of consciousness: Orientation X3 (Person, place, time) ability to move extremities, sensation in all extremities, hand grasps, response to verbal and painful stimuli, pupil size and reaction to light; presence of abnormal posturing; restlessness, anxiety, altered orientation, lethargy, stupor, coma and so on to evaluate neurologic function
- State of hydration and perfusion of skin: (e.g. capillary refill time less than 3 seconds) condition of mucus membrane, sclera, and conjunctive presence of pallor cool, moist skins or warm, flushed skin (septic and anaphylactic shock) cyanosis (later shock) urticarial, rash and angioedema (anaphylactic shock). See Nursing care plan for septic shock (Table 12.3), anaphylactic shock (Table 12.4), hypovolemic shock (Table 12.5)
- Position of trachea: Tracheal deviation may indicate tension pneumothorax
- Presence, location, intensity, duration of pain, what relieves the pain
- Abdominal distension, rigidity, vomiting, hyperactive or diminished bowel sounds
- Circumference of abdomen and or extremities
- Peripheral pulses
- Presence of incarceration, contusions, ecchymoses, petechiae, purpura (also check bruising over flank area)
- Bone deformities
- Presence of medical alert tags or bracelets.

TABLE 12 3 : Nursing care plan for the patient with septic shock

Problems	Objective	Nursing interventions	Rationales
Nursing Diagnosis #1			
Fluid volume deficit related to: 1. Distributional volume loss; shift to interstitial space 2. Increased insensible loss with high fever	Patient will: 1. Maintain adequate circulating blood volume and stable hemodynamic variables: – Heart rate 60–100/min when resting – Systemic arterial blood pressure adequate for tissue perfusion – Normal pulmonary capillary wedge pressure 8–12 mm Hg – Normal central venous pressure 0–8 mm Hg 2. Maintain normal body temperature 3. Maintain adequate urine output > 30 mL/h (mL/kg) 4. Maintain baseline and/or optimal neurological status 5. Maintain fluid and electrolyte balance as demonstrated by laboratory data within normal limits: – Electrolytes – Hemoglobin and hematocrit – BUN and creatinine	• Assess for signs and symptoms of septic shock – Assess for early signs of septic shock: Hyperthermia, warm, dry, flushed skin; chills; weakness; nausea, vomiting, diarrhea – Assess neurological status: 1. Altered level of consciousness 2. Anxiety – Assess cardiovascular status: Hypotension; tachycardia; character of pulse – Observe for ventricular dysrhythmias – Note color and character of the skin: Cool, pale, diaphoretic – Assess renal function: Urine output; urine-specific gravity, urinary sodium – Obtain baseline laboratory data: Cultures: Urine, sputum; wound (if applicable) – Blood cultures—two specimens from different sites by venipuncture – Electrolytes – Coagulation factors and clotting times; fibrin split products – Hemoglobin and hematocrit – White cell count with differential • Assist with the insertion of hemodynamic monitoring devices: – Arterial catheters: Blood pressure; arterial blood gases	• Baseline assessment data is needed to establish the phase of septic shock: Early or late. Baseline data is useful in determining changes in patient status and evaluating response to therapy – Early recognition of septic shock is important in order to institute prompt measures to prevent late or irreversible shock – Neurologic assessment is a way to gauge cerebral perfusion. Orientation and anxiety are indicative of early septic shock, when cerebral perfusion is not as yet compromised. Confusion, disorientation, and coma may indicate decreased perfusion as seen in late septic shock – Dysrhythmias may indicate decreased coronary perfusion, as seen in late septic shock – Cool, pale skin is a sign of decreased perfusion and peripheral vasoconstriction – Reduced renal perfusion will reduce glomerular filtration, causing a decrease in urine output. A decrease in urinary sodium is indicative of hypovolemia secondary to aldosterone release

Contd...

Contd...

Problems	Objective	Nursing interventions	Rationales
		– Pulmonary artery catheter: Central venous pressure; pulmonary artery pressure; cardiac output, SvO_2 (mixed venous gases) • Administer and monitor prescribed fluid replacement therapy: – Monitor hemodynamic variables (as above) – Monitor hourly urine output – Assess respiratory status: Respiratory rate; rhythm of breathing; presence of adventitious breath sounds; crackles, wheezes • Institute measures to control body temperature: – Monitor body temperature every 2 hours if the patient is febrile – Administer antipyretic drugs as ordered; evaluate response to therapy – Apply hypo- or hyperthermia blanket as prescribed: ◆ Manual mode ◆ Automatic cooling mode using rectal probe	– Determination of the portal of entry and focus of infection is crucial to successful treatment. – Bacteremia may be transient. Blood cultures should not be obtained through indwelling venous or arterial catheters, as they may be colonized with bacteria not responsible for the septicemia – These data will be helpful in monitoring fluid replacement therapy and in identifying complications such as DIC – Elevated leukocyte count with a left shift is frequently observed in septic shock; indicative of acute infection • Hemodynamic variables (CVP, PCWP, CO, SVR, SvO_2, A-aDO_2, VO_2) are important in determining the effectiveness of fluid replacement therapy and in determining the phase of septic shock – Reduction in oxygen tension (< 40 mm Hg) in mixed venous gases (SvO_2) is indicative of compromised tissue perfusion – Higher than normal central venous pressure, pulmonary artery pressure, and wedge pressure may indicate a too rapid infusion of fluids and impending fluid overload – Urine output of greater than 30 cc/hour indicates adequate renal perfusion – Tachypnea and crackles may indicate fluid overload • High body temperature increases the metabolic rate of the tissues and may exacerbate tissue ischemia and hypoxia – Insensible fluid loss may increase when the patient is febrile – Continuous measurement of temperature while the patient is on a cooling blanket will prevent excessive cooling and chills
Nursing Diagnosis #2			
Potential impaired gas exchange related to: 1. Hypovolemia resulting in reduced pulmonary perfusion (ventilation/ perfusion mismatch)	Patient will: 1. Maintain acceptable blood gas parameters: – pH 7.35–7.45 – pO_2 > 60 mm Hg – pCO_2 ~ 35–45 mm Hg	• Assess respiratory status – Respiratory rate and rhythm – Breath sounds	• Respiratory distress syndrome may occur in septic shock secondary to decreased perfusion and endotoxin damage to the pulmonary vasculature

Contd...

Contd...

Problems	Objective	Nursing interventions	Rationales
2. Altered alveolar—capillary membrane	2. Maintain baseline and/or optimal neurological status		– Altered respiratory patterns such as hyperventilation and tachypnea occur secondary to fever and sympathetic nervous system stimulation – Development of abnormal breath sounds such as crackles indicate fluid overload and pulmonary edema
Nursing Diagnosis #3			
Ineffective, related to: 1. Tachypnea, hyperventilation	Patient will: 1. Achieve effective alveolar minute ventilation (arterial blood gas values as above) 2. Verbalize ease of breathing	– Monitor arterial blood gases and pH • Maintain patent airway • Administer and monitor oxygen and respiratory therapy – Observe for increase peak inspiratory pressures during mechanical ventilation • Assess neurological status	– Monitor arterial blood gases – Decreased PaO_2 increased $PaCO_2$ > 50 mm Hg (room air) are signs of impending respiratory failure • Patients with septic shock may require endotracheal intubation – In the patient requiring mechanical ventilation, increased inspiratory pressures indicate decreased lung compliance observed in respiratory distress syndrome • Changes in mental status may indicate cerebral hypoxia
Nursing Diagnosis #4			
Alteration in cardiac output: Decreased, related to: 1. Decreased venous return (late septic shock)	Patient will: 1. Demonstrate stable hemodynamic variables: – Blood pressure > 90 mm Hg systolic – Pulmonary capillary wedge pressure 8–12 mm Hg – Cardiac output > 4 L/min – Systemic vascular resistance 800–1400 dyne-seconds/cm^5 3. Maintain adequate urine output > 30 mL/h (mL/kg) 4. Maintain adequate respiratory status: – Respiratory rate < 30/min – Absence of adventitious breath sounds – Arterial blood gases within acceptable limits 5. Demonstrate adequate peripheral tissue perfusion: – Warm, dry skin – Absence of cyanosis – Absence of skin breakdown	• Assess hemodynamic status – Cardiac output – Pulmonary capillary wedge pressure – Systemic vascular resistance • Assess neurological status • Assess respiratory status: – Rate and rhythm of breathing – Adventitious breath sounds • Administer and monitor the effects of prescribed medical interventions: Vasodilators; positive inotropes; antiarrhythmics	• Increase cardiac output and decreased systemic vascular resistance are observed in early septic shock; however, in late septic shock, cardiac output is reduced and systemic vascular resistance is high. Monitoring these variables will determine the effectiveness of therapeutic interventions • Changes in neurological status may indicate decreased cerebral perfusion, secondary to decreased cardiac output • Acute respiratory failure may develop secondary to cardiac failure. Baseline data are needed in order to monitor the effectiveness of therapeutic interventions

Contd...

Contd...

Problems	Objective	Nursing interventions	Rationales
	6. Maintain baseline/optimal neurological function: – Level of consciousness: Oriented to person, place, time – Deep tendon reflexes brisk		
Nursing Diagnosis #5			
Potential impairment of skin integrity, related to: 1. Immobility 2. Decreased tissue perfusion	Patient will: 1. Demonstrate skin integrity as evidenced by the absence of skin breakdown and pressure ulcers	• Assess skin condition frequently • Perform passive range of motion exercises • Provide pressure relief device • Teach the patient to shift position frequently • Establish a turning schedule of every 1–2 hours depending on the patient's condition	• To improve peripheral circulation • Pressure ulcers may be prevented by reducing the amount and duration of pressure to a given area
Nursing Diagnosis #6			
Potential for reinfection	Patient will: 1. Re-establish and maintain normal body temperature 2. Remain without new evidence of infection	• For specific nursing interventions and rationales, refer similar, Nursing Diagnosis mentioned in earlier NCPs	
Nursing Diagnosis #7			
Anxiety related to: 1. Intensive care environment 2. Septic shock	Patient will: 1. State that he/she feels less anxious 2. Verbalize feelings about illness and care in the intensive care unit 3. Perform relaxation techniques	• For specific nursing interventions and rationales, refer similar Nursing Diagnosis mentioned earlier NCPs	
Nursing Diagnosis #8			
Sleep pattern disturbance related to: 1. Intensive care environment 2. Anxiety 3. Assessments and treatments	Patient will: 1. State that he/she feels rested 2. Verbalize feelings about illness	• Plan nursing care activities such as assessment, treatments, and tests to allow for rest periods • Determine the patient's normal sleep pattern • Assess the duration and quality of sleep as perceived by patient • Administer prescribed sedatives and hypnotics – Monitor for signs of respiratory depression: Significantly decreased respiratory rate (< 8 spontaneous breaths/min); evidence of reduced alveolar hypoventilation	• Longer periods of rest can be provided when nursing care is organized • Knowledge of the patient's normal sleep pattern is useful to determine the timing and length of rest periods – Patients in ICU may sleep up to 50 per cent of their limited sleep time during the day; little or no sleep may occur at night due to frequent awakenings and anxiety

TABLE 12.4: Sample of nursing care plan for the patient with anaphylactic shock

Problems	Objective	Nursing interventions	Rationales
Nursing Diagnosis #1			
Airway clearance, ineffective: actual or potential related to: 1. Bronchospasm, laryngospasm 2. Increased pulmonary secretions in response to release of chemical mediators from degranulated mast cells	Patient will: 1. Maintain adequate alveolar ventilation and oxygenation: – $PaCO_2$ ~ 35–45 mm Hg (room air) – PaO_2 > 60 mm Hg – pH 7.35–7.45 2. Verbalize ease of breathing; breath sounds clear on auscultation; absence of adventitious breath sounds 3. Verbalize reduced perform relation exercises: Demonstrate a relaxed demeanor	• Assess respiratory function: – Respiratory parameters: Respiratory rate, rhythm; diaphragmatic excursion; use of accessory muscles – Presence of abnormal or adventitious breath sounds on auscultation – Neurological parameters: Mental status: Orientation to person, place, and date – Cardiovascular parameters: Vital signs – Arterial blood pressure • Implement measures as to assure a patent airway: – Maintain upright position – Place suction and intubation equipment at the bedside – Initiate oxygen therapy as prescribed (e.g. nasal cannula at 2 L/min) – Obtain baseline arterial blood gases (room air) prior to initiating oxygen therapy – Monitor serial arterial blood gas parameters • Administer medication regimen as prescribed: – Anticipate subcutaneous injection of epinephrine – Implement Alupent treatments in conjunction with the Respiratory Therapy department as per physician • Provide restful and calm environment to reduce tension and anxiety: – Spend time at the patient's bedside – Keep abreast of progress – Instruct regarding relaxation exercises – Provide periods of uninterrupted rest and/or sleep	• It is essential to establish baseline function to facilitate evaluating the patient's response to therapeutic measures: – Adventitious sounds are noted with special emphasis placed on the pressure of stridor and wheezing. Inspiratory wheezes and stridor are ominous signs – A deterioration in the level of consciousness may be the first warning sign of inadequate oxygenation and tissue perfusion – Upright position allows for chest wall expansion and diaphragmatic excursion; accessory muscles can be utilized to the fullest – Suction equipment, etc., is needed for prophylactic readiness in case, laryngospasm or edema compromises the airway – Oxygen prevents hypoxia and consequent respiratory acidemia – Monitoring of arterial blood gases provides a direct indication as to the effectiveness of therapeutic measures in assisting the patient to maintain adequate gas exchange – Subcutaneous route may be safer because it is more slowly absorbed. There are fewer adrenergic side effects. Epinephrine will help to control bronchospasm, and improve ventilation – Alupent, a frequently used adrenergic agent, stimulates beta receptors and thus exerts the following effects: Bronchodilation, positive inotropic and chronotropic cardiac activity, and decreased synthesis and release of chemical mediators by most cells
Nursing Diagnosis #2			
Fluid volume deficit, actual or potential, related to: 1. Vasodilation 2. Increased capillary permeability with increased third- spacing (angioedema)	Patient will: 1. Maintain stable vital signs: – Blood pressure within 10 mm Hg of baseline ◆ Heart rate < 100 beats/min 2. Remain without evidence of third-spacing (e.g. no angioedema or pitting edema)	• Monitor vital signs, particularly blood pressure and heart rate • Monitor intake and output hourly • Implement prescribed fluid regimen – Initiate intravenous therapy with lactated Ringer' solution (fluids may need to be infused wide open)	• An increase in blood pressure and decrease in heart rate may be indicative of restoring circulatory volume and cardiac output • Renal function parallels normal cardiac output and normovolemia. Urine output should be maintained at > 30 mL/h

Contd...

Contd...

Problems	Objective	Nursing interventions	Rationales
		– Anticipate repeated doses of SQ epinephrine, followed by intravenous administration if there is no clinical improvement	• Initial fluid challenges must be monitored in relation to patient's clinical status: – Ringer's lactate is the most compatible physiologic (isotonic) solution and can be infused at a rapid rate in an attempt to stabilize intravascular volume – Epinephrine is an endogenous catecholamine that stimulates both alpha and beta receptors. It will increase the heart rate and myocardial contractility; it will increase systemic vascular resistance and thereby increase arterial blood pressure. It may be necessary to give epinephrine intravenously since peripheral perfusion may be inadequate for SQ or IM injection if the shock state progresses. The intravenous route is fast and efficacious, but when this route is unavailable, epinephrine may be instilled directly into the endotracheal tube after intubation (as prescribed)
Nursing Diagnosis #3			
Anxiety related to: 1. Respiratory distress (hypoxia and dyspnea stimulate flight/fight responses and emotional distress) 2. Hypotensive state	Patient will: 1. Verbalize ways to reduce stress and avoid panicking 2. Assume a relaxed demeanor	• Implement measures to assist patient/ family to maintain control and react appropriately in the event of an emergency – Assist patient to assume a position of comfort—may try orthopnea – Allow patient decision-making alternatives – Speak in a calm, soothing voice – Offer optimistic reassurances – Do not leave patient unattended – Keep patient/family informed of treatments and progress – Consider the sedative effects of drugs such as Benadryl to assist in management anxiety	– Facilitates ease of breathing and may relieve respiratory distress – Anxiety may be decreased when patients are permitted decision-making power – Choices facilitate autonomy and self-control – There are positive psychological benefits derived from reassurances – Fear is perpetuated when patient is left alone. The patient's condition may deteriorate rapidly – Fear of the unknown is alleviated – Benadryl can be used as an adjunct epinephrine therapy, after the acute symptoms are controlled
Nursing Diagnosis #4			
Skin integrity, impairment of, related to: 1. Severe urticaria with pruritus	Patient will: 1. Avoid scratching 2. Demonstrate ways to avoid scratching (e.g. massaging with prescribed lotion) 3. Maintain intact skin, with absence of antiedema	• Implement measures to relieve itching and maintain skin integrity: – Apply cool compresses to affected areas, PRN – Remove all unnecessary clothing/ bedding – Instruct patient to avoid scratching: if all else fails, instruct patient to use fingertips rather than nails, and to use a massaging motion	– Cool temperatures reduce the discomfort that coincides with pruritus and angioedema – Removal of clothing sometimes relieves itching and feelings of constriction – Scratching disrupts skin integrity, the first line of defense against infection

Contd...

Contd...

Problems	Objective	Nursing interventions	Rationales
		– Administer Benadryl as prescribed – A prescription may be given upon discharge that includes oral Benadryl and/or a topical cream	– Benadryl competes with histamine for the histamine receptor sites. It effectively controls localized itching – Since some chemical mediators (e.g. SRS-A) have slower and more prolonged action, an antihistamine and local, topical agents may be prescribed to counteract the annoying skin cryptions (urticaria)
Nursing Diagnosis #5			
Knowledge deficit related to: 1. Inability to identify allergen (allergen was disguised as a preservative) 2. Delay in receiving treatment (driving to distant hospital rather than the one nearby; this may have exacerbated the shock-state)	Patient will: 1. Review sources of sulfur preparations 2. Discuss cross-reactivity with allergens 3. Verbalize need to expedite emergency treatment upon exposure to allergen(s)	• Assess patient/family knowledge regarding allergic status: Known allergens; precautions taken to avoid exposure to allergen(s); emergency care with onset of allergic reaction • Assess readiness to learn – Identify support system in family • Implement patient/family education program: – Teach the importance of reading all labels – Reinforce responsibility to notify all health professionals of specific allergies – Encourage patient to wear a "medic alert" tag/bracelet – Recommend an allergy referral – Inform patient/family that treatment must be sought immediately as subsequent reactions may be more severe	• Assessing patient/family knowledge base regarding anaphylaxis assists in determining essential information to include in patient/family instruction; it may also help to discern misunderstandings that might complicate the patient's care • It is imperative that one or more family members be versed in emergency first-aid measures should the patient develop anaphylactic shock – Sulfiting agents (e.g., sulfur, sodium or potassium bisulfate or sodium sulfite) are commonly used as antioxidants and food preservatives. Potatoes, shellfish, and wines are just a few items that contain sulfites – Patients are active participants as well as recipients of interdisciplinary health care – Identification of the allergen or anaphylactoid reaction may be lifesaving, especially if only minutes can be spared – Clients who experience severe systemic reactions need a referral for further evaluation and care – Phase two reactions cause chemical mediators to be released into the blood, since the patient is already sensitized (i.e. has preformed IgE antibody from initial exposure). Treatment must be solicited at nearest hospital, via ambulance if necessary

TABLE 12.5: Nursing care plan for the patient with hypovolemic shock

Problems	Objective	Nursing interventions	Rationales
Nursing Diagnosis #1			
Tissue perfusion, alteration in: Cerebral, renal, and peripheral, related to: 1. Reduced circulating blood volume 2. Fluid volume deficit	Patient will maintain adequate tissue perfusion: 1. Arterial blood pressure within 10 mm Hg of baseline 2. Heart rate less than 100 beats/minute 3. Mental status: Alert; oriented to person, time, and place 4. Skin warm, dry to touch; usual color, good turgor, good capillary refill (<2 seconds) 5. Urinary output greater than 30 mL/h 6. Arterial blood gases within normal range: – PaO_2 > 80 mm Hg – $PaCO_2$ 35–45 mm Hg – HCO_3 22–26 mEq/L – pH 7.35–7.45 7. SVO_2 about 75%	• Assess for signs/symptoms of hypovolemic shock: – Assess cardiovascular function: ◆ Blood pressure (orthostatic) ◆ Heart rate, rhythm ◆ Resting peripheral pulses ◆ Skin color, moisture, temperature, and turgor – Assess neurologic function: ◆ Mental status ◆ Orientation	• A baseline assessment is necessary to establish stage of shock and to determine emergent measures indicated; serves as a measure of the patient's response to therapy – A drop in blood pressure of 10–15 mm Hg from supine to sitting/ standing position suggests blood loss of about 1 liter – Reflects effect of altered intravascular volume on cardiac function – Peripheral pulses, if palpable, may be weak and thready due to decrease in stroke volume and peripheral vasoconstriction – When tissue perfusion is decreased, skin becomes cool and clammy to the touch and pale in color; cyanosis may occur if reduced hemoglobin concentration exceeds 5 g/100 mL – Appropriateness of patient's behavior and responses reflects adequacy of cerebral tissue perfusion
Nursing Diagnosis #2			
Cardiac output, alteration in decreased, related to: 1. Decreased venous return (preload)	Patient will maintain stable hemodynamics: 1. Central venous pressure 0–8 mm Hg 2. Pulmonary artery pressure < 25 mm Hg (systolic) 3. Pulmonary capillary wedge pressure 8–12 mm Hg 4. Cardiac output 4–8 L/min. 5. Systemic vascular resistance (SVR) 800–1200 dynes/sec/cm^{-5}	– Assess renal function: ◆ Urine output ◆ Intake and output – Assess gastrointestinal function: ◆ Bowel sounds, abdominal distention, pain • Establish/maintain 1 or more large-gauge intravenous access sites • Initiate timely and aggressive fluid replacement therapy and monitor response to therapy: – Administer crystalloids, colloids – Transfuse blood/blood products • Initiate hemodynamic monitoring: Arterial, pulmonary artery, and pulmonary capillary wedge pressures – Initiate monitoring of mixed venous blood (SVO_2) • Monitor hydration status during fluid replacement therapy: – Assess respiratory function: ◆ Respiratory rate, rhythm, chest excursion, breath sounds, use of accessory muscles; status of neck veins – Obtain daily weight – Monitor intake and output • Insert Foley catheter to measure hourly urine output	– Reduced circulating blood volume and hypotensive state compromise renal perfusion. Rine output is a reliable indicator of renal perfusion – Decrease in blood flow to fluids and fluid volume expanders and blood and blood products may be necessary to restore circulating blood volume • Rapid administration of fluids and fluid volume expanders and blood and blood products may be necessary to restore circulating blood volume • Insertion of systemic arterial and pulmonary artery catheters in the setting of massive hemorrhage and/or fluid loss with massive fluid volume replacement is essential to accurately follow trends and evaluate patient's response to therapy – Status of mixed venous blood reflects adequacy of peripheral tissue perfusion – Detection of adventitious breath sounds (crackles, rhonchi) in previously clear lungs suggests overhydration

Contd...

Contd...

Problems	Objective	Nursing interventions	Rationales
		• Insert nasogastric tube • Monitor hematology profile: – Hematocrit, hemoglobin, RBCs, platelets	– Most accurate measure of hydration status • Hourly urine outputs reflect status of renal perfusion and underlying hemodynamic status • Decompresses stomach to facilitate respiratory excursion and prevent aspiration of stomach contents, and affords means to monitor for gastrointestinal bleeding • Reflects hemoglobin oxygen-carrying capacity; decrease in hemoglobin levels compromises oxygen delivery to tissues
Nursing Diagnosis #3			
Anxiety, related to: 1. Hemorrhage 2. Transfusion therapy 3. Inherent sympathoadrenal activity (enhanced) 4. ICU setting	Patient will: 1. Verbalize feeling less anxious 2. Demonstrate relaxed demeanor 3. Perform relaxation techniques with assistance 4. Verbalize familiarity with ICU setting	• Assess signs/symptoms of anxiety: – Restlessness, agitation, diaphoresis; tachypnea, tachycardia, palpitations; uncooperative or non-compliant behavior; verbalization of fears and concerns • Examine circumstances underlying anxiety – Manipulate ICU environment to provide calm, restful periods • Assess patient coping behaviors and their effectiveness in dealing with current stressors – Provide positive reinforcement when desired outcome is achieved • Initiate interventions to reduce anxiety: – Relieve pain or other discomfort. ◆ Medication for pain; monitor response ◆ Comfort measures – Monitor effectiveness of ventilation and oxygenation – Serial arterial blood gases – Listen attentively, encourage verbalization, provide a caring touch – Let the patient know it is okay to feel anxious and afraid – Remain with patient during periods of acute stress • Assess readiness to learn and implement the following when appropriate: – Orient patient to environment, ICU equipment and routines, and staff ◆ Explain all procedures and activities involving patient – Involve patient in decision-making regarding care when possible and appropriate – Assist in establishing short-term goals and desired patient outcomes – Instruct patient in relaxation techniques when it is prudent to do so	• Thorough assessment assists in discerning underlying cause of anxiety and provides a basis for therapy. Patients with hypovolemic shock may experience anxiety associated with massive sympathoadrenal output • Removal of precipitating cause may reduce anxiety – Reduction in stimuli is essential to assist patient to relax. This is especially important in the patient at risk of bleeding or rebleeding • Experiencing a bleeding episode can be very distressing – Positive feedback and reassurance nurture self-confidence and confidence in health team – Pain precipitates and/or aggravates anxiety – Inadequate gas exchange, "air hunger," hypoxemia, and/or hypercapnia may cause the patient to experience a "sense of doom" – These nursing activities reassure the patient that he/she is not alone – Reassurance helps patient to focus on feelings and to work them through • Readiness to learn facilitates meaningful learning and a sense of accomplishment: – Knowing what to expect helps to reduce anxiety – Helps patient to maintain some degree of control of health management – Builds and reinforces self-confidence

Contd...

Contd...

Problems	Objective	Nursing interventions	Rationales
			– Use of energy-release techniques allows an outlet for pent up feelings; enables patient to have some control over anxiety
Nursing Diagnosis #4			
Fluid volume, alteration in, related to: 1. Hemorrhage 2. Fluid shifts associated with loss of plasma proteins (hypoproteinemia, hypoalbuminemia)	Patient will: 1. Maintain body weight within 5% of baseline 2. Balance fluid intake and output 3. Exhibit good skin turgor, absence of peripheral edema, absence of jugular venous distention, absence of adventitious breath sounds 4. Maintain serum electrolytes within normal limits	• Maintain fluid and electrolyte balance – Administer prescribed fluid volume – Document intake and output, urine specific gravity – Record daily weight – Monitor serum electrolytes • Monitor hemodynamic parameters: – Arterial blood pressure – Pulmonary artery pressure parameters – Central venous pressure – Cardiac output • Implement nursing measures to improve and/or maintain cardiac output: – Assist patient into positions of comfort that facilitate breathing ◆ Head of bed elevated to 20–30 degrees – Maximize patient activities in accordance with the acuity and limitations of the illness – Provide special care to back and to skin over joints and pressure points – Assist with passive range-of-motion exercises	• Fluid therapy is the mainstay of treatment of hypovolemic shock to restore/maintain tissue perfusion – Close monitoring of urine output helps to evaluate renal perfusion and assess overall hemodynamics – Rapid and massive fluid volume replacement therapy can dilute electrolytes and precipitate electrolyte imbalance • These measures best reflect the patient's status and response to therapy. Rapid administration of crystalloids and colloids may precipitate fluid shift between extracellular and intracellular compartments – Placing patient with hypovolemic shock into Trendelen-burg's position (i.e. the legs higher than the head) may be of little value to hemodynamics or to improvement of cardiac output. Optimal ventilation/perfusion matching occurs in dependent areas of lungs – Nursing interventions are implemented to maximize circulation, prevent pooling or stasis of blood, ensure adequate venous return, and promote comfort – Compromised circulation in a patient with reduced tissue perfusion increases the risk of tissue ischemia and stasis of blood predisposing to venous thrombosis, and reduces venous return and cardiac output

Nursing Diagnoses

The possible potential nursing diagnoses for patient in shock are:

- Ineffective airway clearance
- Ineffective breathing pattern
- Impaired gas exchange
- Altered tissue perfusion: Cerebral, cardiopulmonary, renal, GI, peripheral
- Decreased cardiac output
- Fluid volume deficit
- Altered nutrition: less than body requirement
- Constipation
- Activity intolerance
- Impaired physical mobility
- Sensory/perceptual alteration, visual, auditory, kinetic, olfactory, tactile gestating
- Sleep pattern disturbance
- Impaired or risk for skin integrity
- Self-care deficit, bathing, grooming, dressing, toileting
- Body image disturbance

- Self-esteem disturbance
- Altered role performance
- Personal identity disturbance
- Anxiety, fears, pain and spiritual distress
- Anticipatory grievance.

Planning

Nursing care of the client with shock is complex. Frequent reassessment of the client and nursing activities are essential because the client status often changes rapidly. Specific nursing and medical intervention vary according to individual needs and the setting in which care is delivered. However, these common objectives of the care of the client with shock are:

- Return of tissue perfusion and cellular function to normal
- Meeting metabolic demands
- Preventing further injury
- Effective coping by the client and significant others.

Nursing Intervention

In terms of the patient's cardiovascular status, the recommended position for the treatment of shock (after the chest-X-ray have revealed any neck and spine injury) is supine with the legs elevated to an angle of 45 degrees. The trunk should be horizontal, the head at the level of chest and the knees straight. This Trendelenburg (head down) position should be avoided in shock because it may:

- Initiate aortic and carotid sinus reflexes, causing impaired cerebral blood flow and decreased jugular venous flow
- Cause the abdominal organs to press against diaphragm, thus limiting respiratory excursion and possibly contributing to respiratory distress
- Decrease filling of the coronary arteries causing myocardial ischemia
- Cause an increase in intracranial pressure in the presence of head injury.

This modified Trendelenburg's position promotes increased venous return from the lower extremities without compressing abdominal organs against diaphragm (Further management refer Nursing care plans).

CARDIOGENIC SHOCK

Cardiogenic shock occurs when the heart muscle loses its contractile power. It is a grave condition resulting from sudden and complete loss of cardiac function.

Cardiogenic shock occurs when the hearts ability to pump blood is impaired, leading to an inadequate supply of oxygen for the heart and tissues. The result is a marked reduction in cardiac output, with inadequate perfusion to the heart, brain and kidneys. Causes of cardiogenic shock are either coronary or noncoronary. Coronary cardiogenic shock is more common and is most often in patients with myocardial infarction. Noncoronary causes include tension pneumothorax, severe metabolic problems, such as hypoxemia, acidosis, hypoglycemia, hypocalcemia, cardiac tamponade, cardiomyopathy, valvular damage and dysrhythmias.

Etiology

Absence or inadequate contraction causing cardiac arrest occurs mainly due to: Ventricular fibrillations and occasionally due to ventricular systole. The condition may also result from circulatory collapse with sudden hypotension as in syncope, vasomotor collapse, profound hyperthermia, CNS damage, hypovolemic shock, severe hemorrhage, septicemia, and accidents such as drowning and electrocution. It also occurs from drug or anesthetic overdose and from cardiac catheterization. Extensive damage of the left ventricle due to myocardial infarction commonly initiates a perpetuating 'shock cycle'.

Pathophysiology

Pathological changes occur according to predisposing factors. An impaired contractility causes a marked reduction in cardiac output. This decreased cardiac output results in a lack of blood and oxygen. The lack of blood and oxygen to the heart muscles results in continued damage to the heart muscle, a further decline in contractile power and a continued inability of the heart to provide blood and oxygen to the vital organs. At the end-stage, cardiomyopathy, severe valvular dysfunction, and ventricular aneurysm also precipitate cardiogenic shock.

Clinical Manifestation

- Confusion, restlessness, mental lethargy due to poor perfusion of brain
- Low systolic pressure
- Oliguria-urine output less than 30 mL per hour for at least 2 hours—due to decreased perfusion of kidney - oliguria may lead to acute tubular necrosis
- Cold, clammy skin—The onset is sudden or gradual, but it presents with pale, cold, sweaty skin (due to blood is shunted from the peripheral circulation to perfuse vital organs)
- This condition may give rise to hypotension, tachycardia and heart sound may be difficult to analyze as sinus tachycardia is more than 100 per minute
- Weak thready, peripheral pulses, fatigue, hypotension are due to inadequate cardiac output
- There may be peripheral vasoconstriction leading to peripheral cyanosis or gangrene
- There will be dyspnea, tachypnea, cyanosis due to increased left ventricular pressures resulting in elevation of left atrial and pulmonary pressure, causing pulmonary congestion

- There may be dysrhythmias due to lack of oxygen to heart muscle and sinus tachycardia as a compensatory mechanism for decreased cardiac output
- There may be Cheyne-Stokes respiration, confusion, irritability and an impairment of continuousness
- Chest pain due to lack of oxygen and blood to heart muscle
- There may also be progressive acidosis, visual and cerebral impairment while the cardiac arrhythmias may be intractable
- If late, there may be permanent cerebral damage or loss of peripheral tissue even after recovery
- Hypoxemia is common particularly when there is pulmonary edema
- Neurologic impairment, respiratory distress, renal failure, multiorgan dysfunction syndrome and death are the complications of cardiogenic shock
- Dysrhythmias are common and result from a decrease in oxygen to the myocardium
- Angina pain may be experienced
- Hemodynamic instability
- Classic signs include low blood pressure, rapid and weak pulse
- Cerebral hypoxia manifested by confusion and agitation
- Decreased urinary output and cold, clammy skin.

Diagnosis

Diagnosis of the condition is made on clinical grounds Pulmonary capillary wedge pressure (PCWP), 18 mm Hg or greater, chest X-ray (pulmonary vascular congestion), abnormal laboratory value such as BUN, creatinine and liver enzymes.

Medical Management

Goals of medical treatment include limiting further myocardial damage, preserving the healthy myocardium, and improving the hearts ability to pump effectively. The oxygen needs of the heart muscle are addressed. Hemodynamic monitoring is performed and pharmacologic therapy (e.g. dopamine, nitroglycerin, dobutamine and various antiarrhythmic medications) may be used.

- First-line treatment of cardiogenic shock includes supplying supplemental oxygen, controlling chest pain, administering vasoactive medications, controlling heart rate with medications or pacemakers, and providing selective fluid support
- Mechanical cardiac support, such as intra-aortic balloon counterpulsation, ventricular assist systems, or extracorporeal cardiopulmonary bypass, may be necessary. Coronary cardiogenic shock is treated with thrombolytic therapy, angioplasty, or coronary artery bypass graft surgery
- Noncoronary cardiogenic shock is treated with cardiac valve replacement or correction of dysrhythmia.

Medical Measures

- Use of cardiac glycosides (Digoxin) and positive inotropic drugs (dopamine to stimulate cardiac contractility as prescribed)
- Use of vasodilators to decrease workload of heart and temporary cardiac output
- Use of vasopressors (sometimes it requires)
- Use of diuretics to decrease total body fluid volume and to relieve systemic and pulmonary congestion
- Introducing counterpulsation therapy
- Cardiopulmonary bypass
- Left ventricular assisting device
- Emergency cardiac surgery.

Nursing Management

The nurses should make continuous nursing assessment which includes:

- Identify patients at risk for development of cardiogenic shock
- Assess the early symptoms that are indicative to shock, restlessness, confusion, increasing heart rate, decreasing pulse pressure
- Observe the presence of pulses alternansm (LHF), decreasing urine output, weakness, fatigue, etc.
- Observe the presence of central and peripheral cyanosis
- Observe the development of edema
- Identify signs and symptoms indicative to myocardial infarctions
- Identify patients' and significant others' reaction to crisis situation.

Prevention

- Early on, identify patients at risk for cardiogenic shock
- Promote adequate oxygenation of the heart muscle, and decrease cardiac workload (conserve energy, relieve pain, administer oxygen).

Hemodynamic Monitoring

- Monitor hemodynamic and cardiac status: maintain arterial lines and electrocardiogram (ECG) equipment
- Anticipate need for medications, intravenous fluids, and other equipment
- Document and promptly report changes in hemodynamic cardiac, and pulmonary status.

Fluid Administration

- Provide for safe and accurate administration of intravenous fluids and medications. Neurologic assessment is essential after thrombolytic therapy. Monitor for possible infiltration with intravenous infusions

- Monitor urine output, blood urea nitrogen, and serum creatinine level to detect possible decrease in renal function.

Intra-aortic Balloon Counterpulsation

- Provide ongoing timing adjustments of the balloon pump for maximum effectiveness
- Perform frequent checks of neurovascular status of lower extremities.

The probable nursing diagnosis may be:

- Decreased cardiac output related to impaired contractility due to extensive heart muscle damage
- Impaired gas exchange related to pulmonary congestion due to elevated left ventricular pressure
- Altered tissue perfusion (renal, cerebral, cardiopulmonary gastrointestinal, and peripheral) related to decreased blood flow
- Anxiety related to ICU and threat to death.

Nursing intervention: The condition urgently calls for identification of the primary cause and immediate management. The patient is protected from unnecessary disturbance and is maintained adequate airway. The patient is also given oxygen inhalation and small doses of morphine (IV) for anxiety and pain. For further details see nursing care plan of cardiogenic shock in Table 12.6.

TABLE 12.6: Nursing care plan of cardiogenic shock

Problem	Reason	Objective	Nursing intervention	Evaluation
1. Decreased cardiac output	(Write subjective and Objective data)	Improved cardiac output	• Position the patient properly as directed • Establish continuous ECG monitoring • Monitor hemodynamic parameters continually (PAP, PCWP, CO, CI, SVR) • Administer cautiously drugs as prescribed, i.e. digoxin, IV fluids, vasodilators, diuretics as prescribed • Observe any side effects of drugs • Monitor blood pressure and mean arterial pressure (MAP) • Maintain MAP less than 60 mm Hg • Measure and record urine output every hour • From indwelling catheter and fluid intake • Obtain daily weight • Evaluate serum electrolytes Na^+, K^+ • Be alert to chest pain and report immediately	
2. Impaired gas exchange	"	Improved gas exchange	• Monitor rate and rhythm of respiration every hour • Auscultate lung sound for abnormal sounds • Evaluate arterial blood gas (ABG) • Administer oxygen therapy to increase O_2 tension and improve hypoxia • Elevate the head of bed 20 to 30 degree as tolerated • Reposition the patient to promote ventilation and maintain skin integrity • Observe for frothy pink-tinged sputum and cough • Report abnormality immediately	
3. Altered tissue perfusion	"	Maintain tissue perfusion	• Perform a neurologic check every hour, using Glasgow Coma scale • Report changes immediately • Obtain BUN and creatinine blood levels to evaluate renal function. • Auscultate for bowel sounds every 2 hours • Evaluate character, rate, rhythm and quality of arterial pulses every 2 hours • Mention temperature every 2 to 4 hours • Protect the skin breakdown	
4. Anxiety	"	Reduce anxiety	As state in other NEP	
5. Knowledge deficit related to cardiogenic management	"	Knows management of condition	• Teach the patient on digoxin the importance of medication is prescribed • Teach how to take pulse before digoxin and after reporting any abnormality • Teach the signs of impending heart failure – Increasing edema, shortness of breath, decreasing urine output, increasing pulse and report immediately – Teach specific measures as in MI	

HEART FAILURE

Heart failure occurs when the myocardium is unable to maintain a sufficient cardiac output to meet the metabolic needs of the body. This condition results from systolic dysfunction or diastolic dysfunction.

- Systolic dysfunction results from inadequate pumping of blood from the ventricle. The decrease in pumping power results in a decreased cardiac output. Any process that alters myocardial contractility can produce systolic dysfunction.
- Diastolic dysfunction (stiff heart syndrome) occurs when the ventricle does not fill adequately during diastole. Inadequate filling decreases the amount of blood in the ventricle for cardiac output. Systolic function is often normal or augmented.

Etiology of Heart Failure

The incidence of heart failure increases with advancing age and coronary artery disease. An increase in the number of survivors of MI is in part responsible for the increasing number of patients with heart failure. Additional predictors of heart failure include diabetes, cigarette smoking, obesity and elevated total cholesterol to high density lipoprotein cholesterol ratio, and abnormally high or low hematocrit level and proteinuria.

Heart failure is a life-long diagnosis managed with lifestyle changes and medications to prevent acute congestive episodes. Congestive heart failure is usually an acute presentation of heart failure. Common underlying conditions include coronary atherosclerosis (primary cause), valvular disease, cardiomyopathy, inflammatory or degenerative muscle disease, and arterial hypertension. A number of systemic factors can contribute to the development and severity of cardiac failure. Increased metabolic rate (fever, thyrotoxicosis), hypoxia, and anemia require an increased cardiac output to satisfy systemic oxygen demand. Dysrhythmia decrease the efficiency of myocardial function.

Heart failure, sometimes referred to as congestive heart failure is the inability of the heart to pump sufficient blood to meet the needs of the tissues for oxygen and nutrients. Heart failure is a clinical syndrome characterized by signs and symptoms of fluid overload or inadequate tissue perfusion. The underlying mechanism of heart failure involves impaired contractile properties of the heart (systolic dysfunction) or filling of the heart (diastolic) that leads to a lower-than-normal cardiac output. The low cardiac output can lead to compensatory mechanisms that cause increased workload on the heart and eventual resistance to filling of the heart.

The common causes for chronic and acute heart failure (CCF) are as follows (also see Box 12.9 and 12.10):

Chronic	Acute
• Coronary artery disease	• Acute myocardial infarction
• Hypertensive heart disease	• Arrhythmias
• Rheumatic heart disease	• Pulmonary emboli
• Cor pulmonale	• Thyrotoxicosis
• Cardiomyopathy	• Hypertensive crisis
• Anemia	• Rupture of papillary muscle
• Bacterial endocarditis	• Ventricular septal defect

The common causes for systolic and diastolic dysfunctions are as follows:

Systolic	Diastolic
• Coronary artery disease	• Coronary artery disease
• Hypertension	• Hypertrophy
• Metabolic disorders	• Fibrosis of advanced age constrictive pericarditis
• Myocarditis	• Myocarditis
• Alcohol	• Hypertension
• Cocaine	• Aortic stenosis
• Cardiac valve diseases	• Ventricular remodeling
• Dilated cardiomyopathy	• Collagen diseases
	• Cardiomyopathy

Pathophysiology (Fig. 12.9)

Congestive heart failure may be caused by any interference with normal mechanisms regulating cardiac output. Cardiac output depends on preload, afterload, myocardial contractility, heart rate and metabolic state of the individual. Any alteration in these factors can lead to decreased ventricular function and the resultant of manifestations of CCF; there are some precipitating causes for heart failure. The common precipitating causes for CCF and their mechanism are as follows (Fig. 12.9):

- *Anemia:* Decreases oxygen carrying capacity of the blood, stimulating increase in cardiac output to meet tissue demand.
- *Infection:* Increases oxygen demand of tissues stimulating increase in cardiac output.
- *Thyrotoxicosis:* Increases the tissue metabolic rate, accelerating heart rate and workload of the heart.
- *Hypothyroidism:* Indirectly predisposes to increase atherosclerosis, severe hypothyroidism decreases myocardial contractility.
- *Arrhythmias:* May decrease cardiac output and increase workload and oxygen requirement of myocardial tissue.
- *Bacterial endocarditis:* Increases metabolic demands and oxygen requirements.
- *Valvular dysfunction*: Causes stenosis and regurgitation.

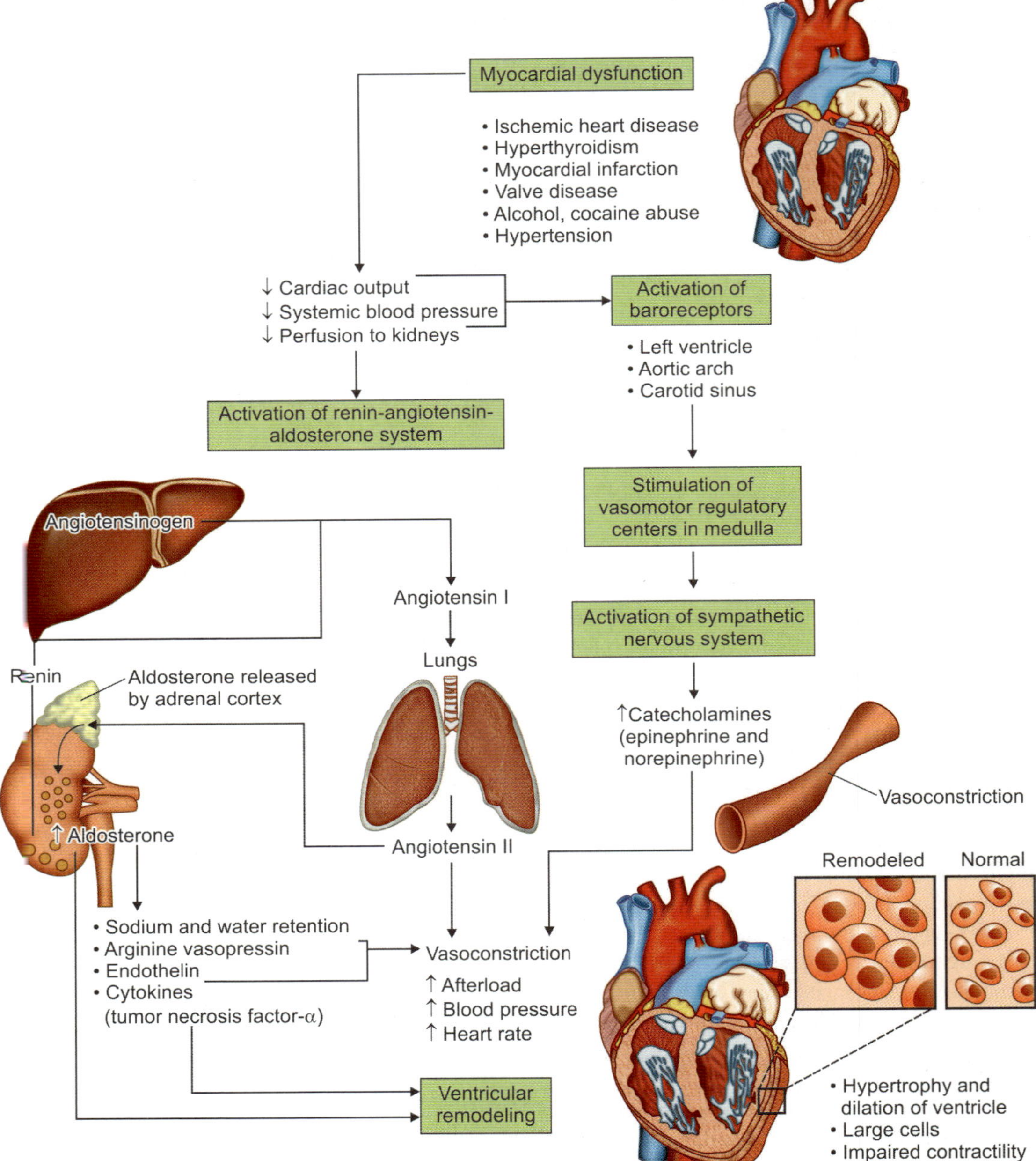

FIG. 12.9: The pathophysiology of heart failure. A decrease in cardiac output activates multiple neurohormonal mechanisms that ultimately result in the signs and symptoms of heart failure

- *Pulmonary embolism:* Increases pulmonary pressure and exerts a pressure load on right ventricle, leading to right ventricle hypertrophy and failure.
- *Pulmonary disease*: Increases pulmonary pressure and exerts a pressure level on the right ventricle, leading to RVH failure.
- *Paget's disease*: Increases work load of the heart by increasing the vascular bed in skeletal muscle.
- *Nutritional deficiencies:* May decrease cardiac function by decreasing myocardial muscles mass and contractility.
- *Hypovolemia:* Increases preload and causes volume load on right ventricle (RV).

Classification of Heart Failure

In addition to above types of heart failure, heart failure can be classified as follows:

1. *Left-Sided versus Right-Sided Heart Failure*

- In left-sided heart failure, left ventricle cardiac output is less than volume received from the pulmonary circulation; blood accumulates in left ventricle, left atrium and pulmonary circulation
- In right-sided heart failure, right ventricle cardiac output is less than volume received from the peripheral venous circulation, blood accumulates in RA, RV and peripheral venous system.

2. *Forward versus backward failure*

- In forward failure, decreased cardiac output results in inadequate tissue perfusion
- In backward failure, blood remains in ventricle after systole, increasing atrial and venous pressure; rise in venous pressure forces fluid out of capillary membrane into extracellular spaces.

3. *High-Output versus Low-Output Failure*

- High output failure occurs in response to conditions that cause the heart to work harder to supply blood; the increased oxygen demand can be met only with an increase in cardiac output; systemic vascular resistance decreases to promote cardiac output
- Low output failure occurs in response to high blood pressure of hypovolemia which, results in impaired peripheral circulation and peripheral vasoconstriction.

4. *Acute versus Chronic Failure*

- Acute failure occurs in response to a sudden decrease in cardiac output which results in rapid decrease in tissue perfusion (Box 12.9)
- So chronic failure, body adjusts to decrease in cardiac output through compensatory mechanisms which results in systemic congestion (Box 12.10).

Recently New York Heart Association classified heart failure as follows:

- Class I: No symptoms tolerate ordinary physical activity.
- Class II: Comfortable at rest, ordinary physical activity results in symptoms.
- Class III: Comfortable at rest, less than ordinary physical activity results in symptoms.
- Class IV: Symptoms may be present at rest, symptoms with any physical activity.

Box 12.9 Acute heart failure

Signs and symptoms	• Rapid respirations with accessory muscle use • Severe dyspnea, orthopnea • Crackles and wheezes • Coughing • Pink, frothy sputum • Anxiety, restlessness • Pale skin and mucous membranes • Clammy, cold skin
Diagnostic test	• Chest X-ray examination • Arterial blood gases • Electrocardiogram • Hemodynamic monitoring
Therapeutic measures	• Oxygen via cannula, mask, or mechanical ventilation • Positioning in high or semi-Fowler's position • IV drugs: Morphine, diuretics, inotropic agents, vasodilators • Frequent vital signs, urinary output • Pulmonary pressures • Daily weights • Treatment of underlying cause

Pathophysiology

In most cases heart failure begins with left ventricular systolic dysfunction. Ventricular failure can be described as:

- A defect in systolic functions that results in impaired ventricular emptying; or
- A defect in diastolic function that causes an impairment in ventricular filling.

It is now recognized that patients with heart failure actually comprise three distinct groups:

i. Those with failure of systolic ejection;
ii. Those with abnormal resistance to diastolic filling; and
iii. Those with mixed systolic and diastolic dysfunction.

- Systolic failure is the most common cause of heart failure. It is a defect in the ability of the cardia myofibrils to shorten, which decreases the muscles' ability to generate enough pressure to eject blood forward through the high-pressure aorta. Inability to move blood forward through the aorta results in:
  - A decreased left ventricular ejection traction (LVET)
  - An acute increase in left ventricular end diastolic pressure (LVEDP)
  - An increase in fluid accumulation in the pulmonary vascular bed (pulmonary congestion).

Systolic failure is due to impaired contractile function (MI), increased after local (HBP) or mechanical abnormalities (valvular disease).

- Diastolic failure is not a disorder of contractility, but of relaxation and ventricular filling. In fact, there is normal

Box 12.10 An overview of chronic heart failure

	Right-sided heart failure	Left-sided heart failure
Signs and symptoms	• Jugular venous distention • Dependent peripheral edema • Ascites • Weight gain • Splenomegaly • Hepatomegaly • GI pain, anorexia nausea • Fatigue, weakness • Tachycardia • Nocturia	• Dyspnea on exertion • Dry hacking cough, especially when supine • Crackles, wheezing • Orthopnea • Paroxysmal nocturnal dyspnea (PND) • Cheyne-Stokes respirations • Cyanosis • Tachypnea, tachycardia • Nocturia
Diagnostic tests	• History and physical examination • Electrocardiogram • Chest X-ray • 2D-echocardiography with Doppler • Exercise stress test • Coronary angiography • Cardiac magnetic resonance imaging • Nuclear imaging studies • Cardiac magnetic resonance imaging • Nuclear imaging studies • Cardiac catheterization • Serum laboratory test: CBC, BNP, electrolytes, BUN, creatinine, liver function test, thyroid-stimulating hormone, fasting blood glucose, lipid profile, ferritin • Arterial blood gases • Urinalysis • Sleep studies • Hemodynamic monitoring	
Complications	• Hepatomegaly • Splenomegaly • Pleural effusion • Left ventricular thrombus and emboli • Cardiogenic shock	
Therapeutic measures	*Noninvasive* • Treat underlying cause • Oxygen by cannula or mask • Drug therapy • Individualized activity plan • Dietary sodium restriction • Fluid restriction • Daily weights *Invasive* • Pacemaker • ICD • Resynchronization therapy • Mechanical assistive devices • Intra-aortic balloon pump • Left ventricular assist device • Total artificial heart • Surgery: CABG, valvuloplasty, heart valve replacement, cardiac transplant	

BNP = brain natriuretic peptide; BUN = blood urea nitrogen; CABG = coronary artery bypass graft; CBC = complete blood count; ICD = implantable cardioverter defibrillator

or hyperdynamic systolic function. Diastolic failure is characterized by high-filling pressure and the resultant venous engorgement in both the pulmonary and systemic systems. The diagnosis of diastolic failure is made on the basis of the presence of pulmonary congestion and pulmonary hypertension in the setting of a normal ejection pattern
- Systolic and diastolic failure of mixed origin is seen in disease state such as dilated cardiomyopathy (DCM), a condition in which poor systolic function is further compromised by dilated left ventricular walls that are unable to relax. This patient often has extremely poor ejection tractions, high pulmonary pressures and biventricular failures.

Heart failures can have an abrupt onset as with acute MI or it can be an insidious process resulting from slow progressive changes. The overloaded heart resorts to certain compensatory mechanisms which include:

- Ventricular dilation
- Ventricular hypertrophy
- Increased sympathetic nervous system stimulation
- Hormonal response.

Dilation is an enlargement of the chambers of the heart. It occurs where pressure in the heart chambers, usually, the left ventricle is elevated over time. The muscle fibers of the heart stretch and thereby increase that contractile force. Initially this increased contraction leads to increased cardiac output and maintenance of arterial blood pressure and perfusion. Therefore, dilation is an adaption mechanism to cope with increasing blood volume. Eventually this becomes inadequate because the elastic elements of the muscle fibers are overstretched and overstrained.

Hypertrophy is an increase in the muscle mass and cardiac wall thickness in response to overwork and strain. It occurs slowly because it takes time for this increased muscle tissue to develop. It generally follows persistent or chronic dilation and then further increases the contractile power of the muscle fibers. This will lead to an increase in cardiac output and maintenance of tissue perfusion. However, hypertrophic heart muscle has poor contractility.

Sympathetic nervous system activation is often the first mechanism triggered in low cardiac output. It is a least effective compensatory mechanism, because there is inadequate stroke volume and CO. There is increased sympathetic nervous system activation resulting in the increased release of epinephrine and norepinephrine. This results in an increased heart rate. Myocardial contractility and peripheral vascular constrictions. This improves cardiac output (CO). However, later, it leads to worsening the ventricular performance with overlooked volume due to peripheral vascular conditions.

Hormonal responses: As the CO falls, blood flow to the kidneys decreases, causing decreased glomerular blood flow. This is interpreted by the juxtaglomerular apparatus in the kidney as decreased volume. The decrease in renal blood flow activates the renin-angiotensin system to correct a perceived hypovolemia. Angiotensin causes the adrenal cortex to release aldesterone which causes sodium retention and increased peripheral vasoconstriction, which increases astral blood pressure. The posterior pituitary senses the increased osmotic pressure and it secretes ADH, which increases water absorption in renal tubules causing water retention and therefore increased blood volume. Therefore, the blood volume is increased in a person who is already volume overloaded.

Clinical Manifestations of Heart Failure

Classic symptoms of heart failure include dyspnea with exertion, orthopnea, nocturnal dyspnea, a dry, hacking cough, and unexplained fatigue. When volume overload contributes to pathology, the following additional symptoms occur: rales, a third heart sound, peripheral edema, unexplained weight gain, jugular venous distention, hepatic engorgements, ascitis and worsening dyspnea. Compensatory mechanism accounts for many of the clinical signs and symptoms of heart failure.

- Symptoms of inadequate tissue perfusion
- Diminished cardiac output with accompanying dizziness, confusion, fatigue, exercise or heat intolerance, cool extremities and oliguria
- Congestion of tissues
- Increased pulmonary venous pressure (pulmonary edema) manifested by cough and shortness of breath
- Dysrhythmia may indicate heart failure or may be noted as a result of the treatment for heart failure
- Increased systemic venous pressure, as evidenced by generalized peripheral edema and weight gain.

Left-sided Heart Failure

Most often precedes right-sided cardiac failure. See Box 12.11 for causes of left sided heart failure

Backward Failure

- Pulmonary congestion; cough; fatigability; tachycardia with an S3 heart sound; anxiety; restlessness
- Dyspnea on exertion (DOE), orthopnea, paroxysmal nocturnal dyspnea (PND)
- Cough may be dry and nonproductive but is most often moist
- Bibasilar crackles advancing to crackles in all lung fields
- Large quantities of frothy sputum, which is sometimes pink (blood-tinged).

Forward Failure

Tachycardia, weak, thready pulse, anxiety, oliguria and nocturia altered digestion, ashen, pale, cool and clammy skin.

Box 12.11 Causes of left sided heart failure

Cause	Primary effect on left ventricular workload
Aortic stenosis	Increased volume to pump from restricted blood outflow
Cardiomyopathy	Increased workload from impaired contractility
Coarctation of the aorta	Restricted outflow and increased resistance from narrowing of aorta
Hypertension	Resistance increased from elevated pressure
Heart muscle infection	Increased workload from damaged myocardium
Myocardial infarction	Increased workload from impaired contractility
Mitral regurgitation	Increased volume to pump from backward blood flow

Box 12.12 Causes of right sided heart failure

Cause	Primary effect on left ventricular workload
Atrial septal defect	Left atrial blood flow into right atrium increases right ventricular volume to pump
Cor pulmonale	Resistance increased from elevated pressure
Left-sided heart failure	Resistance increased from backup of fluid and elevated pressures
Pulmonary hypertension	Resistance increased from elevated pressure
Pulmonary valve stenosis	Increased volume to pump from restricted right ventricular blood outflow

Right-Sided Heart Failure (Box 12.12)

- Congestion of the viscera and peripheral tissues
- Edema of lower extremities (dependent edema), usually pitting edema, weight gain, hepatomegaly
- Distended neck veins (jugular vein distention), ascites, anorexia and nausea
- Nocturia and weakness

The more common symptoms as well as symptoms encountered with progressive heart failure are as follows:

1. Respiratory symptoms
   - Dyspnea
   - Orthopnea
   - Paroxysmal nocturnal dyspnea
   - Persistent hacking cough
   - Alternating periods of apnea and hyperpnea
   - Rales (crackles).
2. Cardiovascular symptoms
   - Angina
   - Jugular venous distention
   - Tachycardia
   - Decrease in systolic blood pressure with increase in diastolic pressure
   - S3 and S4 heart sounds.
3. Gastrointestinal symptoms
   - Enlargement and tenderness in the right upper quadrant of abdomen
   - Ascites
   - Nausea
   - Vomiting
   - Bloating
   - Anorexia
   - Epigastric pain.
4. Cerebral symptoms
   - Altered mental status (confusion, restlessness).
5. Generalized symptoms
   - Fatigue
   - Decrease in activity intolerance
   - Edema (peripheral pitting)
   - Weight gain.
6. Psychosocial
   - Anxiety.

The clinical manifestations specific to right-sided and left-sided heart failure are as follows:

1. Right-sided heart failure.

   Signs
   - Right ventricle heaves
   - Murmurs
   - Peripheral edema
   - Weight gain
   - Edema of dependant body part (sacrum, anterior tibias, pedal edema)
   - Ascites
   - Anasarca (massive generalized body edema)
   - Jugular venous distension
   - Hepatomegaly (liver engorgement)
   - Right-sided pleural effusion.

   Symptoms
   - Fatigue
   - Dependent edema
   - Right upper quadrant pain
   - Anorexia and GI bloating
   - Nausea.
2. Left-sided heart failure

   Signs
   - Left ventricle heaves
   - Cheyne-Stokes respirations
   - Pulsus alternans (alternating pulses: strong, weak)
   - Increased heart rate
   - PMI displaced inferiorly and posteriorly (LV hypertrophy)
   - Decreased PaO_2, slight increased $PaCO_2$ (poor oxygen exchange)
   - Crackles (pulmonary edema)
   - S3 and S4 heart sounds.

Symptoms
- Fatigue
- Dyspnea (shallow respiration up to 32–40/m)
- Orthopnea (Shortness of breath in recumbent position)
- Dry, hacking cough
- Pulmonary edema
- Nocturia
- Paroxysmal nocturnal dyspnea.

Management of Heart Failure

Along with other team members, nurses assess the health status of the patient with heart failure by identifying the clinical manifestations particularly paroxysmal nocturnal dyspnea, orthopnea, new-onset of dyspnea on excretion, fatigue, lower extremity edema, persistent cough and recent weight gain and records, and perform physical assessment which includes third heart sound, respiratory distress, pulmonary rales, elevated jugular venous pressure, increased in daily weight without increased intake, abdominal distension, cool extremities and decreased pulse, alteration in level of consciousness and decreased urine output.

- Evaluation of clinical manifestations (Box 12.13)
- Hemodynamic monitoring

Box 12.13 Assessing for heart failure

Be alert for the following signs and symptoms

General
- Fatigue
- Decreased activity tolerance
- Dependent edema
- Weight gain

Cardiovascular
- Third heart sound (S3)
- Apical impulse enlarged with left lateral displacement
- Pallor and cyanosis
- Jugular venous distention (JVD)

Respiratory
- Dyspnea on exertion
- Pulmonary crackles do not clear with cough
- Orthopnea
- Paroxysmal nocturnal dyspnea (PND)
- Cough on exertion or when supine

Cerebrovascular
- Unexplained confusion or altered mental status
- Lightheadedness

Renal
- Oliguria and decreased frequency during the day
- Nocturia

Gastrointestinal
- Anorexia and nausea
- Enlarged liver
- Ascites
- Hepatojugular reflux

- Cardiac catheterization with radionuclide ventriculography or invasively, by ventriculogram
- Echocardiogram (ejection fraction)
- Chest radiographs, ECG
- Exercise testing to detect coronary artery disease
- Laboratory studies (blood urea nitrogen [BUN], creatinine, thyroid stimulating hormone, complete blood count [CBC] urinalysis)

In addition, nurses also assist in diagnostic test such as ABGs, serum chemistries, liver profile, chest X-ray, hemodynamic monitoring, 12-lead ECG and monitor echocardiogram, nuclear imaging studies and cardiac catheterization.

Nursing diagnosis are determined from analysis of patient's data. The possible nursing diagnosis will include:

- Decreased cardiac output related to alteration in preload, afterload or inotropic changes in heart
- Impaired gas exchange related to alveolar-capillary membrane changes
- Fluid volume excess related to imbalance between O_2 supply and O_2 demand
- Hopelessness related to failing or deteriorating physiological changes.

The objectives of nursing intervention will be:

- Improving cardiac output
- Improving gas exchange
- Restoring fluid volume balance
- Improving activity tolerance
- Supporting the patient experiencing hopelessness
- Educating the patient and family regarding care.

The guidelines for taking care of the person with heart failure are as follows:

1. Support oxygenation
   a. Administer oxygen by nasal cannula at 2 to 6 L/min for oxygen saturation greater than 90 percent
   b. Give oxygen as needed for dyspnea
   c. Patient should be well supported in a semi-Fowler's position
   d. Encourage use of incentive spirometry fourth hourly.
2. Balance rest and activity.
   a. Reinforce importance of conservation of energy and planning for activities that avoid fatigue
   b. Encourage activities within prescribed restriction; monitor for intolerance to activity (dyspnea, fatigue, increased pulse rate does not stabilize)
   c. Assist with ADL as necessary; encourage independence within patient's limitations
   d. Provide diversional activities that assist in conservation of energy
   e. Provide calm and quiet environment.
3. Perform head-to-toe assessment in each shift, including assessment of laboratory values, daily weight, and intake and output.
4. Provide skin care, particularly over edematous areas; use prophylactic measures to prevent skin breakdown.

5. Assist in maintaining an adequate nutritional intake while observing prescribed dietary modifications (offer small meals with supplements).
6. Monitor constipation, give prescribed stool softeners.
7. Give prescribed medications and monitor for adverse effects.
8. Provide patient and family with opportunities to discuss their concerns and time to learn about the diagnosis and plan of care.

See Table 12.7 for nursing care plan of heart failure.

TABLE 12.7: Nursing care plan for the patient with heart failure

Problems	Objective	Nursing interventions	Rationales
Nursing Diagnosis #1			
Cardiac output alteration in, decreased, related to: 1. Impaired myocardial contractile functioning 2. Filling disorders 3. Abnormal volume load 4. Abnormal pressure load	Patient will: 1. Demonstrate signs of hemodynamic stability: – Cardiac output 4–8 liters/minute – Heart rate < 100 beats/min – Systolic blood pressure > 110 mm Hg or within 10 mm Hg of baseline – Pulmonary capillary wedge pressure 8–12 mm Hg (mean) – Absence of S3 and S4 2. Maintain electrophysiologic stability: – Absence of dysrhythmias 3. Maintain state of normovolemia. – Good skin turgor – Absence of peripheral edema – Absence of jugular venous distention – Absence of rales on auscultation – Stable baseline body weight	• Ongoing assessment of signs and symptoms of left ventricular failure: – Rales (crackles) – Bronchial wheezing – Dyspnea – Paroxysmal nocturnal dyspnea – Nocturia – Orthopnea – Anxiety, restlessness, disorientation – Pulsus alternans – Gallop rhythms – Peripheral cyanosis – Central cyanosis – Blood-tinged sputum – Cheyne-Stokes respirations • Ongoing assessment of the signs and symptoms of right ventricular failure: – Jugular venous distention – Peripheral edema – Weight gain – Ascites – Hepatojugular reflux – Anorexia, nausea, vomiting • Identify and correct (if possible) precipitating factors of heart failure • Monitor fluid balance: – Measure weight daily – Document intake and output, urine specific gravity – Maintain fluid restriction as indicated – Use microdrip or infusion pump for fluid administration • Monitor hemodynamic parameters – Arterial blood pressure – Allow for frequent rest periods – Administer oxygen as prescribed – Institute measures to allay anxiety (see *Nursing Diagnosis #4*) • Administer prescribed medication regimen to maximize effects of preload, afterload, and myocardial contractility – Cardiac glycosides – Diuretics: ◆ Monitor I and O; daily weight ◆ Monitor for side effects of diuretic therapy (hypokalemia, hyponatremia, fatigue, muscle cramps, hypotension, tachycardia)	• Provides a systematic approach to data collection to gauge the severity of the disease and the efficacy of therapeutic intervention: – Fluid in alveoli, the result of pressure increases in the pulmonary capillary bed – Bronchiolar constriction from excess fluid – Result of elevation in pulmonary interstitial edema – Serum proteins are at lowest level in early morning; redistribution of volume secondary to recumbent position; nocturnal respiratory depression – Increased renal perfusion secondary to postural redistribution of blood flow – Result of increased venous return from postural redistribution of pulmonary blood flow – Decreased cerebral perfusion and cerebral hypoxia – Secondary to variation in strength of ventricular contraction – S3 associated with increased LVEDP, left atrial pressure, and PCWP – S4 related to decreased ventricular compliance – Secondary to decreased cardiac output and decreased peripheral circulation; blood stays in peripheral tissues longer to extract more oxygen, and when blood reaches distal vascular bed, it has a markedly diminished O_2 content – Results when alveolar edema impairs O_2 diffusion – Rupture of bronchiolar capillaries due to increased hydrostatic pressure in capillaries – Decreased cardiac output causes prolonged circulation time, which in turn causes the respiratory center in the brainstem to be underperfused and under oxygenated

Contd...

Contd...

Problems	Objective	Nursing interventions	Rationales
		– Vasodilators: ◆ Monitor for side effects and efficacy of therapy (headache, dizziness, hypotension, postural hypotension, muscle weakness, syncope; SVR, PCWP, RA pressure, diuresis, increased exercise tolerance, resolution of heart failure symptoms) – Pulmonary capillary wedge pressure – Cardiac output and cardiac intake – Systemic vascular resistance – Right atrial pressure • Monitor laboratory/diagnostic data – Arterial blood gases – Electrolytes – ECG – Chest X-ray – Circulation time – Elevated bilirubin, SGOT, and LDH – Proteinuria, increased specific gravity, increased BUN and creatinine • Implement measures to reduce cardiac work-load: – Place patient in semi-Fowler's position if blood pressure tolerates – Sympathomimetics – Chest X-ray – Circulation time – Elevated bilirubin, SGOT, and LDH – Proteinuria, increased specific gravity, increased BUN and creatinine • Implement measures to reduce cardiac work-load: – Place patient in semi-Fowler's position if blood pressure tolerates – Sympathomimetics • Assess the effects of systemic congestion and decreased cardiac output on drug therapy • Assess medication regimen for drugs with negative inotropic effects; discuss with physician before discontinuing • Monitor for dysrhythmias. – Maintain continuous ECG monitoring – Monitor conditions that precipitate dysrhythmias (hypoxia, acidosis, alkalosis, digoxin toxicity, electrolyte imbalance) and implement corrective action – Document rhythm changes and assess for hemodynamic compromise; notify physician of patient response – Administer treatment to correct dysrhythmias (may include pacing, antiarrhythmics, and/or cardioversion)	– Result of elevated venous pressures – May gain as much as 10–15 lb of extracellular fluid before edema is readily apparent – Pressure on right upper quadrant compresses liver and acts as a temporary fluid challenge; dysfunctional right heart will show a visible increase in pressure in jugular veins; competent right heart will not show a visible increase in pressure – Increased pressure in capillaries of abdominal organs results in edema; nausea is secondary to stretching of liver capsule secondary to edema – Any factor that increases metabolic demand of body stresses the cardiovascular system, which can precipitate the development of heart failure in the patient with cardiac dysfunction. Identification fosters early, more effective intervention • Provide best indication of patient's response to therapy – Decreased systolic pressure or narrowed arterial pulse pressure indicative of decreased cardiac output; increased diastolic blood pressure indicates increased peripheral vascular resistance – Reduces fatigue, decreases myocardial oxygen consumption – Reduces workload of heart and supports cellular energy requirements – Correction of hypoxia related to pulmonary congestion – Myocardial tissue hypoxia predisposes to dysrhythmias and further decreases myocardial contractility – Positive inotropic and negative chronotropic agent—improved cardiac output – Decrease intravascular volume by their direct action on the kidney and by reducing sodium reabsorption; increase venous capacitance, reduce preload to maximize Frank-Starling mechanism

Contd...

Contd...

Problems	Objective	Nursing interventions	Rationales
		• Identify factors that exacerbate structural abnormalities of cardiac function and institute appropriate therapy – Hypertrophic cardiomyopathy: Avoid conditions that increase the degree of obstruction and/or decrease ventricular volume (digitalis, diuretics, nitrates, exercise, sudden postural changes, Valsalva maneuvers, beta-antagonists) – Encourage factors that increase cardiac output (alpha-stimulants, supine or squatting position) • Prepare for insertion of mechanical circulatory assist devices • Maintain properly functioning emergency equipment and ensure its availability on each shift	– Increased venous capacitance provides beneficial effect in patients with left heart failure and pulmonary edema; in patients with right heart failure with vigorous diuresis, this may be detrimental as it contributes to systemic venous pooling, thereby limiting venous return and right ventricular filling and further contributing to a decreased cardiac output – Vasodilators increase cardiac output by decreasing SVR and/or reducing LVEDP by decreasing vascular tone. Vasodilators reduce myocardial oxygen demand, which may help minimize ischemia and infarction size – Pulmonary edema develops when PCWP exceeds plasma osmotic pressure (> 28 mm Hg) – Measure of LVEDP preload; optimal PCWP maximizes contractility via Frank-Starling mechanism. Elevated in aortic stenosis and regurgitation, mitral stenosis and regurgitation, cardiogenic shock, dilated cardiomyopathy, hypertrophic cardiomyopathy, and restrictive cardiomyopathy – Determinant of afterload; increased impedance to left ventricular ejection increases intramyocardial wall tension; result of sympathoadrenergic stimulation; increased SVR increases myocardial oxygen requirements and decreases myocardial contractility – Elevated in pulmonary hypertension, tricuspid and pulmonic stenosis, tricuspid regurgitation right heart failure, and hypervolemia – Increased work of breathing secondary to pulmonary congestion leads to hypoxia and hypercapnia, which further depress myocardial contractility – BUN, Na—reflect hydration status; hypokalemia—diuresis-induced; hyperglycemia—secondary to stress-related catecholamines – May reveal evidence of ischemia, LVH, RVH, dysrhythmias

Contd...

Contd...

Problems	Objective	Nursing interventions	Rationales
			– Presence of pleural effusion, usually right-sided or bilateral (rarely on the left); interstitial pulmonary edema; enlarged cardiac silhouette
			– Prolonged secondary to decreased contractility of ventricles leading to decreased cardiac output
			– Result of hepatic congestion in right heart failure
			– Indicate renal dysfunction as a result of decreased cardiac output and decreased glomerular filtration rate
			– Diminishes venous return and promotes adequate lung expansion
			– Positive inotropic agents that increase cardiac output by increasing stroke volume and contractility; myocardium becomes dependent on circulating catecholamines in heart failure, and sympathomimetic administration provides an exogenous source of catecholamines to support myocardial contractility
			– Presence of pleural effusion, usually right-sided or bilateral (rarely on the left); interstitial pulmonary edema; enlarged cardiac silhouette
			– Prolonged secondary to decreased contractility of ventricles leading to decreased cardiac output
			– Result of hepatic congestion in right heart failure
			– Indicate renal dysfunction as a result of decreased cardiac output and decreased glomerular filtration rate
			– Diminishes venous return and promotes adequate lung expansion
			– Positive inotropic agents that increase cardiac output by increasing stroke volume and contractility; myocardium becomes dependent on circulating catecholamines in heart failure, and sympathomimetic administration provides an exogenous source of catecholamines to support myocardial contractility

Contd...

Contd...

Problems	Objective	Nursing interventions	Rationales
			• Hepatic congestion and renal dysfunction may alter drug metabolism and excretion, predisposing the patient to toxic side effects • Such drugs may cause further compromise of cardiac function but may be controlling dysrhythmias, which may also precipitate a deterioration in patient's condition and in cardiac output – Increased irritability of myocardium predisposes to dysrhythmias – Bradyarrhythmias may decrease cardiac output secondary to decreased stroke volume – Tachyarrhythmias reduce diastolic filling time and increase myocardial oxygen consumption. Loss of atrial kick contributes to a decreased cardiac output – Digitalis, exercise, beta-agonists, and valsalva maneuvers increase contractility and the degree of obstruction should be avoided. Diuretics, nitrates, sudden postural changes decrease ventricular volume
Nursing Diagnosis #2			
Tissue perfusion alteration in, related to: 1. Severely impaired myocardial contractility	Patient will: 1. Demonstrate signs of hemodynamic stability: – Systolic BP > 90 mm Hg – Diastolic BP 60–90 mm Hg – PCWP 8–12 mm Hg (mean) – Cardiac output 4–8 L/min – Heart rate < 100 beats/min – SVR 800–1200 dynes/sec/cm^5 2. Maintain adequate tissue perfusion – Patient awake, alert, oriented – Urine output > 30 mL/h – Skin warm and dry – Absence of peripheral edema – Absence of rales (crackles) on auscultation 3. Maintain electrophysiological stability – Absence of dysrhythmias	• Identify patients at risk of developing cardiogenic shock • Assess signs of inadequate tissue perfusion – Coronary: ◆ Blood pressure ◆ Heart rate ◆ Cardiac output/cardiac index ◆ SVR ◆ MAP ◆ Right atrial pressure ◆ PAP, PCWP ◆ Monitor for signs of left or right ventricular failure and dysrhythmias ◆ Evaluate medication regimen for any treatments that may cause myocardial depression ◆ Assess for signs and symptoms indicative of myocardial ischemia and necrosis – Renal: ◆ Measure urine output hourly; notify physician < 30 mL/h ◆ Measure intake and output ◆ Monitor BUN and creatinine ◆ Assess for increased tolerance to diuretic therapy	• Early recognition and intervention are crucial determinants to patient survival – Decreased pulse pressure, increased diastolic blood pressure, systolic pressure less than 90 mm Hg: Indicative of increased SVR and decreased cardiac output – Compensatory tachycardia – Decreased in heart failure; indicator of tissue perfusion – Measurement of afterload; increased secondary to sympathetic nervous system stimulation – Decreased MAP and increased LVEDP (PCWP) result in decreased coronary artery perfusion potentially resulting in myocardial ischemia and necrosis – Measurement of adequacy of central venous return – Increased secondary to impaired myocardial contractility; maintained slightly higher than normal to maximize Frank-Starling mechanism; serial measurements to evaluate left ventricular function and response to therapy

Contd...

Contd...

Problems	Objective	Nursing interventions	Rationales
	4. Maintain arterial blood gases within normal limits 5. Verbalize anxieties and concerns	– Cerebral: ◆ Assess neurologic status: LOC; restlessness, agitation, confusion, and somnolence; response to verbal and tactile stimuli; EOMs and pupillary responses – Respiratory – Cutaneous: ◆ Assess capillary refill ◆ Assess warmth, color, and moistness of skin ◆ Assess quality of peripheral pulses – Visceral: ◆ Monitor bowel sounds ◆ Assess for abdominal discomfort – Laboratory data (see *Nursing Diagnosis #1*): ◆ Arterial blood gases ◆ Venous blood saturations ◆ Electrolytes ◆ Serum lactate level – Assess for hypovolemia (hydration status) ◆ Intake and output including extrarenal (insensible) losses; urine output; PCWP; and weight changes ◆ Keep physician informed of patient's status ◆ Monitor effects of fluid challenge if ordered ◆ Administer fluid challenge (0.9% normal saline) rapidly: 100 mL every 5–10 minutes ◆ Determine CVP or PCWP after each bolus • Administer medications as prescribed. – Monitor medications for efficacy and toxicity – Monitor hemodynamic parameters to assess efficacy of pharmacologic therapy – Monitor arterial pH • Prepare for use of mechanical circulatory assistance if above measures are ineffective in restoring tissue perfusion • Institute measures to allay anxiety	– *See Nursing Diagnosis #1* – *See Nursing Diagnosis #1* – Refer to discussion of myocardial infarction – Decreased cardiac output results in decreased renal perfusion and function; the afferent arterioles vasoconstriction and glomerular filtration decreases, which results in a decreased ability of the kidneys to filter, excrete, and reabsorb – Decreased cardiac output causes diminished carotid and vertebral artery blood flow. Blood flow to medulla remains normal until late in the stages of shock; midbrain, cerebellum, and cerebral cortex are under-perfused – For respiratory assessment, interventions, and rationales see *Nursing Diagnosis #3*, below – Cool, moist skin indicates decreased perfusion secondary to redistribution of blood flow to central circulation – Weak, thready peripheral pulses are indicative of vasoconstriction – Indicative of decreased perfusion and ischemia to splanchnic area secondary to a profound decrease in cardiac output – Acidosis depresses myocardial contractility; acidosis indicates inadequate tissue perfusion and accumulation of lactic acid – Increased arterial-venous O_2 difference indicates increased O_2 extraction by tissues in response to a decreased cardiac output – Hyponatremia and hyperkalemia are myocardial depressants – Elevated secondary to anaerobic metabolism – Contraindicated for PCWP > 20 mm Hg; CVP > 12 cm H_2O – Ensures intravascular expansion – End points of challenge are hypotension; PCWP at 20 mm Hg; CVP increase by 2 cm H_2O – PCWP > 20 mm Hg increases likelihood of precipitating pulmonary edema – Hypotension, redistribution of blood volume, impaired renal and hepatic perfusion may impair absorption and metabolism – Best indices to LV function and systemic perfusion

Contd...

Contd...

Problems	Objective	Nursing interventions	Rationales
			– Most vasoactive therapy has decreased efficacy in an acidotic or alkalotic environment • Decreases afterload during systole and increases perfusion by increasing aortic pressure during diastole • See *Nursing Diagnosis #4*, below
Nursing Diagnosis #3			
Gas exchange impaired, related to: 1. Pulmonary congestion with increased ventilation/perfusion mismatching, and shunting	Patient will: 1. Demonstrate signs of adequate cerebral oxygenation: Alert mental status; oriented to person, time, and place 2. Demonstrate normal respiratory effort: – Rate < 25/minute; pattern—eupneic 3. Maintain optimal arterial blood gases: – pH 7.35–7.45 – PaO_2 > 60 mm Hg – $PaCO_2$ 35–45 mm Hg 4. Maintain breath sounds clear to auscultation 5. Demonstrate clear lung fields on chest X-ray 6. Maintain effective cardiovascular function: – HR 60–80/min – Cardiac output 4–8 L/min	• Perform ongoing mental status assessment: Confusion, restlessness, anxiety, stupor, loss of consciousness • Monitor respiratory function on ongoing basis – Respiratory rate and rhythm – Dyspnea – Orthopnea – Cough – Status of weakness and fatigue – Secretions: Quality, quantity, presence of blood (frequently pink and frothy secretions) – Cyanosis, pallor – Auscultation of lungs for presence of adventitious sounds: Rales, bronchial and wheezing • Monitor diagnostic tests and studies: – Arterial blood gases – Chest X-ray – ECG • Assess cardiovascular function frequently: – Heart rate – Hemodynamic parameters: ◆ Systemic blood pressure ◆ Cardiac output ◆ PCWP – Jugular venous distention; peripheral edema, sacraledema; presence of S3, S4; gallop rhythm; pulsus alternans; palpitation, chest pain • Implement measures to allay patient anxiety – Assess patient's anxiety – Explain treatment plan and procedures – Maintain calm, reassuring approach to care • Implement measures to increase gas exchange – Administer oxygen as prescribed and monitor response to therapy – Reassure patient of the need for oxygen and its temporary nature – Administer positive pressure as needed – Assess hemodynamic parameters meticulously during positive pressure therapy (PEEP)	• Hypoxemia may predispose to cerebral tissue hypoxia – Reflects work of breathing: Increased work of breathing increases oxygen consumption and myocardial oxygen demand – Secondary to increased pulmonary interstitial edema – Increased venous return secondary to postural redistribution of pulmonary blood flow – Usually nonproductive, periodic, and nocturnal – Secondary to decreased perfusion to skeletal muscles; increased work of breathing further fatigues the patient and predisposes to alveolar hypoventilation with hypercapnia and respiratory acidemia – Result of capillary hydrostatic pressure exceeding pulmonary capillary oncotic pressure, which allows fluid to leak into pulmonary interstitium; when this cannot be reabsorbed via the pulmonary lymphatic system, fluid fills the alveoli – Frequent assessments allow for early intervention, minimizing deleterious effects of respiratory compromise – Reflect effectiveness of gas exchange; decreased PaO_2 result of alveolar flooding; $PaCO_2$ initially decreases secondary to hyperventilation; then it elevates secondary to patient fatigue – Butterfly distribution of pulmonary infiltrates; may take 24 hours after symptoms develop to become apparent on chest X-ray – May reflect signs of myocardial ischemia – Initial tachycardia is the result of sympathetic nervous system stimulation; return of heart rate to baseline may be indicative of resolving pulmonary edema

Contd...

Contd...

Problems	Objective	Nursing interventions	Rationales
		– Initiate intubation and mechanical ventilation as necessary • Implement measures to decrease preload and afterload – Place patient in high Fowler's position with dependent lower extremities if blood pressure allows – Administer morphine sulfate IV ◆ Monitor for respiratory depressant effects; have morphine antagonist at bedside ◆ Monitor blood pressure for hypotension – Administer intravenous vasodilators such as nitroprusside and nitroglycerin. Carefully monitor arterial blood pressure while administering these drugs – Administer intravenous diuretics as ordered (usually potent loop diuretics such as furosemide and ethacrynic acid). Carefully monitor for hypotension and tachycardia, and check for signs of hypokalemia – Apply rotating tourniquets as ordered (automatic tourniquet machine) following appropriate procedure: ◆ Connect to upper portion of arms and legs; only 3 cuffs should be inflated simultaneously ◆ Inflate blood pressure cuffs to 10 mm Hg below the diastolic pressure ◆ Check for presence of peripheral pulses, warmth, and color of extremities ◆ Make certain tourniquets rotate every 15 minutes ◆ When discontinuing tourniquets, remove one by one in a counter clockwise direction every 15 minutes – Assess patient's tolerance to discontinuance of treatment • Implement measures to improve left ventricular contractility – Administer cardiac glycosides as prescribed – Administer dopamine, dobutamine in low doses as prescribed – Administer aminophylline as prescribed (observe for hypotension, dysrhythmias)	– May become hypertensive from sympathetic stimulation – Reflects tissue perfusion – Increased LVEDP reflected back to pulmonary capillary bed, increasing pulmonary intravascular hydrostatic pressure; PCWP > 20 mm Hg – Affords noninvasive evaluation of changes in venous pressure (see *Nursing Diagnosis #1*) • Anxiety causes patient to become tachypneic, which causes him/her to consume more oxygen – O_2 is given to raise PaO_2 above 60 mm Hg when there is hypoxemia without hypercapnia – Hypoxia enhances likelihood of dysrhythmia development, depresses myocardial contractility, and causes pulmonary vasoconstriction, which increases the workload of the right side of the heart; elevating the PaO_2 will minimize and/or reverse these processes – Most patients tolerate administration of oxygen by mask poorly and frequently fear suffocation – Increases mean lung volume (functional lung capacity), allowing more alveoli to participate in gas exchange – Positive pressure can impede venous return, thereby decreasing cardiac output – Dilates peripheral arteries and veins and causes venous pooling, thereby decreasing venous congestion – Reduces patient's anxiety, decreases tachypnea, causes peripheral pooling of blood, decreases preload and afterload – Respiratory depression occurs in approximately 7 minutes – Hypotension, the result of baroreceptors vasoconstrictive reflexes, is inhibited by morphine – Reduce vascular hydrostatic pressure and reduce PCWP; these drugs have systemic venous and arterial vasodilatory properties – Reduce total blood volume and increase venous capacitance – Cause reduction in sodium reabsorption in loop of Henle; direct effect on arterial and venous dilatation

Contd...

Contd...

Problems	Objective	Nursing interventions	Rationales
			– Evidence of circulatory intolerance and potassium wasting is associated with use of these diuretics – Higher pressures will cause fluid loss into the patient's peripheral extravascular spaces – Should not occlude arterial blood flow – Pulse should be palpable with cuff inflated – Avoids excessive increase in venous return • Increased myocardial contractility leads to increased cardiac output with a reduction in LVEDP and PCWP – Stimulate myocardial beta-receptors to enhance contractility – Bronchodilator; also increases myocardial contractility and enhances diuresis
Nursing Diagnosis #4			
Anxiety, related to: 1. Potential for lifestyle modification 2. Powerlessness 3. Intensive care setting 4. Uncertainty related to illness and diagnosis	Patient will: 1. Verbalize anxieties and fears 2. Verbalize feeling and less anxious 3. Demonstrate a relaxed demeanor	• Obtain baseline assessment of anxiety level and coping patterns from patient, family members, or significant others • Assess level of anxiety; include heart rate, blood pressure, increased muscle tension, increased startle response, a change in sleeping patterns, nightmares, irritability, diaphoresis, nausea, diarrhea, repetitive behaviors • Ascertain what the patient or family member is experiencing; eliminate a physiologic basis of symptoms • Determine what the individual's needs are and what resources can be mobilized to decrease feelings of anxiety; provide positive reinforcement when appropriate • Implement therapeutic measures to decrease anxiety – Encourage the patient and/or family to verbalize anxieties and concerns; encourage them to ask questions; listen attentively; provide a caring environment – Explain procedures and limitations to patient/family. Relate to nature of heart disease – Familiarize patient with ICU staff, routines, equipment – Mobilize appropriate resources: ◆ Consult social services, chaplaincy program, financial advisor, or other such services, as appropriate	• Baseline data are essential in evaluating the effectiveness of therapeutic interventions and the patient's ability to cope – Assists in determining the underlying cause of anxiety and provides a basis for intervention • Hypoxemia, hypercarbia, decreased cardiac output, and pain precipitate and intensify feelings of apprehension and anxiety • Positive feedback helps nurture confidence – Helps to create a trusting relationship; reassures patient he/she is not alone – See *Nursing Diagnosis #7*, below – Knowing what to expect will help to reduce anxiety – Removed of multification of precipitating factors may reduce anxiety; social interaction helps modify feelings of depersonalization that accompany hospitalization – Will decrease anxiety by re-establishing sense of control and purpose

Contd...

Contd...

Problems	Objective	Nursing interventions	Rationales
		◆ Modify the environment to decrease anxiety; modify the policy regarding visitors; increase or decrease environmental stimuli as indicated; increase frequency of nurse/patient contacts – Involve patients in their own care within physical limitations	
Nursing Diagnosis #5			
Infection, potential for, related to: 1. Decreased mobility 2. Invasive lines 3. Pulmonary congestion 4. Valvular heart disease	Patient will: 1. Demonstrate absence or resolution of infection as indicated by: – White blood cell count within normal limits – Normal body temperature (37°C, 98.6°F) 2. Demonstrate understanding of importance of antibiotic prophylaxis (as patient's condition warrants) 3. Remain without complications of infectious process (e.g., embolization associated with infective	• Identify patients at high risk of developing an infection: Elderly; rheumatic heart disease; prosthetic heart valves; valvular lesions; intravenous drug abuse; hypertrophic cardiomyopathy; multiple invasive lines; immunocompromised; chronic debilitating diseases • Maintain strict aseptic technique during insertion and changing of hemodynamic monitoring lines; strict adherence to handwashing protocols – Maintain closed system; use sterile stop-cocks with caps – Change pressure tubing and flush solutions every 48 hours or as per unit protocol – Change dressings and observe for signs of infection, as per unit protocol – Record date of insertion of each line; arterial, CVP and PA lines should be changed every 3–4 days, or as per unit protocol – Culture tips of catheters when removed, if indicated • Monitor for signs of infection. – Monitor temperature every 4 hours; report elevation to physician – Monitor WBC count – Observe for tachycardia, chills, or diaphoresis. Keep patient warm and dry • Administer antibiotics and antipyretics as prescribed and monitor response to therapy • Turn every 2 hours while on bed rest • Initiate measures to prevent atelectasis: – Encourage hourly deep breathing while awake and during periods of immobility – Teach use of incentive spirometer if appropriate – Progress activity as tolerated – Note color, quantity, character of secretions (pulmonary) – Auscultate breath sounds every 4 hours and record	• Patients with heart disease are at high risk due to alterations in endothelial integrity on cardiac valves secondary to surgical, congenital, or rheumatic causes. Early detection and treatment may improve prognosis • Minimizes likelihood of airborne and contact organisms entering sterile field – Stopcocks that are not maintained as a closed system contribute to 5–10 percent of the infections associated with intravascular catheters – Has proven sufficient for minimizing incidence of line-related septicemia – Irritation of vessel or endocardium predisposes to thrombophlebitis and infective endocarditis – Fever increases basal metabolic rate and causes tachycardia and increase in cardiac output to meet tissue metabolic demands. This hyperdynamic response is likely to precipitate severe heart failure by markedly elevating myocardial oxygen demand and reducing the time for diastolic filling – Early detection of an inflammatory or infectious process encourages prompt intervention to minimize deleterious effects of the causative organism on the heart and other body processes • To maintain skin integrity and mobilize pulmonary secretions: – Maximizes alveolar inflation and minimizes atelectasis and hypoventilation – Pulmonary edema results in frothy, blood-tinged sputum; pneumonia results in thick, purulent sputum

Contd...

Contd...

Problems	Objective	Nursing interventions	Rationales
		• Assess for potential source of infection: – Urine: Hematuria, cloudy, flank pain – Sputum, character, color, quantity – Monitor cultures and sensitivities • Assess for signs and symptoms of infective endocarditis: – Change in murmur – Fever – Hematuria – Petechiae – Osler's nodes – Roth's spots – Janeway nodes – Nail bed splinter hemorrhages • Assess for complications of embolization: – Change in level of consciousness, visual disturbances, headache – SOB, chest pain, hemoptysis – Hematuria, decreased urine output, increased BUN and creatinine – Dysrhythmias, pericardial friction rub, sudden hemodynamic compromise – Left upper quadrant pain radiating to left shoulder • Instruct patient with valvular heart disease regarding importance of antibiotic prophylaxis	– Assessment for atelectasis, increasing left heart failure, or pneumonia – Assists in assessing response to therapy • Infective endocarditis can precipitate the development of heart failure: – Murmurs are usually absent in patients with right-sided endocarditis, particularly with tricuspid valve involvement – Murmurs that develop with endocarditis are usually regurgitant; vegetative lesion (if large enough) can cause stenotic murmur – New or changing murmur may indicate corrosive complications of valve – *Staphylococcus* is usually associated with acute infectious process and causes temperature elevations with high fever spikes and rigours; *Streptococcus* usually produces a subacute process with moderate temperature elevations – Result of renal emboli and infarction – One of the most frequent signs noted in neck, conjunctivae, clavicles, wrists, ankles, and mucous membranes – Painful, red subcutaneous nodules noted in the pads of the fingers or toes – Retinal hemorrhages with white or pale center, located near optic disc – Non-tender hemorrhagic lesions 1–5 mm in diameter; occur on arms, legs, palms, and soles; intensify when extremity is elevated – In distal one-third of nail; thought to be result of an allergic vasculitis of the arterioles – CNS embolization from left heart endocarditis – Result of right-sided endocarditis causing pulmonary infarction – Embolization to renal vasculature – Left heart endocarditis; result of erosive vegetations. Can cause VSD, fistulas, pericarditis, cardiac tamponade, or myocardial infarction – Spleen is most common site of embolic infarction in bacterial endocarditis • See *Nursing Diagnosis #7*, below

Contd...

Contd...

Problems	Objective	Nursing interventions	Rationales
Nursing Diagnosis #6			
Potential for activity intolerance, related to compromised cardiac reserve	Patient will: 1. Maintain normal muscle tone 2. Maintain highest level of activity that does not produce symptoms of myocardial dysfunction 3. Identify end-points of activity tolerance	• Perform assessment of activity and exercise tolerance: – Age – Weight – Gender – Cardiovascular disorder – Previous activity and motivation • Initiate gradual activity progression in the critical care setting: – Encourage to participate in ADL (feed self, wash hands, shave, active ROM). – Maintain bed rest with commode privileges during acute phase of heart failure. – Prevent complications of immobility. ◆ Assist with frequent position changes. ◆ Provide frequent back care and skin care. ◆ Encourage hourly deep breathing while awake. ◆ Maintain in semi-Fowler's position. • Assess tolerance to activity progression by checking blood pressure, heart rate, and respiratory rate 1 minute and 4 minutes after the activity. Indicators of poor tolerance include dyspnea, syncope, angina, diaphoresis, cyanosis, fatigue, weakness, dysrhythmias; heart rate should return to baseline within 4 minutes. Heart rate should not exceed 20 beats/min above resting heart rate and it should not exceed 110 beats/min: – Monitor systolic blood pressure • Assess readiness to learn and instruct regarding indicators of activity intolerance, as noted above: – Teach patient how to take own pulse – Isometric exercises should be discouraged – Encourage gradual resumption of aerobic activity when free of heart failure – Re-emphasize to patient that activity will be progressed gradually and will be supervised during the initial stages; provide positive reinforcement when appropriate; gradually transfer supervision of tolerance from health care personnel to patient and family	• Initial assessment provides pertinent data that will guide individualized activity prescription from acute to rehabilitative phase: – Physical endurance decreases with age; older patients will tolerate less activity – Obesity increases myocardial burden – Females have more endurance; men can tolerate workload of higher intensity secondary to the increased ratio of muscle mass: total body weight – Cardiovascular history may influence the attitude of the patient to activity (i.e. if angina or palpitations developed on exertion, this may influence the patient's attitude towards exercise) – Identifies patients who may need encouragement to exercise. • Minimizes the deleterious effects of deconditioning, which include a decreased work capacity, tachycardia, orthostatic hypotension, venous thrombosis, and feelings of hopelessness and dependency: – Such activities improve circulation and help to prevent phlebitis or thromboembolism – Physical activity redistributes blood from viscera and kidneys to the skeletal muscle and skin. Bed rest allows for a limited cardiac output and decreases myocardial oxygen demand. However, myocardial oxygen consumption is greater when a patient uses bedpan than during commode use – Maintenance of skin integrity and muscle tone – Minimizes development of atelectasis – Reduces venous return to the heart; increases ability to expand lungs during deep breathing exercises

Contd...

Contd...

Problems	Objective	Nursing interventions	Rationales
			• Physical activity increases venous return to the heart, increases myocardial workload, and increases metabolic heat production, i.e. one-fifth of cardiac output is shunted to skin in thermoregulation and the patient with impaired myocardial function cannot compensate for this with a tachycardia or increased contractile force; symptoms of pulmonary venous congestion and decreased cardiac output intensify: – Fall of 20 mm Hg below resting level and failure of systolic blood pressure to increase above the resting level suggest poor exercise tolerance • Readiness to learn facilitates meaningful learning: – Result in increased blood pressure and cardiac workload; do not improve cardiovascular conditioning – Increases functional capacity and cardiovascular conditioning – Builds and reinforces self-confidence; helps minimize deleterious effects of psycho-physiologic responses to stress (increased myocardial oxygen consumption)
Nursing Diagnosis #7			
Knowledge deficit, related to: 1. Underlying heart disease, treatment, and follow-up	Patient will: 1. Describe underlying disease process and relationship to heart failure 2. Identify own risk factors or precipitating conditions that require modification 3. Identify importance of follow-up care and symptoms requiring medical intervention 4. Describe the importance of medications, diet, and activity to the overall treatment plan 5. Identify signs and symptoms of activity intolerance 6. Identify indications for endocarditis prophylaxis (if patient is in high-risk profile)	• Assess knowledge of heart failure, underlying disease process, and expectations of disease progression • Encourage verbalization of patient/family concerns and their learning needs • Assess readiness to learn • Implement teaching plan, which should include: – Explanation of normal heart function, heart failure, and underlying disease process – Explanation of signs and symptoms and appropriate action regarding their development – Explanation of risk factors and factors that will aggravate the symptoms of heart failure and methods to modify these factors – Explanation of medication regimen (including name, dosage, frequency, action, and side effects) – Explanation of diet modification if indicated – Activity prescription and signs and symptoms of activity intolerance • Assist patient/family in identifying family strengths and resources • Initiate referral to appropriate resources if indicated (social services; community resources)	• Readiness to learn varies because of differences in general education background, intellectual ability, and motivation. Assessment establishes baseline data from which to build or determine need to alter misconceptions • Fosters establishment of open, trusting relationship. Learning is enhanced when patient participates in goal setting. Heart failure affects patient and his/her lifestyle and impacts on the entire family to varying degrees • Readiness facilitates more effective learning • Patient and family have a right to receive information about the disease, treatment, and prognosis; understanding enhances compliance; knowledge allays anxieties and the adverse effects associated with psychophysiologic stress • Engenders self-confidence • It is reassuring to have support services available

Role of Nurses in Medication

Nurses are also responsible for educating the patient as well as family regarding the care of the person with heart failure which include:

1. Monitor for signs and symptoms of recurring heart failure and report these signs and symptoms to the primary provider:
   - Weight gain of 1 to 1.5 kg (2 to 3 lb)
   - Loss of appetite
   - Shortness of breath
   - Orthopnea
   - Swelling of ankles, feet or abdomen
   - Persistent cough
   - Frequent night-time urination.
2. Avoid fatigue and plan activity to allow for rest periods. Incorporate ADL, occupational activity and sexual activity into daily routine by pacing activities.
3. Plan and eat meals within sodium restrictions:
   - Avoid salty foods
   - Avoid drugs with high sodium content (e.g. some laxatives and antacids, Alka-Seltzer—read the labels
   - Eat several small meals rather than three large meals per day.
4. Take prescribed medications.
   - If several medications are prescribed, develop a method to facilitate accurate administration
   - Digitalis: Check own pulse rate daily; report a rate of less than 50/min to primary provider and signs and symptoms of toxicity (Box 12.15)
   - Diuretics (Box 12.14).:
     - Weigh self daily at same time of day
     - Eat foods high in potassium and low in sodium (such as oranges, bananas) if on potassium-depleting diuretics
   - Vasodilators:
     - Report signs of hypotension (light-headedness, rapid pulse, syncope) to physician
     - Avoid alcohol when taking vasodilators.
5. Adopt healthy lifestyle choices; daily routines; develop support groups; smoking cessation; alcohol intake limited to not more than one drink per day and minimize risk of infections.
6. Heart failure signs and symptoms to report to the physician:
   - Shortness of breath
   - Fatigue
   - Dry cough
   - Shortness of breath when lying down (orthopnea)
   - Episodes of sudden awakening with shortness of breath (paroxysmal nocturnal dyspnea)
   - Weight gain of 2 to 3 lb over 1 to 2 days
   - Ankle or foot edema
   - Nocturia
   - Anorexia.
7. Comply with follow-up appointment.
   Thorough evaluation also needed for follow-up scheme.

Box 12.14 Administering and monitoring diuretics

When nursing care involves diuretic therapy for conditions such as heart failure, the nurse to administer the medication and monitor the patient's response carefully, as follows:

- Administer the diuretic at a time conducive to the patient's lifestyle, for example, early in the day to avoid nocturia
- Give supplementary potassium with thiazide and loop diuretics as prescribed to replace potassium loss
- Check laboratory results for electrolyte depletion, especially potassium, magnesium, and sodium; and for electrolyte elevation, especially potassium with potassium-sparing agents
- Monitor daily weights, intake, and output to assess response. Monitor serum blood urea nitrogen and creatinine for increasing levels, which indicate renal dysfunction
- Assess lung sounds, jugular vein distention, daily weight, and peripheral, abdominal, or sacral edema to identify response to therapy
- Monitor for adverse reactions, such as nausea and gastrointestinal distress, vomiting, diarrhea, weakness, headache, fatigue, anxiety or agitation, and cardiac dysrhythmias
- Assess for signs of volume depletion, such as postural hypotension, dizziness, and balance problems
- Monitor for glucose intolerance in patients with and without diabetes mellitus who are receiving thiazide diuretics
- Monitor for potential ototoxicity in patients, especially those with renal failure, who are receiving a loop diuretic
- Advise patients to avoid prolonged exposure to the sun because of the risk of photosensitivity
- Monitor for elevated serum uric acid levels and the development of gout
- Implement nursing actions to facilitate effect of medication, such as positioning patient supine after dose is taken

IDENTIFICATION OF RHYTHM: ARRHYTHMIAS/CARDIAC DYSRHYTHMIAS

Arrhythmias are abnormal cardiac arrhythmias also called as dysrhythmias. The ability to recognize arrhythmias is an essential skill for the nurse. Cardiac monitoring is now used in a wide range of hospital and clinical settings. Prompt assessment of an abnormal cardiac rhythm and patient response to the rhythm is critical.

Cardiac tissue has those properties which enable the conduction system to initiate an electrical impulse that is transmitted through the cardiac tissue stimulating muscle contraction. The four properties are:

- Automaticity, i.e. ability to initiate an impulse spontaneously and continuously
- Contractility, i.e. ability to respond mechanically to an impulse
- Conductivity, i.e. ability to transmit an impulse along a membrane in an orderly manner
- Excitability, i.e. ability to be electrically stimulated.

Box 12.15 Digoxin use and toxicity in heart failure

The therapeutic level of digoxin is usually 0.5 to 2.0 mg/mL. Blood samples are usually obtained and analyzed to determine digitalis concentration at least 6 to 10 hours after the last dose. Toxicity may occur despite normal serum levels, and recommended dosages vary considerably.

Preparations

Digoxin

- Tablets: 0.125, 0.25, 0.5 mg (Lanoxin)
- Capsules: 0.05, 0.1, 0.2 mg (Lanoxicaps)
- Elixir: 0.05 mg/mL (Lanoxin Pediatric elixir)
- Injection: 0.25 mg/mL, 0.1 mg/mL (Lanoxin)

Digoxin toxicity

A serious complication of digoxin therapy is toxicity. Diagnosis of digoxin toxicity is based on the patient's clinical symptoms, which included the following:

- Anorexia, nausea, vomiting, fatigue, depression, and malaise (early effects of digitalis toxicity)
- Changes in heart rate or rhythm; onset of irregular rhythm
- ECG changes indicating SA or AV block; new onset of irregular rhythm indicating ventricular dysrhythmias; and atrial tachycardia with block, junctional tachycardia, and ventricular tachycardia

Reversal of toxicity

Digoxin toxicity is treated by holding the medication while monitoring the patient's symptoms and serum digoxin level. If the toxicity is severe, digoxin immune FAB (Digibind) may be prescribed. Digibind binds with digoxin and makes it unavailable for us. The digibind dosage is based on the digoxin level and the patient's weight. Serum digoxin values are not accurate for several days after administration of digibind because they do not differentiate between bound and unbound digoxin. Because digibind quickly decreases the amount of available digoxin, an increase in ventricular rate due to atrial fibrillation and worsening of symptoms of HF may ensue shortly after its administration

Nursing considerations and actions

1. Assess the patient's clinical response to digoxin therapy by evaluating relief of symptoms such as dyspnea, orthopnea, crackles, hepatomegaly, and peripheral edema
2. Monitor the patient for factors that increase the risk of toxicity
   - Decreased potassium level (hypokalemia), which may be caused by diuretics. Hypokalemia increases the action of digoxin and predisposes patients to digoxin toxicity and dysrhythmias
   - Use of medications that enhance the effects of digoxin including oral antibiotics and cardiac drugs that slow AV conduction and can further decrease heart rate
   - Impaired renal function, particularly in patients age 65 and older. Because digoxin is eliminated by the kidneys, renal function (serum creatinine) is monitored and doses of digoxin are adjusted accordingly
3. Before administering digoxin, it is standard nursing practice to assess apical heart rate. When the patient's rhythm is atrial fibrillation and the heart rate is less than 60 bpm, or the rhythm becomes regular, the nurse may withhold the medication and notify the physician, because these signs indicate the development of AV conduction block. Although withholding digoxin is a common practice, the medication does not need to be withheld for a heart rate of less than 60 bpm if the patient is in sinus rhythm because digoxin does not affect SA node automaticity. Measuring the PR interval for a patient with cardiac monitoring is more important than the apical pulse in determining whether digoxin should be held
4. Monitor for gastrointestinal side effects: Anorexia, nausea, vomiting, abdominal pain, and distention
5. Monitor for neurologic side effects: Headache, malaise, nightmares, forgetfulness, social withdrawal, depression, agitation, confusion, paranoia, hallucinations, decreased visual acuity, yellow or green halo around objects (especially lights), or "snowy" vision

AV, atrioventricular; bpm, beats per minute; ECG, electrocardiogram; HF, heart failure; SA, sinoatrial

The conduction system of the heart is made up of specialized neuromuscular tissues located throughout the heart. A normal cardiac impulse begins in the sinoatrial (SA) node in the upper right atrium. It is transmitted over the atrial myocardium via Bachman's bundle and internodal pathways to the atrioventricular (AV) node. From the AV node, the impulse spreads through the bundle of His and down the left and right bundle branches, emerging in the Purkinje's fibers, which transmit the impulse to the ventricles. A rhythm is classified as 'normal' when it meets the following criteria in ECG.

- Presence of one upright and consistent-appearing P wave before each QRS complex, all PR intervals between 0.12 and 0.20 seconds
- The PR intervals are consistent and the heart rate is between 60 and 100 beats per minute.

Conduction to the point just before the impulse leaves the Purkinje's fibers take place within the time of the PR intervals of the ECG. When the impulse emerges from the Purkinje's fibers, ventricular depolarization occurs, producing mechanical contraction of the ventricles and QRS complex on the ECG. Rates of conduction system are:

- SA node 60–100 times/min
- AV junction 40–60 times/min
- Purkinje's fibers 20–40 times/min

The autonomic nervous system plays an important role in the rate of impulse formation, the speed of conduction, and the strength of cardiac contraction. The components of the autonomic nervous system that affect the heart are this right and left vagus nerve fibers of the parasympathetic nervous system and fibers of the sympathetic nervous system. Stimulation of the vagus nerve causes a decreased rate of firing of the SA node, slaved impulse condition of the AV node and decreased force of cardiac muscle contraction. Stimulation of the sympathetic nerves that supply the heart has essentially the opposite effect on the heart.

Etiology

Cardiac arrhythmias are the result of alterations in impulse formation or propagation. Arrhythmias are often classified by the anatomical site of the dysfunction. For example, sinus dysrhythmias and atrial dysrhythmias. Common causes of arrhythmias include underlying cardiac disease, sympathetic stimulation, vagal stimulation, electrolyte imbalances and hypoxia, which are due to:

- Drug effects of toxicity
- Myocardial cell degeneration
- Hypertrophy of cardiac muscle
- Emotional crisis
- Connective tissue disorders
- Alcohol
- Metabolic conditions (e.g. thyroid dysfunction)
- Coffee, tea, tobacco
- Electrolyte imbalances
- Cellular hypoxia
- Edema
- Acid-base imbalance
- Myocardial ischemia
- Degeneration of conduction system.

Pathophysiology

Alterations in impulse formation and propagation arise from one of the three pathophysiological processes: altered automaticities, altered conduction resulting in delays or blocks and re-entry mechanisms.

i. Altered Automaticity

Automaticity is the ability to depolarize spontaneously without external stimulation, it is a property that normally confines to the cells of the SA node. The SA node usually depolarizes at a faster rate than other potential pacemaker cells because of the steep slope of phase 4, allowing sinus cells to reach threshold at faster rate. A variety of conditions can alter the automaticity of SA node and produce faster or slower than usual heart rates. Vagal stimulation will decrease this slope, resulting in a slower heart rate. Sympathetic stimulation and hypoxia will steepen phase 4 resulting in faster heart rates. If the phase-4 depolarization is found, the AV node or ventricular condition system increases, enhanced automaticity is said to exist. Some causes for enhanced automaticity are hypoxia, catecholamines, hypokalemia, hypocalcemia, atropine, trauma and digital toxicity.

Even cells that do not normally have automaticity may develop abnormal automaticity if the resting membranes potential or threshold potential is altered, increasing the threshold slows the heart rate because it then takes longer to reach threshold. If the resting membrane potential is made, less negative automaticity will increase because it is easier to reach threshold. Altered automaticity may be a consequence of ischemia, infarction, hypokalemia, hypocalcemia or cardiomyopathy. This abnormality is not easily impressed by the activity of the faster pacemakers.

ii. Altered Conductivity

When the rate of amplitude of depolarization decreases, conduction also decreases. Electrolyte imbalances affect the rate of depolarization by altering the resting membrane potential. Hypokalemia causes the resting membrane potential to be positive, decreasing the rate of depolarization and slowing conduction. Any condition decreases the amplitude of the action potential such as ischemia, hypercalcemia, or calcification of the conducting figures can cause cardiac conduction disturbances. Abnormality in conduction occur anywhere in the conduction system, including the SA node, the AV node, and the bundle branches. The severity of impaired conduction ranges from a slight delay to complete cessation or block of impulse transmission.

iii. Re-entry

Re-entry occurs when an impulse is delayed within a pathway of slow conduction, long enough that the impulse is still viable when the remaining myocardium repolarizes. The impulse then re-enters surrounding tissue and produces another impulse. This typically occurs when two different pathways share an initial and final segment. The first impulse travels down the faster pathway, leaving behind its refractory trail. Should a second, early impulse follow, it will be blocked because that path is refractory. The second impulse then enters the slow pathway and can return retrograde through the fast path, initiating a circuitous pattern.

Clinical Manifestation

In most cases with arrhythmias are asymptomatic as long as cardiac output meets the body's metabolic demands. The clinical manifestations associated with most arrhythmias directly relate to decrease in cardiac output from slow or fast heart rates. Significant changes in heart rate may not allow adequate time for the ventricles to fill and empty. The clinical manifestation includes:

i. General

- Palpitations (racing heart, skipped beats)
- Anxiety
- Fatigue.

ii. Altered cardiac output

- Pallor
- Confusion
- Cool and clammy skin
- Dizziness
- Cyanotic
- Weakness
- Shortness of breath
- Presyncope
- Rales
- Syncope with loss of consciousness
- Decreased blood pressure
- Chest pain
- Atrial thrombi (may dislodge to cause systemic emboli).

Management

The diagnosis of arrhythmias begins with the 12-lead ECG. Each arrhythmia exhibits characteristic changes in the ECG tracing. A systematic approach to analyzing the ECG rhythm helps distinguish the different dysrhythmias. The systematic interpretation of ECG tracing are:

- Rale (atrial and ventricular)
- Rhythm (atrial and ventricular)
- Presence or absence of P waves
- PR interval 0.12–0.20 seconds
- QRS complex 0.06–0.12 second
- QT internal less than 0.55 seconds
- Interpretation.

Please note that normal sinus rhythm has an atrial (P) and ventricular (QRS) rate of 60 to 100 beats per minute, a regular rhythm (consistent PP and RR intervals) and a P wave before every QRS.

The other diagnostic tests used in the assessment of arrhythmias include signal-averaged electrocardiomyography, ambulatory holter monitoring and electrophysiological studies.

Medical and nursing management of arrhythmias focuses on alleviating symptoms from altered cardiac output and eliminating or reversing the etiology. Arrhythmia occurring in out- of-hospital setting and present problems of management. Determination of the rhythm by cardiac monitoring is a high priority. Emergency management of arrhythmias indicated where arrhythmias may be due to hypoxia, shock, poisoning, drug ingestion, myocardial infarction, CCF, conduction defects, pulmonary disorders near-drowning, electrolyte imbalances, metabolic imbalances, and electric shock.

During this assessment findings will be:

- Irregular rate and rhythm, palpitations
- Chest, neck, shoulder or arm pain
- Dizziness, syncope
- Dyspnea
- Extreme restlessness
- Decreased level of consciousness
- Feeling of impending doom
- Numbness, tingling of arms
- Weakness and fatigue
- Cold and clammy skin
- Diaphoresis
- Pallor
- Nausea and vomiting
- Decreased blood pressure
- Decreased oxygen saturations.

The nursing intervention will include initially:

- Ensure patient airway
- Administer O_2 via nasal cannula or non-breather mask
- Establish IV access
- Apply cardiac electrodes
- Identify underlying rhythm
- Identify ectopic beats.

Ongoing monitoring includes:

- Monitor vital signs, level of consciousness, O_2 saturation and cardiac rhythm
- Anticipate need for intubation if respiratory distress is evident
- Prepare to initiate CPR, defibrillation or both.

Management of specific arrhythmias according to their types are as follows with their descriptions.

i. Sinus Bradycardia

Sinus bradycardia is characterized by atrial and ventricular rates less than 60 beats per minute. It is a normal sinus rhythm in aerobically trained athletes and in other individuals during sleep. It occurs in response to carotid sinus massage Valsalva's maneuver, hypothermia, increased intraocular pressure, increased vagal tone, and administration of parasympathomimetic drugs. It can be associated with hypothyroidism, increased intracranial pressure, obstructive jaundice and inferior wall MI.

ECG shows the P wave precedes each QRS complex and has normal encounter and a fixed interval (Fig. 12.10A). The clinical significance of sinus bradycardia depends on how the patient tolerates hemodynamically. Hypotension with decrease CO (cardiac output) may occur in some circumstances. An acute MI may predispose the heart to escape arrhythmias and premature beats.

Treatment consists of administration of atrophane (anticholinergic) or isoproterenol is usually effective in increasing HR.

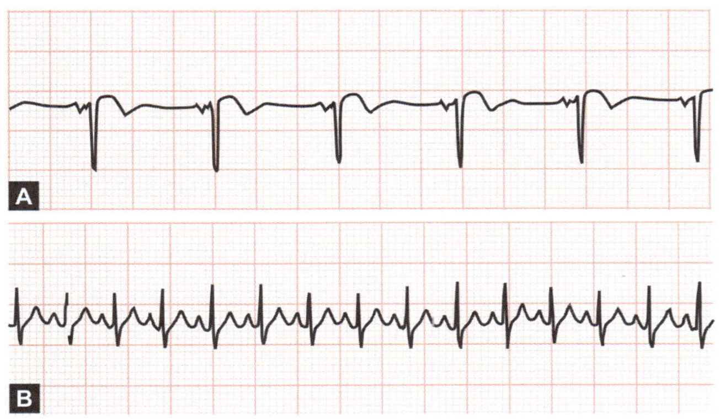

FIGS 12.10A AND B: A. Sinus bradycardia; B. Sinus tachycardia

ii. Sinus Tachycardia

Sinus tachycardia is characterized by an atrial and ventricular rate of 100 beats per minute or more (upper limit 150/m). It is associated with physiologic stressors such as exercise, fever, pain, hypotension, hypovolemia, anxiety, anemia, hypoxia, hypoglycemia, myocardial ischemia, CCF and hyperthyroidism. It can also be occurred by using of drugs such as epinephrine, non-epinephrine, caffeine, atropine theophylline, nifedipine, hydralazine and ingestion of alcohol, caffeine and tobacco.

ECG shows P wave is normal, precedes each QRS complex and has a normal contour and a fixed interval (Fig. 12.10B). It is normal, but HR greater than 100 beat/minute. The clinical significance depends on the patient tolerance on increased heart beat. The patient may complain of palpitations of no symptoms or has symptoms and dizziness and hypotension. In the patient with compromised myocardium, and tachycardia may cause decrease in CO with resultant lightheadedness, chest pain and heart failure.

Treatment is determined by underlying causes. Sinus tachycardia can usually be slowed with digoxin, beta blockers if necessary.

iii. Sinus Dysrhythmia

Sinus dysrhythmia is the most common arrhythmia. It is typically found in young adults and elderly persons. It is an irregular rhythm in which PP intervals are accompanied by changes in RR intervals. The cyclic pattern of changing PP or RR intervals correlates with the pattern of inspiration and expiration. During inspiration, the intervals shorten as the heart rate increases. Conversely, intervals lengthen during expiration. This condition cannot be treated unless the bradycardia phase is marked, causing symptoms that can be treated with administration of atropine.

iv. Sick Sinus Syndrome (SSS)

SSS is one type of tachycardia—bradycardia syndrome, which is characterized by the presence of bradycardia with intermittent episodes of tachydysrhythmias. The episode of tachydysrhythmia often is followed by a long pause before returning to sinus bradycardia. Complication of this inefficient rhythm includes heart failure and CVA resulting from thromboembolism. This condition is associated with ischemia degeneration of SA node, in which (SSS) some patient remain free of symptoms or complain only palpitations. For the patient with severe symptoms, the heart rhythm is stabilized with a permanent implantable pacemaker for the slow phase and administration of digoxin or beta blockers to control the ventricular rate of the tachycardia phase.

v. Sinus Exit Block and Sinus Arrest

Sinus exit block occurs when an impulse originates in the SA node but is blocked immediately. No P wave or QRS complex is generated resulting in a long pause. The next impulse occurs in a time interval representing the normal PP interval. Sinus arrest infers that the SA node never fired; therefore, there is no P or QRS complex. The next impulse is asynchronous to the normal PP interval.

This condition may occur as a result of medication such as digoxin hypoxia, myocardial ischemia and damage or injury to the SA node. The patient is symptomatic from a decrease in cardiac output the pauses or long or frequent. The patient may feel palpitations from the strong stroke volume that accompanies the next beat after the pause. When the patient is symptomatic, atropine may be administered to increase the HR and CO. Definitive therapy includes the insertion of permanent pacemaker.

vi. Premature Atrial Contraction or Beat (PAC or PAB)

PAC or PAB is a contraction originating from an ectopic focus on the atrium in a location other than the sinus node. It originates in the left or right atrium and travel across the atria by abnormal pathway creating a distorted P wave. In normal heart, PAC can result from emotional stress or the use of caffeine, tobacco or alcohol. PAC also occurs in disease state such as infection, inflammation, hyperthyroidism COPD, heart disease (AHD), valvular diseases and others.

ECG shows HR variation with the underlying rate and frequency of PAC and the rhythm is irregular (Fig. 12.11A). The P wave has a different contour from that of a normal P wave. It may be notched to have negative deflection or it may be hidden in the preceding T wave. The PR interval may be shorter or stronger than a normal PR interval originating from the sinus node. But it is within normal limits. The QRS complex is usually normal. A PAC may be a prelude to supraventricular tachycardia.

Treatment depends on the patient's symptoms, withdrawal of sources of stimulation warranted. Drugs such as digoxin, quinidine, procainamide, flecainide and beta-blocker are used.

vii. Wandering Atrial Pacemaker (WAP)

WAP occurs when at least three ectopic sites create the impulse for the cardiac rhythm. ECG shows P waves of different shapes and PR intervals of different lengths. The impulse can originate from the area around the AV node creating inverted P waves from retrograde conduction. Impulses from this lower area may also cause stimulation of the atria at the same time or after the ventricles. The P wave that appear buried in the QRS or occur inverted after the QRS.

WAP usually signifies underlying heart disease or drug toxicity. The patients are asymptomatic unless the HR increases

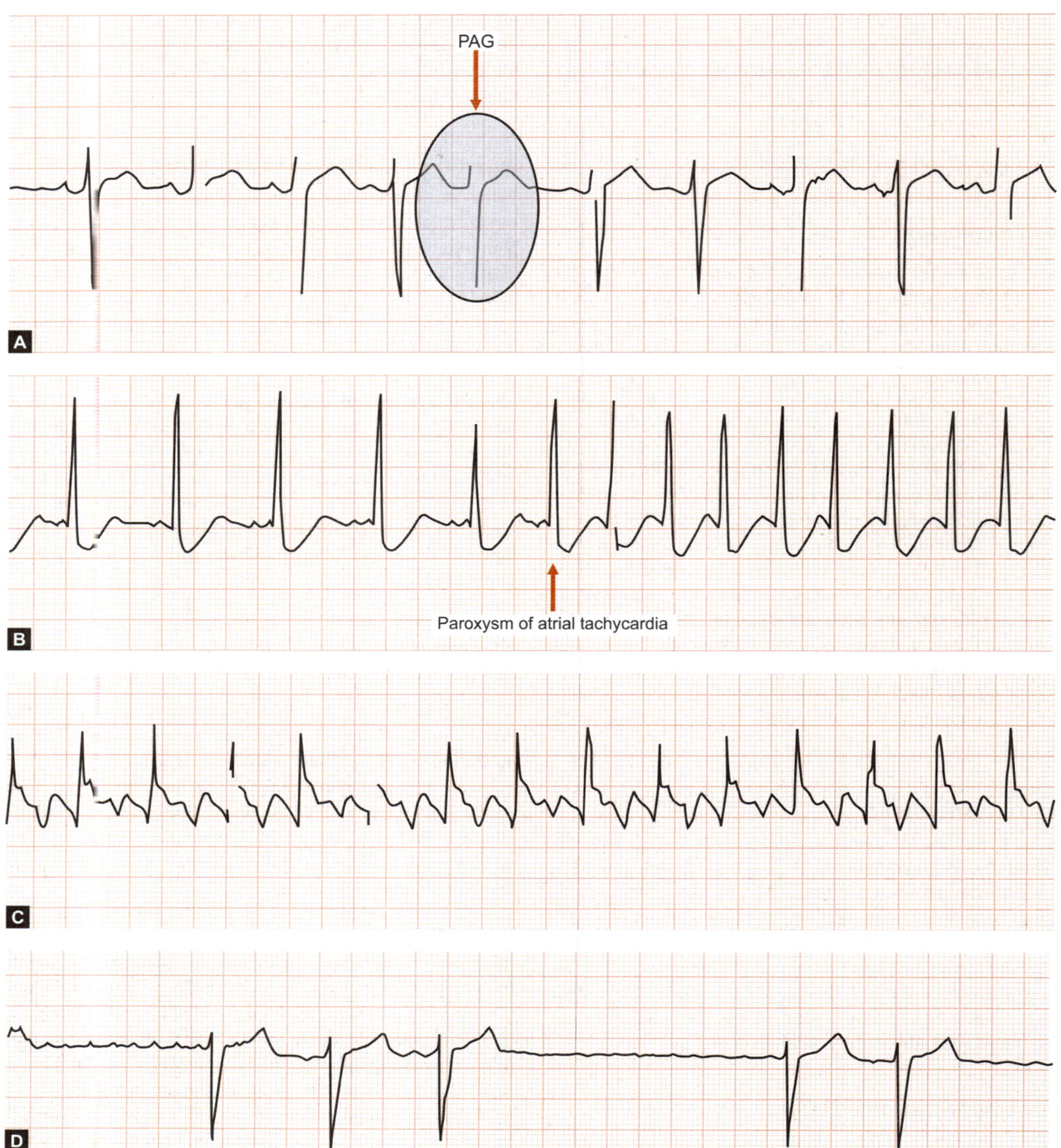

FIGS 12.11A TO D: (A) Normal sinus rhythm with premature atrial contraction; (B) Paroxysmal atrial tachycardia; (C) Atrial flutter; (D) Atrial fibrillation with slow ventricular response (controlled)

or decreases enough to affect cardiac output. The nurse mentions for changes in the rhythm and in the patient's symptoms. Then treat accordingly.

viii. Atrial Tachycardia or Paroxysmal Supraventricular Tachycardia (PSVT or PAT)

PSVT or PAT in an arrhythmia originating in an ectopic focus anywhere above the bifurcation of the bundle of HIS. Paroxysmal refers to an abrupt onset and termination. Termination is sometimes followed by a brief period of asystole. Some degree of AV block may be present (Fig. 12.11B).

In the normal heart, paroxysmal atrial tachycardia (PAT) or PSVT is associated with overexertion, emotional stress, changes in position, deep inspiration and stimulant such as tobacco, or caffeine. It is also associated with RHD, Wolf-Parkinson-White (WPW) syndrome, CAD or cor pulmonale. Transient episodes of PAT may occur in children and young adults in the absence of heart disease.

ECG in PAT, heart rate is approximately 150 to 250 (ranges from 100 to 300) per minute and rhythm is regular. The P waves are present, but may be hidden in the preceding T waves and has an abnormal contour. The PR interval may be prolonged, shortened or normal and QRS complex may have a normal or abnormal contour. The clinical significance of PAT depends on symptoms and heart rate. The prolonged episodes and HR greater than 180 beats/min may precipitate a decreased CO with hypotension and MI.

Treatment includes vagal stimulation and drug therapy. Vagal stimulation induced by carotid massage or Valsalva's maneuver may be used to treat PAT. Administration of adenosine (Adenocard) intravenously is most commonly used to convert PSVT to a normal sinus rhythm. If the rate is unresponsive to adenosine, verapamil, digoxin, diltiazem, or beta blockers may be effective.

ix. Atrial Flutter

Atrial flutter is an atrial tachyarrhythmia identified by recurring regular, saw-tooth-shaped flutter waves. It rarely occurs in normal heart. In disease state, it is associated with CAD, hypertension, mitral valve disorders, pulmonary embolus, cor pulmonale, cardiomyopathy, hyperthyroidism and use of drugs such as digitalis, quinidine, and epinephrine and surgical procedures.

Atrial flutter can be best visualized in leads II, III, and AVF and V on the 12-lead ECG. It is usually associated with a slower ventricular response, because of the refractory characteristic fixed ratio of flutter waves to QRS complexes. The P wave is represented by saw-tooth waves, the PR intervals are variable, and QRS complex is normal in contour. Atrial rate is 250 to 350 beats/minute. High ventricular rates associated with atrial flutter can decrease CO and cause serious consequences such as heart failure (Fig. 12.11C).

Treatment includes electrical cardioversion may be used to convert the atrial flutter to sinus rhythm in an emergency situation. Drugs used include verapamil, diltiazem, digoxin, sotalol, propafenone, quinidine, procainamide and beta-blockers. Ibutilide is effective at terminating atrial flutter in a closely-monitored situation and is used intravenously. Radiofrequency catheter ablation is increasingly being used as curative therapy of atrial flutter.

x. Atrial Fibrillation

Atrial fibrillation is the most rapid atrial dysrhythmia characterized by a total disorganization of atrial electrical activity without effective atrial contraction. Atrial fibrillation may be paroxysmal and transient or chronic. Generally associated with underlying heart disease and typically with pericarditis, thyrotoxicosis, cardiomyopathy, CAD, HHD, Rh. mitral valve disease, cardiac surgery, heart failure and excessive alcohol intake (holiday heart), gastroenteritis and stress.

The ECG demonstrates baseline fibrillatory wave or undulations of variable contour at a rate of 300 to 600 per minute. Atria depolarizes chaotically at rates of 350 to 600 per minute. The baseline is composed of irregular undulations without definable P waves. The QRS complex is usually normal, but the ventricular rhythm is irregularly irregular (Figs 12.11D and 12.12A).

Because of ventricular rhythm irregularity and the loss of synchronous atrial contractions (atrial kick), CO is decreased. Symptoms include fatigue, dyspnea and dizziness. Thrombi may form in the atria and cause emboli, which may lodge in the pulmonary or peripheral blood vessels. The goal of treatment is to prevent complications through control of the ventricular rate and restoration of normal sinus rhythm (NSR). The risk of emboli may necessitate long-term anticoagulation in some patients. Drugs used to control fast ventricular rates include diltiazem, digoxin and beta blockers.

xi. Premature Junctional Beat (PJB)

PJB arises from an ectopic focus either (i) at the junction of atrial and AV nodal tissue or (ii) at the junction of AV nodal tissue and bundle of HIS. If the PJBs arise from the first junction, the P wave will be inverted and premature and will precede the QRS complex. In the second case, the P wave is either hidden in the QRS or is inverted and follows the QRS. The abnormal timing and the inversion of the P wave are caused by depolarization of the atria in a retrograde fashion. The QRS is normal, but the PR interval is less than 0.12 second.

PJB mainly occurs in normal heart. They also may result from digitalis toxicity, ischemia, hypoxia, pain, fever, anxiety, nicotine, caffeine, or electrolyte imbalance. Treatment when needed is directed towards correcting the underlying cause.

xii. Junctional Arrhythmias

Junctional arrhythmias refer to an arrhythmia which originates in the area of AV node. The PJB is one among junctional arrhythmia. Other junctional arrhythmia include junctional escape rhythm (JER), accelerated junctional rhythm (AJR) and junctional tachycardia (JT). JER is often associated with the aerobically trained person who has sinus bradycardia, which may occur with acute MI and dysfunction of SA node. AJR and JT is observed with acute MI digital toxicity and acute Rh, fever during open heart surgery.

Treatment according to the patient tolerance of the rhythm and the patient's clinical condition. Inderal, cardizem and phenytoin are used.

xiii. Premature Ventricular Contraction/Beat (PVC/PVB)

PVC or PVB is contraction originating in an ectopic focus in the ventricles. They are associated with stimulants such as caffeine, alcohol aminophylline, epinephrine, isoproterenol and digoxin. They are also associated with hypokalemia, hypoxia, fever, exercise and emotional stress diseases associated are MI, CHF, CAD and mitral valve prolapse (MVP).

PVC is the premature occurrence of a QRS complex, which is wide and distorted in shape compared with a QRS complex initiated from the supraventricular tissue. The QRS complex is usually wider than 0.12 seconds, and the T wave is generally large and opposite in direction to the major deflection of the QRS complex. Retrograde conduction may occur and the P wave may be seen following the ectopic beat. PVC that are initiated from different foci appear different on contour from each other called multifocal PVCs. When every other beat is a PVC, it is called "ventricular bigeminy" (Fig. 12.12B). When every third beat is PVC, it is called "ventricular trigeminy" two consecutive PVCs are "couplets". Three consecutive PVCs are called "triplets". Ventricular tachycardia occurs when there are three or more consecutive PVCs. When a PVC falls on the T wave of preceding beat, the R on T phenomenon occurs and is considered to be dangerous because it may precipitate ventricular tachycardia or ventricular fibrillation.

ECG finding shows HR variation according to intrinsic rate and a number of PVCs rhythm is irregular because of premature beat. A retrograde P wave is possible. The P wave is rarely visible and is usually lost in the QRS complex of PVC. The PR interval is not measurable. The QRS complex is wide and distorted in shape, more than 0.12 second (Fig. 12.12B).

PVCs are usually a benign finding in the patient with a normal heart PVCs may reduce the CO and precipitate angina and heart failure. PVCs in ischemic heart disease or acute MI represents ventricular irritability. They may also occur as "reperfusion arrhythmias after lysis of a coronary artery clot with thrombolytic therapy in acute MI or following plaque reduction from percutaneous transluminal coronary angioplasty (PTCA).

For treating PVCs, lidocaine is the drug of choice, with an initial IV bolus of 1 to 1.5 mg/kg following by a second bolus of 0.5 to 1.5 mg/kg and continuous lidocaine infusion of 2 to 4 mg/minute. Procainamide in the second drug of choice if lidocaine is ineffective.

xiv. Ventricular Tachycardia

If the SA node and AV junction fail to initiate impulses, a ventricular pacemaking cell will automatically begin to initiate impulses at a rate of 20 to 40 beats per minute. This is known as "idioventricular rhythm". P-waves when seen are not associated with the ventricular rhythm. The QRS complex is greater than 0.12 wide and bizarre. If the rate of ventricular initiated rhythm increases, to 40 to 100 beats per minute, it is known as an "accelerated idioventricular rhythm (AIVR). AIVR may be seen in hypoxic, in digital toxicity, as complication of acute MI and as reperfusions dysrhythmia after thrombolytic therapy.

Ventricular tachycardia (VT) may be sustained (lasting longer than 30 seconds) or non-sustained (lasting 30 seconds or less). VT is associated with acute MI, CAD, significant electrolyte imbalance (e.g. K) cardiomyopathy MVP, long QT syndrome, and coronary reperfusion after therapy.

ECG shown ventricular rate 110 to 250 beats per minute. Rhythm may be regular or irregular. ECG may be taken when a run of three or more PVCs occur. The QRS complex distorted in appearance, with a duration exceeding 0.12 seconds and with the ST-T direction pointing opposite to the major QRS deflection. It occurs when an ectopic focus or foci fire repetitively and the ventricle takes control as the pacemaker. The ventricular rate is 110 to 250; the RR interval may be regular or irregular. AV dissociation may be present, with P waves occurring independently of the QRS complex. VT may cause a severe decrease in CO as a result of ventricular diastolic filling times and loss of atrial contraction. The result may be pulmonary edema, shock and decreased blood flow to the brain. It should be treated immediately (Fig. 12.12C).

Treatment includes, if the patient is hemodynamically stable lidocaine bolus administration. If lidocaine is ineffective, IV procainamide may be tried. The third drug of choice is bretylium IV at a dose of 5 mg/kg for several minutes and increased to 10 mg/kg at 15 to 30 minutes (not to exceed 30 to 35 mg/kg). A continuous infusion of bretylium (1 to 2 mg/min) may be started.

xv. Torsades de Pointes

Torsades de pointes, a variation of ventricular tachycardia, can also progress a ventricular fibrillation if not managed appropriately. It is otherwise known as polymorphic ventricular tachycardia. It is a type of VT characterized by a QRS contour that gradually changes into polarity over a series of beats. It usually occurs when QT prolongation is present.

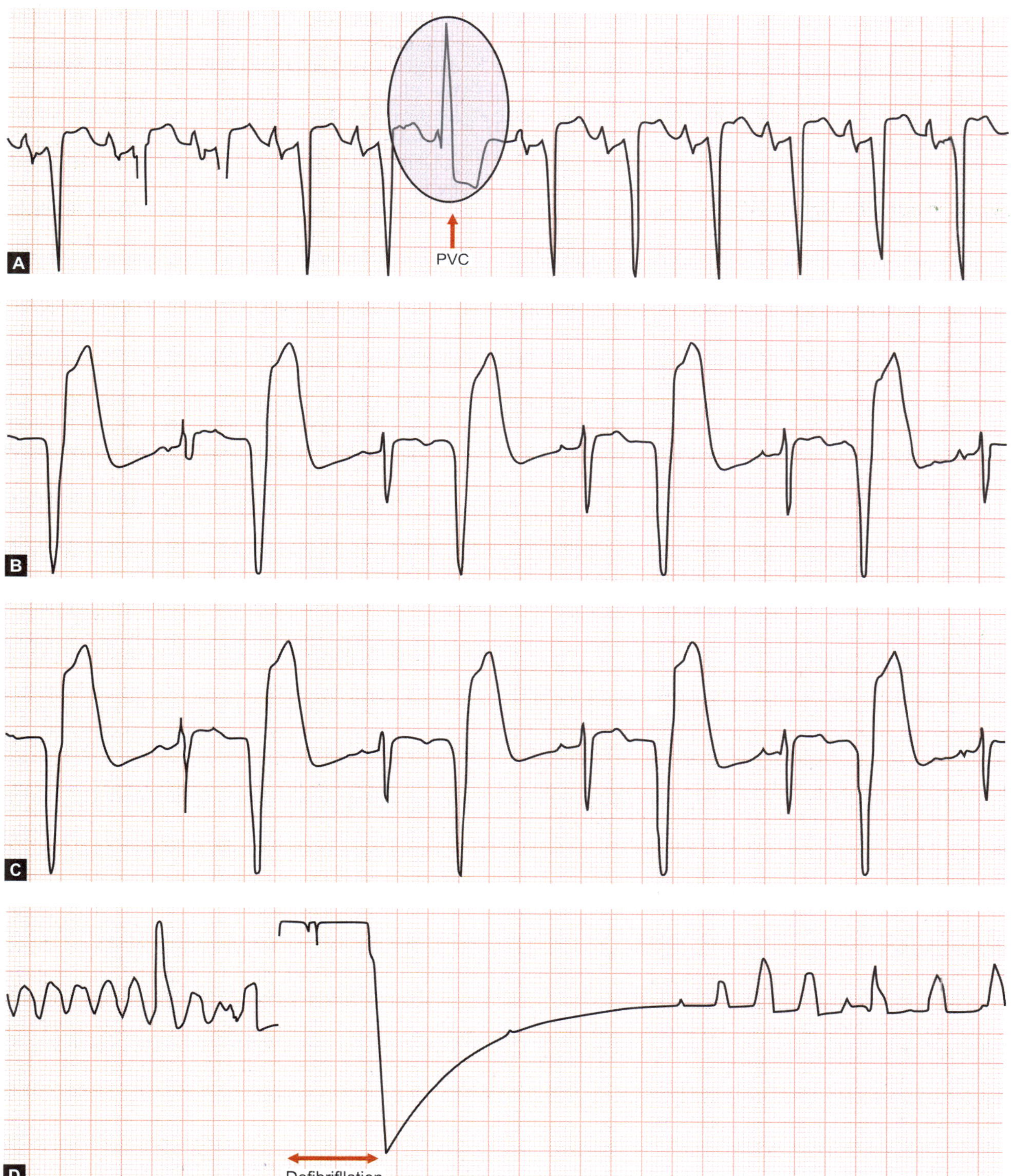

FIGS 12.12A TO D: (A) Normal sinus rhythm with premature ventricular contraction; (B) Ventricular bigeminy; (C) Ventricular tachycardia; (D) Ventricular fibrillation with defibrillation

Magnesium sulfate infusion is the drug of choice for torsade de pointes. Other drugs can be used, are isoproterenol or lidocaine infusion if hemodynamic state is stable. If the patient is unconscious or hemodynamically unstable, immediate cardioversion starting initially with 50 Joules. A defibrillator is used in the synchronized mode of cardioversion.

xvi. Ventricular Fibrillation (VF)

VF is a severe derangement of the heart rhythm characterized on the ECG by irregular undulations of varying contour and amplitude. This represents the firing of multiple ectopic foci in the ventricle Mechanically, the ventricle is simply "quivering" and no effective contraction or CO occurs. VF occurs in acute MI, CAD, myocardial ischemia and cardiomyopathy. It also occurs during cardiac pacing or cardiac catheterization procedure.

ECG shows HR is not measurable. Rhythm is irregular and chaotic. The P wave is not visible and the PR interval and QRS interval are not measurable. VF may result in unconsciousness, absence of pulse, apnea, and seizures, if not intervened, death may occur (Fig. 12.12D).

Treatment consists of immediate initiation of CPR and initiation of advanced cardiac life support (ACLS) measures with the use of defibrillation and definitive drug therapy.

xvii. Asystole

Asystole represents the total absence of ventricular electrical activity. Occasionally P waves can be seen. No ventricular contraction occurs because of depolarization does not occur. This is a lethal arrhythmia that requires immediate treatment. Asystole is usually a result of advanced cardiac disease. Treatment consists of CPR with initiation of ACLS measures which includes intubation and IV therapy with epinephrine and atropine.

xviii. Atrioventricular Block (AV block)

A block to conduction of an impulse may occur at any point along the conduction pathways. One common area in the AV junction. The severity of the block is identified by degrees, i.e. first, second, and third degree AV blocks.

- First degree AV block is present when the PR interval is prolonged to greater than 0.20 second, indicating a conduction delay in the AV node. It is usually found in association with rheumatic fever, digitalis toxicity, acute inferior MI and increased vagal tone. When this occurs in isolation, the patient is asymptomatic and no treatment is needed (Fig. 12.13A)
- Second-degree AV block may be divided into two categories. Type I (Mobitz I or Wenckebach phenomenon) and Type II (Mobitz II) (Fig. 12.13B)
  Type I AV block may result from use of digoxin or beta blockers, and may be associated with cardiac and other diseases that can slow AV conduction. In this atrial rate is normal, but ventricular rate may be slower as a result of dropped QRS complexes. Ventricular rhythm is irregular. The PR interval progressively lengthens before the non-conducted P wave occurs. The P wave has a normal contour. The PR interval lengthens progressively until a P wave is nonconducted and a QRS complex is dropped. The QRS complex has a normal contour of the patient in symptomatic atropine it is used to increase heart rate or temporary pacemaker may be needed (for MI).
  Type II AV block is less common but more serious. It is characterized by non-conducted sinus impulses despite constant PR intervals for the conducted P waves. The nonconducted P waves may occur at random or in patterned ratio (2:1, 3:1). The QRS complexes are widened unless the block is within the bundle of His type II blocks may occur in CAD, MI, RHD, cardiomyopathy and chronic fibrotic disease of the conduction system. For this temporary treatment before the insertion of permanent pacemaker, i.e. temporary pacemaker drugs such as atropine, epinephrine, or dopamine can be tried to increase heart rate until pacemaker therapy is available.
- Third degree AV block is a complete heart block. Here all the sinus atrial impulses are blocked and the atria and ventricle beat independently. The ventricles are driven by either a junctional or a ventricular pacemaker cell. The usual lesion is in the bundle of His or the bundle of branches but may also be at the AV junction. It is associated with fibrosis or calcification of the cardiac conduction system, CAD myocarditis, cardiomyopathy, open heart surgery and some systemic diseases such as amyloidosis and scleroderma. ECG shows the atrial rate usually a sinus rate which is usually a sinus rate of 60 to 100 beats/min artery. The ventricular rate depends on the site of block. The P wave has normal contour. The PR interval is variable and there is no relationship between the P wave and the QRS complex. The QRS complex is normal if escape rhythm is initiated in the bundle of his or above. The third-degree AV block almost always results in reduced CO with subsequent ischemia and heart failure. Syncope from this block may result from severe bradycardia or even episodes of asystole (Fig. 12.13C).
  Treatment includes insertion of temporary pacemaker or an external pacemaker applied on an emergency basis in a patient with acute MI. The use of drug include atropine, epinephrine and dopamine to increase HR and support BP prior to pacemaker insertion.

Management of Arrhythmias

Management of patient with arrhythmias includes diagnosing the specific arrhythmia and its associated etiology and treating the disorders with medications or interventional procedures.

When patient is on medication, the nurse must be knowledgeable about the mechanism of action of specific drugs

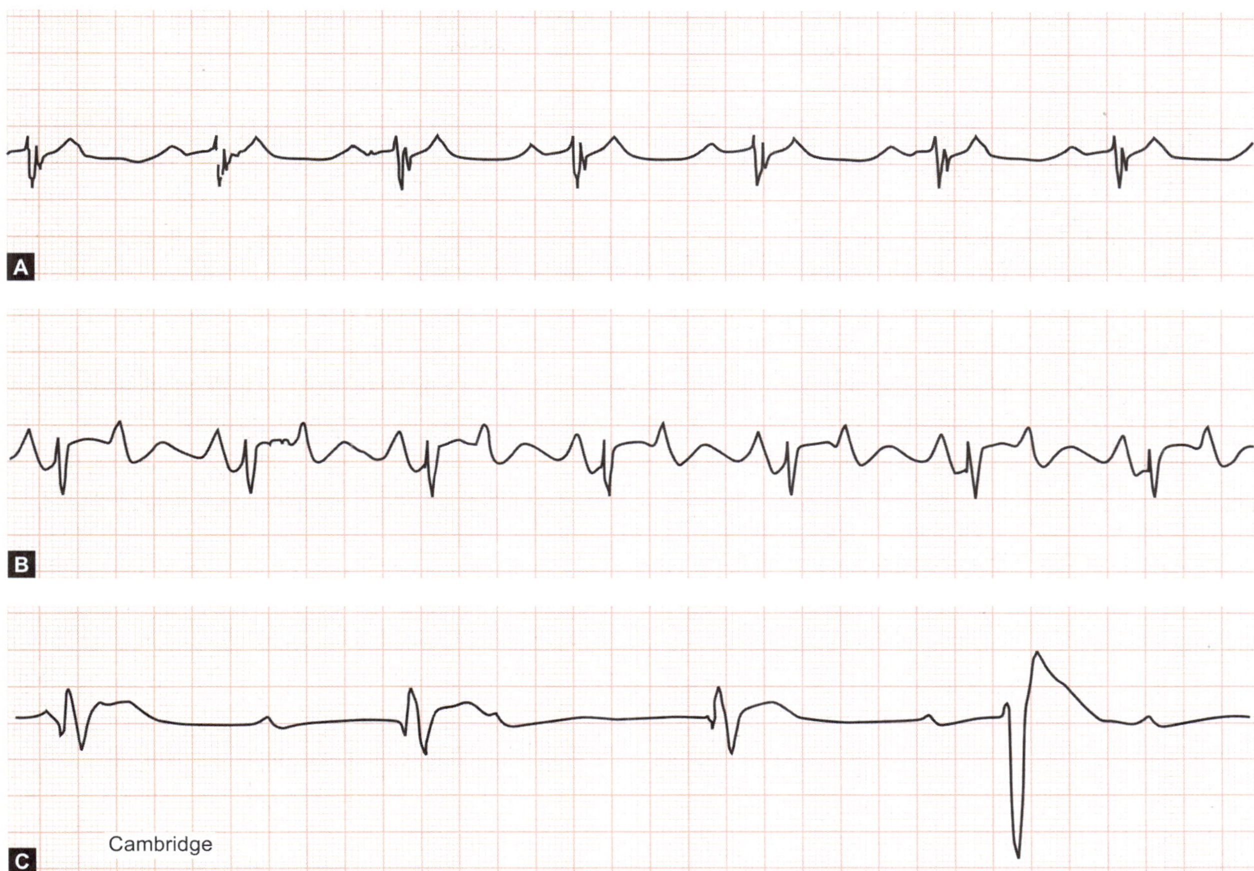

FIGS 12.13A TO C: (A) First-degree AV block; (B) Second-degree AV block (Mobitz 1); (C) Third-degree AV block

and their associated nursing interventions. Careful attention must be given to potential drug interactions and synergetic effects when combination of therapy is used. The metabolism and excretion of medications may be impaired in the elderly and in patients with decreased perfusion to the kidney and liver. The nurse must be aware of new agents approved for the management of cardiac arrhythmia and how to monitor their safe use.

Nursing management of the patient experiencing arrhythmia include interventions to decrease oxygen demand. The nurse spaces activities and encourages frequent rest periods. While medication therapy is being adjusted, patients are on continuous monitoring (telemetry). Rhythms are documented every 4 to 8 hours and as needed. Skin care is provided to minimize the irritation of monitoring electrodes.

The nurse must be alert to changes in a patient's rhythm. Assessment for changes in the cardiac output are documented. Emergency drugs should be available and intravenous access should be ensured. Ancillary equipment such as defibrillators, oxygen suction and temporary pacemaker should be readily available and in good working condition.

Interventions such as cardioversion defibrillation, coronary ablation, pacemaker therapy, automatic implantable cardioverter defibrillators (Fig. 12.14), and CPR are also part of the managements of patients with arrhythmias.

INFLAMMATORY HEART DISEASE

PERICARDITIS (CARDIAC TAMPONADE)

Pericarditis refers to an inflammation of the pericardium, the membranous sac enveloping the heart. It may be primary or may develop in the course of a variety of medical and surgical disorders. Some causes are unknown; others include infection (usually viral, rarely bacterial or fungal), connective tissue disorders, hypersensitivity states, diseases of adjacent structures, neoplastic disease, radiation therapy, trauma, renal disorders, and tuberculosis.

Pericarditis is an inflammatory process of the visceral or parietal pericardium (inflammations of the pericardial sac). It can be acute or chronic and can spread from or to the myocardium.

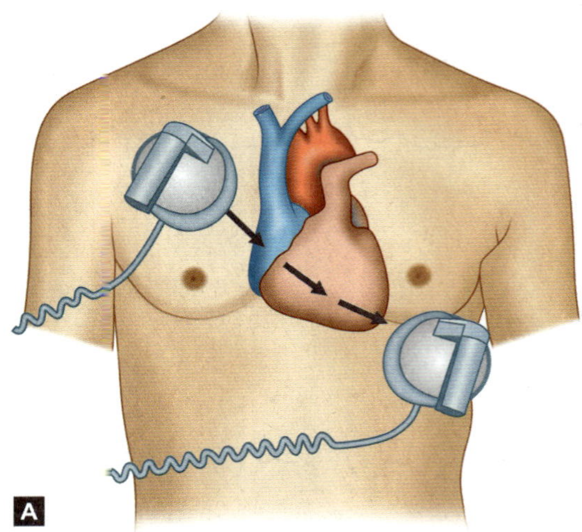

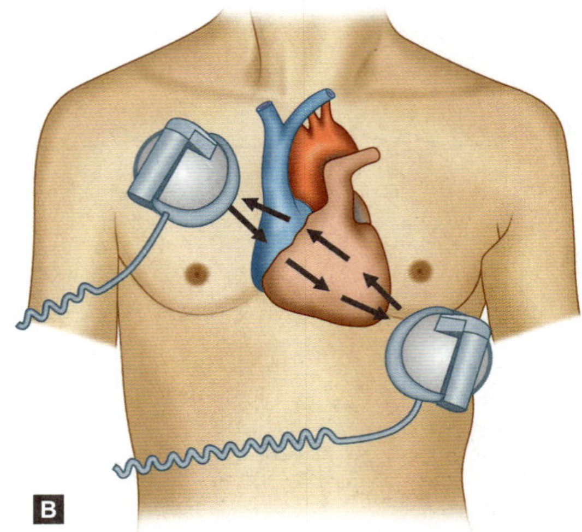

FIGS 12.14A AND B: Paddle placement and current flow in: (A) Monophasic defibrillation and (B) Biphasic defibrillation

Etiology

Pericarditis can occur as a result of bacterial, viral or fungal infection. The causes of pericarditis are as follows:

- Idiopathic or nonspecific causes
- Infection: Usually viral (e.g. human immunodeficiency virus, coxsackievirus, influenza); rarely bacterial (e.g. streptococci, staphylococci, meningococci, gonococci, gram-negative rods); and mycotic (fungal)
- Disorders for connective tissue: Systemic lupus erythematosus, rheumatic fever, rheumatoid arthritis polyarteritis, scleroderma
- Hypersensitivity states: Immune reactions, medication reactions, serum sickness
- Disorders of adjacent structures; myocardial infarction, dissecting aneurysm, pleural and pulmonary disease (pneumonia)
- Neoplastic disease: Caused by metastasis from lung cancer or breast cancer, leukemia, and primary (mesothelioma) neoplasms
- Radiation therapy of chest and upper torso (peak occurrence 5–9 months after treatment)
- Trauma: Chest injury, cardiac surgery, cardiac catheterization, implantation of pacemaker or implantable cardioverter defibrillator (ICD)
- Renal failure and uremia
- Tuberculosis.

i. Infections

- Viral causes including coxsackievirus B, coxsackievirus A, adenovirus mumps, epstein barr vines, varicella zoster and hepatitis B
- Bacterial causes including pneumococci, staphylococci, streptococci septicemia from gram-negative organisms and tuberculosis
- Fungal causes including histoplasma, candida species, infections such as toxoplasmosis and lyme disease.

ii. Non-infections

- Uremia
- Acute MI
- Neoplasms such as lung cancer, breast cancer, Hodgkin's disease and lymphoma
- Trauma after thoracic surgery, pacemaker insertion and cardiac diagnostic procedures
- Radiation
- Dissecting aortic aneurysm
- Myxedema.

iii. Hypertensive or Autoimmune

- Delayed post-myocardial-pericardial injury
- Post-myocardial infarction syndrome (dressler's)
- Postpericardiotomy syndrome
- Rheumatic fever
- Drug reactions (e.g. procainamide and hydralazine).

Pathophysiology

Pericarditis may be acute or chronic and may be classified by the layers of the pericardium becoming attached to each other (adhesive) or by what accumulates in the pericardial sac serum (serous), pus (purulent), calcium deposits (calcific), clotting proteins (fibrinous), or blood (sanguineous). Frequent or prolonged episodes of pericarditis may lead to thickening and decreased elasticity that restrict the heart's ability to fill properly with blood (constrictive pericarditis). The pericardium may also become calcified, which restricts ventricular contraction. Pericarditis can lead to an accumulation of fluid in the pericardial sac (pericardial effusion) and increased pressure on the heart leading to cardiac tamponade.

In acute pericarditis, the membranes surrounding the heart become inflamed. The inflamed membrane rub against each other and produces the classic pericardial friction rub of pericarditis. The friction rub sounds scratching and harsh on the auscultation and lasts throughout systole and diastole. The patient complains of severe precordial chest pain, which may closely resemble that of acute MI. The pain intensifies when the person is lying supine and decreases with sitting. The pain also intensifies when the patient breathes deeply. Patient shows other signs and symptoms (see clinical manifestation).

Chronic pericarditis can be constrictive or adhesive. It usually begins with an initial episode of acute pericarditis (often secondary to neoplasia, radiation, previous surgery, or idiopathic causes) and is characterized by fibrin deposition with clinically undetected pericardial effusion. Organization and resorption of the effusion slowly follows with progression towards the chronic stage of fibrous scarring, thickening of the pericardium from calcium deposition, and eventual obliteration of the pericardial space. The fibrocystic, thickened and adherent pericardium encases the heart, thereby, impairing the ability of the atria and ventricles to stretch sufficiently during diastolic filling. An overview of pericarditis is given in Box 12.16.

Box 12.16 Overview of pericarditis

Signs and Symptoms	Chest pain Dyspnea Low-grade fever Cough Pericardial friction rub
Diagnostic test	Complete blood cell count Electrocardiogram Echocardiogram Magnetic resonance imaging Computed tomography
Therapeutic measures	Surgery, possibly colostomy Radiation Chemotherapy and/or radiation Medications: Analgesics TPN as needed Support and education
Complications	Pericardial effusion Cardiac tamponade

Clinical Manifestations

In acute pericarditis, patient may complain chest pain, dyspnea and a pericardial friction rub. The intense, pleuritic chest pain is generally sharpest over the left pericardium or retrosternally but may radiate to the trapezius ridge and neck (mimicking angina) or sometimes to the epigastrium or abdomen (mimicking abdominal or other non-cardiac pathologic condition).

- Characteristic symptom is pain. Pain, which is felt over the precordium or beneath the clavicle and in the neck and left scapular region, is aggravated by breathing, turning in bed and twisting the body; it is relieved by sitting up (or leaning forward)
- Dyspnea may occur as a result of pericardial compression of the hearts movements
- Other signs may include fever, high white blood cell count and friction rub, or extremely ill appearance.

The pain is aggravated by lying supine, deep breathing, coughing, swallowing and moving the trunk and is eased by sitting up and leaning forward. The dyspnea accompanying acute pericarditis is related to the patients' need to breathe in, rapid, shallow breaths to avoid chest pain and may be aggravated by fever and anxiety. The pericardial rub is a scratching, grating, high-pitched sound believed to arise from friction between the roughened pericardial and epicardial surface. It is best heard with stethoscope.

The two major complications of acute pericarditis induced are pericardial effusion and cardiac tamponade. The accumulation of fluid within the pericardial sac is called "pericardial effusion". The fluid may be serous, purulent, or hemorrhagic. Serous effusion usually accompany heart failure. Purulent effusions indicate underlying disorders such as tuberculosis or neoplasm. Hemorrhagic effusions most often occur from trauma, aneurysm, rupture, coagulation abnormalities. Large effusions may compress adjoining structures. Pulmonary tissue compression can cause cough dyspnea and tachypnea. Phrenic nerve compression can induce hiccups and compression of the laryngeal nerve may result in hoarseness. Heart sounds are generally distant and muffled, although BP is maintained by compensatory mechanism.

The cardiac tamponade develops as the pericardial effusion increases in size compensatory mechanism ultimately fail to adjust to the decreased cardiac output. This can lead to cardiac failure, shock and death. The signs and symptoms of cardiac tamponade include:

- Falling blood pressure, rising venous pressure (distended neck veins), and distant (muffled) heart sounds with pulsus paradoxus
- Anxious, confused and restless state
- Dyspnea, tachypnea and precordial pain
- Elevated central venous pressure (CVP)
- Decrease in systolic BP
- Narrowing pulse pressure

- Pulsus paradoxus (greater than 10 mm Hg)
- Increase in venous pressure and distention of neck veins
- Tachycardia
- Tachypnea
- Possible friction rub
- Muffled heart sounds
- Low voltage EGG
- Rapid enlargement of cardiac heart on chest X-ray
- Peripheral cyanosis
- Anxiety
- Chest pain.

The chronic pericarditis patient may complain of dyspnea and fatigue and exhibits symptom of heart failure as a result of diminished ability of the heart pump.

Management of Acute Pericarditis

To diagnose careful history and physical examination are needed. In addition, auscultation of chest, EGG, chest X-ray, echocardiography, pericardiocentesis, CT scan, nuclear scan of the heart are useful. The management includes:

- Treatment of underlying disease
- Bed rest
- Aspirin
- NSAIDs (non-steroid anti-inflammation drugs)
- Corticosteroids
- Pericardiocentesis (for large pericardial effusion or cardiac tamponade) (Fig. 12.15).

In chronic pericarditis, removal of the pericardium may be necessary to restore cardiac function.

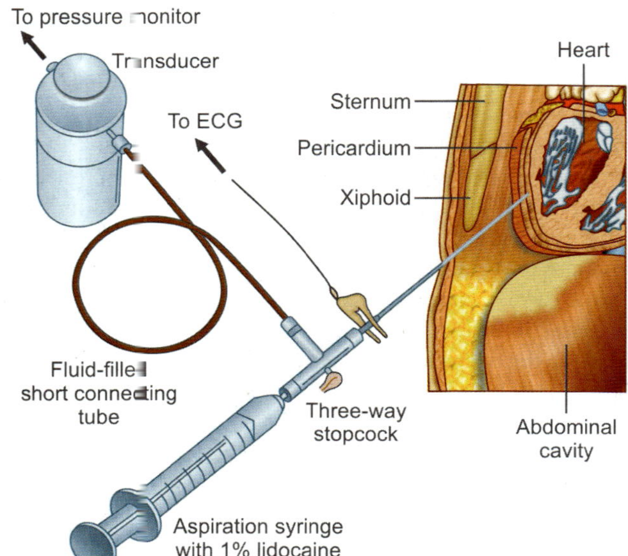

FIG. 12.15: Pericardiocentesis performed under sterile condition in conjunction with electrocardiogram (ECG) and hemodynamic measurements

Nursing Management

Assessment

- Assess pain by observation and evaluation while having patient vary positions to determine precipitating or intensifying factors. (Is pain influenced by respiratory movements?)
- Monitor temperature frequently, because pericarditis causes an abrupt onset of fever in a previously afebrile patient
- Assess pericardial friction rub (a pericardial friction rub is continuous, distinguishing it from a pleural friction rub). Ask patient to hold breath to help in differentiation: audible on auscultation, synchronous with heartbeat, best heard at the left sternal edge in the fourth intercostal space where the pericardium comes into contact with the left chest wall scratchy or leathery sound, louder at the end of expiration and may be best heard with patient in sitting position.

Nursing Diagnoses

Acute pain related to inflammation of the pericardium.

A pericardial friction rub is diagnostic of pericarditis. It has a creaky or scratchy sound and is louder at the end of exhalation. Nurses should monitor for the pericardial friction rub by placing the diaphragm of the stethoscope tightly against the thorax and auscultating the left sternal edge in the fourth intercostal space, the site where the pericardium comes into contact with the left chest wall. The rub may be heard best when a patient is sitting and leaning forward.

Potential Complications

- Pericardial effusion
- Cardiac tamponade.

The major goals of the patient may include relief of pain and absence of complications.

Nursing Interventions

Relieving pain

- Advise bed rest or chair rest in a sitting-upright and leaning-forward position
- Instruct patient to resume activities of daily living as chest pain and friction rub abate
- Administer medications; monitor and record responses
- Instruct patient to resume bed rest if chest pain friction rub recur.

Monitoring and Managing Potential Complications

- Observe for pericardial effusion, which can lead to cardiac tamponade; arterial pressure falls; systolic pressure falls while

diastolic pressure remains stable; pulse pressure narrows; heart sounds progress from being distinct to imperceptible
- Observe for neck vein distention and other signs of rising central venous pressure
- Notify physician immediately upon observing any of the above symptoms, and prepare for pericardiocentesis
- Reassure patient and continue to assess and record signs and symptoms until physician arrives.

The management of the patient's pain and anxiety during acute pericarditis are primary nursing considerations. Assessment and careful observation of pain and attending to it are important and also monitor the anxiety level and take anxiety-reducing measures in addition to regular treatment including care of surgical patients.

In addition, the nurse teaches the patient and their significant others about the nature of the disease and the purposes and correct use of all medications. She teaches measures to decrease fatigue and provides information on how to minimize the risk of complications. The nurse also provides an overview of the signs and symptoms of recurrent pericarditis that would need to be promptly reported to the health care provider.

MYOCARDITIS

Myocarditis, a focal or diffuse inflammation of the myocardium that causes an infiltrate in the myocardial interstitium and injury to an adjacent myocardial cells.

Etiology

Myocarditis may be primary with an unknown etiology or secondary from an identifiable cause such as drug sensitivity or toxicity, connective tissue disease, sarcoidosis, or infection. The inflammation process often develops secondary to infective endocarditis. Myocarditis may be acute or chronic. It has been associated with variety of a etiologic agents including viruses, bacteria, rickettsia, fungi, parasites, radiation and pharmacological and chemical factors. Viral infection is the most common cause. It includes viruses like coxsackievirus B, coxsackievirus A, echovirus, poliovirus, influenza A and B, rubella, mumps, rabies, Epstein-Barr, hepatitis and HIV.

Pathophysiologic

The pathophysiologic mechanisms of myocarditis are poorly understood because there is usually a period of several weeks after the initial infection before the development of manifestations of myocarditis. Immunologic mechanisms may play a role in the development of myocarditis. The majority of infections are benign, self-limiting, and sub-clinical although viral myocardium in infants and pregnant women may be virulent.

Acute myocarditis is an inflammatory process involving the myocardium. When the muscle fibers of the heart are damaged, life is threatened. Myocarditis usually results from an infectious process (e.g. viral, bacterial, mycotic, parasitic, protozoal, or spirochetal). It may be produced in systemic infections, such a rheumatic fever, in patients receiving immunosuppressive therapy, or in patients with infective endocarditis. Myocarditis can cause heart dilation, mural thrombi (on the heart wall), infiltration of circulating blood cells around coronary vessels and between muscle fibers, and degeneration of muscle fibers.

Clinical Manifestation

During the acute viral phase, symptoms are flu-like and include fever, lymphadenopathy, pharyngitis, myalgia and gastrointestinal complaints. Hepatitis, encephalitis, nephritis and orchitis also can occur. The clinical manifestations for patient with myocarditis are variable ranging from a benign course without any overt manifestations to severe heart involvement of sudden death:

- Clinical features depend on the type of infection, degree of myocardial damage, and capacity of the myocardium to recover
- Symptoms may be moderate, mild, or absent
- Patient may report fatigue and dyspnea, palpitations, and occasional discomfort in the chest and upper abdomen
- Patient may develop severe congestive heart failure or sustain sudden cardiac death
- Pericardial friction rub may be heard if myocarditis is associated with pericarditis
- Pulsus alternans may by present
- Fever and tachycardia are common, and symptoms of congestive heart failure may develop.

Usually early cardiac manifestations appear 7 to 10 days after viral infection and include pericardial chest pain with an associated friction rub because pericarditis often accompanies myocarditis. Cardiac signs (S3 crackles, jugular venous distention and peripheral edema) may progress to CHF including pericardial effusion, syncope, and possibly ischemic pain. ECG changes include ST segments, elevation and QT interval prolongation.

Management

Diagnosis can be made through as in pericarditis. In addition, histologic confirmation of myocarditis through endomyocardial biopsy (EMB). The patient with myocarditis are treated with bed rest and digitalis to prevent heart failure and cardiogenic shock. Immunosuppression may be beneficial in reducing inflammation and preventing irreversible myocardial damage. Medical therapy also includes treatment of underlying disease with antibiotics, conventional therapy for CHF and management of arrhythmias.

Medical Management

Appropriate immunizations and early treatment are recommended to decrease the incidence of myocarditis. If myocarditis develops, management involves treating the underlying cause and the following measures:

- Bed rest to decrease cardiac workload and prevent complications
- Continuous cardiac monitoring if dysrhythmia occurs
- Medications to slow the heart rate and augment myocardial contractility (digitalis) when there is evidence of congestive heart failure.

Patients with myocarditis are sensitive to digitalis. Nurses must closely monitor these patients for digitalis toxicity, which is evidenced by dysrhythmia, anorexia, nausea, vomiting, headache, and malaise.

Anti-embolism stockings and passive and active exercises should be used because embolization from venous thrombosis and mural thrombi can occur, especially in patients on bed rest.

Nursing Management

- Because patients with myocarditis are sensitive to digitalis, monitor for digitalis toxicity (dysrhythmia, anorexia, nausea, vomiting, bradycardia, headache, malaise)
- Apply and instruct patient and family in use of, elastic stockings and passive and active exercises to prevent thrombosis
- Instruct patient to increase physical activity slowly and to report any symptoms that occur with increased activity, including rapid heart rate
- Instruct patient to avoid competitive sports and alcohol
- If patient develops heart failure, the management is essentially the same as for all causes of heart failure.

Nursing care includes ongoing monitoring of the patients, physiological status. Patients are commonly anxious about the sudden onset of heart disease and its implications for the future. The nurse provides emotional support and encourages verbalizations of feelings. If EMB is performed, post-biopsy nursing care focuses on the potential for injury that can occur, such as hematoma or bleeding at the cannulation site, cardiac tamponade or pneumothorax. Any alteration should be referred to the physician concerned immediately. Vital signs are monitored closely to assess for continual hemodynamic stability. Monitoring for heart failure is an important consideration. Measure to decrease cardiac workload include frequent rest periods, provisions for a quiet environment, and the use of semi-Fowler's position. The patients and their family members/ significant and others were educated regarding the disease. The nurse encourages slow progression of activities with frequent rest periods and the use of medication with instructions.

INFECTIVE ENDOCARDITIS

Infective endocarditis previously known as bacterial endocarditis is an infection of the endocardial surface with microorganism, present in the lesion. The endocardium, the inner layer of the heart, is contagious with the valves of the heart. Therefore, inflammation from infective endocarditis usually affects the cardiac valves.

Infective endocarditis classified as subacute and acute. The subacute form has a longer clincial course of more insidious onset with less toxicity, and the causative organisms usually of low virulence. In contrast, the acute form has a shorter clinical course with more rapid onset, increased toxicity and more pathogenic causative organism.

Etiology

Etiologic organisms associated with infective endocarditis includes:

- Streptococci
  - Alpha and hemolytic streptococci
  - Enterococci
  - *Streptococcus bovis* and
  - *Streptococcus pneumoniae*
- Staphylococci
  - *Staphylococcus aureus*
  - *Staphylococcus epidermidis*
- Gram-negative bacteria;
  - *Escherichia coli*
  - *Klebsiella* and
  - *Pseudomonas*
- Polymicrobial endocarditis.
  - *Streptococcus agalactiae* and methicillin susceptible *Staphylococcus aureus*
  - *Pseudomonas aeruginosa*, α-hemolytic streptococci and *Micrococcus*
- *Haemophilus*
- *Actinobacillus*
- *Cardiobacterium*
- *Eikenella*
- *Kingella*.

The predisposing conditions to the development of infective endocarditis are as follows:

- Cardiac conditions:
  - Rheumatic heart disease
  - Aortic valve leaflet abnormalities
  - Mitral valve prolapse with murmur
  - Cyanotic congenital heart disease
  - Prosthetic valve
  - Degenerative valvular lesions
  - Prior endocarditis
  - Morton's syndrome
  - Asymmetric septal hypertrophy
  - Idiopathic hypertrophic subaortic stenosis
- Non-cardiac diseases:
  - Associate risks
  - Intravascular devices (leading) bacteremia
- Procedure
  - Associated risks
  - Intravascular devices (leading to nosocomial bacteremia
  - Procedures that require endocarditis antibiotic prophylaxis.

Risk Factors

- Valvular heart disease, rheumatic heart disease, mitral valve prolapse and prosthetic valve surgery
- Age: Infective endocarditis is more common in older people because of their decreased immunologic response, the metabolic changes of aging, and increased invasive diagnostic procedures
- Intravenous drug use: There is a high incidence of staphylococcal endocarditis among intravenous drug users
- Hospitalization: Hospital-acquired endocarditis occurs most often in patients with debilitating disease or indwelling catheters and in those receiving prolonged intravenous or antibiotic therapy
- Immunosuppression: Patients taking immunosuppressive medications or steroids may develop fungal endocarditis.

The patient populations at risk for infective endocarditis are:

High risk
- Prosthetic heart valves
- Previous history of endocarditis
- Complex congenital cyanotic heart disease
- Surgically constructed systemic pulmonary shunts or conduits.

Moderate risk
- Patent ductus arteriosus
- Ventricular septal defect
- Primum atrial septal defect
- Coarctation of aorta
- Acquired valvular dysfunction
- Hypertrophic cardiomyopathy
- Some clinical presentation of mitral valve prolapse.

Pathophysiology

A damaged cardiac valve or a ventricular septal defect produces turbulent blood flow, which allows bacteria to settle on the low pressure side of the valve or defect. The hallmark of endocarditis is the "Platelet fibrin-bacteria mass" on the value called a vegetation. The organism-surround the heart valve become embedded on the valve matrix, and result in vegetative, the primary lesions of the infective endocarditis consist of fibrin, leukocytes, platelets, and microbes that adhere to the valve surface or endocardium. The loss of portions of these friable types of vegetation into the circulation results in embolization. Systemic embolization occurs from left-sided heart vegetation, progressing to organ (particularly brain, kidneys and spleen) and limb infarction. Right-sided heart lesions embolize to the lungs. If the vegetative emboli enter organs, abscesses may form.

The infection may spread locally to cause damage to the valves or to their supporting structures. The resulting valvular incompetence and eventual invasion of the myocardium in the infectious disease result in CHF, generalized myocardial dysfunction and sepsis. Sequential of events of infective endocarditis (Fig. 12.16).

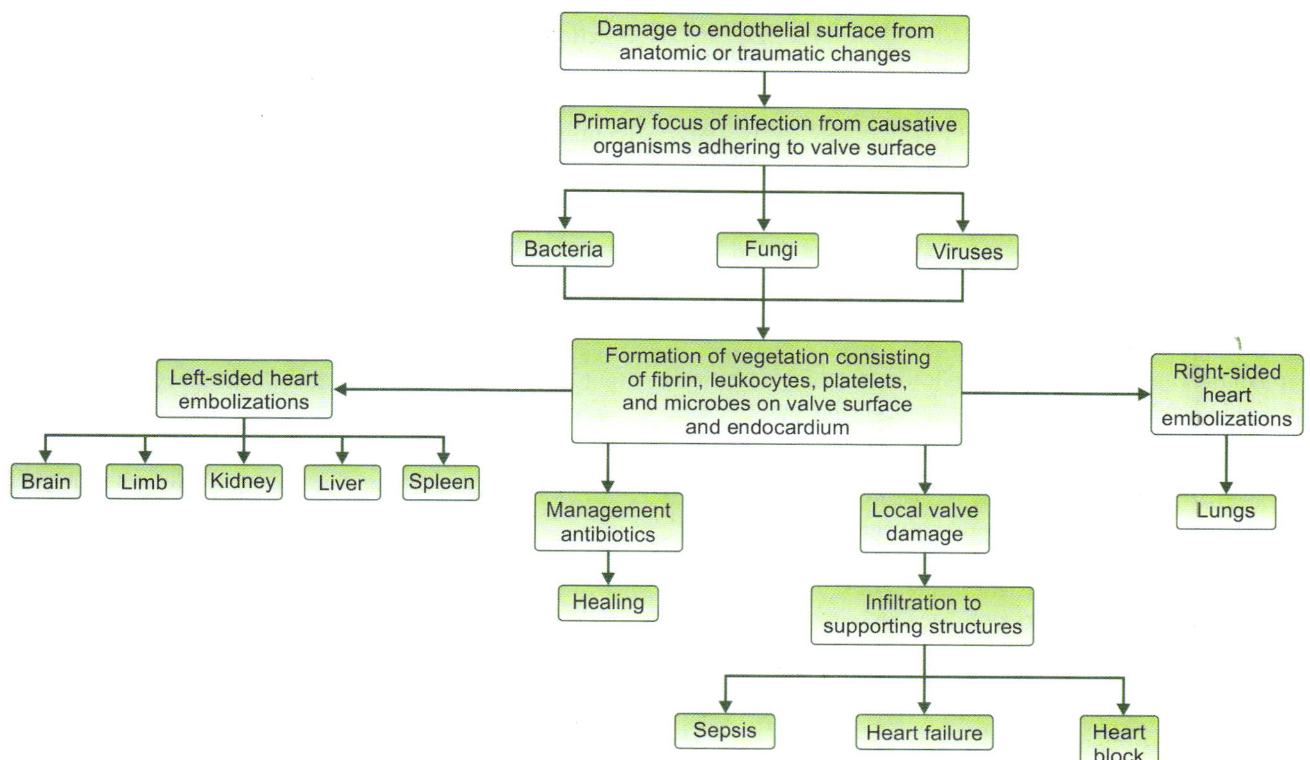

FIG. 12.16: Sequence of events in infective endocarditis

Clinical Manifestations

The onset of SBE (subacute bacterial endocarditis) is gradual and the patient reports malaise and general achiness. Low grade fever is usually present, although a high fever usually occurs with *S. aureus,* infection. The other non-specific manifestations that may accompany fever include chills, weakness, malaise, fatigue, and anorexia. Arthralgia, myalgia, back pain, abdominal discomfort, weight loss and headache, clubbing of fingers may occur in SBE.

- Insidious onset; signs and symptoms develop from toxicity of infection, destruction of heart valves, and embolization of fragments of vegetative growths on the heart
- General manifestations include vague complaints of malaise, anorexia, weight loss, and back and joint pain
- Fever is intermittent; may be absent in patients who are receiving antibiotics or corticosteroids, elderly patients, and patients with heart failure or renal failure
- Splinter hemorrhages under fingernails and toenails and petechiae in conjunctive and mucous membranes
- Hemorrhages with pale centers (Roth's spots) in fundi of eyes
- Small painful nodules (Osler's nodes) in pads of fingers or toes
- Cardiac manifestations: Heart enlargement, heart failure, and heart murmurs (may be absent initially); progressively changing murmurs indicate valvular damage
- Central nervous system manifestations: Headache, transient cerebral ischemia, focal neurologic lesions, stroke
- Emboli involving other organ systems manifest in the lung (recurrent pneumonia, pulmonary abscesses), kidney (hematuria, renal failure), spleen (left upper quadrant pain), heart (myocardial infarction), brain (stroke), and peripheral vessels.

A diagnosis of acute infective endocarditis is made when the onset of infection and resulting valvular destruction are rapid occurring within days to weeks.

- Blood cultures
- Doppler or transesophageal echocardiography.

The Complication Include

Heart failure, cerebral vascular complications, valve stenosis or regurgitation, myocardial damage, mycotic aneurysms.

Vascular manifestation's infective endocarditis includes splinter hemorrhages (black longitudinal streaks) that may occur in nail beds. Petechiae may occur as a result of fragmentation and microembolization of vegetative lesions and are common in the conjunctiva, the lips, the buccal mucosa, the palate, and over the ankles, the feet and the antecubital and popliteal areas osler's nodes (painful, tender, red or purple pea size lesions) may be found in fingertips or toes. Janeway lesions (flat painless, small red spots) may be found on the palms and soles. Fundoscopic examination may reveal hemorrhagic retinal lesions called Roth's spots.

Auscultation reveals murmurs over the affected area and clinical manifestations secondary to embolizations in various body organs may also be present, if embolization of organs and cardinal symptom are as follows:

- Spleen
  - Sharp left upper quadrant pain and splenomegaly, local tenderness and abdominal rigidity
- Kidney
  - Pain in the flank, hematuria and azotemia
- Peripheral
  - Blood vessel of arms and legs may cause gangrene
- Brain
  - Hemiplegia, ataxia, aphasia, visual changes, LOC (level of consciousness) changes
- Pulmonary emboli, occurs in right-sided endocarditis.

Management

For diagnosis obtaining the patient's recent health history is very important particularly inquiry regarding any recent dental urologic, surgical or gynecologic including normal or abnormal obstetric delivery, heart disease diagnostic procedures, infection of skin and respiration or urinary origin are helpful.

In addition to thorough physical examination and routine diagnostic procedures, useful are blood culture and sensitivity, WBC count with differential rheumatoid factor, urine analysis, chest X-ray, ECG, echocardiography and cardiac catheterization.

Medical Management

Objectives of treatment are to eradicate the invading organism through adequate doses of an appropriate antimicrobial agent (continuous intravenous infusion of 2 to 6 weeks at home). Treatment measure include:

- Isolating causative organism through serial blood cultures. Blood cultures are taken to monitor the course of therapy
- Monitoring patients temperature for treatment effectiveness
- After recovery from the infectious process, seriously damaged valves may require debridement or replacement. For example, surgical valve replacement is required if heart failure develops, if patient has more than one serious systemic embolic episode, if infection cannot be controlled or is recurrent, or if infection is caused by a fungus.

The major aim of the therapy is to eliminate all micro-organisms from the vegetative grown and prevent complications. The therapy includes:

- Appropriate antibiotic therapy
- Antipyretics
- Rest
- Repetitions of blood cultures and sensitivity tests
- Surgical valvular repair or replacement (for severe valvular damage).

Nursing Management

- Provide psychosocial support while patient is confined to hospital or home with restrictive intravenous therapy
- Assess heart sounds for new or worsening murmur
- If patient received surgical treatment, provide postsurgical care and instruction
- After surgery, monitor patient's temperature; a fever may be present for weeks
- Monitor for signs and symptoms of systemic embolization, or, for patients with right heart endocarditis, signs and symptoms of pulmonary infarction and infiltrates
- Assess for signs and symptoms of organ damage such as stroke (CVA, brain attack), meningitis, heart failure, myocardial infarction, glomerulonephritis, and splenomegaly
- Instruct patient and family about activity restrictions, medications, and signs and symptoms of infection.
- Reinforce that antibiotic prophylaxis is recommended for patients who have had infective endocarditis and who are undergoing invasive procedures
- Refer to home care nurse to supervise and monitor intravenous antibiotic therapy in the home.

The nurse teaches the patient to avoid excessive fatigue and to stop activity immediately if chest pain, dyspnea, lightheadedness, or faintness occurs. Patients should avoid others with infections. The nurse instructs the patient to inform all primary care providers including physicians, and dentists about history of infective endocarditis, so that appropriate antibiotic therapy can be administered prior to intrusive procedure. American Heart Association recommended following antibiotic prophylaxis of infective endocarditis.

1. For dental, oral, respiratory tract or esophageal procedure, if *Streptococcus viridans* is a pathogen, the antibiotic choice will be:
   - Amoxicillin 2 g 1 hour before procedure, alternative if unable to take oral or if allergic to penicillin
   - Ampicillin IV
   - Clindamycin, oral or IV
   - First-generation cephalosporins—cefazolin IV azithromycin or clarithromycin.
2. For genitourinary and nonesophageal GI, procedures if pathogens is *Enterococcus faecalis*, antibiotic choice will be parenteral ampicillin or amoxicillin, IV/IM gentamicin IV nafcillin, IV vancomycin (for *Staphylococcus*).

In addition, the patient should brush with soft-bristled toothbrush and floss regularly to protect the gums and/or event caries. Good dental hygiene is of utmost importance in decreasing the risk of recurrent infective endocarditis.

Problems

- Activity intolerance related to imbalance between oxygen supply and demand
- Ineffective management related to therapy
- Pain related to arthralgia, myalgia and embolization
- Altered health maintenance
- Emboli related to dislodging vegetation and immobility
- Anxiety related to critical illness.

RHEUMATIC HEART DISEASE

Rheumatic heart disease is an acute inflammatory reaction involving all layers. The resulting damage to the heart from Rh fever is termed "Rheumatic heart disease" a chronic condition characterized by scarring and deformity of heart valves. Rheumatic endocarditis is associated with rheumatic fever caused by group A beta-hemolytic streptococcal infection.

Etiology

Rheumatic fever almost always occurs as a delayed sequela (usually after 2 to 3 weeks) of a group A-beta-hemolytic streptococcal infection of the upper respiratory system. In addition socioeconomic factors, familial factors and presence of an altered immune response have a predisposing role in the development of rheumatic fever.

Pathophysiology

The infectious agent does not invade the tissues but causes a sensitivity phenomenon or reaction in response to hemolytic streptococci. Rheumatic fever affects all bony joints, producing a polyarthritis. The most serious damage occurs in the heart. Rheumatic endocarditis manifests as tiny, translucent vegetations that resemble beads about the size of a pinhead, arranged in a row along the free margins of the valve flaps. The flaps gradually become shorter and thicker than normal, which prevents them from closing the valve orifice completely. The result is valvular regurgitation (leakage); most common is mitral regurgitation. Valvular stenosis may also occur. A few patients become critically ill with intractable heart failure, serious dysrhythmias, and rheumatic pneumonia. The myocardium can compensate for these valvular defects very well for a time. Sooner or later, however, decompensation occurs and is manifested by heart failure.

The inflammation of rheumatic heart disease may involve:

- The lining of the heart or endocardium (endocarditis) including the valves, resulting scarring, distortion and stenosis of the valves
- The heart muscle (myocarditis) or
- The outer covering of the heart (pericarditis), where it may cause adhesions of surrounding tissues.

Clinical Manifestations

The development of symptoms of chronic rheumatic heart disease depends on the involvement of the particular part of the heart.

- Eventually, the heart murmurs characteristic of valvular stenosis, regurgitation, or both become audible on auscultation; "thrills" may be detected on palpation
- Cardiac symptoms depend on which side of the heart is involved. Severity of symptoms depends on size and location of the lesion
- The mitral valve is most often affected, producing symptoms of left-sided heart failure; shortness of breath crackles and wheezes.

Management

Careful history and physical examination are needed to diagnose rheumatic heart disease. In addition, ASO titer (Antistreptolysin O titer) ESR, C-reactive protein, throat culture, WBC count, RBC parameter, chest-X-ray, echocardiography and ECG are useful to identify RHD.

Medical Management

Objectives of medical management are aggressive eradication of the causative organism and prevention of additional complications, such as a thromboembolic event. Prevention is achieved through early and adequate treatment of streptococcal infection in all patients. Long-term antibiotic therapy is the treatment of choice. Parenteral penicillin remains the medication of choice. If valve dysfunction is mild and the disease is quiet, no therapy is required as long as the heart pumps effectively.

Nursing Management

A key nursing role in rheumatic endocarditis is teaching patients about the disease, its treatment, and the steps needed to avoid complications:

- Educate patient and community regarding recognition of streptococcal infections and the need to treat them adequately and to control community epidemics
- Teach susceptible patients that they may require long-term oral antibiotic therapy and may be required to take prophylactic antibiotics before procedures, such as dental checkups. They will also need routine cardiac evaluations
- Emphasize that less common diagnostic procedures, such as cystoscopy also require prophylactic antibiotic therapy.

Prophylactic penicillin is prescribed during acute episodes of rheumatic fever and for several years thereafter lifelong antibiotic prophylaxis may be necessary for persons with significant rheumatic heart disease. Corticosteroids may be prescribed during acute rheumatic fever to decrease the cardiac inflammation If congestive heart failure occurs, bed rest, sodium and fluid restrictions, diuretics, and inotrope usually are prescribed. Antipyretics are also used cautiously.

The nurse emphasizes to the patient and family the importance of rest and adequate nutrition. Additional education to be given as in cardiac diseases.

VALVULAR HEART DISEASE

The heart contains two atrioventricular valves, the mitral and tricuspid, and two semilunar valves, the aortic and the pulmonic which are located in four strategic locations to control unidirectional blood flow. Types of valvular heart diseases are defined according to the valve or valves affected and the two types of functional alterations, stenosis and regurgitation.

1. MITRAL STENOSIS

Mitral stenosis occurs when the blood flow from the left atrium to the left ventricle during ventricular diastole (ventricular filling) is impeded due to thickening or fibrotic changes in the mitral valve (Fig. 12.17).

Etiology

The primary cause is rheumatic fever and carditis, which causes an inflammatory process of the mitral valves chordae tendineae or commissures (leaflets). Less common causes include bacterial vegetation, thrombus formation, calcification of the mitral annulus and atrial myxoma (tumor).

Pathophysiology

Mitral stenosis is the progressive thickening and contracture of the mitral valve leaflets and chordae tendineae that causes narrowing of the orifice and progressive obstruction to blood flow from the left atrium into the left ventricle. Normally, the mitral valve opening is as wide as three fingers. In cases of marked stenosis, the opening narrows to the width of a pencil.

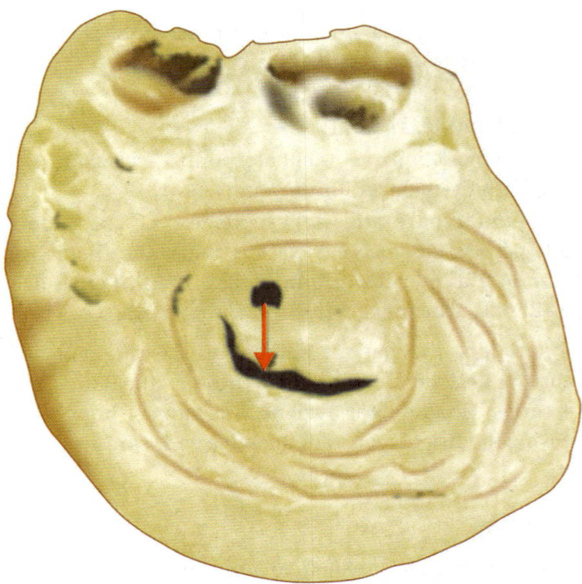

FIG. 12.17: Mitral stenosis with classic "fish mouth" orifice

The left atrium dilates and hypertrophies because it has great difficulty moving blood into the ventricle and because of the increased blood volume the atria must now hold. Because there is no valve to protect the pulmonary veins from the backward flow of blood from the atrium, the pulmonary circulation becomes congested. The resulting high pulmonary pressure can eventually lead to right ventricular failure.

In mitral stenosis, the mitral valve leaflets become thickened and fibrotic from scar tissue formation and calcification. As the valve leaflets become stiff and fused, the valve lumen progressively narrows and becomes immobile. In addition, the chordae tendineae may shorten and thicken. The mitral value of orifice may decrease in size from its normal 4 to 6 cm to less than 1 cm. With progressive mitral stenosis, left atrial pressure elevates as a result of incomplete emptying of the left atrium. Sustained elevated left atrial pressure causes the myocardium to compensate with left atrial dilation and hypertrophy. In addition, high pressures in the left atrium lead to elevated pulmonary venous capillary and arterial pressures. Eventually sustained elevation of the left atrial pressure can produce pulmonary hypertension and subsequent right ventricular hypertrophy. With the increased pressure in the pulmonary vasculature, leakage of fluid across the pulmonary pupillary membrane into the lung interstitium can be produced pulmonary edema. Persons with mitral stenosis also have reduced cardiac output and increases cardiac arrhythmias—(atrial fibrillation), later this may allow thrombus formation and arterial embolization to vital organs.

Clinical Manifestations

- The first symptom is often dyspnea on exertion (due to pulmonary venous hypertension)
- Progressive fatigue (result of low cardiac output), hemoptysis and cough, and repeated respiratory infection may be noted
- Weak and often irregular pulse (because of atrial fibrillation) may also be noted.

The most common cause rheumatic fever. In addition there will be fatigue, weakness. The primary symptoms include dyspnea, an exertion orthopnea, paroxysmal nocturnal dyspnea, predisposing causes to respiratory infections, hemoptysis, pulmonary hypertension and edema. These symptoms may be precipitated by emotional stress, respiratory infections, sexual intercourse or atrial fibrillation. Later neural deficits only associated with emboli (hemiparesis) CVA, ascites, hepatic angina with hepatomegaly, chest pain, palpitations (AF) diastolic murmurs accentuated first heart sound, opening snap. If not treated and right ventricular failure occurs leads to jugular vein distention, pitting edema and hepatomegaly.

Management

Diagnosis of mitral stenosis is established by the clinical symptoms such as an opening snap (best heard at the apex with stethoscope diaphragm) and a low-pitched, rumbling diastolic murmur (best heard at the apex with the stethoscope bell) results from increased velocity of blood flow. If valve calcified no murmur, heard. ECG echocardiogram and cardiac catheterization are also helpful in diagnosis of mitral stenosis. Additional management measures include:

- Prophylactic antibiotic therapy to prevent recurrence of infections; anticoagulant therapy to reduce risk of thrombi
- Treatment of anemia if required
- Cardiotonics and diuretics for treatment of congestive heart failure
- Strenuous exercise restrictions
- Surgical intervention (valvuloplasty, commissurotomy, or replacement of the mitral valve)
- Percutaneous transluminal valvuloplasty for palliation of symptoms.

Mildly symptomatic patient with mitral stenosis are treated with diuretics, and digitalis is used to control heart rate in the event of atrial fibrillations. Anticoagulation therapy is used to prevent embolization. Medical therapy includes antibiotic prophylaxis before dental and surgical procedures to reduce the risk of bacterial endocarditis. Mechanical enlargement of the mitral valve is indicated when the disease causes either loss of exercise capacity or pulmonary hypertension.

- Percutaneous valvuloplasty using balloon dilation provides a non-surgical alternative to repair of mitral stenosis
- Surgical commissurotomy can also be performed while the valve leaflets remain mobile
- Mitral valve replacement using open heart surgery
- Cardiopulmonary bypass is performed when the valve is severely calcified.

Patient who experiences symptoms related to mitral stenosis are prescribed sodium-restricted diet to help prevent fluid retention, and progressive heart failure. Nursing interventions are taken accordingly.

2. MITRAL REGURGITATION

Mitral regurgitation (mitral insufficiency) occurs when the mitral valve fails to completely close during ventricular systole, and consequently some blood flows backward into the left atrium. Mitral regurgitation can be acute or chronic (Fig. 12.18).

Etiology

The causes of mitral regurgitations are numerous and may be inflammatory, degenerative, infective, structural, or congenital in nature. The majority of cases may be attributed to chronic rheumatic heart disease, isolated rupture of chordae tendineae, mitral valve prolapse, ischemic papillary muscle dysfunction and infective endocarditis.

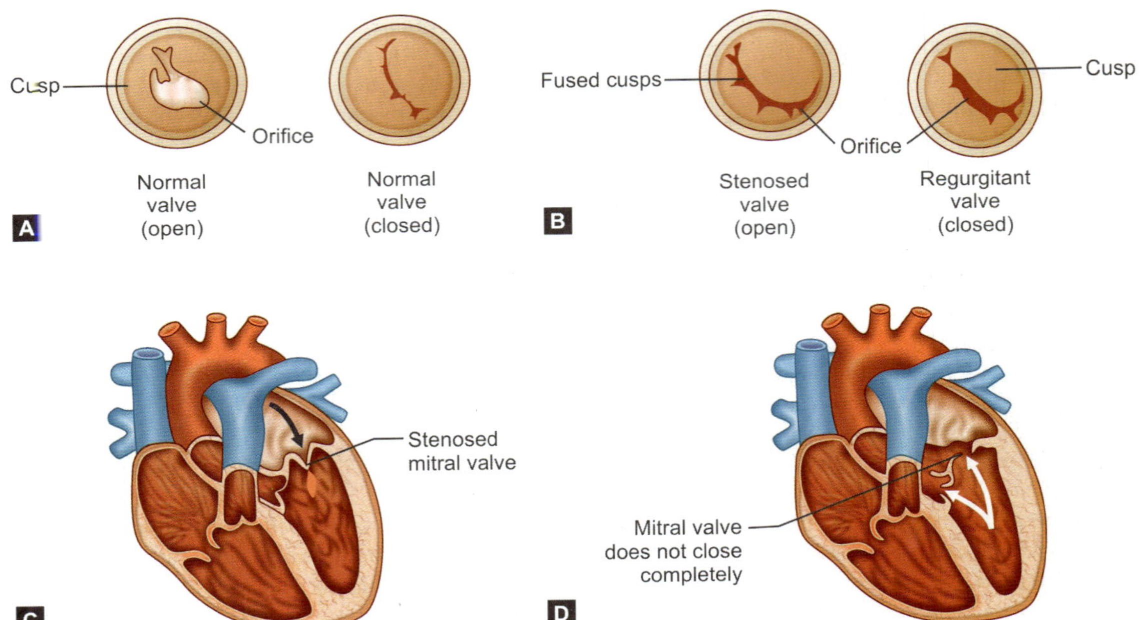

FIGS 12.18A TO D: Valvular stenosis and regurgitation. (A) Normal position of the valve leaflets, or cusps, when the valve is open and closed; (B) Open position of a stenosed valve (left) and position of closed regurgitant valve (right); (C) Hemodynamic effect of mitral stenosis. The stenosed valve is unable to open sufficiently during left atrial systole, inhibiting left ventricular filling; (D) Hemodynamic effect of mitral regurgitation. The mitral valve does not close completely during left ventricular systole, permitting blood to reenter the left atrium

Pathophysiology

Mitral regurgitation results when the margins of the mitral valve are unable to close during systole. There is a problem with one or more of the leaflets, the annulus, or the papillary muscles, preventing closure of the leaflets. At each beat, the left ventricle forces some blood back into the left atrium causing the agent to dilate and hypertrophy. This backward flow of blood from the ventricle eventually causes the lungs to become congested, which adds strain to the right ventricle, resulting in cardiac failure.

The regurgitant mitral orifice is parallel with aortic valve, so that burden imposed on the left ventricle and the left atrium are determined by the etiology, severity and duration of mitral regurgitation. In chronic regurgitation, volume overload on the left ventricle, the left atrium, and the pulmonary bed is created by the backward flow of blood from the left ventricle into the left atrium during ventricular systole, resulting in varying degrees of left atrial enlargement and left ventricular dilation. Acute mitral regurgitation does not result in dilation of the left atrium or left ventricle. Without dilation to accommodate the regurgitant volume, pulmonary vascular pressure rise ultimately, causing pulmonary edema.

Clinical Manifestation

The resultant clinical picture in acute mitral regurgitation is that of pulmonary edema and shock. Patient will have thready, peripheral pulses and cool, clammy extremities. Auscultation findings of a new systolic murmur may be obscured by a low cardiac output.

Chronic mitral regurgitation is often asymptomatic; but acute regurgitation (after MI) usually presents as severe heart failure.

Usual symptoms include dyspnea, shortness of breath on exertion, fatigue, weakness, palpitations of the heart, and cough due to chronic passive pulmonary congestion.

Irregular pulse as a result of either extrasystole or atrial fibrillation may persist indefinitely.

Patient with chronic mitral regurgitation may remain asymptomatic for many years until the development of some degree of LVF. Initial symptoms include weakness, fatigue and dyspnea that gradually progress to orthopnea, paroxysmal nocturnal dyspnea, and peripheral edema, and brisk carotid pulse. Auscultatory findings reflect accentuated left ventricular filling leading to an audible third heart sound (S_3) even in the absence of left ventricular dysfunction. The murmur is a loud pansystolic or holosystolic murmur at the apex radiating to the left axilla.

Management

The diagnosis of mitral regurgitation is made by auscultatory findings. Chest X-ray reveals left atrial enlargement need occasional left ventricular dilation. ECG echocardiogram also is used for diagnosis. Definitive diagnosis is made through cardiac catheterization, which assess left ventricular function and the degree of regurgitation.

Management is the same as for heart failure. Surgical intervention consists of mitral valve replacement of valvuloplasty.

Patient with mild mitral regurgitation are generally managed medically. Acute mitral regurgitation need hospitalization and hemodynamic stabilization. As with other cardiac cases, management of heart failure, arrhythmias, and others by antibiotic prophylaxis, diuretics and digitalis are useful accordingly. The nursing care is also designed accordingly.

3. MITRAL VALVE PROLAPSE (MVP)

Mitral valve prolapse occurs when abnormalities in the mitral valve leaflets, chordae tendineae or papillary muscles allow prolapse of the mitral valve leaflets backward into the left atrium during ventricular systole. It is also known as Barlow's syndrome as well as a "floppy or billowing" mitral valve (Fig. 12.19). Mitral valve prolapse is a dysfunction of the mitral valve leaflets that prevents the mitral valve from closing completely during systole. Blood then regurgitates from the left ventricle back into the left atrium. It occurs more frequently in women.

Etiology

The cause of MVP is unknown but related to pathogenic mecha-nisms of mitral valve apparatus. If incidence is possibly linked to an autosomal dominant inherited trait, and is associated with other inherited connective tissue disorders such as Marfan syndrome, Ehlers-Danlos syndrome and osteogenesis imperfecta. Other causes include endocarditis, CAD, myocarditis, cardiomyopathy, cardiac trauma and hyperthyroidism.

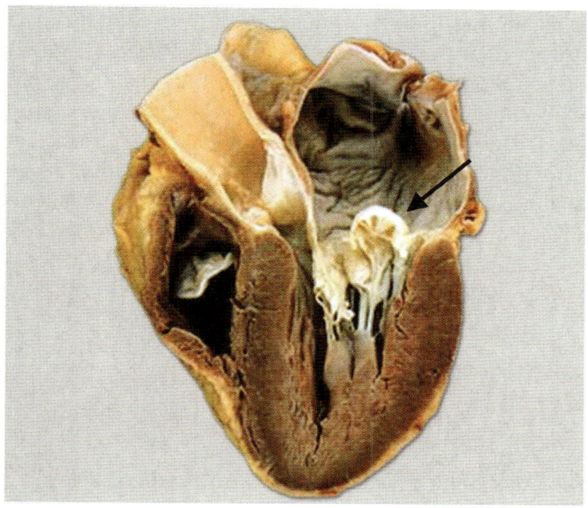

FIG. 12.19: Mitral valve prolapse. In this valvular abnormality, the mitral leaflets prolapsed back into left atrium. They also demonstrate hooding (arrow). The left ventricle is on the right

Pathophysiology

In mitral valve prolapse, the leaflets of mitral valve become enlarged or thickened, and the chordae tendineae may become elongated. These changes permit the valve leaflets to billow upward into the left atrium during ventricular systole. Depending on the degree of prolapse and integrity of the valve leaflets mitral regurgitation may occur. The subsequent pathophysiology parallels that of mitral regurgitation.

Clinical Manifestation

The syndrome may produce no symptoms or may program rapidly and result in sudden death.

- Patients may experience symptoms of fatigue, shortness of breath (not correlated with activity), light headedness, dizziness, syncope, palpitations, chest pain, and anxiety
- Fatigue may be present regardless of the person's activity level and amount of rest or sleep
- During the physical examination, a mitral (systolic) click identified. Presence of a click indicates early valvular incompetence
- The mitral click may deteriorate into a murmur over time the valve leaflets become more dysfunctional
- As the murmur progresses, there may be signs and symptoms of heart failure (not common).

Many cases of MVP are symptomatic. Persons with symptomatic complain of palpitations secondary to arrhythmias and tachycardia, other systems include light-headedness, syncope, fatigue, lethargy, weakness, dyspnea, and chest tightness. In addition, hyperventilation, anxiety, depression, panic attacks and atypical chest pain may occur. Many symptoms are vague, and puzzling and are not necessarily degree of prolapse.

Management

MVP is diagnosed principally by echocardiography, although cardiac angiography may be used to confirm diagnosis. Individuals who experience palpitations require 24 hours ambulatory ECG monitoring to determine severity of arrhythmias.

Medical Management

Medical management is directed at controlling symptoms:

- Antidysrhythmic agents are prescribed
- In advanced stages, mitral valve replacement may be necessary
- Dietary restrictions; avoidance of alcohol and caffeine.

Nursing Management

- Teach patient about antidysrhythmic or antianginal medications, if prescribed
- Explain that alcohol, ephedrine, and epinephrine, which may be in over-the-counter preparations, may stimulate dysrhythmias. Teach patient to read product labels to avoid these agents
- Educate patient about the need for prophylactic antibiotic therapy before undergoing invasive procedures (e.g. dental work, genitourinary procedures, or gastrointestinal procedures). Patient should consult physician if in doubt about need for antibiotics before a procedure.

Teach patient about the diagnosis and the possibility that the disorder is hereditary.

Asymptomatic persons with MVP usually do not require treatment. Symptomatic persons may require medications for the arrhythmias. Beta blockers are the treatment of choice for managing palpitations and chest pain. The drug of choice is atenolol or propranolol. Antibiotic prophylaxis are used to prevent endocarditis. All persons with MVP need regular follow-up and should have an echocardiogram every few years to monitor disease, severity and progression.

Persons with MVP are encouraged to avoid caffeine which may exacerbate the incidence of tachycardia and atrial dysrhythmias.

4. AORTIC STENOSIS

Aortic stenosis (AS) occurs when the aortic valve leaflets become stiff, fused or calcified and impede blood flow from the left ventricle into the aorta during ventricular systole.

Aortic valve stenosis is the narrowing of the orifice between the left ventricle and the aorta. In adults, the stenosis may be congenital, or it may be a result of rheumatic endocarditis or cusp calcification of unknown cause. There is progressive narrowing of the valve orifice over a period of several years to several decades. The heart muscle increases in size (hypertrophy) in response to all degrees of obstruction; clinical signs of heart failure occur when compensatory mechanisms of the heart fail.

Etiology

Aortic stenosis is caused by congenital malformation of the aortic valve inflammatory heart disease (endocarditis) or degenerative disease (calcification). Hypertrophic cardiomyopathy leads to subvalvular lesion that may mimic aortic stenosis.

Pathophysiology

Aortic stenosis results in obstruction of flow from the left ventricle to the aorta during systole. The effect is concentric for left ventricular hypertrophy and increased myocardial oxygen consumption because of the increased myocardial mass. As the disease course progresses and compensatory mechanisms fail, reduced cardiac output leads to pulmonary hypertension.

Clinical Manifestation

The general symptoms is fatigue, dyspnea on exertions, syncope (especially on exertion), pain resembles angina pectoris, bradycardia, dysrhythmias (with heart failure). Systolic murmurs normal or soft S_1, Prominent S_4 crescendo-decrescendo murmur. And there is:

- Exertional dyspnea
- Dizziness and syncope (fainting)
- Angina pectoris
- Blood pressure possibly low but usually normal
- Low pulse pressure (30 mm Hg or less)
- Physical examination: Loud, rough, systolic murmur heard over the aortic area; vibration over the base of the heart.

Management

A diagnosis of aortic valve stenosis is made by clinical symptoms, clinical findings and diagnostic test. Test that help are ECG, Chest X-ray echocardiogram, and cardiac catheterization. Percutaneous balloon valvuloplasty may be used to alleviate aorta stenosis. The definitive therapy for patients with aortic stenosis is valve replacement with a prosthetic aortic valve. In addition, measures to be taken to manage arrhythmias and heart failure. Nursing care is designed accordingly.

Antibiotic prophylaxis is provided to prevent endocarditis. Medications for left ventricular failure or dysrhythmia are administered as needed. Surgical replacement of the aortic valve is the favored definitive treatment. Uncorrected condition can lead to irreversible heart failure. Patients who are symptomatic and are not surgical candidates may benefit from one- or two-balloon percutaneous valvuloplasty procedures.

The diet of persons with aortic stenosis is unrestricted, unless heart failure is present, in which case the nurse instructs patient to restrict their daily intake of sodium and fluid. Activity level must be carefully monitored because patients are at risk for sudden cardiac death. Patients are cautioned against undue physical exertion or stress, which may precipitate heart failure or arrhythmias. Patients and families need ongoing teaching, and support effectively to manage this ongoing challenge in their daily lives. The nurse also reminds patient of the seeking prophylactic antibiotic treatment against endocarditis before any invasive dental procedure or surgery.

5. AORTIC REGURGITATION (INSUFFICIENCY)

Aortic regurgitation occurs when an incompetent aortic valve allows blood to flow backward from the aorta into the left ventricle during diastole.

Aortic insufficiency is the flow of blood back into the left ventricle from the aorta during diastole. The result is left ventricular dilation and hypertrophy. It may be caused by inflammatory lesions that deform the leaflets of the aortic valve. The lesions prevent complete sealing of the aortic orifice during diastole. This disorder may result from endocarditis, congenital abnormalities, or conditions such as blunt chest trauma, syphilis, and dissecting aneurysm that cause dilation or tearing of the ascending aorta.

Etiology

Aortic regurgitation may result in a primary disease of the aortic valve leaflets, the aortic root, or both acute aortic regurgitation may be the result of a primary disease of the aortic valve leaflets, the aortic root, or both. Acute aortic regurgitation is caused by bacterial endocarditis, trauma or aortic dissection and constitute a life-threatening emergency. Chronic aortic regurgitation is generally the syphilis, or chronic rheumatic conditions such as ankylosing spondylitis, or Reiter's syndrome.

Pathophysiology

The basic physiologic consequence of aortic regurgitation is retrograde blood flow from the ascending aorta into the left ventricle resulting in volume overload. The left ventricle initially compensates for chronic aortic regurgitation by dilation and hypertrophy. Myocardial contractility eventually declines and blood volume increases in the left atrium and pulmonary vasculature. Ultimately, pulmonary hypertension and right ventricular failure develops.

Clinical Manifestation

Patients with acute aortic regurgitation have sudden clinical manifestations of cardiovascular collapse. Abrupt onset of profound dyspnea, transient chest pain, progression to shock which need immediate medical attention Patient:

- Develops insidiously (without symptoms in most patients)
- Earliest manifestation: Increased force of heartbeat—that is, visible or palpable pulsations over the temporal arteries (head) and at the neck (carotid)
- Exertional dyspnea and easy fatigability
- Signs and symptoms of left ventricular failure (orthopnea, paroxysmal nocturnal dyspnea)
- Widened pulse pressure
- Water-hammer pulse (pulse strikes the palpating finger with quick, sharp strokes and then suddenly collapses).

Patient with chronic aortic regurgitation have pulses that are of the "water-hammer" or collapsing type with abrupt distension during systole and quick collapse during diastole (Corrigan's pulse). Pistol-shot pulse sounds can be auscultated over the femoral arteries, and some persons demonstrate a typical head bobbing with each heart beat. Auscultatory findings include a soft or absent S_1, presence of S_3 or S_4 and a soft decrescendo and high-pitched diastolic murmur. A systolic murmur also can be heard, i.e. systolic ejection click.

In chronic aortic regurgitation it appear symptomatic for many years and seen with external dyspnea, orthopnea, paroxysmal nocturnal dyspnea only after considerable myocardial dysfunction. Nocturnal angina with diaphoresis and abdominal discomfort may be present.

Management

The diagnosis of aortic regurgitation made by auscultative finding, regular chest X-ray, ECG, and echocardiogram digitalis and diuretic are helpful to persons with heart failure. Aortic valve replacement is indicated for symptomatic persons, after thorough diagnosis. The other measure as in other valvular diseases.

Medical Management

- Antibiotic prophylaxis is used before invasive and dental procedures
- Heart failure and dysrhythmias are treated
- Treatment of choice is aortic valve replacement; surgery is recommended in the presence of left ventricular hypertrophy
- Valve repair (valvuloplasty commissurotomy) may be performed instead of replacement. Repaired valves function longer than replaced valves, and continuous anticoagulation is not required.

Nursing Management

- Teach patient about wound care, diet, activity, medication, and self-care
- Instruct patient on importance of antibiotic prophylaxis to prevent endocarditis
- Reinforce all new information and self-care instructions for 4 to 8 weeks after the procedure.

6. TRICUSPID VALVE DISEASE

Tricuspid stenosis is a restriction of the tricuspid valve orifice that impedes blood flow from the right atrium to the right ventricle during right ventricular diastole (filling). Conversely, tricuspid regurgitation involves an incompetent tricuspid valve that allows blood to flow backward from the right ventricle to the right atrium during ventricular systole.

Etiology

Tricuspid stenosis is extremely uncommon and occurs almost exclusively in patient with rheumatic mitral stenosis. It is also seen in IV drugs users. Tricuspid regurgitation is usually the result of pulmonary hypertension or right ventricular dysfunction.

Pathophysiology

In tricuspid stenosis, right atrial outflow is obstructed, resulting in right atrial enlargement and elevated systemic venous pressures. Volume overload of the right atrium and ventricle occur in tricuspid regurgitation.

Clinical Manifestation

Tricuspid stenosis and regurgitation result in the backward flow of blood into the systemic circulation. Common manifestations are peripheral edema, ascites and hepatomegaly. The murmur of stenosis is presystolic (sinus rhythm) or midsystolic (AF) and pansystolic murmur may be heard in regurgitation. Both types of murmurs dramatically increased in intensity with inspiration.

Management

As in other valvular disease are according to underlying cause.

7. PULMONIC VALVE DISEASE

Tricuspid and pulmonary valve disease all cause similar consequences to cardiac function. Pulmonic valve disease is an uncommon entity and in the case of pulmonary stenosis, it is always congenital. Pulmonary regurgitation as an isolated abnormality has a benign course but it generally is associated with disease of other valves.

To sum up, the management of valvular heart disease includes following measures:

1. Diagnostic measures
   - History and physical examination
   - Chest X-ray
   - ECG
   - Echocardiography
   - Cardiac catheterization.
2. Nonsurgical measures
   - Prophylactic antibiotic therapy to prevent rheumatic fever, infective endocarditis
   - Digitalis
   - Diuretics
   - Sodium restriction
   - Anticoagulant agents—warfarin-dipyridomole
   - Aspirin
   - Antiarrhythmic drugs
   - Oral nitrates
   - Beta-adrenergic blockers
   - Percutaneous transluminal balloon valvulopathy.
3. Surgical measures
   - Valvuloplasty—repair of valve and suturing of torn leaflets
   - Closed commissurotomy (valvotomy dilation of valve; repair of leaflet or commissure, fibrous band or ring)
   - Annuloplasty—repair of ring or annulus of incompetent or diseased valve
   - Valve replacement.

CARDIAC SURGERY

Numerous diseases and conditions may create the need for cardiac surgery. The most common reason for an adult to undergo cardiac surgery is myocardial revascularization (CABG). In addition, patients undergo cardiac surgery for valve repair or replacement, repair of structural defects (acquired or congenital) implantation of devices and cardiac transplantation. The indication for cardiac surgery includes:

- Aneurysm of sinus of Valsalva
- Constrictive pericarditis
- Congenital heart defects
- Coronary artery disease
- Dissecting aortic aneurysm
- Valvular insufficiency or stenosis
- Ventricular aneurysm
- Ventricular septal defect
- Ventricular arrhythmias.

The indications for cardiac surgery and associated procedures are:

- Ischemic heart disease—coronary artery bypass graft (CABP), (Fig. 12.20)
- Repair of structural abnormalities
  - Valve repair
  - Atrial septal defect repair
  - Ventricular septal defect repair
  - Atrial tumor resection
  - Aortic aneurysm (thoracic) repair
- Implantation of devices
  - Automatic implantable cardioverter-defibrillator
  - Ventricular assist device
  - Heart chamber
- Transplantation—replacement of diseased heart with healthy heart.

Cardiac surgery is classified either as an open heart surgery or closed heart surgery, depending on whether the heart is "opened" during the course of the surgery. Cardiac surgery involving the repair of internal structural defects is open heart, whereas revascularization is a closed heart procedure.

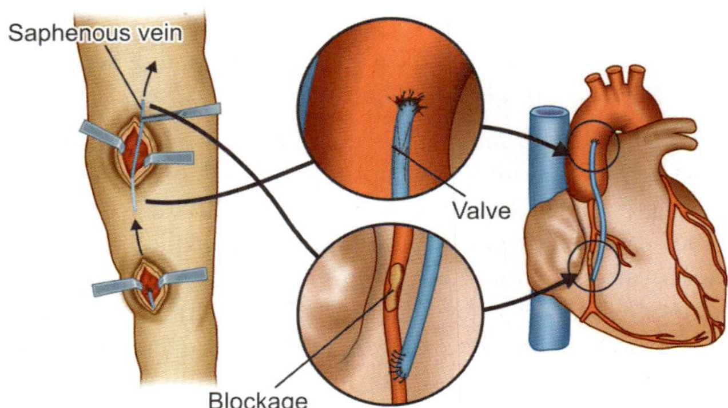

FIG. 12.20: Myocardial reperfusion by coronary artery bypass surgery

Cardiac surgery today provides pain relief, improvement in lifestyle, and improved survival and for the patient undergoing open heart surgical treatment.

Nursing Management

Care of the person undergoing cardiac surgery involves multidisciplinary team approach utilizing the skills of a variety of health care professionals including nurses, physicians, nutritionists and others.

The nurse caring for the cardiac surgery patient provides individualized care that is appropriate for the patient's medical condition, health history and psychosocial history. Important goals for the preoperative period include obtaining an accurate and complete patient history, providing preoperative teaching to the patient and family about the planned surgery and preparation of patients physiologically and psychologically for surgery. The nurse has to take active part in or collect information by required preoperative diagnostic test such as Chest X-ray, cardiac catheterization, coronary angiography, cardiography, stress testing and serum blood analysis as appropriate. A complete-baseline database is documented before surgery. Baseline vital signs including apical and radial heart rates and bilateral arm blood pressure integrity of all pulses (both proximal and distal), neurological status, height, weight, nutritional status, elimination pattern and psychological status are assessed and recorded in the immediate preoperational period. Before surgery, patient continues their normal medical and activity routines. With the exceptions of the withholding aspirin for 1 to 3 days before the day of surgery. Patients remain NPO after midnight before surgery.

Nurse has the main responsibility to perform preoperative teaching to patient undergoing cardiac surgery, which includes the following:

1. General information:
   - Places of care during hospitalization
     - CCU or ICU after surgery
     - Return to general patient care unit in 2 to 3 days
     - Visiting hours and location of waiting rooms.
2. Description of surgery:
   - Simple explanation of anatomy of heart and effect of the patient's cardiovascular disorder (e.g. incompetent valve, CAD)
   - Explanation of surgical procedure including planned incision
   - Definition of any unfamiliar terms: Bypass, extracorporeal
   - Length of time and surgery: 2 to 4 hours
   - Length of time until able to see family (1-1/2 to 2 hours after surgery).
3. Preparation for surgery:
   - Shower or bath at night before surgery with special antimicrobial soap
   - Surgical shave: Shaving the entire chest and abdomen, neck to groin and left mid-axillary line to right
   - Legs shaved in saphenous vein grafts will be used
   - Preoperative medication.
4. Explanation of monitors:
   - Round patches on chest connected to cardiac monitor that record patient's heart beats
   - Monitor makes beeping sound all the time.
5. Explanation of lines:
   - Intravenous routes for fluid and medications
   - Central venous line in neck or chest to monitor fluid status
   - Pulmonary artery catheter in chest or neck to measure pulmonary pressure and monitor fluid status
   - Plastic connector line to obtain blood samples without needle stick.
6. Explanation of drainage tube:
   - Indwelling urinary catheter
   - Chest tube: Bloody drainage expected.
7. Explanation of breathing tube:
   - Tube in windpipe connected to machine called ventilator
   - Unable to speak with tube in place but can mouth words and communicate in writing
   - Tube is removed when patient is awake and stable
   - Secretions in lungs or tube removed by nurse using a suction catheter
   - Food and oral fluids are not permitted until breathing tube is removed.
8. Explanation and demonstration of activities and exercises:
   - Purpose of activity is to promote circulation, keep lungs clear, and prevent infection
   - Activities include turning from side to side in bed; sitting on edge of bed. Sitting on chair at the night or morning after surgery
   - Range of motion exercises
   - Deep breathing using sustained maximal inspiration
   - Tubes and lines will restrict movement to a certain extent but nurse assists.
9. Relief of pain:
   - Some pain will be experienced, but it will not be excruciating
   - Frequent pain medication will be given to relieve pain but patient should inform always when there is pain.

And following guidelines for care of the person who has undergone cardiac surgery (also see Figure 12.21).

1. Monitoring of:
   i. Cardiovascular
      - Blood pressure and pulse (rate, pulse deficit)
      - Pulmonary artery pressure (PAP), pulmonary capillary wedge pressure (PCWD), cardiac output (CO), central venous pressure (CVP) and left atrial-pressure (LAP)
      - ECG for signs of arrhythmias
      - Body temperature
      - Skin color, temperature and capillary filling
      - Signs of hypovolemic shock (decreased CVP, decreased LAP and decreased CO)

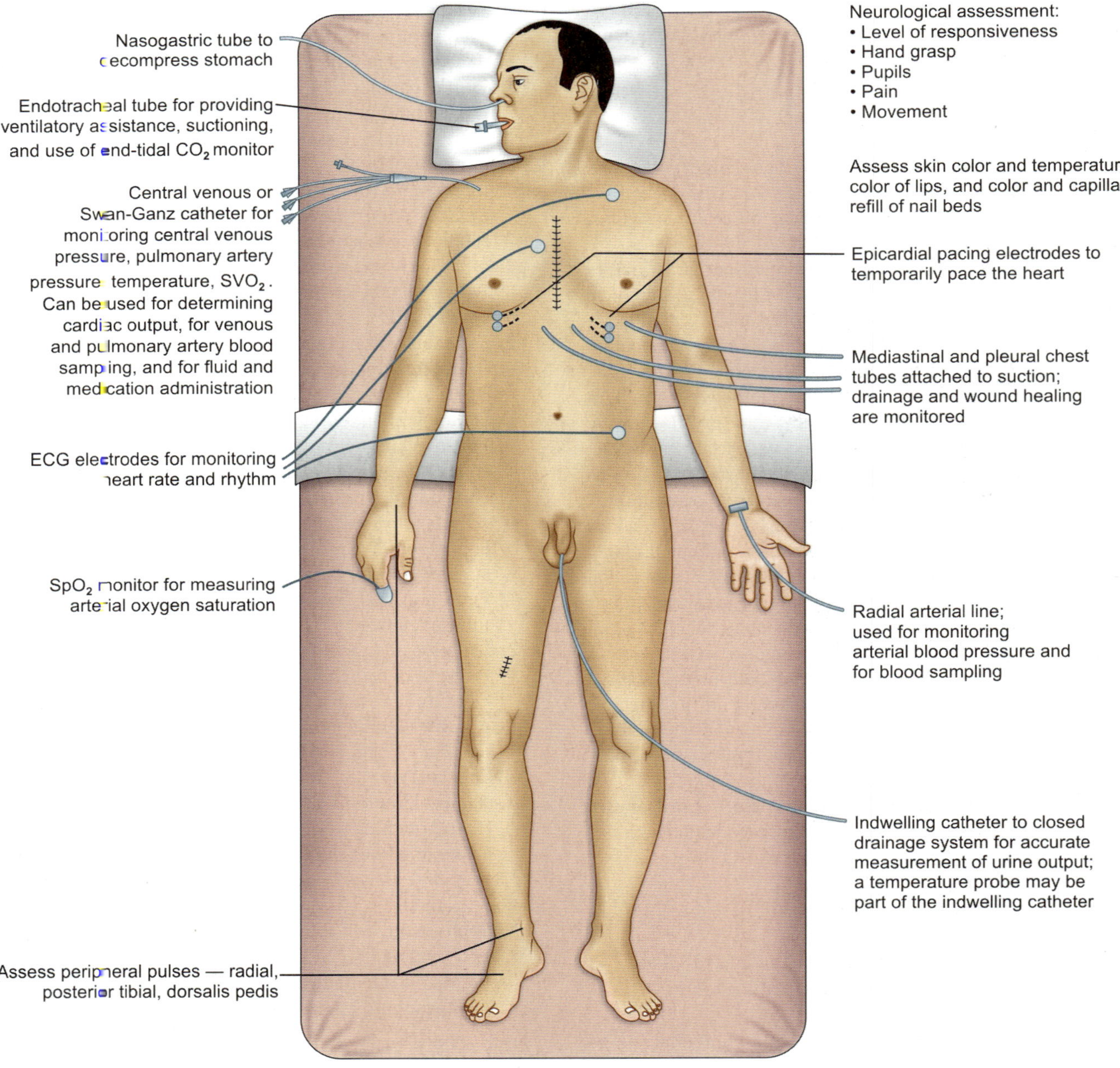

FIG. 12.21: Postoperative care of the cardiac surgical patient requires the nurse to be proficient in interpreting hemodynamics, correlating physical assessments with laboratory progress results, sequencing interventions and evaluating toward desired outcomes

- Signs of cardiac tamponade (cessation of chest drainage) restlessness, increased CVP, PAP and LAP, tachycardial paradoxical pulse, narrowed pulse pressure, diminished or absent point of maximal impulse, diminished heart sound, distended neck vein (CVP).

ii. Respiratory:
- Respirations—rate, depth, quality
- Breach sounds
- Chest tubes for patency and drainage
- Autotransfuse chest tube drainage.

iii. Neurological:
- Level of consciousness
- Pupillary size and reaction
- Orientation
- Movement and sensation of extremities.

iv. Gastrointestinal—nausea, anorexia.
v. Urinary output (amount)—color, pH and specific gravity.
vi. Fluid and electrolytes balance:
  - Intake/output balance
  - Daily weight
  - Serum potassium and calcium levels.
vii. Presence of discomfort-pain, fatigue.
viii. Ability to sleep.
ix. Behavior—repression, fear, disorientation and hallucinations.

2. Promoting oxygen/carbon dioxide exchange:
   - Preoxygenation and suction during intubation—suction as necessary after extubation
   - Position with head only slightly elevated; turn side to side
   - Encourage breathing exercises; incentive spirometry
   - Encourage range of motion exercises and progressive activity.
3. Promoting fluid and electrolytic balance:
   - Record accurate intake and output
   - Maintain prescribed flow rates of parenteral fluid
   - Give prescribed supplemental IV potassium chloride.
4. Promoting comfort:
   - Give narcotic analgesia every 3 hours during first 24 hours then as needed
   - Give frequent mouth care
   - Control environment for comfort
   - Change bed linens when diaphoresis presents (assure patient it is common)
   - Plan activities to permit periods of sleep
   - Provide backrubs for backache
   - Splint incision during coughing
   - Encourage patient to share feelings and experiences
   - Support family visits.
5. Promote activity:
   - Provide for passive than active range of motion exercises
   - Encourage ambulation when permitted.
6. Teaching:
   - Progressive return to physical activity as recommended by the physician
   - Rehabilitation exercise program
   - Sexual activity usually permitted in 3 to 4 weeks
   - Signs of overexertion include fatigue, dyspnea and pain
   - Eat a balanced diet with prescribed modifications (low Na^+, low fat)
   - Medications:
     Name, dosage, schedule action and side effects of prescribed drugs use prescribed education as needed
   - Signs that may persist—dyspnea, pain and night sweats
   - Signs requiring medical attention fever, increasing dyspnea or chest pain with minimal exertion
   - Need for ongoing medical care.

The nurse has to provide discharge instruction for the patient who undergoes cardiac surgery includes:

1. Incision care:
   - Clean twice a day
   - Care of sterile strips staples, sutures
   - Incision massage with cocoa butter after 10 days.
2. Showering:
   - Wash with soap that is unscented, gentle, bactericidal
   - No tube bath until incision is completely healed.
3. Activity:
   - No lifting greater than 10 pounds
   - No driving for 6 weeks
   - No prolonged sitting
   - Activity as tolerated, cardiac rehabilitation if ordered
   - May resume sexual activity when comfort level allows.
4. Nutrition:
   - Low sodium, low-fat and heart-healthy diet
   - Increase protein intake for 4 to 6 weeks.
5. Medications:
   - Pain medications, do not drive or operate machine if taking narcotics.
6. Miscellaneous:
   - Women should wear a bra to help support chest TED stockings
   - Daily weights—notify physician for gain of 6 pounds in 2 days
   - Incentive spirometer three times a day
   - Prevent constipation with fiber, fluids and stool softeners
   - Instruct any adverse symptoms should be reported to physician concerned.

(See also Tables 12.8 and 12.9; Nursing care plan for post-operative care of cardiac surgical patients).

TABLE 12.8: Nursing care plan for preoperative care of the cardiac surgical patient

Problems	Objective	Nursing interventions	Rationales
Nursing Diagnosis #1			
Anxiety, related to: 1. Opening cardiac surgery	The patient will demonstrate decreased anxiety by indicating willingness to discuss the following:	• Teach the patient about the normal function of the heart; underlying disease process including risk factors; the surgical procedure; and the expected outcomes of the surgery	• Teaching provides a basic understanding of the problem, the solution, and what to exepect, thereby decreasing the patient's anxiety. However, not all patients experience a decreased level of anxiety when bombarded with new informations

Contd...

Contd...

Problems	Objective	Nursing interventions	Rationales
	1. Normal function of the heart 2. Disease process, including: a. Risk factors b. Surgical procedure c. Expected outcomes of the surgery	• Use simple terms or explain medical terms used • Utilize posters, models, and handouts/pamphlets • Teach in short blocks if time allows • Observe patient's nonverbal cues • Allow time for questions • Answer questions honestly • Maintain a calm, relaxed, nonrushed atmosphere with little or no interruptions • Have the patient discuss the information in his/her own words • Correct any misconceptions	• Using simple terms or explaining medical terms enhances learning because the patient can understand the explanations. Using medical terms sometimes confuses and overwhelms the patient • Visualization aids learning • Allows assimilation of information before more is added, and thus enhances learning • Enables the nurse to evaluate patient's understanding and anxiety level. The nurse can determine whether to proceed, reiterate, or stop • Relieves anxiety, clarifies information, and prevents misconceptions • Establishes a trusting relationship and attains patient cooperation • Enhances the learning experience • Assists in evaluating what has been learned • Patient knows what to expect, thereby reducing some of his/her anxiety
Nursing Diagnosis #2			
Knowledge deficit regarding preoperative and postoperative expectations	Patient will verbalize an understanding of the preoperative routine: 1. Tests, procedures 2. Medications 3. The night before the surgery 4. The day of the surgery 5. The immediate postoperative care	• Provide information regarding the following: – Tests and procedures that will be performed before surgery – Blood studies: CBC, serum electrolytes, BUN, creatinine, cardiac enzymes, clotting time, prothrombin time, fibrinogen levels, platelets, type and cross-match of blood, arterial blood gases – ECG – Chest X-ray – Urine analysis – Pulmonary function tests (PFTs) – Changes in medication regimen and necessary preoperative medication – Sedation the evening before/prior to surgery – All aspirin, anticoagulants, and anti-inflammatory drugs should be discontinued at least 2 days prior to surgery – Digitalis is usually held 1–2 days prior to the surgery unless the patient is in uncontrolled atrial fibrillation – Propranolol is tapered 24 hours–2 weeks prior to surgery – Diuretics are discontinued 24–48 hours prior to the surgery if congestive heart failure is controlled – Nitroglycerin is kept at the bedside and can be taken for chest pain (as per protocol)	– This is a time when the patient needs and wants to be with family but is frequently interrupted, causing frustration and sometimes anger. Knowing about these studies ahead of time will help in coping with the interruptions – To evaluate baseline values. If any abnormal values are present, treatment can be initiated so as to prevent complications intraoperatively and postoperatively. Patient is typed/cross-matched to ensure, blood is available if needed – Provides a baseline for comparison – To examine for abnormalities; provides a baseline for comparison – To evaluate for signs of infection – To evaluate patient's pulmonary status – Changes in medication regimen can cause anxiety. Understanding of what the changes will help decrease anxiety and enhance patient cooperation – Decreases anxiety, allows a good night's sleep – Prevents bleeding due to altered coagulation studies

Contd...

Contd...

Problems	Objective	Nursing interventions	Rationales
		– Long-acting insulin is changed to regular insulin and patient is placed on a sliding-scale coverage 24 hours prior to the surgery – Potassium supplements are given to maintain the patient's potassium level at 4.0 mEq/L – Norpace may be discontinued 24 hours prior to the surgery – Antidysrhythmics are maintained to control the dysrhythmias – Antihypertensive medications are maintained – Prophylactic antibiotics are given prior to the surgery and continued for 2 days postoperatively – Check the patient for allergies to any medications, especially antibiotics, iodine preparations, or fish • The night before the surgery, the patient will: – Receive a light dinner, then nothing to eat or drink after midnight – Be shaved from the chin to the toes (CABG) or chin to shins (valve replacement) – Shower with an antibacterial agent (i.e., Betadine) • The morning of the surgery, the patient will: – Shower again with the antibacterial agent – Put on a hospital gown – Receive a preoperative sedative – Receive family for a brief visit (according to hospital policy) – Give valuables to the family to take home – Be transferred to a stretcher and transported to the OR • Explain the immediate postoperative care: Inform the patient of the ICU routine: – Patients remain in the ICU for 2–3 days if no complications occur – The unit may be noisy and the lights left on – Patients are checked frequently for vital signs and assessments – Visiting hours are restricted to brief periods – A tour of the unit is offered to those who want it. Patient may be able to meet the nurse who will be taking care of her/him in the ICU • Explain expectations of postoperative period (e.g. equipment/routines). Patient will:	– Digitalis toxicity is a common complication postoperatively, related to low potassium levels. If given to control atrial fibrillation, the patient must be monitored closely for signs of toxicity postoperatively, especially in the immediate postoperative phase – Negative chronotropic and inotropic action postoperatively further decreases the cardiac output. If needed early in the postoperative period, dopamine, epinephrine, isoproterenol, and/or glucagon can be given – Diuretics increase the loss of fluids and potassium, which could cause adverse reactions postoperatively (i.e. hypovolemia, acidemia, hyponatremia, digoxin toxicity) – Relieves chest pain associated with anxiety – Insulin requirements change due to the stress of the surgery and NPO status. Administration of insulin on a sliding scale provides a more precise dosage to meet the patient's needs, thereby preventing hyperglycemia/hypoglycemia – To prevent intraoperative and postoperative complications (i.e. acidemia, digoxin toxicity, dysrhythmias) – Norpace may cause heart failure in the postoperative phase – Prevent further decrease in the cardiac output related to the dysrhythmias; help to prevent serious or life-threatening dysrhythmias – Maintain the patient's blood pressure. Nitroprusside (Nipride) can be given intraoperatively – Prevents infection – Prevents anaphylaxis – Prevents aspiration of the stomach contents – Decreases the possibility of infection since skin and hair harbor bacteria – Decreases the possibility of infection by decreasing the bacteria on the skin – Decreases anxiety and helps the patient to relax

Contd...

Contd...

Problems	Objective	Nursing interventions	Rationales
		– Have an endotracheal tube connected to a ventilator that will help with breathing – Be unable to talk – Experience breathlessness when suctioned • The patient will: – Have a Foley catheter postoperatively – Have peripheral, jugular, and subclavian IVs – Have an arterial line for approximately 1 day – Be connected to a cardiac monitor – Have a rectal temperature probe in place postoperatively until temperature stabilizes (usually 8 hours) – Have chest tubes in place for approximately 2 days • Explain the various suture lines – Advise that postoperatively Ace bandages or elastic stockings are applied	– Allays anxiety of patient and family – There is little room in the ICU for the patient's personal effects. Family will be told what to bring in when it is needed • Knowing what to expect decreases the patient's anxiety and enhances cooperation – The patient should understand that frequent assessments are part of usual ICU protocols. It does not mean that anything is wrong – Awareness of the unit's environment will decrease the anxiety level for some patients. The patient will not become alarmed in response to the noise, frequency of vital signs, and absence of family except during brief visits • Knowledge regarding expectations of care enables the patient to be cooperative and participate in care (e.g. not trying to pull the tubes out, fighting procedures, afraid of moving). The patient needs to know that needs will be anticipated and a method of communication worked out. This serves to reduce anxiety – The endotracheal tube is usually left in place for 8–24 hours – An alternate means of communication should be set up (i.e. mouthing words, finger writing, sign language) – The patient should know that the feeling of breathlessness, should it occur, will last only for a few seconds – The patient should be encouraged to breathe with the ventilator and not to "fight" the ventilator – Allows for an accurate measurement of urine output – Access for emergency medications, fluids, blood and blood products, and plasma expanders as needed. Once stabilized postoperatively, all but one will be discontinued while in the ICU – Access for arterial blood gases and other blood specimens. Allows for continuous monitoring of arterial blood pressure – To monitor heart rhythm and rate

Contd...

Contd...

Problems	Objective	Nursing interventions	Rationales
			– Allows frequent monitoring of the patient's temperature. In the absence of a temperature probe, rectal temperatures can be taken hourly until stabilized – Allows evaluation of bleeding in the chest, which may indicate improper closure of a graft, cardiac tamponade, or coagulation abnormality – The drainage will be bloody initially and then gradually become serous • Patient will have a midline chest incision (medial sternotomy) that will be dressed initially. The dressing is usually removed 24 hours postoperatively. Patient may have some chest discomfort related to the sternum being opened; this pain differs from the chest pain experienced previously. Pain medication will be available • Patient will have an incision in one or both legs. It may extend from the thigh to the knee, the thigh to the ankle, or the knee to the ankle, depending on the amount of graft needed, the surgeon's preference, and the condition of the vein *Note*: When a mammary artery is used as bypass graft, incisions in lower extremities are unnecessary: – Ace bandages/elastic stockings aid in the venous return from the legs; they are also used to prevent thrombi
	Patient will demonstrate activities expected to be performed in the postoperative period: 1. Coughing and deep breathing 2. Splinting the chest incision 3. Use of the incentive spirometer 4. Arm and leg exercises 5. Turning side to side 6. Getting out of bed the day after the surgery	• Demonstrate, and have the patient return the demonstration, activities to be performed postoperatively: – Coughing and deep breathing: Take 4–5 deep breaths, then cough – Pain medication will be given prior to the exercises (as indicated) – Splinting the chest incision – Arm exercises—range of motion and walking up the wall – Leg exercises—ankle range of motion, "ankle pump," and dorsiflexion – Turning side to side every 2 hours – Getting out of bed—splint chest – Inch legs over the side of the bed. Sit up straight on the edge of the bed, then ease the feet down to the floor. Nurses will be present for support and guidance of tubings	• Enhances cooperation in the postoperative activities needed to prevent complications. Ensures that the patient knows what must be done, why, and how it is to be done – Prevent atelectasis and pneumonia – Deep breaths loosen the secretions so they can be mobilized – Decreases the amount of pain so the exercises can be done effectively – Decreases the amount of pain – Prevent frozen shoulder – Increase circulation in the lower extremities and prevent stasis and thrombosis. Range of motion also prevents foot drop – Early ambulation helps prevent many complications, especially pneumonia and thrombosis. It is not as simple a task postoperatively as patients may believe

TABLE 12.9: Nursing care plan for early postoperative care of the cardiac surgical patient

Problems	Objective	Nursing interventions	Rationales
Nursing Diagnosis #1			
Cardiac output, alteration in: Decreased, patient in: 1. Cardiopulmonary bypass 2. Low cardiac output syndrome	Patient will demonstrate stabilization of body functions monitoring and life-supportive systems: 1. Arterial blood pressure within 10 mm Hg of patient's baseline. 2. Stable pulmonary artery pressures: – PAP < 25 mm Hg – PCWP 8-12 mm Hg – CVP 0-8 mm Hg 3. Cardiac output ~5 liters/ minute. – Heart rate > 60 < 100 beats/minute 4. Urine output > 30 mL/hour 5. Alert mental status; oriented to person, place, time 6. Electrolyte balance 7. Acid-base balance: – pH 7.35-7.45 – PaO_2 > 80 mm Hg – $PaCO_2$ 35–45 mm Hg 8. Stable hematology profile: – Hct—male, 45–52%; female, 37–48% – Hgb—male, 13–18 g/100 mL; female, 12–16 g/100 mL – Platelet count: – 150,000–350,000/mm^3	• Monitor vital signs (BP, heart rate, respiratory rate, and temperature) q 5 minutes within limits stable, then q 1 h × 12 • Assess the patient q 1 h until stable, including heart sounds; ECG changes; cardiac rhythm; neck veins; lung sounds; peripheral pulses; capillary refill; skin turgor, color and temperature; movement and sensation • Monitor hemodynamic parameters: Mean arterial pressure (MAP), pulmonary artery pressure (PAP), pulmonary capillary wedge pressure (PCWP), central venous pressure (CVP), or right atrial pressure (RAP), and left atrial pressure (LAP) • Assess the pacemaker concerning type (fixed or demand), the rate it is set at, the milliamperes (mA), and whether it is functioning properly. (Pacing wires are commonly used in valve replacement surgery) – Keep exposed wires wrapped in gauze and place in a plastic covering • Report any abnormalities in vital parameters to physician immediately: – BP: Systolic < 80, > 180 Diastolic > 100 – MAP: < 60, > 100 – CVP: < 5, > 15 – Heart rate: < 60, > 100 – Temperature: Remains hypothermic or rises above 101°F – Excessive or bloody chest tube drainage > 100 mL/h – Urine output < 30 mL/h – Extremities: Cool, moist, mottled, with sluggish capillary refill and poor or absent peripheral pulses – A decrease in movement or sensation – Presence of anginal pain or ECG changes: ST segment elevation or depression; T wave peaked/inverted	• Frequent monitoring of the vital signs allows early detection of abnormalities, and treatment for provable complications • Changes may indicate hemodynamic decompensation or complications. Signs of low cardiac output syndrome include a decrease in arterial pressure, urine output below 30 mL/h, signs of vasoconstriction cool, pale, or cyanotic skin and mucous membranes, tachycardia, dysrhythmias, tachypnea, narrow pulse pressure, weak peripheral pulses, decrease in level of consciousness, restlessness • Parameters will reflect left ventricular function, fluid status, and arterial perfusion • Need to be familiar with equipment in order to use it properly, identify if it is functioning properly, and how to trouble-shoot problems. Pacemaker is usually kept on standby to keep the patient's heart rate above 60 beats/minute and to treat other dysrhythmias – Prevents the possibility of electrical shock or short circuit • Immediate intervention can be ordered to prevent further deterioration/complications: – Pressures below 80 mm Hg could cause graft closure or indicate shock; pressures above 180 mm Hg could cause the graft to "blow," or could cause a CVA – CVP readings below 5 cm H_2O indicate inadequate intravascular fluid; readings above 15 cm H_2O indicate fluid overload – Heart rates below 60 could cause graft closure; rates above 100 will decrease the oxygenation to the myocardium and increase the workload of the heart – Hypothermia prolongs vasoconstriction, adding to low cardiac output syndrome. Temperatures above 101°F may indicate infection – Excessive and/or bloody drainage suggests bleeding at surgical site – Reduced urine output warns of prerenal failure

Contd...

Contd...

Problems	Objective	Nursing interventions	Rationales
			– Signs of decreased peripheral perfusion related to emboli or decreased cardiac output. If accompanied by pain, arterial occlusion of the extremity may have occurred – May indicate possible neurologic involvement or may be due to the effect of the anesthesia – Indicative of myocardial ischemia
Nursing Diagnosis #2			
Breathing pattern, ineffective, related to: 1. General anesthesia 2. Incisional pain with splinting	The patient will maintain: 1. A patent airway 2. Respiratory rate <25–30/ minute; eupneic rhythm 3. ABGs within normal range: – pH 7.35–7.45 – PaO_2 > 80 mm Hg – $PaCO_2$ 35–45 mm Hg – HCO_3 22–26 mEq/L	• Assess respiratory function: Rate, rhythm, pattern, chest excursion, use of accessory muscles; breath sounds; presence of adventitious sounds • Maintain patient on ventilator at prescribed settings – Check the endotracheal cuff for adequate inflation • Administer pain medications to decrease pain and prevent "fighting" the ventilator • Suction prn. Sigh the patient before and after suctioning. (Sigh is a deeper than normal breath with 100 per cent oxygen) – Use hand resuscitator to ventilate and preoxygenate prior to and following each suction pass (some mechanical ventilators have "sigh" capability.) • Monitor ABGs q 1–4 h as the patient's condition warrants; or continuously monitor mixed venous gases (SvO_2) as prescribed • Wean patient off the ventilator as prescribed, when alert, breathing spontaneously, and demonstrating adequate ABGs and appropriate ventilatory parameters (i.e. inspiratory pressure, expiratory pressure, tidal volume, minute volume, and vital capacity) • Administer oxygen through a heated humidified face mask or tent after weaning • Encourage patient to cough and deep breathe hourly; administer chest percussion; encourage the use of the incentive spirometer q 1–2 h while awake – Have respiratory therapist administer IPPB and nebulizer treatments as ordered • Assess breath sounds q 2 h and/or when indicated • Notify the physician of any significant abnormalities in respiratory parameters	• It is essential to establish baseline function with which to compare subsequent findings; assists in following trends • Maintains patient's respirations when the respiratory center is depressed due to the anesthesia and narcotics. Provides adequate oxygenation. Decreases the work-load of the heart – Improper cuff inflation reduces tidal volume and may compromise ventilation • Pain and "fighting" the ventilator can lead to hyperventilation, which may predispose to respiratory alkalosis. Acid-base imbalances can cause dysrhythmias – Tachycardia related to pain can increase workload of the heart • Remove secretions for adequate oxygenation and gas exchange. Sighing the patient before and after expands the alveoli, mobilizes the secretions, and prevents drastic drops in the patient's oxygen levels • Respiratory and metabolic alterations are reflected in the ABGs. Adjustment in the ventilator settings or pharmacologic interventions can be initiated to prevent severe imbalances • The patient must be able to breathe spontaneously with adequate respiratory excursion, tidal volume, minute ventilation, and peak inspiratory pressure • Provides oxygenation with humidification to assist in thinning the secretions and thereby facilitating deep breathing and coughing • Loosens and mobilizes the secretions, thereby preventing atelectasis and pneumonia. Incentive spirometer provides patients with a visual feedback as to how well they are breathing

Contd...

Contd...

Problems	Objective	Nursing interventions	Rationales
			• Decreased breath sounds may indicate atelectasis, pneumonia, or poor breathing technique due to splinting. Absence of breath sounds on one side suggests atelectasis or malpositioning of the endotracheal tube. Endotracheal tube may have slipped down into right bronchus Pneumothorax, if present, is usually accompanied by unequal chest excursion and shifting of trachea to opposite side • Interventions may be taken expeditiously to prevent complications
Nursing Diagnosis #3			
Fluid volume deficit, actual and potential, related to: 1. Surgery-related blood loss or hemorrhage 2. NPO status 3. Peripheral vasodilation associated with rewarming (dis proportion between size of vascular bed and intravascular blood volume)	Patient will: 1. Maintain stable hemodynamic parameters: – BP, pulses, CVP, PAP, PCWP (see Nursing Diagnosis #1, above) 2. Demonstrate adequate peripheral perfusion; peripheral pulses 2+ bilaterally; brisk capillary refill; skin warm, no cyanosis of nail beds or mucous membranes 3. Be alert and oriented 4. Maintain urinary output above 30 mL/ hour with no hematuria 5. Show no sign of hemorrhage (stable vital signs) 6. Maintain a hematocrit above 30%	• Monitor vital signs q 15 minutes while the patient is rewarming • Administer fluids as ordered. (Usually less than 100 mL/h total volume unless the patient is hypovolemic) • Monitor the patient's intake and output carefully. Weigh daily • Monitor urine output q 1 h; specific gravity q 2 h • Monitor BUN and creatinine • Assess skin turgor and mucous membranes for hydration status • Monitor hemodynamic parameters especially when rehydrating the patient • Monitor serum electrolytes and hemoglobin and hematocrit (Hgb and Hct). Administer potassium to maintain level within 3.5–5.5 mEq/liter • Monitor amount and color of chest tube drainage – Observe the dressings and bedding for signs of hemorrhage • Monitor coagulation studies • Administer blood, plasma expanders, and clotting factors as prescribed	• The vascular bed increases during rewarming, causing a disproportion in the vascular volume and the vascular bed size. If the disproportion is great enough the patient will become hypotensive, predisposing to shock. Under these circumstances, there is a risk that the grafts may close off. In response to the hypotension the patient may develop myocardial ischemia with dysrhythmias, prerenal failure, or DIC • Adequate fluids are necessary to prevent hypovolemia; overhydration can cause the patient to develop pulmonary edema • Patient may be retaining fluid if fluid intake is greater than output plus the insensible losses. Daily weighing is a reliable indicator of hydration status (2.2 1b is equal to 1 liter of fluid) • Urine output less than 30 mL/h may, indicate decreased cardiac output, hypovolemia, or renal failure. A decrease in specific gravity indicates hypovolemia • The BUN is an indicator of renal function and fluid status, the creatinine is an indicator of renal function. The physician should be notified of an increase in either, or of any change in BUN/creatinine ratio • Tenting of the skin when pinched indicates dehydration. Edema indicates fluid excess or decreased cardiac output. Dry mucous membranes indicate dehydration; moist mucous membranes indicate adequate hydration

Contd...

Contd...

Problems	Objective	Nursing interventions	Rationales
			• PAP, LAP, and CVP will be decreased in volume depletion. As fluids are administered the pressures also will increase. Pressures will be elevated in fluid overload • Low Hgb and Hct are indicative of blood loss or hemodilution; an elevated Hct is indicative of hemoconcentration • Elevation of potassium may be related to renal failure, cardiopulmonary bypass, or acid-base imbalance. Abnormal potassium levels can cause dysrhythmias • Chest tube drainage greater than 100 mL/h for the first 4 hours is indicative of abnormal bleeding, which could be related to platelet destruction, inadequate reversal of the heparin, inadequate suturing of arteries during the surgery, or diffuse intrathoracic ooze – Bleeding may occur at the suture line. Excessive bleeding may ooze down the patient's side and pool under him • Abnormal coagulation caused by anticoagulants or DIC can cause hemorrhage related to oozing at injection sites, suture lines, insertion sites of IVs • Blood and plasma expanders are given to maintain the intravascular volume. Fresh frozen plasma and cryoprecipitate may be administered to bolster concentration of clotting factors to ensure appropriate blood coagulation and prevent hemorrhaging
Nursing Diagnosis #4			
Tissue perfusion, alteration in peripheral, related to: 1. Low cardiac output syndrome	Patient will: 1. Demonstrate normotension (MAP within 10 mm Hg of patient's baseline) 2. Demonstrate normothermia (98.6°F, 37.0°C) 3. Maintain palpable peripheral pulses and brisk capillary refill 4. Exhibit warm, dry skin, pink in color with good turgor 5. Maintain heart rate >60, <100 6. Maintain urine output > 30 mL/h	• Assess peripheral pulses. Compare right with left. Note characteristics: Rate, rhythm, quality (bounding, weak, and thready), and equality – Mark sites of pulses if difficult to palpate • Assess the skin for temperature, color, capillary refill, breakdown, and sensation • Have patient perform leg and arm exercises as taught in the preoperative phase • Apply elastic stockings or Ace bandages to lower extremities as prescribed – Check size of elastic stockings and apply properly; check pulses q 4 h, administer skin care. Remove stockings once each shift	• Peripheral pulses are indicators of the arterial flow through the extremity. An absence or decrease in the pulse may indicate occlusion of the vessel due to emboli – Marking the sites makes it easier to find the pulse, especially if the pulse is weak • Indicators of peripheral perfusion. A decrease may be indicative of poor perfusion • Exercises increase circulation • Properly applied elastic stockings and Ace bandages assist in venous return, reducing risk of venous stasis • Signs of thrombophlebitis

Contd...

Contd...

Problems	Objective	Nursing interventions	Rationales
		• Assess the patient for calf tenderness, swelling, and a positive Homan's sign • Measure girth of calves and thighs bilaterally • Do not gatch the bed or use pillows under the knee. Discourage the patient from crossing knees and/or ankles	• Often the means of detecting that a deep venous thrombosis is present is by monitoring the circumference • Applies pressure under the knee, thereby decreasing circulation to the lower leg
Nursing Diagnosis #5			
Tissue perfusion, alteration in cerebral, related to: 1. Anesthesia 2. Cardiopulmonary bypass 3. Narcotics 4. Postcardiotomy delirium (PCD)	Patient will: 1. Demonstrate an intact, direct, and consensual pupillary light reflex bilaterally 2. Demonstrate an intact gag reflex 3. Be alert and oriented to person, place, and time 4. Follow commands/ behavior appropriately 5. Speak clearly and understandably 6. Demonstrate movement in all extremities equal to preoperative state	• Assess neurologic status at least every 2–4 h, or when indicated: Pupils—size and equality, reaction to light; level of consciousness; orientation; speech, obeys commands; movement of all extremities • Assess the patient's behavior every shift. Orient to person, place, and time. Provide frequent explanations. Allow family to visit. Reinforce normality of the disorientation (if no other signs of neurologic deficit are present)	• Abnormal neurologic findings may be indicative of permanent or temporary alterations related to the anesthesia, intraoperative stroke, cardiopulmonary bypass machine, hypothermia, decreased cardiac output. Abnormal findings may occur in the immediate postoperative phase but they should gradually return to baseline within the initial 4–8 hours postoperatively • Confusion and disorientation may be indicative of postcardiotomy delirium (PCD).Frequent explanations, reorientation, and visits from family help the patient cope with PCD. Postcardiotomy delirium is associated with cardiopulmonary bypass and is manifested in some patients post-bypass by changes in behavior, confusion, and frank psychosis
Nursing Diagnosis #6			
Infection, potential for, related to: 1. Interruption in integrity of skin barrier (surgical incision) 2. Invasive monitoring 3. Chest tubes, Foley catheter	The patient will remain infection free: 1. Temperature at base-line (98.6°F, 37.0°C) 2. WBC at baseline 3. Incisional area clean, dry, and healing	• Assess incision, IV sites, intravascular lines for signs of infection (warmth, redness, swelling) • Change IV lines and hemodynamic lines per hospital protocol. Maintain sterility of the lines • Change dressings daily or according to hospital protocol • Administer antibiotics as prescribed • Culture any draining wound • Assess breath sounds and appearance of sputum • Maintain the Foley catheter as a closed system. Discontinue as soon as possible • Assess the patient for signs of systemic infection (sepsis): Change in behavior, hyperthermia/hypothermia, chills, diaphoresis • Practice good hand washing technique	• The skin is the first line of defense against infection. Any break in the skin's integrity is prone to infection • These are access sites through which bacteria enter • Dressing changes permit visualization of the surgical site. Redness, warmth, and swelling suggest infection • Timely and accurate administration of antibiotics helps to maintain therapeutic blood levels • Detection of the causative organism is necessary so that appropriate antibiotic therapy can be prescribed • Presence of adventitious sounds and sputum production can signal possible onset of pneumonia • Foley catheters are a common source of infection and can lead to gram-negative sepsis • The first sign of sepsis is a change in behavior. Timely and aggressive intervention is necessary to prevent septic shock and multisystem organ dysfunction • Good hand washing technique is the main way to prevent inspection or its spread

Contd...

Contd...

Problems	Objective	Nursing interventions	Rationales
Nursing Diagnosis #7			
Anxiety, related to: 1. Outcome of surgery 2. Recuperative period 3. Lack of sleep/rest 4. Noisy ICU environment	Patient will verbalize: 1. Feelingless anxious 2. Ability to rest and to sleep 3. Progress made in recuperation 4. Willingness to cooperate in care 5. Desire to make decisions concerning care	• Familiarize with ICU environment: Equipment, procedures, and protocols • Explain condition and treatments. Stress the patient's progress • Administer pain medication as needed. Withhold if the patient is hypotensive, is being weaned off the ventilator, or has neurologic changes • Provide rest periods. Administer sedatives/ pain medication to enhance sleep at night • Allow the patient to take an active part in care; allow patient to make decisions concerning care • Allow the family to visit as much as possible according to unit/hispital policy	• Appropriate explanation decreases anxiety • Reassures the patient. Gives positive reinforcement • Decreasing the pain will decrease the patient's anxiety by breaking the pain-fear-anxiety triangle. Narcotics are not given if they will interfere with assessment or stabilization of the patient • Sleep and rest deprivation causes irritability, which increases anxiety • Decision-making and active participation in care give positive feedback to the patient that he/she is making progress, as well as giving the patient a sense of self-worth • The family is a support system that the patient depends on. Family interaction helps prevent social isolation and gives the patient a sense of being needed

TABLE 12.10: Nursing care plan for early postoperative care of the cardiac surgical patient

Problems	Objective	Nursing interventions	Rationales
Nursing Diagnosis #1			
Alteration in cardiac output, related to pacer malfunction, dysrhythmias	1. Patient will demonstrate clinical behaviors consistent with an adequate cardiac output: – Alert and oriented to person, place and time – Systolic blood pressure greater than 90 mm Hg – Lungs clear to auscultation – Capillary refill less than 2 sec – Urine output greater than 30 mL/hour – Lack of subjective complaints verbalized prior to the pacer insertion (i.e., dizziness, fatigue) – Strong peripheral pulses – Absence of jugular venous distention 2. Patient will not demonstrate pacer malfunction as evidenced by ECG analysis	• Monitor the pacemaker parameters every shift and document: – Sensing ability – Capture frequency – Threshold (check level every day) – Current setting – Mode • Perform comprehensive cardiovascular assessment at least once per shift Include: – Heart rate, rhythm – Quality of peripheral pulses – Heart sounds – Color, temperature of skin – Presence of pulsus paradoxus (a drop of the systolic blood pressure more than the normal 10 mm Hg during inspiration) ◆ Blood pressure ◆ Quantity of urine output ◆ Presence of JVD ◆ Subjective comments ◆ Level of consciousness ◆ ECG strip interpretation • Check pacemaker system every shift including: – Integrity of lead connections – Battery	• Failure of the pacemaker in any one of these functions can jeopardize patient safety – Documentation provides base-line data from which trends in condition can be detected • Baseline assessment will provide data from which comparisons can be made – Development of additional heart sounds may reflect decreased myocardial compliance or incompetence of valves – Decreased or muffled heart sounds, jugular venous distention, and the presence of pulsus paradoxus may reflect tamponade ◆ Quality of pulses, urine output, temperature, color of skin reflect tissue perfusion ◆ Jugular venous distention reflects elevation of right sided heart pressures, which can be associated with tamponade ◆ First symptom of decreased cardiac output may be a change in mentation

Contd...

Contd...

Problems	Objective	Nursing interventions	Rationales
	3. Patient will be free of hemodynamically significant dysrhythmias	– Pacer generator – Pacer settings • Monitor patient for presence of dysrhythmias and document type, patient's response, any associated activity, pacer activity (i.e. inability to sense) • Notify physician at onset of any dysrhythmias. Keep lidocaine at bedside. Ensure patent IV line is present	• Pacemaker function may be closely assessed through strip analysis – Ensure all components of system are functioning appropriately • Dysrhythmias may or may not be hemodynamically significant or related to pacer activity. The pacemaker may need to be adjusted • Physician may want to reposition pacing wire or initiate antiarrhythmic therapy
Nursing Diagnosis #2			
Potential for injury from microshock	1. Patient's environment will be free of microshock hazards 2. Patient will not receive microshock	• Cover any exposed lead wires with rubber gloves, finger cots, or scotch tape • Wear rubber gloves if handling exposed wires • Use only properly-grounded equipment, including the electric bed • Inspect all electric equipment in room for signs of cord fraying • Do not touch patient while handling electrical equipment	• Insulating the lead wires will decrease the risk of conduction • Improperly grounded equipment poses serious threat to patient safety • It is possible for energy to travel through you from the equipment to the patient
Nursing Diagnosis #3			
Anxiety, related to invasive procedure, "heart failure"	1. Patient will demonstrate decreased anxiety as evidenced by: – Subjective comments – Decreased restlessness – Facial expressions – Nonverbal behavior – Ability to concentrate	• Assess patient's understanding of situation, reasons for anxiety • Provide information in supportive manner • Assess patient's understanding of information provided – Observe patient's response • Assess past coping – Establish calm, quiet environment • Provide sedation if needed	• Pattern interventions to patient's level of comprehension • Establishing calm rapport will reassure patient • Patient's level of anxiety may prevent integration of information • Assessing past coping skills will help you develop a more effective plan of care • Sedation may be appropriate if nonpharmacologic interventions are ineffective
Nursing Diagnosis #4			
Knowledge deficit, related to need for pacemaker, procedure for insertion	1. Patient/family will verbalize understanding of: – Need for pacemaker – How pacemaker is helping the heart – Procedure for insertion	• Assess patient/family's level of knowledge with pacemakers • Establish teaching plan, including: – Need for pacemaker – How the pacemaker will help – How long the procedure will take – Sensations of events expected during insertion – Post insertion events • Provide only necessary information • Encourage questions	• Assessing prior level of knowledge will help in developing a more effective teaching plan – Including family will help their understanding of events • Clarification of questions improves understanding
Nursing Diagnosis #5			
Potential for infection: Invasive line placement	1. Patient will be infection-free, as evidenced by: – Normal temperature – Lack of redness, heat, swelling, discharge at insertion site	• Monitor insertion site every day and document findings • Monitor patient's temperature every 8 hours; every 4 hours if an elevation is noted	• Signs/symptoms of infection often begin at local level • Temperature elevation is a clinical sign of the immune system's activity in combating pyrogens

Contd...

Contd...

Problems	Objective	Nursing interventions	Rationales
		• Change dressing using sterile procedure every 24 hours or per unit protocol • Change IV solution every 24 hours if a central line is present – Culture any drainage from site, and notify the physician • Culture all catheter tips if spike in temperature is noted (i.e. central line, pacing catheter) • Do not administer antipyretics for pain	• Frequent sterile dressing changes can prevent infections by providing an aseptic barrier once the skin integrity has become impaired • Changes in IV solution will decrease medium for bacterial growth • Identification of organism involved in the infectious process is vital for determining course of treatment • Antipyretics may mask temperature elevation and signs of infection
Nursing Diagnosis #6			
Alteration in comfort, related to invasive line insertion	1. Patient will verbalize statements of comfort	• Assess patient's level of comfort (verbal and nonverbal cues) • Reposition patient frequently using pillows for support • Rub areas of discomfort with lotion • Provide medication for pain as needed	• Patient may not openly admit discomfort • Repositioning will prevent development of pressure areas and fatigue of dependent sites • Rubbing areas of discomfort promotes relaxation of sore muscle groups and enhances circulation to the area • Medication can provide analgesia necessary to improve the patient's level of comfort

TABLE 12.11: Nursing care plan for the patient with a permanent pacemaker

Problems	Objective	Nursing interventions	Rationales
Nursing Diagnosis #1			
Alteration in cardiac output, related to: 1. Pacemaker malfunction 2. Pacemaker-induced dysrhythmias 3. Electromagnetic interference	1. Patient will demonstrate clinical behaviors consistent with an adequate cardiac output: – Alert and oriented to person, place, and time – Systolic blood pressure greater than 90 mm Hg – Lungs clear on auscultation – Capillary refill less than 2 sec – Urine output greater than 30 mL/h – Lack of the subjective complaints that might have been verbalized before the pacemaker insertion, indicative of low cardiac output (i.e. dizziness, fatigue, nausea) 2. Patient will not demonstrate pacemaker malfunction as evidenced by ECG analysis	Monitor ECG continuously for 24–48 hours after pacemaker insertion for: – Sensing ability – Ability to capture – Firing rate that is consistent with settings – Frequency of pace-assist – Presence of dysrhythmias • Confirm that the pacemaker is firing at the present rate • CV assessment same as temporary pacer • Assess patient's response to dysrhythmias and communicate with physician for appropriate treatment regimen • Rule out any other potential cause of dysrhythmias (i.e. electrolyte imbalance, ischemia and hypoxia) • If cardioversion/defibrillation is required, do not place sternal paddle directly over pulse generator. Keep current approximately 10 cm away from pulse generator at all times. Anteroposterior paddle placement is strongly recommended if possible.	• The pacemaker may "oversense" (i.e. become inhibited by other electrical potential in the body) or it may "undersense" and not recognize intrinsic cardiac activity • Conditions may develop that can increase the threshold and decrease the pacemaker's ability to capture (i.e. fibrosis at the pacing catheter tip, hypoxia, dislodgement of pacing catheter, concurrent drug therapy, electrolyte imbalance) • Determining how frequently the patient's rhythm requires pacemaker assistance will provide you with pertinent clinical information – Foreign object in ventricle can irritate the myocardium and cause dysrhythmias • The pacemaker-induced dysrhythmias may be self-limiting and hemodynamically insignificant, or they might be life-threatening. The physician should be made aware of their occurrence to determine if therapeutic intervention is warranted

Contd...

Contd...

Problems	Objective	Nursing interventions	Rationales
	3. Patient will be free of hemodynamically significant dysrhythmias	• Do not expose patient to any conditions known to cause interference: – Nuclear magnetic resonance – Cautery – Electroconvulsive therapy – Electric razors	• Other variables in the patient's clinical picture may be causing the dysrhythmias and should be excluded before the pacing catheter is implicated • Discharge of high amounts of energy over the electrical circuitry can damage the pacemaker and cause malfunction • Electrical and magnetic fields can alter pacer function
Nursing Diagnosis #2			
Potential for infection, related to the surgical procedure	1. Patient will be infection-free as evidenced by: – Approximation of surgical incision – Lack of elevation of temperature – Lack of redness, swelling, discharge, heat at site of incision	• Monitor incision site and document findings • Cleanse incision with Betadine daily; keep open to air after 24 hours • Monitor patient's temperature every 8 hours, every 4 hours if elevation noted • Do not administer antipyretics for pain	• Signs/symptoms of infection often begin at local level • Washing the wound with antibacterial solution will prevent infection. Keeping the incision open to air will promote granulation of tissue • Temperature elevation is an accurate clinical sign of the immune system's activity in combating pyrogen • Antipyretics may mask temperature elevation and signs of infection
Nursing Diagnosis #3			
Alteration in mobility, related to the surgical procedure	1. Patient will be able to demonstrate full range of motion in affected extremity	• Encourage patient to perform ROM exercises 24–48 hours after the insertion to prevent stiffness of shoulder; provide passive ROM if unable	• Stiffness in affected shoulder occurs because of surgical manipulation of large supportive muscle groups
Nursing Diagnosis #4			
Anxiety, related to surgical procedure	1. Patient will demonstrate decreased levels of anxiety as evidenced by: – Subjective comments – Decreased restlessness – Facial expressions – Non-verbal behavior – Ability to concentrate	• Assess patient's understanding of situation, reasons for anxiety • Provide information in calm, supportive manner – Assess patient's understanding of information provided ◆ Observe patient's response • Assess past-coping behaviors • Establish calm, quiet environment	• Provide sedation if needed • Pattern interventions to patient's level of comprehension • Establishing calming rapport will reassure patient. – Patient's level of anxiety may prevent integration of information • Assessing patient's coping skills will help you develop a more effective plan of care • Sedation may be appropriate if nonpharmacologic interventions are ineffective
Nursing Diagnosis #5			
Potential disturbance in self-concept after dependence on the pacemaker, disfigurement	1. Patient will verbalize acceptance of the pacemaker as integral part of body	Assess patient's level of comfort with the pacemaker. Note comments related to: – Dependence on "a machine" – Fear of malfunction – Insecurity, embarrassment about cosmetic appearance – Loss of self-control and independence	• Patients often have difficulty accepting the pacemaker because it is a continual reminder that they have a cardiac condition and because of its limited lifespan • Many patients have misunderstandings that promote disturbances

Contd...

Contd...

Problems	Objective	Nursing interventions	Rationales
		• Encourage patient to ventilate concerns; reassure and counsel to dispel misconceptions • Assess past coping mechanisms and apply if pertinent – Consult psychiatry if necessary. • Have patient speak with another recipient of permanent pacemaker • Refer to support group (if applicable)	• Past-coping mechanisms will indicate adaptive/maladaptive behavior • Recognition that problems are not unique provides comfort and strength for recovery
Nursing Diagnosis #6			
Knowledge deficit, related to: 1. Indication for permanent pacer 2. How it will function 3. Monitoring pacer function 4. Signs and symptoms of malfunction 5. Return to prior lifestyle 6. Changes in lifestyle 7. Medical alert information 8. Electrical precautions 9. Follow-up care	1. Patient/family will verbalize understanding of: – Indication for permanent pacer – How it will function – Signs and symptoms of malfunction – Monitoring pacer function – Return to prior lifestyle – Changes in lifestyle – Medical alert information – Electrical precautions – Follow-up care 2. Patient and/or family member will demonstrate how to measure pulse rate with 100 per cent accuracy	• Assess patient/family level of knowledge regarding pertinent information • Develop teaching plan specific to their learning needs • Provide written information for reference of the material covered • Explain in layman's terms: – Purpose of conduction system – Why patient needs pacer – How it will work to supplement the patient's cardiac activity ◆ Signs and symptoms of malfunction (relate to signs/symptoms patient presented with if applicable) ◆ Changes in lifestyle required ◆ Need to carry Medic-Alert card with pacer information at all times—use of bracelet or necklace ◆ Follow-up care – Electrical precautions: ◆ Magnetic fields (i.e. store theft devices, some microwaves and radar) ◆ Electrical fields (i.e. electric razors and cautery) Demonstrate to patient/family how to check pulse – Have patient/family do return demonstration with 100% accuracy	• Written materials are helpful references when at home • Understanding will improve patient's ability to care for self – A common misperception is that the pacer is replacing patient's own heart function – Must be able to identify specifics about pacemaker should it malfunction – Magnetic/electrical fields may cause interference with electrical circuitry; ability of pacemaker to function • Patient needs to monitor appropriate functioning of the pacemaker

TABLE 12.12: Nursing care plan for the patient requiring intra-aortic balloon pumping

Problems	Objective	Nursing interventions	Rationales
Nursing Diagnosis #1			
Potential alteration in tissue perfusion, related to myocardial ischemia, peripheral vascular disease and embolic phenomena	1. The patient will demonstrate adequate tissue perfusion as evidenced by: – Absence of angina – Capillary refill of less than 2 seconds – Warm extremities – No change in base-line peripheral pulse quality – Normal respiratory effort	• Check peripheral pulse quality, compare with baseline every hour, and document findings • Place patient in vascular position (reverse Trendelenburg) • Monitor patient for complaints of chest pain, shortness of breath and peripheral pain • Assess color and temperature of extremities with peripheral pulse checks, and compare bilaterally	• Peripheral ischemia or occlusion may occur due to embolization or diminished flow distal to the catheter • Vascular position promotes blood flow to the peripheral bed • Complaints of pain can be indicative of ischemia or embolization – Sudden onset of shortness of breath can indicate development of pulmonary edema or pulmonary embolism

Contd...

Contd...

Problems	Objective	Nursing interventions	Rationales
	– Sensorium alert and oriented	• Avoid flexion of patient at hips • Monitor left radial pulse quality (or arterial pulse, complaints of dizziness • Place a sheet over the leg in which the local is inserted for restraint of movement	• The circulation distal to the IABP catheter is most at risk for compromised flow • This may cause migration of balloon catheter upward in the aorta – If the balloon catheter migrates forward it will occlude the left subclavian or carotid artery, causing diminished flow to the areas they service • This will minimize the possibility of catheter migration cephalad
Nursing Diagnosis #2			
Impaired physical mobility related to cannulation of femoral artery	1. Patient will maintain range of motion in all extremities except cannulated leg	• Position patient with head of bed at 30-degree angle • Encourage patient to perform ROM exercises in all extremities except the cannulated leg • Reposition patient frequently, log-rolling from side to side • Have patient continue ankle and foot exercises in affected leg	• This will permit swallowing and performance of some self-care activities. Elevation of head of bed greater than 30 degrees will cause hip flexion and may encourage migration of the IABP catheter • Maintenance of muscular tone • Repositioning of patient will maintain use of muscle groups. The patient must be log-rolled to maintain alignment of the cannulated extremity • Ankle and foot exercises will help maintain full ROM of these areas without jeopardizing the catheter placement
Nursing Diagnosis #3			
Potential alteration in cardiac output, related to left ventricular dysfunction, dysrhythmias	1. Adequate cardiac output will be maintained as evidenced by: – MAP 70–90 mm Hg – Urine output > 30 mL/hour – Cardiac index > 2.0 liters/minute/m^2 – PCWP < 20 mm Hg – SVR 800–1200 dyne-seconds/cm^{-5}	• Monitor the following hemodynamic parameters every 15–30 minutes: – Systolic and diastolic blood pressure, mean arterial pressure, diastolic blood pressure, mean arterial pressure, diastolic augmentation – Heart rate – Pulmonary artery systolic, diastolic, and mean pressures – Urine output every hour – CVP, PCWP – CO/CI, SVR • Check balloon timing every hour or more frequently with changes in heart rate + 10% • Monitor for dysrhythmias. Note patient's hemodynamic response • If patient is tachycardia (HR greater than 150 bpm) it may be necessary to change IABP frequency to 1:2 • If CPR is required, turn balloon to 1:3 frequency and decrease the volume to minimal level	• Ongoing assessment of clinical data is necessary to detect changes in left ventricular function • Timing must be precise to optimize effects IABP • Dysrhythmias may or may not affect cardiac output • At high heart rate, shuttling of gas and ability of IABP to inflate and deflate may be compromised • It is impossible to coordinate IABP with resuscitative efforts, but the balloon should never remain still in the aorta because of the risk of thrombus formation

Contd...

Contd...

Problems	Objective	Nursing interventions	Rationales
Nursing Diagnosis #4			
Anxiety (patient/family)	1. Patient/family will verbalize feelings of anxiety 2. Patient/family will demonstrate relaxed demeanor as evidenced by verbal and nonverbal clues	• Explain all aspects of treatment or care to patient/family • Explain/describe all expected equipment, sounds before they occur • Maintain interpersonal contact throughout performance of technical care • Approach patient and family with confident, calm and professional behavior	• Understanding of patient care activities minimizes misconceptions and fears • Anticipation of sights and sounds helps prepare the patient • Recognition of human factor amidst technology is vital • Patient/family must have confidence in caregivers
Nursing Diagnosis #5			
Potential alteration in sensory perception, related to sensory overload	1. Patient will demonstrate lucid mentation as evidenced by: – Appropriate conversation – Orientation to person, place, and time	• Maintain quiet, soothing environment • Attempt to preserve day/night sleep cycle • Ensure patient has adequate sleep periods • Restrict traffic around patient's bed; coordinate care to minimize disruptions • Assess patient's mentation • Reorient as necessary	• Interventions are designed to minimize overstimulation, which can contribute to disorientation
Nursing Diagnosis #6			
Potential for infection, related to indwelling catheters	1. Patient will be free of infection as evidenced by: – Lack of temperature elevation – Lack of redness, heat, swelling, or discharge at catheter insertion site	• Maintain meticulous handwashing • Change femoral dressing with aseptic technique – Observe insertion site for signs and symptoms of infection • Monitor temperature every 4–8 hours – Do not administer antipyretics for pain • Meticulous perineal and Foley care	• Handwashing decreases incidence of nosocomial infections • Sterile dressings protect site from organisms • Temperature elevation is an accurate clinical sign of the immune system's activity in combating pyrogens – Antipyretics may mask temperature elevation and signs of infection – Signs and symptoms of infection often begin at a local site • Maintain area free of contamination
Nursing Diagnosis #7			
Potential for physiologic injury: Bleeding, related to: 1. Indwelling arterial catheter 2. Concomitant anticoagulation	1. Patient will not have active bleeding as evidenced by: – Stable hematocrit, hemoglobin levels – Guaiac-free stools. – Absence of hematoma, bruising, or ecchymosis – Stable blood pressure and heart rate	• Monitor laboratory values indicative of bleeding status (PTT, hematocrit, hemoglobin) • Monitor all stools for presence of occult blood • Inspect the patient for oozing and hematoma formation at the catheter insertion site – Inspect the flank area for retroperitoneal ecchymosis. Generally inspect the skin for evidence of bleeding • Apply pressure dressing, direct pressure manually or with a C-clamp if bleeding is noted at the insertion site • Monitor the patient's blood pressure and heart rate for evidence of diminished intravascular volume	• PTT will identify the ability of patient's blood to form clots. The hematocrit and hemoglobin will identify the level of circulating red blood cells • Anticoagulation can promote internal bleeding • Most common site of bleeding is the catheter insertion site – Retroperitoneal ecchymosis may indicate dissection of the iliac artery upon insertion • Stasis of blood can be achieved by application of pressure of the site of bleeding • Unexplained drop in systolic pressure with concurrent rise in heart rate may indicate active bleeding

TABLE 12.13: Nursing care plan for the patient with percutaneous transluminal coronary angioplasty

Problems	Objective	Nursing interventions	Rationales
Nursing Diagnosis #1			
Anxiety, related to upcoming procedure	1. Patient will demonstrate decreased anxiety as evidenced by: – Subjective comments – Decreased restlessness – Facial expressions – Nonverbal behavior – Ability to concentrate	• Assess patient's understanding of the procedure, any past experiences or misconceptions, and reasons for anxiety • Provide information based on assessment in a calm, concise manner • Assess the patient's understanding of the information provided, noting nonverbal cues • Assess patient's past coping behaviors • Establish calm, quiet environment • Provide sedation if needed	• Identifying patient's level of comprehension and contributing factors to anxiety will allow for clarification through provisions of meaningful information • Information will be integrated if it is perceived as meaningful • Patient's anxiety level may prevent integration of information • Assessing patient's coping skills will help you develop a more effective plan of care • Environmental stimuli can add to anxiety level • Sedation may be appropriate to decrease catecholamine release and minimize myocardial oxygen demand if nonpharmacologic interventions are ineffective
Nursing Diagnosis #2			
Potential alteration in comfort, related to: Myocardial ischemia, immobility	1. Patient will remain pain-free as evidenced by lack of verbalization of symptoms of angina 2. Patient will promptly report any symptoms of angina and will verbalize rapid relief after intervention 3. Patient will verbalize comfort during period of immobility	• Instruct patient to report immediately any discomfort. Emphasize the importance of this responsibility • Assess the patient for signs and symptoms of angina • Assess type of discomfort along with associated symptoms and compare with presenting symptoms • Perform stat ECG; note ST segment changes • Notify physician immediately of any complaints of chest pain or changes in condition • Administer sublingual nitroglycerin, procardia, or IV nitroglycerin as per protocol • Instruct patient that although he/she must lie flat during the time interval that the introducer sheaths remain in and for 6 hours after sheaths are removed, there are measures that can be taken to improve his/her comfort level – Place egg crate or air mattress on bed – Elevate head of bed 30 degrees – Reposition patient on side with pillows. Place rolled towel under small of back – Medicate as necessary – Provide diversional activities	• Many patients are afraid or do not understand the implications of chest pain after the procedure • Manifestations of angina may mimic gastric distress • It is important to differentiate pain of cardiac angina • ECG will reflect changes consistent with ischemia – May need to repeat procedure • Vasodilation with nitrates and antispasmodic medication is needed to improve coronary perfusion • Reassurance that this immobility is limited promotes compliance and tolerance – Interventions are patterned to minimize time lying flat on back
Nursing Diagnosis #3			
Potential alteration in tissue perfusion, related to cannulation of femoral artery	1. Patient will demonstrate adequate tissue perfusion of extremities as evidenced by: – No change in peripheral pulse quality from baseline	• Check bilateral pedal pulse quality every 15–30 minutes until sheaths are pulled: – After sheaths are pulled, check pulse quality every 30 minutes for 4 hours then every hour for 6 hours. Mark location of pulse with pen	• The circulation of the extremity distal to the sheath insertion is at high risk for compromise of flow during the period of time that the sheaths remain in and immediately after their removal

Contd...

Contd...

Problems	Objective	Nursing interventions	Rationales
	– No change in color sensitivity, or movement from baseline – Brisk capillary refill (less than 2 seconds)	– Compare findings with baseline. • Place patient in mild vascular position (reverse Trendelenburg) • Remind patient not to bend at waist • Instruct patient to report any pain, tingling, or numbness immediately	• Vascular position promotes flow to lower extremities • Bending at waist could cause puncture of cannulated artery • Pain, tingling, or numbness of the cannulated extremity can indicate vascular compromise and decreased tissue perfusion
Nursing Diagnosis #4			
Potential for physiologic injury: Bleeding, related to: 1. Cannulation of an artery 2. Concomitant anticoagulation	1. Patient will evidence no bleeding at site of sheath insertion or retroperitoneal area	• Check femoral insertion site every 15–30 minutes with pulse checks • Assess the integrity of the sheaths. Ensure that the dilator remains within the arterial cannula • Assess for oozing, hematoma formation • Place 5–1b sandbag over site of insertion • Instruct patient to report any warmth in groin or leg area or sharp flank pain • Monitor PTT levels • Assess patient for retroperitoneal ecchymosis. Notify physician immediately if present • Place direct pressure over site for 20 minutes, or until bleeding stops	• Bleeding frequently occurs at the sheath insertion site • The dilator prevents blood from flowing out of the arterial cannula. If the dilator is not in completely, blood loss can occur • Frank oozing can occur around the cannulae, or hematomas can occur within the subcutaneous tissue • Sandbag promotes hemostasis at insertion site by providing direct pressure • Warmth may indicate unintentional blood flow from the cannulae. Flank pain may indicate iliac dissection, peritoneal bleeding • PTT is indicative of clotting ability and will help direct therapy with heparin. The goal of treatment is to prevent reocclusion of the artery that was dilated • May indicate femoral or iliac dissection, internal bleeding • Direct pressure prevents blood loss and promotes hemostasis
Nursing Diagnosis #5			
Potential alteration in cardiac output, related to: 1. Left ventricular dysfunction 2. Sheath removal 3. Dysrhythmias 4. Orthostatic hypotension	1. Patient will exhibit cardiac output adequate for tissue perfusion as evidenced by: – Systolic blood pressure greater than 90 mm Hg – No change in mentation – Brisk capillary refill time less than 2 seconds – Urinary output greater than 30 mL/hour	• Assess vital signs, rhythm, mentation, capillary refill every 15–30 minutes until sheath removal, then every 30 minutes for 6 hours. Notify physician with status changes • Assess urinary output every hour • Assess peripheral circulation with vital signs • Assess patient's mentation along with vital signs • Encourage fluid intake after procedure • Monitor patient's response to sheath removal, direct groin pressure. Observe for bradycardia, hypotension, complaints of dizziness. Administer normal saline or other rapid volume replacement; place patient in Trendelenburg position and administer atropine, 1 mg IVP, as per protocol	• Urinary output is a consistent noninvasive measure of cardiac output, renal perfusion • Vasoconstriction is a compensatory mechanism for decreased CO • Mentation is one of the most sensitive indicators of altered tissue perfusion • Fluids are important in maintaining intravascular volume • It is common to observe a vasovagal reaction to the removal of femoral arterial sheaths • Orthostatic changes are common after PTCA due to prolonged bedrest, venodilation with nitrates

Contd...

Contd...

Problems	Objective	Nursing interventions	Rationales
		• Check blood pressures in lying and sitting positions once patient is able to get out of bed, and note decrease in systolic blood pressure greater than 20 mm Hg or complaints of dizziness. Return patient to lying position if this occurs • Frequent assessment of patient status promotes detection of subtle changes in condition	
Nursing Diagnosis #6			
Knowledge deficit, related to coronary artery disease post-PTCA expectations	1. Patient/family will be able to verbalize an understanding of: – What CAD is – Why this is a problem for the patient – Purpose of PTCA – Immediate post- PTCA care – Risk factors of CAD that the patient can modity – Name, dosage, and purpose of home going medications – Follow-up care (appointments) – What to do in an emergency	• Determine patient/family understanding of coronary artery disease, and how it affects them • Develop comprehensive teaching plan in conjunction with patient and family, based on learning needs – Utilize diagrams and audiovisuals to enhance understanding of CAD – Supply patient with written instructions for information pertaining to medications, risk factors, expected behavioral changes, and emergent care • Reinforce teaching during care and evaluate level of understanding • Encourage questions and verbalization of feelings	• Identification of baseline level of knowledge is necessary in providing individualized teaching • Mutual agreement on what information is needed is helpful in meeting perceived needs and providing meaningful information – Levels of anxiety during hospitalization as well as quantity of information communicated necessitate written instructions for clarity • It is important to assess patient's understanding after any teaching to identify any misconceptions

TABLE 12.14: Nursing care plan for the patient with disseminated intravascular coagulation

Problems	Objective	Nursing interventions	Rationales
Nursing Diagnosis #1			
Tissue perfusion, alteration in: Decreased cerebral, peripheral, renal, gastrointestinal, related to: 1. Intravascular coagulation with thrombosis in the microcirculation 2. Hypotension	Patient will: 1. Remain alert, and oriented to person, place and date 2. Maintain peripheral pulses that are strong proximally and distally; skin normal pink in color, warm and dry to touch 3. Maintain urine output > 30 mL/hour 4. Maintain negative values for occult blood in body secretions and drainage	• Assess neurologic status – General cerebral functions: Mental status; level of consciousness; monitor for confusion, lethargy, obtundation, coma, seizures, behavioral changes, headache, dizziness – Cranial nerve function: ♦ Assess pupillary reaction to light and accommodation; drooping upper eyelid ♦ Assess for drooping lower eyelid and facial drooping ♦ Ability of patient to talk; presence of protective reflexes: cough and gag – Sensorimotor function: Assess movement and strength of all extremities ♦ Assess for the presence of paresthesias, numbness and tingling	• Ongoing assessment of neurologic status is essential because of risk of possible cerebral emboli/thrombi, intracranial bleeding, cerebral anoxia related to cerebral edema, hypoxemia – Alterations in cranial nerve function reflect brainstem involvement ♦ Signals occulomotor nerve involvement ♦ Signals facial nerve involvement ♦ Reflect function of cranial nerves IX, X. Airway must be protected especially in the compromised patient – Peripheral thrombosis compromises systemic circulation ♦ Deep retroperitoneal bleed may cause pressure on lumbar nerve roots

Contd...

Contd...

Problems	Objective	Nursing interventions	Rationales
Nursing Diagnosis #2			
Cardiac output, alteration in: Decreased, related to: 1. Fluid volume deficit 2. Myocardial infarction 3. Dysrhythmias	Patient will: 1. Maintain stable hemodynamics: – BP within 10 mm Hg of baseline – Heart rate < 100/beats/min – Central venous pressure ~0–8 mm Hg – PAP ~25 mm Hg – PCWP ~8-12 mm Hg – Cardiac output 4–8 liters/min	• Assess cardiovascular status – Assess vital signs: BP and heart rate; heart sounds: gallop rhythms, murmur; CVP, PAP, PCWP, CO; monitor for dysrhythmias – Assess for chest pain – Assess peripheral vascular status: ◆ Degree of peripheral or dependent edema; peripheral pulses; capillary refill – Monitor skin color and temperature of arms and legs. Monitor for signs of thromboemboli: Homan's sign	• Ongoing assessment assists in identifying potential underlying bleeding, and helps to evaluate the patient's response to fluid and blood replacement therapy – Sluggish circulation predisposes to cardiac ischemia ◆ Edema may occur with altered capillary permeability and osmotic pressure dynamics. Note quality of peripheral pulses both proximally and distally; monitor refill time – Presence of acrocyanosis reflects microthrombi within peripheral vasculature
Nursing Diagnosis #3			
Fluid volume deficit, related to: 1. Bleeding/hemorrhaging	Patient will: 1. Remain without signs of re-bleeding: – Without hematemesis, melena – Without hematuria – Without oozing around invasive lines and wounds 2. Maintain balanced intake and output – Skin turgor good; warm to touch 3. Maintain stable laboratory parameters: – RBC and WBC counts. – Hgb: 12–18 g/100 mL – Hct: 37–54% – BUN, creatinine, electrolytes, calcium, and glucose all within acceptable levels 4. Maintain normovolemia – Body weight within 5% of baseline 5. Achieve resolution of impaired coagulation 6. Achieve resolution of underlying cause	• Initiate activities to detect the presence of occult bleeding – Assess skin and mucosal membranes for pallor, cyanosis, jaundice, petechiae: observe sclera and conjunctiva; gingival bleeding? epistaxis? ecchymosis? purpura? – Determine overall status: presence of fatigue, weakness, malaise ◆ Myalgia, hemarthrosis (i.e. bloody effusion into joint cavity) ◆ Presence of visual disturbances – Measurement of blood loss: All body fluids and secretions: Stool (especially if diarrheal), hematochezia (i.e. stool containing red blood); urine; emesis, nasogastric drainage; sputum and/or hemoptysis; diaphoresis, wound drainage, drains. ◆ Bandages and lines should be weighed; sanitary napkins counted – Sequential measurement of extremity circumference as well as abdominal girth ◆ Observe arterial and venipuncture sites for oozing of frank blood – Monitor laboratory parameters: Hemoglobin and hematocrit • Administer prescribed fluid/blood replacement therapy – Administer lactated Ringer's/saline solutions; albumin and other plasma expanders – Blood/blood products replacement therapy ◆ Whole blood, platelets and fresh, frozen plasma may be given for severe depletion of platelets and coagulation factors	– Acrocyanosis reflects microemboli within peripheral circulation; presence of jaundice suggests extensive hemolysis associated with underlying coagulopathy – Bleeding into joint cavities may underlie joint/bone pain – Retinal hemorrhages may underlie vision disturbances – Multi-organ system involvement in some patients with DIC requires a delicate balance between hypovolemic shock on the one hand, and overhydration from overly aggressive fluid/blood replacement therapy on the other. The key to therapy is accurate measure of all fluid and blood losses – Persistent oozing or increase in bloody drainage may indicate a developing/increasing coagulopathy – These parameters are chief indicators as to the presence of bleeding; however, the patient's hydration status must be considered when evaluating these values; blood administration may also alter these values – Early identification of bleeding enables timely initiation of therapy to minimize and/or prevent bleeding

Contd...

Contd...

Problems	Objective	Nursing interventions	Rationales
		◆ Cryoprecipitate is given for depletion of factors V and VIII – Nursing care considerations: Monitor vital signs before, during, and after administrational double-check product with patient's identification, and with donor's type and cross-match – Monitor patient for transfusion reaction. Note: Hives, chills, fever, facial flushing, headache, palpitations, tachycardia, chest pain, dyspnea – Use blood administration set with a filter and large gauge needle (19 gauge). Infuse blood products with normal saline – Allow blood products (e.g. platelets) to warm to room temperature before administering • Initiate actions to prevent further bleeding: – Gentleness is the rule of thumb when caring for the patient with DIC. Use an electric razor – Gentle tooth brushing; cleansing of mouth with cotton swabs – Skin protection through gentle handling; special attention to skin and mucous membranes especially around catheters, endotracheal tubes, and other invasive lines and catheters: ◆ Orotracheal suctioning should be performed only when absolutely essential, and with meticulous aseptic technique ◆ Blood pressure cuffs should be used as infrequently as possible • Administer prescribed medications and monitor response: Oral medications should be given whenever possible; parenteral medications should be administered using the smallest gauge needle and applying pressure to the puncture site for a 5 to 10 minute period – Stool softeners should be given – Aspirin preparations contraindicated: – Heparin therapy via continuous infusion pump or intermittently (via minidose protocol) – Vasopressors (e.g. dopamine) • Monitor hematopoietic function. – Asses the following: Bleeding—estimate loss; presence of petechiae, ecchymosis, purpura, hematoma; note size and location – Monitor hemoglobin, hematocrit, coagulation studies especially platelets, prothrombin time, partial thromboplastin time, fibrin degradation products, and bleeding time	• Adequate tissue perfusion requires an adequate intravascular blood volume: – Massive fluid resuscitation is frequently necessary to maintain intravascular volume at levels to maintain intravascular volume at levels to maintain optimal cardiac output and blood pressure to meet the oxygen and nutrient needs of body tissues – Blood replacement therapy remains controversial. When utilized, it should be initiated after heparin therapy has been administered to prevent rapid consumption of blood products through the underlying disease process – For nursing care considerations and precautions to be taken when administering blood/blood products – Patient should be closely monitored for the initial 30 minutes – Helps to remove injured cells and other debris in blood that may be antigenic. Minimizes injury to red blood cells. Dextrose solutions will cause RBCs to clump – Infusion of chilled blood/ blood products may induce hypothermia. However, blood/ blood products should be administered within 15 minutes of arrival on unit to minimize bacterial contamination/ colonization – Gentle care minimizes injury to fragile tissues, which may predispose to further bleeding – Use of mild saline solution, bicarbonate, and peroxide as a rinse are recommended instead of a mouthwash; if a mouthwash is used, dilute it 1 : 1 – Careful and timely suctioning minimizes injury to mucosal lining, reducing the risk of bleeding and infection – To avoid rupture of superficial capillaries with further bleeding. While an arterial line is invasive, it may be preferred to monitor vital signs and to obtain blood samples – Help to prevent constipation with straining at stool Aspirin interferes with platelet aggregation thus inhibiting coagulation

Contd...

Contd...

Problems	Objective	Nursing interventions	Rationales
			– Controversy regarding use of heparin in treatment of DIC ◆ Heparin is most effective when given early in the course of DIC ◆ Heparin is most effective when given early in the course of DIC ◆ Preferred route of administration is continuous intravenous drip. Doses are adjusted according to patient's overall status – Monitor for exacerbation of bleeding ◆ Heparin therapy is usually continued until clinical and laboratory data indicate patient's condition is stabilizing – Vasopressors may be indicated if blood pressure does not stabilize with full hydration • Changes in laboratory values are indicative of the patient's status and response to therapy; they afford the capability of following trends in the patient's condition that enable timely and appropriate therapy to be instituted – Exacerbation of bleeding in patients receiving heparin therapy longer than eight days may be indicative of antiplatelet antibody formation
Nursing Diagnosis #4			
Gas exchange, impaired, related to: 1. Increased pulmonary capillary permeability, pulmonary embolism, ARDS, with increased pulmonary shunting	Patient will: 1. Maintain respiratory rate < 30/min 2. Maintain adequate ventilation as gauged by the work of breathing and arterial blood gases: – PaO_2 > 60 mm Hg (room air) – $PaCO_2$ ~ 35–45 mm Hg – pH 7.35–7.45 3. Maintain breath sounds clear to auscultation	• Assess pulmonary function – Respiratory rate and breathing pattern – Breath sounds – Adventitious sounds: Rales, rhonchi, stridor – Chest pain: Pleuritic causes – Sputum production; hemoptysis – Monitor arterial blood gases • Initiate precautionary/supportive therapy – Teach patient to cough, sneeze, and blow nose gently – Avoid sudden Valsalva's maneuver – Provide humidified supplemental oxygen – Encourage to breathe deeply at regular intervals ◆ Encourage use of incentive spirometer	• Onset of respiratory distress suggests intravascular clotting and/or bleeding into pulmonary tissues – Tachypnea, orthopnea, tachycardia reflect effort to maintain tissue oxygenation – Hemoptysis suggests possible pulmonary emboli – Altered pulmonary vascular dynamics predisposes to pulmonary shunting with compromised gas exchange and consequent hypoxemia – Reduce risk of dislodging clots and causing rebleeding – Humidification helps to keep secretions moist and easier to mobilize and remove; helps avoid infection ◆ Helps to expand the lungs and prevent areas of atelectasis

Contd...

Contd...

Problems	Objective	Nursing interventions	Rationales
Nursing Diagnosis #5			
Urinary elimination, alteration in, related to; 1. Hematuria 2. Hypovolemia 3. Renal dysfunction associated with microemboli 4. Hemoglobinopathy	Patient will: 1. Maintain urinary output > 30 mL/hour 2. Maintain urine without red blood cells/hemoglobin/ protein 3. Maintain renal function studies at baseline – BUN, creatinine	• Assess renal status. – Hydration: Intake and output; urine specific gravity; body weight – Hematuria – Monitor renal function studies: BUN, creatinine; urine glucose, acetone; renal calculi, if bed rest is prolonged • Monitor urinary function – Assess for hematuria, burning on urination, urgency, frequency – Maintain sterility of closed urinary system if Foley catheter is in place – Use leg strap to secure the tubing to the leg to prevent pulling – Maintain hydration	• Urine output less than 30 mL/hour suggests dehydration, hypovolemic state, or possible microemboli within the kidneys – Oliguria may be associated with renal insufficiency or acute tubular necrosis – Massive fluid resuscitation may be necessary to maintain intravascular volume – Major complication is urinary infection – Tugging on the catheter can cause injury to the urinary meatus and urinary tract
Nursing Diagnosis #6			
Bowel elimination, alteration in, related to: 1. Bleeding potential	Patient will: 1. Remain without signs of intra-abdominal bleeding: – Without abdominal distention and pain – Stable abdominal girth – Without nausea and vomiting – Negative for occult blood in nasogastric drainage, emesis, stools – Bowel sounds appropriate – Vital signs stable	• Assess gastrointestinal function. – Assess for signs of distention and increasing abdominal girth; abdominal cramps or pain; nausea/ vomiting – Assess bowel sounds ◆ Presence of paralytic ileus – Hematest for occult blood: Nasogastric secretions; emesis, stools • Implement precautionary/supportive measures – Maintain good oral hygiene – Avoid loose fitting dentures. Keep lips lubricated – Monitor patient's response to antacid protocol: cimetidine; ranitidine; maalox ◆ Avoid use of rectal temperatures ◆ Avoid use of suppositories ◆ Avoid use of aspirin and steroids. Administer stool softeners as prescribed	– Bleeding into peritoneal cavity should be suspected in the presence of increasing abdominal girth ◆ Presence of microthromboemboli within splanchnic circulation may underlie mesenteric ischemia and/or necrosis – Helps patient to feel good and reduces the risk of infection – Potential for injury to oral mucosa causing bleeding – Reduce secretion and deleterious effects of HCl acid (gastric) – May irritate friable rectal tissues, resulting in bleeding – These drugs compromise hematologic and immunologic functions leading to potential bleeding and infection
Nursing Diagnosis #7			
Nutrition, alteration in: Less than body requirement, related to: 1. NPO status in the presence of potential bleeding 2. Anorexia, fatigue	Patient will: 1. Maintain body weight within 5 per cent of baseline 2. Maintain plasma protein levels 6–8 g/100 mL 3. Maintain triceps skin-fold and mid-arm circumference measurements within acceptable range 4. Maintain blood chemistries within acceptable range – BUN, creatinine – Serum glucose – Serum electrolytes including calcium, phosphorus, magnesium, sodium, potassium, chloride	• Collaborate with nutritionist in assessing nutrition status – Implement prescribed dietary feeding or hyperalimentation. ◆ Maintain strict intake and output – Encourage liquids and soft foods as tolerated ◆ Avoid use of hot, spicy foods/ fluids – Encourage carbonated beverages as tolerated	• Dietary regimen must meet tissue protein needs to promote healing – Avoids oral mucosal irritation and gingival bleeding – Carbonated beverages help to loosen crusts around mouth and oral cavity without bleeding

Contd...

Contd...

Problems	Objective	Nursing interventions	Rationales
Nursing Diagnosis #8			
Mobility, impaired, related to: 1. Pain caused by bleeding into muscle and joints 2. Debilitated state 3. Increased risk of rebleeding	Patient will: 1. Be able to resume pre-illness activity	• Assess mobility – Assess movement of all extremities – Assess for the presence of joint/muscle pain; hemarthrosis. Assess extremities and joints for swelling and tenderness • Institute precautionary measures: – Utilize a bed cradle – Immobilize affected areas – Treat bone/joint pain with hot or cold compresses as prescribed – Maintain proper body alignment – Provide gentle passive range of motion – Utilize extra assistance when moving patient; use draw sheet to lift patient • Monitor all peripheral pulses, color of skin, and temperature of skin	– Thrombosis/bleeding into muscle and joints may necessitate restriction of movement to minimize further trauma • Goal is to protect the patient from further trauma; minor injury/stress may potentiate bleeding – This avoids dragging the patient, as for example, when moving the patient up in bed; such action could cause skin abrasions and other trauma increasing potential for bleeding
Nursing Diagnosis #9			
Skin integrity, impaired, related to: 1. Capillary fragility, bleeding sites 2. Inadequate dietary intake 3. Immobility	Patient will: 1. Maintain skin intact, no breaks, lesions, irritations, or signs of infection; good skin turgor. 2. Without signs of acrocyanosis or tissue necrosis	• Assess integrity of skin and mucous membranes • Institute precautionary measures – Avoid unnecessary intramuscular and subcutaneous injections; if necessary, use small-gauge needle, rotate sites, and apply steady pressure for 5–10 minutes – Implement use of pressure relief device (e.g. air mattress)	– Reduces the risk of bleeding – Reduces pressure points which can predispose to skin breakdown especially in the compromised patient
Nursing Diagnosis #10			
Oral mucous membranes, alteration in	Patient will: 1. Maintain integrity of mucous membranes – Mucous membranes moist – Lips without cracking/fissuring – No evidence of bleeding – No evidence of infection (stomatitis)	– Implement turning and posititoning schedule – Identify pressure areas: Include stage and depth of ulcer if present ◆ Review patient's nutritional status – Keep skin well lubricated ◆ Provide meticulous skin and wound care ◆ Be gentle with patients. Discourage scratching; removing scabs; keep nails trimmed	– Helps to maximize tissue perfusion – Dietary intake should ensure adequate sources of protein for tissue repair – To avoid dryness and cracking which can predispose to skin breakdown and infection ◆ To prevent infection ◆ To avoid trauma
Nursing Diagnosis #11			
Anxiety, fear, related to: 1. Knowledge deficit regarding bleeding and status of condition 2. Altered level of body function and capability for carrying out self-care activities	Patient will: 1. Verbalize fear about bleeding 2. Exhibit relaxed facial expression and overall demeanor 3. Heart rate at baseline for patient	• Assess level of anxiety/discomfort – Signs and symptoms: Verbalization of fear and anxiety; body posture: Clenched fists, restlessness, irritability, insomnia; evaluate pain • Provide comfort measures • Monitor response to pain medication • Promote rest and sleep periods • Offer necessary explanations regarding condition and therapy	• Relaxation affords comfort • Assist in conserving strength • Prevents unnecessary anxiety and concern on the part of patient and family

Contd...

Contd...

Problems	Objective	Nursing interventions	Rationales
Nursing Diagnosis #12			
Coping, ineffective: Individual/family	Patient/family will: 1. Verbalize feelings regarding underlying disease and prognosis 2. Identify strengths and coping mechanisms 3. Make decision of importance to the patient/ family 4. Identify familial and community resources	• Assess patient/family's prior coping methods – Identify family/community resources • Evaluate patient/family's understanding of illness: Anticipate needs; be accessible; make necessary explanations • Provide emotional and psychological support • Assist in self-care activities	• Identifying past coping capabilities may assist patient/family in dealing with current illness; familiarity breeds self-confidence • Knowledge of underlying problem may be especially helpful in coping with a bleeding disorder. The sight of even a little blood can be frightening • Encourages patient/family to assume responsibility for their own health. This is especially important in those instances where the bleeding problem is a chronic problem
Nursing Diagnosis #13			
Potential for infection, related to: 1. Debilitated state 2. Stagnation of blood 3. Open wounds 4. Impaired skin integrity	Patient will remain without signs and symptoms of infection 1. Body temperature at baseline 2. Hematology profile within acceptable limits	• Assess patient for signs and symptoms of possible infection: Monitor temperatures; productive cough with rust-colored or purulent sputum; purulent drainage from open wounds, incisions; redness, swelling, and pain at catheter sites • Implement protocols in the event of infection: Cultures/sensitivity of body secretions and excretions—sputum, blood, urine, wounds and catheter tips	• Patients in a compromised, debilitated state are at increased risk of developing infection and sepsis • Sepsis may be the underlying cause of DIC • See for nursing care considerations in the patient with or at risk of infection

VASCULAR PROBLEMS ARTERIAL DISORDERS

1. ANEURYSMS

Aneurysms are outpouchings or dilation of the arterial wall and are a common problem involving aorta. Aneurysm is a Greek word meaning "widening". Aneurysms are points of weakness, dilation of outpouching of arteries to at least 1.5 times their normal size. Aneurysm occurs most commonly on the aorta but they can occur in any artery of the body. The other common sites include the femoral and popliteal artery.

Etiology

The exact cause of aneurysm is unknown. The several factors are associated with developments of aneurysm, including hypertension, smoking, atherosclerosis, trauma, syphilis, congenital abnormalities of the vessel infection, (TB) and connective tissue disorders that cause weakness on the wall of the vessel. Abdominal aortic aneurysms are more common among patients between the ages of 60 and 90 years. Risk factors include genetic predisposition, smoking, and hypertension. If surgical complications are expected to be life-threatening, repair may be delayed until the aneurysm is about 5.5 cm (2 in) wide.

A dissecting aneurysm of the aorta is caused by rupture in the intimal layer, resulting in blood dissecting the vessel layers. It is often associated with poorly controlled hypertension and is there times more common in men between ages 50 and 70. Early diagnosis is difficult because of a variable clinical picture. An overview of aneurysm is given in Box 12.17.

Pathophysiology

An aneurysm is a localized sac or dilation of an artery formed at a weak point in the vessel wall. The most common cause is atherosclerosis. Saccular and fusiform are the most common forms of aneurysm. Saccular aneurysms project from one side of the vessel only; fusiform aneurysms involve dilation of an entire arterial segment. Mycotic aneurysms are small aneurysms due to local infections. Aortic aneurysms are usually classified as thoracic, abdominal, or dissecting. Other causes include trauma to the wall of the artery, infection (pyogenic or syphilitic), and congenital defects of the artery wall. Men are affected more often than women. Rupture can lead to hemorrhage and death.

Thoracic aortic aneurysms occur most frequently in men between the ages of 40 and 70 years. The thoracic area is the most common site for the development of a dissecting aneurysms. About one third of patients die from rupture.

Most aneurysms are found in the abdominal aorta below the level of renal arteries. The aortic wall weakens and dilates with the turbulent blood flow. The growth rate of aneurysm is unpredictable, but the larger the aneurysm, the greater the risk

Box 10.17 Overview of aneurysm

Signs and symptoms	Back pain Flank pain Abdominal fullness Nausea Pulsating mass in abdomen Severe sudden back pain with rupture Shock from blood loss
Diagnostic test	Ultrasound Chest X-ray MRI CT scan Aortography
Therapeutic measures	Observe for growth of aneurysm Maintain blood pressure Surgical repair and graft
Complications	Rupture Shock Hemorrhage

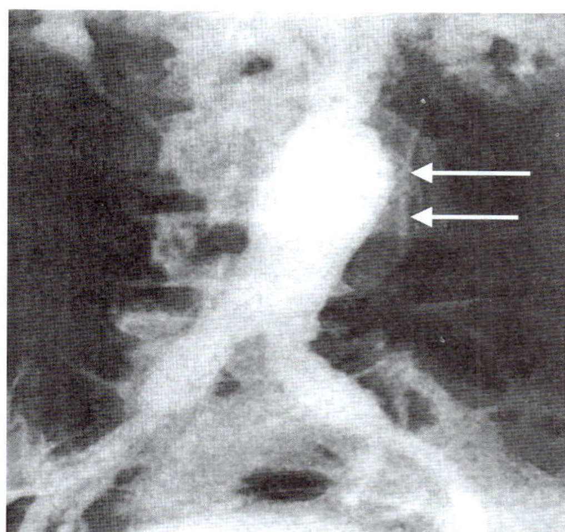

FIG. 12.22: Angiography demonstrating fusiform abdominal aortic aneurysm. Note calcification of the aortic wall (arrows) and extension of the aneurysm into the common iliac a-teries

of rupture. Thrombi are deposited on the aortic wall and can embolize. There are three types of aneurysm.

- A fusiform aneurysm involves a circumferential dilation of the vessel well and is relatively uniform in shape (Figs 12.22 and 12.23)
- A saccular aneurysm is pouch-like with a narrow neck connecting the bulge to one side of the arterial wall
- A dissecting aneurysm develops from a tear in the time of the artery that causes an accumulation of blood in the newly formed cavity between the intima and the media. They further classified according to type of tear and degree of hematoma.

A cause of aortic aneurysm is atherosclerosis with plaques composed of lipids, cholesterol, fibrin, and other debris deposited beneath the intima or lining of the artery. This plaque formation causes degenerative changes in the media (middle layer of arterial wall), leading to loss of elasticity, weakening and eventual dilation of aorta.

Clinical Manifestation

Patients with aneurysm are commonly asymptomatic. Abdominal aneurysm may be felt as a palpable mass and a systolic bruit may be heard. The patient may complain of abdominal or back pain. If the aneurysm leaks or ruptures, the patient will develop severe pain signs of shock, decreased RBCs count, and increased WBCs count.

Symptoms of thoracic aneurysm vary and depend on the size and placement of the aneurysm and its effect on the surrounding structures. Most patients may experience anterior chest wall, back, flank or abdominal pain or may develop signs of shock if the aneurysm leaks. Symptoms such as dyspnea, cough, wheezing may develop if the aneurysm puts pressure on the trachea or bronchi.

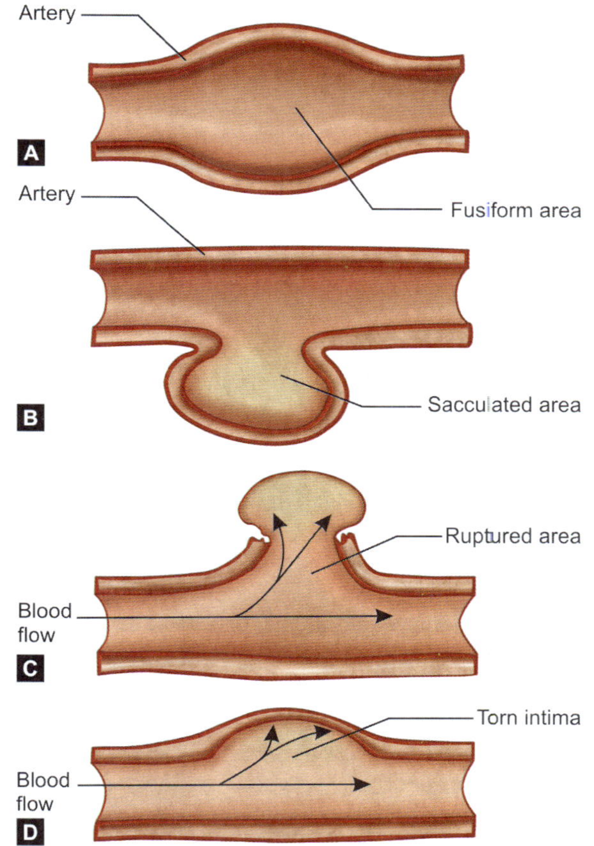

FIGS 12.23A TO D: (A) True fusiform abdominal aortic aneurysm; (B) True saccular aortic aneurysm; (C) Aortic dissection; (D) False aneurysm or pseudoaneurysm

Symptoms are variable and depend on how rapidly the aneurysm dilates and affects surrounding intrathoracic structures.

Thoracic Aortic Aneurysm

Some do not produce symptoms.

- Constant, boring pain, which may occur only when supine (prominent symptom)
- Dyspnea, cough (paroxysmal and brassy), or stridor
- Hoarseness, weak voice or aphonia (complete loss of voice)
- Dysphagia
- Dilated superficial veins on chest, neck or arms
- Edematous areas on chest wall
- Cyanosis
- Unequal pupils.

Abdominal Aortic Aneurysm

- Patient complains of "heart beating" in abdomen when lying down or a feeling of an abdominal mass or abdominal throbbing
- Possibly, "blue-toe syndrome" (occlusion of a digital vessel) if aneurysm is associated with thrombus
- Severe back pain or abdominal pain is a sign of impending rupture.

Dissecting Aneurysm

- Sudden onset with severe and persistent pain described as "tearing" or "ripping" in anterior chest of back, extending to shoulders, epigastric area, or abdomen (may be mistaken for acute myocardial infarction)
- Pallor, sweating and tachycardia
- Blood pressure elevated or markedly different from one arm to the other
- Death usually caused by external rupture of the hematoma.

Management

Most aneurysms are found on routine physical or X-ray examinations (chest and abdomen), ECG, CT scan, and MRI may also be used to diagnose and assess the severity of aneurysms.

- Chest radiograph, angiogram, transesophageal echocardiography and magnetic resonance imaging (MRI)
- Duplex ultrasonography or computed tomography (CT) scan to determine size, length, and location of aneurysm
- In abdominal aortic aneurysms, a pulsatile mass in middle and upper abdomen; a systolic bruit may be auscultated over the mass.

Medical Management

Medical or surgical treatment depends on the type of aneurysms. For a ruptured aneurysm, prognosis is poor and surgery is performed immediately. When surgery can be delayed, medical measures include:

- Strict control of blood pressure and reduction in pulsatile flow
- Systolic pressure maintained at 100 and 120 mm Hg with antihypertensive drugs, such as nitroprusside
- Pulsatile flow reduced by medication that reduce cardiac contractility, such as propranolol.

Surgical Management

Removal of the aneurysm and restoration of vascular continuity with a graft (resection and bypass graft or endovascular grafting) is the goal of surgery and the treatment of choice for abdominal aortic aneurysms larger than 5.5 cm (2 inches) in diameter or those that are enlarging. Intensive monitoring in the critical care unit is required (Figs 12.22 and 12.23).

Examples

Aortography: Anatomic mapping of the aortic system by contrast imaging is not a reliable method, but it helps the surgeon with accurate information about the visceral, renal or distal vessels.

The goal of management is to prevent rupture of the aneurysm. Therefore, early detection and prompt treatment of the patient are imperative. Once an aneurysm is suspected, studies are performed to determine its exact size and location. A careful review of all body systems is necessary to identify and coexisting disorders, especially of the lungs, heart or kidney because they may influence the patient's risk of surgery.

The choice of treatment is surgery. The surgical technique involves:

i. Incising the diseased segment of the aorta
ii. Removing intraluminal thrombus or plaque
iii. Inserting a synthetic arterial graft (Dacron or Polytetrafluoroethylene) which is sutured to the normal aorta proximal or distal to the aneurysm; and
iv. Suturing the native aortic wall around the graft so that it will act as a protective cover.

Prior to surgery, every effort is made to bring the patient into best possible state of hydration and electrolyte balance. Any abnormalities in coagulation and blood cell count are corrected. The patients may receive antibiotics and baths with antiseptics before surgery. If aneurysm has ruptured immediate, surgical intervention is needed. All aneurysm resections require cross-clamping of the aorta proximal or distal to aneurysm. When aneurysms are repaired electively, the patient is systematically anticoagulated with IV heparin before cross clamping aorta. This prevents clotting of pooled blood distal to the aneurysm. If surgery is emergent, no anticoagulative is indicated.

Bifurcated endovascular stent (Figs 12.24 and 12.25).

Nursing Management

Preoperative Assessment

- Assessment is guided by the fact that the aneurysm may rupture (signs include persistent or intermittent back or abdominal pain that may be localized in the middle or lower abdomen or lower back)
- Establish functional capacity of all organ systems, recognizing possible cerebral, cardiovascular, pulmonary and renal impairment due to atherosclerosis
- Implement medical therapies to stabilize patient.

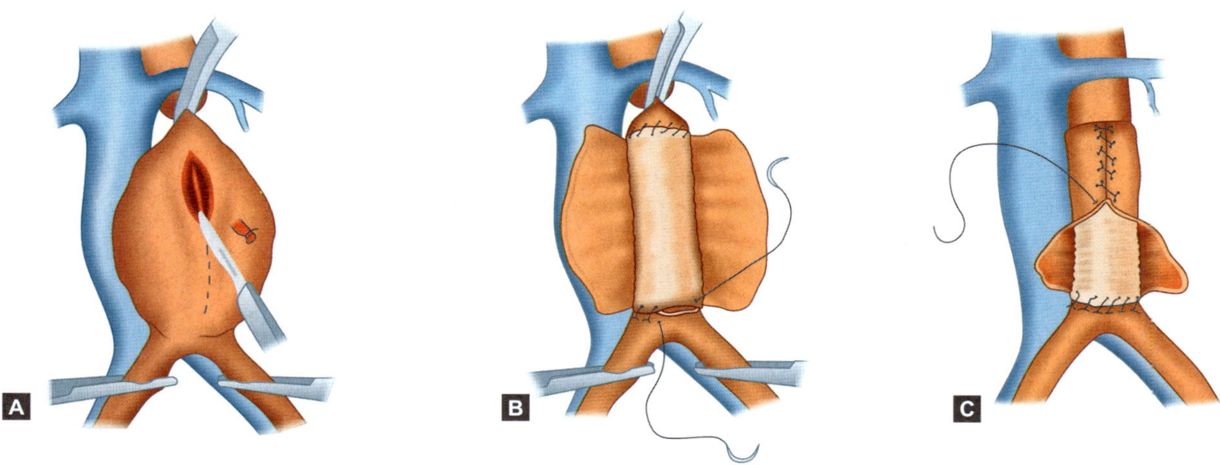

FIGS 12.24A TO C: Surgical repair of an abdominal aortic aneurysm. (A) Incising the aneurysmal sac; (B) Insertion of synthetic graft; (C) Suturing native aortic wall over synthetic graft

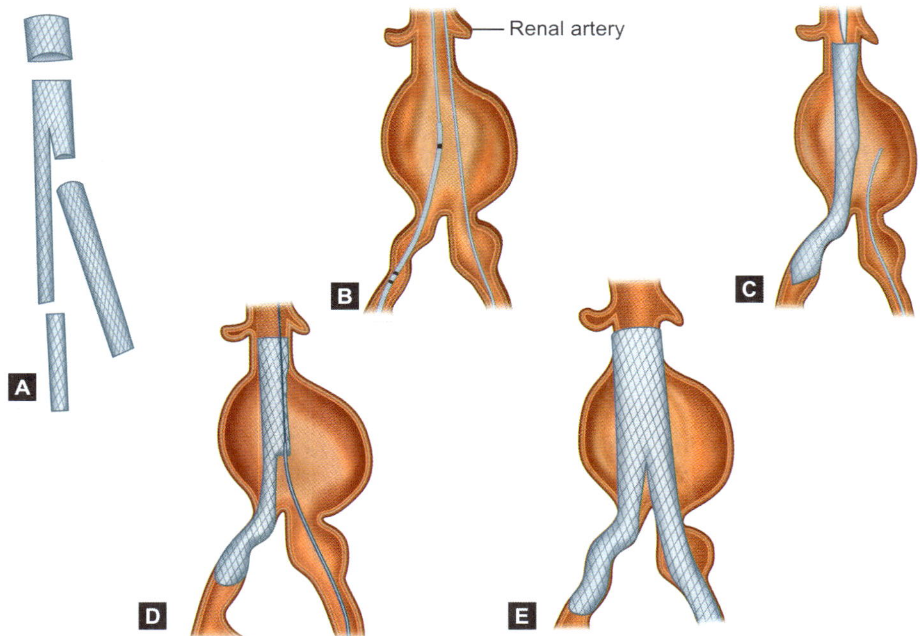

FIGS 12.25A TO E: Bifurcated (two branched) endovascular stent grafting of an aneurysm. (A) The insertion of a woven polyester tube (graft) covered by a tubular metal web (stent); (B) The stent graft is inserted through a large blood vessel (e.g. femoral artery) using a delivery catheter. The catheter is positioned below the renal arteries in the area of the aneurysm; (C) The stent graft is slowly released (deployed) into the blood vessel. When the stent comes in contact with the blood vessel, it expands to a preset size; (D) A second stent graft can be inserted in the contralateral (opposite) vessel if necessary; (E) Fully deployed bifurcated stent graft

Postoperative Assessment

- Intensely monitor the pulmonary, cardiovascular, renal and neurologic systems
- Monitor for complications: Arterial occlusion, hemorrhage, infection, ischemic bowel, renal failure and impotence
- Prescribe an exercise schedule after the acute recovery phase
- Discourage prolonged sitting.

Constant intense back pain, falling blood pressure, and decreasing hematocrit are signs of a rupturing abdominal aortic aneurysm. Hematomas into the scrotum, perineum, flank, or penis indicate retroperitoneal rupture. Rupture into the peritoneal cavity is rapidly fatal.

All patients undergoing aneurysmectomy should be placed in an intensive care unit with appropriate support services and equipment. The nursing role during the preoperative period should include teaching, providing support for the patient and family, and carefully assessing all body systems. It is imperative that problems be identified early and proper intervention instituted. In addition to maintaining adequate respiratory function, fluid and electrolyte balance, and pain control in the postoperative period, the nurse must monitor graft patency and renal perfusion. The nurse can also assist in preventing ventricular arrhythmias, infections and neurologic complications. Nursing care plan for preoperative and postoperative cardiac surgical patient see Tables 12.8 and 12.9.

Aortic Dissection

Aortic dissection, occurring most commonly in the thoracic aorta, is a longitudinal splitting of the medial layer of the artery by a column of blood.

Etiology

Exact cause is unknown; but most people with aortic dissection problem have hypertension, or Marfan's syndrome.

Pathophysiology

Aortic dissection results from a small tear in the intimal lining of the artery, allowing blood to "track" between the intima and media and creating a false lumen of blood flow. As the heart contracts each systolic pulsation causes increased pressure on the damaged area, which further increases dissection. As it extends proximally, distally, it may occlude major branches of the aorta, cutting of blood supply to the areas such as the brain, abdominal organs, kidneys, spinal cord, and extremities. Occasionally a small tear develops distally and the blood flow re-enters the true vested lumen. Aortic dissection differs from an aortic aneurysm. Aortic dissections are usually classified as Type I, II, and III.

- Type I involves the ascending aorta and descending thoracic aorta
- Type II involves the ascending aorta only and
- Type III involves the aorta distal to the subclavian artery.

Clinical Manifestation

The patient with acute aorta dissection usually has sudden severe pain in the back, chest, or abdomen. The pain is described as "tearing" or "ripping". The severe pain resembles MI. As the dissection progresses pain may be located both above and below the diaphragm. Dyspnea may also be present.

Management

The diagnostic studies used to assess dissection of aortas are history and physical examination, ECG, Chest X-ray, CT scan, transesophageal echocardiography, MRI, and aortography. The goal of therapy for aortic dissections without complications is to lower the BP and myocardial contractility to diminish the pulsatile forces within the aorta. The use of trimethaphan and nitroprusside IV reduces BP and IV beta blockers may be used. Propranolol is used to decrease the force of myocardial contractility. Supportive treatment directed towards pain relief, blood transfusion and management of heart failure is indicated. Surgery is indicated when drug therapy is ineffective or when complications are present. Surgery involves resection of the aortic segment containing intimal tear and replacement with synthetic graft material.

The nursing intervention includes:

- Bed-rest—keep patient in semi-Fowler's position and maintain quiet environment
- Administrate narcotic or tranquilizers as ordered to reduce anxiety
- Continuous IV administration of anti-hypertensives
- ECG monitoring
- Monitoring of vital signs, level of consciousness (LOC)
- Preoperative care
- Postoperative care.

ACUTE ARTERIAL OCCLUSIVE DISORDERS

The arteries are thick-walled vessels that transport blood and oxygen from the heart to the tissues. Arterial disease can affect any artery of the body and can manifest itself as an acute or chronic condition. Disruption of the arterial blood flow can be caused by narrowing or complete obstruction of the wall of the vessels.

Acute arterial occlusion occurs suddenly without warning signs. An arterial embolus is a vascular occlusion. It arises most commonly from thrombi that develop in the chambers of the heart as a result of arterial fibrillation, myocardial infraction, infective endocarditis, or chronic heart failure.

Arterial thrombosis is a slowly developing clot in a degenerated vessel that can itself occlude an artery. Thrombi also become detached and carried from the left side of the heart into the arterial system, where they cause obstruction. The immediate effect is cessation of distal blood flow. Secondary vasospasm can contribute to ischemia. Emboli tend to lodge at arterial bifurcations and areas of atherosclerotic narrowing (cerebral, mesenteric, renal and coronary arteries). Acute thrombosis frequently occurs in patients with preexisting ischemic symptoms.

Etiology

Acute arterial occlusion caused by embolism, thrombosis of the already narrowed artery, or trauma, embolization of a thrombus from the heart or an atherosclerotic aneurysm is the most frequent cause of acute arterial occlusion. Heart condition in which thrombi are prone to develop include infective endocarditis, MI, mitral valve disease, chronic atrial fibrillation, cardiomyopathic and prosthetic heart valves.

Pathophysiology

The thrombi becomes dislodged and may travel to the lungs if they originate in the right side of the heart or to anywhere in the systematic circulation if they originate in the left side of the heart. Arterial emboli tend to lodge at sites of arterial branching or in areas of atherosclerotic narrowing. An acute arterial occlusion causes the blood supply distal to the embolus to decrease. The degree and extent of symptoms depend on the size and location of the obstruction, the occurrence of clots fragmentation with embolism to smaller vessels, and the degree of peripheral vascular disease already present. Sudden local thrombosis may occur at the location of an atherosclerotic plaque. Traumatic injury to the extremity itself may produce partial or total occlusion of a vessel from compression and shearing or laceration.

Clinical Manifestation

The symptoms of arterial emboli depend primarily on the size of the embolus, the organ involved, and the state of the collateral vessels.

- Symptoms can generally be described as the six "Ps"—pain, pallor, pulselessness, paresthesia, poikilothermia (coldness) and paralysis
- The part of the limb below the occlusion is markedly colder and paler than above as a result of ischemia.

Signs and symptoms of an acute arterial occlusion usually have an abrupt onset. Clinical manifestation of it includes the six "Ps". Pain, pallor, pulselessness, paresthesia, paralysis and poikilothermia (adaptation of ischemic limb to its environmental temperature, most often cool). Without immediate intervention, ischemia may progress to tissue necrosis and gangrene within hours. Paralysis is a late sign.

The nurse should note the symptoms that occur suddenly and are severe as follows:

Pain: When the obstruction is complete, the pain is severe and constant and is not relieved by rest.

Pallor: The limb typically appears pale and mottled.

Pulselessness: Numbness, tingling and burning in the extremity are common when ischemia is severe.

Poikilothermia: The limb is typically cool, if not frankly cold to the touch.

Paralysis: Mobility of the part in limited. The development of frank paralysis is an ominous sign because it may indicate the ischemic death of nerves in the extremity.

If perfusion is not rapidly restored, the limb will develop signs of necrosis and gangrene often is a matter of hours.

Management

Diagnosis of acute occlusion is primarily established through physical assessment of affected limb, Doppler ultrasonic studies, ABI measurement, MRI and angiography if indicated.

- Sudden or acute onset of symptoms and apparent source for the embolus is diagnostic
- Two-dimensional echocardiography, transesophageal echocardiography, chest X-ray, ECG, noninvasive duplex and Doppler ultrasonography, and arteriography might be used.

Medical Management

- In cases of acute embolic occlusion, heparin therapy is initiated immediately, followed by emergency embolectomy as the surgical procedure of choice only if the involved extremity is viable. Percutaneous thrombectomy devices, which require inserting a catheter into the obstructed artery, may also be used
- When collateral circulation is affected, the anticoagulant heparin is administered intravenously. Intra-arterial thrombolytic therapy may be administered with agents such as streptokinase, reteplase, staphylokinase, or urokinase and other. Contraindications to thrombolytic therapy are internal bleeding, stroke, recent major surgery, uncontrolled hypertension, and pregnancy

Nursing Management

- Encourage movement of the leg to stimulate circulation and prevent stasis
- Continue anticoagulants to prevent thrombosis of the affected artery and to diminish development of subsequent thrombi
- Assess surgical incision frequently for potential hemorrhage.

Drug therapy by immediate initiation of anticoagulant through continuous IV heparin. A few long-term measures, i.e. procedure used and treatment includes:
- Percutaneous balloon angioplasty
- Intravascular ultrasound
- Laser-assisted balloon angioplasty (LABA)
- Peripheral atherectomy
- Intravascular stents

The options for surgical repairs of acute arterial occlusion are:
- Endarterectomy: A direct opening is made into the artery to remove the obstruction
- Embolectomy: Removal of embolus from artery
- Femoral-femoral bypass: A graft from one femoral artery to other.
- Axilla-femoral bypass: A graft from axilla artery to femoral.
- Femoral-popliteal bypass (Fig. 12.26A).
- Aortoiliac bypass.
- Femoral posterior tibial bypass (Fig. 12.26B)

The patient may be undergoing varieties of emergency tests and procedures and will have extensive needs of teaching and support. Preoperative care focuses on the physical, emotional and psychosocial preparation of severely-stressed patient. The nurse is an important mediator between the patient and the rest of the treatment team and attempts to keep the channel of communication open while taking care of the person with acute arterial occlusion are as follows:

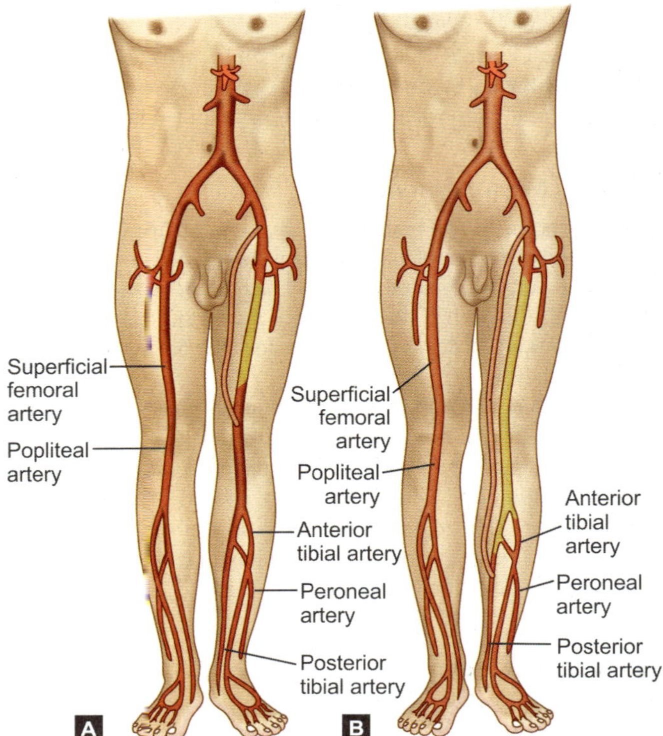

FIGS 12.26A AND B: (A) Femoral- popliteal bypass graft around an occluded superficial femoral artery; (B) Femoral-posterior tibial bypass graft around occluded superficial femoral, popliteal, and proximal tibial arteries

- Monitor the patient for any change in circulatory status to the affected limb. Monitor temperature, color, sensation and pain. A change in these parameters may indicate worsening occlusion
- Monitor peripheral pulses bilaterally for presence, strength, quality and symmetry
- Keeping the extremity warm, but do not apply direct heat or heat lamps
- Avoid chilling
- Maintain bed rest unless activity is specifically ordered
- Keep the extremity flat or in a slightly dependent position to promote perfusion
- Use an overbed cradle to protect a painful extremity from the pressure of linens
- Use sheepskin and 4-inch forum mattress beneath the extremity
- Do not use the knee gatch on the bed; instruct the patient not to cross the legs at the knee or ankle
- Do not apply any restraint to the affected limb
- Keep the head of the bed low to support circulation to the lower extremities
- Monitor the effects of anticoagulant and thrombolytic therapy
- Monitor prothrombin time, partial thromboplastin time, platelets and other studies
- Assess for local and systematic bleeding.

The patient receives meticulous general surgical care. The complications of vascular surgery can affect virtually any organ system. The more invasion procedure, the greater the risk of complication. Potential complications include bleeding, infection at graft site, cardiac failure, myocardial injury to the adjacent organs and tissues (e.g. ureters and nerves). The nurse is responsible for meticulous postoperative monitoring of all the body systems and supporting circulation and perfusion, preventing respiratory complication, supposing fluid balance, and promote wound healing and providing discharge instruction to the patient. The discharge instructions after bypass graft surgery includes:
- Shower daily, clearing the incision gently with a mild or antibacterial soap without lotion of perfume added. Pat dry. Use a shower chair or stool to prevent falling if any instability. Avoid tube baths until healing is complete
- Monitor the incision daily for signs of infections-redness, swelling, increased pain, discharge of suture or staple separation. Report any of these symptoms to surgeon promptly
- Advance activity gradually as tolerated initiate a daily walking regime. Expect to feel fatigued and plan for rest periods throughout the day. Avoid lifting anything heavier than 10 pounds until approved by the surgeon

- Resume a low-fat, low-cholesterol diet as tolerated. Use supplements as needed to ensure adequate calories, proteins and vitamin C during the healing period. Four to six small meals a day are often better tolerated than three large ones
- Avoid constipation and straining at stool. Eat a high-fiber diet with plenty of fluids to avoid constipation. Remain active. Take a stool softener daily plus a bulk-forming laxative if constipation cannot be managed through diets and fluids
- Use prescribed pain medication as needed to ensure adequate rest and activity. Take oral medication with food to prevent gastric irritation.

CHRONIC ARTERIAL OCCLUSIVE DISEASE

Chronic peripheral arterial occlusive disease involves progressive narrowing and degeneration and eventual obstruction of the arteries to the extremities occurring predominantly in the legs. It may affect the aortoiliac, femoral, popliteal, tibial, peroneal vessels or any combinations of these areas. Arteriosclerosis obliterans is the most common form of chronic arterial occlusive disease (Fig. 12.27).

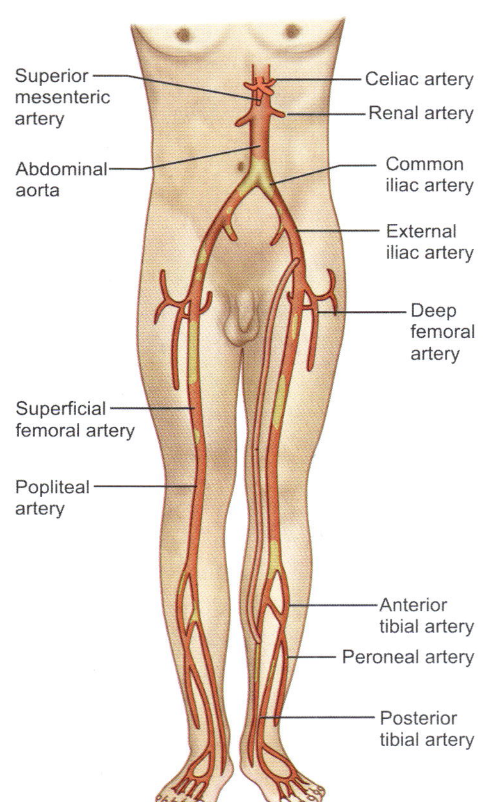

FIG. 12.27: Common anatomic locations of atherosclerotic lesions; yellow of the abdominal aorta and lower extremities

Arteriosclerosis, or "hardening of the arteries", is the most common disease of the arteries. It is a diffuse process whereby the muscle fibers and the endothelial lining of the walls of small arteries and arterioles become thickened.

Atherosclerosis primarily affects the intima of the large and medium-sized arteries, causing changes that include the accumulation of lipids (atheromas), calcium, blood components, carbohydrates, and fibrous tissue on the intimal layer of the artery. Although the pathologic process of arteriosclerosis and atherosclerosis differ, rarely does one occur without the other. The terms are used interchangeably. The most common direct results of atherosclerosis in the arteries include narrowing (stenosis) of the lumen and obstruction by thrombosis, aneurysm, ulceration, and rupture; ischemia and necrosis occur if the supply of blood, nutrients and oxygen is severely and permanently disrupted.

Atherosclerosis can develop anywhere in the body but is most common in bifurcation or branch areas of blood vessels. The fibrous plaques are predominantly found in the abdominal aorta and coronary, and internal carotid arteries.

Etiology

The leading cause of chronic arterial occlusion is the atherosclerosis a gradual thickening of the intima and media, which leads to narrowing of the vessel of lumen. Atherosclerosis primarily affects large arteries. The involvement is generally segmental with normal segments, interspersed between involved ones. The femoral-popliteal area is the site most commonly affects in the non-diabetic persons. The patient with diabetes tend to develop disease in the arteries below the knee (specifically the anterior tibial, posterior tibial and peroneal arteries). In advanced stages, multiple level of occlusions are seen.

The risk factors of peripheral vascular disease (PVD) include-increased age, smoking, hypertension, atherosclerosis, obesity, diabetes mellitus, stress, family history of PVD or atherosclerosis, sedentary lifestyle, hyperlipidemia.

Pathophysiology

Atherosclerosis, the build-up of cholesterol and triglyceride plaque within the arteries, combines with process of diffuse arteriosclerosis is calcification produced widespread, slowly progressive and narrowing of the arteries. Chronic arterial obstruction leads to progressively inadequate oxygenation of the tissues supplied by the obstructed arteries. The pain attributable to ischemia is produced by end products of anaerobic cellular metabolism, such as lactic acid. This usually occurs in the larger muscle groups of the legs (buttocks, thighs and calves) during exercise. Once the patient stops exercising the metabolites are and pain subsides. As disease process becomes advanced, pain develops at rest. "Rest pain" most often occurs in the feet or toes and indicates insufficient blood flow to the nerve supplying the distal extremity. The patient may notice rest pain more often at night and achieve partial relief by lowering the limb below heart level (e.g. dangling the leg over the side of the bed). The clinical manifestations depend on the site and extent of the obstruction and the extent and the amount of collateral circulation. Figure 12.27 shows common anatomical locations of atherosclerotic lesion.

Clinical Manifestation

Clinical features depend on the tissue or organ affected: heart (angina and myocardial infarction due to coronary atherosclerosis), brain (transient ischemic attacks and stroke due to cerebrovascular disease), peripheral vessels (includes hypertension and symptoms of aneurysm of the aorta, renovascular disease atherosclerotic lesions of the extremities). See specific condition for greater detail.

- Intermittent claudication in:
  - Buttocks and upper thigh due to occlusion of aortoiliac arteries
  - Calves due to occlusion of femoral or popliteal artery
  - If disease extends internal iliac artery results impotence and sexual dysfunction occurs in aortoiliac artery occlusion
- Rest pain in advanced diseases-precipitated by a predictable amount of exercise, relieved by resting and reproducible (rest ischemia)
- Diminished hair growth on affected extremities
- Thick, brittle and slow-growing nails
- Shiny, thin, fragile, taut skin, dry and scaly
- Cool temperature
- Diminished or absent pulses
- Palees blanched appearance with extremity elevation
- Reddish discoloration: Rubor with extremity in dependent position
- Reactive hyperemia
- Decreased motor function
- Ulcer formation with advanced disease
- ABI (Ankle-Brachial Index) of 0.5–0.95.

The complication of chronic occlusion disorder is that ischemia leads to atrophy of the skin and underlying structure which in turn leads to decreased ability to heal, infection and necrosis and may result from even minor trauma (e.g. diabetes). Ischemic ulcer and gangrene are the most serious complications, may result in lower extremity amputation if blood flow is not restored.

Management

Various tests have been used to diagnose arterial occlusive disorder. Non-invasive tests include ultrasonography, segmental limb pressure, pulse volume recordings and exercise testing. In addition, Doppler ultrasound studies, duplex imaging, angiography, magnetic resonance angiography are also used.

Traditional management of atherosclerosis includes risk factor modification, medication administration, a controlled exercise program, interventional or surgical graft procedures (inflow or outflow procedures), and nursing measures related to the resulting disease.

Several radiologic techniques are important adjunctive therapies to surgical procedures. They include arteriography, percutaneous transluminal angioplasty, stents and stent grafts, and rotational atherectomy.

The conservative therapy includes projecting the extremity from trauma, slowing the progression of atherosclerosis, decreasing vasospasm, preventing and controlling infection, and improving collateral circulation. The patient's risk factors should be assessed and proper intervention should be begun regarding cessation of smoking, weight reduction (if indicated) and control of lipid disorders. Hypertension should also be properly managed. The nurse should assist in teaching diet modification to reduce the intake of animal fat and refined sugars, proper care of the feet, and the avoidance of injury to the extremities. The patient with family history of cardiac, diabetes and vascular disease should be encouraged to obtain regular follow-up case.

The common drugs used for arterial occlusive diseases include antiplatelets (aspirin, ticlopidine, dipyridamaole) Xanthine derivative (Pentoxifylline) dihydropyridine (Nifedipine), isradipine, felodipine and vasodilators (hydralazine, minoxidil). The nurse should know the action of drugs and monitor the effects and side effects of the drugs and monitor the effect of claudication and exercise tolerance. Monitor BP and Pulse.

The patient with atherosclerosis should be taught and encouraged to do the following:

- Adjust calorie intake so that optimum weight can be achieved and maintained
- Decrease dietary cholesterol to less than 200 mg/day
- Substantially reduce saturated dietary fat
- Restrict sodium to 2 g per day if edema is present.

The procedure/therapy used for acute care of the person with chronic arterial occlusive disease including:

- Percutaneous transluminal angioplasty with or without stent
- Atherectomy
- Arterial bypass
- Patch graft angioplasty, often in conjunction with bypass
- Thrombolytic therapy/anticoagulation
- Endarterectomy (done rarely, with localized stenosis)
- Amputation required, if gangrene is extensive.

BUERGER'S DISEASE

Buerger's disease is an obstructive vascular disorder caused by segmental inflammation in the arteries and veins of the upper or lower extremities. It is also known as thromboangiitis obliterans (TAO).

Buerger's disease is a recurring inflammation of the intermediate and small arteries and veins of the lower or rarely the upper extremities. It results in thrombus formation and occlusion of the vessels. It is believed to be an autoimmune vasculitis. It occurs most often in men between the ages of 20 and 35 years and has been reported in all races in many areas of the world. There is considerable evidence that heavy smoking or chewing tobacco is either a causative or aggravating factor. Involvement is generally bilateral and symmetric with focal lesions. Superficial thrombophlebitis may be present.

Etiology

It typically occurs in men between the ages of 20 and 40 years but rare in women. The basic cause is unknown. But incidences are strongly associated with cigarette smoking—the disease does not occur in non-smokers.

Pathophysiology

Buerger's disease causes an inflammatory response in the arteries, veins and nerves. There is infiltration of white cells and the area becomes fibrotic as healing occurs, which can result in vessel occlusion. Occlusion of the vessel occurs when development of collateral circulation around areas of obstruction. Necrotic lesions form at the tips of fingers and toes and recurrent superficial thrombophlebitis commonly occurs in both upper and lower extremities.

Clinical Manifestation

Symptoms include slowly developing claudication, cyanosis and coldness which can progress necrosis and gangrene. Rest pain is common. The risk of gangrene increases with the presence of collagen disease or atherosclerosis and in response to cold weather. The other symptoms may include color and temperature changes in the affected limb or limbs, paresthesia thrombophlebitis, and cold sensitivity, painful ulceration and gangrene.

- Pain is the outstanding symptom. Patients complain of cramps in the feet, particularly the arches, after exercise (instep claudication). Pain is relieved by rest. Involvement is usually bilateral and symmetric
- Burning pain aggravated by emotional disturbances, nicotine, or chilling; digital rest pain (fingers or toes); and a feeling of coldness or sensitivity to cold may be early symptoms
- Various types of paresthesia may develop; radial and ulnar artery pulses are absent or diminished
- Color changes (rubor) of the feet progress to cyanosis (in only one extremity or certain digits) that appears when the extremity is in a dependent position
- Eventually ulceration and gangrene occur.

Management

Buerger's disease is difficult to treat and management is focussed on assisting the patient to quit smoking and avoidance of trauma to the extremity. Patients are often told that they have choice between their cigarettes/bidis and their legs. They cannot have both. In addition to cessation of smoking efforts, the patient has to avoid exposure to cold and protect the extremities from injury and trauma. Supportive psychotherapy and pharmacologic treatment of underlying anxiety disorders are sometimes helpful in assisting the patient to stop smoking. Although this disorder is difficult to treat, anticoagulants and vasodilator therapy have been used. A sympathectomy may help to eliminate vasospasm, but it must be performed early in the disease process. Amputation generally below the knee may be necessary in advanced cases.

Medical Management

Main objectives are to improve circulation to the extremities, prevent progression of the disease, and protect extremities from trauma and infection. Treatment measures include:

- Completely stopping use of tobacco
- Regional sympathetic block or ganglionectomy produces vasodilation and increases blood flow
- Conservative debridement of necrotic tissue is used in treatment of ulceration and gangrene
- If gangrene of a toe develops, usually a below-knee amputation, or occasionally an above-knee amputation, is necessary. Indications for amputation are worsening gangrene (especially if moist), severe rest pain, or sepsis secondary to gangrene
- Vasodilators are rarely prescribed (cause dilation of healthy vessels only).

RAYNAUD'S DISEASE

Raynaud's disease (arteriospastic disease) is an episodic vasospastic disorder of the small cutaneous arteries, usually involving the fingers and toes. First described by Maurice Raynaud (1802). Raynaud's disease is a form of intermittent arteriolar vasoconstriction that affects the fingers and toes. The cause is unknown but episodes may be associated with immunologic disorder (scleroderma, systemic lupus erythematosus, rheumatoid arthritis, obstructive arterial disease). Episodes may be triggered by emotional factors or by unusual sensitivity to cold. Raynaud's disease is most common in women between the ages of 16 and 40 years and is seen much more frequently in cold climates and during the winter months. The term "Raynaud's phenomenon" as opposed to Raynaud's disease, is currently used to refer to localized, intermittent episodes of vasoconstriction of small arteries of the feet and hands, causing color and temperature changes. It is generally unilateral and affects only one or two digits. It is always associated with an underlying systemic disease. The prognosis for Raynaud's disease varies: some patients slowly improve some grow slowly worse, and other show no change.

Etiology

The exact cause is not known. Associated disorder includes systemic sclerosis, systemic lupus erythematosus, rheumatoid arthritis, hematological disorders, trauma, and arterial obstruction, other contributing factors include occupation-related trauma and pressure to the fingertips (e.g. typists, pianists and workers who use handheld vibrating equipments). Symptoms are commonly precipitated by exposure to cold, emotional upset, caffeine ingestion and tobacco use.

Pathophysiology

Vasoconstriction is regulated by alpha-2 receptors. Sympathetic stimulation or cold exposure causes the release of noradrenaline which activate the alpha-2 receptors and cause vasoconstriction and vasospasm. Persons with Raynaud's disease may have increased number of alpha-2 receptors. They may also have a decreased is beta-receptors and calcitonin which are responsible for vasodilation. The pathological sequence is not completely understood.

Clinical Manifestation

- Coldness, pain, and pallor brought on by sudden vasoconstriction followed by cyanosis followed by vasodilation and hyperemia (exaggerated reflow) with a resultant red color (rubor); the progression follows the characteristic color change white, blue, red
- Numbness, tingling, and burning pain occur as color changes
- Involvement tends to be bilateral and symmetric.

The symptoms are symmetrical and bilateral. The vasospasm confined to the digits and does not usually thumb. Only the tip of the finger distal to the metacarpophalangeal joint is typically affected. Toes may also be affected in same pattern. The disorder is characterized by three color changes (white, red and blue). Initially the vasoconstrictive effect produces pallor (white), followed by cyanosis (bluish purple). These changes are subsequently followed by rubor (red) or hyperemia. The patient usually describes cold and numbness in the vasoconstrictive phase and throbbing aching pain; tingling and swelling in the hyperemic phase. This type of episode usually lasts only for minutes but in severe cases, may persist for several hours. Complications include punctuate (small hole) lesions of the fingertips and superficial gangrenous ulcers in advanced cases.

See Figure 12.28 for Raynaud's phenomenon.

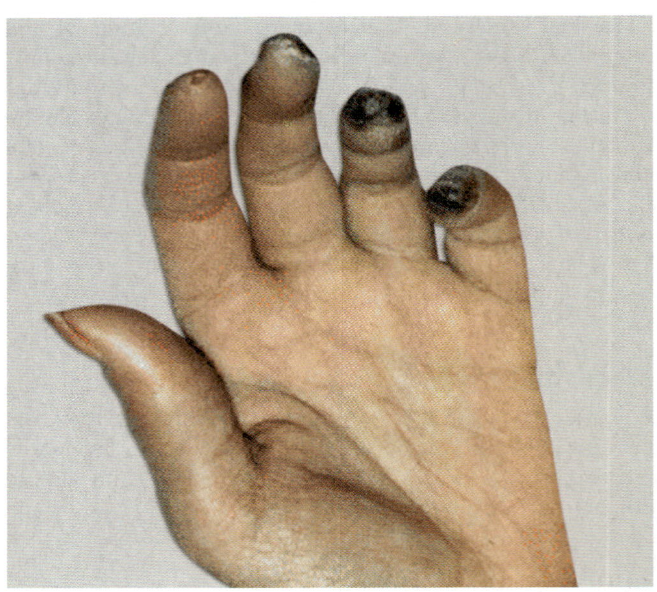

FIG. 12.28: Raynaud's phenomenon

Management

The prime objective in controlling Raynaud's disease is having the stimuli (cold, tobacco) that provoke vasoconstriction.

Calcium-channel blockers may be effective in relieving symptoms. *Sympathectomy* (interruption of sympathetic nerves by removal of sympathetic ganglia or division of their branches) may be helpful.

Mild cases do not require any treatment. Patients are advised to have protection from cold by wearing loose, warm clothing or gloves when handling refrigerator, extreme should also be avoided and advised to stop smoking, avoid caffeine. Advise to immerse hands in warm water to decrease spasm. The drugs used are calcium channel blockers and beta-adrenergic blocking agents may help to some extent. Sympathectomy is considered only in advanced cases.

Nursing Management

- Instruct patient to avoid situations that may be upsetting, stressful, or unsafe
- Reassure patient that serious complications (gangrene and amputation) are not usual
- Emphasize the importance of avoiding nicotine (smoking cessation without use of nicotine patches); assist in finding support group
- Advise patient to minimize exposure to cold, remain indoors as much as possible, and wear protective clothing when outdoors during cold weather
- Advise patient to handle sharp objects carefully to avoid injuring the fingers
- Caution about postural hypotension (results from drugs and is increased by alcohol, exercise, and hot weather).

AMPUTATION AND ITS MANAGEMENT

Amputation is a surgical intervention commonly used in the treatment of peripheral vascular disease. It is the last resort of treatment when other medical and surgical measures have failed to save the limb. Amputation, although radical and traumatic for the patient, it can provide relief of chronic pain, the potential to walk against with the use of prosthesis and an improved quality of life.

The possible causes for indications or factors responsible for amputation are diabetes with pathology, peripheral vascular disease, birth defects, trauma and malignancy. Chronic tissue ischemia that results in necrosis and then gangrene is the most common pathological sequence that results in amputation.

The goal of amputations is to preserve as much of the functional length of the extremity as possible while removing all infected of ischemic tissue. Lower extremity amputations are roughly classified as follows:

1. Below-the-knee amputation (BKA).
2. Above-the-knee amputation (AKA).
3. Amputation of the foot and ankle (Symes).
4. Amputation of the foot between metatarsus and tarsus (Hey's or Lisfracs).
5. Hip disarticulation—removal of the limb from the hip joint.
6. Hemicorporectomy—removal of half of the body from pelvis and lumbar areas.

Preoperative Care

The preoperative period focuses on the careful evaluation and preparation for surgery include carrying out routine diagnostic measure as indicated according to the underlying disease. Stabilization of patient from infection, diabetes and others. The nurse focuses on teaching and patient support in the preoperative period. Amputation can have tremendous psychological implication. This radical change in body image can evoke feelings of loss, anger, fear, shock and denial, so that psychological preparation of the patients in very essential preoperative teaching emphasizes care that will be provided in the postoperative period, pain management strategies, plans for prosthesis fitting, and a basic introduction to stump care routines. The patient should be told to anticipate the occurrence of phantom limb sensation, a sensation of aching, tingling or simple awareness of the amputated part. In addition, other routine for surgery performed by the nurses.

The nursing care of the person after amputation includes:

1. Assess stump and monitor drainage for color and amount, report signs of increased drainage.
2. Position of the patient with no flexion at hip or knee to avoid contractures and encourage prone position.
3. Maintain patient in low-Fowler's or flat position after AK.
4. Support stump with pillow for first 24-hours (according to physician or Surgeon's preference and avoiding flexion); place rolled bath blanket.
5. Encourage exercises to prevent thromboembolism:
   - Active ROM of unaffected leg, ankle rotations and pumps
   - Use of overhead trapeze when moving in bed
   - Push-ups from sitting position in bed
   - Quadriceps sets
   - Lifting stump and buttocks off bed while lying flat on back to strengthen abdominal muscles.
6. Teach care of stump:
   - Inspect for redness, blister and abrasions
   - Wash stump with mild soap, rinse with water, and pat dry
   - Avoid use of alcohol, oils and creams
   - Remove stump bandage or stump sock and reapply as needed; use firm smooth figure of -8 ace wrapping to reduce swelling and shape stump (if rigid dressing not used).
7. Encourage patient to ambulate using correct crutch walking-techniques.
   - Keep elbows extended, limit elbow flexion to 30 degrees or less
   - Avoid pressure on axilla
   - Bear weight on palms of hands, not on axilla
   - Maintaining upright posture (head up, chest up, abdomen in, pelvis in foot straight).
8. Monitor patient's ability to use a prosthesis.

VENOUS DISORDERS/DISORDERS OF VEINS

DEEP VEIN THROMBOSIS/ THROMBOPHLEBITIS (DVT)

The most common venous disorder, results from incompetent valves in the veins and obstruction of venous return to the heart usually results in a thrombus. The formation of thrombus (clot) in association with inflammation of the veins is called "Thrombophlebitis".

Although the vein disorders described here do not necessarily present an identical pathology, for clinical purposes these terms are often used interchangeably. The exact cause of venous thrombosis remains unclear, although three factors (Virchow's triad) are believed to play a significant role in its development—stasis of blood, injury to the vessel wall, and altered blood coagulation.

Thrombophlebitis is an inflammation of the walls of the veins, often accompanied by the formation of a clot. When a clot develops initially in the veins as a result of stasis or hypercoagulability, but without inflammation, the process is referred to as phlebothrombosis.

Etiology

Venous thrombosis typically results from at least one element of Virchows triad: Venous stasis, damage to the endothelial lining of the vein, and hypercoagulopathy. The patients at risk for the development of thrombophlebitis usually has predisposing conditions to these three disorders. Venous thrombosis can occur in any vein but is most frequent in the veins of the lower extremities. Both superficial and deep veins of the legs may be affected. Damage to the lining of blood vessels creates a site for clot formation, and increased blood coagulability occurs in patients who abruptly stop taking anticoagulant medications and also occurs with oral contraceptive use and several blood dyscrasias. The danger associated with venous thrombosis is that parts of a clot can become detached an produce and embolic occlusion of the pulmonary blood vessels. Venous thrombosis is less common in the upper extremity than in the lower extremity.

Risk Factors

- Obesity
- Advanced age
- Oral contraceptive use

Risk factors for deep vein thrombosis are as follows:

- Advanced age—the elderly typically have a number of risk factors.
- Gender—DVT occurs more often in women
- Positive history of thromboses
- Immobility/stasis
  - Surgery, bed rest, paralysis, fractured hip, spinal cord injury
  - Prolonged sitting (automobile or air travel)
  - Obesity and pregnancy.
- Increased viscosity (Hypercoagulable stumps)
  - Dehydration, fever and malnutrition
  - Polycythemia vera and severe anemias.
- Intimal damage
  - Central and peripheral IV catheters, pacemaker wires, IV therapy
  - IV drug abuse
- Associated conditions/disorders
  - Malignancy
  - Varicose veins
  - Inherited coagulation disorder
  - Hemolytic anemia (sickle cell anemia).
- Trauma
  - Fractures especially involving the pelvis and long bones
  - Burns.
- Use of oral contraceptives (risk primarily related to estrogen content)
- Chronic lung and heart disease (CHF, cerebrovascular disease)
- Cigarette smoking
- Venous cannulation or catheterization).

Pathophysiology

Thrombi develop from platelets, fibrin and both red and white cells. They typically form in areas where the blood flow is slow or turbulent. The major elements of stasis increased coagulability, and intimal damage dramatically accelerate the process. Muscle spasm and changes in the intravascular pressure can cause the developing thrombus to dislodge and move towards the heart and lungs. The lungs are rich in heparin and plasmin activators and can effectively dissolve some thrombi. However, if the thrombus is not successfully dissolved, it can lodge in an artery and obstruct perfusion to the lung segment causing problems.

Clinical Manifestation

- Half of all patients have no symptoms; signs and symptom are nonspecific
- Edema and swelling of the extremity resulting from obstruction of deep veins of the leg
- Skin over the affected leg may become warmer; superficial veins may become more prominent (cordlike venous segment)
- Bilateral swelling may be difficult to detect (lack of size difference)
- Tenderness occurs later and is detected by gently palpating the leg
- Homans' sign (pain in the calf after sharp dorsiflexion of the foot) is not specific for deep vein thrombosis (DVT) because it can be elicited in any painful condition of the calf
- In some cases, signs of a pulmonary embolus are the first indication of DVT
- Thrombus of superficial veins produces pain or tenderness redness, and warmth in the involved area
- In massive iliofemoral venous thrombosis (phlegmasia cerulea dolens), the entire extremity becomes massively swollen, tense, painful, and cool to touch.

Clinical manifestation of the thrombophlebitis varies according to the size and location of the thrombus and the adequacy of collateral circulation. The patient with superficial thrombophlebitis may have a palpable firm, subcutaneous cord-like vein. The area surrounding the vein may be tender to the touch, reddened, and warm. A mild systemic temperature elevation and leukocytoses may be present. Edema of the extremity may occur or may not occur.

The patient with deep thrombophlebitis may have no symptoms or have unilateral leg edema, pain, warm skin, and temperature greater than 38°C. If the calf is involved, tenderness may be present on palpation. Homan's sign, pain on dorsiflexion of the foot when the leg is raised is a classic but unreliable sign because it is not specific for DVT. If the inferior vena cava involved, the lower extremities may be edematous and cyanotic. If the superior vena cava is involved, the upper extremities, neck, back and face may be edematous and cyanotic.

The most serious complication of DVT are pulmonary embolism, chronic venous insufficiency and phlegmasia cerulea dolens.

Management

Various diagnostic studies are used to determine the site or location and extent of the thrombus or embolic which includes chest X-ray, APTT (activated partial thromboplastin time), PT (prothrombin time) venous studies, venogram of the affected limb (rarely), lung scan and pulmonary angiogram.

- History revealing risk factors such as varicose veins or neoplastic disease
- Doppler ultrasonography, impedance plethysmography, duplex imaging
- ^{125}I-labeled fibrinogen scanning, contrast phlebography (venography)

Prevention

Prevention is dependent on identifying risk factors for thrombus and on educating the patient about appropriate interventions.

Medical Management

Objectives of management are to prevent the thrombus from growing and fragmenting, resolve the current thrombus, and prevent recurrence.

Pharmacologic Therapy

- Heparin is administered for 5 to 7 days by intermittent or continuous intravenous infusion. Dosage is regulated by partial thromboplastin time (PTT), international normalized ratio (INR), and platelet counts. Low-molecular-weight heparin is given in one or two injection daily, it is more expensive than unfractionated heparin but safer
- Oral anticoagulants (e.g. warfarin [Coumadin]) are given with heparin theapy
- Thrombolytic (fibrinolytic) therapy is given within the first 3 days after acute thrombosis. Drugs such as streptokinase, urokinase, and tissue plasminogen activator are used
- Throughout therapy, PTT prothrombin time, hemoglobin, hematocrit, platelet count, and fibrinogen level are monitored frequently. Drug therapy is discontinued if bleeding occurs and cannot be stopped
- Fondaparinux given subcutaneously for prophylaxis during major orthopedic surgery (hip replacement, etc.).

The patients with DVT are treated with complete bed rest, because the patient on traditional heparin therapy will be on bed rest for 5 to 7 days. Patient on low-molecular-weight heparin can be out of bed after 24 hours if pain level permits. Patient can be treated with the use of local heat to extremity when inflammation is acute, fit the patient carefully for graduated compression stockings and teach correct use.

Patients are on anticoagulant therapy should be taught the action, dosage and side effects of medication, and they are advised to eat dark green and yellow leafy vegetables moderately because these are rich in vitamin K, which can counteract the effect of Coumadin (Warfarin) and advise them to use alcohol only in moderation because it increases the anticoagulant effect. In addition, patient should be taught the following:

- Risks and complications of DVT, signs and symptoms of complication
- Risk, complications of heparin administration, signs and symptoms and complications
- Bleeding precautions
- Need for ongoing laboratory follow-up of anticoagulation levels after discharge.

The conservative treatment includes:

- Continuous IV heparin
- Bed rest with bathroom privileges
- Elevation of legs above the heart level
- Anticoagulant therapy and heparin, warfarin
- Elastic compression stockings
- Measurement and charting of size of both thighs and calves every morning
- Mild oral analgesics such as aspirin and codeine
- NSAIDs.

Surgical Management

Thrombectomy is the treatment of choice when anticoagulant or thrombolytic therapy is contraindicated, the danger of pulmonary embolism is extreme, and permanent damage to the extremity will probably result. A vena cava filter may be placed to trap emboli and prevent pulmonary complications.
Surgical procedure if indicated include:

- Intracaval filter insertion
- Venous thrombectomy (rarely done).

The primary option is transvenous filtration device placed in the vena cava to trap emboli before they reach the heart and pulmonary vessels. Two types are currently in use; the Greenfield filter and bird's nest filter. Both filters are permanently implanted and rarely become dislodged or occluded. The nursing care of the patient with a vena caval filter includes:

- Assess venipuncture site for signs of bleeding or infection. Maintain an adhesive covering over the insertion site
- Immobilize the extremity after the procedure per institution protocol or physician's order
- Assess peripheral pulses, temperature, color and sensation in affected extremity per protocol. Assess for pain and presence of positive Homan's sign

- Assess respiratory status and monitor pulse oximetry or blood gases as indicated. Position is partial or high-Fowler's position
- Implement bleeding precautions and associated safety measures if systemic anticoagulation is to be continued. Monitor appropriate laboratory test results (PTT, HB, Hct, INR)
- Teach the patient to monitor for signs of infection at insertion site. Signs of systemic bleeding (e.g. blood in stool, urine, gums, nosebleed easy bruises); bleeding precaution for home use, if anticoagulation is continued (e.g. use of soft toothbrush, electric razor, stool softener), symptoms to report to the health care provider (bleeding and infection) DVT. Pulmonary embolism-swelling and warmth in extremity, sudden chest pain, dyspnea, tachypnea, restlessness, filter occlusion
- Localized pain, venous stasis, or swelling and unusual symptoms.

Nursing Management

Assessment (Fig. 12.29)

- Assess for early signs of venous disorders in lower extremities
- Take history of varicose veins, hypercoagulation, neoplastic disease, cardiovascular disease, or recent major surgery or injury. Obese people elderly people, and women taking oral contraceptives are at risk
- Question patient about leg pain, heaviness, and any functional impairment or edema
- Inspect legs from groin to feet, noting asymmetry and measuring and recording calf circumference (one early indication of edema is engorgement of the space behind the ankle)
- Note any increase in temperature in the affected leg
- Identify areas of tenderness and any thromboses
- Advise patient to remove elastic stocking for a brief interval at least twice daily and at night; to inspect skin for signs of irritation; to examine calves for possible tenderness; and to report any skin changes or signs of tenderness and see Figure 12.30.

Nursing Interventions

Providing Comfort

- Intermittent pneumatic compression devices can be used with elastic stocking for prevention of DVT. Ensure that prescribed pressures are not exceeded, and assess for comfort
- Recommend bed rest. Advise patient to elevate affected extremity. Provide elastic stockings, and administer analgesic agents for pain. For DVT advise bed rest for 5 to 7 days after diagnosis
- Use elastic stocking when patient begins to ambulate apply and monitor carefully to prevent it from rolling down to form a tourniquet (which restricts circulation)
- Encourage walking (better than standing or sitting for long periods)
- Recommend bed exercises, such as dorsiflexion of the foot against a footboard

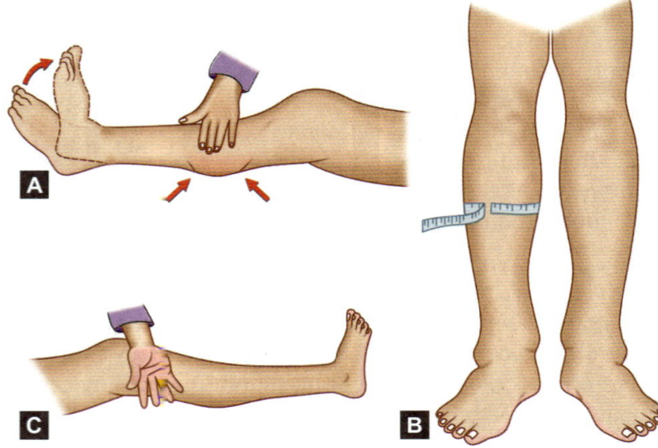

FIGS 12.29A TO C: Nursing assessment for deep vein thrombosis. (A) Pain and tenderness in the calf of the affected extremity, especially on dorsiflexion of the foot (Homan's sign); (B) The affected extremity may have a larger circumference than the unaffected extremity caused by edema; (C) The affected extremity will be warm to touch compared to the unaffected extremity

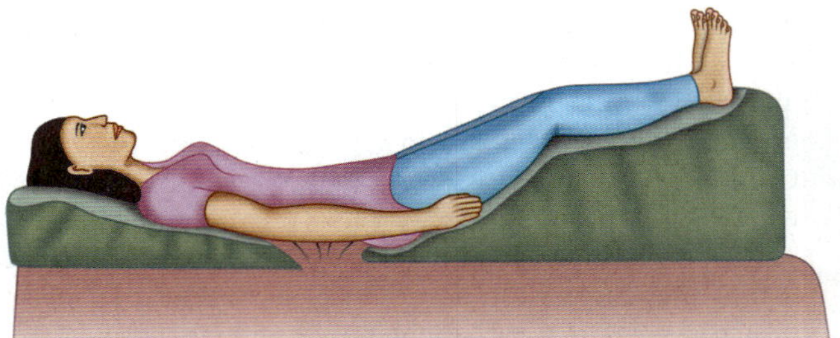

FIG. 12.30: This leg elevator is of foam construction with a removable cotton cover that may be machine washed. It is clamped to the lower end of the mattress. This position is anatomically correct and provides adequate support to all parts of the leg edema and stasis of the lower extremities can be controlled

- Apply warm, moist packs to affected extremity to reduce discomfort
- Provide additional pain relief with mild analgesic agents as prescribed.

Elderly patients may be unable to apply elastic stockings properly. Teach the family member who is to assist the patient to apply the stocking so that they do not cause undue pressure on any part or the feet or legs.

Positioning the Body and Encouraging Exercise

- Elevate feet and lower legs periodically above heart level when on bed rest
- Perform active and passive leg exercises, particularly those involving calf muscles, to increase venous flow preoperatively and postoperatively
- Provide early ambulation to help prevent venous stasis
- Encourage deep-breathing exercises because they produce increased negative pressure in the thorax, which assists in emptying the large veins.

Monitoring and Managing Potential Complications

- Monitor urinalysis for hematuria (first sign of anticoagulant toxicity)
- Monitor anticoagulant therapy closely and regularly. Prepare to reverse anticoagulant effects by administering protamine sulfate for heparin or vitamin K and fresh-frozen plasma for warfarin
- Monitor for heparin-induced thrombocytopenia. Note platelet counts regularly and report counts less than 100,000/mL or a greater than 25 percent decrease in platelet count. Report the need for increasing doses of heparin to maintain therapeutic levels. Note thromboembolic or hemorrhagic complications. Report a patient history of heparin sensitivity
- Closely monitor the medication schedule, because oral anticoagulants interact with many other medications and herbal and nutritional supplements.

Teach patient which medications potentiate oral anticoagulants; salicylates, anabolic steroids, chloral hydrate, glucagon, chloramphenicol, neomycin quinidine, vitamin E, and phenylbutazone (Butazolidin). Medications that decrease the anticoagulant effect include phenytoin, barbiturates, diuretics, and estrogen. Identify medication interactions for patients taking specific oral anticoagulants.

Teaching Patients Self-Care

- Teach patient how to apply elastic stockings. Any type of stocking can inadvertently become a tourniquet if applied incorrectly (i.e. rolled tightly at the top). In such instances, the stockings produce rather than prevent stasis. For ambulatory patients, graduated compression stocking are removed at night and reapplied before the legs are lowered from the bed to the floor in the morning
- Instruct patient on the purpose and importance of medication (correct dosage at specific times) and need for scheduled blood tests to regulate medications.

VARICOSE VEINS

Varicose veins or varicosities are prominent, abnormally dilated, tortuous subcutaneous veins most frequently occur in saphenous system, most oftenly in the lower extremities because of the effects of gravity on venous presence.

Etiology

The etiology of varicose veins is unknown. The increased venous pressure may result from congenital weakness of the vein structure, obesity, pregnancy, venous obstruction resulting from thrombosis or extrinsic pressure by tumors or occupations that require prolonged standing (e.g. police constable, OT nurse, etc.). It may be hereditary and effects chronic diseases such as cirrhosis or CHF.

Pathophysiology

As the veins enlarge, the valves are stretched and become incompetent allowing blood flow to be reversed. As back pressure increases and the calf muscle pump (muscle movement that squeezes venous blood back towards heart) fails. Further venous distention results. The increased venous pressure is transmitted to the capillary bed and edema develops.

Clinical Manifestation

Discomfort from varicose veins varies dramatically among people and tends to be worsened by superficial thrombophlebitis. In addition, many patients voice concern about cosmetic disfigurement. The most common symptom of varicose veins is an ache or pain after prolonged standing, which is relieved by walking or by elevating the limb. Some patients feel pressure or a cramp-like sensation. Swelling may accompany discomfort nocturnal leg cramps, especially in calf area occurs. The common complication is superficial thrombophlebitis. Ulceration may develop as a result of skin infections or trauma.

Management

A duplex ultrasound can detect obstruction and reflux in the verities system with considerable accuracy. Treatment is not indicated if varicose veins are only a cosmetic problem. If incompetency of venous system develops, the care involves rest with the affected limb elevated, compression stocking and exercise such as walking. Sclerotherapy is a technique used in the treatment of unsightly superficial varicosities. Direct IV injection of a sclerosing agent such as sodium tetradecyl induces inflammation and results in eventual thrombosis of vein. After procedure leg is wrapped with an elastic bandage for 24 to 72 hours to maintain persons over the vein- local tenderness subsides within 2 to 3 weeks and eventually thrombosed vein disappears. After this patients are advised to wear compression stockings to prevent further varicosities.

The nurse should instruct patients to avoid sitting or standing for long time, maintain ideal body weight, take precautions against injury to the extremities and avoid wearing constrictive clothing. After vein ligation, the nurse should encourage deep breathing for promoting venous return. The extremities should be checked regularly for color, movement, sensation, temperature, presence of edema and padal pulses. Postoperatively the extremities are elevated at a 15 degree angle to prevent development of various stasis and edema. Some other measures are also important which have to take care.

VENOUS STASIS ULCER

Chronic venous insufficiency can lead to venous stasis ulceration, which may occur as a result of previous DVT.

Etiology

Leg ulcers can be caused by many conditions including venous hypertension, infection, diabetes mellitus, malignancy, connective tissue disorders, rheumatoid arthritis and damage through DVT or VS, external injuries such as trauma, pressure, and insect bites.

Pathophysiology

The basic dysfunction is incompetent valves of the deep veins. As capillaries rupture, RBCs breakdown and release hemosiderin causing a brownish discoloration of the skin due to the deposition of melanin, and hemosiderin. The venous stasis ulcers usually develop around the ankles, especially in the area of the medial malleoli. Loss of epidermis occurs, and portions of the dermis may also be involved, depending on the degree of venous stasis.

Clinical Manifestation

The skin of the lower leg is leathery, with a characteristic brownish or "brawny" appearance. Edema has usually been present for a prolonged period. The ulcer is concave lesion below the margin of skin surface. Pain may occur when the limb is in a dependent position or during ambulation. Pain is usually relieved by elevation of the foot. If the ulcer is not treated, infection may occur. Scar tissue is formed around the rim of the ulcer. Poor hygiene, debilitation, and inadequate nutritional status contribute to severity of ulcer.

Management

- Elevation of affected limb to reduce venous stasis and V. hypertension and edema
- Extrinsic compression methods—Stocking's elastic bandages and hydrocolloid dressings
- Routine prophylactic antibiotic therapy (culture and sensitivity if needed)
- Protein—Vitamin supplementation
- Calorie limitation for weight reduction
- Surgery—Excision of ulcer.

PULMONARY EMBOLISM

Pulmonary embolism is the most common complication in hospitalized patients. Pulmonary embolism refers to the obstruction of the base of one more branches of the pulmonary arteries by a thrombus (or thrombi) that originates somewhere in the venous system or in the right side of the heart. Gas exchange is impaired in the lung mass supplied by the obstructed vessel. Massive pulmonary embolism is life-threatening and can cause death within the first 1 to 2 hours after the embolic event. It is a common disorder associated with trauma, surgery (orthopedic, major abdominal pelvic, gynecologic), pregnancy, oral contraceptive use, congestive heart failure, age older than 50 years, hypercoagulable states and prolonged immobility. Most thrombi originate in the deep veins of the legs.

Etiology

Thrombi in the deep veins can dislodge spontaneously. However, more common mechanism is jarring of the thrombus by mechanical forces, such as sudden standing, and changes in the rate of blood flow such as those that occur with Valsalvas maneuver. In addition, less common causes include fat emboli, (from fractured long bones), air emboli (from improper IV therapy) and amniotic fluids and tumors.

Pathophysiology

Most pulmonary emboli arise from thrombi in the deep veins of the legs. Other sites of origin include right side of the heart, upper extremities (rarely) and the pelvic veins (after surgery or childbirth). Lethal pulmonary emboli originate most commonly in the femoral or iliac veins. Emboli are mobile clots that generally do not stop moving until they lodge at a narrowed part of the circulatory system. The lungs are an ideal location for emboli to lodge because of their extensive arterial and capillary network. The lower lobes are more frequently affected because they have higher blood flow than the other lobes. Occasionally, the presence of deep vein thrombosis is unsuspected until pulmonary embolism occurs.

Clinical Manifestation

Symptoms depend on the size of the thrombus and the area of the pulmonary artery occlusion:

- Dyspnea is the most common symptom. Tachypnea is the most frequent sign
- Chest pain is common, usually sudden in onset and pleuritic in nature; it can be substernal and may mimic angina pectoris
- Fever, tachycardia, apprehension, cough, diaphoresis, hemoptysis, syncope, shock, and sudden death may occur
- Multiple small emboli in the terminal pulmonary arterioles simulate symptoms of bronchopneumonia or heart failure.

The severity of clinical manifestation depends on the size of the emboli and the size and number of blood vessels occluded. Most common are the sudden onset of unexplained dyspnea, tachypnea, or tachycardia. Other manifestations are cough, chest pain, hemoptysis, crackles, fever accentuation of the pulmonic heart sound, and sudden change in mental status as a result of hypoxemia. Massive emboli may produce sudden collapse of the patient with shock, pallor, severe dyspnea, and crushing chest pain. Some patients may have no pain. The complications of pulmonary embolism are pulmonary infarction and pulmonary hypertension.

- Ventilation-perfusion scan, pulmonary angiography, chest X-ray
- Electrocardiogram (ECG) to assess PR interval and T-wave changes, peripheral vascular studies, impedance plethysmography, and arterial blood gas (ABG) analysis hypoxemia).

Prevention

- Ambulation or leg exercises in patients on bed rest
- Anticoagulant therapy before abdominothoracic surgery and every 8 to 12 hours until discharge from hospital
- Application of sequential compression devices.

Management

Medical Management

Immediate objective is to stabilize the cardiorespiratory system:

- Nasal oxygen is administered immediately to relieve hypoxemia, respiratory distress, and cyanosis
- An infusion is started to establish an intravenous route for drugs or fluids
- In some circumstances pulmonary angiography, spiral CT, perfusion lung scans, hemodynamic measurements, and ABGs are performed
- An indwelling urethral catheter is inserted to monitor urinary output, if embolism is massive and patient is hypotensive
- Hypotension is treated by infusion of dobutamine or dopamine
- ECG is monitored continuously for dysrhythmias and right ventricular failure
- Digitalis glycosides, intravenous diuretics, and antiarrhythmic agents are administered when appropriate
- Blood is drawn for serum electrolyte, complete blood count, and hematocrit analyses
- Patient is placed on a volume-controlled ventilator if clinical assessment and ABGs indicate
- Small doses of intravenous morphine are given to relieve anxiety, alleviate chest discomfort, help patient tolerate endotracheal tube, and ease adaptation to mechanical ventilator.

Anticoagulation Therapy

- The partial thromboplastin time (PTT) is maintained at 1.5 to 2.0 times normal, or an INR of 2.0 to 2.5
- Heparin is administered for 5 to 7 days
- Warfarin (Coumadin) is begun within 24 hours following the start of heparin therapy and continued for 3 to 6 months.

Thrombolytic Therapy

- Thrombolytic therapy may include urokinase alteplase, anistreplase, reteplase, and streptokinase (tissue plasminogen activator). It is reserved to pulmonary embolism affecting a significant area and causing hemodynamic instability
- Bleeding is a significant side effect; nonessential invasive procedures are avoided.

Surgical Management

- Embolectomy by means of thoracotomy with cardiopulmonary bypass technique
- Transvenous catheter embolectomy with or without insertion of an inferior vena caval filter (e.g. Greenfield).

Diagnosis measures of pulmonary emboli include in addition to routine history need physical assent; venous studies, chest X-ray, continuous ECG monitoring, ABGs, CBC, lung scan, and pulmonary angiography treatment measures include:

- Oxygen by mask on Cannula
- Establishment of IV route for drugs and fluids
- Continuous IV heparin
- Bed rest
- Narcotics for pain relief
- Thrombolytic agents in certain patients
- Vena cava filter
- Pulmonary embolectomy in life-threatening situation.

Nursing Management

The major goals include adequate oxygenation, absence of additional thrombus, effective pharmacologic therapy, minimal chest pain and anxiety, positive postoperative status, and effective home and community care.

Nursing Interventions

Providing General Care

- Ensure understanding of need for continuous oxygen therapy
- Provide nebulizers, incentive spirometry, or percussion and postural drainage
- Encourage deep-breathing exercises.

Preventing Thrombus Formation

- Encourage early ambulation and active and passive leg exercises
- Instruct patient to move legs in a "pumping" exercise
- Advise patient to avoid prolonged sitting, immobility, and constrictive clothing
- Do not permit dangling of legs and feet in a dependent position
- Instruct patient to place feet on floor or chair and to avoid crossing legs
- Do not leave intravenous catheters in veins for prolonged periods.

Monitoring Anticoagulant and Thrombolytic Therapy

- Advise bed rest, monitor vital signs every 2 hours, limit invasive procedures
- Measure PT or activated PTT every 3 to 4 hours after thrombolytic infusion is started to confirm activation of fibrinolytic system
- Perform only essential ABG studies on upper extremities with manual compression of puncture site for at least 30 minutes.

Minimizing Chest Pain, Pleuritic

- Place patient in semi-Fowler's position; turn and reposition frequently
- Administer analgesics as prescribed for severe pain.

Alleviating Anxiety

- Encourage patient to express feeling and concerns
- Answer questions concisely and accurately
- Explain therapy, and describe how to recognize untoward effects early.

Managing Oxygen Therapy

Assess for hypoxia (pulse oximetry), deep breathing, incentive spirometer, nebulizer therapy, percussion, and postnasal drainage.

Providing Postoperative Nursing Care

- Measure pulmonary arterial pressure and urinary output
- Assess insertion site of arterial catheter for hematoma formation and infection
- Maintain blood pressure to ensure perfusion of vital organs
- Encourage isometric exercises, antiembolism stockings, and walking when permitted out of bed; elevate foot of bed when patient is resting
- Discourage sitting; hip flexion compresses large veins in the legs.

Promoting Home and Community-based Care

Teaching Patients Self-Care

- Before discharge and at follow-up clinic or home visits, teach patient how to prevent recurrence and which signs and symptoms should alert patient to seek medical attention
- Teach patient to look for bruising and bleeding when taking anticoagulants and to avoid bumping into objects. Advise patient to use a toothbrush with soft bristles to prevent gingival bleeding
- Instruct patient not to take aspirin (as anticoagulant) or antihistamine drugs while taking warfarin sodium (Coumadin)
- Advise patient to check with physician before taking any medication, including over-the-counter drugs
- Advise patient to continue wearing antiembolism stocking as long as directed
- Instruct patient to avoid laxatives, which affect vitamin K absorption (vitamin K promotes coagulation)
- Teach patient to avoid sitting with legs crossed or for prolonged periods
- Recommend that patient change position regularly when traveling, walk occasionally, and do active exercises of legs and ankles
- Advise patient to drink plenty of liquids
- Teach patient to report dark, tarry stools immediately
- Recommend that patient wear identification stating that he or she is taking anticoagulants.

Procedure 12.1: Central venous pressure (CVP) monitoring

Equipment

- Venous pressure tray, arm-board (for antecubital insertion).
- Cut-down tray
- Infusion solution/infusion
- Heparin flush system/pressure bag [if transducer Carpenter's level (for establishing zero point) to be used] IV pole
- Sterile dressing tape
- Gowns, masks, caps and set with CVP manometer sterile gloves.
- ECG monitoring

Steps of procedure

Nursing action	Rationale
Preparatory phase	
1. Assemble equipment according to manufacturer's directions	1. Evaluate patient's PT, PTT and CBC
2. Explain the procedure to the patient and obtain informed consent a. Explain to the patient how to perform the Valsalva's maneuver b. NPO 6 hours before insertion	2. Procedure is similar to an IV, and the patient may move in bed as desired after passage of catheter a. The Valsalva's maneuver performed during catheter insertion and removal decreases chance of air emboli
3. Position patient appropriately a. Place in supine position i. Arm vein—extend arm and secure on arm-board ii. Neck veins—place patient in Trendelenburg's position, place a small rolled towel under shoulders (subclavian approach)	3. Provides for maximum visibility of veins Trendelenburg's position prevents chance of air emboli. Anatomic access and clinical status of the patient are considered in site selection
4. Flush IV infusion set and manometer (measuring device) or, prepare heparin flush for use with transducer (Fig. 12.31) a. Attach manometer to IV pole. The zero point of the manometer should be on a level with the patient's right atrium b. Calibrate/zero transducer and level port with patient's right atrium	4. Secure all connections to prevent air emboli and bleeding a. The level of the right atrium is at the 4th intercostal space midaxillary line b. Mark midaxillary line with indelible ink for subsequent readings
5. Place patient on ECG monitor	5. Dysrhythmias may be noted during insertion as catheter is advanced

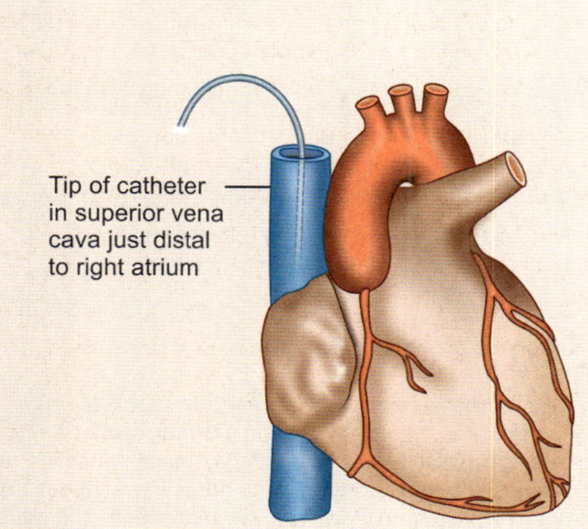

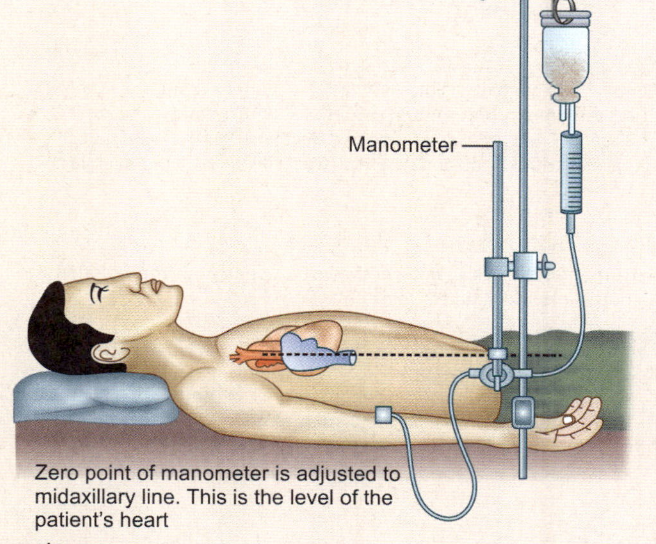

FIG. 12.31: Central venous pressure

Nursing action	Rationale
Insertion phase (by physician)	
1. Physician dons gown, cap, and mask	1. VP insertion is a sterile procedure
2. The CVP site is surgically cleansed. The physician introduces the CVP catheter percutaneously or by direct venous cut-down	2. Patient may be asked to perform Valsalva's maneuver to protect against chance of air embolus
3. Assist patient to remain motionless during insertion	

Contd...

Contd...

Nursing action	Rationale
4. Monitor for dysrhythmias as catheter is threaded to great vein or right atrium	
5. Connect primed IV tubing/heparin flush system to catheter and allow IV solution to flow at a minimum rate to keep vein open (25 mL maximum)	5. Catheter placement must be verified before hypertonic or blood products can be administered
6. The catheter should be sutured in place	6. Prevents inadvertent catheter advancement or dislodgement
7. Place a sterile occlusive dressing over site	
8. Obtain a chest X-ray	8. Verify correct catheter position
To measure the CVP	
1. Place the patient in a position of comfort. This is the baseline position used for subsequent readings	
2. Position the zero point of the manometer at the level of the right atrium (see accompanying figure). Central venous pressure	2. The zero point of baseline for the manometer should be on a level with the patient's right atrium. The middle of the right atrium is the midaxillary line in the 4th intercostal space
3. Turn the stopcock so the IV solution flows into the manometer, filling to about the 20 to 25 cm level. Then turn stopcock to solution in manometer flows into patient	
4. Observe the fall in the height of the column of fluid in manometer. Record the level at which the solution stabilizes or stops moving downward. This is the central venous pressure. Record CVP and the position of the patient	4. The column of fluid will fail until it meets an equal pressure (i.e. the patient's central venous pressure). The CVP reading is reflected by the height of a column of fluid in the manometer when there is open communication between the catheter and the manometer. The fluid in the manometer will fluctuate slightly with the patient's respirations. This confirms that the CVP line is not obstructed by clotted blood
5. The CVP catheter may be connected to a transducer and an electrical monitor with either digital or calibrated CVP wave readout	
6. The CVP may range from 5 to 12 cm H_2O (Absolute numerical values have not been agreed on) or 2 to 6 mm Hg	6. The change in CVP is a more useful indication of adequacy of venous blood volume and alterations of cardiovascular function. The management of the patient is not based on one reading, but on repeated serial readings in correlation with patient's clinical status
7. Assess the patient's clinical condition. Frequent changes in measurements (interpreted within the context of the clinical situation) will serve as a guide to defect whether the heart can handle its fluid load and whether hypovolemia or hypervolemia is present	7. CVP is interpreted by considering the patient's entire clinical picture hourly urine output, heart rate, blood pressure, cardiac output measurements a. A CVP near zero indicates that the patient is hypovolemic (verified if rapid IV infusion causes patient to improve) b. A CVP above 15 to 20 cm H_2O may be due to either hypervolemia or poor cardiac contractility
8. Turn the stopcock again to allow IV solution to flow from solution bottle into the patient's veins	8. When readings are not being made, flow is formed a very slow microdrip to the catheter, bypassing the manometer
Follow-up phase	
1. Observe for complications a. From catheter insertion, pneumothorax, hemothorax, air embolism, hematoma, and cardiac tamponade b. From indwelling catheter infection, and air embolism	1. Patient's complaints of new of different pain must be assessed closely. a. Signs/symptoms of air embolism include; severe shortness of breath hypotension, hypoxia, rumbling murmur, cardiac arrest b. If air embolism is suspected, immediately place patient in left lateral Trendelenburg's position and administer oxygen. Air bubbles will be prevented from moving into the lungs and will be absorbed in 10 to 15 minutes in the right ventricular outflow tract
2. Carry out ongoing nursing surveillance of the insertion site and maintain aseptic technique a. Inspect entry site twice daily for signs of local inflammation/ phlebitis. Remove immediately if there are any signs of infection b. Change dressings as prescribed c. Label to show date/time of change d. Send the catheter tip for bacteriologic culture when it is removed	*Nursing focus* A CVP line is a potential source of septicemia

Procedure 12.2: Measuring pulmonary artery pressure by flow-directed balloon-tipped catheter (Swan-Ganz catheter)

Equipment:

- Swan-Ganz catheter, set
- ECG, monitor and display unit with paper recorder
- For SVO_2 monitoring, fiberoptic
- PA catheter, optical module, and microprocessor unit
- Defibrillator
- Pressure transducer (disposable/reusable)
- Cut-down tray
- Sterile saline solution.
- Pressurized bag
- Heparin infusion in plastic bag
- Continuous flush device
- Local anesthetic
- Skin antiseptic
- Transparent/gauze dressing
- Tape.

Steps of procedure

Nursing action	Rationale
Preparatory phase (by nurses)	
1. Explain procedure to the patient and family/significant others. Obtain informed consent	1. Explain that patient may feel the catheter moving through veins, and this is normal
2. Check vital signs and apply ECG electrodes	
3. Place patient in a position of comfort, this is the baseline position	3. Note the angle of elevation of patient cannot be lied flat, as subsequent pressure readings are taken from this baseline position to ensure consistency. Patient may need to be in Trendelenburg's position briefly if the jugular or subclavian vein is used
4. Set up equipment according to manufacturer's directives a. The pulmonary artery catheter requires a transducer, recording, amplifying and flush systems b. Flush system according to manufacturer's directions	4. a. Monitoring systems may vary greatly. The complexity of equipment requires an understanding of the equipment in use. A constant microdrip of heparin flush solution is maintained to ensure catheter patency b. Flushing of the catheter system ensures patency and eliminates air bubbles
5. Adjust transducer to level of patient's right atrium (phlebostatic axis 4th intercostal space, midaxillary line) (Fig. 12.32)	5. Differences between the level of the right atrium and the transducer will result in incorrect pressure readings, the phlebostatic axis is at the level of the right atrium
6. Calibrate pressure equipment (especially important when reusable transducers are employed)	6. A known quantity of pressure is applied to the transducer (usually by mercury manometer) to ensure accurate monitoring of pressure readings
7. Clip excess hair prepare skin over insertion site	7. The catheter is inserted percutaneously under sterile conditions
Performance phase (by the physician)	
1. Physician dons sterile gown and gloves, and places sterile drapes over patient	1. Sterile field is established to prevent chance of infection
2. The balloon is inflated with air understerile water or saline to test for leakage (bubbles). The catheter may be flushed with saline at this time	2. To ensure that the balloon is intact and to remove air from catheter
3. The Swan-Ganz catheter is inserted through the internal jugular, Subclavian, or any easily accessible vein by either percutaneous puncture or venotomy (Fig. 12.32)	3. The internal jugular vein establishes a short route into the central venous system
4. The catheter is advanced to the superior vena cava. Oscillations of the pressure wave forms will indicate when the tip of the catheter is within the thoracic cavity. The patient may be asked to cough	4. Catheter placement may be determined by characteristic wave forms and changes. Coughing will produce deflections in the pressure tracing when the catheter tip is in the thorax
5. The Catheter is then advanced gently into the right atrium and the balloon inflated with air	5. The amount of air to be used is indicated on the catheter
6. The inflated balloon at the tip of the catheter will be guided by the flowing stream of blood through the right atrium and tricuspid valve into the right ventricle. From this position, if finds its way into the main pulmonary artery. The catheter tip pressures are recorded continuously by specific pressure wave forms as the catheter advances through the various chambers of the heart	6. Watch ECG monitor for signs of ventricular irritability as catheter enters the right ventricle. Report any signs of dysrhythmia to the physician

Contd...

Contd...

Nursing action	Rationale
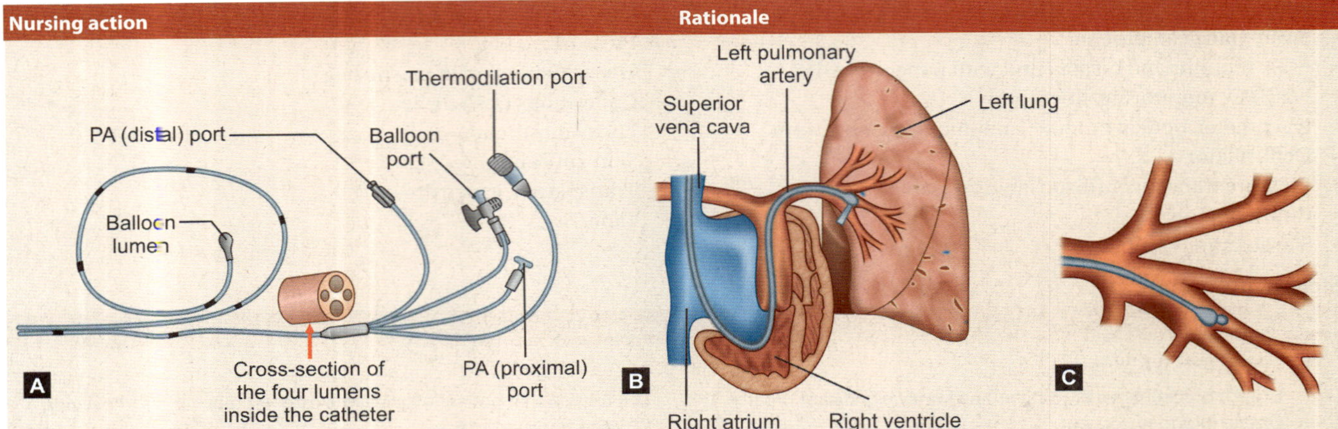 **FIGS 12.32A TO C:** (A) Swan-Ganz catheter; (B) Location of the Swan-Ganz catheter within the heart. The catheter enters the right atrium via the superior vena cava. The balloon is then inflated, allowing the catheter to follow the blood flow through the tricuspid valve, through the right ventricle, through the pulmonic valve, and into the main pulmonary artery. Wave form and pressure readings are noted during insertion to identify location of the catheter with the heart. The balloon is deflated once the catheter is in the pulmonary artery and properly secured; (C) Pulmonary capillary wedge pressure (PCWP). The catheter floats into a distal branch of the pulmonary artery when the balloon is inflated, and becomes "wedged." The wedged catheter occludes blood flow from behind, and the tip of the lumen records pressures in front of the catheter. The balloon is then deflated, allowing the catheter to float back into the main pulmonary artery	
7. The flowing blood will continue to direct the catheter more distally into the pulmonary tree. When the catheter reaches a pulmonary vessel that is approximately the same size or slightly smaller in diameter than the inflated balloon, it cannot be advanced any further. This is the wedge position, called pulmonary capillary wedge pressure (PAWP)	7. With the catheter in the wedge position, the balloon blocks the flow of blood from the right side of the heart towards the lungs. The sensor at the tip of the balloon detects pressures distally, which results in the sensing of retrograde left a trial pressures. The PCWP is thus equal to left atrial pressures a. Normal PCWP is 8–12 mm Hg. Optimal LV function appears to be at a wedge between 14–18 mm Hg b. Wedge pressure is a valuable parameter of cardiac function. Filling pressures less than 8–10 mm Hg may indicate hypovolemia and in an acutely injured heart are often associated with reduction in cardiac, output, hypotension, and tachycardia. Filling pressures greater than 20 mm Hg are associated with left ventricular failure, pulmonary congestion, and hypervolemia
8. The balloon is deflated, causing the catheter to retract spontaneously into a larger pulmonary artery. This gives a continuous pulmonary artery systolic, diastolic, and mean pressure	8. The normal systolic pulmonary pressure rangers are 20–30 mm Hg, and the diastolic pulmonary artery pressure (average pressure in pulmonary artery throughout the entire cardiac cycle) is 15–20 mm Hg
9. The catheter is then attached to a continuous heparin flush and transducer	9. A low-flow continuous irrigation ensures that the catheter remains patient. The transducer converts the pressure wave into an electronic wave that is displayed on the oscilloscope
10. The catheter is sutured in place and covered with a sterile dressing	
11. A chest X-ray is obtained after. Swan-Ganz insertion if fluoroscopy was not used to guide insertion	11. To confirm catheter position and to provide a baseline for future reference
To obtain a wedge pressure reading	
1. Note amount of air to be injected into balloon, usually 1 mL. Do not introduce more air into balloon than specified	
2. Inflate the balloon slowly until the contour of the pulmonary arterial pressure changes to that of pulmonary wedge pressure. As soon as a wedge pattern is observed, no more air is introduced a. Note the digital pressure recordings on the monitor (an average of pressure waves is displayed, but these waves are not taken at end expiration) b. Obtain a strip of the pressure tracing c. Determine PCWP from strip at end expiration	2. The transducer converts the pressure wave into an electronic wave that is displayed on a screen a. PCWP should be determined at end expiration because respiratory variation of the wave form occurs due to changes in intrathoracic pressures b. A calibrated oscilloscope or graph paper is needed to read pressures at end expiration

Contd...

Contd...

Nursing action	Rationale
3. Deflate the balloon as soon as the pressure reading is obtained. Do not draw back with force on the syringe because too forceful a deflation may damage the balloon	3. Segmental lung infarction may occur if the catheter balloon is left inflated for long periods. Pulmonary, capillary wedge pressures are only measured intermittently. Do not allow catheter to remain in wedge position when patient is unattended or when not directly making the measurement
4. Record PCWP reading and amount of air needed to obtain wedge reading. Document recorded wave form is placing a strip of the waveform in patient's chart showing wedge tracing reverting to pulmonary artery waveform	4. Overinflation of the balloon may cause a "superwedge" wave form and data obtained will be inaccurate. Overinflation of balloon may cause balloon to lose elastic properties and rupture. The strip provides documentation that catheter was not left in wedge position
To obtain a SvO_2 reading:	
1. Before insertion, perform a preinsertion calibration of the catheter	1. This calibrates the catheter to light intensity in the environment
2. After insertion, perform a calibration for light intensity and an *in vivo* calibration every 8 hours	2. The in vivo calibration ensures that there is minimal difference, or "drift" between the actual SvO_2 value and the value displayed on the monitor. The light calibration adjusts for changes in light in the environment
Nursing focus Also perform *in vivo* calibration if the optical module is disconnected at the catheter junction, if calibration data are lost, or if the SvO_2 is + 4% of the SvO_2 value calculated from mixed various values obtained from the pulmonary artery catheter	
3. Monitor SvO_2 at frequent intervals. Values of 60–80% are normal	3. Causes of an SvO_2 60% include: a. Decrease in cardiac output b. Decrease in SaO_2 c. Decrease in hemoglobin d. Increase in Q_2 consumption Causes of an SvO_2 80% include;: a. Increase in SaO_2 b. Decrease in O_2 consumption
4. If the SvO_2 changes + 10% from the prior value, confirm that the change reflects a change in patient condition	4. The value displayed may not be accurate if fibrin or a clot is obstructing the catheter tip (low-intensity signal), if the catheter is touching the vessel wall or in a wedged position (high intensity signal), or if the catheter is no longer calibrated accurately
5. If the catheter is not functioning properly, initiate steps to resolve the problem	5. These steps may include aspiration to determine if a clot is obstructing the catheter or notifying the physician of the need to reposition the catheter
6. If no catheter malfunction is identified, report changes to the physician, initiate therapy based on standards of care	6. Prompt intervention can restore normal tissue oxygen delivery before untoward effects occur
Follow-up phase	
1. Inspect the insertion site daily. Look for signs of infection, swelling, and bleeding	1. A foreign body (catheter) in the vascular system increases the risk of sepsis
2. Record date and time of dressing change and IV, tubing change	
3. Assess contour of waveform, frequently and compare with previous documented waveforms	3. Catheter may move forward and become lodged in wedge position or drift back into right ventricle. Turn patient to left side and ask him to cough (may dislodge catheter from wedge position). If not dislodged notify physician
4. Assess for complications, pulmonary embolism, dysrhythmias, heart block, damage to tricuspid valve, intracardiac knotting of catheter, thrombophlebitis, infection, balloon rupture and rupture of pulmonary artery	4. Blood coming back into syringe indicates balloon rupture. Notify physician immediately
5. When indicated, the catheter is removed without excessive force or traction, pressure dressing is applied over the site	5. The site should be checked periodically for bleeding

Procedure 12.3: Measurement of cardiac output (CO) by thermodilution method

Equipment:

- Flow directed thermodilution
- Catheter in place.
- CO set, which includes IV tubing
- 10 mL syringe and three-way stopcock
- Normal saline or D5W solution bag
- Cardiac monitor with CO computation capability or stand-alone CO computer
- Temperature sensor cable.

Steps of procedure

Nursing action	Rationale
1. Explain procedure to patient	
2. Connect IV solution bag and CO set maintaining aseptic technique	
3. If you do not have a prepackaged CO set, attach IV solution bag to IV tubing connect a three-way stopcock to the end of the tubing, connect a 10 mL syringe to the middle part of the three-way stopcock	
4. Attach the three-way stopcock to the proximal injectate port of the thermodilution catheter. This port should be reserved solely for determination of CO. No medications	4. The proximal injectate port should have its distal end in the right atrium. If medications are infusing in this port, they will be flushed through in bolus form when CO measurements are taken
5. Another three-way stopcock may be used to allow for IV solution to run at a keep open rate	5. Once the CO set is connected, the system should remain closed
6. Connect temperature sensor cable to the thermistor port of the thermodilution catheter	6. When solution is injected through catheter, it mixes with the blood in the right side of the heart and flows to the pulmonary artery where blood temperature is detected by the thermistor
7. Set cardiac monitor to CO computation format. If using a stand-alone CO computer, enter the temperature of the injectable solution and the code number for the size of thermodilution catheter in use (code will be located on the thermodilution catheter packaging)	7. The injectate solution should be 15–20 degrees cooler than the patient's body temperature. Room temperature injectate is usually adequate
8. Fill 10-mL syringe with injectate solution by turning stopcock off to patient and open to syringe and solution	
9. Turn off IV keep open solution if present	9. Need closed system from syringe to catheter
10. Turn stopcock off to injectate solution and open to patient and syringe	
11. Press inject button on the CO computer or monitor and inject 10 mL, rapidly (within 4 seconds) and smoothly into the proximal port)	11. Delay will interfere with results
12. Wait for computation to be complete. Repeat the procedure two or three times to obtain an average	12. Same monitors display a waveform for the injectate dispersal to evaluate the adequacy of dispersal and temperature sensing
13. Turn stopcock off to the syringe and injectate and allow keep open IV fluid to infuse through the proximal port	

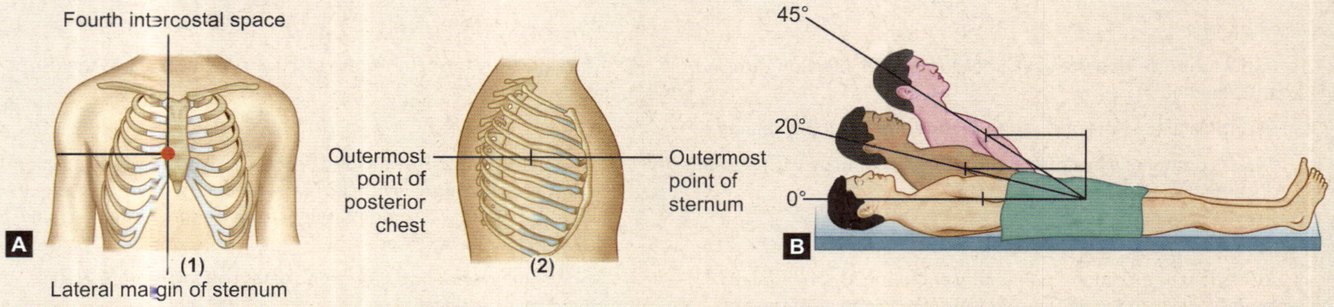

Fourth intercostal space

Outermost point of posterior chest

Outermost point of sternum

(1) Lateral margin of sternum

(2)

45°

20°

0°

FIGS 12.33A AND B: The phlebostatic axis and the phlebostatic level. (A) The phlebostatic axis is the crossing of two reference lines: (1) A line from the fourth intercostal space at the point where it joins the sternum, drawn out to the side of the body beneath the axilla; (2) A line midpoint between the anterior and posterior surfaces of the chest; (B) The phlebostatic level is a horizontal line through the phlebostatic axis. The transducer or the zero mark on the manometer must be level with this axis for accurate measurements. As the patient moves from the flat to erect positions, the chest moves and therefore the reference level; the phlebostatic level stays horizontal through the same reference point

Procedure 12.4: Transcutaneous cardiac pacing

Equipment

- Disposable electrode pads
- External pacing module
- Resuscitative equipment.

Steps of procedure

Nursing action	Rationale
Preparatory phase	
1. Explain procedure to patient	1. Allays anxiety
2. Explain sensation of discomfort with external pacing	2. Discomfort is felt with each firing, but can be relieved with analgesics
Performance phase	
1. Place electrodes as follows: a. Anterior/posterior. The negative electrode is placed on the anterior chest at the V3-V1 position, the positive electrode is placed on the back to the left of the spine b. Anterior/anterior, the negative electrode is placed under the right clavicle and the positive electrode is placed at the V6 position	1. Electrodes must be placed so the current passes through as much of the myocardium as possible with the least distance between the pads
2. Ensure that pacing module is off or on standby and that milliamp output is set at the minimal level before connecting electrodes to external module	2. Prevents accidental shock on connection
3. Connect pacing electrodes to external module	
4. Determine rate setting according to instructions and/or patient condition. If patient HR is consistently too low to maintain adequate cardiac output, set rate at 70–80, If the patient's HR falls only intermittently and the pacemaker will be utilized in the demand mode, set rate at 60	4. Can be set at a fixed rate or on demand, to pace only if heart rate falls below 60 (or other rate)
5. Gradually increase milliamp output, until a pacing spike and corresponding QRS complex are seen. Palpate pulse to ensure adequate response to electrical event	5. If using the demand mode, set the rate higher than the patient's rate to establish the correct output and capture, then return the rate to 60
6. Check pad placement frequently	6. Patient perspiration may cause pads to loosen or slip
Follow-up phase	
1. Check vital signs at least every 15 minute, while continuous pacing is employed	1. To determine if cardiac output is adequate
2. Monitor ECG continuously for pacer functioning	2. To detect malfunction (may occur due to electrodes loosening)
3. Assure patient that treatment is temporary	3. Should only be used continuously for 2 hours
4. Prepare patient for transvenous or permanent pacemaker insertion as indicated	

Procedure 12.5: Direct current defibrillation for ventricular fibrillation

Equipment:

- DC defibrillator with paddles (Fig. 12.34)
- Interface material (disposable conductive get pads, electrode gets and pastes)
- Resuscitative equipment.

Steps of procedure

Nursing action	Rationale
Performance phase	
1. Monitored patient—if ventricular fibrillation recognized with 2 minutes, give precordial thump, assess rhythm and carotid pulse, and expose anterior chest. Unmonitored patient-expose anterior chest	

Contd...

Contd...

Nursing action	Rationale
2. Unmonitored patient—start cardiopulmonary resuscitation Immediately Monitored patient—if within 2 minutes of detection of ventricular fibrillation, defibrillate before initiating cardiopulmonary resuscitation. Beyond 2 minutes, start resuscitation efforts immediately	2. This procedure should be carried out immediately after ventricular fibrillation is detected to minimize cerebral and circulatory deterioration Cardiopulmonary resuscitation, is essential before and after defibrillation to ensure blood supply to the cerebral and coronary arteries
3. Apply interface material to the patient (gel pads) or to the paddles (gel, paste). The electrode paddles should be in firm contact with the patients skin	3. The interface material helps provide better conduction and prevents skin burns. Do not allow any paste on the skin between the electrodes. If the paste areas touch, the current may short circuit (severely burning the patient and may not penetrate the heart. Saline pads are not recommended because the saline can easily drip, forming a path for the current
4. Remove oxygen from immediate area	4. Prevents danger of fire or explosion
5. A second person should turn on the defibrillator to the prescribed setting. The American Heart Association recommends that initial defibrillation should be 200–300 watt-seconds of delivered energy. A second attempt at same level should be given if first attempt unsuccessful. A third attempt within increase of energy level to 360 watt-seconds should be attempted. Allow only approximately 5 seconds between the successive attempts to assess rhythm and pulse	5. The shock is measured in joules or Watt-seconds (the dose is 2 Joules kg in paediatric, patients based on estimated body weight). The ideal energy dose for defibrillation remains controversial
6. Apply one electrode just to the right of the upper sternum below the clavicle and the other electrode just to the left of the cardiac apex or left nipple (Fig. 12.35). About 20–21 lb of pressure is applied to paddles to ensure good contact with the patient's skin	6. The paddies are placed so that the electrical discharge flows through as much myocardial mass as possible. If anteroposterior paddies are used, the anterior paddle is held with pressure on the middle sternum while the patient lies on the posterior paddle under the left infrascapular region. In this method the countershock more directly traverses the heart
7. Grasp the paddles only by the insulated handles	

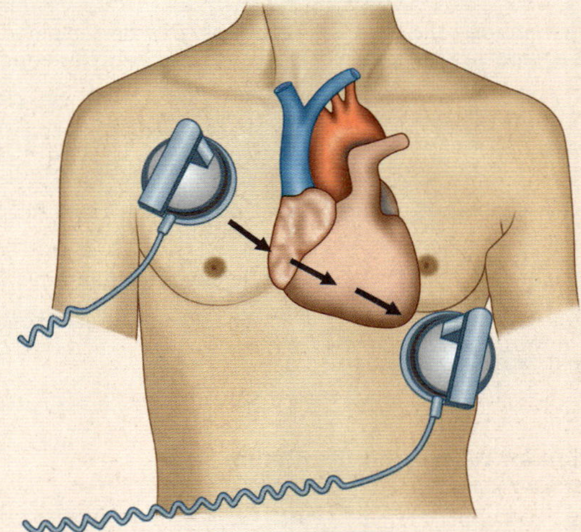

FIG. 12.34: Placement of defibrillator paddles on chest

Nursing action	Rationale
8. Charge the paddles, once paddles are charged. Give the command for personnel to stand clear of the patient and the bed. Look quickly to make sure all are away from the patient and bed	8. If a person touches the bed, he or she may act as a ground for the current and receive a shock, especially if there are electrolyte solutions on the floor
9. Push the discharge buttons in both paddles simultaneously	
10. Remove the paddles from the patient immediately after the shock is administered (unless monitoring leads are in the paddles)	
11. Resume cardiopulmonary resuscitation efforts until stable rhythm, spontaneous respirations, pulse, and blood pressure return	11. After the third attempt to countershock, CPR efforts should be resumed, total delay should be no more than 5 seconds to oxygenate the patient and restore circulation

Contd...

Contd...

Nursing action	Rationale
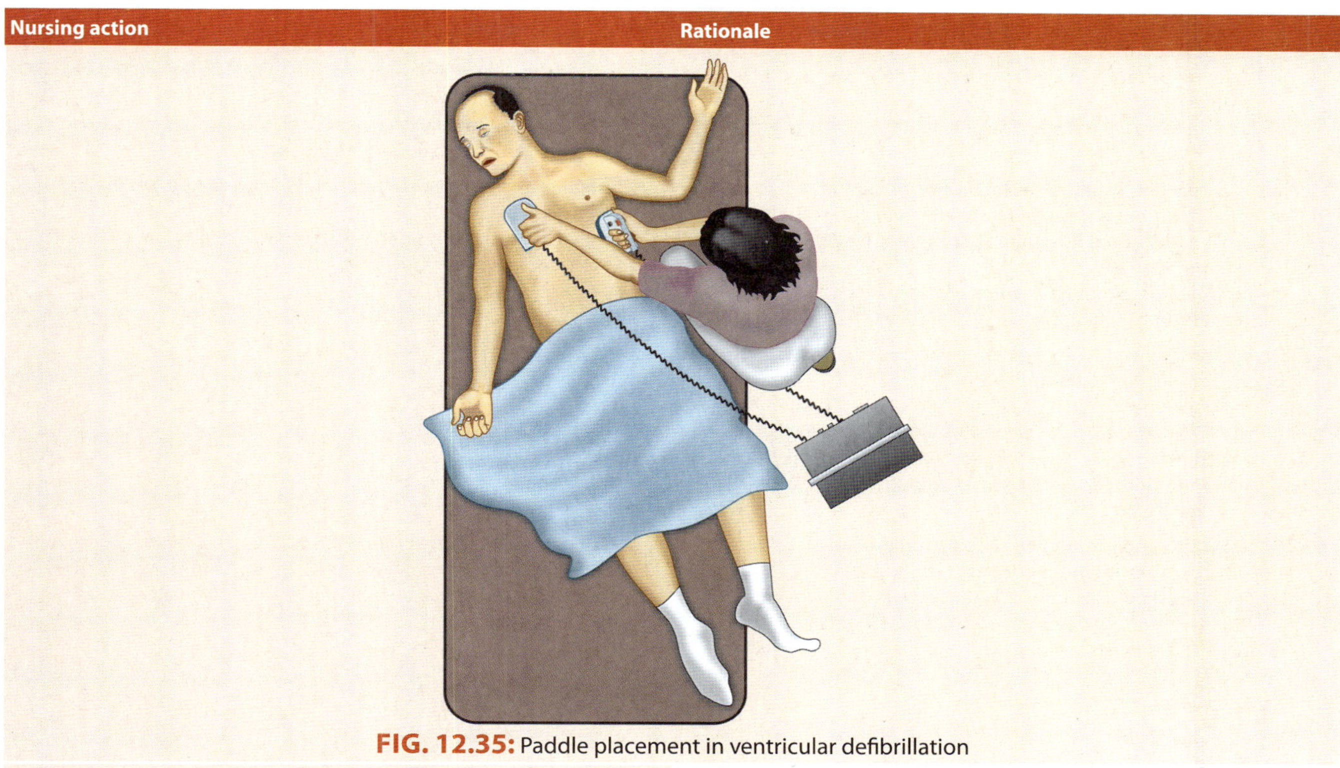 FIG. 12.35: Paddle placement in ventricular defibrillation	
12. Look at the ECG monitor to determine the specific therapy for the resultant electrical mechanism. Further high energy counter shocks may be necessary	
Paddle placement in ventricular defibrillation	
Follow-up phase	
1. After the patient is defibrillated and rhythm is restored, indochine is usually given to prevent recurrent episodes	1. Any resultant dysrhythmia may require appropriate drug intervention

Procedure 12.6: Synchronized cardioversion

Equipment

- Cardioverter (Fig. 12.36) and ECG machine
- Conduction jelly or gel pads and cardiac medications
- Resuscitative equipment.

Steps of procedure

Nursing action	Rationale
1. If the procedure is elective. It is advisable to have the patient "NPO" 12 hours before the cardioversion a. Reassure the patient and see that informed consent has been obtained b. Make sure the patient has not been taking digitalis and that the serum potassium is normal	1. During sedation or the procedure the patient may vomit and aspirate if the stomach is full a. Do not use word "shock" because this will increase the patient's apprehension b. Low potassium may precipitate post-shock dysrhythmias
2. Make sure IV line is secure	2. An IV line may be necessary for administration of emergency medications
3. Obtain a 12-lead ECG before and after cardioversion with the ECG machine. The ECG machine wires are best left on the patient, because the ECG printout is of much better quality than that of the monitor. This fact is especially important when one is trying to dissect complicated dysrhythmias	3. An ECG is taken to ensure that the patient has not had a recent myocardial infarction (either just before or after the cardioversion)

Contd...

Contd...

Nursing action	Rationale
4. a. Allow the patient to receive oxygen before and after cardioversion b. Do not give oxygen during the procedure	4. a. Oxygen will help prevent unwanted dysrhythmias after cardioversion b. An explosion could occur if a spark from the paddles should ignite the oxygen during the procedure
5. Place the paddles in one of the following two positions: a. Anterior posterior position. One paddle-left infrascapular area. Other paddle-upper sternum at 3rd interspace b. Anterior position One paddle-just to right of sternum at 2nd interspace. Other paddle-just under left nipple	a. If the electrical discharge hits the T wave. Ventricular fibrillation may occur b. Synchronization is not used for ventricular fibrillation if the synchronization mode is on
6. Determine if the machine's synchronization mechanism is working before applying the paddles a. The discharge should hit near the peak of the R wave b. The R wave usually must be of substantial height. If it is not, adjust the gain (sensitivity) or change in the lead. On many machines the R wave must be upright before there is synchronization	
7. If using paste, apply to all of the paddle surface, but make sure there is no excess around the edges of the paddles a. The paste should be rubbed on the skin very thoroughly; this allows more electricity to penetrate the body surface b. Make sure paddles are clean because surface material will interfere with the flow of electricity c. Apply firm pressure to the paddle	7. If there is excess paste around the paddles, the discharge may run onto the skin, causing a burn. If there is not firm contact between the paddle and skin, a burn may occur, also electricity is lost from the heart

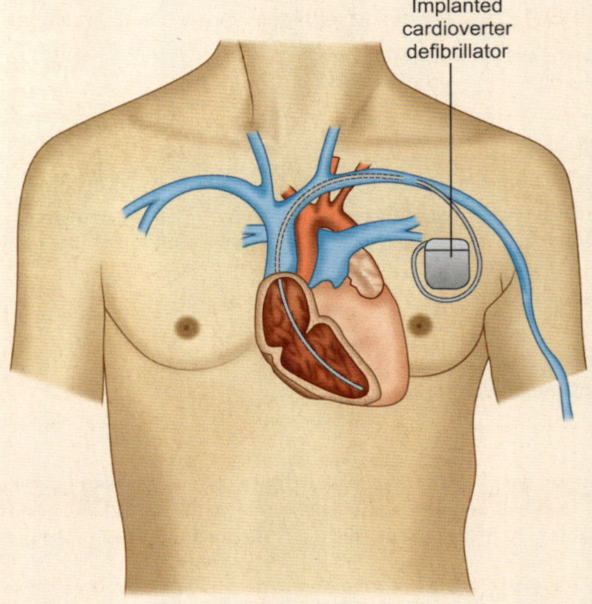

FIG. 12.36: An implanted cardioverter defibrillator in place

Nursing action	Rationale
8. If using gel pads, place pads where paddles are to be positioned	8. Excessive energies may cause unnecessary discomfort to the patient
9. Set dial for lowest level of electrical energy that can be expected to convert the dysrhythmia. Some dysrhythmias (such as atrial flutter) can be converted with very low energies, such as 25 watt-seconds (Joules)	9. This helps, produce amnesia concerning the cardioversion
10. A short acting sedative such as midazolam (versed) should be given if the patient is conscious	

Contd...

Contd...

Nursing action	Rationale
11. After the patient is in a light sleep from the IV medication and when no one is touching the bed of patient, discharge the cardioverter. If cardioversion does not occur, proceed to a higher energy level	11. The patient may revert to previous dysrhythmias after conversion
12. Monitor the ECG after conversion occurs, blood pressures should be recorded about every 15 minutes until the preshock blood pressure is reached	

Procedure 12.7: Assisting the patient undergoing pericardiocentesis (Figs 12.37 and 12.38)

Equipment

- Pericardiocentesis tray
- Intracatheter set
- Skin antiseptic 1–2 percent Lidocaine
- Sterile gloves
- ECG for monitoring purposes
- Sterile ground were to be connected between pericardial needle and V lead of ECG (use alligator clip type connectors)
- Equipment for cardiopulmonary resuscitation.

Steps of procedure

Nursing action	Rationale
Preparatory phase	
1. Medicate the patient as prescribed	
2. Start a slow intravenous drip of saline or glucose	2. This preserves a route for intravenous therapy in the event of an emergency
3. Place the patient in a comfortable position with the head of the bed or treatment table raised to a 45 degree angle	3. This position makes it easier to insert weedle into pericardial sac
4. Apply the limb leads of the ECG to the patient	4. The patient is monitored during the procedure by ECG
5. Have defibrillator available for immediate use	5. In case the procedure has severe adverse effect
6. Have pacemaker available	
7. Open the tray using aseptic technique	

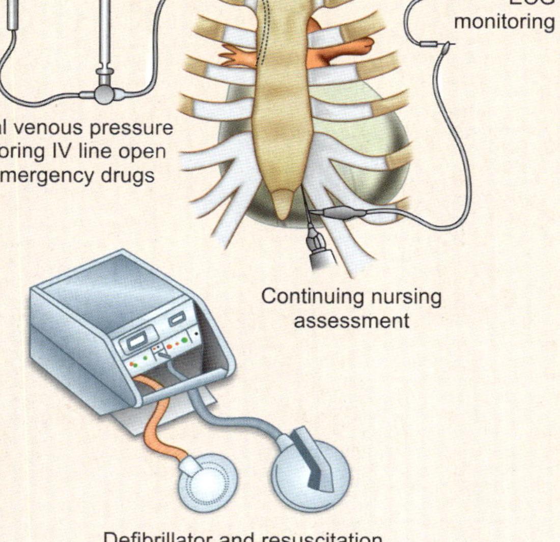

FIG. 12.37: Nursing support of the patient undergoing pericardiocentesis (small circles indicate sites for pericardial aspiration)

Contd...

Contd...

Nursing action	Rationale
Performance phase (by physician)	
1. The site is prepared with skin antiseptic, the area is draped with sterile towels and injected with anesthetic	
2. The pericardial aspiration needle is attached to a 50 mL, syringe by a three-way stopcock. The V lead (precordial lead wire) of the ECG is attached to the hub of the aspirating needle by a sterile wire and alligator clips or clamp	2. There is danger of laceration of myocardium/coronary artery and of cardiac dysrhythmias
3. The needle is advanced slowly until fluid is obtained	3. Fluid is generally aspirated at a depth of 2.5–4 cm (1–1½ inches)
4. When the pericardial sac has been entered, a hemostat is clamped to the needle at the chest wall just where it penetrates the skin. Pericardial fluid is aspirated slowly	4. This prevents movement of the needle and further penetration while fluid is being removed. Aspirated fluid may be cloudy, clear or bloody
5. Monitor the patient's ECG blood pressure, and venous pressure constantly	5. a. The ST segment rises if the point of the needle contacts the ventricle, there may be ventricular ectopic beats b. The PR segment is elevated when the needle touches the atrium c. Large, erratic QRS complexes indicate penetration of the myocardium
6. If a large amount of fluid is present, a polyethylene catheter may be inserted through a needle (an intracath) and left in the pericardial sac	6. An indwelling catheter left in the pericardial space permits further slow drainage of fluid and prevents recurrence of cardiac tamponade
7. Watch for presence of bloody fluid. If blood accumulates rapidly, an immediate thoracotomy and cardiorrhaphy (suturing of heart muscle) may be indicated	7. Bloody pericardial fluid may be due to trauma. Bloody pericardial effusion fluid does not clot readily, whereas blood obtained from inadvertent puncture of one of the heart chambers does clot
Follow-up phase	
1. Monitor patient closely a. Watch for rising venous pressure and falling arterial pressure b. Auscultate the area over the heart	1. After pericardiocentesis, careful monitoring of blood pressure, and heart sounds will be necessary to indicate possible recurrence of tamponade, repeated aspiration is then necessary
2. Prepare for surgical drainage of pericardium if. a. Pericardial fluid repeatedly accumulates, or b. The aspiration is unsuccessful, or c. Complications develop	2. In the presence of these sign the patient is probably experiencing cardiac tamponade
3. Assess for complications. Inadvertent puncture of heart chamber Dysrhythmias Puncture of lung, stomach or liver Laveration of coronary artery or myocardium	3. Listen for decrease in intensity of heart sounds indicating recurring cardiac tamponade

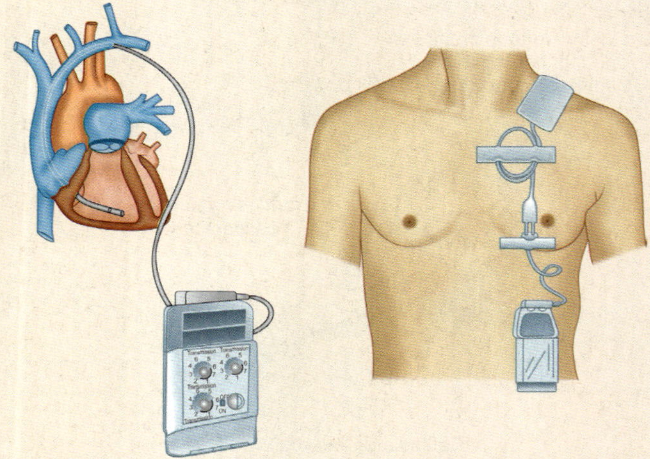

FIG. 12.38: Temporary transvenous pacer wire with external pulse generator